CLINICAL CARDIOVASCULAR IMAGING

■ ■ ■ A Companion to Braunwald's Heart Disease

Martin G. St. John Sutton, MBBS, FRCP, FACC
John W. Bryfogle Professor of Medicine, University of Pennsylvania
Director, Cardiovascular Imaging Program
Director, Cardiovascular Fellowship Program
Hospital of the University of Pennsylvania
Philadelphia, Pennsylvania

John D. Rutherford, MB, ChB, FRACP, FACC
Vice President for Clinical Operations
Professor of Internal Medicine
Gail Griffiths Hill Chair in Cardiology
University of Texas Southwestern Medical Center
Dallas, Texas

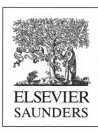

ELSEVIER
SAUNDERS

ELSEVIER
SAUNDERS

The Curtis Center
170 S Independence Mall W 300E
Philadelphia, Pennsylvania 19106

Clinical Cardiovascular Imaging: ISBN 0-7216-9068-8
A Companion to Braunwald's Heart Disease

NOTICE

Medicine is an ever-changing field. Standard safety precautions must be followed, but as new research and clinical experience broaden our knowledge, changes in treatment and drug therapy may become necessary or appropriate. Readers are advised to check the most current product information provided by the manufacturer of each drug to be administered to verify the recommended dose, the method and duration of administration, and contraindications. It is the responsibility of the licensed prescriber, relying on experience and knowledge of the patient, to determine dosages and the best treatment for each individual patient. Neither the publisher nor the author assumes any liability for any injury and/or damage to persons or property arising from this publication.

Library of Congress Cataloging-in-Publication Data
Clinical cardiovascular imaging: a companion to Braunwald's Heart disease / [edited by] Martin G. St. John Sutton, John D. Rutherford.– 1st ed.
    p. ; cm.
  Includes bibliographical references and index.
  ISBN 0-7216-9068-8
  1. Heart–Diseases. 2. Cardiovascular system–Diseases. 3. Heart–Imaging. 4. Cardiovascular system–Imaging.
  [DNLM: 1. Diagnostic Imaging–methods. 2. Heart Diseases–diagnosis. 3. Cardiovascular Diseases–diagnosis. WG 141 C6413 2004] I. St. John Sutton, Martin, 1945-II. Rutherford, John D. III. Heart disease.
RC681.H36 2001 Suppl.
616.1'20754–dc22
2003066014

Publisher: Anne Lenehan
Editorial Assistant: Vera Ginsburg
Project Manager: Mary Stermel

Printed in United States of America

Last digit is the print number: 9 8 7 6 5 4 3 2 1

This book is dedicated to our families

Clare, Eleanor and Eugenie St. John Sutton

Evelyn Magali and Claire Helene St. John Sutton

Cynthia Rutherford

Matt, JJ, and Maya Rutherford

Anna Rutherford and Brendan Everett

The dramatic reductions in cardiovascular mortality and morbidity during the past three decades represent one of the major triumphs of twentieth-century medicine. Striking advances in three major areas are responsible – diagnosis, therapy, and prevention. The first of these, cardiac diagnosis, has leapt forward almost entirely as a consequence of the spectacular developments in cardiac imaging. During the past five years, in particular, the technologies available for cardiac imaging have progressed exponentially, and the contributions made by non-invasive or minimally invasive cardiac imaging to every aspect of cardiac care have expanded with unexpected rapidity.

The public expectations of the medical profession are increasing. Patients, their families, and those who pay for medical care require first and foremost an accurate clinical assessment and an estimation of prognosis – not merely a diagnosis. In the case of patients with cardiac disease, both anatomic and functional evaluations are required, and clinicians now have a broad array of cardiac imaging techniques available to them for accomplishing these tasks. *Clinical Cardiovascular Imaging* presents cardiologists, cardiovascular radiologists, cardiovascular surgeons and especially trainees in these fields with an understanding of the physical principles of cardiovascular imaging. It also provides the information required to use and interpret the entire gamut of contemporary imaging modalities and serves as a helpful guide to the use of these complex and sometimes costly techniques to solve a broad array of clinical problems. In an era of cost conscious medicine, it is essential to select the appropriate technique without paying for unnecessary or redundant information.

This book compares the various imaging techniques in the quantification of ventricular function and myocardial perfusion and in assessing cardiac metabolism. It also emphasizes the use of imaging in diagnostic decision making and the approach to assessment of the cost effectiveness of these important techniques.

We congratulate the editors, Drs. St. John Sutton and Rutherford, and their talented authors, true experts in their respective fields, on providing this fine companion to *Braunwald's Heart Disease: A Textbook of Cardiovascular Medicine*.

Eugene Braunwald, M.D.
Douglas P. Zipes, M.D.
Peter Libby, M.D.
Robert O. Bonow, M.D.

Imaging is an integral part of clinical care and problem solving for most cardiovascular diseases, and both cardiovascular specialists and non-specialist healthcare professionals provide this care. Traditional imaging text books have had a technical emphasis and have usually been subdivided into specific imaging techniques describing instrumentation and physical principles and then have discussed an array of topics associated with the individual techniques. *Heart Disease, A Textbook of Cardiovascular Medicine*, Edited by Braunwald, Zipes and Libby, describes the major imaging techniques in introductory chapters and discusses their use in specific diseases. However, because of space limitations, a comprehensive description of specific diseases is not included.

Clinical Cardiovascular Imaging: A Companion to Heart Disease has a greater emphasis on imaging of specific cardiovascular diseases. The aim of this text is to provide a disease specific, problem-oriented approach to the use of diagnostic imaging for cardiologists, cardiac and vascular surgeons, "imagers" and also for non-cardiovascular specialists.

The text has been divided into two major parts. The first section of the book describes imaging modalities and the cost-effectiveness of imaging techniques. The second major section of the book focuses on the investigation of various diseases with imaging technology. Because no individual is likely to have expert knowledge about each of the imaging modalities available, or needed, to investigate a particular aspect of cardiovascular disease, the chapters each have a lead author and co-authors with complementary expertise. This format has provided significant challenges to the book editors, and lead authors, in providing a well-organized, coherent, readable text. Most chapters begin with a detailed outline to facilitate finding information on specific subjects. We have tried to emphasize the optimal selection of the imaging techniques for accurate and expeditious diagno-

sis in all aspects of cardiovascular disease and where possible have tried to adhere to the logical order of clinical decisions. While practice guidelines for medical therapy are highly developed in many aspects of cardiovascular disease, they are less well developed with respect to the choice of various imaging techniques. We believe, during the next decade, with rising healthcare costs and the increasing limitations on resources that comprehensive imaging guidelines will emerge.

With the acquisition of W.B. Saunders Company by Elsevier Science, we were encouraged to make some changes in the format of the text in the process of publication. Specifically, we became convinced that with the easy availability of electronic reference material exhaustive numbers of references in the chapters were unnecessary, and accordingly, the editors accepted responsibility for focusing on a relatively small number of references. This has been a large, new project and despite our best efforts the reader may find areas of omission, or have suggestions for improvement, and we encourage communication with either one of us by E-mail (*suttonm@mail.med.upenn.edu* or *john.rutherford@utsouthwestern.edu*).

We hope that this textbook will be clinically useful to healthcare providers and trainees in cardiovascular medicine. The editors acknowledge the commitment, and dedication, of the expert contributors. We thank Anne Lenehan and her team at Elsevier Science for their dedication and assistance, and Tracy Grace at Kolam, Inc. For administrative support we remain indebted to our assistants, Shirley Crook, Doris Matthews, and Catharine Kelly. Last, we hope that *Clinical Cardiovascular Imaging: A Companion to Braunwald's Heart Disease* will provide a stimulus for better patient care and further exploration in cardiovascular disease.

Martin G. St. John Sutton
John D. Rutherford

Luis I. Araujo, M.D.
Associate Professor, Department of Radiology and Medicine, University of Pennsylvania; Director, Department of Nuclear Cardiology, Hospital of the University of Pennsylvania, Philadelphia, Pennsylvania
Physical Principles of Cardiovascular Imaging

Gerard P. Aurigemma, M.D.
Professor of Medicine and Radiology, Department of Medicine, Division of Cardiovascular Medicine, University of, Massachusetts Medical School; Director, Noninvasive Cardiology, Department of Medicine, Division of Cardiovascular Medicine, University of Massachusetts Medical Center, Worcester, Massachusetts
Chronic Coronary Heart Disease

Thomas M. Bashore, M.D.
Professor of Medicine, Division of Cardiology, Duke University Medical Center, Durham, North Carolina
Quantitation of Ventricular Function

Joshua A. Beckman, M.D., M.S.
Instructor of Medicine, Department of Internal Medicine Harvard University School of Medicine; Associate Attending, Cardiovascular Division, Brigham and Women's Hospital, Boston, Massachusetts
Peripheral Arterial, Aortic, Renal Artery, and Carotid Artery Diseases

Steven R. Bergmann, M.D., Ph.D.
Professor of Medicine, Albert Einstein College of Medicine; Adjunct Professor of Medicine, Cardiovascular Division, College of Physicians and Surgeons of Columbia University; Chief, Division of Cardiology, Beth Israel Medical Center, New York, New York
Quantitation of Myocardial Perfusion

David A. Bluemke, M.D., Ph.D.
Associate Professor and Clinical Director, MRI, Department of Radiology and Radiological Sciences, Johns Hopkins University School of Medicine; Johns Hopkins Hospital, Department of Radiology, Baltimore, Maryland
Cardiac Imaging of Masses, Tumors, and Thrombi

Ignasi Carrio, M.D.
Professor and Director, Department of Radiology, Autonomous University; Director, Department of Nuclear Medicine, Hospital Sant Pau, Barcelona, Spain
Imaging of Myocardial Antigens, Receptors, Hypoxia, Necrosis, Apoptosis, Metabolism, and Viability

Joaquin E. Cigarroa, M.D.
Associate Professor of Medicine; Director of Cardiac Catheterization Labs, Department of Cardiology, University of Texas Southwestern Medical Center, Dallas, Texas
Coronary Heart Disease—Acute Coronary Syndromes

Mark A. Creager, M.D.
Professor of Medicine, Harvard Medical School; Director, Vascular Center; Simon S. Fireman Scholar in Cardiovascular Medicine, Cardiovascular Division, Brigham and Women's Hospital, Boston, Massachusetts
Peripheral Arterial, Aortic, Renal Artery, and Carotid Artery Diseases

Roger Andrew O. de Freitas, M.D.
Assistant Professor, Departments of Pediatrics and Medicine, Northwestern University School of Medicine; Director of Adult Congenital Cardiac Program, Department of Cardiology, Children's Memorial Hospital; Staff Cardiologist, Department of Cardiology, Northwestern Memorial Hospital, Chicago, Illinois
Imaging of the Adult with Congenital Heart Disease

Vibhas S. Deshpande, Ph.D.
Department of Radiology and Department of Biomedical Engineering, Northwestern University, Chicago, Illinois; Siemens Medical Solutions, Los Angeles, California
Quantitation of Myocardial Perfusion

Marcelo F. Di Carli, M.D., F.A.C.C.
Assistant Professor, Department of Radiology, Harvard Medical School; Chief, Director of Nuclear Cardiology, Department of Radiology, Brigham and Women's Hospital, Boston, Massachusetts
Quantitation of Myocardial Perfusion

Sharmila Dorbala, M.B.B.S.
Instructor, Department of Radiology, Harvard Medical School; Associate Director, Nuclear Cardiology, Department of Radiology, Brigham and Women's Hospital, Boston, Massachuetts
Quantitation of Myocardial Perfusion

Andrew C. Eisenhauer, M.D.
Assistant Professor of Medicine, Radiology and Surgery, Harvard Medical School; Director, Interventional Cardiovascular Medicine Service, Brigham and Women's Hospital, Boston, Massachusetts
Peripheral Arterial, Aortic, Renal Artery, and Carotid Artery Diseases

Kirsten E. Fleischmann, M.D., M.P.H.
Assistant Professor in Residence, Department of Medicine, University of California, San Francisco; University of California San Francisco Medical Center, San Francisco, California
Cost-Effectiveness of Imaging Techniques in the Medical Marketplace

Albert Flotats, M.D.
Associate Professor, Department of Nuclear Medicine, Autonomous University of Barcelona; Physician, Department of Nuclear Medicine, Hospital Sant Pau, Barcelona, Spain
Imaging of Myocardial Antigens, Receptors, Hypoxia, Necrosis, Apoptosis, Metabolism, and Viability

Bernhard L. Gerber, M.D., Ph.D.
Assistant Professor of Medicine, Department of Cardiology, Université Catholique de Louvain; Department of Cardiology, Cliniques Universitaries St. Luc, Brussels, Belgium
Physical Principles of Cardiovascular Imaging; Cardiac Imaging of Masses, Tumors, and Thrombi

Marie Gerhard-Herman, M.D.
Assistant Professor, Department of Medicine, Harvard Medical School; Medical Director, Vascular Diagnostic Laboratory, Department of Medicine, Cardiovascular Division, Brigham and Women's Hospital, Boston, Massachusetts
Peripheral Arterial, Aortic, Renal Artery, and Carotid Artery Diseases

Raymond J. Gibbons, M.D.
Arthur M. and Gladys D. Gray Professor of Medicine, Mayo Medical School; Co-Director, Nuclear Cardiology Laboratory, Mayo Clinic, Rochester, Minnesota
Evidence-Based Medicine: A Guide to Cardiac Imaging

C. Michael Gibson, M.D., M.S.
Associate Professor of Medicine, Harvard Medical School; Associate Chief of Cardiology, Department of Medicine, Beth Israel Deaconess Medical Center; Director, Thrombolysis in Myocardial Infarction Data Coordinating Center and Core Laboratory, Brigham and Women's Hospital, Boston, Massachusetts
Quantitation of Myocardial Perfusion

Satyendra Giri, M.D., M.P.H., M.R.C.P. (UK), F.A.C.C., F.S.C.A.I.
Assistant Professor, Division of Cardiology, The University of Texas Health Science Center at Houston Medical School, Houston, Texas; Director, Department of Cardiovascular Services, Redding Medical Center, Redding, California
Peripheral Arterial, Aortic, Renal Artery, and Carotid Artery Diseases

Lee R. Goldberg, M.D., M.P.H.
Assistant Professor of Medicine; Medical Director Heart-Lung Transplant Program, Cardiovascular Medicine Division, Heart Failure and Cardiac Transplant Program, University of Pennsylvania; Attending Physician, Cardiovascular Medicine Division, Hospital of the University of Pennsylvania, Philadelphia, Pennsylvania
Heart Failure

Samuel Z. Goldhaber, M.D.
Associate Professor of Medicine, Harvard Medical School; Director, Venous Thromboembolism Research Group; Director, Anticoagulation Service; Staff Cardiologist, Cardiovascular Division, Department of Medicine, Brigham and Women's Hospital, Boston, Massachusetts
Pulmonary Embolism, Pulmonary Hypertension, and Cor Pulmonale

Paul A. Grayburn, M.D.
Professor of Medicine, Department of Internal Medicine, Baylor University Medical Center; Clinical Professor of Medicine, Department of Internal Medicine, University of Texas Southwestern Medical Center, Dallas, Texas
*Quantitation of Ventricular Function
Quantitation of Myocardial Perfusion*

Gary V. Heller, M.D., Ph.D., F.A.C.C.
Professor, Department of Medicine and Nuclear Medicine, University of Connecticut School of Medicine, Farmington, Connecticut; Associate Director, Department of Cardiology; Director, Nuclear Cardiology Laboratory Hartford Hospital, Director, Cardiovascular Fellowship Program, Hartford Hospital/University of Connecticut, Hartford, Connecticut
Chronic Coronary Heart Disease

Howard C. Herrmann, M.D.
Professor of Medicine, Cardiovascular Division, Department of Medicine, University of Pennsylvania School of Medicine; Director, Interventional Cardiology and Cardiac Catheterization Laboratories, University of Pennsylvania Medical Center, Philadelphia, Pennsylvania
Valvular Heart Disease

Bonnie L. Hiatt, M.D.
Interventional Cardiology Fellow, Department of Cardiology, Stanford University Medical Center, Stanford, California
Coronary Heart Disease—Acute Coronary Syndromes

Karen M. Horton, M.D.
Associate Professor of Radiology, The Russell H. Morgan Department of Radiology and Radiological Science, Johns Hopkins Medical Institutions, Baltimore, Maryland
Cardiac Imaging of Masses, Tumors, and Thrombi

Martin G. Keane, M.D.
Assistant Professor of Medicine, Cardiovascular Division; Associate Scholar, Department of Biostatistics and Epidemiology, University of Pennsylvania School of Medicine; Attending Physician, Cardiovascular Division, Hospital of the University of Pennsylvania, Philadelphia, Pennsylvania
Heart Failure

Jorge R. Kizer, M.D., M.Sc.
Assistant Professor, Department of Medicine and Public Health, Weill Medical College of Cornell University; Assistant Attending Physician, Department of Medicine, New York-Presbyterian Hospital, New York, New York
Heart Failure

Michael J. Landzberg, M.D.
Director, Boston Adult Congenital Heart (BACH) Group, Departments of Internal Medicine, Pediatrics and Surgery, Brigham and Women's Hospital and Children's Hospital, Harvard University, Boston, Massachusetts
Imaging of the Adult with Congenital Heart Disease

David P. Lee, M.D.
Assistant Professor of Medicine; Associate Director, Cardiac Catheterization and Coronary Intervention Laboratories, Department of Cardiovascular Medicine, Stanford University, Stanford, California
Coronary Heart Disease—Acute Coronary Syndromes

Jeffrey A. Leppo, M.D.
Professor of Medicine and Radiology, Department of Medicine and Radiology, University of Massachusetts Medical School; Director of Nuclear Medicine and Nuclear Cardiology, Department of Medicine and Radiology, University of Massachusetts Memorial Hospital Center, Worcester, Massachusetts
Chronic Coronary Heart Disease

Debiao Li, Ph.D.
Associate Professor, Department of Radiology and Biomedical Engineering, Northwestern University, Evanston, Illinois
Quantitation of Myocardial Perfusion

Joao A.C. Lima, M.D., M.B.A.
Associate Professor of Medicine, Radiology and Epidemiology Director, Cardiovascular Imaging in Cardiology, Department of Medicine, Johns Hopkins University, Baltimore, Maryland
Physical Principles of Cardiovascular Imaging;
Cardiac Imaging of Masses, Tumors, and Thrombi

Evan Loh, M.D., F.A.C.C.
Assistant Vice President, Department of Clinical Research and Development, Wyeth Pharmaceuticals, Collegeville, Pennsylvania
Heart Failure

Jamshid Maddahi, M.D., F.A.C.C.
Professor, Department of Molecular and Medical Pharmacology (Nuclear Medicine) and Radiological Sciences, David Geffen School of Medicine at UCLA; Director of Cardiac Imaging, Nuclear Medicine, and PET, Biomedical Imaging Institute, Los Angeles, California
Chronic Coronary Heart Disease

Mahadevappa Mahesh, MS, Ph.D.
Assistant Professor of Radiology, The Russell H. Morgan Department of Radiology and Radiological Science, Johns Hopkins University; Chief Physicist, Department of Radiology, Johns Hopkins Hospital, Baltimore, Maryland
Physical Principles of Cardiovascular Imaging

John J. Mahmarian, MD
Professor of Medicine, Section of Cardiology, Department of Medicine, Baylor College of Medicine; Medical Director, The Methodist DeBakey Heart Center Nuclear Cardiology Laboratory, The Methodist Hospital; Medical Director, Nuclear Cardiology Laboratory, Baylor Heart Clinic, Houston, Texas
Chronic Coronary Heart Disease

Carina Mari, M.D.
Research Fellow, Cardiovascular Nuclear Medicine, Radiology, Nuclear Medicine Division, Stanford University Medical Center, Palo Alto, California
Imaging of Myocardial Antigens, Receptors, Hypoxia, Necrosis, Apoptosis, Metabolism, and Viability

Gerald Ross Marx, M.D.
Associate Professor, Department of Pediatrics, Harvard Medical School; Senior Associate in Cardiology, Department of Cardiology, Boston Children's Hospital, Boston, Massachusetts
Imaging of the Adult with Congenital Heart Disease

Jagat Narula, M.D., D.M., Ph.D.
Professor of Medicine; Associate Dean; Chief, Division of Cardiology, Department of Medicine, University of California, Irvine College of Medicine, Orange, California
Imaging of Myocardial Antigens, Receptors, Hypoxia, Necrosis, Apoptosis, Metabolism, and Viability

Prasad M. Panse, M.D.
Resident in Radiology, Department of Radiology, University of Florida Shands, Jacksonville, Florida
Quantitation of Myocardial Perfusion

Georgios I. Papaioannou, M.D.
Cardiovascular Fellow, Department of Cardiology, University of Connecticut School of Medicine; Cardiovascular Fellow, Department of Cardiology, Hartford Hospital, Hartford, Connecticut
Chronic Coronary Heart Disease

Alan S. Pearlman, M.D., F.A.C.C., F.A.S.E., F.A.H.A.
Professor of Medicine, Division of Cardiology, Department of Medicine, University of Washington School of Medicine; Director, Echocardiography, UW Medicine Regional Heart Center, University of Washington Medical Center, Seattle, Washington
Chronic Coronary Heart Disease

Dudley Pennell, M.D., M.R.C.P., F.A.C.C., F.E.S.C.
Professor of Cardiology, National Heart and Lung Institute, Imperial College; Director, Cardiovascular Magnetic Resonance Unit, Royal Brompton Hospital, London, United Kingdom
Chronic Coronary Heart Disease

Ronald M. Peshock, M.D.
Professor of Radiology and Internal Medicine; Associate Dean for Informatics, University of Texas Southwestern Medical Center, Dallas, Texas
Coronary Heart Disease—Acute Coronary Syndromes

Ted Plappert, C.V.T.
Center for Quantitative Echocardiography, University of Pennsylvania Medical Center, Philadelphia, Pennsylvania
Valvular Heart Disease

Eric D. Popjes, M.D.
Assistant Professor of Medicine, Department of Medicine, Pennsylvania State University Milton S. Hershey Medical School; Assistant Professor of Medicine, Department of Medicine and Cardiology, Pennsylvania State University, Milton S. Hershey Medical Center, Hershey, Pennsylvania
Heart Failure

Gilbert L. Raff, M.D., F.A.C.P., F.A.C.C.
Director of Cardiac MRI Research, Department of Cardiology, William Beaumont Hospital, Royal Oak, Michigan
Quantitation of Myocardial Perfusion

Sharon Coplen Reimold, M.D.
Associate Professor of Medicine, Department of Internal Medicine, University of Texas Southwestern Medical Center, Dallas, Texas
Coronary Heart Disease—Acute Coronary Syndromes; The Role of Cardiac Imaging and Hemodynamic Assessment in Pericardial Disease

Boaz D. Rosen, M.D.
Visiting Scholar, Department of Cardiology, Johns Hopkins Hospital; Medical Doctor, Department of Cardiology, Johns Hopkins Hospital, Baltimore, Maryland; Medical Doctor, Clinical Investigator, and Staff Cardiologist, Heart Institute, Wolfson Medical Center, Holon and Sackler School of Medicine, Tel Aviv University, Israel
Physical Principles of Cardiovascular Imaging

John A. Rumberger, M.D., Ph.D.
Clinical Professor of Medicine, Department of Cardiovascular Diseases, The Ohio State University; Medical Director, Healthwise Wellness Diagnostic Center, Columbus, Ohio
Cardiac Imaging of Masses, Tumors, and Thrombi

John D. Rutherford, M.B. Ch.B., F.R.A.C.P., F.A.C.C.
Vice President for Clinical Operations, Professor of Internal Medicine, Gail Griffiths Hill Chair in Cardiology, University of Texas Southwestern Medical Center, Dallas, Texas
Coronary Heart Disease—Acute Coronary Syndromes

J. Sanford Schwartz, MD
Professor of Medicine and Health Management and Economics, The University of Pennsylvania School of Medicine and The Wharton School, The University of Pennsylvania, Philadelphia, Pennsylvania
Diagnostic Decision Making

Piotr S. Sobieszczyk, M.D.
Fellow in Cardiovascular Medicine, Department of Medicine, Cardiovascular Division, Brigham and Women's Hospital, Boston, Massachusetts
Peripheral Arterial, Aortic, Renal Artery, and Carotid Artery Diseases

Martin G. St. John Sutton, M.B.B.S., F.R.C.P., F.A.C.C.
John W. Bryfogle Professor of Medicine, University of Pennsylvania; Director, Cardiovascular Imaging Program, Director, Cardiovascular Fellowship Program, Hospital of the University of Pennsylvania, Philadelphia, Pennsylvania
Physical Principles of Cardiovascular Imaging; Valvular Heart Disease

H. William Strauss, M.D.
Clinical Director, Department of Nuclear Medicine, Memorial Sloan Kettering Cancer Center, New York, New York
Imaging of Myocardial Antigens, Receptors, Hypoxia, Necrosis, Apoptosis, Metabolism, and Viability

Nagara Tamaki, M.D., Ph.D.
Professor and Chairman, Department of Nuclear Medicine, Hokkaido University Graduate School of Medicine; Director, Department of Nuclear Medicine, Hokkaido University Hospital
Sapporo, Japan
Imaging of Myocardial Antigens, Receptors, Hypoxia, Necrosis, Apoptosis, Metabolism, and Viability

Susan E. Wiegers, M.D., F.A.C.C.
Associate Professor of Medicine, Director of Clinical Echocardiography, The Hospital of the University of Pennsylvania, Philadelphia, Pennsylvania
Valvular Heart Disease

Norbert Wilke, M.D.
Associate Professor of Radiology, Associate Professor of Medicine, Chief, Cardiovascular MR and CT, University of Florida, Shands, Jacksonville, Florida
Quantitation of Myocardial Perfusion

Du Wayne L. Willett, M.D., M.S.
Associate Professor, Department of Internal Medicine, University of Texas Southwestern Medical Center, Dallas, Texas
Coronary Heart Disease—Acute Coronary Syndromes

Alan C. Yeung, M.D.
Associate Professor of Medicine, Chief, Division of Cardiovascular Medicine, Stanford University Medical Center, Redwood City, California
Coronary Heart Disease—Acute Coronary Syndromes

CONTENTS

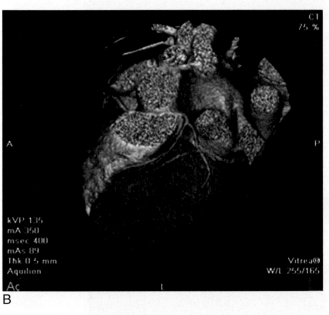

FIGURE 1-7. B, 3D CT image.

Gated ⁹⁹ᵐTc Sestamibi

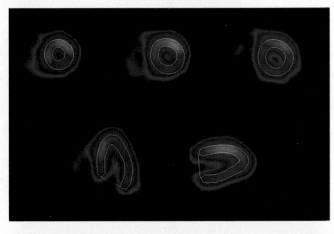

End diastole

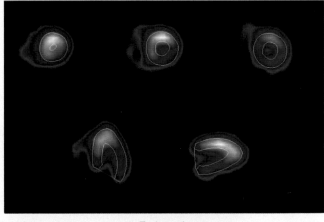

End sysole

FIGURE 1-37. ⁹⁹Tc sestamibi–gated SPECT images with a prior infero-lateral myocardial infarction. Note that brightness (apparent radioactivity) increases at end-systole because of myocardial thickening, which improves the recovery coefficient caused by partial volume effect. The inferolateral segments do not increase the brightness, because those segments do not thicken because of the prior myocardial infarction.

Effect of Attenuation Correction on a Uniform Cylindrical Phantom

No correction   With correction

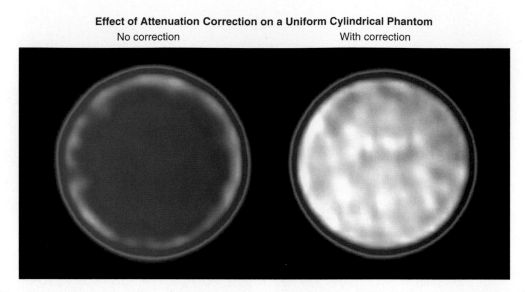

FIGURE 1-38. The effect of photon attenuation on the tomographic images of a uniform cylinder filled with water containing ^{99m}Tc. Note that apparent tracer concentration in the centers is lower than in the periphery. This is due to the attenuation of the gamma rays originating in the center of the cylinder as they travel through water. After applying attenuation correction, the apparent radioactive ^{99m}Tc reflects the uniform radioactive distribution present in the cylinder.

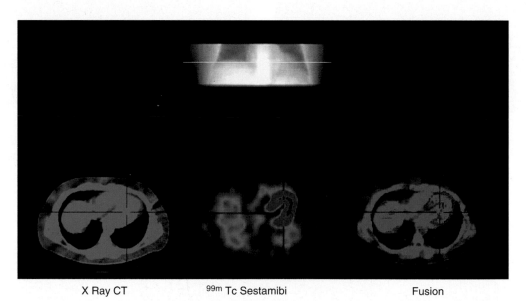

X Ray CT ^{99m} Tc Sestamibi   Fusion

FIGURE 1-39. Example of a myocardial perfusion study with attenuation correction using X-ray CT to create a attenuation map.

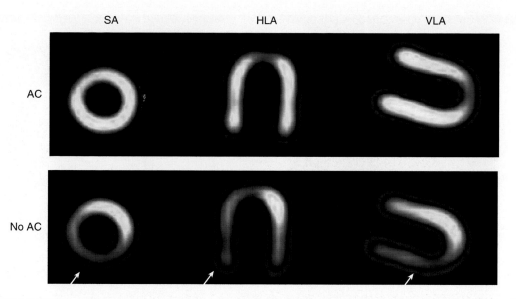

FIGURE 1-40. Short-axis (SA), horizontal long axis (HLA), and vertical long-axis (VLA) views of a heart phantom filled with a uniform solution of ^{99m}Tc in water. Note the lower intensity in the "inferior" wall in the uncorrected images. Attenuation correction (AC) images demonstrate more uniform distribution.

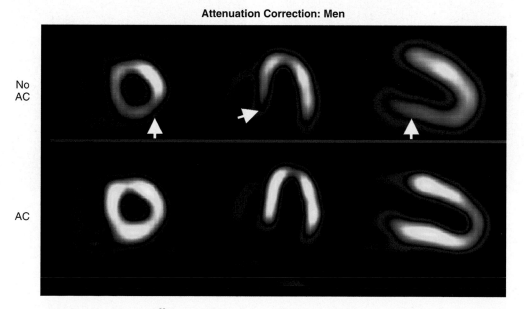

FIGURE 1-41. Representative example of a normal ^{99}Tc sestamibi study in a man with no attenuation correction (No AC) and with AC. Tracer uptake is more uniform in those images with correction.

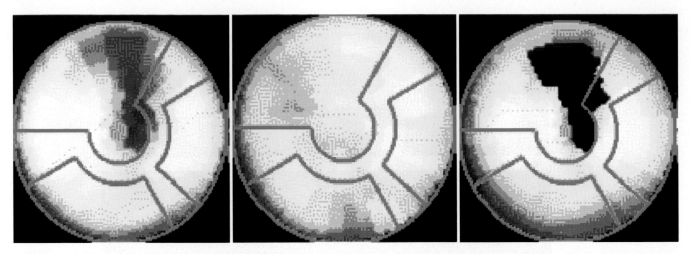

FIGURE 1-42. Polar map graph of a ^{99m}Tc sestamibi study at stress and rest. The left graph represents myocardial tracer uptake after exercise, the center graph represents myocardial tracer uptake at rest, and the graph on the right represents the extent of the defect. Note that a perfusion defect is present on the images after stress, indicating stress-induced ischemia in the territory of the left anterior descending coronary artery.

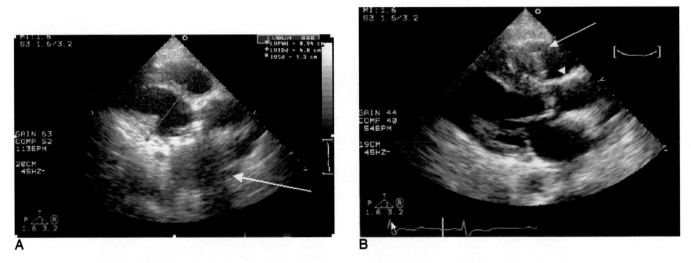

FIGURE 1-58. Examples of artifacts commonly encountered in cardiac imaging. **A,** Acoustic shadowing from a prosthetic aortic valve; **B,** reverberation artifact originating from a pacemaker electrode. The "true" electrode *(arrow)* is the echogenic object close to the transducer. The artifact is located deeper *(arrow head)*.

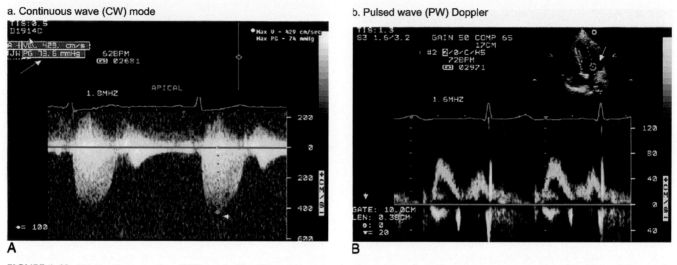

FIGURE 1-63. (**A**) Continuous wave (CW) mode. The US wave is transmitted continuously, without interruptions, and received by a different element in the transducer. The transducer is oriented through the tricuspid valve. The flow measured is a jet of tricuspid regurgitation *(arrowhead)*. The peak gradient through the tricuspid valve can be calculated (73.6 mmHg) by measuring the peak velocity of the regurgitant jet and using the Bernoulli rule. (**B**) Pulsed-wave (PW) Doppler. A short wave is sent. Doppler-shifted echoes may be received only when the range gate is open. When the gate is closed, all the echoes are discarded. This figure shows a normal pattern of blood flow through the mitral valve. Note the sampling volume in the 2D image, located adjacent to the tips of the mitral leaflets *(small arrow, upper right)*. Sampling depth and its length are indicated (arrowhead, lower left).

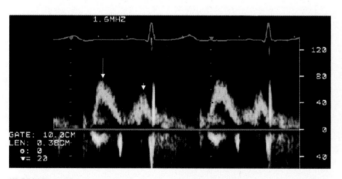

FIGURE 1-65. A standard display of the Doppler instruments that includes Doppler shifts and their magnitude as a function of time (x-axis). Amplitude is displayed as *brightness* on a gray scale, and each time point in the cardiac cycle is represented by a *vertical line*. As the flow in a certain time point is more organized, the FFT spectrum is narrower and the vertical line is shorter. Positive and negative shifts indicate movement toward and away from the transducer, respectively. A normal transmitral flow pattern is shown in the figure. Note the organized flow characterized by short vertical lines and two peaks indicating early (E wave) *(arrow)* and late diastolic filling (A wave) *(arrowhead)*.

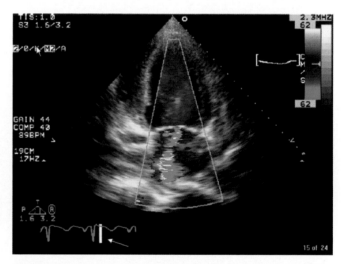

FIGURE 1-67. Color Doppler. ECG tracing is shown below and time of sampling during systole is indicated *(small arrow)*. Note the marked blood flow from the left ventricle toward the left atrium, indicating severe mitral regurgitation. On this color scale, brighter colors indicate higher velocities.

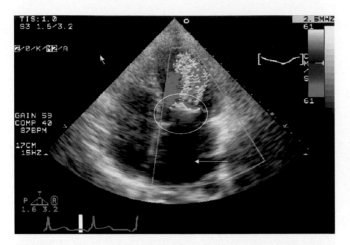

FIGURE 1-68. Aliasing in color Doppler. Diastolic flow (note ECG tracing below) through a severely stenotic mitral valve. Note the sphere with orange, yellow, and blue layers *(circled)*, indicating aliasing caused by acceleration proximal to the mitral valve, and the highly turbulent flow manifested as a mosaic of multiple colors. The area of the proximal sphere is termed the proximal isovelocity surface area (PISA). Note also the dilated left atrium *(arrow)* characteristic of mitral stenosis

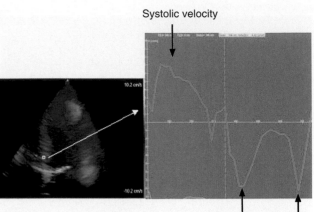

Systolic velocity

Em wave Am wave

FIGURE 1-71. Tissue velocity imaging in a normal volunteer. Myocardial velocity in the basal septum is interrogated (see arrow). Myocardial velocity in the myocardium is color encoded. Red color indicates motion toward the transducer, and blue indicates movement away from the transducer. On the right, a plot representing myocardial motion is shown. Movement toward the transducer (systole) is above baseline, whereas movement away from the transducer is located below baseline. Note Em and Am waves indicating early and late filling, respectively. (See Color Insert.)

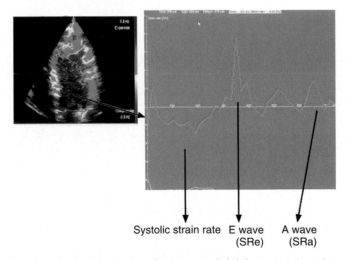

Systolic strain rate E wave   A wave
                      (SRe)   (SRa)

FIGURE 1-72. Strain rate imaging in a healthy volunteer. Strain rate reflects myocardial deformation along the cardiac cycle. Positive values indicate myocardial elongation, whereas negative values indicate shortening. On the left side, strain rate imaging is shown. Blue color indicates elongation (positive strain rate), and yellow and red colors indicate myocardial shortening. On the right side, a plot reflecting strain rate measured from the septum is shown. Note the negative systolic wave, reflecting longitudinal shortening and positive waves during diastole, implying early and late myocardial elongation (SrE and SrA, respectively). (See Color Insert).

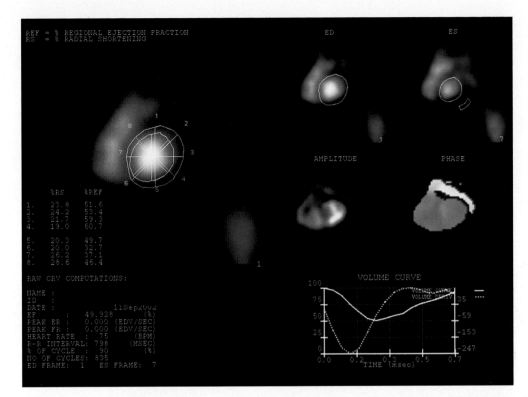

FIGURE 2-16. Radionuclide angiogram by MUGA technique. At the upper right, regions of interest are drawn around the left ventricle in a left anterior oblique projection at end-diastole (ED) and end-systole (ES). A volume-time curve showing radioactive counts during the cardiac cycle is shown at bottom right. The global LVEF is 50%. At upper left is a polar map showing percent radial shortening and percent ejection fraction in each of eight segments. (Courtesy of Michael Brophey, MD.)

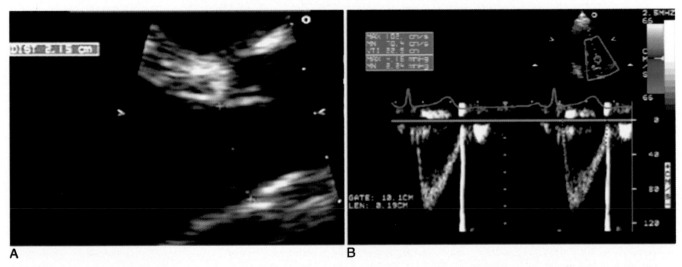

A   B

FIGURE 2-19. Doppler method of measuring cardiac output at the aortic annulus. *Left panel,* Parasternal long-axis view using zoom mode to magnify the measurement of the LV outflow tract diameter at the base of the aortic leaflets. *Right panel,* Pulsed Doppler velocity signal from the LV outflow tract. The modal velocity is traced to display the velocity-time integral in centimeters. This value is equal to the stroke distance or the distance that the heart would propel a single red blood cell. The product of stroke distance and LV outflow tract cross-sectional area is the stroke volume. (Courtesy of Brad Roberts, RDCS.)

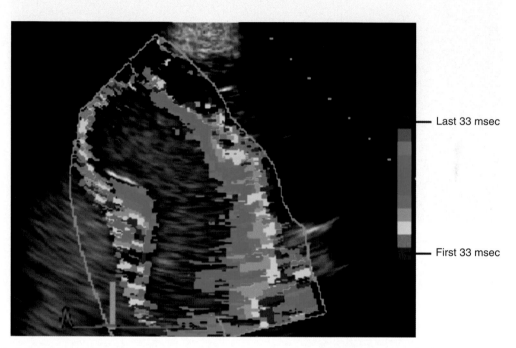

Last 33 msec

First 33 msec

FIGURE 2-27. Color kinesis images from a patient with apical akinesis *(arrows)*. Each color shown in the color bar represents endocardial motion during systole. Orange represents the first 33 ms and each subsequent 33-ms period is represented by a different color; bright blue represents the final 33 ms of systole (Courtesy of Brad Roberts, RDCS).

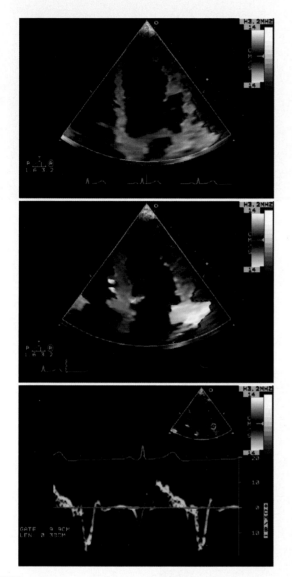

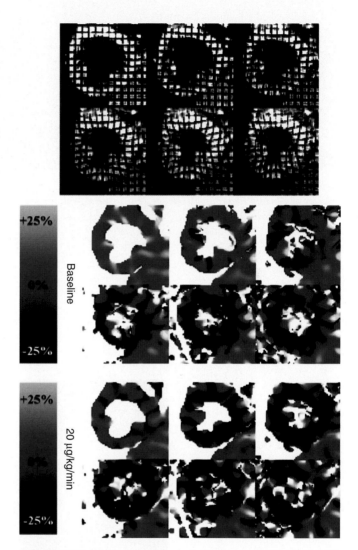

FIGURE 2-28. Tissue Doppler images. *Left panel,* 2D color tissue Doppler image in an apical four-chamber view. T*op panel,* Tissue Doppler image of myocardial velocities during systole in the apical four-chamber view. The red signal indicates diastolic tissue motion toward the transducer. *Middle panel,* Tissue Doppler image of myocardial velocities during diastole. The blue signal indicates diastolic tissue motion away from the transducer. *Bottom panel,* Spectral tissue Doppler display of velocities at the lateral mitral annulus. Systolic motion (S) is displayed above the baseline; early diastolic (E′) and atrial contraction (A′) velocities are below the baseline. (Courtesy of Brad Roberts, RDCS.)

FIGURE 2-30. Spatial modulation of magnetization (SPAMM) CMR images illustrating the concept of tracking the motion of CMR tags, seen as dark lines overlying the images in the upper panel (see text). By measuring the spatial and temporal motion of the tags, 3D strain and strain rate can be determined accurately. The middle panel shows myocardial strain on a pixel-by-pixel basis at baseline; the bottom panel shows myocardial strain during dobutamine infusion. (Reprinted with permission from Garot J, Bluemke DA, Osman NF, et al. Fast determination of regional myocardial strain fields from tagged cardiac images using harmonic phase CMR. *Circulation* 2000; 101:981.)

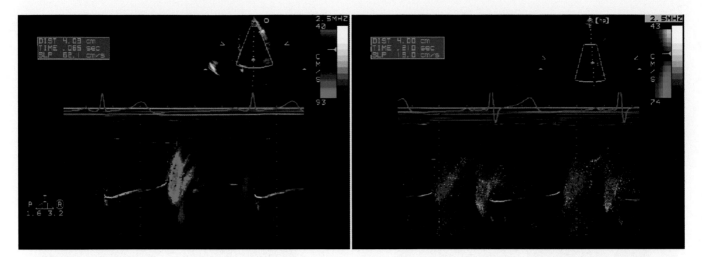

FIGURE 2-34. Color M-mode flow propagation as a measure of LV filling. *Left panel,* Tracing from a normal subject showing a flow propagation velocity of 62 cm/s. *Right panel,* Tracing from a patient with isolated LV diastolic dysfunction and a propagation velocity of 9 cm/s. (Courtesy of Brad Roberts, RDCS.)

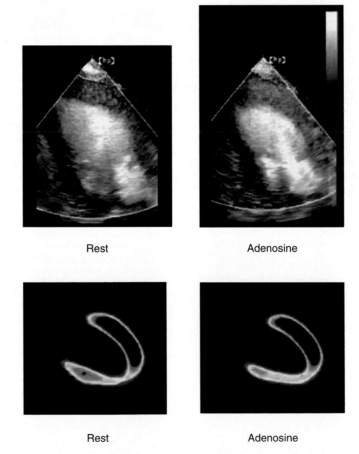

Rest   Adenosine

Rest   Adenosine

FIGURE 3-4. *Top panel,* Harmonic power Doppler images from an apical two-chamber view at rest *(left)* and during adenosine infusion *(right).* There is normal perfusion of the anterior wall but a fixed defect in the inferior wall. *Bottom panel,* SPECT sestamibi images confirm the fixed inferior defect in the same patient.

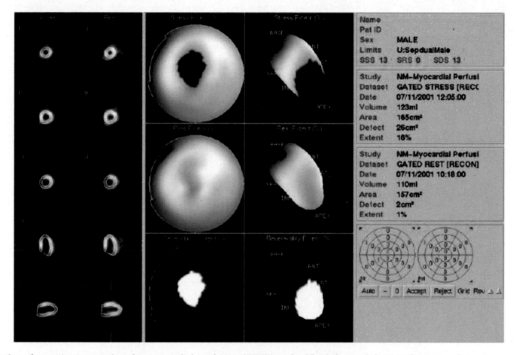

FIGURE 3-6. Display of quantitative results of a myocardial perfusion SPECT study. The left panel depicts the rest and stress myocardial slices used for quantitative analysis. The 2D *(middle panel)* and 3D *(right panel)* polar maps depict the relative quantitative tracer uptake during stress *(top)*, at rest *(middle)*, and their difference *(bottom)* reflecting the amount of defect reversibility. In the 2D polar maps, the left ventricular apex is represented at the center, the septum is to the left, the anterior wall is on the top, the lateral wall is to the right, and the inferior wall is at the bottom. The blackout regions in the polar maps reflect the extent of the perfusion abnormality, and the white color in the reversibility polar map reflects the amount of stress-induced ischemia. This example demonstrates a moderately large area of inducible ischemia in a patient with significant stenosis in the mid left anterior descending coronary artery.

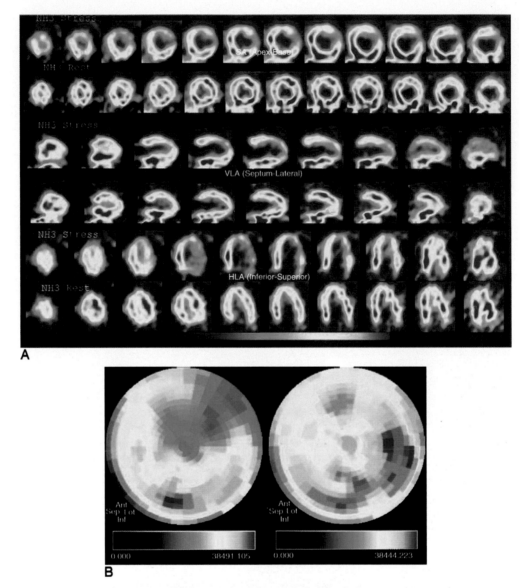

FIGURE 3-18. A, Short- and long-axis images of a patient with coronary artery disease obtained after adenosine stress *(top)* and rest *(bottom)* using $^{13}NH_3$. There is a large anterolateral perfusion defect. **B,** Polar map of the stress perfusion image *(left)* and rest image *(right)*.

SPECT

Stress

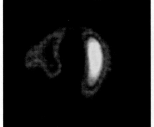

PET

Perfusion ($^{13}NH_3$)

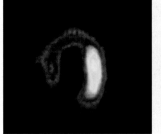

24 Hours

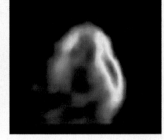

Metabolism (^{18}F-FDG)

IVUS: Unstable angina

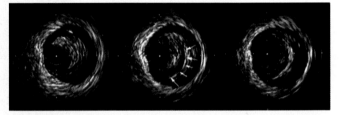

FIGURE 3-22. Image taken from a patient showing discrepancies between perfusion obtained with SPECT and that obtained with PET. On the left are stress, 4-hour, and 24-hour redistribution images obtained after administration of ^{201}Tl. To the right are analogous images obtained after administration of $^{13}NH_3$ and FDG. Areas of apparent decreased flow in the septum are actually caused by tissue attenuation in the SPECT scan, and analysis of a SPECT perfusion vs. PET FDG scan would result in a false-positive assessment of hibernating myocardium. Thus, caution must be used when performing interpretation obtained with SPECT and PET because of differences in tracer attenuation and attenuation correction.

FIGURE 8-5. Coronary intravascular ultrasound images of a patient who presented with unstable angina. *Panel 1,* Intravascular ultrasound image proximal to an angiographic stenosis, illustrating an eccentric plaque with a fair amount of echogenicity. This is consistent with fibrofatty plaque. *Panel 2,* Intravascular ultrasound image of the stenosis. The arrows illustrate the interface between plaque and intraluminal thrombus. *Panel 3,* Intravascular ultrasound image of the distal lesion.

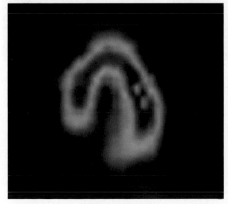

SAX - Apex

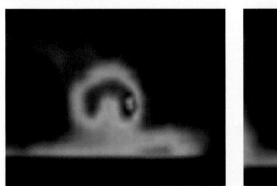

SAX - Base

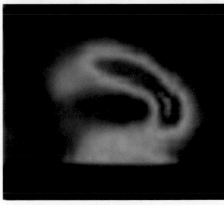

Horizontal LAX

Vertical LAX

FIGURE 8-9. Sestamibi imaging of a patient with atypical chest pain. A 67-year-old woman was seen in the emergency room with atypical chest pain and an electrocardiogram with a left bundle-branch block pattern. A sestamibi scan revealed an inferior wall perfusion defect. Subsequent coronary angiography showed 99% stenosis of the proximal right coronary artery, which was successfully revascularized by percutaneous coronary intervention. SAX, short axis; LAX, long axis.

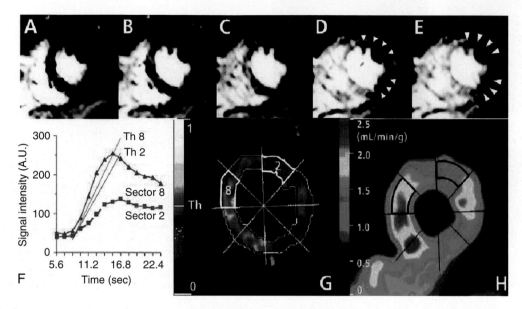

FIGURE 8-12. Perfusion imaging. **A-E,** In this patient with stenoses in the left anterior descending coronary artery and the right coronary artery, the transit of contrast material through the left ventricular myocardium during hyperemia demonstrates delayed wash-in in both the subendocardial and subepicardial layers of both arteries *(arrowheads)*. **F,** Representative signal intensity–time curves are shown for normal myocardium (sector 8) and hypoperfused myocardium (sector 2). On the parametric slope map **G,** pixels below/above the threshold (Th) are encoded in shades of blue/red, respectively. On the PET image **H,** reduced hyperemic flow is demonstrated in corresponding sectors. (Adapted from Schwitter J, Nanz D, Kneifel S, et al. Assessment of myocardial perfusion in coronary artery disease by magnetic resonance. A comparison with positron emission tomography and coronary angiography. *Circulation* 2001; 103:2230.)

Vulnerable Plaque

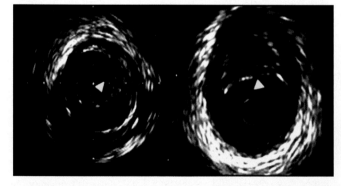

FIGURE 8-13. Intravascular ultrasound images of a highly remodeled coronary plaque with features of vulnerable plaque. There is an echolucent core and a thin fibrous cap *(arrows)*.

Red Clot and White Clot

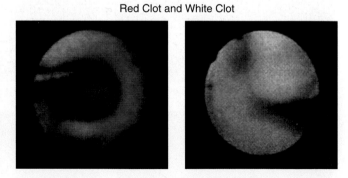

FIGURE 8-14. Angioscopy of two plaques in patients with a acute coronary syndrome. The left panel shows a plaque that is rich in red cells and probably fibrin. The right panel shows a plaque that is rich in platelets. (Reprinted from Abela et al. *Am J Cardiol* 1999; 83:94, with permission from Excerpta Medica Inc.)

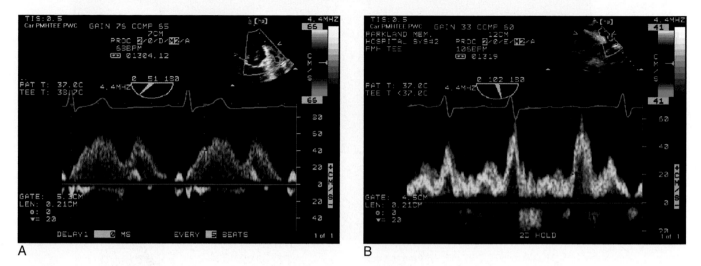

A

B

FIGURE 8-15. Pulmonary venous inflow patterns. **A,** Normal pulmonary venous flow depicted with antegrade flow in systole and diastole. Normally the systolic velocity and velocity time integral exceed the respective diastolic components. **B,** In the abnormal state, diastolic flow velocities exceed systolic flow velocities. This may be seen in individuals with low cardiac output, significant mitral regurgitation, or elevated left atrial filling pressures.

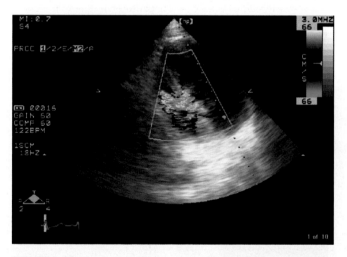

FIGURE 8-16. Echocardiographic imaging of a ventricular septal defect. A loud systolic murmur developed in this patient 4 days after an inferior myocardial infarction. **A,** A large defect is seen in the inferior septum from this modified apical projection. **B,** Color flow Doppler demonstrates left to right flow consistent with a postmyocardial infarction ventricular septal defect.

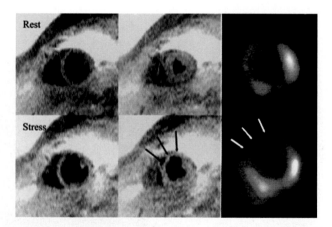

FIGURE 9-7. Dipyridamole CMR in a patient with left anterior descending artery disease. In the top row are short axis images before dipyridamole with postdipyridamole images in the lower row. End-diastole is in the left column, and end-systole is in the middle column. Left ventricular contraction is normal before vasodilatation but reduced in the anteroseptal region after dipyridamole *(black arrows).* The stress-induced contraction abnormality is closely matched by the defect seen during dipyridamole thallium myocardial perfusion tomography *(white arrows on the color maps in the right column),* which shows full reversibility. (Reproduced with permission from reference 29.)

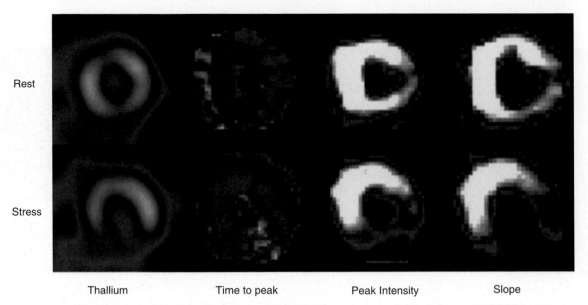

Rest

Stress

Thallium   Time to peak   Peak Intensity   Slope

FIGURE 9-8. Parametric map analysis for representation of perfusion CMR in a patient with an inferolateral reversible defect, with the corresponding thallium images *(first column)*. Columns 2 through 4 show the time to peak CMR myocardial signal intensity, the peak signal intensity, and the peak slope of the signal intensity vs. Time curves. There is good correlation between the CMR maps and the thallium scan. (Reproduced with permission from reference 31.)

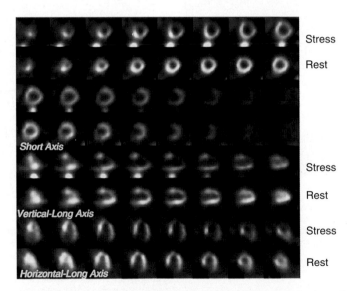

Stress

Rest

Short Axis

Stress

Rest

Vertical-Long Axis

Stress

Rest

Horizontal-Long Axis

FIGURE 9-10. High-risk scan: Demonstration of exercise ^{99m}Tc-sestamibi myocardial perfusion imaging in multiple views (short-axis, vertical long-axis, horizontal long-axis; stress images on top of each row with test images on the bottom). Stress images demonstrate transient cavity dilation and extensive ischemia involving the anterior, anteroseptal, anterolateral, and anteroapical distribution. Rest images reveal normalization of the cavity size and elimination of the perfusion abnormalities. These findings predict a high risk for future cardiac events for the particular patient.

N-13 Ammonia

^{18}F-deoxyglucose

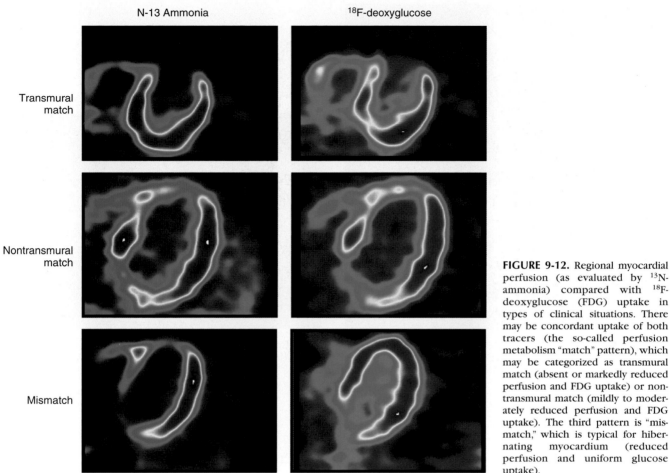

Transmural
match

Nontransmural
match

Mismatch

FIGURE 9-12. Regional myocardial perfusion (as evaluated by ^{13}N-ammonia) compared with ^{18}F-deoxyglucose (FDG) uptake in types of clinical situations. There may be concordant uptake of both tracers (the so-called perfusion metabolism "match" pattern), which may be categorized as transmural match (absent or markedly reduced perfusion and FDG uptake) or nontransmural match (mildly to moderately reduced perfusion and FDG uptake). The third pattern is "mismatch," which is typical for hibernating myocardium (reduced perfusion and uniform glucose uptake).

Stress Tc-99m Sestamibi SPECT

Rest FDG SPECT

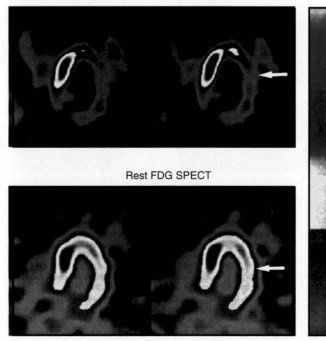

FIGURE 9-13. Patient study demonstrating "mismatch" of FDG (glucose metabolism) and sestamibi (perfusion) performed on a SPECT imaging camera (not a dedicated PET camera). There is decreased perfusion in the posterior lateral wall, but glucose uptake is preserved (viable myocardium).

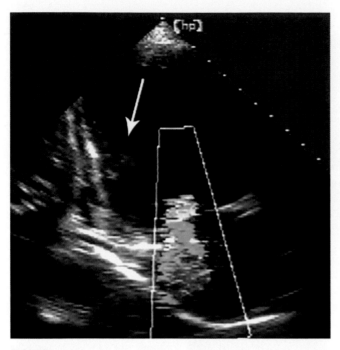

FIGURE 10-1. Apical two-chamber view demonstrates eccentric, posteriorly directed mitral regurgitation. The inferior wall and posteromedial papillary muscle *(arrow)* are scarred from prior myocardial infarction. Restricted systolic motion of the posterior mitral valve leaflet results in an overriding anterior mitral leaflet and eccentric regurgitation.

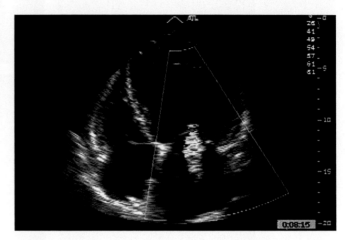

FIGURE 10-5. Atrial and ventricular cavity enlargement result in uniform dilation of the mitral annulus, with central malcoaptation of the mitral valve leaflets. This results in centrally oriented mitral regurgitation.

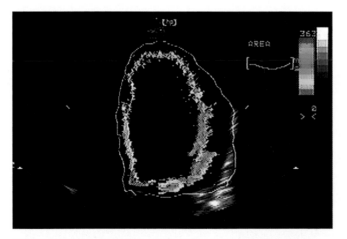

FIGURE 10-16. Color kinesis display of the left ventricular long axis.

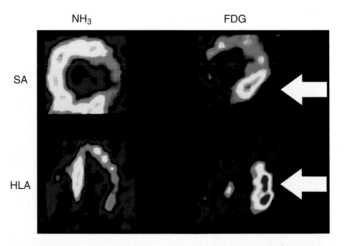

FIGURE 10-17. PET scan from a patient with angina and heart failure. Echocardiogram demonstrated LV ejection fraction of 30% with lateral akinesis. ^{18}F-fluorodeoxyglucose scan shows significant metabolic activity in the lateral wall *(arrow)*, but ^{13}N-ammonia uptake is minimal in this region. This perfusion-metabolism mismatch is consistent with hibernating myocardium. After redo bypass of the circumflex, LV ejection fraction increased to 65%, with return of lateral wall function (SA, short axis; HLA, horizontal long axis). (Courtesy of Luis Aruago, University of Pennsylvania.)

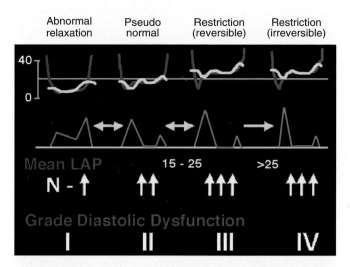

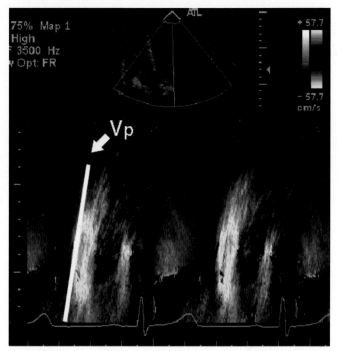

FIGURE 10-22. Diagrammatic display of pulsed-wave Doppler of mitral inflow patterns from the apical position. Normal diastolic filling is characterized by a velocity of the early filling wave of 0.8 to 1.0 cm/s, which is higher than the atrial wave velocity. **I**, Diastolic dysfunction pattern. The early filling wave velocity is lower than the A wave, and the deceleration time of the E wave has increased compared with normal **II**, Pseudonormalized pattern. Increased left atrial pressure results in increased early driving force for transmitral flow. The E wave again becomes prominent, despite impaired relaxation. **III**, and **IV**, Restrictive patterns. The E wave demonstrates a rapid deceleration time because of restrictive disease. The A wave is diminutive in this case because of atrial systolic failure. (Adapted from Tajik.)

FIGURE 10-25. Color Doppler M-mode recording of mitral inflow. The normal early filling wave propagates rapidly toward the apex. The slope of the color signal demonstrated by the straight line on the second filling pattern is the velocity of propagation of early filling. Note that the velocity of the early wave is higher than the A wave and reaches farther into the LV cavity.

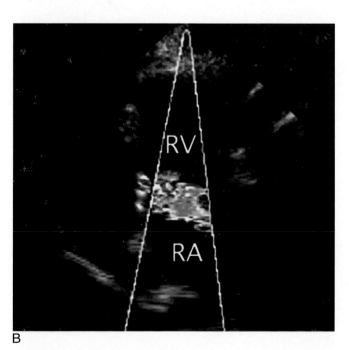

B

FIGURE 10-27. (B). The perforation results in a wide-based color Doppler jet of tricuspid regurgitation.

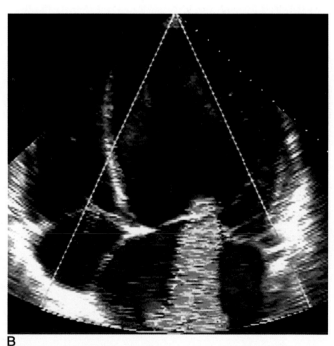

B

FIGURE 11-14. B, Similar view in the same patient with color Doppler flow imaging in systole. A large color jet of mitral regurgitation extends to the posterior wall of the left atrium. The mitral regurgitation begins in the left ventricle at the level of the mitral leaflet tips, more apically displaced than is normal. A jet of tricuspid regurgitation is incompletely visualized in the right atrium (RA).

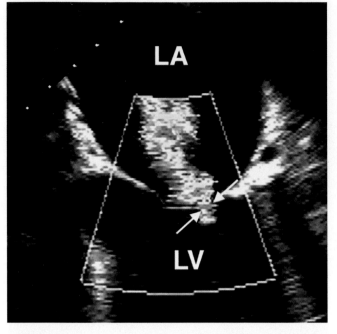

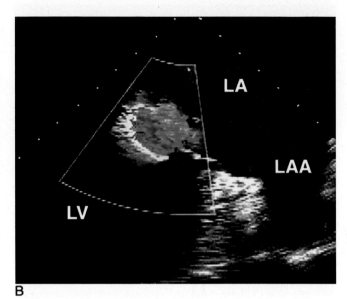

FIGURE 11-16. Transesophageal color flow Doppler image from the transverse plane in a patient with moderate mitral regurgitation. The vena contracta *(indicated by arrows)* is the narrowest area of the jet as it passes just beyond the mitral valve leaflets. The vena contracta in this patient is approximately 0.4 mm, consistent with moderate mitral regurgitation.

FIGURE 11-17. B, Demonstration of PISA phenomenon in a patient with severe mitral regurgitation caused by a flail anterior leaflet. The jet is very eccentric, and its course cannot be visualized in the left atrium in this plane (LAA, left atrial appendage).

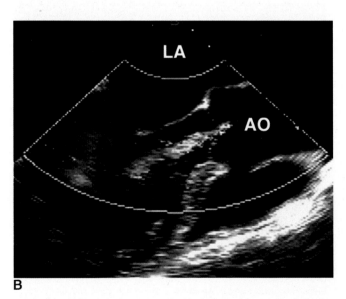

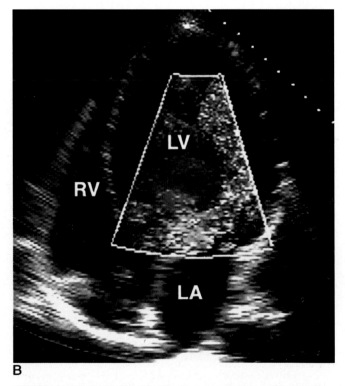

FIGURE 11-27. B, Transesophageal echocardiogram from the same transducer position. A high-velocity turbulent jet of aortic regurgitation arises from the aortic leaflets and extends into the left ventricular outflow tract. The ratio of the jet width immediately below the valve leaflets to the outflow tract diameter is much less than 25%, which is diagnostic of mild aortic regurgitation.

FIGURE 11-33. B, Similar view in the same patient with color flow Doppler imaging. The high-velocity, turbulent jet of aortic regurgitation extends almost to the apex of the dilated ventricle.

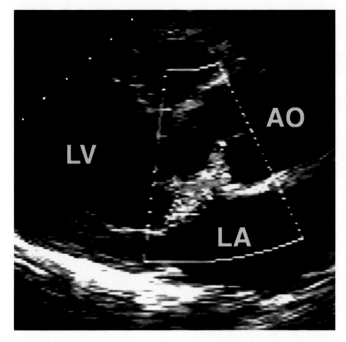

FIGURE 11-35. Parasternal long-axis view in diastole. There is eccentric aortic regurgitation that is directed posteriorly along the anterior mitral valve leaflet. The width of the jet immediately below the aortic valve leaflets is difficult to measure, because the jet runs parallel to the leaflets. The degree of regurgitation was moderate. The mitral valve appears closed in this diastolic frame, but filling was normal. The patient has a dilated root and had mitral valve prolapse in systole (not shown). These findings are consistent with the diagnosis of Marfan's syndrome.

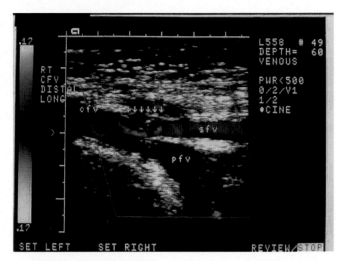

FIGURE 12-5. Longitudinal axis view of a color Doppler ultrasound examination demonstrating an extensive superficial femoral vein thrombosis. The "superficial" femoral vein, despite its name, is a deep vein. The superficial femoral vein (SFV) and the profunda femoral vein (PFV) join to form the common femoral (CF) vein. (From Dr. Goldhaber's private collection.)

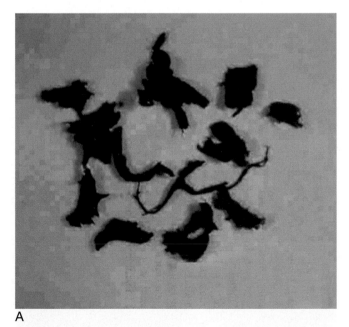

A

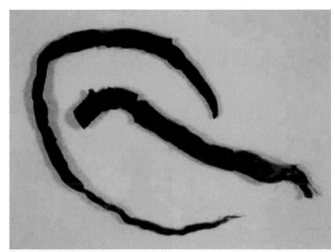

B

FIGURE 12-17. This 34-year-old woman was initially seen with chest discomfort, shortness of breath, and left arm discomfort and numbness. Chest CT scan suggested both pulmonary embolism and aortic thrombus. Further workup included transesophageal echocardiography, which showed moderately severe right ventricular dysfunction, bidirectional color flow across the interatrial septum, and a thrombus at the proximal origin of the left subclavian artery. We diagnosed pulmonary and paradoxical arterial thromboembolism and referred her for urgent embolectomy. At surgery, a 15- to 20-mm patent foramen ovale was closed with two layers of sutures. **A,** Multiple fragments of acute pulmonary embolus were removed from both proximal pulmonary arteries. The thromboembolus measured 4 × 3 × 2 cm in aggregate. **B,** Two large arterial thromboemboli, measuring 11 cm and 16 cm, were then removed. The 11-cm embolus extended from the left subclavian artery to the descending aorta. The 16-cm embolus extended from the left subclavian artery to the right subclavian artery by way of the innominate artery. (From Dr. Goldhaber's private collection.)

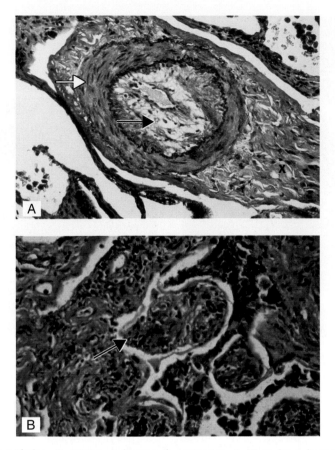

FIGURE 12-20. Characteristic lung pathology in primary pulmonary hypertension. **A,** Muscular pulmonary artery with medical hypertrophy *(white arrow)*, luminal narrowing by intimal proliferation *(black arrow)*, and proliferation of adventitia *(X)*. **B,** Characteristic plexiform lesion from an obstructed muscular pulmonary artery *(arrow)*. (Reproduced with permission from Gaine SP, Rubin LJ. Primary pulmonary hypertension. *Lancet* 1998; 352:719.)

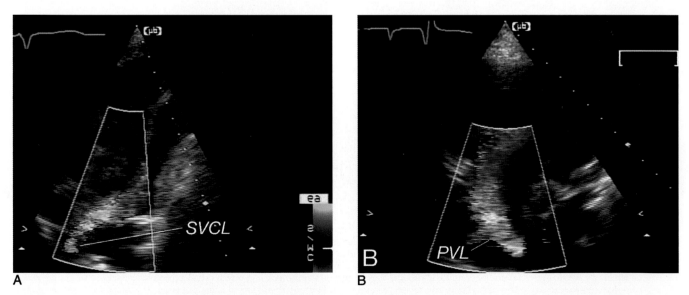

FIGURE 14-23. Color-flow Doppler imaging of a Mustard baffle. Because transthoracic windows are usually very limited, baffle pathways may be visualized only with color-flow Doppler interrogation, which demonstrates the SVC limb **(A)** and the pulmonary venous chambers **(B)**.

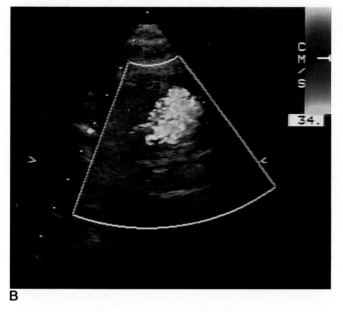

B

FIGURE 14-26. B, Color-flow Doppler is used to assess for flow acceleration indicating possible stenoses.

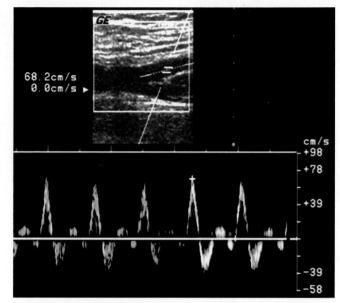

FIGURE 16-4. Duplex ultrasound recording of the common femoral artery bifurcation with pulse Doppler velocity analysis of the superficial femoral artery. This normal pulse velocity waveform demonstrates rapid forward flow during systole, transient flow reversal during early diastole, and antegrade flow at a low velocity during the remainder of diastole.

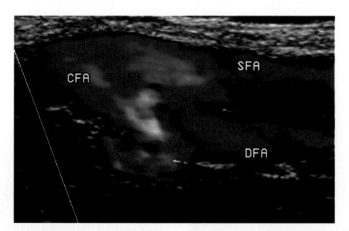

FIGURE 16-5. Color duplex ultrasound examination of a normal common femoral artery bifurcation. The homogeneous red color is indicative of laminar flow.

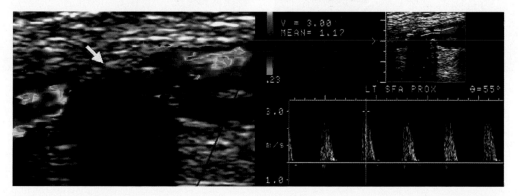

FIGURE 16-6. Duplex ultrasound examination of the proximal portion of a superficial femoral artery. Acoustic shadowing is indicative of a calcified atherosclerotic plaque *(arrow) (left panel).* The pulse Doppler velocity profile is 300 cm/s, greater than twofold more than that recorded in a more proximal normal section of this artery *(right panel).* This finding is consistent with a stenosis of at least 50%.

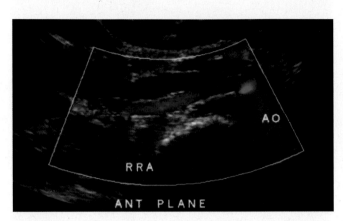

FIGURE 16-25. Color duplex ultrasound examination of the right renal artery. (Courtesy of Dr. Jeffrey Olin, Mt. Sinai Medical Center, New York, NY.)

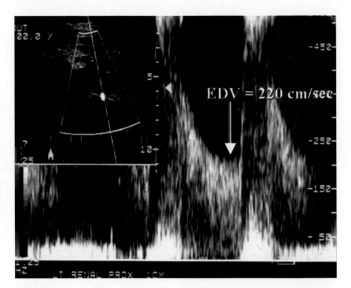

FIGURE 16-26. Continuous-wave Doppler interrogation of a stenosed left renal artery. The peak systolic velocity is >450 cm/s, and the end-diastolic velocity is 200 cm/s, each indicative of a severe stenosis. (Courtesy of Dr. Jeffrey Olin, Mt. Sinai Medical Center, New York, NY.)

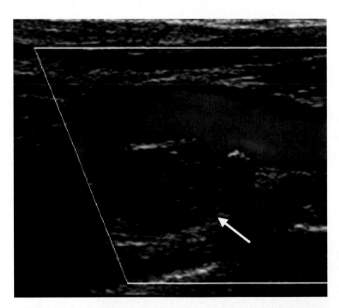

FIGURE 16-35. Duplex ultrasound of the carotid bifurcation. The arrow indicates the carotid body tumor posterior to the carotid artery.

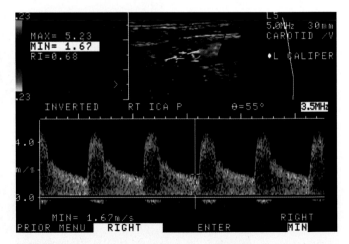

FIGURE 16-36. Duplex ultrasound of a right internal carotid artery. Color Doppler is used to identify areas of turbulence and aliasing. The spectral waveform is notable for the elevated peak systolic velocity of 523 cm/s and the end-diastolic velocity of 167 cm/s. These findings indicate diameter reduction of 95% or greater.

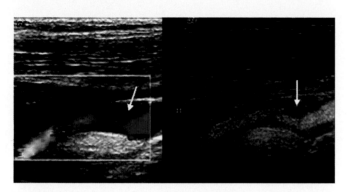 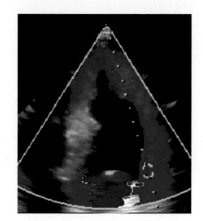

FIGURE 16-37. Blood flow to vessel wall interface of the same vessel evaluated with color Doppler *(left)* and B flow *(right)*. Relatively hypoechoic plaque (P) is evident on the near wall in both images. The color Doppler is written over the gray scale image, resulting in less definition of the blood flow vessel wall interface than is evident in the B flow image. The B flow image is a gray scale image that uses very high pulse repetition frequency. The internal jugular vein (IJ) is seen above the carotid.

Cover Art 02

Physical Principles of Cardiovascular Imaging

Bernhard L. Gerber
Boaz D. Rosen
Mahadevappa Mahesh
Luis I. Araujo
Martin G. St. John Sutton
João A. C. Lima

BACKGROUND

The development of invasive coronary angiography ushered in a revolution in the practice of cardiovascular medicine four and one-half decades ago. The power of imaging to guide the diagnosis and treatment of cardiovascular diseases was further advanced by the development, validation, and widespread implementation of echocardiography in valvular heart disease and nuclear methods to assess myocardial perfusion and viability. By the end of the 1980s, diagnostic and treatment strategies in cardiology had already become heavily dependent on the use of imaging modalities, and this fueled their further development. Advances in imaging technology also contributed significantly to the progress achieved by cardiologists, cardiac surgeons, and cardiovascular scientists in reducing morbidity and mortality caused by diseases of the heart and circulation.

The accelerated technological development that characterized the 1990s in the fields of computer science, synthetic materials, and applied electronics enabled the adaptation of powerful tomographic imaging modalities such as cardiac magnetic resonance (CMR) imaging and computed tomography (CT) to study the heart and cardiovascular system. New information obtained with these novel imaging methods has resulted in their increased use in the current practice of cardiovascular medicine. Concomitant with the introduction of CMR and CT for cardiovascular imaging, new advanced technologies have been developed in echocardiography and nuclear cardiology that have enhanced noninvasive diagnostic capabilities and had an impact on clinical treatment algorithms. The development of positron emission tomography, Doppler echocardiography, transesophageal echocardiography, and intravascular ultrasound has transformed the clinical approach to patients with cardiovascular disease. In addition, epidemiological studies have defined the role of electron beam CT and carotid ultrasound in assessing atherosclerotic burden and the risk for clinical manifestations of vascular disease. Future developments in cardiovascular imaging include the capability of imaging coronary vessels noninvasively with CMR or CT, which will impact on clinical decision making.

The technological advancement in cardiovascular imaging over the past decade has created the need for novel types of knowledge and expertise, so that cardiologists and cardiovascular physicians involved in the care of patients with heart disease are faced with decisions regarding the choice of imaging studies and the need to understand their interpretation. In this regard, a basic understanding of the physical principles underlying imaging methods as applied to the cardiovascular system is important for optimal use of these technologies. This chapter is designed to provide a concise description of the basic physical principles and instrumentation involved in current cardiovascular CT, CMR, nuclear, and ultrasound imaging techniques.

PHYSICAL PRINCIPLES OF MULTIPLE-ROW DETECTOR AND ELECTRON BEAM COMPUTED TOMOGRAPHY

The introduction of rapid CT techniques enabled noninvasive assessment of coronary atherosclerosis in individuals at risk for myocardial infarction or angina pectoris. The possibility of obtaining reliable coronary angiograms in patients with suspected coronary artery disease noninvasively has recently propelled CT to center stage.

Cardiovascular imaging began with fluoroscopic techniques of the heart and later the coronary arteries. Imaging of the heart and coronary arteries was the stimulus for the development of therapeutic methods that revolutionized the practice of cardiovascular medicine, including coronary artery bypass surgery, surgical valve repair/replacement, and more recently percutaneous transluminal coronary angioplasty (PTCA) with stent deployment. However, conventional projection X-ray imaging is limited because of the loss of detail from superimposition of three-dimensional (3D) structural information on to a two-dimensional (2D) surface, which occurs despite the very high spatial resolution (five line-pairs/mm) and very short acquisition times (10-100 ms) sufficient to freeze cardiac motion. The latter capability is critical to imaging moving organs with minimal degradation from motion artifacts. Small differences in X-ray attenuation by various tissues are not readily detectable on X-ray film or on fluoroscopic display modalities. Therefore, a large percentage of the radiation detected is scattered within the patient, thus reducing the signal-to-noise (S/N) ratio. Since its introduction in 1972, X-ray CT has evolved into an important diagnostic imaging tool, because it greatly minimizes these problems, providing the clinician with an accurate tool for the noninvasive examination of internal structures of the body. Dramatic improvements in image quality, acquisition speed, and patient throughput have resulted from recent technical developments in helical and, more recently, multiple-row detector technologies (MDCT). This evolution in CT technology has greatly enabled cardiac imaging and evaluation of cardiac function with unprecedented accuracy and specificity.

In the 1970s, imaging the heart by CT techniques was limited by temporal resolution. The parallel development of electron beam CT (EBCT) methods placed EBCT technology as the diagnostic imaging modality of choice in the 1980s and 1990s, when important strides were made to validate CT techniques for quantification of coronary artery calcification with disease. The introduction of MDCT scanners with improved temporal resolution and high spatial resolution led several investigators to examine its potential for imaging the heart at similar speeds as EBCT. The latter interest was fueled by the widespread availability of MDCT scanners worldwide. In this chapter, several important technical aspects of CT are described, with special emphasis on MDCT and EBCT, the CT modalities primarily used to image the cardiovascular system. First, a brief description is provided of the basic principles of CT along with different generations of CT scanners. This is followed by a description of spiral CT principles that led to the development of MDCT scanners. Because EBCT is an established modality for most CT imaging of the heart, briefer descriptions of the technology and its applications are given. Finally, instrumentation requisite for the essential image quality parameters, including radiation dose pertinent to cardiac imaging, are discussed, as well as the strengths and weaknesses of MDCT and EBCT methods. It is important to emphasize that only the basic principles of CT are described, with the aim of providing the practicing cardiologist and cardiovascular scientist (the consumers) with sufficient basic knowledge to critically appraise CT imaging of the cardiovascular system. The reader is referred to a list of references (1-13) for an in-depth description of the physical principles involved in CT imaging.

Basic Principles of CT

CT is fundamentally a method for acquiring and reconstructing an image of a thin cross-section of an object.[1] It differs from conventional projection imaging in two important ways: first, CT forms a cross-sectional image, eliminating the superimposition of structures that occurs in plane film imaging because of compression of 3D body structures onto the 2D recording system. Second, the sensitivity of CT to subtle differences in X-ray attenuation is at least a factor of 10 higher than normally achieved by film screen recording systems because of the virtual elimination of scatter. Thus CT is based on measurements of X-ray attenuation through the section using many different projections. The CT scanner makes many measurements of attenuation through the plane of a finite thickness cross-section of the body. The system uses those data to reconstruct a digital image of the cross-section in which each pixel in the image represents a measurement of the mean attenuation of a box-like element (voxel) extending through the thickness of the section. An attenuation measurement quantifies the fraction of radiation removed in passing through a given amount of a specific material of thickness (x as shown in Figure 1-1, A. Attenuation is expressed as:

$$I_t = I_o e^{-\mu 1 \Delta x} \qquad (1)$$

where, I_t and I_o are the X-ray intensities measured with and without the material in the X-ray beam path, respectively, and μ is the linear attenuation coefficient of the specific material. To illustrate CT principles, any material can be considered as a stack of voxels along the beam path (Figure 1-1, B). Each attenuation measurement is called a ray sum, because attenuation along a specific straight-line path through the patient from the tube focal spot to a detector is the sum of the individual attenuations of all materials along the path. Assuming that the ray path through the tissue is broken up into incremental voxel thicknesses Δx, the transmitted intensity is

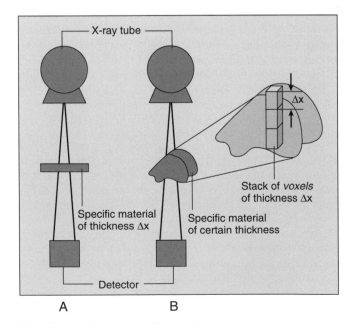

FIGURE 1-1. Illustration of CT principles. X-ray attenuation through (**A**) specific material of finite thickness (Δx) (refer to Eq. 1). **B,** Material considered as a stack of voxels with each voxel of finite thickness (Δx) (refer to Eq. 2).

given by:

$$I_t = I_o e^{-\sum_{i=1}^{k} \mu_i \Delta x} \qquad (2)$$

Expressed as the natural logarithm (ln):

$$\ln\left[\frac{I_0}{I_t}\right] = \sum_{i=1}^{k} \mu_i \Delta x \qquad (3)$$

The image reconstruction process derives the average attenuation coefficient (μ) values for each voxel in the cross-section by use of many rays from many different rotational angles around the cross-section.[2] The specific attenuation of a voxel (μ) increases with the density and the atomic numbers of tissues averaged through the volume of the voxel and declines with increasing X-ray energy.

Mathematically, the attenuation (μ) value for each voxel can be solved algebraically with a very large number of simultaneous equations using all ray sums that intersect the voxel. A more elegant and simpler method called *filtered back-projection* was used in the early CT scanners and remains in use today.[3] Rays are collected in sets called *projections* that are made across the patient in a particular direction through the section plane. There may be from 500 to 1000 or more rays in a single projection. To reconstruct the image from the ray measurements, each voxel must be viewed from multiple different directions. A complete data set requires many projections at fine rotational intervals of 1 degree or less around the cross-section. Back-projection effectively reverses the attenuation process by adding the attenuation value of each ray in each projection back through the reconstruction matrix. Because this process generates a blurred image, the data from each projection are mathematically altered (filtered) before back-projection, eliminating the intrinsic blurring effect.[3] Several advanced reconstruction techniques are currently used in the CT image reconstruction process, but detailed descriptions of these methods are beyond the scope of this chapter.

As a final process, the individual voxel attenuation values are scaled to more convenient integers and normalized to voxel values containing water (μ_w). CT numbers are computed as:

$$CT\# = K\left|\frac{\mu_m - \mu_w}{\mu_w}\right| \qquad (4)$$

where μ_m is the measured attenuation of the material in the voxel and K (1000) is the scaling factor. The attenuation coefficient of water is obtained during calibration of the CT machine. Voxels containing materials that attenuate more than water (e.g., muscle tissue, liver, and bone) have positive CT numbers, whereas materials with less attenuation than water, such as lung or adipose tissues, have negative CT numbers. With the exception of water and air, the CT numbers for a given material will vary with changes in the X-ray tube potential and from manufacturer to manufacturer.

Technical Characteristics of CT Scanners

Conventional CT Generations

In 1979, Sir Godfrey N. Hounsfield and Alan M. Cormack were awarded the Nobel Prize in medicine for the "development of computer assisted tomography." The mathematical principles of image reconstruction date earlier to Radon in 1917. A variety of CT geometries have been developed to acquire the X-ray transmission data for image reconstruction. These geometries are commonly called *generations* and remain useful in differentiating scanner designs.[1,2]

First-Generation CT Scanners

The EMI Mark I scanner, the first commercial scanner invented by Hounsfield, was introduced in 1973. This scanner acquired data with an X-ray beam collimated to a narrow "pencil" beam directed to a single detector on the other side of the patient; the detector and the beam were aligned in a scanning frame. A single projection was acquired by moving the tube and detector in a straight-line motion (translation) on opposite sides of the patient (Figure 1-2, *A*). To acquire the next projection, the frame rotated 1 degree then translated in the other direction. This process of translation and rotation was repeated until 180 projections were obtained. The earliest versions required about 4.5 minutes for a single scan and thus were restricted to regions where patient motion could be controlled (head). Because procedures consisted of a series of scans, procedure time was reduced somewhat by using two detectors, so that two parallel sections were acquired in one scan. Although contrast resolution of internal structures was unprecedented, images had poor spatial resolution (on the order of 3 mm for a field of view of 25 cm and 80 × 80 matrix) and very poor z-axis resolution (~13-mm section slice thickness).

Second-Generation CT Scanners

The main impetus for improvement was in reducing scan time, so that regions in the trunk could be imaged. The addition of detectors angularly displaced enabled several projections to be obtained in a single translation. For example, one early design used three detectors each displaced by 1 degree. Because each detector viewed the X-ray tube at a different angle, a single translation produced three projections. Hence the system could rotate 3 degrees to the next projection rather than 1 degree and had to make only 60 translations instead of 180 to acquire a complete slice (Figure 1-2, *B*). Thus, scan times were reduced by a factor of 3. Designs of this type had up to 53 detectors and were ultimately fast enough (10s of seconds) to permit acquisition during a single breath hold and were the first designs to permit scans of the trunk of the body. Because rotating anode tubes could not withstand the wear and tear of rotate-translate motion, this design required a relatively low-output stationary anode X-ray tube. The power limits of stationary anodes for efficient heat dissipation were improved with the use of asymmetrical focal spots (smaller in scan plane than in z-axis direction), but this resulted in higher radiation doses because of poor beam restriction to the scan plane. Nevertheless, these scanners required slower scan speeds to obtain adequate X-ray flux at the detectors when scanning thicker patients or body parts.

Third-Generation CT Scanners

Design engineers realized that if a pure rotational scanning motion could be used, it would be possible to use higher power, rotating anode X-ray tubes, and thereby improve scan speeds in thicker body parts. One of the first designs to do so was the so-called third-generation or rotate-rotate geometry. In these scanners, the X-ray tube is collimated to a wide fan-shaped X-ray beam and directed toward an arc-shaped row of detectors. During scanning, the tube and detector array rotate around the patient (Figure 1-2, *C*), and different projections are obtained during rotation by pulsing the X-ray source or by sampling the detectors at a very high rate. The number of detectors varied from 300 in early versions to 700 or so in modern scanners. Because the slam-bang trans-

lation motion was replaced with smooth rotational motion, higher output rotating anode X-ray tubes could be used, which greatly reduced scan times. One aspect of this geometry is that rays in a single projection are divergent rather than parallel to each other as in earlier designs. Beam divergence required some modification of reconstruction algorithms, and sampling considerations required scanning an additional arc of one fan angle beyond 180 degrees, although most scanners rotate 360 degrees for each scan. Nearly all current helical scanners are based on modifications of rotate-rotate designs. Typical scan times are on the order of a few seconds or less, and recent versions are capable of sub-second scan times.

Fourth-Generation CT Scanners

This design evolved almost simultaneously with third-generation scanners and eliminated translate-rotate motion. In this case only the source rotates within a stationary ring of detectors (Figure 1-2, *D*). The X-ray tube is positioned to rotate about the patient within the

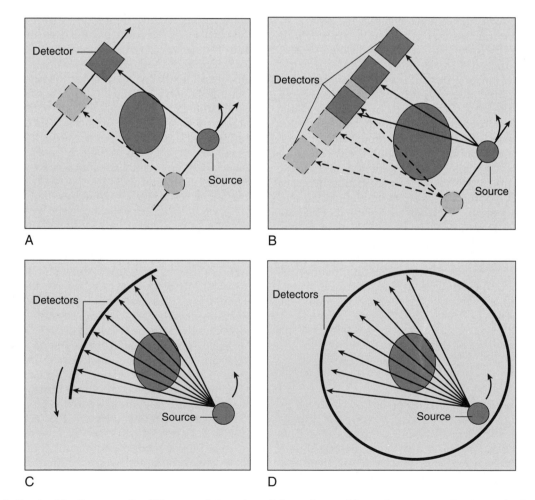

A

B

C

D

FIGURE 1-2. A, Sketch of the first-generation CT scanner that used parallel x-ray beam with translate-rotate motion to acquire data. **B,** Sketch of a second-generation CT scanner with translate-rotation motion to acquire data. **C,** Schematic representation of a third-generation CT scanner, which acquires data by rotating both the x-ray source (with a wide fan beam geometry) and detectors around the patient, and hence the geometry is referred to as rotate-rotate motion. **D,** Schematic representation of a fourth-generation CT scanner that uses a stationary ring of detectors positioned around the patient. Only the x-ray source rotates by use of a wide fan beam geometry, whereas the detectors are stationary; hence, it is referred to as rotate-stationary motion.

space between the patient and the outer detector ring. One clever version, which is no longer in production, moved the X-ray tube out of the detector ring and tilted the ring out of the X-ray beam in a wobbling *(nutation)* motion as the tube rotated. This design permitted a smaller detector ring with fewer detectors for a similar level of performance. Early fourth-generation scanners had some 600 detectors and later versions up to 4800 detectors. Within the same period, scan times of fourth-generation designs were comparable to those of third-generation scanners. One limitation of fourth-generation designs is the less efficient use of detectors, because less than one fourth is used at any point during scanning. These scanners are also more susceptible to scatter artifacts than third-generation types, because they cannot use antiscatter collimators. CT scanners of this design are no longer commercially available except for special-purpose applications.

Until 1990, CT technology had evolved to deliver scan plane or axial plane resolutions of one to two line pairs per millimeter, but *z*-axis or longitudinal resolution remained poor, and interscan delay was problematic because of the stop-start action necessary for table translation and for cable unwinding, both of which resulted in longer examination times. The *z*-axis resolution was limited by the choice of slice thickness, which ranged from 1 to 10 mm. For thicker slices the partial volume averaging between different tissues led to partial volume artifacts. These artifacts were reduced to some extent by scanning thinner slices. In addition, even though it was possible to obtain 3D images by stacking thin sections, inaccuracy dominated because of inconsistent levels of inspiration from scan to scan. Also, the conventional method of slice-by-slice acquisition produced misregistration of lesions between sections caused by involuntary motion of anatomy in subsequent breath holds between scans. Several investigators have attempted to use conventional CT for dynamic studies of the heart, lung, and circulation.[4] However, conventional CT was inadequate for true dynamic structural or functional studies of moving organs, because they either ignored motion with deleterious effects on image resolution, or they used gating techniques to reduce motion artifacts, which also resulted in image degradation. Acquisition of multiple sections during a single breath hold improved the ability to image lesions in moving organs such as the heart. However, this required some technological advances, which led to the development of helical CT scanners.

Principles of Helical CT Scanners

The development of helical or spiral CT[5] around 1990 was a truly revolutionary advancement in CT scanning that finally allowed true 3D image acquisition within a single breath hold. The technique involves the continuous acquisition of projection data through a 3D volume of tissue by continuous rotation of the X-ray tube and detectors with simultaneous translation of the patient through the gantry opening (Figure 1-3). Three technological developments were required: slip-ring gantry designs, very high-power X-ray tubes, and interpolation algorithms to handle the non-coplanar projection data.

Slip-Ring Technology

Slip rings are electromechanical devices consisting of circular electrical conductive rings and brushes that transmit electrical energy across a moving interface. All power and control signals from the stationary parts of the scanner system are communicated to the rotating frame through the slip ring. The slip-ring design consists of sets of parallel conductive rings concentric to the gantry axis that connect to the tube, detectors, and control circuits by sliding contractors (Figure 1-3, *A*). These "sliding contractors" allow the scan frame to rotate continuously with no need to stop between rotations to rewind the system cables. This engineering advancement resulted initially from the desire to reduce interscan delay and improve throughput. Reduced interscan delay increased the thermal demands on the X-ray tube; hence, tubes with much higher thermal capacities were required to withstand continuous operation over multiple rotations.

High-Power X-ray Tubes

Compared with any other diagnostic X-ray application, CT X-ray tubes are subjected to far higher thermal loads. In first- and second-generation CT scanners, stationary anode X-ray tubes were used, because the long scan times meant the instantaneous power level was low. Long scan times also allowed for heat dissipation. Shorter scan times in later versions of CT scanners required high-power X-ray tubes and the use of oil-cooled rotating anodes for efficient thermal dissipation. Heat storage capacities varied from 1 to 3 MHU in early third-generation CT scanners. The introduction of helical CT with continuous scanner rotation placed new demands on X-ray tubes. Several technical advances in component design have been made to achieve these power levels and deal with the problems of target temperature, heat storage, and dissipation. For example, the tube envelope, cathode assembly, anode assemblies including anode rotation, and target design have been redesigned. Because scan times have decreased, anode heat capacities have increased by as much as a factor of 5, preventing the need for cooling delays during most clinical procedures, and tubes with capacities of 5-8 million heat units are available. In addition, improvement in heat dissipation rate (KHU/min) has increased the heat storage capacity on modern X-ray tubes. The large heat capacities are achieved with thick graphite backing of the target disks and anode diameters of 200 mm or more, improved high-temperature rotor bearings, and metal housings with ceramic insulators (Figure 1-3, *B*) among other factors. The working life of tubes used to date ranges from 10,000 to 40,000 hours compared with 1000 hours, which is typical of conventional CT tubes. Because many of the engineering changes serve to increase the mass of the tube, much of the recent design effort was also dedicated to reduce the mass to better withstand increasing gantry rotational rates required by ever faster scan times.

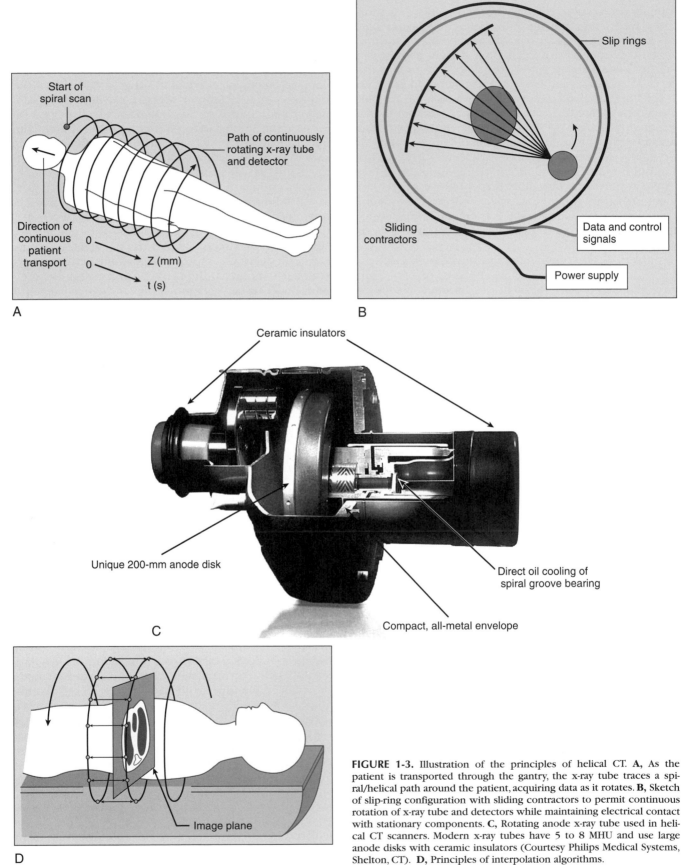

FIGURE 1-3. Illustration of the principles of helical CT. **A,** As the patient is transported through the gantry, the x-ray tube traces a spiral/helical path around the patient, acquiring data as it rotates. **B,** Sketch of slip-ring configuration with sliding contractors to permit continuous rotation of x-ray tube and detectors while maintaining electrical contact with stationary components. **C,** Rotating anode x-ray tube used in helical CT scanners. Modern x-ray tubes have 5 to 8 MHU and use large anode disks with ceramic insulators (Courtesy Philips Medical Systems, Shelton, CT). **D,** Principles of interpolation algorithms.

Interpolation Algorithms

Conventional scanners stepped the patient through the gantry to provide a series of contiguous sections, but it was soon realized that if acquisition could be achieved with continuous table motion, a much more satisfactory result would be obtained. The problem with continuous tube and table motion was that projections precessed in a helical motion around the patient and did not lie in a single plane. This meant that conventional reconstruction algorithms could not be used. Development of interpolation methods[5,6] to generate projections in a single plane so that conventional back-projections could be used alleviated this problem. There were several important benefits to this development. First, the reconstruction planes could be placed in any arbitrary position along the scanned volume encompassed by the table traverse during multiple rotations (Figure 1-3, C), so that sections could be overlapping along the scan axis, thus greatly improving data sampling and making 3D reconstructions practical. Second, because images can be acquired in a single breath hold, the 3D reconstructions are free of the misregistration artifacts caused by involuntary motion that bedevil conventional CT. True 3D volumes could be acquired that can be viewed in any perspective, making the promise of true 3D radiography a practical reality.[7] A final benefit was that because overlapping slices were generated by mathematical methods rather than overlapping X-ray beams, the improved z-axis sampling was obtained without increased radiation dose to the patient. A number of advanced interpolation algorithms were developed,[6] with differing effects on image quality, but these are beyond the scope of this chapter.

During helical scans, the table motion causes displacement of the fan beam projections along the z-axis; the relative displacement is a function of the table speed and the beam width. The ratio of table increment per 360-degree rotation to section thickness is termed *pitch*, an important dimensionless quantity with implications for patient dose and image quality. For example, a pitch less than 1 implies overlapping of anatomy, hence higher patient dose, whereas pitches greater than 1 imply extended imaging and lower patient dose.

Capabilities of Single-Row Detector Helical CT

Considerable progress was made toward faster CT scans with the advent of helical CT. Complete organs could be scanned in about 30 to 40 seconds, and artifacts caused by patient motion and tissue misregistration from involuntary motion were virtually eliminated. It became possible to generate slices in any arbitrary plane through the scanned volume. Significant improvements in z-axis resolution were achieved because of improved sampling, because slices could be reconstructed at intervals less than the section width along the z-axis. Near isotropic resolution could be obtained with the thinnest (~1 mm) section widths at a pitch less than 1, but this can only be obtained over relatively short lengths because of tube and breath hold limitations.[8] Higher power tubes capable of longer continuous operation coupled with faster rotation speeds can scan larger lengths with higher resolution. The practical limit on such brute force approaches, however, became the length of time a sick patient could reliably breath hold, which is between 15 and 30 seconds. Even though the z-axis resolution for helical CT images far exceeds that of conventional CT images, the type of interpolation algorithm and pitch still affects the overall image quality. Several cardiac calcification studies that used helical CT scanners have shown good agreement with EBCT findings; however, cardiac imaging became more feasible with the introduction of multiple-row detector CT technology.[9]

Multiple-Row Detector Helical CT

One of the most dramatic improvements in CT technology has been the introduction of multiple-row detector helical CT.[10] Development of high-power X-ray tubes with impressive heat storage and heat dissipation capacity, per the demand of the single-row detector (SDCT), is used efficiently with wider beam collimation. However, opening up the collimator to improve X-ray tube use decreases spatial resolution with increasing slice thickness. On the other hand, by replacing the single row of detectors used in helical CT with a thin multiple row of detectors, X-ray tube use and spatial resolution are improved, and a large volume of the patient's anatomy is covered by each X-ray tube rotation.

Principles of MDCT

The principal difference between single- and multiple-row detector helical scanners is illustrated in Figure 1-4.[11] In both cases, the X-ray tube and the detectors rotate around the patient to collect multiple projection data (similar to third-generation conventional CT scanners), while the patient table is translated simultaneously through the CT gantry. The differences are in the number of detector rows in the z-direction of the patient and the number of multiple slices obtained at the isocenter. The basic idea actually dates from the very first EMI Mark I scanner that had two parallel detectors and acquired two slices simultaneously. The first helical scanner to use this idea, the Elscint CT Twin, was launched in 1992. By late 1998, all major CT manufacturers had multiple-row detector CT scanners capable of providing at least four slices/section per rotation with minimum gantry rotation times of 0.5 second. This enabled acquisition of volumetric data eight times faster than the SDCT with 1-second scan time. A number of novel image reconstruction algorithms have been developed to handle the large-volume data sets.[12,13] The improved z-axis resolution, along with improved temporal resolution caused by electrocardiographic (ECG) gating, provides a scan technique well suited for CT imaging of the heart and other moving organs,[14-16] with comparable sensitivity and specificity with regard to cardiac scoring by EBCT scans.[17,18]

Several manufacturers adopted various multiple-row detector designs in the first-generation MDCT scanners. Irrespective of the number of detector rows in the z-direction, all designs yielded up to a maximum of four slices at isocenter. This is mainly due to the number of

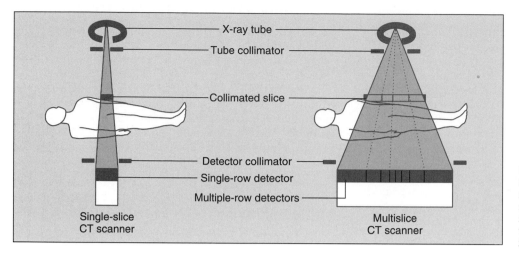

FIGURE 1-4. Sketch illustrating the difference between single-slice and multislice CT design. The multiple-row detector array shown is asymmetrical in design and represents the design of one particular manufacturer.

data acquisition channels available to collect the projection data from respective detector elements. The detectors in first-generation MDCT scanners are differentiated on the basis of the array design and can be grouped as *uniform element arrays, non-uniform element arrays,* and *hybrid element arrays,* respectively (Figure 1-5, *A*).[11] A brief description of the various multiple-row detector array designs is given in the following.

Uniform Element Arrays

In this type of detector array designs, several small solid-state detectors of the same dimension are arranged in rows of identical thickness (e.g., 16 rows of 1.25 mm). The image acquired depends on the X-ray beam width, selec-

tion of detector rows, and how the two are coupled. It is possible to acquire four simultaneous slices of 1.25 mm each or to increase the slice thickness by coupling rows of detectors (e.g., coupling two, three, and four detector rows together) to obtain four slices of 2.5-, 3.75-, and 5-mm thick, respectively.

Non-Uniform Element Arrays

In this type of detector array, the detector width gradually increases in thickness as it moves away from the center of axis of rotation. The two detector rows in the center of the array are 1 mm each, whereas the detectors adjacent to the central row are of increasing thickness, with the outermost detector row 5 mm thick.

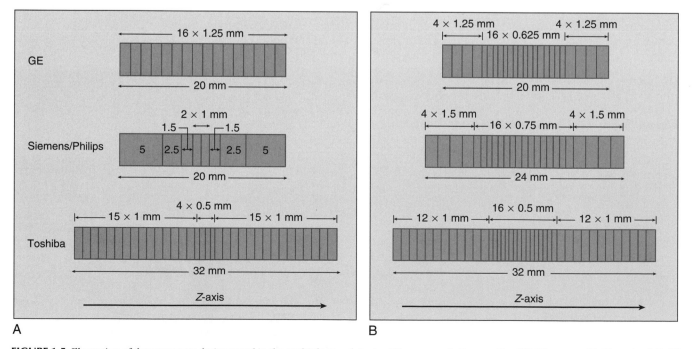

A

B

FIGURE 1-5. Illustration of detector array designs used in the multiple-row detector CT scanners. **A,** Four-section MDCT systems; **B,** 16-section MDCT systems.

Hybrid Element Arrays

The third type of design incorporates features of uniform and non-uniform design. This detector array is composed of 4 thin detectors of 0.5 mm at the center and 15 detectors 1-mm wide on either side of the central detectors for the total z-axis coverage of 32 mm per X-ray tube rotation around the gantry.

With rapid image acquisition, thinner slices acquired at a shorter scan time yield increased scan volume coverage, improved longitudinal resolution, and increased temporal resolution. In single-row detector helical CT designs, scan volume can be increased by increasing pitch at the expense of poorer z-axis resolution, whereas z-axis resolution can be preserved in multiple-row detector designs. For example, if a 10-mm collimation were divided into four 2.5-mm detectors, the same scan length could be obtained in the same time but with a z-axis resolution improved from 10 mm to 2.5 mm. In another example, a multiple-row detector scanner with four 5-mm detectors and a beam width of 20 mm reduces the scan time by a factor of 4 to 15 seconds for the same z-axis resolution. By increasing the number of CT detector rows in the z-direction, data acquisition capability dramatically increases, and at the same time the X-ray tubes are used more efficiently. For cardiac imaging with MDCT, either of the two scanning modes, namely sequential or helical scan modes, is routinely used.

Sequential or Axial Scan Mode

The sequential or axial scan mode is similar to conventional "step-and-shoot" scanning, in which after each tube rotation, the patient is translated to the next position for subsequent scans. Compared with SDCT scanners, the volume of data acquired with each rotation is enhanced nearly four to eight times with 0.5-second rotation time scanners. Thicker slices can be reconstructed retrospectively by use of data from multiple data channels. Reconstructing thicker slices has the inherent advantage in situations required to avoid streak artifacts caused by partial volume averaging and to improve low-contrast detection with improved image noise. For most cardiac imaging, in first-generation MDCT scanners, sequential scanning of the heart is performed with gating techniques at 4×1 mm or 4×2.5 mm and then reconstructed into slices 1-mm or 2.5-mm thick. With X-ray tube rotation at 0.5 second and anatomical coverage of 10 mm per rotation, cardiac scans are significantly faster than SDCT scanners, with enhanced capability to perform coronary studies with results comparable to EBCT scans.

Spiral or Helical Scan Mode

The spiral or helical scan mode is analogous to the SDCT helical scanning mode, with four data channels simultaneously obtaining data as the patient is translated into the gantry. The data from all four channels contribute to each of the four reconstructed slices. The interpolation algorithms can be adjusted to trade off longitudinal resolution against noise and artifacts. One can reconstruct different slice thicknesses by adjusting the slice profiles retrospectively, according to the desired image quality.

For example, scanning at 4×2.5-mm mode, one can reconstruct slices of thickness equal to or greater than 2.5 mm retrospectively.

To minimize motion artifacts and preserve high spatial resolution in all directions, most cardiac imaging studies are obtained either with retrospective ECG gating or with prospective ECG gating.[19] In retrospective gating, the projections at various angles of view are assembled for reconstruction after the scan, on the basis of the ECG recorded during the scan. In prospective gating, the scan is performed at preselected points within the cardiac cycle. In both methods, collection of several angles of view to achieve reasonable resolution in the reconstructed transaxial image requires data acquisition over several cardiac cycles and during several rotations of the X-ray source. The advantage of retrospective gating is that different sets of projection data can be assembled after the continuous data acquisition to reconstruct the same cross-section of the heart at different points within the cardiac cycle. On the other hand, the radiation dose to the patient is reduced with prospective gating, because X-ray exposure is required only during the portion of the cardiac cycle that is of interest during successive cardiac cycles.

Despite the advances of first-generation MDCT scanners, additional challenges remain for ECG-gated MDCT examinations of the heart and the coronary arteries: adequate visualization of stents and severely calcified coronary arteries and examination of a patient with higher heart rates and patients who cannot breath hold for at least 30 seconds. Also, in MDCT, the projection of the X-ray beam on the detectors creates "cone angles," because the X-ray beam falls perpendicular on the central detectors and at a divergent angle on the peripheral detectors. This results in widening of imaged structures projected on the peripheral detectors compared with central detectors. Without correcting for cone beam divergence, slices obtained at the peripheral detectors are slightly wider than those obtained at the center of the detector array. Therefore, data obtained at the peripheral detectors are often discarded during reconstruction. Several cone beam correction algorithms are being developed to correct this slice widening. The second-generation MDCT scanners offer simultaneous acquisition of up to 16 sub-millimeter slices and gantry rotation times shorter than 0.5 second and have the potential to overcome some of these limitations.[20,21]

With the intention of obtaining very thin slices to attain isotropic resolution, all the major manufacturers have migrated toward hybrid detector designs (Figure 1-5, *B*). The number of data acquisition channels has increased from 4 to 8 to 16, with increased number of submillimeter detectors in the center of the beam. With increased data channels and submillimeter size detectors, it is now possible to acquire an increased number of thin slices (12 to 16) per X-ray tube rotation. In addition, specialized software packets are developed by most CT manufacturers to perform cardiac imaging. Partial scan rotation with retrospective ECG gating and with segmental reconstruction methods have enabled MDCT scanners to provide temporal resolutions in the order of 150 to 250 ms.[22]

Helical Pitch

With single-slice helical CT scanners, the concept of *pitch* is straightforward. Referring to Figure 1-6, with the X-ray beam width given by W (in millimeters) and the table increment per gantry rotation defined as I (in millimeters), *pitch,* and more specifically the *beam pitch,* is defined as:

$$\text{Beam pitch} = \frac{I}{W} \qquad (5)$$

With the introduction of multiple-row detector CT scanners, ambiguity arises in terms of the definition of pitch, because different manufacturers use different definitions of pitch, resulting in much confusion.[23] Consequently, beam pitch needs to be distinguished from *detector pitch,* which is defined as:

$$\text{Detector pitch} = \frac{I}{T} \qquad (6)$$

where T is the width of single data acquisition system/channel (DAS) in millimeters (Figure 1-6). If the X-ray beam is collimated to "N" DAS channels in a multiple-row detector CT scanner, the relationship between beam and detector pitch is as shown below:

$$\text{Beam pitch} = \frac{\text{Detector pitch}}{N} = \frac{I}{N*T} \qquad (7)$$

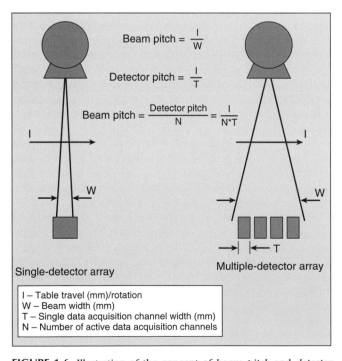

Beam pitch $= \dfrac{I}{W}$

Detector pitch $= \dfrac{I}{T}$

Beam pitch $= \dfrac{\text{Detector pitch}}{N} = \dfrac{I}{N*T}$

Single-detector array

Multiple-detector array

I – Table travel (mm)/rotation
W – Beam width (mm)
T – Single data acquisition channel width (mm)
N – Number of active data acquisition channels

FIGURE 1-6. Illustration of the concept of *beam pitch* and *detector pitch. Beam pitch* is consistent with the previous definition of *pitch* used in single-slice helical CT and may also be applied to multiple-row detector CT scanners. Beam pitch is simply named pitch to maintain consistency between the single-row detector and multiple-row detector helical CT.

Adopting the use of *beam pitch* would be applicable equally to both SDCT and MDCT systems. According to the IEC agreement,[24] consensus among all CT manufacturers has been reached to adopt this definition of beam pitch and calling it simply "pitch." This aims to eliminate existing confusion between the relationship of radiation dose and various manufacturers' definition of pitch.

Advantages of Multiple-Row Detector CT

The clinical advantages of multiple-row detector technology for cardiac imaging can be broadly divided into three categories: (1) The ability to obtain a large number of thin slices resulting in higher spatial resolution in both axial and longitudinal direction. This is important in terms of obtaining isotropic spatial resolution (i.e., cubic voxels), wherein the images are equally sharp in any plane traversing the scanned volume. This capability is reasonably obtained with multiple sections of submillimeter thickness. Ideally, the true 3D radiograph would have cubic voxels of <1 mm, over large volumes, acquired with very short times within a reasonable breath hold. Cardiac imaging, which was possible with the SDCT scanners, became practical with multiple-row detector scanners. (2) The speed can be used for fast imaging of a large volume of tissue with variable slice thickness. This is particularly useful in studies when patient motion is a limiting factor. With a four-slice system and a 0.5-second rotation, the volume data can be acquired eight times faster than with the single-slice, 1-second scanner. With 16-slice systems and rotation times of less than 0.5 second, the volume data are acquired at an even higher rate than that of first-generation MDCT scanners. (3) The other main advantage of multislice systems is their ability to cover large volumes in short scan times. The volume coverage and speed performance in MDCT scanners is better than its counterpart SDCT without compromising image quality. The fast rotation times and large volume coverage provides improved multiplanar reconstruction and 3D images (Figure 1-7) with reduced image artifacts.[22]

Electron Beam CT

Because third- and fourth-generation conventional CT scanners became popular by the early 1980s, many investigators attempted cardiac imaging using the scanners but to no avail. Numerous technical limitations, such as long scan times, X-ray tube heating, and others, precluded imaging of the beating heart without major motion artifacts. In the early 1980s, Boyd and colleagues designed and built the very first ultrafast CT scanner, which is familiarly known as EBCT, which made CT imaging of heart and coronary arteries practical. The technology differed from conventional CT system with the immovable X-ray source that enabled fast data acquisition in the order of 50 to 100 ms.

Principles of EBCT

EBCT uses an electron gun and stationary rings of tungsten "targets" rather than a stationary X-ray tube to gen-

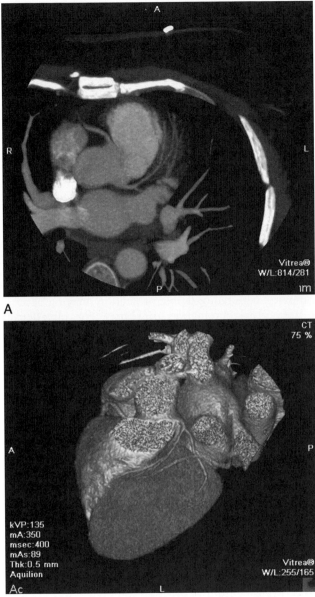

A

B

FIGURE 1-7. Cardiac CT images obtained from 16-section MDCT scanner. **A,** Transaxial CT image; **B,** 3D CT image. See also Color Insert.

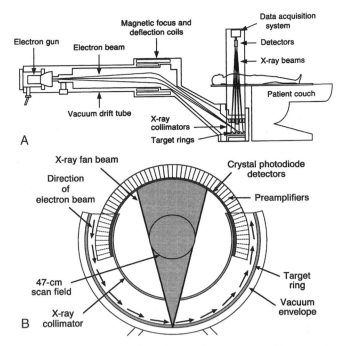

A

B

FIGURE 1-8. Illustration of an electron beam computed tomography scanner. (From McCollough CH, Morin RL. The technical design and performance of ultrafast computed tomography. *Radiol Clin North Am* 1994;32:521, with permission.)

breath-holding sequences and are triggered by the ECG signal set to a certain portion of the cardiac cycle (R-R interval), near end-diastole before atrial contraction. The rapid image acquisition time virtually eliminates motion artifact related to cardiac contraction.

The main strength of EBCT technology is the ability to acquire cross-sectional X-ray images in times as short as 50 or 100 ms, which is unmatched even by the current MDCT systems. However, the EBCT technology is technically complex, and these scanners have remained dedicated for cardiac imaging. With the arrival of MDCT scanners, many new cardiac protocols have been developed for MDCT systems as they are more widely available and the technology is less complex.

Critical Imaging Parameters for Cardiac Imaging

Spatial Resolution

Spatial resolution is defined as the ability of the system to resolve small objects adjacent to each other in space. In CT, the spatial resolution is defined in both axial and in longitudinal (z-axis) direction and is characterized by examining the limiting high-contrast spatial resolution. Limiting resolution is typically measured with a phantom with line-pair patterns of varying spatial frequencies. The axial plane resolution has always been high (10 to 20 lp/cm) compared with longitudinal resolution even with conventional CT and is further improved with the MDCT scanners. Alternately, longitudinal spatial resolution is poor in conventional CT (1 lp/cm) but is improved significantly with helical CT. Longitudinal spatial resolution is described by slice sensitivity profile,

erate X-rays, thus permitting very rapid scanning times (Figure 1-8).[25] X-rays are produced by sweeping a highly focused electron beam around the semicircular tungsten target. The 210-degree target ring centered below the patient at a radius of 90 cm from scanner isocenter acts as the source for X-ray production. A stationary detector ring is centered above the patient and forms a 216-degree arc opposite the target ring. The X-rays produced around the tungsten ring are captured by the ring of detectors, which are then transmitted to computers for reconstruction. The detector ring is composed of two detector arrays, one having nearly half of the detector elements of the other. Single or multiple slices are obtained by focusing electron beams on single or multiple target rings. Serial axial images are obtained in 50 to 100 ms with thickness of 3 to 6 mm. Thirty to 40 adjacent axial scans are usually obtained during one to two

and in spiral CT it is affected by beam collimation, table speed, pitch, and the type of interpolation algorithm. With submillimeter multiple-row detectors in MDCT scanners, it is now possible to obtain high spatial resolution (5 to 10 lp/cm) in the longitudinal direction. With high spatial resolution in all directions, it is now possible to obtain 3D images with isotropic resolution. The introduction of 16-slice CT scanners made it possible to obtain spatial resolution as high as 0.5 mm $\times 0.5$ mm $\times 0.5$ mm. On the other hand, with EBCT scanners, the spatial resolution is usually of the order of 1.5 to 4.0 line pairs per cm (Table 1-1).

Temporal Resolution

Temporal resolution is the ability of the system to resolve events occurring within short intervals. Because heart rates are on the average 60 to 90 pulses per second, to freeze the anatomical motion it is critical for the imaging system to have the capability to acquire data in very short intervals. This is achieved with EBCT technology with an immovable X-ray source, wherein the temporal resolution is as low as 50 to 100 ms (Table 1-1); that has been the "gold standard" for cardiac imaging. Temporal resolution is one of the key image quality parameters that current MDCT technology is striving to achieve. The temporal resolution obtained by MDCT scanners depends on many factors, including scan speed, size of the field of view, position of the field of view in the entire scan field, image reconstruction, and postprocessing algorithms. Scan data from half a gantry rotation and the fan beam angle are needed for reconstruction of a single tomographic image. Therefore, the temporal resolution of the fastest currently available MDCT scanners is approximately 250 ms or more. This can be sufficient to obtain images of the beating heart during diastole (when cardiac motion is minimal) that are free of apparent motion artifact if the heart rate is low (<60 bpm). Because radiation exposure scales increase linearly with

■ ▦ ■

TABLE 1-1 SPATIAL RESOLUTION AND TEMPORAL RESOLUTION FOR MDCT AND EBCT SCANNERS

	SPATIAL RESOLUTION	
Modality	Direction	Spatial resolution (lp/cm)*
MDCT	Axial[†]	10-20
	Longitudinal[‡]	7-8
EBCT	Axial	1.9-3.9
	TEMPORAL RESOLUTION	
Modality	Scan time (ms)	Temporal resolution (ms)[§]
MDCT	400-500	400-500
		105-210[2]
EBCT	50-100	50-100

*Spatial resolution reported in number of line pairs resolvable per centimeter.
[†]In the x-y plane or in the plane of gantry also known as transaxial plane.
[‡]In the z-axis direction, perpendicular to axial plane.
[§]Temporal resolution reported in milliseconds (1/1000th of a second).
[2]Achieved with partial scan and segmented reconstruction method (tradeoff with spatial resolution, image noise, and artifacts).

exposure time, short exposures result in a decrease in the number of X-ray photons measured by the detectors and an increase in image noise levels. Thus, a tradeoff between image noise and temporal resolution is necessary, and the choice depends on the specific clinical application. The need for shorter scan time has resulted in the use of higher tube current, which is possible with MDCT scanners, because X-ray tube loading is no longer the limitation.

Contrast Resolution

Contrast resolution is the ability of an imaging system to image objects of very low contrast (i.e., when the CT number of the object differs by only a small amount from that of the surrounding background material). It is measured by imaging objects of varying sizes embedded in a tissue-equivalent phantom and is defined by the diameter of the smallest low-contrast object visualized. In general, the low-contrast detectability is relatively high compared with radiographic projection imaging because of the virtual elimination of scatter. For high-density objects the contrast resolution is high irrespective of the slice thickness or image noise. However, for a less dense object compared with background, because the differences are small, low-contrast detectability is affected by choice of slice thickness, image noise, and other factors. Increasing slice thickness improves contrast resolution at the cost of spatial resolution. Increasing X-ray photons improves image noise, hence low-contrast resolution but at the cost of increased radiation dose to the patient. Thus, there is always a tradeoff between image noise, spatial resolution, and contrast resolution. The low-contrast resolution is usually higher in MDCT than in EBCT.

Image Noise

The statistical fluctuation of CT numbers in the image of a uniformly dense object is directly related to the number of photons used in creating the image. In CT, image noise is measured as the standard deviation of pixel values within a region of interest located at the center of a uniform object.

Radiation Dose

With recent advances in technology, the use of X-rays for imaging the heart is increasing rapidly. There has also been increased awareness regarding radiation dose from CT examinations. A number of things have contributed to this, including an increasing number of new protocols, widespread availability of CT scanners, and an increasing number of screening examinations despite their unproven track record. This has put increasing demand on CT users such as radiologists and cardiologists to understand the basics of radiation dose, how it is measured, and what it means.

The radiation dose distribution in patients is markedly different with MDCT and EBCT compared with other X-ray imaging modalities, and there are inherent differences even between the two modalities as a result of geometry.

The biological risks from radiation are similar for both imaging modalities, because X-rays of similar beam energies are used. This section briefly discusses the various concepts of radiation dose encountered in CT and provides references for further detail.[26-30]

In cardiac imaging, the emphasis to stop cardiac motion demands faster data acquisition. This is achieved in both EBCT and MDCT by acquiring either single or multiple sections at a time by use of techniques such as prospective ECG triggering or retrospective ECG gating. With prospective triggering, the X-rays are only produced during a predetermined instant of the cardiac cycle. In retrospective gating, radiation is produced, and image data are acquired continuously throughout the cardiac cycle, although images are usually reconstructed only during ventricular diastole. The continuous production of radiation throughout the cardiac cycle causes the radiation dose of retrospectively gated studies to be higher than those of prospectively triggered studies for the same degree of image quality in both type of studies.

In practice, CT studies consist of multiple slices/sections through the regional anatomy of interest with a prescribed slice thickness at a prescribed interval. Ideally, the radiation dose is confined to the slice thickness of the anatomy; however, the radiation dose profile seems to have a central "peak" and "tails" on either side (Figure 1-9). With multiple slices/sections, the radiation dose is greater than any individual section. The radiation dose to a specific location is delivered by the scan positioned at that location and by the neighboring scans.

The fundamental radiation dose parameter in CT is the computed tomography dose index (CTDI). CTDI[26] provides the magnitude of the dose that would result from an infinite series of abutted slices. This is measured with thermoluminescent dosimeters in a very labor-intensive method. A more convenient method of measurement is $CTDI_{100}$, obtained with an ionization chamber placed in round polymethylmethacrylate (Plexiglas) phantom of 16-cm or 32-cm diameters. The $CTDI_{100}$ is measured at the center of the Plexiglas phantom, as well as at peripheral locations to represent the spatial distribution of the radiation exposure. These measurements demonstrate the marked difference between the EBCT and MDCT because of their geometry. In MDCT, with the X-ray tube rotating around the patient, the radiation dose is uniformly distributed and maximum on the surface and decreases toward the center (Figure 1-10, A). By contrast, in EBCT the maximal radiation dose distribution is imparted at the edge of the object closest to the radiation source (tungsten rings), decreases substantially toward the top of the object, and is symmetrical from left to right (Figure 1-10, B). For this reason, the average breast dose for a single-slice multiple scan examination using EBCT is about 25%[27] of the dose delivered to the posterior surface of a supine patient.

To represent an approximation of average radiation dose to a cross-section of the patient's body, the $CTDI_w$ parameter is defined. The $CTDI_w$[28] is the weighted average of the $CTDI_{100}$ measurements at the center and the peripheral locations of the phantom and is calculated as follows:

$$CTDI_w = \left[\frac{2}{3} CTDI_{100}\,(periphery) + \frac{1}{3} CTDI_{100}\,(center) \right] f \quad (8)$$

where f is the conversion factor between the absorption of radiation in air and the absorption in the phantom.

Because CT examinations consist of multiple slices/section, the average radiation dose over a central scan of a CT study consists of multiple parallel sections, which is defined as the multiple scan average dose (MSAD) index. Typically MSAD is higher than the peak of the radiation dose profile of a single scan by a factor of 2 to 3 (Figure 1-11). The value of MSAD is directly related to the spatial separation of successive scans. This spatial separation is dependent on the advance of the patient table, especially during a helical CT examination. As described earlier, the advance of the patient table is quantified by a dimensionless quantity "pitch," which has an impact on the radiation dose during heli-

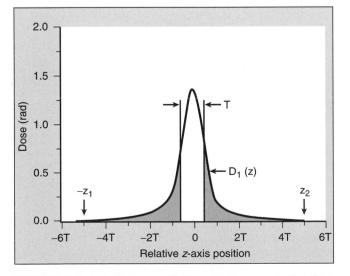

FIGURE 1-9. Typical CT dose profile for a single scan with slice thickness T. (From Shope TJ. *Med Phys* 1981; 8[4]:488-495).

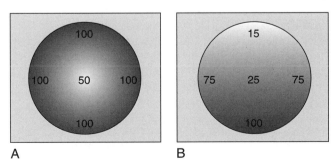

A   B

FIGURE 1-10. Radiation dose distribution within a circular acrylic phantom 32 cm in diameter. **A,** In multiple-row detector CT scanners, the maximal radiation dose is distributed uniformly on the surface of the circular object and decreased toward the center of the object. **B,** In electron beam CT, the maximal radiation dose is imparted to the edge of the object closest to the radiation source. The radiation dose decreases substantially toward the top of the object and is symmetrical from left to right.

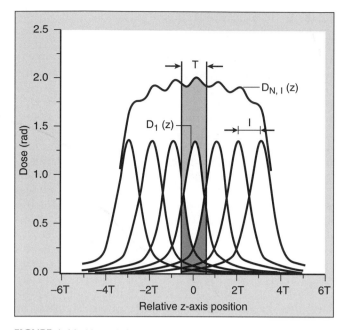

FIGURE 1-11. Typical dose profile resulting from summation of several scans separated by a distance I equal to the slice thickness T. (From Shope TJ. *Med Phys* 1981; 8[4]:488-495.)

cal scans. With the introduction of MDCT, several definitions of pitch have been used that have resulted in considerable confusion, as discussed earlier. However, an international consensus[24] has resolved this by defining pitch as the ratio of table travel per gantry rotation to the total X-ray beam width. This is applicable to both MDCT systems and to its predecessor SDCT systems. For example, if the table advance during one gantry rotation is less than the total beam width (pitch <1), scans overlap, resulting in an increased radiation dose. This is the case in cardiac imaging with CT, because the demand for minimizing motion artifact and greater image quality restricts cardiac protocols to use lower pitch values (0.2-0.4). Lower pitch values means greater tissue overlap and hence increased radiation dose.

The volume CTDI ($CTDI_{vol}$) is a new radiation dose parameter, which is a derivative of CTDI and can be used to express the average dose delivered to the scan volume for a specific examination. The $CTDI_{vol}$[28] is useful in designing CT imaging protocols and comparing the radiation doses among different protocols. The $CTDI_{vol}$ is defined as:

$$CTDI_{vol} = \left[\frac{N * T}{I} \right] CTDI_w = \left[\frac{I}{Pitch} \right] CTDI_w \qquad (9)$$

The $CTDI_{vol}$ is currently the preferred expression of radiation dose in CT, and most current scanners can display the value on the operator's console.

These measured parameters by themselves have limited use in explaining the biological risks from radiation. When a patient asks "what's my dose?" they really mean "what's my risk?" In that regard, the preceding measured dose parameters have limited use in explaining the risk. The parameter to express the radiation risk from CT examination is "effective dose," which provides a quantity that is equivalent in risk to a uniform exposure of the entire body of that magnitude. Effective dose is useful in assessing and comparing the potential biological risk from a specific examination. It reflects the non-uniform radiation absorption of partial-body exposures relative to a whole-body radiation dose and allows comparisons of risk among different radiological examinations. The effective dose is calculated from measured parameters such as $CTDI_{vol}$ and information about dose to individual organs and relative radiation risk assigned to each organ. Typical effective dose values for a number of CT examinations are listed in Table 1-2.[29,30] Because several data sets and calculation methods exist, the results can vary, depending on the method used in estimating effective dose for a particular protocol.

Future Directions

CT technology has evolved considerably over the past 30 years. With the development of multiple-row detector CT, clinical scanners capable of producing 8 to 32 slices per second are now available. The next logical step is to increase the number of detector arrays. However, cone beam artifacts become problematic with the current reconstruction methods. Future developments in the directions of cone beam reconstructions are underway, and the next-generation CT scanners will adopt this method, so that large area detectors can replace multiple-array detectors. Area detectors such as flat panel detectors currently introduced in general radiography will find applications in CT. With substantial z-axis coverage, it will be possible to scan most organs in one or two rotations. Scan times may be further reduced to 150 msec, because the gantry is redesigned to withstand very high centrifugal force. The days of single rotation of the

■ ■ ■

TABLE 1-2   EFFECTIVE DOSE OF SELECTED CT EXAMINATIONS

GENERAL CT PROCEDURES		
Procedures	**Modality**	**Effective dose (mSv)**
Head CT		1-2
Chest CT		5-7
Abdomen and pelvis CT		8-11
CARDIAC CT PROCEDURES		
Calcium scoring*	EBCT	1.0-1.3
	MDCT	1.5-6.2
CT-Coronary angiography*	EBCT	1.5-2.0
	MDCT	6.7-13.0
OTHER RADIOLOGICAL PROCEDURES FOR PERSPECTIVES		
PA and lateral chest x-ray		~0.05-0.1
Diagnostic coronary angiogram		2-10
AVERAGE ANNUAL BACKGROUND RADIATION IN US IS ~3.6 MSV		

*From Hunold P, et al. *Radiology* 2003;226:145-152.

gantry resulting in coverage of almost the entire body are not too distant. This can lead into far-reaching applications such as comprehensive screening examinations. Image reconstruction times will continue to decrease, partly from the pressure of the vast number of images that will be generated by CT examinations. With increased awareness about the radiation dose encountered during CT scan, strategies are underway to develop real exposure control to reduce radiation dose without loss of image quality by measuring patient attenuation during scanogram/scout scans and thereby adjusting tube current during each gantry rotation.

Conclusions

Cardiac imaging with CT is evolving rapidly with recent advances in CT technology. Widespread availability and increasing numbers of studies demonstrating high sensitivity and specificity in diagnosing early onset of cardiovascular diseases will enable MDCT systems to play significant roles in diagnosis and follow-up of treatment for cardiovascular diseases in the near future.

PHYSICAL PRINCIPLES OF CARDIOVASCULAR MAGNETIC RESONANCE IMAGING

CMR is a tomographic technique that produces images of the body using the principles of nuclear magnetic resonance (NMR). The impact of this imaging technique on diagnostic radiology has been revolutionary because of its ability to produce high-quality, fiducial anatomical images. Although CMR has been available clinically for imaging most other organs for approximately 15 years, only recent progress has allowed imaging of the moving heart. CMR is a versatile technique that can provide information about myocardial anatomy, function, perfusion, and metabolism. One of the most exciting perspectives of CMR is the potential for direct submillimeter coronary artery imaging. These various techniques can be combined and have resulted in CMR being regarded as a "one stop shop" for cardiac imaging.

CMR is not yet a "push-button" technique. The use of different pulse sequence schemes may produce different image characteristics and differing contrast between structures that may reveal different diseases. Adequate knowledge of the parameters involved in different pulse sequences is crucial for optimal use of the technique and to ensure maximum image quality. Thus, an understanding of the physics of CMR is the keystone for the successful use of CMR. The purpose of this section is to provide a simplified introduction to the physics of CMR and a summary of the available pulse sequences to the cardiologist and other clinical consumers of this exciting new technique for cardiac imaging. This section is divided into three parts. In the first part, the general principles of CMR are outlined. The second part describes how CMR is adapted specifically for cardiac imaging. The third part briefly discusses the typical pulse sequences that are currently used for CMR.

General Principles of CMR

Nuclear Magnetic Resonance (NMR): Magnetic Spin and Nuclear Magnetism

NMR is based on the feature that certain atoms have the physical property called *magnetic spin*. These nuclei present a charge, and because of the rotation of the nucleus, this charge generates a magnetic field called *spin*. Magnetic spin has an angular momentum with both magnitude and direction that can be represented in a simplified way as a spinning gyroscope in a magnetic field (Figure 1-12). Atoms with an even mass number and even charge (i.e., ^{14}C, ^{16}O) have no magnetic spin. Nuclei with an odd mass number (such as ^{1}H, ^{13}C, ^{19}F, and ^{31}P) have half-integral spin (either $-1/2$ or $+1/2$). Nuclei with an even mass number and uneven charge (such as ^{23}Na, ^{17}O) have integral spin. Each spin corresponds to specific energy levels. The number of energy states a nucleus can adopt is given by $2S + 1$. Nuclei with a spin $S = 1/2$ can have two energy states ($S = -1/2$ and $+1/2$) corresponding to the direction of their spin: Some nuclei spin about their axis ($-1/2$), others in the opposite way ($+1/2$). Nuclei with spin 3/2 or 5/2 have more than two energy states (i.e., ^{13}N with a spin of 3/2 has four energy states ($-3/2$, $-1/2$, $+1/2$, and $+3/2$). Table 1-3 provides a glossary of abbreviations and acronyms used. Because the ^{1}H hydrogen nucleus in present in the largest quantities within the human body (more than 60% of the body weight is water, representing more than 1 thousand trillion ^{1}H nuclei), it gives the strongest MR signal and is therefore the main atom of interest for in vivo CMR. The other nuclei are present in much smaller quantities in the human body. Therefore their signal in vivo is much weaker than the ^{1}H signal, and these nuclei are of interest for spectroscopic rather than for imaging purposes.

Atoms with nuclear spin present *nuclear magnetism* when placed in an external magnetic field. In the resting state (before applying a magnetic field), the spins of all nuclei are oriented in random order. When an external magnetic field is applied, the nuclei align their direction of spin to the orientation of the magnetic field. This can best be compared with the alignment of compass needles placed in a magnetic field (Figure 1-13). At the

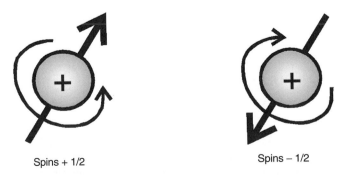

Spins + 1/2   Spins − 1/2

FIGURE 1-12. Magnetic spin. Charged nuclei, such as this water proton, present an angular momentum called *magnetic spin*. The proton has half-integral spin and can adopt two directions of spin ($-1/2$ and $+1/2$) corresponding to two different energy levels.

■ ■ ■

TABLE 1-3   GLOSSARY OF ABBREVIATIONS AND ACRONYMS

FID	Free induction decay
FOV	Field of view
HR	Heart rate
MRI	Magnetic resonance imaging
NMR	Nuclear magnetic resonance
S/N	Signal to noise
TE	Echo time
TR	Repetition time

atomic level, some of the protons align with the field, and some actually align against the field canceling each other out. A slight excess of protons will align with the external magnetic field (B_0). This excess number of protons in the higher energy state is known as the net magnetization of the substance (M_0). This net magnetization is the magnetization that becomes altered during CMR. The net magnetic field of the substance increases in direct proportion with the strength of the external field. This explains why higher field magnets provide stronger MR signals and better imaging quality.

Magnetic Resonance, Larmor Frequency, and Free Induction Decay

When placed in an external magnetic field, atoms with magnetic spin exhibit *magnetic resonance*. Indeed all objects can vibrate at a certain frequency, known as their natural or resonant frequency. When they are excited at the same frequency as their natural or resonant frequency, the energy causing the object to resonate is absorbed and subsequently released. Atoms with magnetic spin will precess around their axis with a given natural frequency when placed in an external magnetic

A) Before application of an external magnetic field

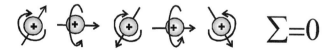

B) After application of an external magnetic field

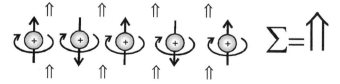

FIGURE 1-13. Behavior of nuclei with magnetic spin in an external magnetic field. When no external magnetic field is present (**A**), the orientation of the spins of all protons is random, and the sum of all spins is zero. When placed in an external magnetic field (**B**), the direction of the spins will align to the direction of the external magnetic field. This is called *nuclear magnetism*. The effect of the alignment of spins is the production of a net magnetic field vector moment that will tend to reduce the external field.

field. This is similar to the precession of a spinning top. Like all other vibrating objects, atoms with magnetic spin can resonate when excited by an energy level corresponding to their resonant frequency of precession. The resonant frequency of atoms with magnetic spin is known as the *Larmor frequency* and is given by the *Larmor equation* $\varpi = \gamma \cdot B_0$, where ϖ is the Larmor frequency, γ the gyromagnetic ratio of the atom, and B_0 the magnetic field. As illustrated by this formula, the Larmor frequency depends on the field strength of the external magnetic field, as well as the gyromagnetic ratio of the nucleus, which is a constant for each nucleus (45 MHz/G for protons). The Larmor frequency of protons and other spinning atoms in magnetic fields obtained by CMR magnets corresponds to the wavelength of FM radiowaves (3-100 MHz, 63 MHz for protons at 1.5 T). Such exciting radiowaves are emitted by the *transmitting coil* of the MR magnet. When excited by a radiowave of the appropriate energy (corresponding to their resonant Larmor frequency), the energy delivered by the photons of the radiofrequency (RF) wave causes the proton to precess in a different direction. This change in orientation of the magnetic axes causes the protons to "jump" to a higher energy state (Figure 1-14). Thus the net magnetization (M_0) of the tissue is altered, which results in a change in orientation of the nuclear magne-

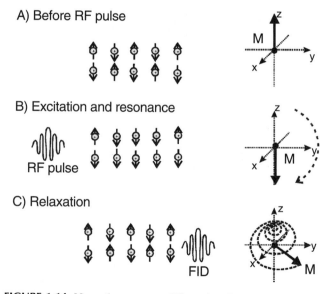

FIGURE 1-14. Magnetic resonance. When placed in an external magnetic field, the protons will align with the external field (**A**). Magnetic resonance can be induced by exciting the protons by a radiofrequency (RF) wave of the same wavelength as their natural frequency (Larmor frequency) (**B**). When they are excited, the protons will absorb the energy of the RF wave and change their direction of spin. Thereby they will adopt a state of higher energy. When the exciting RF wave is stopped (**C**), the protons will fall back to their initial state of lower energy. The energy difference will be released in the form of another RF wave of the same wavelength. This RF wave can be captured as the free induction decay (FID). The right panel shows the changes in the net magnetization vector of the tissue during these phenomena. At baseline, the net magnetization of the tissue is aligned with the external field. During excitation by a RF wave of sufficient energy, the net magnetization is flipped by 180 degrees. During relaxation, the net magnetization vector will return to baseline. This can be observed as a slowly declining spiral by an outside observer.

tization away from its equilibrium state. The net amount of rotation of the nuclear magnetization vector depends on the strength and duration of the applied excitation RF pulse. If the excitation of the RF pulse has a certain duration, the net magnetization of the tissue (Mo) can be completely reversed by 180 degrees. This is known as a 180-degree RF pulse. A shorter RF pulse can cause a 90-degree rotation of the net magnetic field and is known as a 90-degree pulse. Thus, the net magnetic direction can be changed by any degree using an adequate pulse duration and intensity (Figure 1-15). It is important to understand that the degree of rotation refers to the overall effect of the net magnetization direction of the tissue and not to individual protons (i.e., each proton does not rotate 90 degrees during a 90-degree pulse, but the net magnetization direction/vector rotates by 90 degrees).

When the RF pulse is switched off, the opposite phenomenon of magnetic resonance occurs, and the excited nuclei gradually realign themselves with the external magnetic field and return to their net magnetic direction. This phenomenon is called relaxation. The relaxation of the bulk magnetization occurs by two time constants known as T1 and T2 relaxation times (Figure 1-16). The return of the magnetization along the longitudinal axis M_z (i.e., along the direction of the external magnetic field) occurs along an exponential curve with the rate constant *T1*. This time is also known as *spin lattice time,* because it refers to the time it takes for the spins to give back the energy to the surrounding lattice. At the same time, the transverse magnetization (along the *x-y* axis) decreases by another time constant known as *T2* (the *transverse or spin-spin relaxation time*). This transverse relaxation has its origin in the dephasing of spins between the individual protons. The magnetic field of one proton affects the proton next to it, causing it to slightly change its precessional frequency. Thus the magnetic field of one proton will cause the neighboring protons to slightly alter their precessional frequency over time. Over time, all protons will spin at slightly different precessional frequencies than their neighbors. Although the differences in the magnetic environment are small, the small changes in the precessional frequency of the individual protons cause a

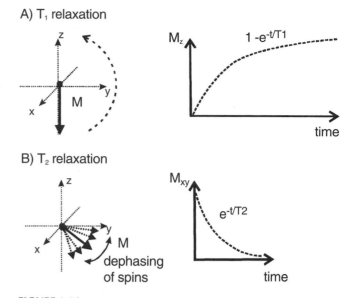

FIGURE 1-16. Nuclear magnetic resonance relaxation: T1- and T2-time constants. Relaxation occurs by two phenomena. The buildup of longitudinal magnetization (M_z) occurs by a slow time constant T1 (**A**). The decrease of transverse magnetization in the x-y plane occurs by rapid spin-spin dephasing by a time constant T2 (**B**).

dephasing of the sum of the individual magnetization vectors that form the net X-Y magnetization vector. The net X-Y magnetization of the tissue, which is externally recorded, will rapidly decrease, much faster than the increase of the Z magnetization to its initial state. Thus, the T2 relaxation time in most tissues is much shorter than the T1 relaxation time of the tissue.

T1 and T2 are inherent properties of the tissue and depend on the magnetic environment of the ^1H protons. They vary with the tissue type and field strength but are fixed for a specific tissue at a given magnetic field strength. For example, T1 is much shorter for fat than for solid tissue, but is still shorter than for water. This is because T1 relaxation time depends on the motional frequencies of the protons. The motional frequency is influenced by physical state of the tissue and is influenced by the atoms the protons are attached to in the molecules. The motional frequencies of small molecules like water are higher than for large solid tissues like proteins. In fat the motional frequencies of the protons are highest. Therefore the T1 relaxation time is shortest for fat, intermediate for water, and longest for proteinaceous tissues.

The T2 relaxation time by opposition is long for water, intermediate for fat, and short for solid tissues. This is because in water the protons are relatively distant. Therefore the spin–spin interaction between these protons is minimal. By contrast, in the proteinaceous structure of solid tissues, the water protons are more compactly packed. Therefore their spin–spin interaction is more important, resulting is shorter T2 relaxation time.

The return of the net magnetization that occurs during the relaxation of the spins of the ^1H protons to their equilibrium state is accompanied by a release of the energy in the form of radiowaves at the same

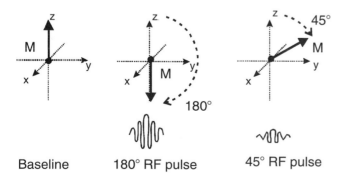

FIGURE 1-15. Concept of flip angle. By applying radiofrequency (RF) waves of different energy or duration, the net magnetization of the tissue can be altered by different degrees. If the RF wave is of sufficient energy, the net magnetization is flipped by 180 degrees. RF waves of shorter duration or energy may change the net magnetization vector by lesser degrees. This defines the so-called *flip angle* of the RF pulse.

wavelength as the resonant frequency of the ¹H protons. The emitted radio energy can be externally recorded and is known as the *free induction decay (FID)*. The FID is the signal recorded by the *receiving coil* of the MR magnet and is precessed to produce the CMR signal. The received FID is a RF signal of short duration (Figure 1-14) emitted at the Larmor frequency, which decreases rapidly in time. In fact, it decreases by a time constant slightly greater than T2. The magnetic field of the MR magnet is not perfect but has small inhomogeneities. These inhomogeneities of the external magnetic field also cause small changes in the Larmor frequency of protons in different locations and accentuate the dephasing of the different protons caused by their spin–spin interaction. The effect of small imperfections of the magnet adds to the spin–spin relaxation time T2 and causes the received signal to decrease by a time constant called *T2**, which is slightly higher than the T2 time of the tissue itself.

T1 and T2 relaxation times are important determinants of image contrast that can also be used to characterize tissue in vivo. Although typically T1 and T2 times are not directly measured in typical MR images, the images can be weighted either for T1 or T2 time or for the average density of protons (proton weighted).

Signal Generation with the Spin-Echo Pulse Sequence and T1 and T2 Weighting

The simplest MR pulse sequence is represented by a spin-echo sequence (Figure 1-17, *A*). This sequence consists of applying a 90-degree *(saturation pulse)*, which nulls the magnetization in the z plane (Figure 1-17). After application of the saturation pulse, the tissue magnetization slowly increases from total saturation to partial saturation before finally returning to its equilibrium state. This occurs according to an exponential curve with the time constant T1. If more saturation pulses are applied after a time TR *(repetition time)*, while the tissue is still partially saturated, the magnetization of the tissue will reach a steady state of magnetization in the z plane. This steady state depends on the repetition time and the T1 constant of the tissue. If the repetition time is short, the steady state is very much dependent on the T1 time of the tissue. A tissue with short T1 is able to rapidly recover its longitudinal magnetization. By contrast, a tissue with long T1 would not have had the time to increase its longitudinal magnetization when the next saturation pulse occurs. Therefore its partial saturation would be lower and its signal intensity less than a tissue with short T1. If TR would be long, the effect of T1 would be much less on the steady state reached and thus on sig-

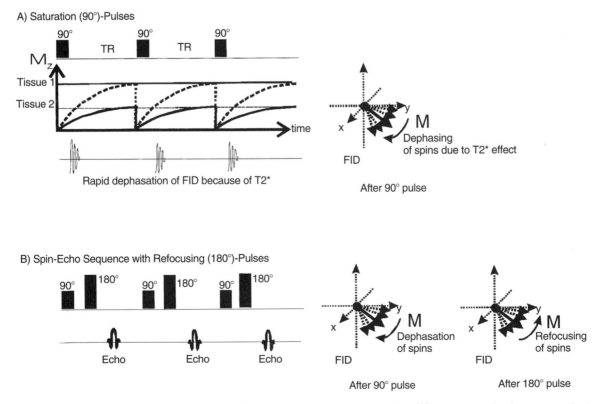

FIGURE 1-17. Spin-echo sequence. The sequence uses sequential 90-degree (saturation) pulses **(A)** to saturate the tissue magnetization in the Z-axis. The time between the saturation pulses is called the repetition time (TR). Tissues will reach a steady state of magnetization depending on their T1 relaxation time and the TR interval. Theoretically, a FID could be recorded after every 90-degree pulse; however, this FID would be very short because of the rapid dephasing of spins caused by the T2* effect. To overcome this dephasing, the spin-echo sequence **(B)** uses a 180-degree pulse to refocus the spins (refocusing pulse). If the time between the 90 degrees and the 180 degrees was called τ, the spins would all be in phase again at 2* τ. At this time an echo will form. Therefore the time 2* τ is called the echo time (TE).

nal intensity. The application of such a sequence that uses several saturation pulses would allow an FID immediately after each saturation pulse and allow characterization of the T1 times of the tissue. Yet this FID, which would be recorded by a simple saturation pulse scheme, would be very difficult to record, because the magnetization in the x-y plane decreases much faster because of dephasing of spins in the transverse plane. This occurs with the time constant T2*. The FID after the initial saturation pulse will rapidly decrease because of dephasing of spins in the x-y plane because of T2* effect. To avoid this, the spin-echo sequence (Figure 1-17, *B*) uses a 180-degree pulse *(refocusing pulse)* a certain time τ after the 90-degree pulse. This refocusing pulse inverts the magnetization in the x-y plane, reversing the direction of dephasing of the spins in the horizontal plane. Therefore at a time 2τ all the spins will have returned to phase. At that time the FID will reform as an echo. Therefore the time 2τ is also called *echo-time (TE)*. After the spins have refocused, they defocus again in the opposite direction. By applying additional refocusing pulses at times $3, 5, 7, \tau$, they can be refocused again to record further echoes at times $4, 6, 8, \tau$ (2, 3, 4 TE). Because this refocusing plane eliminates the decrease in spin–spin magnetization caused by external magnetization inhomogeneity (T2*) but by spin–spin interaction (T2 effect), the FID recorded at the different TE times will decrease according to a time constant $e^{-t/T2}$. If long TE times are chosen, the signal in tissues with short T2 time will have rapidly decreased, whereas the magnetization in tissues with long T2 times will still be present. Image contrast will thus be heavily dependent on T2 times of tissue. By contrast, for short TE times, the effect will be much less, because magnetization for both tissues with long and short TE will not have had the time to decrease.

Thus in a spin-echo image sequence, two parameters affect imaging contrast: TR and TE times. When short TR times are used, the signal strength and thus the image contrast will be heavily dependent on the T1 times of the tissue. The images will thus be *T1 weighted*. Long TE times will cause image contrast to depend on T2 times. The images will thus be *T2 weighted*. Intermediate TR and TE will cause image contrast to depend neither very strongly on T1 nor on T2 times. The images will thus be essentially *proton density weighted*.

Imaging With NMR–Slice Selection–Spatial Encoding

Ideally, when a human body is placed in the magnetic field of the MR magnet, all nuclei in the human body are subjected to the same field strength. All protons in the body would precess at the same Larmor frequency. Thus the external signal recorded after an excitation pulse would not differentiate between different parts of the body but would reflect the total signal of all protons of the body. To be able to produce images using NMR, it is necessary to obtain different signals from protons located in different parts of the body. To be able to achieve this aim, local magnetic field gradients are added to the static magnetic field, allowing resolution of the RF signal spatially. Spatial encoding is performed in two ways. First, the magnetic resonance excitation can be applied selectively

to certain slices. This is performed by adding a perpendicular gradient field to the static magnetic field at the time of excitation (the so-called *slice selection gradient Gz*). This external gradient will increase or decrease the net magnetic field strength in different parts of the body. This will increase or decrease the Larmor frequency of the protons as a function of their respective position to the slice selection gradient. By applying a selective RF pulse of a certain frequency and bandwidth, only a thin plane will have its Larmor frequency correspond to the exciting RF pulse and resonate. The slice position at which NMR is induced can be specifically controlled by changing the frequency of the RF pulse or by changing the strength of the gradient. The width of the excited slice depends on the bandwidth of the pulse and the slope of the slice selective gradient. Proton excitation and slice selection can be performed selectively at any spatial location by varying the gradient strength and slope, as well as the frequency and bandwidth of the excitation pulse (Figure 1-18).

The second method by which information necessary for imaging is resolved spatially is during the readout of the MR signal. This is performed by encoding in two directions to obtain a 2D image. If another gradient *Gx, the frequency encoding gradient,* is applied during the time the FID echo is received, the local magnetic field of the resonating protons will be slightly increased or decreased by the gradients. This will slightly modify the precessional frequency of the resonating protons linearly along the gradients (Figure 1-19, *A*). The received FID signal is the sum of the resonant FID from all protons in the excited slice. Because of the change of the precessional frequency caused by the frequency encoding gradients, the FID will no longer be fixed at one specified frequency but will become a signal at varying frequencies in a given bandwidth, corresponding to the different Larmor frequencies along the frequency encoding gradi-

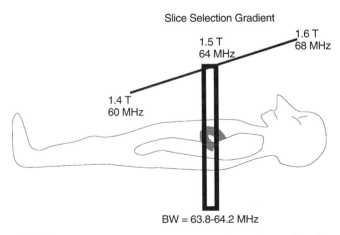

FIGURE 1-18. Magnetic resonance imaging and spatial encoding: slice selection. Slice selection is performed by adding a gradient to the static magnetic field at the time of excitation. The gradient will add or decrease the static field in a linear fashion, which will modify the Larmor frequency of the protons in a linear direction. An RF pulse with a specified bandwidth will only excite the protons in a 2D slice of a specified width in the body. The location and width of this slice will depend on the bandwidth of the pulse and the slope of the gradients used.

A) Frequency Encoding

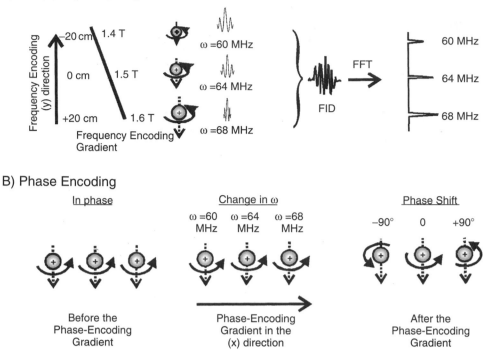

B) Phase Encoding

FIGURE 1-19. Magnetic resonance imaging and spatial encoding: frequency and phase encoding. Frequency encoding is performed by applying a frequency-encoding gradient during the time the FID echo is received. This gradient will alter the precessional frequency of the resonating protons linearly along the gradients. The FID received will contain the sum of all frequencies. Fourier transformation of the spectrum allows one to resolve this information spatially and to encode the position of the protons corresponding to the spatial position of the individual protons in the y-axis. Phase encoding is performed by applying another gradient, before the read out this time. The phase-encoding gradient will induce a phase shift of all the protons at a given spatial location. By use of different phase-encoding gradients, it is thus possible to encode in the second direction (along the x-axis).

ent. The different frequencies in the FID will reflect protons at different levels along the frequency-encoding gradient. The spatial encoding provided by the shift in frequencies of the FID can be easily resolved with Fourier transformation. However, frequency encoding only allows spatial encoding in one direction. To be able to resolve for the second direction, it is necessary to apply another gradient in the opposite direction. This gradient is called *Gy, the phase-encoding gradient.* The phase-encoding gradient is usually applied between the 180 and 90 RF or between the 180 pulse and the echo readout in a spin-echo experiment. The phase-encoding gradient will induce a phase shift of all the protons at a given level. In fact, before the application of the phase-encoding gradient, all the protons are in phase (Figure 1-19, *B*). When the phase-encoding gradient is applied to the protons, they will slightly increase or decrease their precessional speed according to the increase or decrease in the net magnetic field strength gradients. When the gradient is turned off, all protons will return to the same precessional speed. However, the protons will be out of phase according to their spatial position in the phase-encoding gradient. Those that were in the middle of the gradient and will not have had any modification in their precessional speed will still be at the same phase as before application of the gradient. The protons that will have experienced a slight increase in their precessional frequency during the application of the phase-encoding gradient will have advanced in their oscillatory movement compared with those that had no change in precessional frequency. Therefore, they will have a slight advance in phase compared with the other protons. By contrast, those protons that had their precessional frequency decreased during the application of the phase-encoding gradient will have experienced a slight delay in

their oscillatory movement and will have a slight delay in phase. By applying the phase-encoding gradient in a direction perpendicular to the frequency gradient, it is possible to change the phase of protons according to their spatial position. The phase shift of each row of protons is directly related to its spatial position in the phase direction. To determine the phase shift of the next row, it is necessary to repeat the read out with a slightly altered phase-encoding gradient. It is clear from the previous discussion that with phase and frequency encoding, it is only possible to read out one line at the time but not an entire 2D image. One FID allows the image information relating to one line in space to be read out. It takes a number of *phase-encoding steps* (i.e., successive excitations) to obtain all successive 1D lines to complete the 2D space that encodes the image (Figure 1-20).

K Space Sampling

The theory of *K space* may be the most misunderstood concept in CMR. K space is a digital data space in the memory of the computer in which the FID resulting from the different excitations needed to form the MR image are sampled. The raw data in K space are sampled typically line by line from the different excitation pulses by applying frequency and phase encoding as previously outlined (Figure 1-21). Once K space is completely filled in, it is Fourier transformed to form the actual MR image. K space is thus the raw data of the MR image before its reconstruction by a Fourier transformation. Understanding the properties of K space and how it is sampled is the keystone for understanding the different MR pulse sequences and how potential artifacts may occur. The entire K space consists of the phase- and frequency-encoded data from the different excitation pulses.

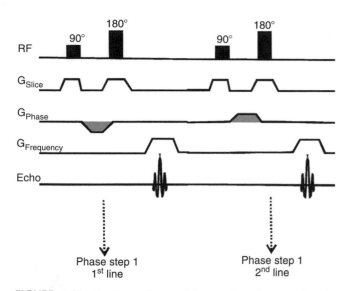

FIGURE 1-20. Gradients for spatial encoding. In typical pulse sequences, every echo will produce one frequency-encoded FID, which represents one line of data encoded in the frequency (y) direction. To resolve the MRI information for the second spatial direction (the *x* or phase-encoded direction), it is necessary to acquire several echoes, each encoded with different phase-encoded gradients. It thus requires several phase-encoded steps to reconstruct a 2D image.

Sampling of the K space can be performed in different ways. Mathematically, the final image looks exactly the same, irrespective of the way data are sampled in K space.

In most cases, the K-space sampling is performed linearly, that is line by line (Figure 1-22, *A*). In instances in which the K space (and the actual MR image) is not acquired all at once but in small pieces related to the different excitation pulses, each excitation pulse fills one line in the frequency direction of K space. However, it takes several phase-encoding steps (typically 128 to 256, although any number may be specified in the imaging protocol) to acquire the entire K space and thus the complete images. It requires a certain time to acquire all the phase-encoding pulses to totally fill up K space and to acquire one image. Depending on the type of pulse sequence, this time may be quite substantial, on the order of several minutes, to acquire one image.

Other ways to sample K space exist. Echo-planar imaging, which will be discussed later, acquires several lines of K space in one excitation shot (Figure 1-22, *B*). This is performed by rapidly inverting the readout gradients while applying a phase-encoding gradient. By this means, several FIDs may be acquired for each excitation shot. The advantage of such a technique is substantial reduction of imaging time, because several lines of K space may be sampled in the phase direction for each excitation pulse, allowing for the reduction of the number of excitation shots required to fill up K space. Spiral imaging is another imaging method in which all K space is sampled after only one excitation pulse (Figure 1-22, *C*). An alternate approach, known as radial sampling, reads lines rotating around the center of K space (Figure 1-22, *D*). Instead of performing linear K-space sampling in a 2D plane, it is possible to sample a 3D K space by adding another phase-encoding gradient in the Z direction. Pulse sequences that use this type of K-space sampling are called 3D imaging.

K space has several important properties that are related to the Fourier transformation. It is important to understand that K space does not look like the actual image, because it is the inverse Fourier transformation of the image and looks rather like a series of concentric rings, which correspond to the oscillations of the acquired FID. The Fourier transformation of this infor-

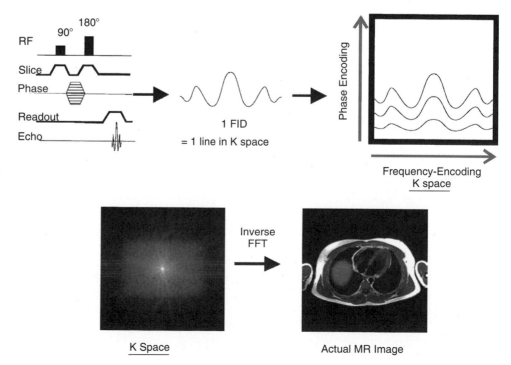

FIGURE 1-21. K space. K space is the digital data space in which the information from the FID is sampled. In typical pulse sequences, every echo will produce one phase- and frequency-encoded FID that represents one line in K space. To fill up all lines in K space, it requires several FIDs, each encoded with different phase-encoding steps. Once all the phase-encoding steps are acquired, the MR image can be formed from the data in K space. The sampled data in K space look different from a typical image (lower left) and require an inverse Fourier transformation to form the final MR image (lower right).

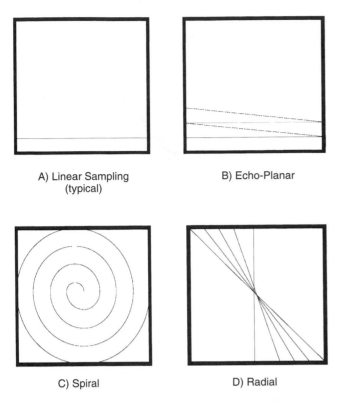

A) Linear Sampling (typical)

B) Echo-Planar

C) Spiral

D) Radial

FIGURE 1-22. Different sampling techniques for K space. In most typical pulse sequences, 2D K space is sampled linearly, line by line (A). In echo-planar imaging, several lines in K space can be read per excitation (B). Spiral imaging reads the entire K space in one shot, starting at the center of K space and progressing to the periphery (C). Radial sampling reads lines rotating around the center of K space. These latter two techniques are applied for certain specific applications only (coronary imaging, etc.). The final image will look the same, regardless of the K-space sampling method used.

mation allows resolution of the spatial information encoded in the phase and frequency direction and reconstructs the actual image. There is a one-to-one relation between K space and the actual MR image. Furthermore, it is important to note that different parts of K space encode for different features of the image. The center of the K space represents the maximum signal of the image. The outer parts of the K space contribute to the detail and resolution of the image. Thus the image center will be encoded by low-resolution K-space data, whereas the image edges are encoded by high-resolution K-space data. This property may be useful for certain purposes; for example, when the shot duration of the image is long and when it is desirable to avoid motion artifacts, it might be more appropriate to encode the parts of K space that encode for high resolution of the image first. In other circumstances it may be more appropriate to acquire the periphery of K space first. For instance, when using a prepulse, which alters the magnetization properties of the tissue, it is important to sample the center of the image first if the prepulse is to be as short as possible, because the important time to affect image contrast is the time from the prepulse to the center of the K space. Another interesting property of K space is that it is symmetrical in both the frequency and phase direction, because the information contained in K space represents small wavelets from the FID, and like all waves they behave symmetrically. The symmetry of K space along its two directions allows for the fact that it is possible to acquire only part of the K space and still reconstruct the entire image. Theoretically, it is possible to use only one quarter of the entire K space to reconstruct the entire image (i.e., half of the information of K space in frequency direction and half of the phase direction). However, because of the presence of small phase errors in the data, in practice it is necessary to acquire a little more than 50% of the K space in any direction to reconstruct an artifact-free image. Reduced K-space sampling is a technique to reduce image acquisition time. Reduction of sampling in the frequency direction may reduce the sampling time of the FID and reduce TE. More often, sampling of K space is reduced in the phase direction, because this may reduce the number of phase-encoded steps required to reconstruct the image and thereby significantly reduce image acquisition time. The tradeoff of reduced K-space sampling is reduction in S/N in the image. S/N decreases by a factor of $\sqrt{2}$ when half the K space is sampled. Further details of reduced K-space sampling are discussed later. Similar to all waves, the Nyquist limit also applies to MR imaging and to undersampled MR images. If the image is undersampled relative to its actual size, this will cause a so-called wraparound artifact, in which the part of the image outside of the field of view is aliased (wrapped) on top of true imaging signal. Wraparound in cardiac imaging occurs typically from structures such as the chest wall or the patients' arms overlapping on top of the heart.

Finally, a further important property of K space is that actually two dimensions of K space can be sampled. The FID that is sampled has two dimensions, a frequency and a phase direction. In imaginary numbers, therefore, K space will have two dimensions: a real and an imaginary component. The real component corresponds to the magnitude of the image. The imaginary component corresponds to the phase shift of the image. We usually look at magnitude images, which are the familiar MR images. However, the phase information can be used to obtain information about the velocity of the moving spins, which can be used to construct the so-called *phase contrast images,* which encode for the flow velocity of the displacement of the moving spins that may be used to calculate flow and velocity of moving blood in the heart and great vessels.

Signal to Noise (S/N)

S/N is one of the major limiting factors for imaging small structures such as coronary arteries using MR images. Similar to all imaging modalities including MR imaging, S/N depends on the size of the voxel, which gives the signal used in the actual image. Decreasing voxel size will reduce S/N, whereas increasing voxel size will increase S/N. With MR imaging, S/N will depend on the size of the 3D voxel, in the X, Y, and Z directions. Thus, decreasing the field of view by half, or increasing the image resolution by a factor of 2 and thereby decreasing the pixel size by the same amount, will reduce the S/N by a factor of $\sqrt{2}$. S/N is also affected linearly by slice thickness.

Increasing slice thickness by a factor of 2 will increase S/N by the same amount. S/N in CMR depends on a multitude of other factors. First, S/N increases linearly with field strength. Therefore the S/N in a 1.5-T system is three times greater than S/N in a 0.5-T system. Signal strength and S/N decreases exponentially with distance to the receiving coil. S/N is largest when the coil is placed directly on the region to be imaged. For cardiac imaging, surface coils are generally placed directly on the chest wall. S/N also depends on coil design, being greater for phased-array coils than single loop coils. Yet S/N also decreases with the depth from the coil. For example, the S/N of the posterior wall of the heart is less than the S/N of the anterior wall. S/N is less for obese than for thin patients because of the greater distance of the heart from the coil. S/N also depends on a number of pulse sequence–related parameters. S/N primarily depends on the flip angle used, being lower for smaller flip angles and highest for flip angles approaching 90 degrees, although this relationship is complex and nonlinear. Many other pulse sequence- related parameters, such as TR and TE, influence S/N. Of particular importance for cardiac imaging is that the use of reduced K-space sampling strategies, such as those used to increase acquisition speed, result in reductions of S/N by a factor of $\sqrt{2}$ when the image is undersampled. For example, reduction of voxel size to 75% of original value reduces the S/N ratio to 56% of the original S/N ratio. Partial K-space sampling, by undersampling the phase direction by 25%, results in a reduction of the S/N to 75% of the original value. These relationships are important considerations when optimizing pulse sequence parameters in cardiac imaging.

Adaptation of MR to Cardiac Imaging

The use of CMR for cardiac imaging is technically more challenging than MR imaging of other organs because of the complex dynamic motion caused by both cardiac contraction and respiration. This motion, if unaccounted for, causes major artifacts on conventional cardiac MR images. Several strategies can be applied to decrease these motion artifacts. To minimize artifacts caused by cardiac motion, it is necessary to gate imaging to the cardiac cycle with either an ECG or a pulse signal. Different strategies may be used to avoid respiratory motion artifacts. One common method involves suspending diaphragmatic motion during imaging using sequential breath holds (Figure 1-23). Alternatively, newly developed respiratory navigator sequences or multiple excitations may be used to minimize respiratory motion. Ultrafast real-time imaging is a newer strategy, in which imaging is performed at such speeds that cardiac and respiratory motion artifacts are greatly decreased.

These motion correction strategies for cardiac imaging typically require fast imaging and are available only on newer generation scanners with higher gradient strengths, which are specifically designed for cardiac imaging. In general, CMR should be performed on high-field (1.5-T) scanners with dedicated surface coils for cardiac or thoracic imaging to maximize S/N ratio and image quality.

Fast Imaging Techniques

Because of the rapid and dynamic motion of the heart, cardiac imaging requires fast imaging techniques to minimize motion artifacts and to allow imaging to be performed during single breath holds. Several strategies are used to shorten image acquisition time in CMR.[31-33]

Low Shot–Gradient Echo Imaging Techniques

Gradient echo (GRE) imaging, also known as gradient refocused acquisition in the steady state (GRASS) or fast field echo (FFE) imaging, was the first fast imaging technique available for fast cardiac imaging. Similar to the basic spin-echo technique (previously described), a single RF pulse is used to produce an echo signal. The major difference between spin-echo and fast GRE techniques is that to form the echo, the 180-degree rephasing pulse is replaced by refocusing gradients. The use of refocusing gradients instead of 180-degree rephasing pulses allows the use of smaller flip angle excitations (10-20 degrees) and a steady state in longitudinal imaging with short (5-10 ms) TR can be reached. The use of such short TR allows significant acceleration of image acquisition speed. Because of the small flip angles used, this technique is also called fast low-shot angle (FLASH).

Echo-Planar

Echo-planar imaging (EPI) is another high-speed imaging technique in which sequences are characterized by a series of rapid gradient reversals by the readout gradient. Similar to gradient echo imaging, each of these gradient reversals produces an echo signal, and each echo is acquired with a different phase encoding. This enables readout of multiple lines in K space per excitation pulse (TR), which accelerates imaging by the factor of lines read per excitation (the echo-planar factor). Typically four to eight lines can be read, and image acquisition speed can thus be accelerated by a factor of four to eight times. Echo-planar readout may be combined with a

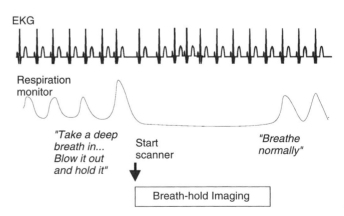

FIGURE 1-23. Breath-hold scheme for cardiac imaging. The patient is instructed to take a deep inspiration and then to hold his or her breath after reaching a comfortable end expiration. Scanning is started when the patient is in stable apnea. The patient is allowed to breathe normally after completion of the acquisition of the image. Then the next image is acquired.

number of pulse sequence schemes such as spin-echo or low-shot excitation pulses to form hybrid pulse sequences. The advantage of echo-planar readout is a significant acceleration of image readout. However, because of the multiple refocusing gradients, echo-planar imaging is very sensitive to T2* effects caused by field inhomogeneity effects, for instance, caused by the presence of foreign metal objects. In addition, the presence of small inhomogeneities in the field may cause phase shifts from one direction of readout to the next, commonly known as zipper artifacts.

Spiral Imaging

Spiral imaging is a special type of EPI. Similar to conventional EPI, rapid gradient reversals are used to read K space rapidly. For spiral imaging, these gradient reversals are used in two directions simultaneously. Two increasing sinusoidal gradients are used, so that K space is traversed in a spiral fashion. This technique requires only one excitation to acquire the entire K space. Compared with conventional EPI, spiral imaging is less sensitive to phase shifts, because the central part of K space is measured early in the sequence and because the two directions of sampling compensate each other. The disadvantages of spiral imaging acquisitions include artifacts caused by off-resonance effects and time-consuming image reconstruction, which requires the spiral data to be interpolated to the rectangular grid of the K space. Thus, spiral imaging is only rarely used for clinical cardiac imaging at present.

Partial K-space Sampling Techniques

Partial K-space sampling is a technique that is frequently used to increase acquisition speed for cardiac imaging. K space is symmetrical in both the phase-encoding and frequency-encoding direction, and only part of K space (slightly more than one half [50%] in each direction) can be used to reconstruct the entire image. For cardiac imaging, the number of phase-encoding steps is reduced to about 60% to 70% to increase imaging speed by 30% to 40%. The disadvantage of reduced K-space sampling is reduction in S/N. A frequent problem with reduced K-space sampling is the possibility of aliasing, resulting in wraparound or foldover artifacts. This problem may be attenuated by increasing the field of view or by carefully choosing the direction of phase encoding. For instance, because the thorax is asymmetrical and usually larger in width than in height, foldover artifacts often occur if the phase-encoding direction is chosen parallel to the chest wall. In this case, aliasing of signal from the arms may occur. This effect may be resolved by reversing the frequency and phase-encoding directions, so that phase encoding is performed perpendicular to thoracic wall, where less tissue signal is produced that may cause these foldover artifacts.

Parallel Imaging Techniques

Parallel imaging techniques (SMASH [SiMultaneous Acquisition of Spatial Harmonics) and SENSE (SENSitivity Encoding]) are the most recent technical advances for increasing imaging acquisition speed.[34,35] Both these techniques explore information inherent in the geometry of a phased-array surface coil system. Simply stated, the phased-array coil system uses several coils arranged linearly over the chest to acquire signal from the heart. The magnitude of signal of each individual coil varies with respect to its proximity to the object to be imaged. The parallel imaging techniques make use of this property. A sensitivity map of the organ of interest is acquired first, which permits information about the origin of the signal to be resolved. With this method, both SENSE and SMASH allow acquisition of several lines of K space for each excitation shot, which reduces the number of phase-encoding steps required to reconstruct the image, thereby significantly reducing imaging time. The greater the number of coils in the surface coil array, the larger the time saved. This method may be used in addition to other fast imaging techniques, such as partial K-space sampling. Current coils allow acceleration factors of approximately 2. In common with all techniques, the tradeoff for reducing imaging time is a reduction in S/N by a factor of $\sqrt{2}$.

Methods to Compensate for Cardiac Motion: Cardiac Gating

Motion of the heart and the great vessels causes degradation of the images. When this motion is uncompensated, it is nearly impossible to image the heart with any degree of clarity. Several strategies exist to overcome these limitations.

Cardiac gating is the most common method by which cardiac motion artifacts can be prevented during cardiac MR imaging. Simply stated, cardiac gating synchronizes the MR acquisition protocol to the cardiac cycle. Gating can be performed either using an ECG or pulse pressure signal.

ECG Gating

ECG gating is the current form of cardiac gating. Three or four ECG leads are placed on the patient's chest, and a single lead or vector-cardiographic signal is derived to trigger the MR scanner on the Q wave of the ECG. To avoid burns by current induction in the leads during the gradient application, the ECG leads must have high impedance. One of the major problems of ECG gating is alteration in morphology of the ECG within the magnetic field caused by the motion of the protons of the blood. This is known as the magneto-hydric effect, which occurs with increasing field strength. Typically, T waves become much larger, and Q waves become depressed compared with ECG recordings outside the magnetic field. These abnormalities may cause significant difficulties in ECG recognition, which limit the use of ECG changes for detection of ischemia, such as during CMR stress testing. The high-field gradients used in cardiac gating may add significant noise to the ECG signal and cause problems with ECG gating. Sophisticated filters and precessing algorithms are used in CMR systems to remedy these potential problems.

Pulse Pressure Gating

Because of the problems inherent in ECG gating, pulse pressure gating can be used as alternative method. To this end, an oxygen saturation pulse sensor can be placed on the fingertip of the patient and the cyclical waveform used to trigger cardiac gating. The advantage of such a system is that it is unaffected by alterations in the ECG, does not run the risk of burns, and is not influenced by the effects of the gradients. However, this method also has several disadvantages. The most important problem with pulse pressure gating is that this type of gating does not provide a distinct trigger at the beginning of cardiac systole. The maximum pulse wave is reached typically in mid-systole, end-systole, or in diastole, depending on the vascular impedance of the patient. Although this is not a problem if static imaging (i.e., T1- or T2-weighted) is performed, it precludes cine imaging with a fixed reference point to the cardiac cycle. Pulse pressure recording is also sensitive to the motion of the patient and is prone to artifacts caused by arrhythmia, which cause important variations in the height of the waveform.

Arrhythmia Rejection

Irregular heart rhythms such as atrial fibrillation or frequent premature beats can be problematic in gated cardiac MR studies because of varying cardiac cycle lengths. In gated cardiac studies varying cardiac cycle length may cause artifacts by assembling K space belonging to different phases of the cardiac cycle. To avoid these problems, cardiac MR scanners use different types of arrhythmia rejection schemes. These schemes reject information when cycle duration falls outside a prespecified range. For instance, all information from cardiac cycles that are either 10% shorter or 10% longer than the average cycle length may be rejected. The cost of arrhythmia rejection schemes is an increase in scan duration, which may introduce problems if imaging is performed during breath holds, because breath-hold duration may increase to unsustainable levels. Furthermore, cardiac cycle length actually changes during breath-hold imaging (i.e., at the beginning of breath hold, cycle length usually shortens because of the Valsalva reflex, and when a breath hold is significantly prolonged, heart-rate typically increases because of oxygen desaturation and carbon dioxide accumulation in the blood, triggering reflex tachycardia.

Methods to Compensate for Respiratory Motion

Breath-hold Imaging

One of the simplest techniques to avoid breathing motion on cardiac imaging is to perform imaging during breath holds. Before starting each acquisition, the patient is instructed to take a deep breath, exhale, and hold his breath until imaging is completed. Most patients can suspend respiration better in expiration than in inspiration, so that imaging during expiration is preferred for repeated breath holds. Breath-hold imaging requires patient cooperation and may therefore be difficult in some patients, especially in young children, patients with pulmonary disease, or very ill patients. Young healthy volunteers can usually hold their breath for more than 30 seconds, whereas most patients can only hold their breath for 10 to 15 seconds. This relatively short duration requires breath-hold imaging to be rapid. This may be achieved by reducing the total number of phase-encoding steps, with the disadvantage of reducing spatial resolution. Alternatively, breath-hold duration may be shortened by increasing the number of phase-encoding steps acquired during each heartbeat. However, the drawback of this approach is that the "shot" duration is increased, which reduces temporal resolution. The quality of breath-hold imaging is greatly improved by proper patient instruction before entering the MR scanner and by adapting the breath-hold duration to the capability of the individual patient. Typically, the quality of the breath holds is monitored by recording a chest wall signal and instructing the patient to improve his or her technique according to this signal. In our experience, more than 90% of patients are able to perform good quality breath-hold imaging when breath-hold duration is <10 seconds; however, success decreases when breath-hold duration is >15 seconds.

Respiratory Gating

To overcome the problems of breath-hold imaging or to perform cardiac imaging in patients unable or unwilling to hold their breath, MR imaging may also be respiratory gated. This is performed in similar fashion as cardiac gating. A flexible pneumograph (PEAR) is placed on the abdomen or chest wall of the patient to record respiratory motion patterns, and imaging is triggered on end-inspiration chest expansion. Because this only represents a small fraction of the respiratory cycle, respiratory gating significantly increases the duration of the imaging protocol by a factor of between fourfold to fivefold. In addition, the chest wall signal and motion of the heart are not temporally related, especially when respiration is irregular. Respiratory signal quality is affected by patient motion, so that respiratory-gated cardiac imaging is typically inferior to image quality during breath holds or with respiratory navigator gating. Respiratory gating is usually insufficient to avoid motion-free imaging of small structures such as the coronary arteries.

Respiratory Navigator

To overcome the limitations of respiratory gating, respiratory navigator gating was developed. The respiratory navigator is a linear CMR pulse of a predetermined width that is positioned on the diaphragm and read only in a 1D direction (Figure 1-24). It provides a 1D image of the interface between the high-signal liver and low-signal lung that can be used to determine the position of the diaphragm. The navigator produces an interval of stable end-expiratory positions, and the navigator pulse is performed immediately before every shot of the actual imaging pulse. Use of navigators is associated with gating efficiency approaching 50%, so that imaging time is only increased twofold, which is significantly better than chest wall respiratory gating. Newer techniques are being developed to increase navigator efficiency, for example, selected K-space sampling may be coupled with the navigator data.

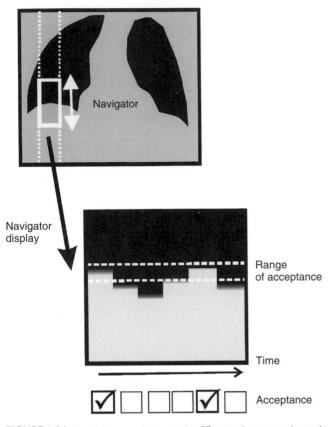

FIGURE 1-24. Respiratory navigator gating. The respiratory navigator is a linear CMR pulse of a determined width that is positioned on the diaphragm and provides a 1D (M-mode) readout of the diaphragm, lung interface *(top).* According to its position, subsequent imaging pulses are accepted or rejected for imaging *(bottom).*

This means that the periphery of K space, corresponding to the high-resolution data, may be acquired during the time when the position of the diaphragm is most stable, whereas the center of K space, which is less sensitive to motion, is acquired during phases of the respiratory cycle when motion is slightly greater. The position of the respiratory navigator correlates better with the actual position of the heart than respiratory chest wall position. Therefore respiratory navigator gating has fewer motion artifacts than respiratory chest wall gating. One particular problem with respiratory navigator gating is drift of diaphragmatic position, which means that end-expiratory positions may change over time. Another limitation of respiratory navigator gating is that it is incompatible with cine imaging, in which the entire cardiac cycle must be sampled for image acquisition.

Typical Cardiac MR Pulse Sequence Schemes

Several pulse sequences that are used typically for cardiac imaging techniques are described.

Anatomical Spin-Echo Imaging: Double-Inversion Black Blood

Detailed morphological information of the heart, great vessels, and adjacent structures is usually obtained using spin-echo imaging. At present, breath-hold gated turbo-spin echo (RARE) is the preferred technique.[36] Compared with conventional spin-echo, it provides higher acquisition speed and avoids respiratory motion artifacts. The breath-hold turbo–spin-echo sequences make use of a double-inversion recovery pulse to eliminate signal from the blood pool in the imaged slice ("black blood imaging"), facilitating the differentiation of the cardiac structures from the blood-filled cavities. The double-inversion pulse sequence consists of two sequential 180-degree pulses (Figure 1-25, *A*). The first inversion pulse is non-slice selective and inverts the magnetization in the entire body. The second inversion pulse is slice selective and restores the magnetization in a region slightly larger than the slice to be imaged. The black blood pulse is applied a certain time before the actual spin echo imaging. This inversion time is calculated to null the signal intensity of the blood when the actual spin-echo imaging is performed (approximately 300 ms). The double-inversion pulse inverts the magnetization of all protons situated outside the slice while leaving the overall magnetization of tissue unchanged in the slice to be imaged. Because the flowing blood entering the slice from either side has its magnetization inverted, it appears black (Figure 1-25, *B*). The spin-echo sequences are gated to the ECG (i.e., the TR is determined by the R-R interval of the ECG). Multiple echoes are read per excitation (16 to 24, depending on the desired image matrix and breath-hold duration) using multiple 180-degree pulses after the initial 90-degree pulse. Typically a single slice is acquired during a breath hold lasting 12 to 16 heartbeats. Only part of the Fourier domain (HASTE) may be acquired to reduce breath-hold duration. Breath-hold duration can be further reduced (six to eight heartbeats) by the use of parallel imaging techniques (SENSE/SMASH). Field of view and foldover artifacts can be reduced by outer presaturation bands.[37] For cardiac gated turbo-spin echo acquisitions, TR must always be a multiple of the R-R interval of the patient. To obtain T1 weighting, a relatively short repetition time of one RR interval (approximately 800-1000 ms depending on heart rate) and the shortest possible excitation time (TE) (<20 ms) is selected. To obtain T2 weighting, a longer TR (two to four RR intervals [i.e.] 2000-4000 ms]) and longer TE (80-100 ms) are used. T1-weighted images have excellent imaging contrast and high S/N and are therefore used to obtain images for evaluating cardiac anatomy. Compared with T1-weighted imaging, T2-weighted images have increased image contrast but less S/N ratio. Use of T1 and T2 weighting allows some degree of tissue characterization, for instance, in characterizing cardiac masses or the content of pericardial effusion. Additional tissue differentiation can be obtained with the use of fat-suppression techniques. Fat suppression may be obtained by adding a short inversion recovery pulse (STIR) to a T1-weighted turbo–spin-echo sequence.[38] Because of the third inversion pulse, the sequence is often also termed triple-inversion recovery. Application of this short inversion recovery pulse allows signal nulling of fat but not of tissues with longer T1. Alternately, fat suppression may be obtained by use of the chemical shift technique (i.e., to exclude the fat peak in the acquired spectrum).

Gated Multislice Cine Imaging

Cine imaging sequences are useful for assessing regional and global cardiac function. Cine images are typically acquired during short breath holds in a multiphase mode. This means that each breath hold allows acquisition of a single slice in cine format, that is, a series of consecutive images covering the entire cardiac cycle (starting at the R wave of ECG, and covering the systolic and diastolic phases of the cardiac cycle). To obtain images in a cine multiphase mode, segmented K space is acquired in several groups or segments after each ECG trigger.[39] RF excitation "shots" are delivered continuously during the entire cardiac cycle and are then reordered according to the number of phases desired. Yet within each cardiac cycle, only part of the K space for each cardiac phase is acquired. K space is filled phase by phase over several cardiac cycles. For instance, in the first cardiac cycle, the first eight excitations are used to acquire the first eight lines in K space of the first phase image (Figure 1-26). The following eight excitations, which occur somewhat later in the cardiac cycle, are used for the next phase images. They will be used to read the first eight lines in K space of the second phase image, and so forth, during the second heartbeat, the first eight excitations will fill lines 9 to 16 of the first phase; the next excitations will fill the same lines in K space for the second phase. Thus, several car-

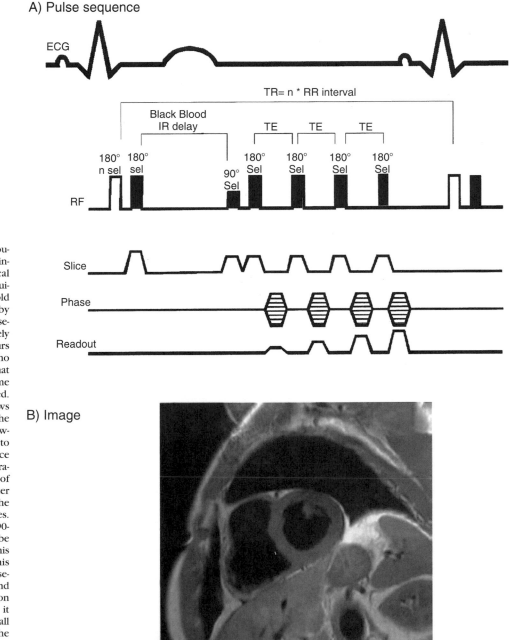

A) Pulse sequence

B) Image

FIGURE 1-25. Illustration of the double inversion black blood turbo–spin-echo sequence for anatomical imaging. The technique allows acquisition of one slice during breath-hold imaging. Black blood is obtained by using two inversion pulses. A nonselective pulse is followed immediately by a slice-selective pulse. This occurs at a delay before the actual spin-echo sequence, which is chosen so that the blood will be nulled at the time the spin-echo images are acquired. The double-inversion pulse allows blood to be saturated outside of the imaging slice and will cause inflowing blood in the imaging slice to appear black. The spin-echo sequence consists of one 90-degree saturation pulse and a sequence of 180-degree refocusing pulses, after which the echo will form. TE is the time between the refocusing pulses. TR is the time between the 90-degree saturation pulses and must be a multiple of the R-R interval (in this example, 1 R-R interval). In this example, if the number of phase-encoding steps would be 192 and the number of echoes per excitation (echo-train length) would be 24, it would take 8 heartbeats to fill up all K space. This would thus be the breath-hold duration. Example of a T1-weighted spin-echo image (TR= 1 RR, TE = 5 ms).

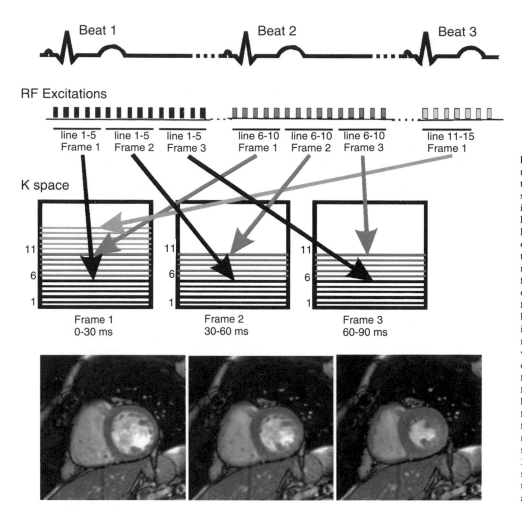

FIGURE 1-26. Illustration of segmented K-space cine imaging. The technique allows acquisition of one slice in a cine imaging mode by sharing the information over several heartbeats. The illustration shows how subsequent excitations are allocated to the different cine frames. In this example, TR is 6 ms, and the number of phase-encoding steps per frame is 5. This allows a temporal resolution of 30 ms/frame. Thus, the first five excitations in the first heartbeat will be used to fill the five lines in K space of the first frame (0-30 ms). The following 5 lines in K space will be used to fill lines 1 through 5 of the next frame (30-60 ms), and so forth. In the following heartbeat, the first 5 excitations of the next heartbeat will fill lines 6 through 10 for frame 1, then lines 6 through 10 frame 2. In this example, if the total number of phase-encoding steps is selected to be 96, it will take 96/5 = 20 cardiac cycles to complete the K space of all cine frames. This would thus be the breath-hold duration to acquire one slice in cine mode.

diac cycles are required to fill up all the lines of K space of all cine images. To allow such segmented K-space imaging, TR must be short, and low-shot flip angles are used. Cine imaging may be performed either with gated gradient echo techniques or with newer steady-state free precession (SSFP) sequences, which are somewhat faster. Both gradient echo and SSFP images are characterized by bright signal intensity in the blood pool because of the inflow of nonexcited protons (they are therefore also called "bright blood" images).

FLASH–FFE–Gradient Echo

As previously described, fast low-shot angle (FLASH) or fast field echo (FFE) imaging uses small flip angles (10-20 degrees) to allow short repetition times and fast image acquisition. The basic FLASH technique uses a single RF pulse to produce an echo signal. A magnetic field gradient is used to focus the protons to produce an MR signal. This technique is also known as gradient echo imaging (Figure 1-27, A). Improvement in gradient strength has allowed further shortening of TR and acceleration of the sequences called turbo-FLASH or turbo-FFE. Current fast gradient echo sequences have a repetition time (TR) of 5 to 7 ms, which typically allows the acquisition of one cine slice with a 256 × 160 matrix and a temporal resolution of 40 to 50 ms within one breath hold of a 12- to 16-cardiac cycle duration.

Because of the inflow of nonexcited protons from adjacent regions, gradient echo sequences demonstrate bright blood and myocardial tissue signal is intermediate, allowing excellent differentiation of the cardiac boundaries (Figure 1-27, A, lower panel). Overall, gradient echo images are characterized by lower soft tissue contrast, making them less valuable for imaging anatomical abnormalities, such as cardiac masses or infarction, than spin-echo techniques. In addition, gradient echo images are more prone to paramagnetic susceptibility artifacts within the imaged slice than spin-echo images, because T2* effects are not refocused with a 180-degree RF pulse.

Several variations of gradient echo imaging exist: Spoiling (SPGR) may be used to return transverse magnetization to null. This may be achieved by varying the phase of the RF excitation pulse or by applying gradient pulses to spoil transverse magnetization. Spoiling allows acquisition of more T1-weighted images. If spoiling is not used, the residual transverse magnetization may be maintained, such as in refocused gradient echo images. In this case, the images are more T2*-weighted. Finally, gradient echo sequences may also be combined with echo-planar readout to increase acquisition speed and acquire several lines of K space per excitation.[40] These types of hybrid sequences have significantly faster imaging speed but are more sensitive to T2* effects because of field inhomogeneity artifacts.

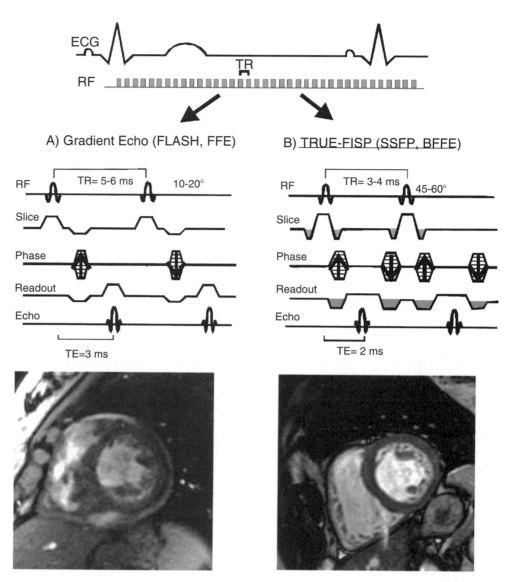

FIGURE 1-27. Illustration of the gradient echo and SSFP (true Fisp) pulse sequences. Both these sequences are typically used in combination with segmented K space to obtain cine imaging. Both type of sequences use gradients to refocus the spins, allowing formation of the echo. TR is very short, and one echo per excitation is obtained. SSFP **(B)** differs from gradient echo **(A)** by the fact that all the slice-encoding, phase-encoding, and read out gradients are balanced by applying refocusing gradients (shown in gray) that will return the total magnetization to zero. This allows a steady state of transverse magnetization, higher flip angles, and shorter TR, permitting greater S/N and faster imaging.

SSFP (BFFE–True FISP– FIESTA)

SSFP (product names: True FISP (Fast Imaging with Steady-state Precession), BFFE (Balanced Fast Field Echo), FIESTA (Fast Imaging Employing STeady-state Acquisition) sequences[41,42] are gradient echo sequences in which refocusing gradients are balanced. This means that refocusing gradients along all three axes are applied after each slice-selective and readout gradient, so that the total gradient moment returns to null at each TR. When TR is in the order of T2, a steady state of both the longitudinal and transverse magnetization is reached. This implies that SSFP imaging can be run at very short TR without compromising S/N. Therefore SSFP allows further shortening of image acquisitions (TR 2-3 ms and typical breath-hold duration of six to eight heartbeats for a temporal resolution of 40 to 50 ms per image, Figure 1-27, *B*). For SSFP imaging, the signal intensity is determined by T2/T1 times of tissues. Therefore the myocardial signal on SSFP sequences is very low, and SSFP sequences show very high contrast between the darker myocardium and the bright flowing blood (Figure 1-27, *B*, lower panel).

Because SSFP sequences rely on a steady state of constant excitation, factors that tend to disrupt this steady state (field inhomogeneities, eddy currents, and the presence of metal foreign bodies) result in off-resonance effects that are manifest as dark stripes or ghosting of flow. Because of their short echo times, for SSFP sequences water and fat are largely out of phase. Thus, SSFP sequences are more prone to chemical shift artifacts at interfaces between fat and water (for instance at the pericardial fat interface) than conventional gradient echo sequences. SSFP sequences are approximately twice as fast as GRE sequences. In addition, SSFP sequences allow better definition of the myocardial border and give typically higher quality cardiac images than GRE sequences. Therefore SSFP is currently emerging as the preferred cine imaging sequence for cardiac imaging.

Tagging

Tagging relies on the application of a pattern of selective presaturation pulses to the myocardium at end-diastole, just after the ECG signal.[43] Multiple tags are applied simultaneously in a parallel, evenly spaced stripe pattern using a sequence of nonselective RF pulses separated by magnetic field gradient (SPAtial Modulation of Magnetization technique: Dante-SPAMM).[44,45] Tags may be also be applied in a grid pattern by applying a second SPAMM pulse in an orthogonal direction. The tags are thus linear regions where the magnetization of the tissue is saturated. Because of the relaxation of the tissue, they persist for a period of approximately 500 ms on the myocardium and can be visualized as black bands on subsequent cine gradient echo images during systole. Because the tags represent a material property of the tissue, they move and deform with the motion of the myocardium during the cardiac cycle. Deformation of tag lines can thus allow the differentiation of contractile from noncontractile tissue. By use of algorithms of deformation and tracking of the tags, the regional deformation or strain of the myocardium may be calculated.[46,47]

Real-Time Cardiac Imaging

An intriguing method to avoid motion artifacts caused by cardiac and respiratory imaging is real-time imaging. This requires imaging to be performed in a frame-by-frame mode at a rate rapid enough that the image itself is not affected by cardiac and respiratory motion. The method does not require either cardiac gating or breath-hold imaging. This goal can be achieved in current state-of-the-art scanners by use of different fast imaging strategies such as SSFP, gradient echo, or EPI modes. For instance, with SSFP with a TR of 3 ms, an image encoded with 76 phase-encoding steps can be obtained in 200 ms. Temporal resolution would thus be 200 ms or approximately 5 frames/second. By use of parallel imaging techniques, temporal resolution may be halved to 100-120 ms (10 frames/second). EPI with an echo train length (ETL) of seven to nine may allow even higher temporal resolution of up to 50 ms (20 frames/second). This temporal resolution may, however, not be sufficient to follow cardiac contraction completely, especially in patients with elevated heart rates. The gain in temporal resolution, however, is offset by a reduction in spatial resolution (i.e., imaging with only 80 phase-encoded steps in a reduced field of view of 28 cm requires a reduction in pixel size resolution to about 3 to 4 mm). Thus, real-time imaging is currently used for purposes such as rapid slice localization for subsequent high-resolution imaging. It may also be used for monitoring purposes, such as the real-time assessment of regional wall motion during dobutamine stress testing.

Perfusion Imaging

Perfusion imaging is typically used to follow the passage of an intravenous bolus injection of a gadolinium-based contrast agent through the myocardium. The technique seeks to demonstrate perfusion defects in the cardiac muscle either at rest[48] or during pharmacological vasodilatation, for instance after dipyridamole infusion.[49-51] Perfusion sequences have two basic requirements: first, they must have a heavy T1 weighting to be able to reveal the subtle changes in signal intensity that occur in the myocardium after the injection of the contrast agent. Second, these sequences must image the heart with a high temporal resolution to better evaluate the brief period during which the perfusion defect appears with the first pass of the contrast bolus. Typically, a temporal resolution of one image every two heartbeats or greater is required. It is also important that the sequences have the capability to image several cardiac slices, so that perfusion defects in several coronary territories may be assessed. A number of sequences have been proposed for cardiac perfusion imaging. All use dynamic multiphase acquisitions that are repeated every single or second heartbeat for the duration of the passage of the contrast bolus (about 1 minute). Most sequences use a saturation pulse to obtain T1 weighting (Figure 1-28, A). After a delay, these sequences then acquire a given number of cardiac slices before being repeated on the next or second heartbeat. Either Turbo-FLASH or hybrid EPI sequences have been used. The various pulse sequences differ in their spatial and temporal resolution and by the use of a shared or a slice selective T1 prepulse. All sequences acquire the entire K space of one slice using several shots, followed by the next slice, and so forth (Figure 1-28, B). By use of a hybrid EPI sequence with a matrix of 128×96 pixels, an EPI factor of 4 and a TR of 10 ms, it would take 96/4 phase-encoding steps to fill K space, and thus each image would take 240 ms to acquire. If the patient has a heart rate of 60 beats per minute, it would be possible to acquire four slices every cardiac cycle.

Viability and Infarct Imaging

Viability imaging is a newer technique that delineates the extent of infarcted and noninfarcted (viable) myocardium regardless of the age of the infarction.[52] Imaging is performed several minutes (generally 15-20) after injection of Gd-based extravascular (conventional) contrast agents (such as Gd-DTPA or Gd-DOTA) demonstrate significant accumulation of the contrast agent in the infarcted myocardium.[48] This occurs because there is increased distribution volume to the extravascular contrast agent relative to normal myocardium both in the acute and chronic phase of infarction. The identification of infarcted (nonviable) myocardium is facilitated by sequences with high T1 weighting. Currently, the best identification is provided by segmented turbo-FLASH (gradient echo) sequences with inversion recovery preparation.[53] This sequence provides high signal contrast between infarcted and noninfarcted myocardium by making use of an inversion recovery (180-degree) prepulse that inverts the longitudinal magnetization in the entire tissue (Figure 1-29, A). After application of this pulse, the longitudinal magnetization slowly recovers according to the T1 time of the tissue. Because the infarct has a greater concentration of Gd, its T1 recovery will be faster than that of noninfarcted myocardium. Maximum contrast and thus best identification of infarcted from noninfarcted myocardium can be obtained by choosing an inversion time between the application of the inversion pulse and the image acquisition, so that the normal myocardium passes through the

A) Pulse sequence

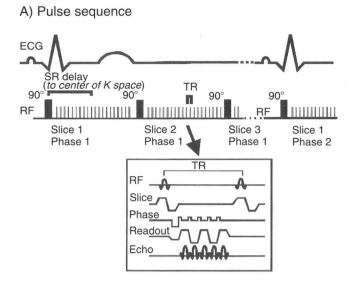

B) Example

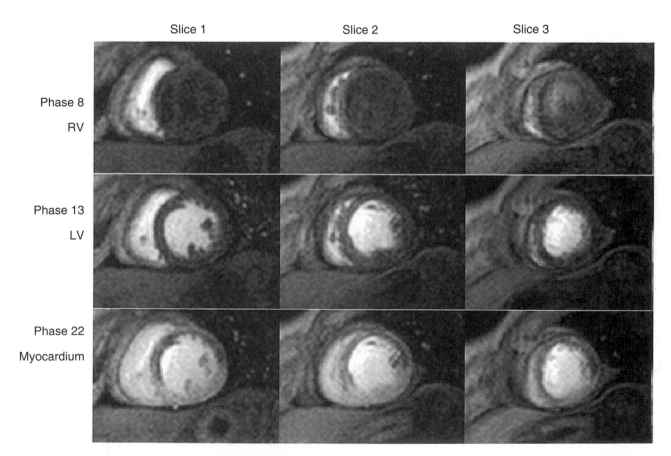

FIGURE 1-28. Example of a saturation recovery prepared perfusion hybrid gradient echo–EPI pulse sequence. This is an example of a typical sequence that can be used for multiphase first-pass perfusion imaging. Other types of sequences exist, however. In this example, a 90-degree saturation pulse is used to achieve T1 weighting. A specified time for saturation preparation is allowed, then a hybrid gradient echo–EPI pulse sequence is used to acquire the images. In this example, the EPI factor is 5, therefore five lines in K space would be read for every excitation. Excitations are repeated until the entire K space for one image is filled up. If the image were constituted out of 96 phase-encoding steps and TR were 11 ms, it would thus take 20 shots and 20 × TR or 220 ms to fill K space and to acquire one image. The completion of this image is followed by a new saturation pulse and acquisition of the next slice. The illustrated pulse sequence could thus acquire four slices every heartbeat if the R-R interval was 1000 ms (for a heart rate of 60/min). Example of a perfusion image with the previous pulse sequence.

A) Pulse sequence

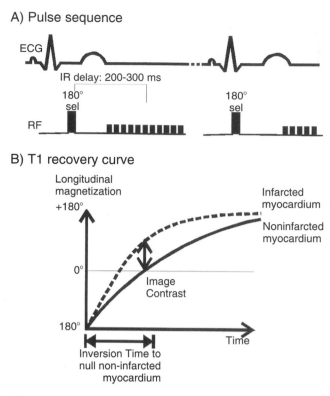

B) T1 recovery curve

C) Images

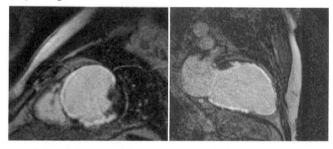

FIGURE 1-29. Example of an inversion recovery prepared gradient echo for infarct imaging. The pulse sequence uses a slice-selective inversion pulse. An inversion time is selected so that the noninfarcted myocardium is nulled. Imaging is performed with standard gradient echo readout. Magnetization recovery curves of the infarcted and non-infarcted myocardium. Because of higher Gd concentration, the infarcted myocardium has a shorter T1 than the noninfarcted myocardium and recovers its magnetization more rapidly. The inversion time is chosen so that the noninfarcted myocardium is nulled. This allows maximum contrast between the infarcted and noninfarcted myocardium. Image contrast depends on correct selection of this inversion time. Example of a short-axis and a two-chamber view image from a patient with anterior and inferior infarction. The infarct appears bright relative to the noninfarcted myocardium.

"null-point" of the curve (Figure 1-29, *B*). This allows the normal myocardium to appear black on images, whereas the infarcted myocardium, which has already recovered more of its longitudinal magnetization, will appear bright (Figure 1-29, *C*).

Different modifications of the sequence have been applied, and it is now possible to image the entire heart by use of a 3D acquisition. Alternatively, it is possible to combine the sequence with respiratory navigators, eliminating the need for breath-hold imaging.

Flow/Phase Contrast Imaging

Phase contrast imaging[54,55] is a method that allows quantitative measurement of blood flow velocity by CMR. The phase contrast method makes use of a gradient in either the slice encoding or the frequency-encoding direction (Figure 1-30, *A*). As protons (spins) move with a specific velocity along this gradient, such as during the movement of flowing blood, there is a shift in their angular position relative to the nonmoving stationary spins. This is called the spin phase shift and is proportional to the velocity of the moving spins. The phase contrast method resolves this phase shift in the Fourier transformation to reconstruct phase-encoded and magnitude-encoded images (Figure 1-30, *B*). The phase-encoded images are reconstructed, so that the grey level within each pixel is coded for the velocity of the relative pixel.

A) Phase Contrast Pulse Sequence

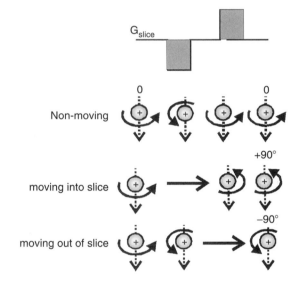

B) Images

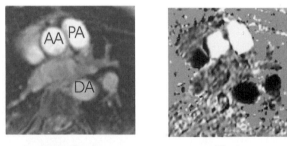

Magnitude   Phase

FIGURE 1-30. Phase contrast imaging. The phase contrast method is based on the use of a bipolar flow-encoding gradient. This gradient induces a positive and then a negative phase shift. Stationary protons will undergo both phase shifts and therefore have no net change of spin. Protons moving into or out of the slice will undergo a change of phase proportional to their velocity, because the effect of the two phenomena will be unbalanced. Example of a magnitude and phase-encoded image at the level of the aortic root. Images are encoded with a phase shift perpendicular to the image plane. Forward flow in the ascending aorta (AA) and pulmonary artery (PA) appears white. Reverse flow in the descending aorta (DA) appears black.

The phase contrast information is incorporated in standard cine sequences, which allows measurement of the velocity and direction of blood flow within each pixel over time. The phase contrast method is comparable to Doppler echocardiography and can be used to calculate pressure gradients from flow acceleration velocities in stenotic orifices by means of the Bernoulli equation. New phase contrast sequences have been accelerated, allowing phase contrast imaging to be performed during single breath holds, thereby reducing motion artifacts. In addition, motion sliding correction may be applied to correct for valvular motion during the cardiac cycle.[5]

MR Angiography

MR angiography (MRA) allows the selective visualization of the great vessels of the body by enhancing the signal of intravascular blood. Two basic methods exist: time of flight and contrast-enhanced MRA. Time of flight angiography does not require administration of a contrast agent but makes use of saturation techniques using short TR to suppress the stationary tissue in the imaging volume. Flowing blood entering the slice will be unsaturated and appear bright. Time of flight angiography is used mainly for angiography of the brain and for assessment of peripheral arterial disease. Because of the motion artifacts induced by respiratory and cardiac motion, it cannot be used to image the intrathoracic great vessels. Contrast-enhanced CMR is currently the preferred technique[57,58] because of its higher acquisition speed and excellent depiction of vessel borders (Figure 1-31). Contrast-enhanced CMR is performed after intravenous bolus injection of Gd-DTPA contrast. Shortly thereafter, a 3D gradient echo sequence is acquired while the patient holds his or her breath for approximately 20 seconds. Typical sequences are noncardiac-gated 3D T1-weighted turbo FLASH (GRE) sequences with short TR (5-6 ms) and TE (2-3 ms) and with a field of view of about 350 mm and a matrix of $256 \times 160 \times 16$, resulting in a pixel resolution of about $2 \times 2 \times 3$ mm for adult patients. The problem with contrast-enhanced MRA is the timing of the acquisition with respect to the start of the injection. This timing is crucial for optimal imaging quality and may vary largely between individuals because of differing transit times. Modern CMR scanners have therefore been equipped with bolus tracking sequences. These are very rapid low-resolution real-time sequences that detect the time of the peak bolus either semiautomatically or fully automatically, which triggers the start of the high-resolution 3D scan.

MR Coronary Imaging

Noninvasive coronary imaging is one of the most attractive clinical applications of cardiac CMR.[59,60] The technical challenges to meet this goal are multiple: The coronary arteries are small and move with high velocity during cardiac contraction. In addition, their course in the heart is complex and often curvilinear. Therefore, to image the coronary arteries, it is necessary to obtain images with high spatial resolution and with submillimeter resolution with high S/N. Several techniques have been proposed,

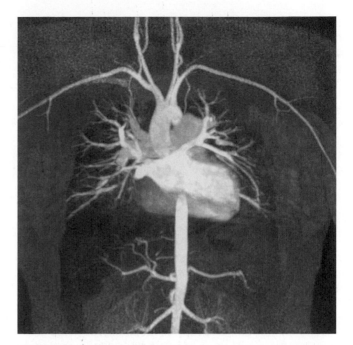

FIGURE 1-31. Example of a 3D contrast-enhanced angiogram. A time-resolved contrast-enhanced 3D magnetic resonance angiogram (MRA) of the chest and upper abdomen is shown in the late venous/midarterial phase. The 3D data set is collected as a series of contiguous thin slabs in the coronal plane, then reformatted to an oblique maximal intensity projection image. This image represents an oblique slab through a 3D MRA data set following the reformatting technique, which permits reorientation of the data set from the strict coronal (original) plane to an oblique coronal view. The method depicts the course of the intravenous contrast bolus from the right heart and lungs (light gray area in the midchest) to the pulmonary veins and left ventricle, and into the great vessels and descending aorta (bright white vessels in the upper and lower thirds of the figure).

some incorporating breath-hold techniques. These methods can acquire only a few 2D slices or a relatively low-resolution 3D stack within a single breath-hold duration. Spiral imaging has been proposed to increase imaging speed, and others have proposed 3D imaging techniques combined with respiratory navigators. These techniques allow high-quality images to be obtained in patients without the need for breath holds; however, they are relatively slow, taking about 7 to 10 minutes to acquire a high-resolution 3D stack for one coronary artery. Both black-blood spin-echo and bright-blood 3D gradient echo techniques have been used for coronary imaging; however it is currently not clear which technique is preferable. Because the relatively limited S/N ratio of current coronary imaging techniques constrains the resolution to about 0.7- to 0.9-mm pixel size, MR coronary imaging is not yet sufficient to accurately quantify stenosis severity or to image smaller branch arteries compared with invasive coronary angiography. Further improvement in coil design and parallel imaging techniques will minimize these limitations, making MR coronary imaging a more promising clinical technique for noninvasive coronary imaging in the near future.

MR Spectroscopy

The detailed description of spectroscopy is beyond the scope of this chapter. Spectroscopy makes use of the

NMR principle of nuclei with nuclear magnetism in the body other than ^1H. These nuclei have Larmor frequencies different from ^1H, and therefore their resonant frequency is different from that of ^1H. Because these nuclei are about 1000 less abundant than ^1H in the body, their signal is significantly smaller than the proton image. Therefore the technique is not generally used for cardiac imaging but instead to acquire spectra in a given region of interest. This technique provides information about regional or global metabolic phenomena by use of the relative abundance of the different spectral peaks. The resonant frequencies of some atoms may be affected by their chemical state, for example the phosphorous (^{31}P) spectrum for adenosine triphosphate (ATP), adenosine diphosphate (ADP), and free P has different, but characteristic, spectral peaks that may be used to measure their relative abundance. Their individual concentrations may be affected by phenomena such as ischemia and by intracellular pH. In vivo, ^{31}P spectroscopy was used to detect viability in infarcted myocardium,[61] as well as myocardial ischemia.[62] Other potential nuclei for cardiac imaging include ^{23}Na.[63] Imaging applications are possible with ^{23}Na, because the intracellular sodium concentration in normal (viable) myocytes is low because of the Na-K pump. After myocardial infarction, sodium rapidly accumulates in the myocytes because of cell membrane rupture. ^{23}Na spectroscopy and imaging have been used to identify the presence of myocardial infarction in humans.

PRINCIPLES OF NUCLEAR CARDIOLOGY IMAGING

Diagnostic cardiovascular nuclear imaging techniques are well-established tools in current clinical cardiovascular practice. In the United States alone, more than 3 million studies were performed in 2001, a 20% increase compared with studies performed in 1999 and one of the highest growth rates in cardiovascular noninvasive imaging modalities. By contrast, less than 1 million stress echocardiograms were performed in 2002 compared with 900,000 studies performed in 1997 (growth rate of 5%). Most nuclear imaging tests are performed to assess myocardial perfusion, but radionuclide angiography and the assessment of myocardial viability are diagnostic techniques used in specific clinical conditions.

In this section, the basic principles involved in cardiac nuclear imaging are described. This includes a description of the radioactive materials, the instruments used to image this radioactive material, and the radiopharmaceuticals used for the assessment of physiological cardiac function. In the following sections the two major components of cardiac nuclear imaging, radiopharmaceuticals and the imaging instruments, are described.

Radiopharmaceuticals

Radiopharmaceuticals are radioactive substances used for therapeutic or diagnostic purposes. These radioactive substances have two components, a carrier molecule and a radionuclide. The carrier molecule has a specific affinity and kinetics for an organ whose function is to be explored, and the radionuclide is the unstable element that transmutes by generating radioactivity that is detected by an appropriate instrument. A typical example used in nuclear cardiology practice is ^{99m}Tc sestamibi, in which the radionuclide that emits the gamma rays is the unstable ^{99m}Tc, and the carrier molecule is sestamibi. Sestamibi is a highly lipophilic molecule that freely diffuses through the myocyte cell membrane and is retained inside the cell. The radionuclide component of this radiopharmaceutical is ^{99m}Tc, which emits gamma rays that are externally detected by a gamma camera that processes the data and generates an image that represents relative myocardial perfusion.

Radionuclides

Radionuclides are elements with an unstable nucleus that release energy in the form of radioactivity in an attempt to reach a stable condition.

Elemental atoms have a central nucleus that contains positively charged particles, protons, and neutral particles called neutrons. Electrons are smaller negatively charged particles surrounding the nucleus. The stability of the atom results from the balance of the forces of the nuclear particles. An unstable atom resulting from an imbalance of forces in the nuclear particles, that is, a relative excess of protons or neutrons, will attempt to reach a stable condition by emitting particles (alpha or beta radiation) or electromagnetic radiation (X-rays or gamma rays).

The time required for half of the atoms in any given quantity of a radionuclide to decay is the half-life of that isotope. This is an exponential function described by the following equation $A(t) = A(0)e^{-\lambda t}$, where $A(t)$ is the activity at a time t, $A(0)$ is the initial activity, and $e^{-\lambda t}$ is the decay factor that can be expressed as $DF = e^{-0.693t/T1/2}$, where t is the time elapsed from $A(0)$ to $A(t)$ and $T1/2$ is the radionuclide half-life. Each isotope has its own half-life, for example, the half-life of ^{99m}Tc is 6 hours.[6] In addition, each gamma-emitting radionuclide has its own energy, that is, the energy released to a more stable status of the element. The energy is an important characteristic that has to be adequately set and periodically monitored in the gamma camera for optimal image acquisition.

All nuclear imaging techniques use radionuclides that are gamma-emitting elements. The most commonly used radionuclide in diagnostic techniques is ^{99m}Tc followed, in the case of cardiac imaging, by ^{201}thallium.

Positron-emitting radionuclides decay by emitting from the nuclei a small particle, positron, which has the same mass as an orbital electron but is positively charged. This type of decay is known as beta decay. Once the positron is released from the nuclei, it travels through the matter, where it quickly collides with orbital electrons generating two gamma rays of 511 KeV of energy that are directed 180 degrees apart (Figure 1-32).

This pair of gamma rays of the same energy that travel in opposing directions is characteristic of the positron-emitting isotopes and allows special radiation detection called coincidence counting. Most of the positron-emitting radionuclides used in clinical nuclear imaging are

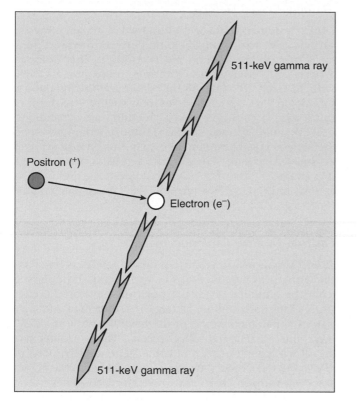

FIGURE 1-32. Schematic representation of the annihilation reaction between a positron and an ordinary electron. Note that a pair of gamma rays with the same energy but opposite directions is emitted.

produced in particle accelerators called cyclotrons and are characterized by a very short radioactive half-life. An example of this group is ^{18}F (half-life = 120 minutes), which is used when attached to deoxy-glucose (FDG) for the assessment of myocardial metabolism with positron emission tomography (PET).

Some positron-emitting radionuclides can be obtained from generators for which a cyclotron is not necessary, for example ^{82}rubidium (^{82}Rb), which is obtained from the decay of ^{82}strontium (^{82}Sr) contained in a generator. ^{82}Rb (half-life =76 seconds) is a potassium analog similar to thallium that is used for the assessment of myocardial perfusion with PET.

Radiation Detection

When radiation interacts with a material, it transfers energy to the atoms of the material causing two effects: ionization or excitation. Ionization occurs when the energy is sufficient to produce release of an orbital electron, leaving an ion pair. When the energy transferred is insufficient to dislodge an electron but enough to alter the normal particle arrangement, it causes excitation. Radiation detection is based on the interaction of radiation with the material used in the detector systems. There are gas-filled detectors, semiconductor detectors, and scintillation detectors.

Gas-filled detectors detect the ionization that radiation produces on a gas. Gas ionization creates an electrical current that can be measured as voltage difference between two electrodes. Gas-filled detectors include the ionization chamber, the proportional counter, and the Geiger-Mueller counter. Two important instruments used in a nuclear cardiology laboratory, the dose calibrator and the survey meter, are gas-filled detectors. The dose calibrator is used to assay syringes and vials containing radioactivity administered to patients, and survey meters are used to monitor the radioactivity level for radiation protection purposes.

Semiconductor detectors are essentially solid-state–filled gas ionization chambers. Silicon or germanium is the most commonly used material. These detectors are characterized by high-energy resolution, but their small size and high cost have limited their application in clinical nuclear imaging. New positron emission tomographs use this type of detector.[65]

Scintillation detectors emit light on interaction with radiation. The most common crystal used in current nuclear imaging equipment is thallium-activated sodium iodide NaI(Tl). When a gamma ray interacts with the crystal, a light photon is emitted and is transformed and magnified to an electrical pulse by a photomultiplier tube coupled to the crystal. The photomultiplier tube output is very low voltage and is optimized by a preamplifier. This signal is amplified from a low-level signal (in the mV range), transformed into a reshaped pulse (in the V range) and subsequently analyzed by a pulse-height analyzer (PHA). In scintillation detectors in which NaI(Tl) crystal is used, the signal amplitude is proportional to the energy of the gamma ray detected. Thus, by choosing signals of the same amplitude, it is possible to select the counting of specific gamma ray energy. This is the function of the PHA, which is critical in a nuclear cardiology laboratory to select the specific energies of the radionuclides used for imaging. If the radiopharmaceutical used for myocardial perfusion imaging is ^{99m}Tc sestamibi, the scanner should be adjusted to the specific energy of ^{99m}Tc, which is 140 keV. In many laboratories, a dual-radionuclide technique is used in which resting perfusion scans are performed with ^{201}Tl, and the stress scans are performed with ^{99m}Tc compounds. In this example, the PHA of the scanner should be set for the appropriate energy for these two radionuclides, which is 80 keV for ^{201}Tl and 140 keV for ^{99m}Tc. In the current instrumentation, multiple-channel PHA are available, allowing the simultaneous acquisition of multiple-energy windows. This technique can be applied for scatter or attenuation correction described later.

The Gamma Camera

Basic Design

Hal Anger described the first design of a gamma camera in the early 1950s. The basic components of a gamma camera are shown in Figure 1-33. A gamma ray image is projected by a collimator on a large NaI(Tl) crystal that scintillates proportionally to the radioactivity distribution of the organ being imaged. The light output produced by the scintillator crystal is transmitted to an array of photomultiplier tubes, where it is transformed to electrical pulses, which are subsequently magnified. An electronic circuit position system determines the precise

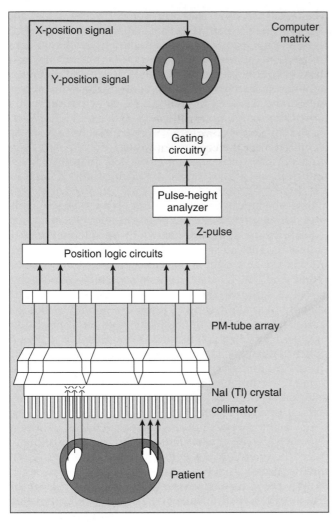

FIGURE 1-33. This schematic depicts the basic components of a gamma camera. Once the event position is determined, the data are stored in a computer for further processing, display, and analysis.

location of the events as they occur in the crystal. Events are also analyzed by a PHA that accepts pulses of specific height (that is, of a specific energy) and provides a specific X-Y location in a computer matrix or display.

The Detector

Single Crystal Detectors

Most current scanners are equipped with a 6-mm thick variable rectangular-sized single NaI(Tl) crystal. This crystal thickness is well suited for low-energy gamma ray imaging such as for ^{99m}Tc or ^{201}Tl. For imaging higher energy radionuclides, such as positron-emitting isotopes, the crystal has to be thicker (12.5 mm). An example of this situation would be when a SPECT scanner is used to image ^{18}FDG to assess myocardial viability. Most new scanners are equipped with two or three detectors that permit acquisition of more information over the same time frame. The main advantage of the single crystal technology is that it provides better spatial resolution but at a lower sensitivity than multiple crystal detectors.

Multiple Crystal Detectors

Other designs consist of multiple small crystal arrays of various sizes with lead shielding between them to minimize intercrystal gamma ray scattering. This detector array is coupled to a photomultiplier tube system (PMT) with an elaborate "light piping" scheme, allowing the use of a single PMT per eight or more crystals. The result of this design is a scanner with high count rate capabilities, however, with a lower spatial resolution compared with the single crystal scanner. Typically, this type of scanner is used when fast dynamic image acquisition is required; for example, for first-pass radionuclide angiography at rest and stress to determine left ventricular systolic function.

Positron-Emitting Radionuclide Detectors

Detection of positron-emitting radionuclides is based on the principal characteristics of the gamma rays derived from the annihilation of the positrons and orbital electrons of the surrounding matter. These gamma rays are a pair of simultaneous rays of the same energy (511 KeV) traveling 180 degrees apart. Because these gamma rays are of a higher energy than that generated by ^{99}Tc or ^{201}Tl, the type of crystal required must have a higher stopping power than that necessary to detect low-energy gamma rays. Although NaI(Tl) crystals can be used, greater crystal thickness is necessary. Bismuth germanate, gadolinium SO and Ba are the compounds used as detectors in current PET scanners.

The distinguishing feature of the PET scanners is coincidence counting, which is the ability to detect simultaneous events by opposing crystals within a very narrow time window. Coincident counting allows rejection of random events and increases the ability of the scanners to detect more events per unit of radioactive tracer than conventional gamma cameras.

Collimators

To obtain an image with a gamma camera, it is necessary to "project" incoming gamma rays onto the detector surface by using the principle of absorptive collimation by which only gamma rays arriving at a specific angle from the source are allowed to reach the detector. Those gamma rays traveling in a different direction are absorbed by the lead lining of the collimator before they reach the detector crystal. Collimators are designed with small holes arranged in a specific geometry to allow the passage of gamma rays. There are several types of collimators, but the basic ones are pinhole collimators, parallel hole collimators, and divergent and convergent collimators.

Pinhole collimators consist of a small pinhole in a lead or other heavy-metal material located typically 20 to 25 cm from the detector. This collimator inverts and magnifies the image if the source of radioactivity is close to the pinhole of the collimator. Pinhole collimators are seldom used in clinical nuclear medicine except for thyroid imaging.

Parallel-hole collimators are the most frequently used collimators in nuclear cardiology clinical practice.

These collimators project the gamma ray image of the same size as the radioactive source distribution onto the detector. A variant of the parallel-hole collimator is the slant collimator, in which the holes are parallel but at an angle, typically 25 degrees, from perpendicular. Currently, these collimators are used to acquire transmission scans from external radioactive sources that are used for attenuation correction.

Performance Characteristics

Image Linearity and Uniformity

A problem arising from the detector and electronic imperfections is image nonlinearity. Nonlinearity occurs when a linear source of gamma rays appears as a curved image, which can result from the variable performance of the photomultiplier (PM) tubes. Modern gamma cameras have digital automatic PM tuning systems that make the linearity a more stable performance parameter. However, testing the linearity of a scanner is one of the basic quality assurance procedures that should be performed periodically in every laboratory (Figure 1-34).

When a detector is exposed to a uniform source of gamma rays, the image obtained should be uniform in a normally functioning scanner. Even in an optimally functioning scanner, uniformity may not be perfect and may need to be corrected. The sources of non-uniformity are usually related to the performance of PM tubes. One problem arises from small differences in the pulse height of different tubes, and a second problem relates to the different efficiency of the PM tubes detecting light pulses in the center of the PM tube or when the pulses are in between PM tubes. The efficiency is higher when

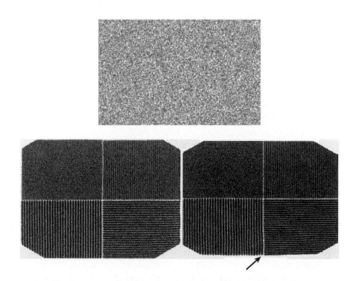

FIGURE 1-34. The top panel shows flood images obtained with a uniform flat radioactive source. The purpose of this image is to assess uniformity of the scanner. Images in the bottom panel were obtained by interposing a bar phantom between a flat radioactive source and the scanner. Bar phantoms are used to test scanner linearity and spatial resolution. Lead bars are spaced at 3.5, 3, 2.5, and 2 mm in each quadrant. The image on the left demonstrates good linearity and resolution, whereas the image on the right shows an area of curved lines. Nonlinearity will impact on the final resolution of the tomographic images.

the light is detected in the center of the PM tube, resulting in an image with apparent "hot spots" located in the center of the PM tubes with apparent cold spots in areas distant from the center of the PM tubes. Digital tuning of the PM in conjunction with the acquisition of calibration tables is currently available and adjusts the individual PM tube gains, thus compensating for non-uniformity. The initial calibration is usually performed after construction of the scanner is completed, but periodic calibrations are required after the equipment installation.

Spatial Resolution

The entire system spatial resolution, that is, the ability of the system to detect sharp edges or small point sources of radiation, is determined by a number of factors, important among which are the intrinsic resolution, collimator resolution, scattered radiation, and septal penetration. The limit of achievable spatial resolution by the detector and the electronics is called intrinsic resolution. Intrinsic resolution is limited by two factors. The first factor is related to multiple scattering of photons within the detector, which occurs when a photon originating from the radioactive source interacts with the crystal and generates a scattered photon that interacts with the crystal at a very short distance from the original event. These two events are recorded as a single event that is located somewhere between them. The second and more important factor that reduces the intrinsic resolution is related to the statistical fluctuation in the distribution of light photons between PM tubes from one scintillation event to the next. Intrinsic resolution also depends on the thickness of the detector crystal. The thicker the crystal, the greater spreading of the scintillation light reaching the PM tubes, which is why gamma cameras have a relatively thin crystal. Intrinsic resolution is also affected by the energy of the gamma ray, because low-energy gamma rays produce smaller numbers of light photons, leading to a greater statistical fluctuation in the light collected at the PM tubes resulting in blurring in the recorded image. This is one of the reasons that imaging with ^{201}Tl (80 keV) has a lower spatial resolution than ^{99m}Tc (140 keV). However, the main limitation to intrinsic resolution is the use of collimators. The collimator "projects" the object's radioactive distribution to the crystal. Collimators are built with heavy metals that have the capacity to absorb gamma rays. Collimators only allow passage of gamma rays traveling in the proper direction through small holes while absorbing gamma rays that are not traveling in the appropriately oriented direction. This absorption takes place in the septa that separate the collimator holes. The septa thickness should be as small as possible to avoid obstructing the crystal, but needs to be thick enough to stop the differently oriented gamma rays. For example, the septa thickness of a lead, low-energy collimator is in the order of a few tenths of 1 mm. Thus, for imaging high-energy gamma rays, thicker collimator septa are required. Collimators for high-, medium-, and low-energy gamma rays are available for clinical use. Lower energy collimators have an upper limit of about 150 keV and medium-energy collimators approximately 400 keV. Currently, special collimators used for imaging positron-emitting radionuclides (511 keV) with gamma cameras are available.

The use of collimators is somewhat inefficient, because a significant part of the gamma rays originated in the object are absorbed, which limits the counting statistics. Collimator efficiency is referred to as the fraction of gamma rays striking the collimator that actually pass through it to project the image onto the detector. This collimator characteristic is an important determinant of the system sensitivity.

Another important characteristic of a collimator is the collimator spatial resolution, which is the ability to project sharp detail of small objects onto the crystal. This is a function of the geometry of the collimator holes, specifically their diameter, length, and shape. The preferred shape of the holes to maximize the exposed area of the detector for a given septal thickness is hexagonal or round. The diameter of the hole is a major determinant of the collimator resolution, in that the smaller the hole, the higher the resolution. A larger number of small holes for a given septal thickness results in a higher projected image on the detector, but the smaller holes diminish the amount of gamma rays passing though the collimator. Thus, there is a tradeoff between collimator resolution and efficiency. For a given septal thickness (related to the energy of the gamma ray) collimator resolution is improved at the expense of decreased collimator efficiency. This compromise has clinical implications when choosing a collimator for a specific type of study. For example, to acquire a first-pass radionuclide ventriculography in which high efficiency is required because of the short transit time of the radioactive bolus through the cardiac chambers, a high-sensitivity collimator should be used. However, this collimator will have a low resolution. Conversely, for the acquisition of a stress perfusion scan with ^{99m}Tc sestamibi, a high-resolution collimator is used, because time is not as important as for the first-pass study. Thus, for the perfusion study, higher spatial resolution is selected at the expense of low collimator efficiency.

Dead Time

Gamma cameras experience counting losses at high-count rates. Counting losses occur when two gamma rays are detected so close together in time that they are perceived by the electronic circuit as a single event. This results in an underestimation of the true radioactivity present in the field of view. Dead time losses are not important when acquiring typical static images such as rest or stress perfusion images with ^{99m}Tc sestamibi, because the count rate does not reach the dead time of most systems. However, counting losses can be relevant in dynamic acquisitions in which high radioactive concentration is in the field of view as occurs in a first-pass study to assess left ventricular function. Dead time artifacts may be manifest as loss of contrast in the final image.

Principles of Tomography

A single gamma camera image represents a 2D projection of a 3D radioactive tracer distribution. Images of a specific organ or structure of interest may be obscured by overlying and underlying radioactivity. However, this information can be obtained by acquiring multiple planar images from different projections around the patient. A typical example is the former commonly used planar acquisitions for thallium images in which the standard protocol included anterior, left anterior oblique, and lateral views. An alternative method is tomographic imaging in which images are 2D representations of structures lying within a selected plane or depth of a 3D object.

Tomographic imaging was originally developed in diagnostic radiology and later applied in nuclear medicine. In contrast with X-ray CT, which uses transmitted radiation, nuclear medicine techniques are generally referred to as emission computed tomography (ECT). Current techniques, including single photon emission tomography (SPECT) and PET, use projection data obtained with detectors that rotate (SPECT) or are placed around the subject (PET), and mathematical algorithms are used to reconstruct images of selected planes. Tomograms or cross-sectional images demonstrate structures in depth and avoid confusing superimposition of organs. Tomograms are created by mathematically combining a series of planar images obtained at various degrees of an orbit around the patient's region or organ of interest. For SPECT cardiac imaging, the gamma camera rotates around the thorax, and images are acquired either every 3 or 6 degrees over 180- or 360-degree orbits.[66,67] These planar images or projections are then reconstructed in tomograms or cross-sectional images of the chest. The basic reconstruction process is achieved by a method called filtered back-projection. Projection or planar images do not indicate the depth or distance from the scanner of the source of radioactivity imaged. A first approximation of the source distribution can be obtained by back-projecting the data from each of the planar images or projections acquired across the entire image plane. Increasing the number of views improves the tomographic effect, but even with infinite angular views the resulting images will be blurred. To compensate for blurring a filtering function is applied to the process (Figure 1-35).

Alternative reconstruction methods incorporate additional corrections to compensate image degradation from photon attenuation. Iterative reconstruction methods generate an estimate of a cross-sectional image, which is reprojected and compared with the actual projection or planar images. In each iteration, the process attempts to minimize the difference between the created projections and the actual data. One method of iterative reconstruction uses a statistical algorithm of expectation maximization and is referred to as EM reconstruction. The advantage of iterative reconstruction is that it can be used for attenuation correction to reduce noise from relatively low statistics images. Iterative reconstruction techniques are computer-intensive processes, but with current optimized algorithms like ordered sectors expectation maximization (OSEM) and greater computer power, they are more commonly used in modern scanners.[68-70]

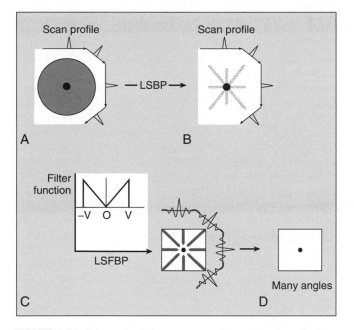

FIGURE 1-35. Schematic of linear superposition of back-projections (LSBP) and filtered back-projections. Scan profiles are obtained from the individual projections (the series of planar views acquired around the radioactive source or patient). Linear superimposition of back-projections produces an approximation of the actual activity distribution. The filter function eliminates the blurring. (From Sorensen and Phelps, in *Physics in Nuclear Medicine*, ed 2, p 399.)

Quantitative Aspects of Computed Tomography

Spatial Resolution

The spatial resolution of SPECT and PET scanners has two components, the in-plane resolution, measured in the imaging plane, and the axial resolution, measured perpendicular to the imaging plane. The *in-plane resolution* is determined by a number of factors, including the intrinsic resolution (detector and electronics of the equipment), collimator resolution, angular sampling (i.e., number of projections in a given orbit), reconstruction filter function, scattered radiation, and image display matrix. Axial resolution depends on the slice thickness, which is determined by the detector resolution in the axial direction.

Patient motion reduces spatial resolution, which is why it is important to minimize patient motion during the study acquisition to respiratory and cardiac motion. Electrocardiographic gating of image acquisition to the cardiac cycle reduces blurring of the images resulting from cardiac motion.

Partial Volume Effect

The resolution volume of a tomographic system is defined by two times the in-plane resolution and two times the axial resolution. Imaging objects of this size or larger results in tomograms that reflect the amount and the concentration of radioactivity. However, if smaller objects are imaged, the actual concentration will be sys-

tematically underestimated. If the concentration of a tracer is kept constant, the apparent concentration in the image decreases as the size of the object decreases. The ratio of apparent concentration over true concentration is the "recovery coefficient" RC.[71] The relation between RC and object size is shown in Figure 1-36. This so-called partial volume effect is an important consideration for quantitative or qualitative image interpretation and has practical implications in cardiac imaging. The most frequent study performed in nuclear cardiology is myocardial perfusion imaging, hence the myocardial wall is the target organ. Myocardial perfusion defects are assessed on ungated images, so the resulting image represents the average apparent tracer distribution during the cardiac cycle. In addition, gated SPECT images can also be obtained to assess regional wall motion. Myocardial wall thickness is less than 10 mm in diastole and no more than 15 mm in systole, well under the 2 × spatial resolution of most SPECT scanners. On the basis of the partial volume effect described earlier, at a constant tracer concentration throughout the cardiac cycle, the apparent tracer concentration observed in the myocardial wall image is less in diastole than in systole because of the change in myocardial thickness. This is translated into a brighter systolic image compared with the diastolic images. In this case, the apparent change in tracer concentration during the cardiac cycle is proportional to the thickening of the left ventricular wall. This constitutes the basis for assessment of regional wall motion with gated SPECT imaging. When a segment of myocardium is severely hypokinetic, the myocardial wall thickness does not change from diastole to systole; hence, the apparent tracer concentration (manifested visually as brightness) remains unchanged (Figure 1-37).

Partial volume effect is important when interpreting myocardial perfusion images in the early assessment of

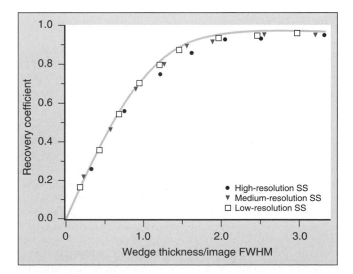

FIGURE 1-36. This graph shows the relationship between the recovery coefficient and the object size. Note that the recovery coefficient, a ratio between the observed activity over the true activity, is lower in thinner objects. (From Hoffman EJ. et al. Quantitation in positron emission computed tomography. 1. Effect of object size. *J Comput Assist Tomogr* 1979;3:299.)

Gated ^{99m}Tc sestamibi

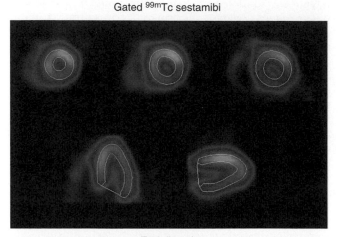

End-diastole

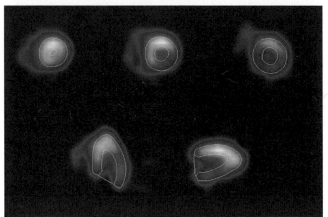

End-systole

FIGURE 1-37. ^{99}Tc sestamibi–gated SPECT images with a prior infero-lateral myocardial infarction. Note that brightness (apparent radioactivity) increases at end-systole because of myocardial thickening, which improves the recovery coefficient caused by partial volume effect. The inferolateral segments do not increase the brightness, because those segments do not thicken because of the prior myocardial infarction. See also Color Insert.

patients with acute coronary syndromes without evidence of acute myocardial infarction in whom revascularization was performed. Under these circumstances, an apparent perfusion defect can occur in the area at risk because of decreased perfusion in that territory, but it can also be the result of the presence of severe hypokinesis in that territory (stunned myocardium). Diminished or absent regional wall thickening of the affected myocardial segments causes a decrease in the wall average thickness compared with the normal remote areas. If the radionuclide tracer concentration is the same in both normal and abnormal segments, the tracer concentration will appear to be less in the myocardial segment with the thinner wall thickness. This "perfusion defect" at rest is likely to become normal as the contractile function recovers.

In summary, it is important to consider partial volume effect in cardiac imaging, because the myocardial thickness is well below the volume resolution of the SPECT scanners.

Effects of Photon Attenuation

Attenuation of a monochromatic photon beam is described as $I = I_0 e^{-\mu x}$, where I is the transmitted intensity, I_0 is the initial intensity, x is the path length through the absorber, and μ is the linear attenuation coefficient of the absorber for the energy of the incident radiation. Body tissues absorb a significant amount of radiation, creating distortion of the reconstructed images. It is important to compensate for photon attenuation so that the image is more representative of the true tracer distribution. A simple representative attenuation artifact is shown in Figure 1-38. A cylinder filled with uniformly distributed ^{99m}Tc in water is shown. Note that the distribution of radioactivity seems to be predominantly in the periphery of the cylinder. After attenuation correction, the distribution more closely resembles the uniform concentration of the tracer in water.

Attenuation correction may be performed by several methods. Most SPECT systems have an algorithm for calculated attenuation correction that can be applied to the filtered backprojection reconstructed images known as the Chang algorithm.[72] This method estimates attenuation coefficients of the thorax to derive correction factors that are then applied to the tomographic image. The variable densities of the thorax and the variation among individuals preclude use of this method for cardiac imaging, because it can generate significant attenuation correction artifacts. Thus, a critical factor for all attenuation correction methods is the acquisition of an accurate attenuation map that is representative on a pixel-by-pixel basis of the actual density of each individual imaged.[73-75] As opposed to the calculated attenuation coefficients, all the current methods involve the acquisition of transmission scans that are used to create an attenuation map of each individual patient, which is used to correct each pixel of the emission scan (e.g., a ^{99m}Tc sestamibi). Current SPECT scanners perform attenuation correction by use of transmission scans with either an external source of gamma rays or an X-ray CT system. Examples of transmission scans are shown in Figures 1-39 and 1-40. The most commonly used radionuclide for

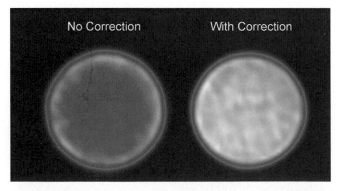

FIGURE 1-38. The effect of photon attenuation on the tomographic images of a uniform cylinder filled with water containing ^{99m}Tc. Note that apparent tracer concentration in the centers is lower than in the periphery. This is due to the attenuation of the gamma rays originating in the center of the cylinder as they travel through water. After applying attenuation correction, the apparent radioactive ^{99m}Tc reflects the uniform radioactive distribution present in the cylinder. See also Color Insert.

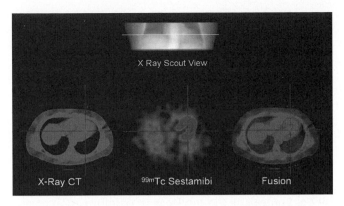

FIGURE 1-39. Example of a myocardial perfusion study with attenuation correction using X-ray CT to create a attenuation map. See also Color Insert.

acquiring transmission images is ^{153}Gd (energy = 90 keV; half-life, 253 days). Gadolinium gamma rays can be acquired simultaneously with ^{99m}Tc gamma rays by setting the acquisition with energy windows to acquire 90-keV gamma rays (transmission scans) and 140-keV gamma rays (emission scans). One of the disadvantages of the simultaneous acquisition with these radionuclides is the potential contamination (scatter from the higher energy to the lower gamma rays). Scatter correction methods have been developed and used to reduce cross-contamination between these two radionuclides.[76] Scatter is avoided by use of an X-ray CT method. However, a potential source of error may result from patient motion between the emission and X-ray CT acquisition when these two scans are performed sequentially. This leads to misregistration of the transmission and emission scans and errors in the attenuation correction.

Attenuation artifacts are common in cardiac imaging and lead to a decreased diagnostic accuracy of heart disease. This is particularly relevant in myocardial perfusion imaging. Myocardial perfusion is uniform throughout the left ventricular wall. However, the myocardial perfusion images most commonly obtained in the average nuclear cardiology laboratory present areas of apparent reduction of tracer uptake ranging from 10% to 30% because of attenuation artifact that is variable from patient to patient, depending on the individual thorax configuration. Inferior wall attenuation artifacts occur frequently in men, and anteroapical artifacts are present in women because of the effect of breast attenuation. Images with attenuation correction render more uniform perfusion scans, thus improving the diagnostic accuracy of perfusion imaging for diagnosing coronary artery disease[77-79] (Figures 1-40 and 1-41).

Image Noise

Image noise is usually described in terms of S/N ratio, as the relevance of the noise in relation to the magnitude of the signal. The noise (or standard deviation of the measurement) is given by $\sqrt{N}$, where N is the number of counts. For example, for measurement of 100 counts, the S/N ratio is 10 or the noise level is 10% (S/N$^{-1} \times 100$), and for measurement of 1000 counts, the S/N ratio is 31.62 or the noise level is 3.16%. This concept applies to planar images, but when tomography is used, the noise is propagated because of the number of mathematical operations performed during the reconstruction process among all the pixel elements along a sampling line. The noise propagation is greater for longer paths through the body and also increases as the number of pixels along the line increases (higher spatial resolution.) The S/N in tomography is given by $\sqrt{12N/\pi^2}(D/d)^3$, where N is the number of counts, D is the diameter of the body section, and d is the linear sampling distance. Thus, the greater the number of counts acquired in a scan, the better S/N ratio will be achieved. Acquiring images with a high-count density is an important prerequisite for obtaining high-quality images. To obtain high-density count images and high resolution, a high-resolution collimator has to be used. As discussed previously, a high-resolution collimator has decreased sensitivity. Therefore, to acquire high-count density images with the same radionuclide dose, the acquisition time has to be prolonged. This is often in conflict with patient throughput; however, it is imperative to maintain high image quality.

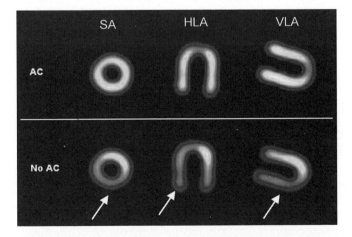

FIGURE 1-40. Short-axis (SA), horizontal long axis (HLA), and vertical long-axis (VLA) views of a heart phantom filled with a uniform solution of ^{99m}Tc in water. Note the lower intensity in the "inferior" wall in the uncorrected images. Attenuation correction (AC) images demonstrate more uniform distribution. See also Color Insert.

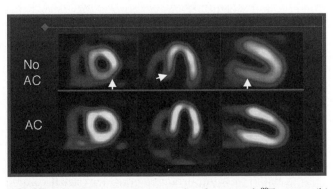

FIGURE 1-41. Representative example of a normal ^{99}Tc sestamibi study in a man with no attenuation correction (No AC) and with AC. Tracer uptake is more uniform in those images with correction. See also Color Insert.

Capabilities of Modern Gamma Cameras

Most modern gamma cameras are multiple-detector scanners that can be equipped for attenuation correction. Basic components of a modern scanner are the detector heads, the gantry, the patient table, acquisition and processing computers, and electronic modules.

The addition of attenuation correction capabilities requires additional hardware and software to generate and process the gamma or X-ray transmission scans necessary to create attenuation maps.

The basic systems are as described previously in the section on radiation detection. Most current scanners consist of a rectangular NaI(Tl) detector, a digital system that directly converts the photomultiplier tube (PMT) output to a digital signal located in the head of the scanner, that is used to analyze the energy and position of the events using digital electronics. The advantage of the digital capabilities is improvement of the PMT, which increases both uniformity and resolution. Each of the detectors is attached to a low-energy high-resolution parallel hole collimator that is suitable for imaging the most frequently used radionuclides in nuclear cardiology, namely ^{99m}Tc (energy, 140 keV) and ^{201}Tl (energy, 80 keV). The detectors, collimators, and electronics are packaged in single-head, two-head, or three-head scanners. Most of the current manufacturers use a dual-head configuration. The main advantage of multiple-head scanners is their greater sensitivity, that is, the ability to acquire more counts in the same time for a given amount of radioactivity in the field of view. Increased sensitivity allows the acquisition of higher density images rendering a better S/N ratio. Higher resolution images can be acquired with the use of higher resolution collimators. In addition, the greater sensitivity of the multiheaded scanners allows the acquisition of multiple gates or frames during a cardiac cycle using the R wave of the ECG to synchronize the acquisition. Typically,, the cardiac cycle can be acquired in 8 or 16 gates from end-systole to end-systole, which can be displayed in a cine format that enables simultaneous assessment of left ventricular function and myocardial perfusion.

Heads are attached to a gantry, which contains all the mechanics to control the head motion and positioning, as well as the electronics. The gantry gives stability to the heads, constitutes the largest part of the scanner, and determines the space necessary to install the equipment. The size and weight are characteristics that need to be considered during the planning phase before scanner installation.

Patient tables are currently designed with carbon fiber for strength, low weight, and low attenuation to gamma rays. In addition to their physical properties, modern tables have a computer-controlled motion mechanism to coordinate the most accurate patient position in relation to the gantry and detectors. For example, a specific system (Phillips Medical systems) moves the table during the scanning acquisition to maintain the patient as close as possible to the scanner head to preserve optimal resolution. Another example is a feature present in one of the newer models (General Electric Medical Systems) in which the patient table moves automatically from the position for the emission scan to the exact position to record the X-ray CT scan, which is obtained immediately after the emission scan. Strict control is necessary to avoid patient motion that can lead to significant imaging artifacts.

Computers are the other important component of the scanners. Computers have two main functions, one is the acquisition and the second is processing the raw data to generate the final images that are stored, displayed, and subsequently analyzed.

Most new scanners have a separate computer to accomplish these two functions.

The acquisition computer interfaces with the scanner receiving position of scintillations from the detectors, as well as controlling a complex array of information regarding position of the scanner heads in the gantry and patient table position and motion. Computers also accept a trigger signal originated from the patient ECG to acquire gated SPECT images. The raw data that arrived into this computer are stored for further processing.

The functions of the processing workstation involve image reconstruction, image filtering, image reorientation, image display, and data storage.

Image Acquisition

SPECT images are typically acquired by rotating the scanner heads around the patient's chest over a 180- or 360-degree orbit. The scanner records a projection for a variable time, typically 12 to 18 seconds, and moves to the next position to record the next projection known as a step and shoot mode. The number of projections depends on the acquisition protocol used. Acquisitions using 180-degree orbits are the most frequently used protocols, largely because of a shorter scan duration and because they were developed and used in the past when multiple-head scanners were not available and use of the lower energy thallium was the norm. The acquisition begins in a 45-degree right anterior oblique to 45-degree left posterior oblique angle, imaging a projection every 3 degrees of rotation. These images have the least attenuation, scatter, and loss of resolution with distance because the detector is close to the heart. However, because the tomographic reconstruction is not truly complete because 180-degree arc projections are missing, there are occasional artifacts with the 180-degree acquisition. Multiple-headed scanners and the use of higher energy gamma rays radionuclide such as ^{99m}Tc allow image acquisition through a 360-degree orbit in a shorter time and with the full set of projections to be used for the image reconstruction. The orbits may be circular or noncircular. The circular orbit was used in the past, because the head and gantry motion was limited. The main disadvantage is that the head is at a variable distance from the patient's body in different angles, and, consequently, the resolution differs from projection to projection. To avoid this problem and improve the resolution, noncircular orbits are used, which also keeps the head closer to the patient. This involves a more complex motion and motion control of the heads and gantry. Elliptical orbits are better than circular orbits, and automated body contours are even better, because the detectors are kept closest to the patient in each angle. This is achieved, for example, by using an array of laser beams in each head that detect the patient's contour and adjust the head position in each angle.

Special Features Related to Cardiac Imaging

Gated Imaging

Ungated cardiac SPECT studies may be blurred as a result of heart motion, resulting in lower spatial resolution. In addition, ungated SPECT scans represent an averaged image throughout the cardiac cycle, including the variation in left ventricular wall thickness from systole to diastole. Because the apparent tracer uptake is related to left ventricular wall thickness, the ungated images represent myocardial perfusion and relative myocardial thickness. This may result in apparent regional differences in myocardial perfusion. For example, a region that has the same tracer concentration but is severely hypokinetic will appear less bright on the ungated SPECT scan, because the average myocardial thickness is lower in the hypokinetic segments than in normally contracting myocardium.

As briefly discussed previously, image acquisition can be synchronized with the ECG to obtain a gated SPECT study. The basic concept is to generate a series of SPECT scans throughout the cardiac cycle to minimize the effect of heart motion. The ECG is used to determine the duration of the cardiac cycle and the end-diastolic period. Typically, the R-R interval is divided into 8 or 16 frames, and counts are collected in each of these frames in every projection. The end result is a gated study of 8 to 16 images through the cardiac cycle, which are the sum of several hundred beats. Gated images can be reviewed in cine format and information on regional wall thickening derived from the change of apparent tracer concentration from diastole to systole (brightening). Automated algorithms to detect the "endocardial edge" can be applied to the gated images to calculate left ventricular volumes and ejection fraction.

Gated SPECT images minimize the blurring effect from cardiac motion, which are therefore more suitable for interpreting myocardial perfusion defects.[80,81] However, several limitations remain, including the low count density and the absence of attenuation correction. A number of important and practical considerations exist regarding gated SPECT imaging. First, gated SPECT images have a significantly lower S/N ratio, and images are of much lower quality than the ungated SPECT. Because the cardiac cycle is divided into 8 or 16 frames, the gated images will have 1/8 or 1/16 of the count density of the ungated scan for the same scanning time. Longer scanning time and higher radiotracer dose can partially offset the low count rate. Gated SPECT images may not be obtainable in patients with highly variable R-R intervals as occurs with atrial fibrillation or multiple premature ventricular contractions. During gated acquisitions, an average cardiac cycle length is calculated, and future cardiac cycles are accepted if the duration is within a certain window that can be predetermined to ensure that the final gated images represent a cardiac cycle of similar duration. If the R-R interval is too variable, too many beats will be rejected, rendering an unacceptably low count image. In these circumstances, gated SPECT image acquisition is best avoided, and high-quality ungated SPECT studies should be acquired.

Perfusion Image Quantification

The myocardial tracer uptake in the left ventricular wall can be quantified and thus permit estimation of the presence, extent, and severity of myocardial perfusion defects. In addition, the location and the relative change between rest and stress myocardial perfusion images can be automatically quantified. Most methods generate a 2D graph of the 3D set of images to estimate the tracer distribution of an individual set of images and then compare them to a "normal" distribution.

The generation of the graph known as a polar map or bull's-eye graph is based on the extraction of circumferential profiles from a series of short-axis views of the left ventricular wall. A circumferential profile is a graph of the maximal count values against the angle at which they are encountered. All values are normalized to the maximum count value obtained in the entire left ventricle for each individual, and all the profiles are rescaled to a standard value of 100.

Polar maps are a method of viewing all circumferential profiles arranged in color-coded images. The points on a circumferential profile are assigned a color on the basis of normalized count values, and the colored profiles are shaped into concentric rings. The most apical ring forms the center of the graph, and each profile from successive short-axis views is added seriatim so that the outermost profile represents the most basal short-axis slice. These graphs represent the tracer distribution and identify the presence and location of a perfusion defect (Figure 1-42). Comparison of the polar maps obtained at rest and with stress identify regional differences in myocardial perfusion that are not present at rest, indicating myocardial ischemia caused by flow-limiting epicardial coronary artery stenoses.[82]

Quality Control

Strict quality control of all the scanner components is required to avoid errors in the scanning procedures that could lead to nondiagnostic examinations or at worst, false-positive or false-negative results that SPECT is supposed to help prevent.

Quality control procedures are directed to test the performance of the gamma camera as a single detector for planar imaging and for the SPECT system especially, because a system that produces 3D images should be tested in three dimensions.

Quality Control for Gamma Cameras

One important daily quality control procedure is to assess the correctness of the energy peak to ensure that the scanner is selecting the correct energy setting for the radionuclide being imaged. When the scanner is not at peak energy for the respective radionuclide, significant artifacts may occur in the reconstructed images. The energy peak is tested with a flat source of a known radionuclide, and the energy setting is investigated.

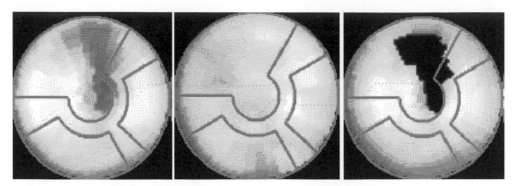

FIGURE 1-42. Polar map graph of a ^{99m}Tc sestamibi study at stress and rest. The left graph represents myocardial tracer uptake after exercise, the center graph represents myocardial tracer uptake at rest, and the graph on the right represents the extent of the defect. Note that a perfusion defect is present on the images after stress, indicating stress-induced ischemia in the territory of the left anterior descending coronary artery. See also Color Insert.

Typically a flat source of ^{53}Co is used to assess energy peak and uniformity. Uniformity is another important daily quality control procedure that evaluates the performance of the scanner. This test provides information about the scanner overall and is invaluable for detecting changes in the performance of the PMT energy peak setting that may result in a non-uniform radiation source. There are two methods to measure uniformity. One is called intrinsic uniformity, which is measured without the collimator by use of a point source of radiation, and the second is called extrinsic uniformity, which is measured with the collimator in place by use of a flat source of radioactivity. There are advantages and disadvantages of both methods, but in clinical practice the extrinsic uniformity is more frequently used. Typically, the same flat ^{53}Co source is used for the assessment of the energy peak and uniformity. The uniformity scans should be visually inspected and quantified. Uniformity is usually assessed by computer software determining the standard deviation in the entire image, as well as in the center of the field of view. Additional daily quality control is required in those scanners that have X-ray CT. Uniformity and resolution are tested daily by use of a specifically designed phantom.

Linearity is a measure of how accurately the scanner is able to image a straight line. Poor linearity will cause decreased spatial resolution on the 3D reconstructed images. Linearity can be assessed by use of a bar phantom that consists of a number of different size lead bars placed at different distances. Typically, this phantom has four quadrants with different-sized lines and spaces that also allow assessment of the spatial resolution of the scanner. This test should be performed weekly.

Spatial Resolution

Spatial resolution of the scanner can be assessed at various levels. Intrinsic resolution is measured without the collimator and represents the resolution achieved by the crystal and electronics attached to the detector. Extrinsic resolution represents the intrinsic resolution and the collimator resolution. The extrinsic resolution is the more commonly evaluated, because it corresponds to the actual resolution used during clinical settings.

Center of Rotation

The x and y axes of the scanner must correspond to x and y axes of the computer matrix. Special calibrations are use to ensure that the axis of rotation falls in the center of the computer matrix, which is of pivotal importance for the correct tomographic image reconstruction. If the center of rotation is offset, a reconstructed image of a point source will appear as a ring artifact. Modern scanners have more stability than the older equipment and thus require less frequent testing of the center of rotation.

Gating

Most cardiovascular nuclear studies are gated acquisitions. This is a technical procedure that synchronizes image acquisition to the patient's ECG. The gating equipment transforms the R wave of the ECG into a square pulse that is recognized by the scanner and is used to set a number of frames to divide the cardiac cycle. Failure to recognize all or some of the R waves causes suboptimal acquisition that may preclude interpretation of the image. Simple visualization of the ECG signal is usually sufficient. However, the entire gating system can be tested with an ECG simulator. It should be noted that counts should be identical in all frames. Gated SPECT image acquisition should be tested using a 3D phantom.

Quality Control for SPECT

Mechanical motion of the gantry, patient table, and response to instructions from the computer need to be examined. Most modern scanners have an automated mechanism for minimizing the distance between the collimator and the patient. This is achieved by adjusting the heads or by moving the patient table. All these motions have a safety mechanism to prevent injury to the patient. These safety mechanisms have to be thoroughly tested by running the camera to an immovable object to ensure that the motion stops.

Sensitivity, Uniformity, Linearity, Resolution, Attenuation Correction, and Volume Calibration

After assessing the performance of a scanner in a planar function, its performance in two or three dimensions must be tested. To reduce the number of time-consuming pretests, phantoms have been designed to test several functions simultaneously.

A watertight cylindrical phantom filled with a solution with a known concentration of ^{99m}Tc and containing a number of solid inserts can assess several functions during a single image acquisition. For example, there is a segment with uniform tracer concentration to assess uniformity and sections with spherical or cylindrical compartments to assess volumes and spatial resolution. Quarterly phantom imaging is sufficient for monitoring SPECT performance.

Quality Control for Clinical Studies

It is important to monitor quality control when reviewing patient studies. A logical sequence is to follow the actual steps in the process of image acquisition and processing.

Examining the raw data (projection images) in cine mode estimates the degree of patient motion and would account for artifacts in the reconstructed image. Correct positioning of the heart in the center of the field of view is essential. Complications from skin contamination with radioisotope are some of the additional information that can be obtained by reviewing the raw data. The reconstructed transaxial images should be examined, and these images should be consistent with the count density observed in the raw data. Degradation of the count density suggests an error in the reconstruction process. The adequacy of the filtering should also be evaluated. The presence of arcs or ring artifacts may indicate non-uniformities or center of rotation artifacts. Degradation of the spatial resolution may occur for a number of reasons, including problematic gantry motion, too large or variable a distance between the patient and collimator, center of rotation, camera being off energy peak, etc. In scanners equipped with attenuation correction, the transmission scan needs to be evaluated for motion and image quality as described earlier. It is important to evaluate motion or misregistration between the transmission and emission scans that may cause significant image artifacts. If significant motion is detected between the transmission and emission scans, the uncorrected images should be interpreted and the attenuation correction ignored.

In summary, although SPECT imaging is more accurate in determining the true tracer distribution in three dimensions, the complexity of the procedures involved in the acquisition, processing, and evaluation of the images necessitates rigorous quality control.

PET

Positron-Emitting Radionuclides

Positron-emitting radioisotopes decay by releasing a positron (β+ particle) from the nucleus. This particle traverses the surrounding matter until it collides with an electron that has the same mass but negative charge. This collision generates two gamma rays with the same energy (511 keV) but traveling in opposite directions.

Positron-emitting radionuclides characteristically have relatively short half-lives, ranging from 76 seconds for ^{82}rubudium (^{82}Rb) to 120 minutes for ^{18}fluorine (^{18}F).

The short half-life has advantages in that background activity is minimal, so that repeat tracer dosage can be administered if required. For example, myocardial perfusion images can be obtained at rest and after stress with two separate administrations of ^{82}Rb, because the half-life of ^{82}Rb is only 76 seconds, and therefore there will be no background activity remaining at the time of the second administration. This is in contrast to the more commonly used Tc-labeled compounds for SPECT imaging, which require a significantly higher dose of radionuclide for the second administration to override the background activity present in the myocardium after the first tracer administration (same-day rest stress ^{99m}Tc sestamibi protocols). The main disadvantage of most of these tracers, with the exception of ^{18}F, is that they have to be produced on site by a particle accelerator (cyclotron). Positron-emitting radionuclides can be classified into those produced in a cyclotron and those produced in a generator (Table 1-4). The latter category does not require a cyclotron close to the imaging center.

The most common cyclotron-produced radionuclides are ^{15}oxygen, ^{13}nitrogen, ^{11}carbon, and ^{18}fluorine. ^{15}Oxygen can be used to label water and can be used as a myocardial perfusion tracer. ^{13}Nitrogen can be used to label ammonia and also as a myocardial perfusion tracer, and ^{11}C is used to label acetate for assessing myocardial oxidative metabolism and labeling false neurotransmitters, for example, ^{11}C pseudoephedrine to assess myocardial adrenergic innervation. ^{18}Fluorine, perhaps the most frequently used radionuclide, is used to label deoxyglucose for assessing myocardial glucose metabolism. ^{82}Rubidium is not the only generator-produced positron-emitting radionuclide,

■ ■ ■

TABLE 1-4 POSITRON-EMITTING RADIONUCLIDES AND RADIOPHARMACEUTICALS USED FOR PET OF THE HEART

CYCLOTRON PRODUCED			
Name	Half-life	Radiopharmaceutical used in cardio-vascular imaging	Function
^{15}Oxygen	2.1 min	^{15}O water	Perfusion volume
		C^{15}O	Blood
		^{15}O$_2$	Oxygen metabolism
^{13}Nitrogen	10 min	^{15}N ammonia	Perfusion
^{11}Carbon	20.4 min	^{11}C acetate	Metabolism
		^{11}C palmitate	Metabolism
		^{11}C hydroxyephedrine	Adrenergic innervation
		^{11}C microspheres	Perfusion
^{18}Fluorine	120 min	^{18}F fluorodeoxy glucose (FDG)	Metabolism
		^{18}F fluoromisonidazole	Myocardial hypoxia
GENERATOR PRODUCED			
^{82}Rubidium	1.26 min	^{82}Rb	Perfusion
^{68}Gallium	68 min	^{68}Ga microspheres	Perfusion
^{62}Copper	9.7 min	^{62}CuPTSM	Perfusion

PTSM, Pyruvaldehyde bis(N^4-methylthiosemicarbazone).

but it is the most commonly used and currently commercially available. Rubidium is a potassium analog used for assessing myocardial perfusion.

The Scanners

On the basis of the decay characteristics of positron emission radionuclides that generate two gamma rays of the same energy but traveling in opposite directions, a special detection system consisting of opposite detectors is used. By limiting the detectors with a narrow time window to acquire events that occur simultaneously, the system will be able to detect coincident events and reject random ones. This constitutes an electronic collimation without the lead collimators used in gamma cameras. The absence of lead collimators results in a much higher sensitivity of the PET scanners compared with SPECT cameras. The higher energy of the gamma rays requires a different detector material with higher stopping power. When NaI(Tl) is used as a detector, a thicker crystal is necessary. Other materials used in PET scanners include bismuth germanate, cesium fluoride, barium fluoride, and a new generation of crystals like gadolinium SO.[65]

Most PET scanners consist of a detector array of 360 degrees with an axial field of view ranging from 15 to 30 cm. All scanners are equipped for attenuation correction with either gamma or more recently X-rays. As described for the gamma cameras, the basic components of the PET scanners are similar to the gamma camera and consist of a gantry containing the detectors, PMTs and the corresponding electronics, the patient table, computers, and electronics.

Cardiovascular PET imaging is currently used clinically for the assessment of myocardial perfusion or metabolism.

Basic Principles of Commonly Used Radiopharmaceuticals Used in Cardiovascular Nuclear Imaging

Myocardial Perfusion

Myocardial perfusion imaging is one of the most frequently used nuclear techniques in cardiovascular medicine. The extensive use of stress nuclear imaging has resulted from its improved diagnostic accuracy for detection of coronary artery disease compared with routine stress electrocardiography. Unlike invasive techniques, which evaluate the coronary anatomy and provide estimates of blood flow through the large epicardial arteries, nuclear imaging evaluates blood flow at the myocardial level.

Myocardial Perfusion Tracers Retained in the Myocardium

Myocardial perfusion tracers access the myocardium by way of the blood circulation, and the uptake of tracer is proportional to myocardial blood and the tracer first-pass extraction (tracer uptake = MBF*E). High first-pass extraction kinetics is a prerequisite for any radionuclide tracer used to assess myocardial perfusion. For example, microspheres are almost totally extracted during the first pass through the myocardial capillaries.

Myocardial perfusion tracers could be classified into two categories on the basis of their kinetic characteristics. The first category is those tracers that are retained in the myocardium, and the second category is tracers that are freely diffusible (Box 1-1). Tracers that are retained in the myocardium can be in turn subdivided according to whether they are retained within the myocardial wall. Thus, there are tracers that are mechanically retained within the myocardium, such as microspheres that are retained in the capillaries because of their size. Microspheres are particles of at least 15 μ in diameter (twice as big as a red blood cell) that are not able to cross the capillaries. Microspheres are extracted from the circulation almost entirely, except a small percentage that pass into the venous circulation through arteriovenous shunts. Thus, because the extraction fraction is close to 1, the concentration of microspheres in the myocardium reflects myocardial blood flow (tracer uptake = MBF*1). Although microspheres are a reliable myocardial blood flow tracer and the "gold standard" for measuring myocardial blood flow, microspheres have to be injected into the left atrium or left ventricle to allow good mixing in arterial blood and to access the coronary circulation. ^{99m}Tc or ^{11}C albumin microspheres were used in humans, but this technique is no longer used clinically, because it is invasive and because of concern regarding potential organ damage from occlusion of terminal arterioles in the brain, retina, and kidney microcirculations.

The other group of radionuclide tracers used for routine myocardial perfusion imaging is retained in the myocardium as the result of a cellular metabolic process. This group of tracers has been named "chemical microspheres." The typical example of this group of tracers is ^{201}Tl, which is a potassium analog that is retained in the myocardium in proportion to the Na/K pump. Thallium first-pass extraction is approximately 60%; thus, the initial thallium uptake reflects mostly myocardial blood flow (thallium uptake = +MBF*0.6). Another radionuclide tracer retained through a metabolic process is ^{13}N ammonia. This myocardial perfusion tracer is used with PET, because ^{13}N is a cyclotron-produced radionuclide with a 10-minute half-life. ^{13}N ammonia freely diffuses through the cell membrane and is converted to glutamine by the glutamine synthase activity within the cell. ^{13}N glutamine has none or minimal back-diffusion to the circulation. ^{99m}Tc compounds like ^{99m}Tc sestamibi and ^{99m}Tc tetrofosmin are retained in the myocardium by means of a different mechanism.

■ ■ ■

BOX 1-1   MYOCARDIAL PERFUSION TRACERS

Tracers that are retained in the myocardium
a. Mechanically retained: Microspheres: ^{99m}Tc or ^{11}C albumin
b. Metabolically retained: Potassium analogs: ^{201}Tl, ^{82}Rb, or ^{13}N ammonia
c. Mitochondrial membrane electrical gradients: ^{99m}Tc sestamibi or ^{99m}Tc tetrofosmin
Diffusible tracers
a. Hydrophilic: ^{15}O water
b. Lipophilic: ^{15}O butanol
^{99m}Tc teboroxime

^{99m}Tc sestamibi (^{99m}Tc hexakis 2-methoxyisobutryl isonitrile) is a cation that is sufficiently lipophilic to cross the cell membranes and is retained in the mitochondria in proportion to membrane potential with no or minimal back-diffusion into the circulation. ^{99m}Tc tetrofosmin is similar to ^{99m}Tc sestamibi in that it is concentrated in the mitochondria. Unlike microspheres, tracers retained in the myocardium through a metabolic process have a variable first-pass extraction, because the retention mechanism can be saturated. Thus, first-pass extraction decreases with higher blood flow, and, consequently, the tracer uptake is not linearly related to myocardial blood flow. Most of these types of tracers underestimate myocardial blood greater than 2 mL/g/min by different degrees (Figure 1-43). Because normal resting myocardial blood flow is approximately 1 mL/g/min and most of the patients undergoing exercise stress double resting flow rates, these tracers accurately reflect myocardial blood flow. However, in patients undergoing pharmacological stress with coronary vasodilation, myocardial blood flow increases by three to four times the resting values in myocardium with normal coronary arteries. It is possible that myocardial blood flow is underestimated under these conditions. The potential clinical implication is that there may be less contrast between the normal territory (in which uptake is not increasing as much as blood flow) and a territory of moderate coronary stenosis (in which blood flow will increase between 1.5 to 2 times the resting values).

Diffusible Myocardial Perfusion Tracers

Diffusible tracers are those that traverse freely to and from the myocardial cell in proportion to blood flow. Freely diffusible tracers can be hydrophilic or very lipophilic. The typical example of hydrophilic tracer is ^{15}O water that is imaged with PET. This tracer freely diffuses through the sarcolemma in proportion to blood flow. Because it is not retained in the myocardium, fast dynamic imaging is required to generate time activity curves and apply tracer kinetic analysis. Although these procedures are more complex, they do enable true quantification of regional blood flow. These techniques are more accurate than SPECT imaging for quantification but are difficult to apply clinically, because a PET center with a cyclotron and significant expertise are required. An example of a diffusible lipophilic tracer is butanol, which can be labeled with ^{15}O for PET imaging. Another lipophilic tracer that can be used with SPECT imaging is ^{99m}Tc teboroxime, which freely diffuses into the myocardial cells and rapidly diffuses back to the circulation. Because of their rapid clearance from the myocardium, these radionuclide tracers are difficult to use for exercise stress testing. This is one of the limitations of this group and one of the reasons why teboroxime is not widely used in the clinical laboratories.

Advantages and Disadvantages of Tracers Retained in the Myocardium

The main advantage of the perfusion tracers retained in the myocardium derive from the fact that once the tracer is taken up in the tissue, it is retained and remains unchanged for a period of time after intravenous administration. This characteristic allows more time for imaging and hence more counts. No change of myocardial tracer concentration makes the following features of myocardial perfusion imaging possible:

1. A single static image acquisition is sufficient to assess myocardial perfusion as opposed to multiple dynamic scans necessary when diffusible tracers are used. The acquisition of a single image is simple to process, evaluate, and store.
2. Images can be acquired some time after the tracer administration. This is important when the tracer is administered during a stress test so the stress and the imaging portions of the study can be performed sequentially instead of simultaneously. This facilitates the logistics of studying a series of patients with stress testing and imaging. Simultaneous tracer administration and image acquisition is required when a diffusible tracer is used.
3. Higher resolution collimators and therefore higher resolution images are possible.
4. Synchronization of the image acquisition to the patient's ECG.

This procedure enables the acquisition of gated SPECT images. Gated images enable assessment of myocardial perfusion, as well as the assessment of regional wall motion and the estimation of left ventricular ejection fraction with the same study.

One disadvantage of this group of tracers is that the extraction fraction is not constant, and therefore tracer uptake varies in a nonlinear fashion with myocardial blood flow. As discussed previously, most of these tracers underestimate myocardial blood flow when it is double the resting blood flow. This is a limitation of true myocardial blood flow quantification when evaluation of mild to moderate coronary stenoses is desired.

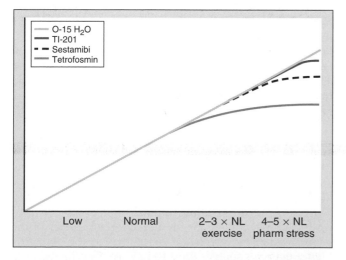

FIGURE 1-43. Graph shows the relationship between myocardial perfusion tracers and true myocardial blood flow situations. Note that tracers that are retained in the myocardium underestimate high blood flow rates.

Advantages and Disadvantages of Diffusible Tracers

Diffusible radionuclide tracers allow true quantification of myocardial blood flow, because counts vary linearly with perfusion over a wide range of myocardial blood flows. A typical example of this group of diffusible tracers is ^{15}O water. ^{15}O is a cyclotron-produced radionuclide with a half-life of 2.1 minutes. The short half-life enables multiple sequential images to be acquired over a short time without the problem of background from the preceding image (for example, rest stress images). However, because of its very short half-life, a cyclotron is necessary for almost continuous radionuclide production. In addition, because the nature of the tracer, rapid dynamic imaging is necessary to create myocardial time activity curves by use of tracer kinetic modeling to estimate myocardial blood flow. Although this technique produces accurate estimates of myocardial blood flow, the complexity of radiopharmaceutical production, imaging, and processing required is such that this technique is impractical and thus is not used clinically. This technique is mainly used as a clinical research tool but is one of the few methods available for reliable quantification of regional myocardial blood flow in humans.

Differences Between ^{201}Tl-Labeled and ^{99m}Tc-Labeled Compounds

Thallium has been extensively used for more than two decades, and a substantial body of clinical information has demonstrated its usefulness as a perfusion tracer. However, since the development of ^{99m}Tc-labeled compounds, there has been a shift away from thallium to ^{99m}Tc-labeled compounds for assessment of myocardial perfusion.

Tracer Kinetics

Thallium is a potassium analog that is taken up by the myocardium in proportion to myocardial blood flow because of its high first-pass extraction. Thallium quickly redistributes between the intracellular and extracellular compartments to reach equilibrium after 6 to 8 hours. The initial thallium uptake and the clearance rate from the myocardium are both proportional to myocardial blood flow. Thallium uptake correlates linearly with myocardial blood flow over a wide range of flows, but because tracer is retained in the myocardium, thallium tends to underestimate high flow rates, but less so than ^{99m}Tc-labeled tracers. This kinetic has practical implications when thallium imaging is used for the diagnosis of coronary artery disease during stress testing. Because of its relatively rapid redistribution, thallium imaging has to be obtained immediately after intravenous administration at peak stress. Excessive delay of the image acquisition allows tracer redistribution, which minimizes the contrast between the normal and the abnormal regions (Figure 1-44). Alternately, redistribution allows acquisition of the delayed images as a resting perfusion scan, so that with a single tracer administration stress-redistribution images can be acquired.

The characteristic tracer kinetics of the potassium analogs also permits assessment of myocardial viability, because the delayed images (at equilibrium) reflect the ability of the myocardial cell to concentrate thallium (through the Na/K pump). Thus, the rest-redistribution thallium study provides information regarding resting myocardial blood flow in the initial images and myocardial membrane functional integrity in the delayed images.

^{99m}Tc sestamibi and ^{99m}tetrofosmin are lipophilic cations that diffuse freely through the sarcolemma and are retained in the mitochondria with very little or no significant back-diffusion to the intravascular compartment. Lack of redistribution is the major difference in kinetics between the lipophilic (sestamibi and tetrofosmin) and thallium (Figure 1-45). Myocardial perfusion imaging at rest and stress therefore requires two separate tracer administrations. The best possible protocol is to perform the rest and stress images on separate days to avoid background activity and optimize the administered dose. However, this strategy is impractical, because it requires two visits to the nuclear laboratory. A single-day protocol is also possible, administering a low dose for the first images (preferably the resting image) and a higher dose for the second image to override the existing background radioactivity (typically three times the resting dose).

^{99m}Tc sestamibi and ^{99m}Tc tetrofosmin are taken up by the myocardium in proportion to blood flow because of their relatively high first-pass extraction; however, both underestimate high blood flows, ^{99m}Tc tetrofosmin more so than ^{99m}Tc sestamibi. Both tracers are excreted by the liver and biliary system; the hepatic clearance of ^{99m}Tc tetrofosmin is greater than ^{99m}Tc sestamibi. Because of the liver excretion of these tracers, a delay in the acquisition is necessary to avoid spillover activity from liver to the inferior left ventricular wall, which may lead to erroneous interpretation of perfusion defects in the territory of the right coronary artery. The lack of redistribution in combination with the physical properties of ^{99m}Tc allows more time for imaging and gating the acquisition to the ECG. This type of acquisition permits the simultaneous evaluation of myocardial perfusion and left ventricular wall motion. The use of myocardial perfusion images to evaluate acute chest pain syndromes is also possible with these compounds, because immediate image acquisition after the tracer administration is not required. The tracer administration can be performed in the emergency department, and the images acquired later in the nuclear cardiology laboratory.

Physical Properties

Thallium decays by electron capture to ^{210}mercury by electron capture emitting, mostly (94% abundance) 83-keV gamma rays with a physical half-life of 73 hours. The energy of the thallium gamma rays is relatively low, posing a disadvantage for the detection efficiency of the gamma cameras, which are better suited for detecting higher energies such as the 140 keV of ^{99m}Tc. In addition, the low-energy gamma rays are more affected by the surrounding tissue attenuation, leading to higher prevalence of attenuation artifacts on the myocardial perfusion images. The relatively long half-life limits the amount of

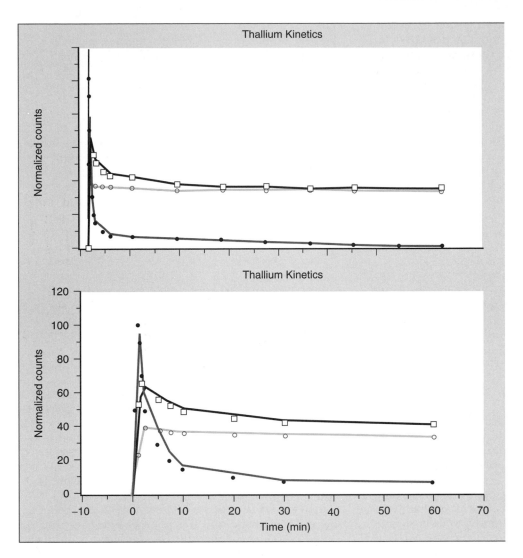

FIGURE 1-44. Schematic represents ^{210}Tl kinetics. Thallium's initial distribution is highly related to myocardial blood flow because of the high first-pass thallium extraction. In this example, the open squares represent normal myocardium, the open circles represent ischemic myocardium, and the closed circles represent arterial tracer concentration. Note the tracer redistribution as it reaches equilibrium. Stress images are normally acquired within 15 minutes after the tracer injection, and delayed images are acquired 4 hours later.

thallium administered to patients to equivalent radioactive exposure for shorter lived radionuclides. The effect of administering lower doses is the lower photon flux, resulting in a lower S/N ratio on the final perfusion images.

^{99m}Tc gamma rays have 140-keV gamma rays, which are more favorable for imaging with the standard gamma cameras. The higher energy gamma rays are less attenuated by surrounding chest tissue, and its shorter half-life (6 hours) permits the use of greater radionuclide

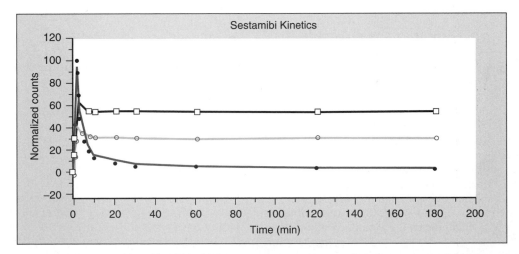

FIGURE 1-45. Schematic of ^{99m}Tc sestamibi or tetrofosmin. In this example, the open squares represent normal myocardium, the open circles represent ischemic myocardium, and the closed circles represent arterial tracer concentration. Note the lack of redistribution like thallium. Tracers remain in the myocardium with the same concentration after the initial uptake.

administration. The combination of greater photon flux with a higher energy and the tracer kinetics characteristics described previously, make these compounds suitable for imaging and convenient for the routine running of a busy clinical nuclear cardiology laboratory.

In summary, ^{99m}Tc-labeled compounds are better suited for myocardial perfusion imaging because of their more ideal physical properties, including their lack of redistribution. Thallium has the advantage that as a potassium analog it has well-known tracer kinetics and provides information on myocardial perfusion, as well as the integrity of the sarcolemma of the myocytes, which makes this tracer better suited for assessment of myocardial viability.

Tracers Used for the Assessment of Myocardial Metabolism

The most commonly used techniques are to evaluate myocardial glucose use and oxidative metabolism. Under resting and fasting conditions, two thirds of the energy in the myocardium is derived from free fatty acids. Circulating free fatty acids freely diffuse through the sarcolemma. Intracellular free fatty acids are involved in a number of metabolic pathways, including formation of structural lipoprotein, storage as triglycerides when energy requirements are low, or oxidation to yield high-energy phosphates.

The other important energy substrate for myocardial energy generation is glucose. Glucose is transported by the membrane carrier insulin-sensitive Glut 4 and is phosphorylated by hexokinase to glucose-6-phosphate in the cytosol. Glucose-6-phosphate is a potential substrate for several metabolic pathways. Glucose-6-phosphate can be stored as glycogen, enter the pentose shunt pathway, or enter the anaerobic glycolysis pathway to form pyruvate. In turn, pyruvate is transformed in acetyl coenzyme A (CoA) and enters the oxidative metabolism pathway within the mitochondria. During hypoxia or ischemia, the energy substrate use changes. Free fatty oxidation decreases because of a decreased level of oxidative metabolism in the mitochondria, such that free fatty acids may accumulate in the cytosol as triglycerides. There is

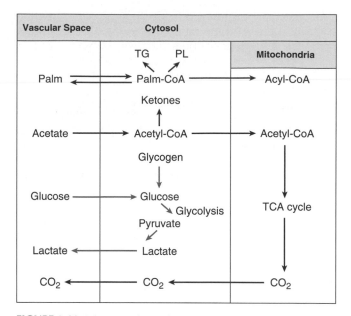

FIGURE 1-46. Schematic shows the energy substrate use changes associated with myocardial ischemia. Note the decreased lipid oxidation and the relative increment of anaerobic glucose use with release of lactate.

concomitant acceleration of glycolysis with use of glucose from the intracellular stores and glycogen (Figure 1-46). In summary, during ischemia there is a shift of energy substrate use from free fatty acids to glucose. A number of radiopharmaceuticals have been used to assess these changes, but the most commonly used tracers are [18]FDG and ^{11}C acetate.

The carrier of glucose also transports FDG through the cell membrane, and it is phosphorylated by hexokinase to FDG-6-phosphate. FDG-6-phophate is not a substrate for further metabolic pathways in the cell and therefore accumulates in proportion to the glucose transport and rate of phosphorylation (Figure 1-47). [11]C acetate is a short-chain fatty acid that freely diffuses into the cell and enters the oxidative metabolic pathway at the level of acetyl CoA. The clearance rate of this tracer

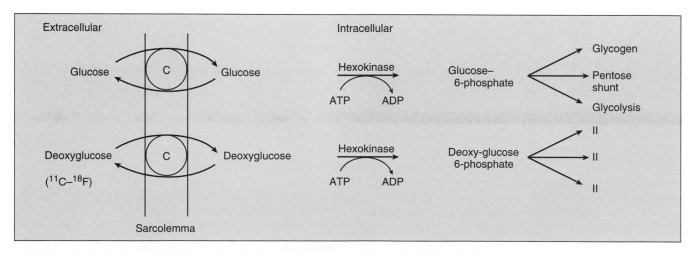

FIGURE 1-47. Schematic showing the tracer characteristics of ^{18}F deoxyglucose (FDG). FDG-6-phosphate is not a substrate for any of the glucose-6-phosphate metabolic pathways and accumulates in the cytosol.

represents the rate of oxidation. FDG has been used to identify increased metabolic activity after ischemic episodes in patients with myocardial ischemia and for assessment of myocardial viability in patients with coronary artery disease and segmental left ventricular dysfunction. In these patients, regions with hypocontractile function and decreased perfusion may be further characterized by their glucose uptake. Decreased perfusion and normal FDG uptake indicate the presence of ischemic, but viable, myocardium, whereas decreased perfusion and proportionally decreased FDG uptake indicate segments with scar tissue. Similarly, the presence of residual oxidative metabolic activity indicates the presence of ischemic but viable myocardium in segments with decreased contractile function. Accurate differentiation between ischemic but viable myocardium vs. scar tissue is of critical importance, because revascularization of viable dysfunctional myocardium improves clinical outcome in this high-risk patient population.

Future Developments

Imaging the Atherosclerotic Plaque

Basic investigation is currently being undertaken to develop new tracers to identify various components of the atherosclerotic plaque. Proliferating smooth muscle cells are being targeted with several tracers, for example, ^{99}Tc-labeled endothelin-1 or diadenosine diphosphate.[83] Ongoing studies are assessing the presence of activated macrophages using FDG, because these cells have an avid anaerobic glucose metabolism. Preliminary studies demonstrated increased FDG uptake in the atherosclerotic plaques of large arteries.[84] In addition, the apoptotic process could be imaged using [99m]Tc Annexin, which binds to the cell surface of the cells undergoing apoptosis. This new tracer has also been used for the noninvasive assessment of cardiac rejection after heart transplantation.[85]

ECHOCARDIOGRAPHY: PHYSICAL PRINCIPLES AND INSTRUMENTATION

Echocardiography uses ultrasound (US) to form images of the heart. High-quality tomographic images of the anatomy of the cardiac chambers and great vessels can be acquired in real time for assessment of global and regional myocardial function. Blood flow velocities within the heart can also be measured with Doppler US to quantify intracardiac hemodynamics and assess valvular function.

Echocardiography is noninvasive (transesophageal echo is considered a semiinvasive procedure) and is used extensively, because it is portable, widely available, and without hazardous bioeffects at intensities used for diagnostic imaging.

A prerequisite for obtaining optimal echocardiographic images is an understanding of the fundamental physical principles of US and familiarity with the technical and instrumental aspects of image formation and precessing.

Physical Principles of Sound

Sound is a wave of mechanical energy that is transmitted through a medium as local pressure variations. Sound waves create vibrations in the particles and cyclic variations in particle density along the path of propagation. Sound waves have peaks (compressions) and troughs (rarefactions) that depend on the presence of a medium and cannot propagate in a vacuum. Propagation of sound waves obeys the same physical principles for electromagnetic waves (Figure 1-48).

Wavelength (λ) is the distance that one cycle travels. One cycle includes one peak and one trough. *Frequency* is the number of cycles per unit of time, usually expressed in Hertz units (1 Hertz = 1 cycle/second, 1 kilohertz = 1000 cycles/second, 1 megahertz = 10^6 cycles/second). Sound includes the range of frequencies perceived by the human ear (20 Hz-20 KHz). US is defined as frequencies >20 KHz. The frequency range of standard transducers in cardiac imaging is between 1 and 10 MHz.

The *velocity* of sound differs according to the medium through which it travels. Velocity of sound waves is greater in stiffer, noncompressible tissues. The average velocity of sound in "soft" biological tissue is 1540 m/sec compared with approximately 300 m/sec in air.

The velocity of sound (C) is the product of frequency and wavelength:

$$F \times \lambda = C$$

The velocity of sound is constant in a specific medium, so that wavelength is inversely proportional to frequency. Because the propagation velocity of sound is constant in soft tissues, the time of return of the echo can be used to calculate the distance between the transducer and the region of interest.

The *amplitude* of a sound wave is defined as the height of the peak compression or peak rarefaction above the average and describes the energy content or "loudness" of the sound wave. Sound waves consist of compressions and rarefactions and therefore can be measured in units of pressure (mmHg).

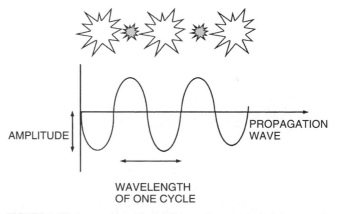

FIGURE 1-48. Propagation of sound wave. Propagation of the wave is characterized by peaks (compressions) and nadirs (rarefactions). Amplitude is defined as distance between the peak and baseline. Wavelength is defined as traveling distance of one cycle (one cycle equals on peak and one trough). During the time of peak, there is compression of the particles in the medium.

Pulse length is the time for one pulse to occur. *Pulse duration* is the time of the occurrence of one cycle multiplied by the number of cycles. As the frequency of the signal increases, pulse duration is decreased if the number of cycles remains the same. Usually pulses of 2 to 3 cycles are used for clinical US imaging compared with the 5 to 20 cycles pulses used for pulsed wave Doppler.

Pulse repetition frequency (PRF) is the frequency that the pulses are sent out from the transducer. Because it takes time for sound to travel from the transducer to the object of interest and back again (roundtrip time 13 μs/cm), the next pulse is transmitted only after the previous echoes are received.

To avoid misregistration of structures and range ambiguity in the image, all echoes received by the transducer must be processed before the next pulse is sent.[86]

Acoustic energy is the energy included in a sound wave. *Acoustic power* is the energy emitted in unit time measured in watts (1 watt = 1 Joule/sec). *Intensity* is the acoustic power divided by the cross-sectional area (units, watts/cm^2), and perceived as loudness or sound volume that is also measured in units of decibels (dB). Decibel is defined as the logarithm of sound intensity divided by the minimum intensity perceived by the human ear. Decibel units are used in measuring intensities in US instruments.

Reflection, Scattering, and Refraction

The US beam encounters a variety of tissue interfaces along its route. When the beam encounters an interface between tissues with different acoustic impedances, a portion of the beam is absorbed in the tissue as thermal energy, and another part is reflected. The difference between the acoustic impedances of the two media determines the proportion of the sound waves that are reflected. The two major factors that affect acoustic impedance are the density of the medium and the velocity of sound propagation in the medium. The direction of the reflected beam is equal to the angle at which the transmitted beam strikes the interface between the two media (angle of incidence). As the angle between the beam and the interface increases, the portion of the beam that returns to the transducer is increased and is maximal when the interface is perpendicular to the beam. Reception of the reflected waves (echoes) produces a signal that is displayed as an image (Figure 1-49). When the beam encounters a large (relative to wavelength), smooth interface, it is reflected backward and produces a *specular echo*. If the surface is relatively small or irregular, the transmitted sound will be reflected in all directions and produce *scattered echoes*, so that only a small fraction of the transmitted US energy returns to the transducer. Scattered echoes are produced when the US beam encounters small objects such as red blood cells (RBCs), and this interaction is the basis of the Doppler signal from moving RBCs (Figure 1-50). The remainder of the sound waves continue traveling forward through the tissue. If the beam passes through two media, with differing acoustic impedances, the sound waves are refracted. The magnitude of *refraction* depends on the difference between the acoustic impedances of the two media and

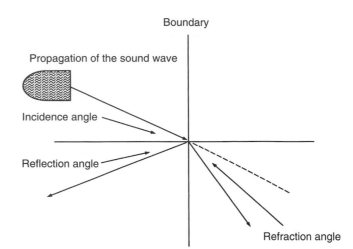

FIGURE 1-49. Reflection and refraction. When a sound wave strikes a large, smooth surface between two media, it is partially reflected. Another portion continues to travel forward, but in a different direction (refraction). Incidence angle equals the reflection angle.

the angle of incidence. When the incident angle is 90 degrees, refraction does not occur. Thus, for image formation it is important to direct the US beam perpendicular (or close to perpendicular) to the object of interest.

When US travels through tissue, it loses intensity because of reflection, scattering, absorption, and divergence. This loss of intensity is termed *attenuation* and depends on the distance the beam travels and the density of tissue it traverses. The intensity of sound decreases exponentially with the distance traveled. Attenuation is also dependent on the attenuation coefficient of the medium through which it travels. Attenuation coefficient is expressed in terms of half-power distance, which is the distance the beam travels before it reaches half its original intensity. Air and bone have short half-power distances (0.08 cm and 0.7-0.2 cm, respectively). The US beam during cardiac imaging may encounter both air (lung) and bone (ribs and sternum) that may occasionally preclude adequate image acquisition. To compensate for attenuation of US returning from cardiac structures deep within the thorax, a *time-gain compensation* (TGC) function is used. As the time from the signal transmission increases, the returning echo is amplified, equalizing the intensity of echoes from distant structures to echoes from closer tissues.[86]

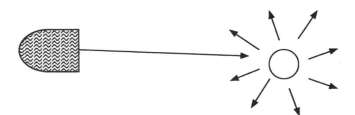

FIGURE 1-50. Scattering. When the US wave strikes a small object (relative to its wavelength) or a rough surface between two media, the wave is reflected to all directions. The resultant signal (scattered echo) is much weaker and not angle dependent.

Structure of the Echocardiographic Scanner

The echo scanner consists of four integrated components: a transducer, a beam former, an image/signal processor, and a display system (Figure 1-51). The transducer converts electrical pulses to mechanical vibrations that generate US waves. The transducer also receives returning US waves and translates them back into electrical current. The transducer is linked to a beam former that controls times of transmission and the rate of the scanning, respectively; an analog to digital converter (ADC converter); and a pulse-delay circuit. The US signal is passed through the image processor and finally displayed on a cathode ray tube (CRT).[87]

The Transducer

The main component of the transducer (Figure 1-52) is the piezoelectric element. Piezoelectric (pressure-electric) substances deform and emit US waves in response to an electric current, and, conversely, when they are physically deformed, they produce an electric current. The substances used in transducers include ceramics such as barium titanate or lead zirconate titanate. The frequency at which the element deforms or vibrates in response to electrical current equals the frequency of the US. The beam former controls the rate of the current change and the rate of the element vibration. The operating frequency of the transducer is determined by the thickness of the element, which equals half the wavelength of the transmitted US. Transducers may be constructed from a single circular crystal or from multiple elements. The element can be formed as a series of rings as in annular array transducers. The most common transducers in use currently are phased-array elements.

Manufacture of a transducer involves placement of a "matching layer" in front of the element, with an acoustic impedance between the high impedance of the solid element and the relatively low impedance of soft tissues (skin). The purpose of this matching layer is to reduce the reflection and refraction of the transmitted US before it enters the skin. Air has very low impedance and can reflect all the transmitted sound waves. During clinical scanning, a coupling medium (gel) is used to exclude the

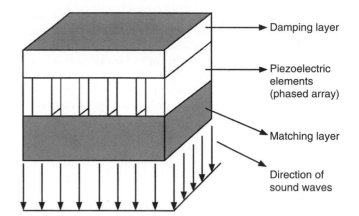

FIGURE 1-52. Structure of a transducer. The piezoelectric element is the key component of the transducer. In the transducers in use today, it is set in a phased array. Behind the piezoelectric element, there is a damping layer for improving spatial resolution. In front of the element, there is a matching layer.

air interface between the transducer and the patient to facilitate propagation of the US beam. A "damping material" is positioned behind the piezoelectric element to serve as a "shock absorber" to absorb the ringing responses of the vibrating element and produce a pulse with a shorter duration and spatial length (spatial length = λ × number of cycles). A pulse with shorter spatial length improves spatial resolution, which is the minimum distance between two adjacent objects that can be distinguished as different objects.

The US beam from a single element has an hourglass shape with three zones (Figure 1-53): a conical converging *near zone*, a *transition zone* that includes the focal zone, and a *far zone* in the form of a diverging cone. The length of the near field is equal to the square of the transducer radius divided by the wavelength. The divergence of the beam in the far field is inversely proportional to the radius of the transducer. To extend the near field and reduce beam divergence, the *size* of the element and/or the *operating frequency* must be increased. The size and shape of the beam are important, because these factors determine the intensity of the signal and the lateral resolution. The narrower and more focused the beam, the stronger its intensity and the greater the lateral resolution.

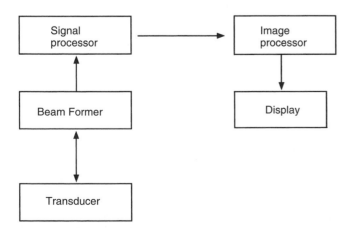

FIGURE 1-51. Structure of an echo device (From Kremkau. Figure 4-1a, page 103).

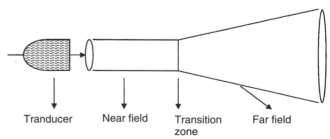

FIGURE 1-53. The configuration of a simple US beam created by a single-element transducer. Near field is a cylindrical region located close to the transducer. As the beam diverges, it forms a field with a cone shape (far field zone). Between these fields, there is a transition zone.

Beam focusing can be achieved by an acoustic lens or appropriate timing of the firing of the multiple elements in a phased-array transducer. The beam can be focused at a predetermined distance from the transducer surface where the optimal resolution is desired. The distribution of the acoustic intensity is not homogenous, and the boundaries of the beam are not precisely demarcated. The intensity of the beam is reduced as the distance from its center increases. In the near field, because of complex interference, the decrease in intensity is in the form of multiple oscillations manifested as side lobes of the primary beam. In the far field, the intensity reduction is simpler and is in the configuration of a bell shape (Figure 1-54). Beam width is measured where the beam reaches half of the maximal intensity in the central axis of the beam. In reception mode, higher gain settings are required to image peripheral regions where the intensity is low, because with low gain, only the central portions of the returning beam are imaged.[86]

Methods of Scanning

When a US beam strikes an object along its course, an echo is reflected back to the transducer. The magnitude of reflection depends on the size of the object and its impedance (relative to the impedance of the previous medium). The reflected echo reaches the transducer element and causes a mechanical vibration, which is translated into an electrical current. The time interval between the pulse transmission and its return to the transducer correlates directly with the distance between the object and the transducer (depth). The echo can be displayed in several formats (Figure 1-55).

1. Amplitude (A mode): As the degree of the reflection from the object in the scanning pathway increases, the amplitude of mechanical vibration sensed by the element increases, and this is displayed on a CRT as a voltage spike with a magnitude proportional to the amplitude of the reflection. The position of the spike is proportional to the distance between the object and the transducer. This display of a series of spikes of various magnitudes and locations is no longer used in cardiology.

2. Brightness (B mode): The location of the object is depicted along the scan line in relation to the depth of the object. The degree of the reflection from the object is registered as brightness. This format is used in cross-sectional imaging. B-mode is displayed as a series of points in different locations with varying degrees of brightness along the scanning line (or lines).

3. Motion display (M mode): M mode is a modification of B mode. In M mode the points are displayed in different positions with differing brightness. The difference from B mode is that the tracing moves. Thus, all the dots along the scanning lines appear as *lines* with differing degrees of brightness for different depths. If the object does not move (or moves perpendicular to the beam), it appears as a straight line. If it moves and changes its *depth* along the beam line, it is shown as a line that runs periodically up and down. This mode adds *time dimension* to the scanning. The temporal resolution of M mode is excellent. However, it is limited, because it shows only points along one fixed scanning line and does not provide a spatial image.

2D B-mode Display

To construct a 2D image, multiple scanning lines are required to display the returning echoes simultaneously. The reflecting objects are displayed as dots on the screen. Depth is determined by the echo return time, and its lateral position corresponds to the characteristics of the scanning line (position and orientation). The brightness of the dot reflects the intensity of the echo (B-mode). To display multiple lines simultaneously, the dots should remain bright until the entire field is scanned and constructed. In all 2D cross-sectional images, the beam should move (sweep), which is achieved in three basic formats (Figure 1-56).

1. Linear scan: Origins of the scanning beam move, but the multiple scan lines remain parallel to each other.
2. Sector scan: Origin of the beam is fixed, but the beam is gradually swept through an arc with a predetermined angle. Therefore, the orientation of the beam progressively changes.

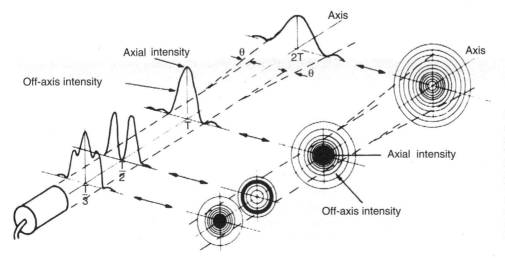

FIGURE 1-54. Configuration of a sound beam in the near field and far field. Note that in the near field, the wave consists of prominent side lobes, whereas in the far field, side lobes are diminished, and the sound beam acquires a bell-shaped configuration. (From Weyman, AE Principles and Practice of Echocardiography. 2nd edition. Lea and Febiger, 1994. Reproduced with permission. Figure 1-9, page 8.

Instrumentation

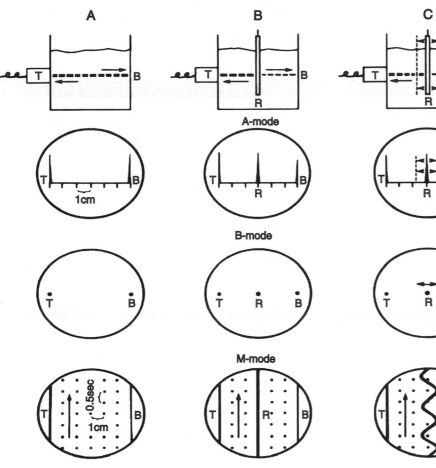

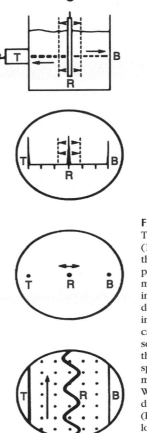

FIGURE 1-55. Scanning modes. Three basic scanning modes include: (1) A-mode (amplitude). In this mode, the signal intensity is reflected in the peak of the displayed spike. (2) B-mode (brightness). Signal intensity is indicated by the brightness of the dot. (3) M-mode (motion). The signal intensity of a specific site is indicated by its brightness. In M-mode scanning, the tracing is moving. Note that the flat plate is displayed as a spike in the A-mode, as a dot in B mode, and as a line in the M mode. When the plate starts to move, it is displayed as multiple oscillations. (From Feigenbaum, H., Echocardiology. 4th edition. Lea and Febiger, Philadelphia, 1986, figure 1-16, p. 9.

3. Arc scan: Origin of the beam (the position of the transducer) constantly moves. However, the beams are oriented to a fixed position.

The linear scan covers a large area, and its lateral resolution is homogenous (since the distance between the lines is constant regardless of the distance from the transducer). This mode of scanning is mainly in use in abdominal and gynecological imaging of relatively

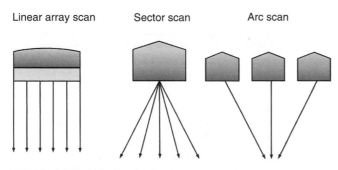

FIGURE 1-56. Methods of 2-D scanning. In a linear array scan, the beams are parallel. In sector scanning, the origin of the beams is constant. However, the beams are gradually tilted in a defined angle. In arc scan, the transducer moves, but the beams are oriented to a predefined target. Because of acoustic window limitations, sector scanning in used in cardiac imaging.

static organs. The main limitation is that it requires a large transducer aperture to cover a sufficient field. The thoracic acoustic window for cardiac imaging is limited by the sternum, ribs, and lungs, and satisfactory images can only be acquired by *sector scanning*.

Scanning Systems: Mechanical vs. Electronic Sweeping, Phased-array Transducers

Beam sweeping can be performed mechanically and electronically. Mechanical transducers have a motor that either rotates or oscillates the piezoelectric element. A rotating scanner may have three to four rotating elements, and when the element is parallel to the surface of the transducer, it sends a pulse. The oscillating transducer is tilted through a predetermined angle. When the element reaches a certain point, it sends and receives signals. A third type of mechanical transducer, rarely in use today, includes a fixed element with rotating or oscillating mirrors.

Nowadays, most of the transducers use *electronic beam* sweeping rather than *mechanical beam* sweeping. The transducer consists of multiple piezoelectric elements arranged in a matrix. Each of the elements can be programmed to send a pulse independent of the other elements. When a group of elements is activated and fires signals, the wavelets from each element summate to form a large wavefront. When elements aligned in a row fire simultaneously, they form a signal with a longitudinal front. After the wave returns, the second row is activated and so on. This activation sequence forms parallel beams with a linear scanning pattern referred to as a *linear array*. To increase the line density (and lateral resolution), there may be an overlap between the activated rows (the first sequence includes element lines (1-2-3-4-5), and the second sequence may include lines (2-3-4-5-6). This mode is known as *grouped linear array*. The maximal line density correlates with the number of elements included in the transducer. The beam formed by this mode is rectangular. Changing the beam angle is achieved by controlling the time sequence of firing of the individual elements and delaying the activation of particular elements, such that wavelet formation is delayed. The summated wavefront of both early and delayed wavelets is tilted. The angle of the beam can be changed by controlling the time delay of activation of the individual elements, so that a sweeping beam is formed. This format constitutes the *phased-array transducer*, which is the most extensively used for cardiac imaging (Figure 1-57). Beam focusing is controlled by changing the time delay of the electrical activation of the individual elements. A converging beam is produced by activating the most peripheral elements first, and, after a programmed delay, the central elements are activated. The depth of focus of the beam is varied by the changing activation time intervals. Electronic sweeping requires control of the sequence of activation by the *beam former*.

The beam former consists of a pulser, which generates the pulses of voltages that activate the elements. These activating voltages are passed through electric circuits that cause delay in activation of the individual elements (delay generator). Phase delay takes into account the time that the echo is received, so that time of travel is translated into distance from the transducer. The beam former consists of digital delay lines (echo delays) that compensate for the time delay during transmission.[88-90] The wavefront in phased-array transducers is composed of several scanning lines from the individual elements activated with some time delay. Building a single scan line takes time and results in *decreased frame rate* and *decreased temporal resolution*. Thus, there is a tradeoff between resolution, size of the scanned area, and temporal resolution (frame rate).

Beam Processor

The components of the US system receiving the echo (receive mode), the image processor, and display mode are described in this section. The transducer usually functions in pulsed mode, sending a pulse of US waves in a phased-array form and then switching to "receive mode" (an important exception is continuous wave Doppler in which the pulse of US is sent continuously). Continuous mode Doppler requires two transducers, one for transmitting pulses and a second for receiving echoes. In pulsed Doppler mode, the same elements participate in both processes, transmission and reception. The beam former participates in both processes. In the "transmit mode," the beam former generates voltages that drive the transducer elements. The generated voltages are relayed though "pulse delay" channels. The "pulse delay" component generates the phased-array form described in the previous section. Pulse transmission takes 1 to 2 μs. After completing the transmission process, a transmission/ reception (T/R) switch switches the transducer to *receive mode*.

The receive mode component includes amplifiers connected to individual elements (or to a set of elements functioning synchronously). The amplifier increases the signal from a few millivolts to the order of hundreds of millivolts. Increase in amplitude is defined as *gain* and is expressed in decibels. A ratio of received/ amplified signal amplitude of 1.0 indicates gain of 0 dB; a ratio of 3.2 implies gain of 10 dB, and a ratio of 10^5 indicates gain of 100 dB. The amplifier includes a time gain compensation function (TGC). Delayed echoes originating from deeper structures receive enhanced amplification. TGC compensates for signal attenuation during the transmission and returning phases. In the current echo scanners, amplification can be further increased by the gain controls. A brighter image is obtained by increased amplification. By increasing the gain, the noise is also amplified, and S/N ratio decreases. Objects with low signals may be obscured by the noise and may not appear in the display. After passing through the amplifier, the echoes reach the ADC. The returning

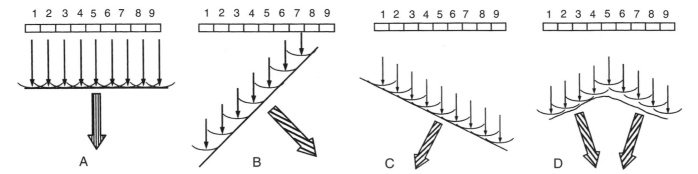

FIGURE 1-57. Phased-array transducer. The beam is obtained by multiple small wavelets generated from individual elements included in the phased array. All the wavelets summate to form a large beam. The orientation of the beam is changed progressively by changing the time delay between the pulses. A delay generator included in the beam former controls the time delay. **A,** All the elements are activated simultaneously, and a perpendicular front is formed. **B,** A gradual activation of the individual elements (elements 1 to 3 are activated earlier, and their pulses travel to a greater distance than elements 5 to 7). Therefore the wavefront is tilted to the right. **C,** An opposite activation sequence. **D,** Peripheral elements are activated before the central elements, comprising a focused wavefront.

echoes are in the form of *analog signals* (voltages). ADC converts analog signals to *digital*. The signal amplitudes are translated into binary numbers, which are processed and stored in the computer.

After "receiving a binary number" in the ADC, the signals proceed to the echo delay component, which compensates for time delays caused by beam sweeping and dynamic focusing. This compensation enables building a logical image. After the signal has traveled through all these components, it reaches the "summer." The summer combines all the signals received during a predetermined time and adds them to build a single data line.

Signal Processing[86,88]

Signal processing involves three basic functions: filtering, demodulation/detection, and compression. The received signal is defined by its frequency and amplitude. The signal includes echoes returning from the object and noise. The filtering process eliminates the signals outside a defined bandwidth. (Bandwidth is the range of frequencies received by the transducer.) The rejected signals are presumed to include more noise; thus S/N ratio and image quality can be improved.

The second function is *demodulation* or *detection*. RF signals are processed so that only the peak amplitudes are retained for further processing. The processed signal is integrated so that the area under the curve correlates with its amplitude. When B-mode is used, the area under curve correlates with *signal brightness*.

A third process is *dynamic compression*. The amplifiers in the receiving transducer handle a huge range of voltages corresponding to amplitude range of 100 dB. The signal amplitude and intensity in the B-mode is displayed as shade differences on a gray scale (strongest signals are bright, and weakest signals are black). The dynamic range that human vision can detect is approximately 20 dB.[86] To accommodate for such a huge difference without missing important data, the signals are compressed to a smaller range. Compression is performed on a logarithmic scale. Signals below a certain level are assigned as zero (dark spots), and signals above a predefined value are assigned as a maximal signal (white). Values falling inside the dynamic range are assigned to various shades of gray. Dynamic range compression is an operator-dependent function. Dynamic range is the range between minimal and maximal signal intensity that can be registered as difference in shades. The shades scale is limited (256 colors on a gray scale). Therefore, as the dynamic range decreases, contrast resolution *improves*. Dynamic range can be set manually.

Image Processing

From the signal processor, the scanning line is transferred to the scan converter in a compressed and filtered form. The scan converter prepares the individual lines for display by analyzing the lines according to their direction and the returning echoes according to their depth, which correlates with return times. Individual lines and points are assigned a specific location in image memory. All lines of data obtained in one passage of the beam over the scanned object are defined as a field. A frame is defined as all the lines of data that are obtained until the beam returns to its original position. In current scanning methods, one frame consists of two fields. Before entering image memory, the signal undergoes preprocessing. One of these steps involves persistence. Persistence includes averaging several frames to obtain a smoother image.

Image Memory[86,88]

After processing, frames are stored in the image memory. A frame is stored as a *matrix* divided into small units called pixels (picture elements). The standard matrix used in the United States includes 256×512 or 512×512 pixels. Each pixel corresponds to the direction of the data line and the position of the echo within this data line. A binary number that correlates with the signal intensity fills each pixel. With an increasing number of gray shades in the gray scale, the required memory for storage is larger. (For two shades, black and white, two numbers are needed, 0 or 1). This requires $2 \times 512 \times 512$ bits if a 512×512 matrix is used. Therefore, one frame requires 524,288 bits or 65,536 bytes (1 byte = 8 bits). For 256 shades, 8 binary numbers are needed to define each pixel ($2^8 = 256$). Therefore, a matrix with 256 shades of gray requires $512 \times 512 \times 8 = 2,097,152$ bits or 262,144 bytes = 262.144 KB for one frame, which is a huge amount of memory.

Image Magnification/Writing Zoom

This is a preprocessing technique in which a smaller region of interest is represented by a similar or a larger number of pixels. In this process, the region of interest is magnified, and its spatial resolution is increased. Writing zoom is a preprocessing step that is performed before the signals are stored as digital memory.

Postprocessing and Display

After the echo signals are stored in memory, they are transformed back to analog format by a digital to analog converter (DAC) to display them as an image. Before analog conversion, images may undergo postprocessing steps. Postprocessing includes all the image processing applied to the image after it was stored. These steps include assigning different numbers to signals in different pixels (number is equivalent to signal intensity or brightness), magnifying the entire image (reading zoom), or changing the color scale. Edge enhancement can be performed in postprocessing to emphasize the boundaries between the structures. A further function is designed to measure distances. The matrix can be calibrated by the pixel size.[88,89]

Display

The echo signals pass through DAC to the display on a CRT. The CRT produces an electron beam that strikes a fluorescent surface. This layer contains phosphor particles that illuminate when the beam strikes them. The intensity of the electron beam correlates with the voltage generated by the signal. In a B-mode display, this correlates with the brightness of the spot.

The electron beam moves across the screen from the left side to the right side. After completing one line, it moves downward and scans the next line. In this way, an image is created from the left upper corner to the right lower corner. The position of the spot in the image corresponds to its position and depth in the scanned object. After the beam completes its reading along the lines on the screen, it moves back to its original spot. The time it takes for the beam to finish one cycle is called *refreshing time*. On a standard computer monitor display, refreshing frequency is 60 times per second. The rapid processing time enables image display at the same rate of acquisition except for a slight time delay and is termed *real-time imaging*.

To create an image, the bright dots must continue to illuminate through all the frame time, otherwise the image fades and is erased from the screen. *Persistence* is an intrinsic property of the phosphor particles that enables continuous presentation of the image. Occasionally, a strong signal (calcification, prosthetic valve) may introduce an artifact by persisting for several frames (persistence artifact).

TV Screen

Scanning and display formats should fit to the television system standard (PAL/SECAM or NTSC, which is the system used in the United States). In the NTSC system, each frame includes 525 lines, and its scanning is completed within 1/30 second (each field is completed within 1/60 second). This frame rate is relatively slow. To avoid flickering of the screen, the scanning lines are read in a special way. First, the odd lines are read, and then even lines are read. Each set of lines comprises a field (odd/even field), and *both fields* are included in one frame.

Color Display

In several scanning modes (color-Doppler, and color B-mode) different colors are used. Color display is made by a color CRT. A color CRT is composed of three cathodes, and the screen includes three types of phosphorous particles close to each other. Each of the particles converts to a different color (red/green/blue) when struck by an electron beam. Various combinations of the colors create the entire color spectrum.

Basic Tradeoffs

Real-time imaging implies reliable display of moving structures. Data should be presented rapidly, with a frame rate that allows movement of the structures to be displayed. Motion of the structure would be incorrectly represented, or appear static, if the frame rate was less than the rate that the structure moves. This is especially important in rapidly moving structures such as the heart.

Temporal resolution is the ability to distinguish between two events occurring close in time and is determined by the time it takes to present one frame. Frame time is inversely related to the frame rate. As frame time decreases, the frame rate increases, and temporal resolution improves. The time to prepare a frame is determined by the time it takes to transmit and receive a pulse and create a single scan line; the second factor is the number of lines created in a single frame. To avoid range ambiguity and misregistration of returning pulses, all the echoes created by one pulse must return before the next pulse is transmitted. Thus, the maximal frequency that pulses may be sent pulse repitition frequency (PRF) is determined by the time it takes for a pulse to do a roundtrip in the tissue scanned. Because each line is created by a distinct pulse, and each frame is built by a determined number of lines, there is a *limit* to the frame rate.

In a normal adult scan, the back of the heart is approximately 17 cm from the sternum and 20 cm from the apex (in obese patients it is longer, and in children it is shorter). To send and acquire one line takes 13 µs $\times$ 17 = 221 µs or 0.221 ms in parasternal view and 260 µs or 0.260 ms from an apical view), where 13 µs is 1 cm roundtrip time of the US beam. Usually, 60 to 100 lines per frame are created, and it takes about 0.221 $\times$ 60 = 13.26 ms or 22.1 ms to obtain a frame from the parasternal and apical views, respectively. The frame rate that can be achieved is 1000/13.26 or 1000/22.1 = 73.5 or 45.25 frames/second, and the temporal resolution is 13.26 ms or 21.2 ms. Temporal resolution may be improved either by shorter scanning lines or by reducing the line number (or the number of focal zones) in a frame. However, reduction in the length of scanning line is usually not feasible without affecting image quality because of the distance between the heart and the transducer. Reducing the scanning lines per frame decreases lateral resolution.

Lateral resolution is the minimal distance between two points located side by side that can be distinguished as two discrete points. The ability to distinguish between two adjacent points depends on the line density (lateral distance between one line and the next one). If line density is reduced, lateral resolution decreases. Because of the configuration of the sector beam as a fan, the distance between the lines increases, and their density decreases as the beam moves farther away from the transducer. Therefore, as the distance between the object and the transducer increases, lateral resolution is reduced. The width of the US beam that creates one scanning line also affects lateral resolution; as the beam width decreases, lateral resolution increases. Optimal lateral resolution is close to the beam focus.

The standard line density is one or two lines per degree, and the usual PRF is 3000 to 5000 pulses per second. To obtain optimal resolution at different depths, more than one focus can be used, but this compromises temporal resolution, because each line must be rescanned for each additional focus. A simple method to retain lateral resolution without compromising temporal resolution is to decrease the number of lines by reducing the scanning angle, thus limiting the image to the region of interest.

Axial resolution is the ability to distinguish between two points located on the same scan line. That is the minimal distance between two echoes returning from two adjacent points that can be distinguished as two discrete points. Axial resolution equals one half of the pulse length.

Pulse length equals wavelength (λ) × number of cycles. As wavelength decreases and frequency increases, axial resolution improves. One of the most important factors that determine axial resolution is the frequency of the beam; but as frequency increases, attenuation is enhanced and, therefore, the intensity of the returning signal is reduced. Thus, there is a limit to the frequency at which the signal can be transmitted so that the returning echo will have a sufficient intensity. When the distance between the heart and the transducer is smaller, there is less attenuation, and higher frequency transducers may be used to gain higher resolution images. In standard adult transducers, the common operating (fundamental) frequency is 3.5 MHz. In pediatric cardiology 5 to 10 MHz transducers are used. Transesophageal echocardiography (TEE) probes usually use 5 MHz transducers. Intravascular US probes with a frequency of at least 15 MHz are used. By use of a higher frequency, the ability to obtain high-resolution images is improved. A second factor that determines spatial pulse length is the number of cycles in the pulse. The damping layer reduces the number of the cycles in one pulse. The usual number of cycles in an imaging pulse is 1 to 3 (pulses designed to acquire Doppler shifts are longer and include 5 to 20 cycles).

Contrast Resolution

Contrast resolution is the ability to distinguish between two close signal intensities as two different shades of color in the display. Different intensities of the returning echoes are registered as different binary numbers in each pixel. As the number of possible shades is increased, more memory is required for storage. Usually, 256 gray shades are used for the standard echo scanner. As the dynamic range (the range between the lowest and the highest intensity) is decreased, contrast resolution is improved, because signals with smaller intensity difference are registered by different shades. Because the range between maximum intensity and minimal intensity is reduced, more echoes (high intensities and low intensities) will be registered as bright or dark areas.

Echo scanning to obtain high-quality images is based on a series of "tradeoffs" related to the physical properties of sound in that improving one parameter can only be achieved by compromising a different parameter (or set of parameters). The ultrasonographer has to decide what is required to obtain the maximum information: improving axial/lateral or temporal resolution, increasing frame size, sector angle, or depth. Familiarity with the possible tradeoffs and manipulations in these parameters enables acquisition of the highest quality images.

Artifacts in Echo[86]

Artifacts result from an inadequate display of the scanned object or function (motion). Artifacts may include presentation of nonexistent objects; failure to display objects; or improper display of size, shape, location, brightness, or motion. Artifacts may impose an important obstacle to correct diagnosis or even result in erroneous diagnoses.

There are multiple types of artifacts that may be encountered. The most frequent and relevant ones are discussed in the following.

Limitation in axial and lateral resolution may produce artifacts by failing to differentiate two small discrete objects that are close in space.

Noise

Electronic devices close to the transducer can introduce a significant amount of noise to the image. These artifacts are usually repetitive and relate to the operating frequency of the electronic device. This type of artifact is common in monitored environments such as the intensive care units (ICU) or operating rooms when electrocauterization is used while intraoperative TEE is performed. The transducer itself may introduce substantial noise in the scanned region because of high-amplitude vibrations and voltages, which are displayed as a bright area close to the position of the transducer (located at the frame apex). This artifact is called *near-field clutter*.

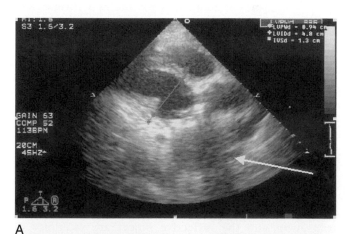

A

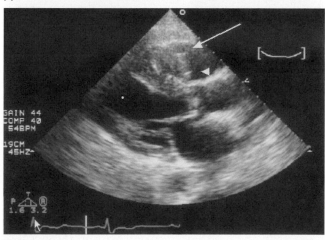

B

FIGURE 1-58. Examples of artifacts commonly encountered in cardiac imaging. **A,** Acoustic shadowing from a prosthetic aortic valve; **B,** reverberation artifact originating from a pacemaker electrode. The "true" electrode (arrow) is the echogenic object close to the transducer. The artifact is located deeper (arrow head). See also Color Insert.

Acoustic Shadowing

Acoustic shadowing is a common artifact in cardiac imaging. When there is a highly reflective object in the path of the US beam, such as prosthetic valve, calcified mass, catheter, or electrode, most of the beam is reflected back to the transducer. As the beam travels distally, it loses intensity and amplitude. This is manifested as a dark area behind the reflective object and tissues located in this area are masked (Figure 1-58, A). The opposite phenomenon is *enhancement*. When a beam passes through soft tissues, it is normally attenuated. This attenuation is compensated for by the time-gain compensation (TGC). If the beam passes through a liquid medium such as blood, there will be less attenuation relative to the surrounding tissues. The intensity of the US beam that strikes a structure behind the less attenuating area will be higher than expected, and, as a result, the intensity of the reflected echo will be also increased. Therefore, structures distal to a less attenuating or hypoechoic region will appear brighter and more reflective.

Acoustic Speckling

The texture of normal soft tissue is relatively homogenous and appears granular, with multiple bright and dark spots that do not represent the true nature of the tissue. Acoustic speckling occurs because of positive and negative interferences of the US beams, which is important in harmonic imaging.

Reverberation

Reverberation (Figure 1-58, B) is produced by multiple reflections from a single interface. When a US beam encounters a highly reflective object, an echo is reflected back toward the transducer, and an image is created. The transducer may act as a second interface and reflect the beam back toward the object, receive the reflected beam, and so on. Traveling times between the transducer and the reflective object are multiples of the original roundtrip time. Because roundtrip time is registered in the display as distance from the transducer, reverberation appears as a series of lines located at equal distances behind the true object. Reverberation requires a highly reflective object, because the returning echo from a less reflective object is too weak to produce additional echoes. Reverberation artifact is common in the presence of nonbiological materials such as catheters or electrodes.

Side Lobes and Grating Lobes

A single-element transducer creates side lobes, whereas grating lobes are produced by phased-array elements. *Side lobes* are components of the US beam generated by the edges of the piezoelectric element. *Grating lobes* are components of the US beam created because of interactions (interferences) between the beams generated by the individual elements in a phased-array transducer. Both side lobes and grating lobes are located at predetermined distances and angles along the sides of the main beam. The secondary beams are weaker than the primary beam, but if they encounter a highly reflective object, an echo will result. The echo is received by the transducer and perceived and processed as if it originated from the *main beam* and will be presented in the display as if it came from a different location. Later, the main beam will encounter the same object, and its true location will be registered. In this way, the same object will be registered twice and represented in two positions: one by the side lobe (or grating lobe) and the second by the main beam. Grating lobe artifacts are seen especially in hypoechoic regions (such as blood-filled cavities). Side-lobe artifacts can also be reduced by decreasing gain.

Refraction

When a US beam encounters a boundary with two different acoustic impedances at an angle of incidence < 90°, it changes its direction on passing through the boundary. This results in an object that is not in the direction of the original beam path being encountered and incorrectly displayed. Refraction may cause distortions and/or duplications of objects.

Range Ambiguity

Transducers usually function in a pulsed mode (except in continuous wave Doppler), transmitting short-duration signals (usually 1 to 2 μs). All the reflected echoes from the objects encountered along its path are received and analyzed before the next signal is transmitted. However, echoes from distant objects returning after the next pulse is sent are perceived as if the echo came *shortly after the second pulse*. The object will be displayed close to the transducer, although it is quite distant. This phenomenon is known as *range ambiguity artifact*. Pulse repetition frequency is automatically reduced when deeper structures are scanned. Pulse repetition frequency is the main factor that determines the rate that the frame can be built. To obtain high-quality images of moving cardiac structures, a high temporal resolution is required (30-60 frames/sec); thus an optimal balance between PRF and frame depth must be achieved. An alternative means of achieving depth without compromising frame rate is by reducing the number of scanning lines or by reducing the sector angle.[86]

Spectral Doppler and Color Doppler

The Doppler effect was first described by the Austrian mathematician and physicist Christian Johann Doppler in 1842. Doppler effect describes a phenomenon that when a source sends a wave (sound/electromagnetic wave such as light) and either the source, target, or both move in relation to each other; the frequency of the returning wave perceived by the source is different from the frequency of the transmitted wave. The difference between the frequency of the transmitted wave and the frequency of the reflected wave perceived by the source is known as the *Doppler shift*. If the source or the target move toward each other, the frequency perceived by the source will be higher than the frequency of the transmitted wave (positive Doppler shift), and if the source (or the target) move away from each other, the frequency perceived by the source will be lower than the transmitted frequency (a negative Doppler shift). Thus the sign (positive or negative) of the Doppler shift in frequency provides directional information regarding wave propagation. The magnitude of the Doppler shift is proportional to the velocity of the moving reflector (if the source is stationary).

Velocity can be calculated from the Doppler shift by the following formula:

$$Fd = \frac{2FoVcos\theta}{C}$$

or:

$$V = \frac{C\,Fd}{2\,FoVcos\theta}$$

where *Fd* is Doppler shift; *V* is the relative speed of the scanned object (such as red blood cells [RBCs]), $\tilde{\theta}$ the angle between the directions of the wave and the moving object; *C* the velocity of the sound (usually 1540 m/sec); and *Fo* the frequency of the transmitted wave (operating frequency of the transducer) (Figure 1-59).

The *angle* between the transmitted wave and the direction of the scatterer has a very important function in the equation. The Doppler shift is maximal when the direction of the beam is *parallel* to the direction of scatterer movement and is dependent on the cosine function (cos $\tilde{\theta}$ = 1), and it is 0 when the direction of the scatterer is perpendicular to the beam (cos $\tilde{\theta}$ = 0). Measurement of blood flow velocity during cardiac scanning requires that the angle between the US beam and the direction of blood flow be as close to zero degrees as possible. Provided that the angle is less than 20 degrees, the magnitude of error in velocity estimation is approximately 6% (cos 20° = 0.94).

Doppler technology is an obligate component of all echocardiographic instruments for measuring blood flow velocities in which the RBCs perform the function of moving scatterers. Measurement of blood velocities by Doppler is an integral part of every echocardiographic study.

Doppler ultrasound can provide qualitative and quantitative information about the dynamics of the blood flow and cardiac function. Doppler is most often used to determine blood flow velocity. *Blood flow velocity* is the distance RBCs travel per unit time. *Blood flow* refers to the volume of blood that passes a certain point per unit time. Blood flow is dependent on the cross-sectional area of the vessel in which it travels. In a closed system in which there is no change in volume flow, reduction in the cross-sectional area of the blood vessel results in increased blood flow velocity. Blood flow between two points is related to the pressure gradient and resistance between the two points:

Flow = Pressure gradient/Resistance

Blood flow increases directly with pressure gradient and inversely with resistance. Resistance of a vessel is dependent on its radius, length, and fluid viscosity. The major determinant of resistance is the fourth power of the radius of the vessel:

Poiseuille's equation: Volume flow rate =

$$\frac{\text{Pressure gradient} \times \pi \times (\text{radius})^4}{8 \times \text{length} \times \text{Viscosity}}$$

Blood flow may exhibit several different flow profiles as described in the following (Figure 1-60):

1. *Laminar flow:* Flow in which the layers of the blood move in parallel. The velocity of the most central layers or core is greater than the layers in close proximity to the vessel wall. The flow front profile is parabolic. Laminar flow typically occurs in distal blood vessels.

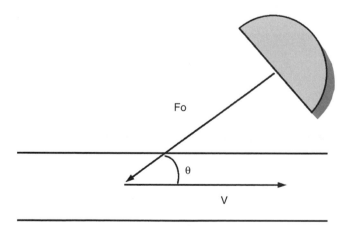

FIGURE 1-59. Relationship between Doppler shift, velocity, speed of sound, beam frequency, and its angle. By measuring the Doppler shift, velocity can be calculated by the following formula:

$$V = C\,Fd/2FoV\,cos\theta$$

where *V* is the relative speed of the scanned object (RBC); *Fd* is the Doppler shift; θ is the angle between the direction of the wave and the moving object; *C* is the speed of sound (usually 1540 m/sec); and *Fo* is the frequency of the sent wave (operating frequency of the transducer).

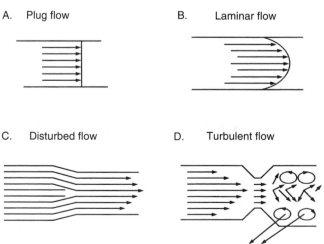

A. Plug flow   B. Laminar flow

C. Disturbed flow   D. Turbulent flow

Eddi flows

FIGURE 1-60. Flow profiles seen in blood vessels. **A** and **B**, show Laminar flow. Note the parallel movement of the various layers and the parabolic configuration of the flow profile in laminar flow as opposed to a flat profile in plug flow. **C** and **D**, Disturbed flow and turbulent flow. Note the chaotic pattern in a turbulent flow. Flows in multiple directions and eddies are seen.

2. *Plug flow:* Fluid moves in a tube as a unit. The layers close to the wall move at the same speed as the central layer. The flow front profile of is typically flat. This type of flow occurs in the heart chambers and large blood vessels.
3. *Disturbed flow:* Pattern of flow that occurs in blood vessel bifurcations, curved or torturous vessels, or at stenoses. The parallel layers of flow become curved.
4. *Eddy flow:* Circular movement of the fluid that occurs at arterial bifurcations.
5. *Turbulent flow:* A pattern of chaotic flow with multiple small eddies. In this type of flow, RBCs move at random speeds and multiple directions, although the general flow direction is *forward*. This flow is typical in vascular obstructions or in valvular stenosis. The value that determines existence of a turbulent flow is called Reynold's number. Factors that determine Reynold's number are velocity of the blood, its viscosity, density, and the size of the blood vessel.

Calculation of blood volume flow is complicated, because flow is pulsatile, and velocity varies with the cardiac cycle. Despite these and other potentially confounding factors, estimates of flow and pressures by Doppler echocardiography correlate with measurements made by catheterization.

Bernoulli's Law

Moving blood has kinetic and potential energy. The movement of blood and its density determine its kinetic energy. Potential energy is determined by the hydrostatic pressure that the moving fluid blood exerts on the ves-

sel walls. The law of energy conservation states that the total energy of a fluid in a certain point (potential energy + kinetic energy) is equal to its energy at other points along the vessel. This relationship is described in *Bernoulli's equation* (Figure 1-61):

$$P_1 - P_2 = \tfrac{1}{2}\,\rho(V_2{}^2 - V_1{}^2) + \rho_1 \int_{1}^{2} f^2\,dV/dT \times DS + R\,(V)$$

where $V_2{}^2 - V_1{}^2$ is convective acceleration, dV/dT is flow acceleration, $R(V)$ is vicious friction, P_1 is the pressure proximal to the obstruction, V_1 is the velocity proximal to the obstruction, P_2 and V_2 are pressure and velocity distal to the obstruction, and ρ is the ~ blood density. Blood velocity can be determined by the Doppler shift, which is described in the following. In estimation of blood flow in the human heart and blood vessels, the flow acceleration and viscous friction terms are inconsequential and are disregarded, and because $V_1 \ll V_2$, the preceding equation above can be simplified to:

$$P_1 - P_2 = 4V_2{}^2$$

This is the modified Bernoulli equation that is used routinely for noninvasive estimation of pressure gradients across stenotic valves or obstructions. Excellent correlations have been demonstrated between transvalvular pressure gradients determined by the modified Bernoulli equation and pressure gradients measured at catheterization.

Continuity Equation

The continuity equation can be used for calculations of luminal size or valve area. It is based on the principle

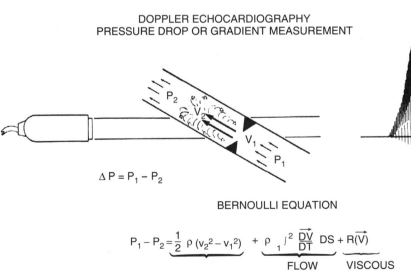

DOPPLER ECHOCARDIOGRAPHY
PRESSURE DROP OR GRADIENT MEASUREMENT

$\Delta P = P_1 - P_2$

BERNOULLI EQUATION

$$P_1 - P_2 = \frac{1}{2}\,\rho\,(v_2{}^2 - v_1{}^2) + \rho_1 \int^2 \frac{\overrightarrow{DV}}{DT}\,DS + R\overrightarrow{(V)}$$

FLOW ACCELERATION   VISCOUS FRICTION

$$P_1 - P_2 = \frac{1}{2}\,\rho\,(v_2{}^2 - v_1{}^2)$$

V_1 MUCH $< V_2$ ∴ IGNORE V_1

ρ = MASS DENSITY OF BLOOD = 1.06 10^3 KG/M^3

∴ $\Delta P = 4V_2{}^2$

FIGURE 1-61. Bernoulli equation. Measurement of pressure gradients is possible by using a modified Bernoulli equation. The assumptions are that pressure gradient caused by viscous friction and flow acceleration can be ignored and $V_2 \gg V_1$. (From Feigenbaum, Figure 1-64, page 36). H. Feigerbaum. Echocardiography. 4th Edition. Lea and Febiger, Philadelphia, 1986.

of *mass conservation*. If a fluid flows through a vessel or an obstruction, the same volume flow occurs proximal and distal to the obstruction as through the region of the obstruction. Blood volume flow is calculated as the product of the flow velocity time integral and the cross-sectional area of the flow stream (Figure 1-62).

V_1, V_2, and V_3 are velocities in segments 1, 2, and 3 and can be measured by Doppler. A_1, A_2, and A_3 are cross-sectional areas of segments 1, 2, and 3, which can be determined by 2D echocardiology (Figure 1-62).

The mathematical expression of the continuity equation is:

$$A_1 \times V_1 = A_2 \times V_2 = A_3 \times V_3$$

If segment 2 represents a stenotic valve or obstructed vessel, the cross-sectional area (A_2) of which is unknown, it can be calculated if V_1, V_2, and A_1 are known:

$$A_2 = A_1 \times V_1/V_2$$

If it is assumed that the cross-sectional area is close to circular (such as left ventricular outflow tract, or a blood vessel), *area* can be calculated by the formula:

$$Area = \frac{\pi (D)^2}{4}$$

where *D* is the left ventricular outflow tract diameter or diameter of the vessel proximal to the obstruction.

Spectral Doppler Instrumentation

Spectral Doppler includes two modes: continuous wave (CW; Figure 1-63, *A*) and pulsed-wave (PW; Figure 1-63, *B*), both of which are combined in one phased-array transducer. The CW transducer is composed of separate transmitting elements and receiving elements so that US is transmitted and received continuously. The continuous transmission of US in CW mode precludes spatial resolution along the beam path but allows measurement of an unlimited range of velocities. The PW Doppler transducer uses the same elements to transmit and receive echoes and is primarily used to assess blood flow velocities at specific regions of interest. Thus, PW Doppler is combined with an anatomical cross-sectional echocardiographic image, so that the operator can select the location of the region of interest and the size of the sample volume to be interrogated. Thus, in PW (in contrast to CW) the location of the source of the Doppler shifted fre-

a. Continuous wave (CW) mode

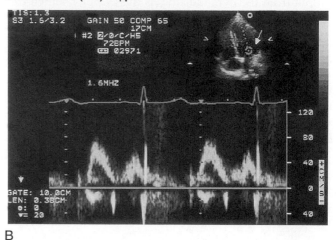

A

b. Pulsed wave (PW) Doppler

B

FIGURE 1-63. (A) Continuous wave (CW) mode. The US wave is transmitted continuously, without interruptions, and received by a different element in the transducer. The transducer is oriented through the tricuspid valve. The flow measured is a jet of tricuspid regurgitation (arrowhead). The peak gradient through the tricuspid valve can be calculated (73.6 mmHg) by measuring the peak velocity of the regurgitant jet and using the Bernoulli rule. (B) Pulsed-wave (PW) Doppler. A short wave is sent. Doppler-shifted echoes may be received only when the range gate is open. When the gate is closed, all the echoes are discarded. This figure shows a normal pattern of blood flow through the mitral valve. Note the sampling volume in the 2D image, located adjacent to the tips of the mitral leaflets (small arrow, upper right). Sampling depth and its length are indicated (arrowhead, lower left). See also Color Insert.

quencies can be precisely determined. However, the return trip of the US waves to the region of interest takes a finite period of time, and thus there is a limit to the magnitude of velocity that can be measured by PW Doppler.

CW Doppler System

The transmitting and the receiving elements are separate in CW Doppler. The transmitted wave is generated continuously by an oscillator. Its frequency is usually in the range of 2 to 10 MHz. The received echo is transferred to a Doppler detector in which the voltage originated by the echo is first amplified by a *RF amplifier*. (Amplification is

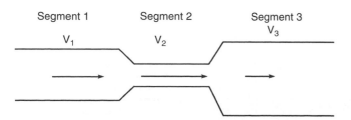

FIGURE 1-62. Continuity equation. The flow in each segment of the blood vessel remains similar. V_1, V_2, and V_3 are the velocities in segments 1, 2, and 3. A_1, A_2, and A_3 are the cross-sectional areas of these segments.

essential, because the magnitude of the received signal is very low.) The amplified echo is passed to a *demodulator* in which the returning echoes are mixed with the output from the oscillator. The output consists of a wave with the original transmitted frequency. Depending on the channel that the waves entered, the mixed waves are either summed or subtracted. The summed waves are filtered out. If the wave returns from a motionless structure or scatterer, it will not generate a Doppler shift, and its frequency will be equal to the oscillator frequency. Therefore, it will be eliminated in the subtraction procedure. If the echo returns from a moving scatterer, its frequency will be either higher or lower than the original frequency. The difference between the frequencies equals the Doppler shift and correlates with the velocity of the scatterer. The Doppler-shifted frequencies are amplified. Audio signals may be generated, and their pitch correlates with the magnitude of the Doppler shift. The output from the demodulators is the Doppler-shifted frequency. However, the *direction* of the movement is unknown. Directional information is extracted by several techniques, including signal side band filtering, heterodyne demodulation, or quadrature phase demodulation. Quadrature phase demodulation is the most commonly used technique, in which the Doppler-shifted echo (now transformed to voltage) runs in two parallel channels: the direct channel and the quadrature channel. In each channel, the Doppler-shifted signal is *mixed* with the original voltage from the oscillator. In the direct channel, it is mixed with the original voltage; and in the quadrature phase channel, it is mixed with a *delayed phase voltage* (delay is 90 degrees or quarter phase). A further 90-degree delay is introduced into both the direct and the quadrature channels. After the second delay, the original voltages from the direct channel (before the delays were introduced) are mixed with the voltage from the quadrature

channel and vice versa. In this way, the negative shifted waves cancel each other in the direct channel, and only positive shifts will be present. As a result, only positive Doppler shifts are present in the direct channel and negative shifts in the quadrature channel.

The signal obtained by the Doppler detector is a complex waveform that includes multiple Doppler-shifted frequencies, each with magnitude and directional information that requires further analysis. The most important step is *spectral analysis* by which all the frequencies included in the waveform are separated and organized. The mathematical method used for the spectral analysis is *fast Fourier transform (FFT)*. The waveform is separated by FFT into its frequency components and arranged in increasing order, so that each frequency has its own amplitude. The frequency denotes the Doppler shift frequency, which reflects the velocity of the scatterer(s). The amplitude (power) expresses the number of scatterers moving with a certain velocity causing the particular Doppler shift (Figure 1-64).

A simple spectral analysis presents only the frequency shifts and magnitude. However, blood flow is pulsatile, so it is important to display flow as a *function of time*. The standard display of the Doppler instruments includes Doppler shifts and their magnitude as a function of time (Figure 1-65). Amplitude is displayed as the *brightness* on a gray scale, and each time point in the cardiac cycle is represented by a *vertical line* that reflects the FFT spectrum. If blood flow at a certain time point is more organized, the FFT spectrum is narrower, and the vertical line is smaller. As the flow becomes more turbulent and disorganized, the Fourier spectrum widens and includes more frequency shifts displayed as a longer vertical line at this time point. In this format, positive Doppler shifts caused by objects moving toward the transducer are by convention depicted as shifts above baseline, whereas

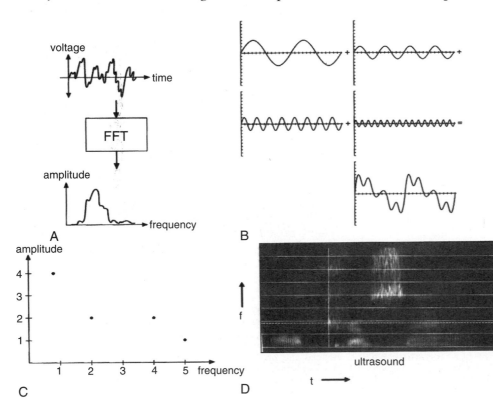

FIGURE 1-64. Fast Fourier transform (FFT). The waveform is separated into its frequency components and arranged in an increasing order, and each frequency has its own amplitude. Frequency denotes the Doppler shift frequency, reflecting velocity. Amplitude (power) expresses the number of scatterers moving in a certain velocity causing the particular Doppler shift. The initial signal (**A**) is separated into its individual components (**B**). Each component includes a different frequency and amplitude. In the next step, the frequencies are arranged in an increasing order, each frequency with its own amplitude (**C**). (**D**) FFT of the sound of the word "ultrasound."

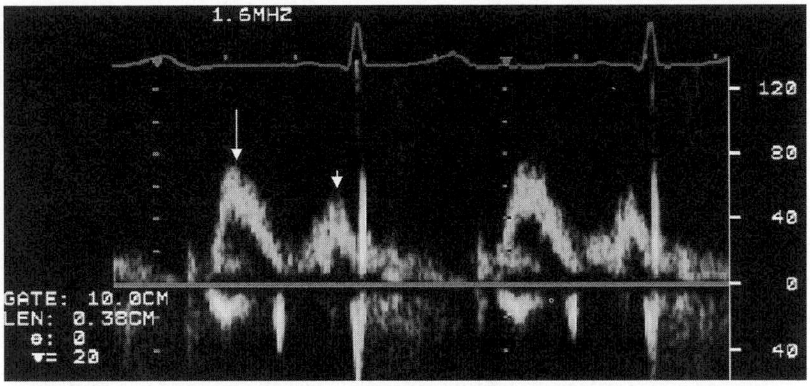

FIGURE 1-65. A standard display of the Doppler instruments that includes Doppler shifts and their magnitude as a function of time (x-axis). Amplitude is displayed as *brightness* on a gray scale, and each time point in the cardiac cycle is represented by a *vertical line*. As the flow in a certain time point is more organized, the FFT spectrum is narrower and the vertical line is shorter. Positive and negative shifts indicate movement toward and away from the transducer, respectively. A normal transmitral flow pattern is shown in the figure. Note the organized flow characterized by short vertical lines and two peaks indicating early (E wave) (arrow) and late diastolic filling (A wave) (arrowhead). See also Color Insert.

negative Doppler shifts (objects moving away from the transducer) are presented as signals below baseline.

PW Doppler System

The PW Doppler instrument transmits pulses (Figure 1-63) each consisting of 5 to 20 cycles that are longer than the imaging pulses (2 to 3 cycles). After a pulse is transmitted, the transducer is silent and waits for the returning echoes. At a specific operator-controlled time, the range gate opens, and returning signals are allowed to be received. Range gating allows that only Doppler shifts from a defined depth will be presented. After a certain period, a second pulse is transmitted. Pulse repetition frequency (PRF) is the frequency with which the individual pulses are sent.

The basic design of the PW Doppler transducer is similar to the CW transducer. However, it is modified so that it functions in a pulsed mode for transmitting and receiving. PW includes a master clock that opens the transmitting gate and after a certain delay, opens the receiving gate to the desired depth; after a predefined interval, the range gate is closed. PW Doppler, in contrast to CW Doppler, does not analyze the entire signal of the Doppler shift. PW Doppler is a *sampling system* so that each transmitted pulse obtains only a *sample* of the Doppler-shifted frequency. To define the Doppler shift accurately, *at least two samples should be taken from each cycle.* When the number of samples is inadequate, an artificially low frequency shift will be displayed with directional ambiguity. This phenomenon is called *aliasing* (Figure 1-66). As the velocity of the moving object increases, a higher Doppler shift will result. A higher Doppler frequency shift requires an increased number of samplings, and if there is undersampling, aliasing will result. The maximal Doppler shift frequency that can be detected without aliasing is defined by the Nyquist limit.

$$\text{Nyquist limit} = \text{PRF}/2$$

Aliasing precludes estimation of peak velocity and assessment of flow direction. This phenomenon is common when measurement of high-velocity flows is attempted (for example, in stenotic or regurgitant valves).

There are several ways to avoid aliasing:

1. The simplest method is to change baseline. The entire signal will be included either above or below baseline if the velocity is not too high.

2. Increasing the angle θ between the transducer and the presumed direction of the scatterer, so that the obtained Doppler shift will *decrease*. This may introduce an inaccuracy in the measurements (as the angle is larger, the range of error also

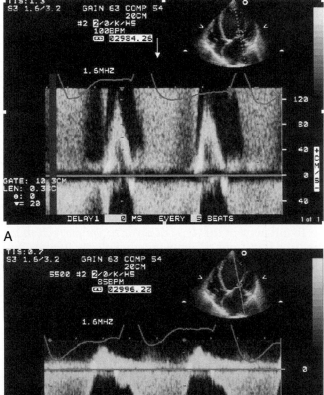

A

B

FIGURE 1-66. A, Aliasing in spectral Doppler (PW) in a patient with severe mitral regurgitation. Note the positive and negative Doppler shifts (signal above and below the baseline), reflecting an ambiguous detection of flow direction. Also the measured speed is not accurate. Aliasing is common when high-velocity flows are evaluated and can be noticed only on PW Doppler. **B,** Correction of aliasing. In this image, the acquisition mode was changed to CW Doppler to prevent aliasing, the baseline was raised, and the velocity range was increased to include higher velocities.

increases) and is not recommended in clinical practice.

3. Increasing PRF increases the sampling frequency, so that PW Doppler is able to measure higher velocities before reaching the Nyquist limit. There is a limit to the maximal PRF, because it may introduce range ambiguity artifact. As the distance between the transducer and the object (depth) increases, the maximal PRF that can be achieved without causing range ambiguity decreases. In circumstances in which there are a number of stenoses in series occasions with high velocities, *high PRF* PW Doppler may be useful. One of the sampling windows is moved to a location where a high velocity is not expected, and the second window is set to sample the high-velocity region. In this wayhigh velocities causing increased Doppler shifts can be measured without aliasing.

4. Doppler shift is dependent on the operating frequency of the transducer. If a lower frequency is used, higher velocities may be detected with lower Doppler shifts. However, spatial resolution is compromised. Changing frequency usually requires a different transducer.

5. The use of CW Doppler because sampling is continuous, and, therefore, CW Doppler may detect high velocities of any magnitude.

Underestimation of Velocity

A potential problem with Doppler systems (CW and PW) is underestimation of the Doppler shift. Because the Doppler shift is angle dependent, the maximal (most accurate) shift is obtained when the beam is parallel to the direction of the scatterer. As the angle increases, Doppler shift decreases, and the calculated velocities become increasingly inaccurate. When the angle is less than 20 degrees, the "error" range is relatively small (approximately 6%).

To circumvent this type of error, *angle correction* can be used but is not recommended clinically, because usually the angle itself cannot be estimated accurately in three dimensions. In clinical practice this problem is minimized by recording velocity signals from different windows and measuring the maximal velocity (which is obtained at the smallest angle).

Color Doppler

In color Doppler (Figure 1-67), the two main applications of the echo, imaging and flow, are combined. The display includes both structural data as cross-sectional imaging and velocity information in *real time*. The importance of color Doppler is that it shows both normal and abnormal directional flow in relation to cardiac anatomical location. From these images, abnormal flows can be located and analyzed in detail.

The requirements from the system to generate a color Doppler image are enormous, because both a cross-sectional image and Doppler shifts from multiple points have to be integrated to create an image. Color Doppler systems operate in pulsed mode and are subject to the same tradeoffs, including spatial resolution, range, line density, angle, PRF, frame rate, and accuracy, of Doppler

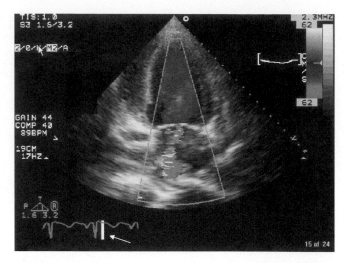

FIGURE 1-67. Color Doppler. ECG tracing is shown below and time of sampling during systole is indicated (small arrow). Note the marked blood flow from the left ventricle toward the left atrium, indicating severe mitral regurgitation. On this color scale, brighter colors indicate higher velocities. See also Color Insert.

shift detection. To overcome the conflict between spatial resolution (when higher frequency transducers are advantageous) and the accuracy of detecting Doppler shifts (where low-frequency transducers are needed), a dual-frequency transducer has been developed.

The colors in a color Doppler instrument represent flow direction and speed. Red indicates movement toward the transducer, blue represents movement away from the transducer, and black indicates lack of movement. The magnitude of the shifted frequency (indicating velocity) is depicted in hues of red and blue. Brighter hues of red toward orange and yellow indicate higher velocity toward the transducer, and lighter shades of blue represent higher velocities away from the transducer. The *amplitude* of the signal (number of RBC moving in the same speed) is expressed by the color brightness. Low-amplitude signals are pale. *Variance* is noted by multiple colors in a small area. Multiple colors indicate multiple velocities as occurs with turbulent flow (mosaic pattern). Another method of demonstrating increased variance is by a green color.

Instrumentation

Echoes reflected from stationary structures are processed and used for constructing a 2D cross-sectional image in the same way as conventional echo. The echoes reflected from moving objects are Doppler shifted. The Doppler-shifted echoes are passed to a signal processor, where they undergo a complex procedure termed *autocorrelation*. In the process of autocorrelation, velocity, amplitude (power), direction, and variance of every Doppler shifted echo from multiple sample volumes is determined and encoded in colors and stored in memory until the whole frame is analyzed before the full color Doppler image is presented. The Doppler data and the data from the amplitude channel from the stationary tissues are *combined* to yield a full color-flow and 2D image. Usually the first data array that is constructed is the tissue data plane. After the gray-scale image is constructed, the Doppler data are interrogated, color-encoded, and inserted into empty (dark) or low-amplitude pixels (where no structure is supposed to exist). This algorithm (tissue or amplitude priority) prevents inserting flows into regions where solid structures exist or a spillover of flow from the heart or blood vessels.

Color at a certain point in the scanning line reflects a Doppler-shifted frequency. Because of autocorrelation, three pulses are needed for each point. The number of pulses used to interrogate one scanning line is called *ensemble length*. Usually the ensemble length ranges from 3 to 20, but it can be as high as 32 pulses per line. A large ensemble length provides a more complete flow image, with a better resolution of Doppler shifts and colors. The compromise is a *lower frame rate*.

Limitations and Artifacts in Color Doppler

Color Doppler has more limitations and restrictions than a conventional image, because for each scanning line in a conventional image one pulse is needed. By contrast, to display Doppler-shifted images in color, 3 to 20 pulses are required, depending on the ensemble length and the minimal line density needed (1.5 to 2 scanning lines per degree). All these limitations are reflected in a *slower frame rate* (20-30 frames/sec) and a lower temporal resolution. A higher frame rate and better temporal resolution can be achieved by reducing the scanning (sector) angle and thereby the number of scan lines. An alternative strategy is to reduce the ensemble line, but in so doing the quality of the color image declines. Range reduction is not possible because of the unchanging depth of the region of interest.

Color-Doppler is *angle dependent*, and the maximal measured velocity (and the most accurate measurement reflecting the actual velocity of the scatterer) is obtained when the beam is parallel to the direction of the scatterer (cos θ = 1). Therefore, the color reflects both the flow velocity and direction.

Frequency resolution achieved by color Doppler is *less* than the resolution gained by spectral Doppler. This is apparent by the more uniform appearance of colors in the color Doppler compared with that expected if spectral analysis were performed in any individual sample volume. This is due to multiple steps of image processing, including signal averaging and smoothing algorithms.

Aliasing is more common in color Doppler than spectral PW Doppler, because a portion of the pulses is assigned to obtain cross-sectional images, and, therefore, the actual number of pulses deployed for Doppler sampling in a color Doppler mode is less than the total number of pulses provided by the PRF. Therefore, aliasing occurs in color Doppler at lower velocities compared with PW Doppler in which all the pulses are assigned to sample Doppler shifts. Aliasing in color Doppler images appears as sequential red and blue bands. These bands reflect directional ambiguity, where red represents movement toward the transducer and blue away from the transducer. The boundaries between blue and red bands have a *brighter hue*, reflecting increasing velocities. This is equivalent to the wrap-around image seen in spectral Doppler, with a simultaneous appearance of the signal above and below baseline (Figure 1-68). A true directional change and aliasing can be differentiated by the appearance of the boundaries between the red and blue layers. In true directional change, the boundary is dark, whereas in aliasing, the hue changes to a light color (light blue or yellow) and then flips to a color indicating the opposite direction.

Aliasing is commonly seen in color Doppler, and it may aid in diagnosis and evaluation of abnormal flows in lesions such as valvular stenosis and regurgitation. When the blood approaches a stenotic or a regurgitant valve, it accelerates because of the reduced size of its orifice. When the blood accelerates, its speed produces a Doppler shift exceeding the Nyquist limit, and aliasing occurs. Aliasing is noted as a series of small spherical surfaces with multiple blue and red bands. The surface area of the aliasing sphere is called the proximal isovelocity surface area (PISA). The surface area of the sphere designates the maximal blood velocity before it passed the Nyquist limit. Measurement of the radius of the sphere and use of the continuity equation enable the size of the regurgitant orifice to be determined and regurgitant volume to be calculated (see Chapter 11).

New Methods of Imaging

Tissue Harmonic Imaging[91]

Conventional imaging by echo is based on receiving and analyzing echoes at the same frequency as the original pulses (fundamental frequency). When a sound wave propagates through a tissue, it does not retain its original form. A new wave conformation arises with additional frequency components. The additional frequency components are multiples (harmonic frequencies) of the transmitted wave (fundamental frequency). Usually the second harmonic, which equals twice the fundamental frequency, is used for harmonic imaging.

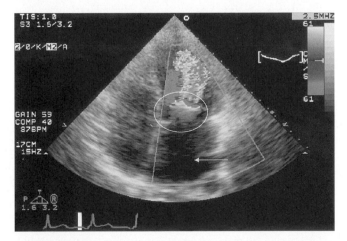

FIGURE 1-68. Aliasing in color Doppler. Diastolic flow (note ECG tracing below) through a severely stenotic mitral valve. Note the sphere with orange, yellow, and blue layers (circled), indicating aliasing caused by acceleration proximal to the mitral valve, and the highly turbulent flow manifested as a mosaic of multiple colors. The area of the proximal sphere is termed the proximal isovelocity surface area (PISA). Note also the dilated left atrium (arrow) characteristic of mitral stenosis. See also Color Insert.

The intensity of an echo with harmonic frequencies tends to increase with propagating distance. Therefore, structures close to the transducer such as skin and chest wall produce weak harmonic signals, and the signals from more distant structures (heart) tend to be stronger. A second important attribute of harmonic frequency is that the effect of the fundamental frequency on the harmonic intensity is nonlinear. Weaker fundamental signals generate a very weak harmonic echo. Thus, signals that are usually weak but produce artifacts in fundamental echo, such as scatters, reverberations, or grating lobe artifacts, are not evident with harmonic imaging. The requirements of an instrument operating in tissue harmonic imaging are a wide dynamic range, a narrow transmitting bandwidth (that does not include harmonic frequency), and a sharp filter.

High-quality cardiac images can be obtained with tissue harmonic imaging, with clearer delineation of the valves and endocardial contours and with less noise. High-quality images may be obtained even in technically difficult cases (obese patients, during stress). In modern echocardiography, tissue harmonic imaging is used routinely.

3D Imaging

The most recent development in echocardiography is the development of *3D imaging* (Figure 1-69).[92,93] The first step was to acquire multiple 2D tomographic slices that were registered spatially. Series of 2D slices in multiple planes were either acquired by angulation of the transducer (as tilting a fan), thus obtaining a pyramidal scanning field (tilting can be performed electronically in

a phased array), or rotating the transducer through 360 degrees (usually, rotation is performed in steps of 2-3 degrees). Registration of the spatial location and orientation of the slice relative to other slices is achieved by special locator-sensor systems. All the slices are stored in the computer and undergo complex processing steps, including interpolation (filling in the missed data), filtration, and fitting. Eventually, the sets of slices are integrated into a complete 3D structure. Each plane is registered in a different cycle. Therefore, ECG and respiratory gating are required, so that only corresponding images (in time and location) are used in reconstructing the 3D image. Today, there are echo devices capable of performing real-time 3D imaging, which obviates the need for gating.

3D reconstruction may be performed with TTE or with multiplanar TEE. 3D imaging yields important information about anatomical structures that is unattainable by 2D echocardiography. This is especially useful in congenital heart and valvular heart diseases. Complex congenital malformations difficult to interpret from 2D images can be seen in 3D. Even with apparently "simple" anomalies such as atrial septal defect or ventricular septal defect, knowledge of the 3D relations may assist the surgeon in planning the operation. 3D imaging helps in decision making regarding whether closure of an atrial septal defect is optimal by percutaneous device or surgery. In acquired valvular disease, detailed anatomy of the mitral and aortic valve can be obtained with 3D echocardiographic imaging, which has clarified the mechanism of mitral regurgitation and likelihood of successful mitral valve repair.

Quantitative 3D echocardiography will allow quantitation of left ventricular volumes, myocardial mass, global, and regional function without any geometric assumptions about ventricular shape. These are only a few of many potential uses of 3D echocardiography.

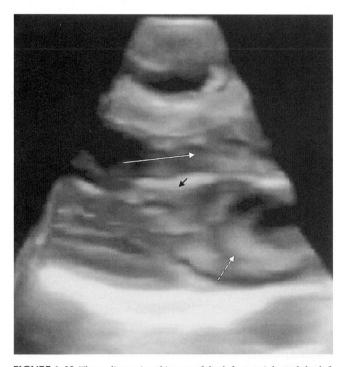

FIGURE 1-69. Three-dimensional image of the left ventricle and the left atrium in early diastole from the parasternal view. The black arrowhead marks the anterior mitral leaflet, and the white arrow is directed to the left ventricular outflow tract. The broken line is directed to the left atrium.

Contrast Echocardiography[94,95] (Figure 1-70)

Contrast echocardiography is an application that was developed initially to improve image quality in technically difficult patients. Contrast solutions consist of microbubbles comparable in size to RBCs (4-7 μm) that pass through the pulmonary capillaries to the left heart chambers. These microbubbles need to be relatively stable with a uniform size, because the signal returning from a bubble is proportional to the sixth power of its radius.

The first contrast used (still in use today) was agitated saline. However, this yields unstable bubbles because of a rapid diffusion of the air out of the bubbles, and after a few cardiac cycles, the microbubbles disappear. The first generation of commercially produced echo-contrast agents consisted of air-filled microbubbles made by sonication (exposure of the solution to a constant US energy) of albumin or dextrose solutions (Albunex [Mallinckrodt] and Levovist [Schering/Berlex], respectively). However, air-filled microbubbles are unstable and tend to dissolve rapidly when exposed to water.

The second-generation bubbles include sonicated albumin or dextrose plus surfactant in the presence of high molecular weight and nondiffusible gases such as

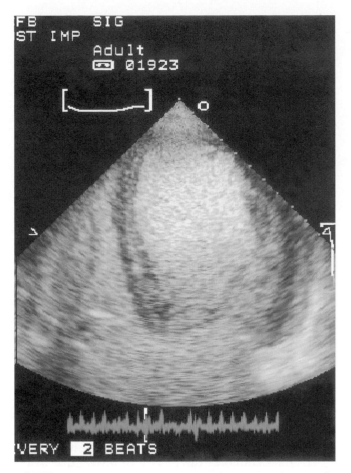

FIGURE 1-70. Contrast echo in a patient with dilated cardiomyopathy from the apical four-chamber view. The contrast within the cavity enables a clear distinction between the left ventricular cavity and the endocardium. All cardiac chambers are filled with contrast.

fluorocarbons (Optison [Mallinckrodt] and Echogen [Sonus], respectively). Of these, only Albunex and Optison are approved by the Federal Food and Drug Administration.

Because of their size and compressibility, the bubbles function as *scatterers* of US. After intravenous injection, the bubbles opacify right-sided and then left-sided cardiac chambers. Ventricular opacification provides an improved delineation of endocardial contours that is especially useful for assessment of left ventricular size, global and regional myocardial function during rest, and stress echocardiography. Contrast can also be used to enhance Doppler signals for assessing valvular stenosis or regurgitation and for detecting intracardiac shunts.

Myocardial contrast enhancement (MCE) is an emerging use of contrast for assessment of myocardial perfusion. The signal from the microbubbles in the myocardial microvasculature can be enhanced by several techniques (signal subtraction, pulse-inversion, and harmonics). The concentration of the microbubbles correlates with the regional myocardial blood flow, and, therefore, MCE can provide information relating to myocardial perfusion and microvascular integrity. Contrast enhancement enables improved endocardial definition and assessment of regional function and perfusion, and as such has emerged as a powerful diagnostic tool in ischemic heart disease. In addition, intracoronary injection of contrast demonstrates perfusion territory, area of myocardium at risk, and no-reflow phenomenon.

Echoes returning from the microbubbles include different frequencies, which are usually multiples (harmonics) of the original frequency (fundamental). Harmonic signals obtained from the microbubbles are *stronger* than the harmonic signal generated by the imaged tissues. Therefore, harmonic imaging with echo-contrast yields higher quality images than without contrast. Microbubbles tend to be destroyed and disappear within several cardiac cycles. Larger bubbles are entrapped in the pulmonary microcirculation. The main cause of disappearance of microbubbles is disruption by the energy of the US beam. Disruption of the microbubbles can be attenuated by reducing the *power* of the US beam, increasing its frequency (low-frequency beams cause more destruction), or by intermittent imaging with gating to specific phases in the cardiac cycle. Echo-contrast studies of myocardial perfusion imaging have greater temporal and spatial resolution than radionuclide imaging (SPECT and PET). However, despite its excellent resolution, the main clinical indication for the use of echo-contrast is to improve endocardial definition to enable assessment of global and regional myocardial function in patients with technically limited images.

Echo-contrast is not devoid of adverse effects. Intravenous or intracoronary injection of echo-contrast may cause transient hemodynamic changes in the systemic and coronary circulation and a reduction in coronary blood flow.

Tissue Doppler Imaging, Strain, and Strain Rate[96,97] (Figures 1-71 and 1-72)

Tissue Doppler imaging (TDI) is a relatively new application of 2D echo-Doppler. TDI permits direct measurement of myocardial velocities and assessment of regional and global myocardial function. The techniques and instrumentation of TDI are similar to routine Doppler methods used for measurements of blood velocity. With TDI, Doppler frequency shifts are received, and velocities are calculated. In contrast to conventional Doppler measurements, TDI focuses on high-amplitude low-frequency Doppler shifts obtained from myocardial motion (TDI lacks a high-frequency pass filter). Both pulsed-wave and color-coded Doppler are used in TDI.

Myocardial velocity is an indicator of systolic and diastolic myocardial function. Global systolic function can be assessed by measuring the motion of the mitral anulus by color or PW Doppler. During systole, the base of the heart (including the annulus) moves toward the apex, so that a positive deflection is obtained (S). After the short period of isovolumic relaxation, a rapid filling phase occurs that results in a large negative deflection (E′). The rapid filling phase is followed by a period of diastasis, after which a second negative peak occurs because of atrial contraction (A′). Filling periods (E′ and A′) are noted as negative deflections, because the basal regions move away from the transducer, whereas the apex remains relatively stationary. An excellent correlation

Systolic velocity

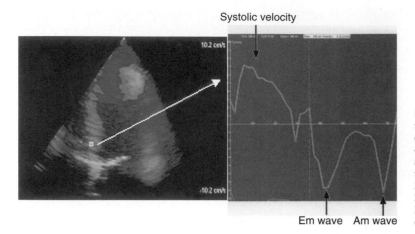

Em wave   Am wave

FIGURE 1-71. Tissue velocity imaging in a normal volunteer. Myocardial velocity in the basal septum is interrogated (see arrow). Myocardial velocity in the myocardium is color encoded. Red color indicates motion toward the transducer, and blue indicates movement away from the transducer. On the right, a plot representing myocardial motion is shown. Movement toward the transducer (systole) is above baseline, whereas movement away from the transducer is located below baseline. Note Em and Am waves indicating early and late filling, respectively. (See Color Insert.)

was found between the peak systolic mitral annular velocity and EF obtained by radionuclide ventriculography ($r = 0.86$). Mitral annular velocity of more than 5.4 cm/sec by color-coded Doppler (average of six sites) was highly predictive of ejection fraction of >50%.[98] DTI is currently being evaluated for assessing regional myocardial function during dobutamine-stress echo for ischemia and viability.

Diastolic function can be evaluated by measuring E′ and A′. Previous studies have shown that E′ is reduced when diastolic function is impaired, similar to peak transmitral E wave. E′ was less affected by loading conditions than early transmitral inflow.

Although there are a number of emerging applications for tissue-velocity imaging, there are also important limitations to assessment of tissue velocity. The most important limitation is that TDI cannot differentiate between velocity obtained by the contractile myocardial function and the global cardiac movement or translation motion. A second limitation is that the velocities in the basal regions are higher than the apical regions (both in systole and in diastole), and despite similar contractile function, there is a velocity gradient between the base and the apex of the left ventricle. A third limitation inherent in all the devices that use the Doppler principle is angle limitation. TDI can measure only velocities parallel to the transducer. To overcome the first two limitations, a

new application was recently developed, strain and strain rate imaging (SRI). SRI detects the degree of tissue deformation: longitudinal elongation/ shortening and radial thickening/thinning. Because of the geometric considerations described previously, there is a spatial gradient of velocities. This velocity gradient can be measured and expressed as strain rate.

$$\text{Strain rate} = V_1 - V_2 / \Delta L$$

ΔL is the distance between the two points where the velocities were measured (V_1 and V_2).

Strain is the time integral of strain rate divided by the distance that both points moved one in relation to the other. Strain connotes the degree of myocardial deformation, whereas strain rate implies the deformation rate.

The wave of myocardial longitudinal elongation of the myocardium during early diastole starts at the base of the heart and propagates toward the apex. Therefore, the velocities at the base of the heart are *higher* than at the apex. The same pattern is seen in the myocardial radial contraction/and thinning. Velocity of the *endocardium* is *faster* than that of the epicardium. Therefore, a *velocity gradient* can be demonstrated across the short axis of the ventricle and measured in terms of strain, which is *independent* of cardiac movement and the motion of adjacent myocardial tissues.[99]

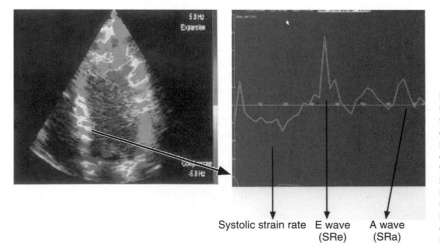

Systolic strain rate   E wave   A wave
                        (SRe)   (SRa)

FIGURE 1-72. Strain rate imaging in a healthy volunteer. Strain rate reflects myocardial deformation along the cardiac cycle. Positive values indicate myocardial elongation, whereas negative values indicate shortening. On the left side, strain rate imaging is shown. Blue color indicates elongation (positive strain rate), and yellow and red colors indicate myocardial shortening. On the right side, a plot reflecting strain rate measured from the septum is shown. Note the negative systolic wave, reflecting longitudinal shortening and positive waves during diastole, implying early and late myocardial elongation (SrE and SrA, respectively). (See Color Insert).

Because of angle limitations, only limited types of strains can be analyzed. In the apical four-chamber and two-chamber views, only longitudinal strains can be measured from lateral, inferoseptal, anterior, and inferior walls, respectively. From parasternal short axis, radial strains can be obtained from the anterior and posterior walls and circumferential strains from the lateral and septal walls.

Longitudinal strain rate during systole is negative because of systolic shortening, whereas longitudinal SR during diastole shows two positive deflections analogous to E′ and A′. Normal radial strain is positive during systole because of radial thickening.

Increases in preload enhance propagation of the velocity of left ventricular lengthening, thereby increasing SR. Impairment in diastolic function causes a reduction in peak early diastolic strain rate (SR-E′) and in the propagation velocity of SR during early diastole.[99]

SR in Myocardial Ischemia

SR has been measured in patients with unstable angina undergoing PTCA. Balloon occlusion of the coronary artery causes rapid reduction in systolic velocity and decreased systolic SR in the ischemic regions. SR and end-systolic strain have a higher diagnostic accuracy than systolic velocity for detecting ischemia in regions with a baseline wall motion abnormality.[100] An important feature of left ventricular diastolic dysfunction during ischemia is late/postsystolic compression (PSC).[101] SR imaging is also useful for detecting viable myocardium. In a study comparing low-dose dobutamine echo and PET scan for assessment of viable myocardium, measurements of regional systolic strain allowed an accurate detection of regional myocardial viability. Results of SR measurements were more accurate than 2D echo or tissue velocity in detecting viable myocardium.[102] An excellent correlation was demonstrated between myocardial strains measured by both echo and CMR in healthy volunteers, patients after acute myocardial infarction, and patients undergoing dobutamine stress imaging for suspected coronary artery disease.[103]

Transesophaged Echocardiography[104,105] (Figure 1-73)

The chest wall and air in the lungs pose an obstacle to acquisition of optimal transthoracic cardiac images in some patients. Imaging is further limited in patients with chronic pulmonary disease, obesity, after trauma, and

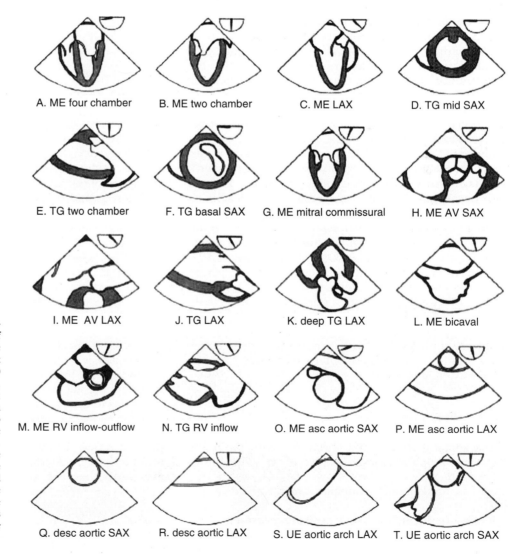

FIGURE 1-73. Recommended transesophageal views. Note the angle of the indicator (when it points to the left, it indicates 0 degrees; when it points downward, it indicates 90 degrees). ME, midesophageal; UE, upper esophageal; TG, trans gastric; SAX, short axis; LAX, long axis. In A-C and H, the structure closest to the probe is the left atrium. Note the left atrial appendage in B and E. In H, note the trileaflet aortic valve in the middle of the image. In I, the left ventricular outflow tract and the aortic and mitral valves can be seen. In the short-axis TG view, the posterior wall of the left ventricle is closest to the probe. (From *J Am Soc Echo* 1999;12[10]:887.)

A. ME four chamber   B. ME two chamber   C. ME LAX   D. TG mid SAX

E. TG two chamber   F. TG basal SAX   G. ME mitral commissural   H. ME AV SAX

I. ME AV LAX   J. TG LAX   K. deep TG LAX   L. ME bicaval

M. ME RV inflow-outflow   N. TG RV inflow   O. ME asc aortic SAX   P. ME asc aortic LAX

Q. desc aortic SAX   R. desc aortic LAX   S. UE aortic arch LAX   T. UE aortic arch SAX

those on a mechanical ventilator. These obstacles are overcome by TEE, which provides exquisite images of the heart and great vessels. TEE is a semiinvasive procedure and requires special preparations, staff, and expertise.

The transducer of a TEE probe is mounted on a tip of modified flexible endoscope. The tip of the probe can be manipulated in four directions (anteflexion, retroflexion, right, and left). A high-frequency phased-array transducer is used (usually 5.0-7.0 MHz or multiple frequencies (from 3.0-7.0 MHz) to provide better spatial resolution together with full Doppler capabilities including color and spectral Doppler (PW and CW).

The first TEE probe was monoplane in which the position and the orientation of the transducer were fixed, so that only horizontal (transverse) images could be acquired.

The second generation was a biplane transducer that could provide both horizontal and longitudinal images. There are two types of biplane probes: stacked transducers in which two orthogonal arrays are located, one proximal to the other; and matrix transducers in which both orthogonal arrays are at the same level. By manipulating the TEE probe, short-axis, long axis, and four-chamber images can be obtained, but this required numerous maneuvers. Orthogonal images of the left ventricle can be obtained with the stacked transducers only by advancing and withdrawing the probe.

The multiplane TEE probe is most commonly used today. Multiplane (or Omniplane) TEE probes include a phased-array transducer mounted on the tip so that the US beam can be rotated through 180 degrees. Changing the orientation of the beam enables acquisition of images from multiple transitional planes, thus increasing the number of contiguous images of the cardiac structures without moving the probe.

Contraindications to TEE include recent upper gastrointestinal surgery (esophagus and stomach), esophageal strictures, tumors, and diverticula. Patients with dysphagia and odynophagia should be excluded from undergoing TEE until evaluated by a gastroenterologist. Bleeding esophageal varices, acute hematemesis, and swallowing abnormalities are relative contraindications to TEE. Risk/benefit ratio should be considered carefully in these patients. Extreme caution should be exercised in patients with cervical spine diseases. Bleeding diatheses pose additional risk. Anticoagulation or antiplatelet therapy should not be interrupted before TEE. TEE can be performed safely in ventilated patients. Antibiotic prophylaxis for infective endocarditis before TEE is not recommended by the AHA/ ACC guidelines.[106]

Multiplane TEE

A detailed description of the sequence and orientation of the anatomical structures visualized with the multiplane transesophageal probe is beyond the scope of this chapter.

Several fundamental principles are observed during TEE.

Vital signs including blood pressure, heart rate, oxygenation, ECG, and clinical status are monitored continuously throughout the transesophageal examination, and the procedure is terminated if the patient's hemodynamic or respiratory status is compromised.

TEE should be "problem-oriented," that is, provide an answer to a specific predefined clinical problem, for example, "rule out vegetative endocarditis."

The study should be performed in a systematic order, because unexpected findings may be encountered. Images are acquired from two basic locations: the esophagus and stomach. Maneuvering the TEE probe should be minimized by use of the transducer tip flexion and angle rotation functions.

The various anatomical images from different planes and regions of interest are acquired in conjunction with the color and spectral Doppler velocity signals.

Orientation

When the TEE probe is in the esophagus or stomach, the posterior and inferior cardiac structures are located closest to the transducer. This is in contrast to transthoracic echo (TTE) in which the anterior cardiac structures are closest to the transducer. Structures closest to the transducer are in the upper part of the display. In most of the midesophageal views, the chamber closest to the transducer (in the apex of the sector) is the left atrium. In transgastric short-axis images, the posterior left ventricular wall is closest to the transducer, and the anterior wall is the most distant.

Angles (Figure 1-73)

The TEE transducer elements can be rotated to 180 degrees. Rotation of the transducer provides multiple cross-sectional images with standard and transitional images. At 0 degrees, horizontal cross-sectional images are displayed (right-sided structures are displayed on the left side of the screen). In transgastric view, serial short-axis views of the left ventricle are visualized. The short-axis view at midpapillary level is used for assessment of left ventricular function. The short-axis view at the base of the left ventricle is useful for evaluating the mitral valve leaflets and commissures. At the midesophageal level, a four-chamber view can be obtained, and at 45 degrees, an image similar to the standard parasternal short-axis view, which shows the three leaflets of the aortic valve, left atrium, right atrium, and right ventricular outflow tract, can be seen.

The 90-degree midesophageal angle provides a longitudinal axis of the left ventricle in a two-chamber view, which also is important for evaluating the left atrial appendage. At 135 degrees, a long-axis view of the left ventricle and the left ventricular outflow tract are obtained, analogous to the parasternal long axis view in TTE.

Serial short-axis images of the descending thoracic aorta are obtained when the transducer is rotated posteriorly at 0 degrees by withdrawing the probe from the lower esophagus. At 90 degrees, with the probe oriented posteriorly, the aorta is visualized in long axis.

Clinical Applications

TEE is not a substitute for TTE, because in most patients (>90%) TTE yields the required information. TEE is justi-

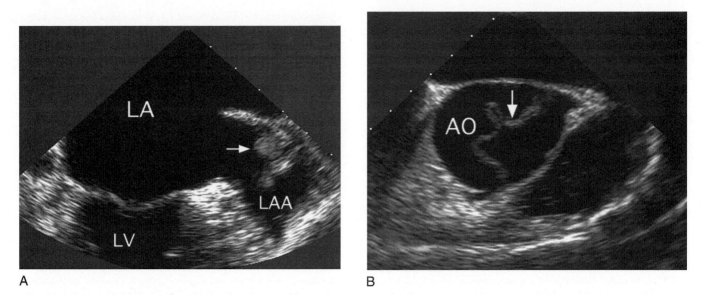

FIGURE 1-74. TEE images. **A,** A thrombus in the left atrial appendage (LAA, small arrow). A common source of systemic embolism in patients with atrial fibrillation. The left atrium (LA) and left ventricle (LV) are also seen in this midesophageal long-axis view. **B,** Dissection of the ascending aorta (AO). Note the flap separating the true and the false lumens (arrow).

fied only when TTE cannot or does not provide the required diagnostic information for optimal patient management. There is a small subset of patients (5%) in whom imaging by TTE is suboptimal because of structural deformities, obesity, pulmonary disease, or in ventilated patients. A major advantage of TEE compared with other diagnostic imaging modalities is its accessibility and portability. TEE can be performed as a bedside procedure in the emergency room, operating room, or intensive care unit in hemodynamically unstable and ventilated patients.

In a subset of cardiovascular disorders, TTE cannot provide a definitive diagnosis, and primary TEE is the imaging modality of choice. These include causes of cardioembolism such as left atrial appendage thrombus, atherosclerotic aortic plaques, acute aortic dissection, patent foramen ovale, and vegetative endocarditis (Figure 1-74). Patent foramen ovale (PFO) is an important potential source for paradoxical emboli and cryptogenic stroke, especially if associated with atrial septal aneurysm.[107] The yield of TEE for diagnosing PFO is higher than TTE even with contrast and physiological maneuvers. A further important application of TEE is in detecting left atrial thrombi and factors that predispose to thrombus formation (spontaneous contrast) before elective cardioversion in patients with atrial fibrillation, a therapeutic strategy that curtails the need for oral anticoagulation.[108]

Prosthetic valve malfunction and complications of endocarditis are frequently difficult to establish by TTE because of their echogenicity and acoustic shadowing. Accurate diagnosis can be unequivocally elucidated by TEE. An indisputable role for TEE that cannot be substituted for by TTE is intraoperative imaging, because it does not interfere with the operative field and provides high-quality images. Intraoperative TEE images of the mitral valve before instituting cardiopulmonary bypass are invaluable for determining the mechanism of mitral regurgitation and assessing whether repair of the native valve apparatus is feasible. Postbypass TEE allows assess-

ment of valve competence and left ventricular contractile function with transient increases in preload and/or afterload.

Complications

The complication rate of TEE in a series of 7134 studies was 2.8%. Most of these complications were mild, including transient hypotension or hypertension, hypoxemia, supraventricular tachycardia, transient bradycardia, bloody sputum, hoarseness, and sore throat. Severe complications such as laryngospasm, aspiration pneumonia, sustained ventricular tachycardia, exacerbation of congestive heart failure, and perforation of the esophagus vary from 0.18% to 0.5%.

Bioeffects and Safety of US Imaging

There are no confirmed biological effects on patients or the ultrasonographer caused by exposures from present diagnostic US instruments.[109,110] However, human tissues absorb US energy, and the effects of the propagating US wave are thermal (excessive heating) and mechanical effects (cavitations). Thus, there are potential bioeffects, and prudent use of diagnostic US should be concordant with the "as low as reasonably achievable" *(ALARA)* concept. ALARA recommends that during US studies, patients experience the least amount of exposure for minimal time without compromising the study quality.

REFERENCES

1. Bushberg JT, Siebert JA, Leidholdt EM, Boone JM. *The Essential Physics of Medical Imaging.* Baltimore: Lippincott Williams & Wilkins, 2002.
2. Ramachandran GN, Lakshminarayanan AV. Three-dimensional reconstruction from radiographs and electron micrographs: application of convolutions of Fourier transforms. *Proc Natl Acad Sci* 1971; 68:2236.

3. Shepp LA, Logan EC. The Fourier reconstruction of a head section. *IEEE Trans Nucl Sci* 1974; 21:2.

4. Wexler L, Brundage B, Crouse J, et al. Coronary artery calcification: pathophysiology, epidemiology, imaging methods, and clinical implications. A statement for health professionals from the American Heart Association. Writing Group. *Circulation* 1996; 94:1175.

5. Kalender WA, Seissler W, Klotz E, Vock P. Spiral volumetric CT with single-breath-hold technique, continuous transport, and continuous scanner rotation. *Radiology* 1990; 176:181.

6. Hsieh J. A general approach to the reconstruction of X-ray helical computed tomography. *Med Phys* 1996; 23:221.

7. Fishman EK, Kuszyk B. 3D imaging: musculoskeletal applications. *Crit Rev Diagn Imaging* 2001; 42:59.

8. Kalender WA. Thin-section three-dimensional spiral CT: is isotropic imaging possible? *Radiology* 1995; 197:578.

9. Becker CR, Schoepf UJ, Reiser MF. Methods for quantification of coronary artery calcifications with electron beam and conventional CT and pushing the spiral CT envelope: new cardiac applications. *Int J Cardiovasc Imaging* 2001; 17:203.

10. Hu H, He HD, Foley WD, Fox SH. Four multidetector-row helical CT: image quality and volume coverage speed. *Radiology* 2000; 215:55.

11. Mahesh M. Search for isotropic resolution in CT from conventional through multiple-row detector. *Radiographics* 2002; 22:949.

12. Taguchi K, Aradate H. Algorithm for image reconstruction in multi-slice helical CT. *Med Phys* 1998; 25:550.

13. Hui H, Pan T, Shen Y. Multislice helical CT: image temporal resolution. *IEEE Trans Med Imaging* 2000; 19:384.

14. Jakobs TF, Becker CR, Ohnesorge B, et al. Multislice helical CT of the heart with retrospective ECG gating: reduction of radiation exposure by ECG-controlled tube current modulation. *Eur Radiol* 2002; 12:1081.

15. Klingenbeck-Regn K, Flohr T, Ohnesorge B, Regn J, Schaller S. Strategies for cardiac CT imaging. *Int J Cardiovasc Imaging* 2002; 18:143.

16. Nieman K, van Ooijen P, Rensing B, Oudkerk M, de Feyter PJ. Four-dimensional cardiac imaging with multislice computed tomography. *Circulation* 2001; 103:E62.

17. Becker CR, Knez A, Leber A, et al. Detection of coronary artery stenoses with multislice helical CT angiography. *J Comput Assist Tomogr* 2002; 26:750.

18. Fayad ZA, Fuster V, Nikolaou K, Becker C. Computed tomography and magnetic resonance imaging for noninvasive coronary angiography and plaque imaging: current and potential future concepts. *Circulation* 2002; 106:2026.

19. Gerber TC, Kuzo RS, Karstaedt N, et al. Current results and new developments of coronary angiography with use of contrast-enhanced computed tomography of the heart. *Mayo Clin Proc* 2002; 77:55.

20. Flohr T, Stierstorfer K, Bruder H, Simon J, Polacin A, Schaller S. Image reconstruction and image quality evaluation for a 16-slice CT scanner. *Med Phys* 2003; 30:832.

21. Flohr T, Prokop M, Becker C, et al. A retrospectively ECG-gated multislice spiral CT scan and reconstruction technique with suppression of heart pulsation artifacts for cardio-thoracic imaging with extended volume coverage. *Eur Radiol* 2002; 12:1497.

22. Flohr TG, Schoepf UJ, Kuettner A, et al. Advances in cardiac imaging with 16-section CT systems. *Acad Radiol* 2003; 10:386.

23. Mahesh M, Scatarige JC, Cooper J, Fishman EK. Dose and pitch relationship for a particular multislice CT scanner. *Am J Roentgenol* 2001; 177:1273.

24. IEC. Medical Electrical Equipment. *Part 2-44: Particular Requirements for the Safety of X-ray Equipment for Computed Tomography*. IEC Publications No. 60601-2-44. Geneva, Switzerland, 2002.

25. McCollough CH, Morin RL. The technical design and performance of ultrafast computed tomography. *Radiol Clin North Am* 1994; 32:521.

26. Shope TB, Gagne RM, Johnson GC. A method for describing the doses delivered by transmission X-ray computed tomography. *Med Phys* 1981; 8:488.

27. McCollough CH, Zink FE, Morin RL. Radiation dosimetry for electron beam CT. *Radiology* 1994; 192:637.

28. Nagel HD (ed). *Radiation Exposure in Computed Tomography: Fundamentals, Influencing Parameters, Dose Assessment, Optimisation, Scanner Data, Terminology*. Hamburg: COCIR, 2002.

29. Morin RL, Gerber TC, McCollough CH. Radiation dose in computed tomography of the heart. *Circulation* 2003; 107:917.

30. Hunold P, Vogt FM, Schmermund A, et al. Radiation exposure during cardiac CT: effective doses at multi-detector row CT and electron-beam CT. *Radiology* 2003; 226:145.

31. Pettigrew RI, Oshinski JN, Chatzimavroudis G, et al. CMR techniques for cardiovascular imaging. *J Magn Reson Imaging* 1999; 10:590.

32. Sakuma H, Takeda K, Higgins CB. Fast magnetic resonance imaging of the heart. *Eur J Radiol* 1999; 29:101.

33. Chen Q, Stock KW, Prasad PV, et al. Fast magnetic resonance imaging techniques. *Eur J Radiol* 1999; 29:90.

34. Pruessmann KP, Weiger M, Scheidegger MB, et al. SENSE: sensitivity encoding for fast CMR. *Magn Reson Med* 1999; 42:952.

35. Sodickson DK, Griswold MA, Jakob PM. SMASH imaging. *Magn Reson Imaging Clin North Am* 1999; 7:237.

36. Stehling MK, Holzknecht NG, Laub G, et al. Single-shot T1- and T2-weighted magnetic resonance imaging of the heart with black blood: preliminary experience. *MAGMA* 1996; 4:231.

37. Le Roux P, Gilles RJ, McKinnon GC, et al. Optimized outer volume suppression for single-shot fast spin-echo cardiac imaging. *J Magn Reson Imaging* 1998; 8:1022.

38. Simonetti OP, Finn JP, White RD, et al. "Black blood" T2-weighted inversion-recovery MR imaging of the heart. *Radiology*. 1996; 199:49.

39. Edelman RR, Wallner B, Singer A, et al. Segmented turboFLASH: method for breath-hold MR imaging of the liver with flexible contrast. *Radiology* 1990; 177:515.

40. Reeder SB, Atalar E, Faranesh AZ, et al. Multi-echo segmented k-space imaging: an optimized hybrid sequence for ultrafast cardiac imaging. *Magn Reson Med* 1999; 41:375.

41. Miller S, Simonetti OP, Carr J, et al. MR Imaging of the heart with cine true fast imaging with steady-state precession: influence of spatial and temporal resolutions on left ventricular functional parameters. *Radiology* 2002; 223:263.

42. S, Resnick D, Bundy JM, et al. Cardiac function: MR evaluation in one breath hold with real-time true fast imaging with steady-state precession. *Radiology* 2002; 222:835.

43. Zerhouni EA, Parish DM, Rogers WJ, et al. Human heart: tagging with MR imaging—a method for noninvasive assessment of myocardial motion. *Radiology* 1988; 169:59.

44. Axel L, Dougherty L. MR imaging of motion with spatial modulation of magnetization. *Radiology* 1989; 171:841.

45. Mosher TJ, Smith MB. A DANTE tagging sequence for the evaluation of translational sample motion. *Magn Reson Med* 1990; 15:334.

46. Moore CC, O'Dell WG, McVeigh ER, et al. Calculation of three-dimensional left ventricular strains from biplanar tagged MR images. *J Magn Reson Imaging* 1992; 2:165.

47. Osman NF, Kerwin WS, McVeigh ER, et al. Cardiac motion tracking using CINE harmonic phase (HARP) magnetic resonance imaging. *Magn Reson Med* 1999; 42:1048.

48. Lima JA, Judd RM, Bazille A, et al. Regional heterogeneity of human myocardial infarcts demonstrated by contrast-enhanced CMR. Potential mechanisms. *Circulation* 1995; 92:1117.

49. Al Saadi N, Nagel E, Gross M, et al. Noninvasive detection of myocardial ischemia from perfusion reserve based on cardiovascular magnetic resonance. *Circulation* 2000; 101:1379.

50. Eichenberger AC, Schuiki E, Kochli VD, et al. Ischemic heart disease: assessment with gadolinium-enhanced ultrafast MR imaging and dipyridamole stress. *J Magn Reson Imaging* 1994; 4:425.

51. Wilke N, Jerosch-Herold M, Wang Y, et al. Myocardial perfusion reserve: assessment with multisection, quantitative, first-pass MR imaging. *Radiology* 1997; 204:373.

52. Kim RJ, Wu E, Rafael A, et al. The use of contrast-enhanced magnetic resonance imaging to identify reversible myocardial dysfunction. *N Engl J Med* 2000; 343:1445.

53. Simonetti OP, Kim RJ, Fieno DS, et al. An improved MR imaging technique for the visualization of myocardial infarction. *Radiology* 2001; 218:215.

54. Firmin DN, Nayler GL, Klipstein RH, et al. In vivo validation of MR velocity imaging. *J Comput Assist Tomogr* 1987; 11:751.

55. Nayler GL, Firmin DN, Longmore DB. Blood flow imaging by cine magnetic resonance. *J Comput Assist Tomogr* 1986; 10:715.

56. Kozerke S, Schwitter J, Pedersen EM, et al. Aortic and mitral regurgitation: quantification using moving slice velocity mapping. *J Magn Reson Imaging* 2001; 14:106.

57. Leung DA, McKinnon GC, Davis CP, et al. Breath-hold, contrast-enhanced, three-dimensional MR angiography. *Radiology* 1996; 200:569.

58. Prince MR, Narasimham DL, Stanley JC, et al. Breath-hold gadolinium-enhanced MR angiography of the abdominal aorta and its major branches. *Radiology* 1995; 197:785.

59. Manning WJ, Li W, Edelman RR. A preliminary report comparing magnetic resonance coronary angiography with conventional angiography. *N Engl J Med* 1993; 328:828.

60. Kim WY, Danias PG, Stuber M, et al. Coronary magnetic resonance angiography for the detection of coronary stenoses. *N Engl J Med* 2001; 345:1863.

61. Bottomley PA, Weiss RG. Non-invasive magnetic-resonance detection of creatine depletion in non-viable infarcted myocardium. *Lancet* 1998; 351:714.

62. Weiss RG, Bottomley PA, Hardy CJ, et al. Regional myocardial metabolism of high-energy phosphates during isometric exercise in patients with coronary artery disease. *N Engl J Med* 1990; 323:1593.

63. Constantinides CD, Kraitchman DL, O'Brien KO, et al. Noninvasive quantification of total sodium concentrations in acute reperfused myocardial infarction using 23Na CMR. *Magn Reson Med* 2001; 46:1144.

64. Sorensen JA, Phelps MR. Radioactive decay. *Physics in Nuclear Medicine*, ed 2. Philadelphia: Saunders, 1987, p 41.

65. Muehlehner G. Karp JS. Surti S. Design considerations for PET scanners. *Q J Nucl Med* 2002; 46:16.

66. Maublant JC, Peycelon P, Kwiatkowski F, et al. Comparison between 180° and 360° data collection in technetium99m MIBI SPECT of the myocardium. *J Nucl Med* 1989; 30:295.

67. Liu YH, Lam PT, Sinusas AJ, Wackers FJ. Differential effect of 180 degrees and 360 degrees acquisition orbits on the accuracy of SPECT imaging: quantitative evaluation in phantoms. *J Nucl Med* 2002; 43:1115.

68. Shepp LA, Vardi Y. Maximum likelihood reconstruction for emission tomography. *IEEE Trans Med Imaging* 1982; 1:113.

69. Lalush DS, Tsui BM. Performance of ordered-subset reconstruction algorithms under conditions of extreme attenuation and truncation in myocardial SPECT. *J Nucl Med* 2000; 41:737.

70. Narayanan MV, Byrne CL, King MA. An interior point iterative maximum-likelihood reconstruction algorithm incorporating upper and lower bounds with application to SPECT transmission imaging. *IEEE Trans Med Imaging* 2001; 20:342.

71. Hoffman EA, Huang S-C, Phelps ME. Quantitation in positron emission computed tomography. 1. Effect of object size. *J Comput Assist Tomogr* 1979; 3:299.

72. Chang LT. A method for attenuation correction in radionuclide computed tomography. *IEEE Trans Nucl Sci* 1978; 25:638.

73. Laurette I, Zeng GL, Welch A, Christian PE, Gullberg GT. A three-dimensional ray-driven attenuation, scatter and geometric response correction technique for SPECT in inhomogeneous media. *Phys Med Biol* 2000; 45:3459.

74. LaCroix KJ, Tsui BM, Frey EC, Jaszczak RJ. Receiver operating characteristic evaluation of iterative reconstruction with attenuation correction in 99mTc-sestamibi myocardial SPECT images. *J Nucl Med* 2000; 41:502.

75. Narayanan MV, Byrne CL, King MA. An interior point iterative maximum-likelihood reconstruction algorithm incorporating upper and lower bounds with application to SPECT transmission imaging. *IEEE Trans Med Imaging* 2001; 20:342.

76. Pretorius PH, Narayanan MV, Dahlberg ST, Leppo JA, King MA. The influence of attenuation and scatter compensation on the apparent distribution of Tc-99m sestamibi in cardiac slices. *J Nucl Cardiol* 2001; 8:356.

77. Araujo LI, Jimenez-Hoyuela JM, McClellan JR, Lin E, Viggiano J, Alavi A. Improved uniformity in tomographic myocardial perfusion imaging with attenuation correction and enhanced acquisition and processing. *J Nucl Med* 2000; 41:1139.

78. Duvernoy CS, Ficaro EP, Karabajakian MZ, Rose PA, Corbett JR. Improved detection of left main coronary artery disease with attenuation-corrected SPECT. *J Nucl Cardiol* 2000; 7:639.

79. Hendel RC, Corbett JR, Cullom SJ, DePuey EG, Garcia EV, Bateman TM. The value and practice of attenuation correction for myocardial perfusion SPECT imaging: a joint position statement from the American Society of Nuclear Cardiology and the Society of Nuclear Medicine. *J Nucl Cardiol* 2002; 9:135.

80. Sharir T, Berman DS, Waechter PB, Areeda J, Kavanagh PB, Gerlach J, Kang X, Germano G. Quantitative analysis of regional motion and thickening by gated myocardial perfusion SPECT: normal heterogeneity and criteria for abnormality. *J Nucl Med* 2001; 42:1630.

81. Links JM, DePuey EG, Taillefer R, Becker LC. Attenuation correction and gating synergistically improve the diagnostic accuracy of myocardial perfusion SPECT. *J Nucl Cardiol* 2002; 9:183.

82. Germano G, Kavanagh PB, Waechter P, Areeda J, Van Kriekinge S, Sharir T, Lewin HC, Berman DS. A new algorithm for the quantitation of myocardial perfusion SPECT. I. Technical principles and reproducibility. *J Nucl Med* 2000; 41:712.

83. Tepe G, Duda SH, Meding J, et al. Tc-99m-labeled endothelin derivative for imaging of experimentally induced atherosclerosis. *Atherosclerosis* 2001; 157:383.

84. Yun M, Yeh D, Araujo LI, Jang S, Newberg A, Alavi A. F-18 FDG uptake in the large arteries: a new observation. *Clin Nucl Med* 2001; 26:314.

85. Narula J, Acio ER, Narula N, Samuels LE, Fyfe B, Wood D, Fitzpatrick JM, Raghunath PN, Tomaszewski JE, Kelly C, Steinmetz N, Green A, Tait JF, Leppo J, Blankenberg FG, Jain D, Strauss HW. Annexin-V imaging for noninvasive detection of cardiac allograft rejection. *Nat Med* 2001; 7:1347.

86. Kremkau FW. *Diagnostic Ultrasound. Principles and Instruments*, ed 6. Philadelphia: Saunders, 2002, p 17.

87. Leonardo Massoti. Basic principles and advanced technological aspects of ultrasound imaging, in Guzzardi R (ed): *Physics and Engineering of Medical Imaging*. Dordrecht: The Netherlands: Martinus Nijhoff Publishers, 1987, p 263.

88. Hedrick WR, Hykes DL, Strachman DE. *Ultrasound Physics and Instrumentation*. St. Louis: Mosby, 1995, p 71.

89. Kremkau FW. *Diagnostic Ultrasound. Principles and Instruments*, ed 6. Philadelphia: Saunders, 2002, p 61.

90. Karrer E. Phased array acoustic imaging systems, in Guzzardi R (ed): *Physics and Engineering of Medical Imaging*. Dordrecht, The Netherlands: Martinus Nijhoff Publishers, 1987.

91. Thomas JD, Rubin DN. Tissue harmonic imaging: why does it work? *J Am Soc Echocardiogr* 1998; 11:803.

92. Lange A, Palka P, Burstow DJ. Three dimensional echocardiography: historical development and current applications—review article. *J Am Soc Echocardiogr* 2001; 14:403.

93. Mele D, Maehle J, Pendini I, Alboni P, Levine R. Three dimensional echocardiographic reconstruction: description and applications of a simplified technique for quantitative assessment of left ventricular size and function. Am J Cardiol 1998; 81(12A):107G.

94. The American Task Force on Standards and Guidelines for the Use of Ultrasonic Contrast in Echocardiography. Contrast Echocardiography: Current and Future Applications. ASE Position Paper. *J Am Soc Echocardiogr* 2000; 13(4):331.

95. Kaul S. Myocardial contrast echocardiography. Basic principles. *Prog Cardiovasc Dis* 2001; 44:1.

96. Gorcsan J III. Tissue Doppler echocardiography. *Curr Opin Cardiol* 2000; 15:232.

97. Pislaru C, Abraham TP, Belohlavek M. Strain and strain rate echocardiography. *Curr Opin Cardiol* 2002; 17:443.

98. Gulati VK, Katz WE, Follansbee WP, Gorcsan J III. Mitral annular descent velocity by tissue Doppler echocardiography as an index of global left ventricular function. *Am J Cardiol* 1996; 77:979.

99. Stoylen A, Slordahl S, Skjelvan GK, Heimdal A, Skjaerpe T. Strain rate imaging in normal and reduced diastolic function: comparison with pulsed Doppler imaging of the mitral annulus. *J Am Soc Echocardiogr* 2001; 14:264.

100. Kukulski T, Jamal F, D'Hooge J, Bijnens B, De-Scheerder I, Sutherland GR. Acute changes in systolic and diastolic events during clinical coronary angioplasty: a comparison of regional velocity, strain rate and strain measurement. *J Am Soc Echocardiogr* 2002; 15:1.

101. Belohlavek M, Pislaru C, Bae RY, Greenleaf JF, Seward JB. Real time strain rate echocardiographic imaging: temporal and spatial analysis of postsystolic compression in acutely ischemic myocardium. *J Am Coll Echocardiogr* 2001; 14:360.

102. Hoffman R, Altiok E, Nowak B, Hussen N, Kuhl H, Kaiser H-J, Bull U, Hanrath P. Strain rate measurement by Doppler echocardiography allows improved assessment of myocardial viability in patients with depressed left ventricular function. *J Am Coll Cardiol* 2002; 39:443.

103. Edvardsen T, Gerber B, Garot J, Bluemke DA, Lima JAC, Smiseth O. Quantitative assessment of intrinsic regional myocardial deformation by Doppler strain rate echocardiography in humans. *Circulation* 2002; 106:50.

104. Seward JB, Khandheria BK, Freeman WK, Oh JK, Enriquez-Sarano M, Miller FA, Edwards WD, Tajik J. Multiplane transesophageal echocardiography: image orientation, examination technique, and clinical applications. *Mayo Clin Proc* 1993; 68:523.

105. Shanewise JS, Cheung AT, Aronson S, et al. ASE/SCA guidelines for performing a comprehensive intraoperative multiplane transesophageal echocardiography examination: recommendations of the American Society of Echocardiography and the Society of Cardiovascular Anesthesiologists task force for certification in perioperative transesophageal echocardiography. *J Am Soc Echocardiogr* 1999; 12:884.

106. Bonow RO, Carabello B, Leon AC, Edmunds LH, Fedderly BJ, Freed MD, Gaasch WH, McKay CR, Nishimura RA, O'Gara PT, O'Rourke RA, Rahimtoda SH. Management of patients with valvular heart disease: ACC/AHA practice guidelines. *J Am Coll Cardiol* 1998; 32(5):1486.

107. Mas JL, Arquizan C, Lamy C, Zuber M, Cabanes L, Derumeaux G, Coste J, for the Patent Foramen Ovale and Atrial Septal Aneurysm Study Group. Recurrent cerebrovascular events associated with patent foramen ovale, atrial septal aneurysm, or both. *N Engl J Med* 2001; 345:1740.

108. Klein AL, Grimm RA, Murray RD, et al. Use of transesophageal echocardiography to guide cardioversion in patients with atrial fibrillation (ACUTE study). *N Engl J Med* 2001; 344:1411.

109. American Institute of Ultrasound in Medicine (AIUM). Official statements October 1982, approved March 1997. (www.aium.org/consumer). AIUM, Laurel, MD.

110. American Institute of Ultrasound in Medicine: Medical Ultrasound Safety. Part one: Bioeffects and biophysics. Part two: Prudent Use. Part Three: Implementing ALARA. Copyright 1994 by the AIUM, Laurel, MD.

Quantitation of Ventricular Function

Thomas M. Bashore
Paul A. Grayburn

This chapter focuses on the optimal use of cardiac imaging methods to quantify ventricular function. The most commonly used imaging methods, including contrast angiography, echocardiography (both transthoracic and transesophageal), magnetic resonance imaging (CMR), and radionuclide angiography, are discussed as they relate to the clinical assessment of ventricular function. The technical details of these imaging modalities have already been described in Chapter 1. The aim of this chapter is to provide a clinically oriented practical guide to the use of these methods for the quantification of ventricular systolic and diastolic function.

To understand the images that are derived from these methods, this chapter will initially describe the basic anatomical features and function of each cardiac chamber. The method involved in determining the volumes of each cardiac chamber is reviewed. Finally, the methods for quantifying global and regional wall motion are addressed with emphasis on the clinical usefulness of the available methods.

BASIC CARDIAC ANATOMICAL FEATURES

General Cardiac Anatomy

The average heart weight is approximately 300 g in the normal adult man and 250 g in the normal adult woman. The heart is enclosed by the pericardium, which covers the ascending aorta, pulmonary trunk, and the superior vena cava (SVC). The pericardium is similar to a balloon with the heart pressed into it. Thus the visceral pericardium directly covers the surface of the heart and great vessels, and the parietal and visceral layers are separated by the serous pericardial space. The heart is tethered to the diaphragm inferiorly by the pericardiophrenic ligament. Sternopericardial ligaments hold the pericardium anteriorly to the sternum, and loose connective tissue secures it posteriorly. Where the aorta and pulmonary

trunk exit the heart, a transverse pericardial space or sinus is present, which is bounded by the right ventricle (RV) anteriorly, the left atrium (LA) posteriorly, and superiorly by the right pulmonary artery (RPA). The SVC, inferior vena cava (IVC), and the pulmonary veins (PV) enter the heart posteriorly, and in this region an oblique pericardial sinus is present. This posterior sinus is bound by the pericardial reflections, and thus one cannot pass a digit through this sinus.

The heart is oriented obliquely in the chest. The atrial and ventricular septal structures are aligned virtually through the middle of the heart, at a 45-degree angle to the sagittal plane. The planes of the mitral and tricuspid valve are oriented approximately 90 to 120 degrees to each other. The right atrium (RA) is located to the right and both anterior and inferior to the LA. The RV is an anterior structure, extending below the left ventricle (LV) anteriorly and to the left and superior to the aortic valve. The LA is posterior, and the LV forms the lateral and apical portion of the cardiac contour.

The Left Ventricle

The LV is designed as a pressure-generating pump. It is an ellipsoid-shaped structure with wall thickness three times thicker than that of the RV (Figure 2-1). The LV has fewer trabeculae than the RV and two discrete papillary muscles. Blood flow into the LV enters through the mitral valve, turns a full 180 degrees, and is then ejected through the LV outflow tract. The flow of blood in the RV and LV is shown diagrammatically in Figure 2-2. The mitral valve is situated about 45 degrees to the sagittal plane of the heart with a slight forward tilt. The mitral, tricuspid, and aortic valve orifices all share the central fibrous body. The mitral annulus encircles the orifice of the mitral valve, except where the mitral and aortic valves share the intervalvular fibrosa. Thus, a calcified mitral valve annulus appears radiographically as a "hook" shape rather than a circular shape. The anterior leaflet is the larger, sail-like leaflet that attaches to one third of the mitral annulus. It also forms the lateral wall of the LV outflow tract. The anterior leaflet directs LA flow in diastole toward the LV apex. The posterior mitral leaflet attaches to the remaining two thirds of the annulus and is separated into anterolateral, middle, and posteromedial scallops.

Two major papillary muscles (the anterolateral and posteromedial) are well defined and send chordae to both leaflets of the mitral valve. When LV contraction

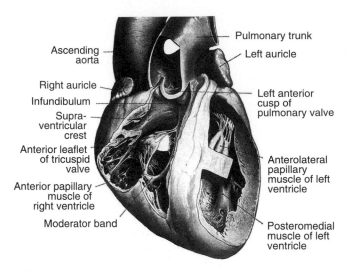

FIGURE 2-1. Left ventricular (LV) anatomy compared with right ventricular (RV) anatomy. The much thicker LV is designed as a pressure-generating pump. (From Gabella G. Cardiovascular system, in Williams PL, Bannister LH, Berry MM, Collins P, Dyson M, Dussek JE, et al (eds): *Gray's Anatomy*. New York: Churchill Livingstone, 1995, p 1484.) See text for discussion.

occurs, the papillary muscles contract initially and pull the mitral leaflets into parallel alignment with each other. As contraction proceeds, the papillary muscles continue to contract with annular contraction reducing the orifice by as much as 20% to 40%. LV systolic pressure tends to hold the two coapted mitral leaflets

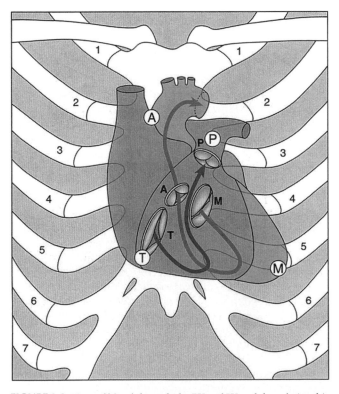

FIGURE 2-2. Flow of blood through the RV and LV and the relationship to the cardiac valve positions. (From Gabella G. Cardiovascular system, in Williams PL, Bannister LH, Berry MM, Collins P, Dyson M, Dussek JE, et al (eds): *Gray's Anatomy*. New York: Churchill Livingstone, 1995, p 1491.)

together (referred to as the keystone effect, similar to the keystone in the center of an archway). All these components of the mitral apparatus prevent prolapse of the mitral valve into the LA during ventricular systole.

Accessory chordae are occasionally attached to the LV endocardium and result in incomplete coaptation of the mitral leaflets and mitral regurgitation. When the LV outflow tract is narrowed, such as in hypertrophic cardiomyopathy, the mitral valve may be drawn into the LV outflow tract during systole (systolic anterior motion).

The LV itself resembles an ellipsoid of revolution whose axis spans from the mitral valve plane at the base to the apex. The LV wall is composed primarily of muscle bundles wound around the chamber, with some encompassing the RV as well. The LV wall thickness is much greater at its mid portion than at the apex, where circular fibers are no longer present. Because wall thickness is inversely proportional to wall tension, the wall tensions throughout the ventricle are least at the mid-wall surface and greatest at the apex. Because of this, most of the stroke volume ejected results from short-axis shortening rather than long-axis shortening. This has important implications for assessing LV systolic function.

The aortic valve is situated at the end of the smooth LV outflow tract. It is composed of three equal-sized semilunar cusps supported by the three sinuses of Valsalva. There is no true annulus, although functionally the fibrous semilunar attachments perform this role. The cusps are partially attached to the aortic wall and partially to the LV. There is a shared attachment to the anterior leaflet of the mitral valve.

The Right Ventricle

The right ventricle is designed as a volume pump and is almost pyramidal in shape (Figure 2-1). It forms most of the anterior surface of the heart, as well as the inferior border. For clinical purposes, it has three components: an inlet portion, a trabeculated apical portion, and an outlet portion. The inlet and outlet portions surround the tricuspid valve and are separated at the roof of the RV by the prominent crista supraventricularis, a muscular high-arched structure. The RV inlet is trabeculated, whereas the outlet is not. A moderator band containing the right bundle branch of the conduction system crosses the RV chamber from the septum to the free wall.

The tricuspid valve is divided into anterior, inferior, and septal leaflets, the anterior being the largest. Its plane is about 45 degrees to the sagittal plane of the heart and slightly inclined toward the vertical plane. Chordae attach from the free edges, as well as the ventricular surface (underneath), of the valve leaflets to three papillary muscles (anterior, posterior, and septal), which in turn insert into the RV endocardial surface. This latter feature results in displacement of the tricuspid valve when the RV dilates, frequently causing tricuspid regurgitation. The septal surface of the RV is divided into a basal portion, a muscular trabeculated region, and an infundibular area. RV trabeculations tend to be more coarse and straighter than those in the LV.

The pulmonary valve is separated from the tricuspid valve by the muscular infundibulum, and this characteristic is critical in distinguishing the morphologic RV from the LV in congenital heart disease. Continuity of the semilunar valve with the atrioventricular valve is not seen on the right side of the heart, whereas aortic-mitral continuity is characteristic of the left heart chambers. The plane of the pulmonic valve faces superiorly, to the left, and slightly posteriorly. The leaflets attach to the infundibular wall of the RV and partly to the pulmonary trunk. Although there is no true circular pulmonary annulus per se, the base of the valve is often referred to as such.

From an imaging standpoint, the general shapes of each of the cardiac chambers might be described as spherical for the RA, pyramidal for the RV, oval for the LA, and ellipsoidal for the LV. Human casts of the RA and RV (Figure 2-3) and the LA and LV (Figure 2-4) provide visual evidence for these assumptions. Corresponding representative contrast and cardiac magnetic resonance imaging (CMR) angiograms are shown in Figure 2-5 for the RV and Figure 2-6 for the LV.

FUNCTIONAL-ANATOMICAL RELATIONSHIPS

Atrial Contraction and Function

The extra boost of volume into the ventricles from atrial contraction contributes substantially to ventricular preload and stroke volume, and its loss might adversely affect cardiac output, especially in patients with diastolic dysfunction. Atrial performance includes reservoir, conduit, and pump functions, with the motion of the annulus toward the ventricular apex in ventricular systole and toward the atrium in ventricular diastole. The left atrial appendage appears to be more distensible than the rest of the left atrium and might help modulate pressure elevations that occur in the LA.

Left Ventricular Contraction and Function

The LV is a complex structure with heterogeneous contraction and relaxation patterns. Some of the vagaries in assessing LV motion and function have recently been reviewed by Spotnitz.[1]

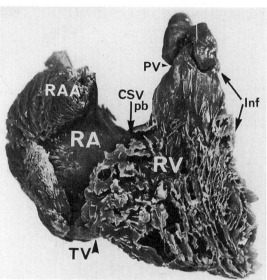
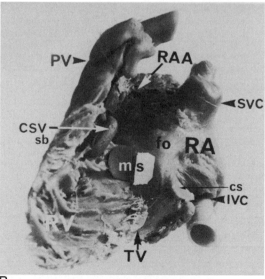

FIGURE 2-3. Human casts of the RA and RV. Anterior view (top panel) and lateral view (bottom panel). RAA = right atrial appendage, PV = pulmonary vein, Inf = infundibulum, CSV = crista supraventricularis, SVC = superior vena cava, TV = tricuspid valve, fo = foramen ovale, IVC = inferior vena cava. The area in the middle of **B** is the membranous septum with the dark area (m) the intraventricular component beneath the tricuspid septal leaflet, and the white area (s) the component above the tricuspid leaflet separating the LV from the RA. (From Hartnell GG, Raphael MJ. Cardiac anatomy and enlargement, in Grainger RG, Allison D, Adam A, Dixon AK (eds): *Diagnostic Radiology. A Textbook of Medical Imaging.* New York: Churchill Livingstone, 2001, p 675.)

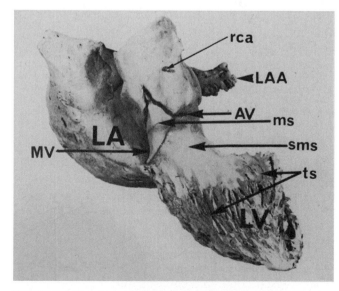

FIGURE 2-4. Human casts of the LA and LV chambers in the AP view. LAA = left atrial appendage, MV = mitral valve, AV = aortic valve, rca = right coronary artery, ts = trabeculated muscular septum, sms = smooth muscular septum, ms = membranous septum, apm = anterior papillary muscle. (From Grainger RG, Allison D, Adam A, Dixon AK (eds). *Diagnostic Radiology. A Textbook of Medical Imaging.* New York: Churchill Livingstone, 2001, p 677.)

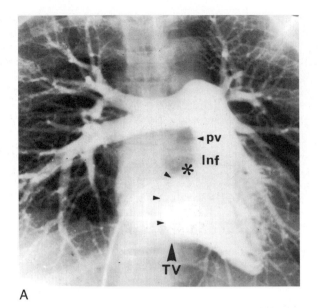

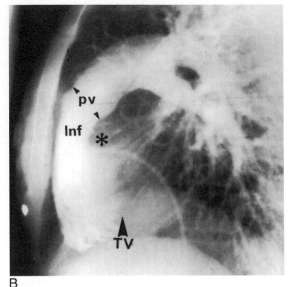

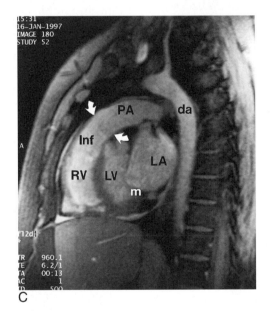

FIGURE 2-5. RV angiogram in AP view (left panel) and lateral view (middle panel) compared with a single image from a cardiac magnetic resonance imaging (CMR) study in the lateral view (right panel). pv = pulmonic valve, TV = tricuspid valve, Inf = RV infundibulum, LA = left atrium, LV = left ventricle, da = descending aorta, m = mitral valve. The asterisk indicates the body of the crista supraventricularis. (From Grainger RG, Allison D, Adam A, Dixon AK (eds). *Diagnostic Radiology. A Textbook of Medical Imaging.* New York: Churchill Livingstone, 2001, p 676.

During LV systole the ventricle shortens, twists, squeezes on itself, and thickens. The walls thicken radially in relation to the long axis, whereas the apex-to-base length shortens in a meridional manner along curved lines parallel to the long axis. Shortening also occurs circumferentially along the curved lines in the short-axis plane. In addition, the apex twists relative to the base, and it does so in the opposite direction (the apex twists counterclockwise and the base clockwise).[2] This twisting or torsion reverses itself rapidly in early diastole. Given that the LV walls are much thicker at the waist than at the apex, wall tension is significantly less at the waist (Tension = [Pressure × Radius]/[2 × Wall thickness]). This reduced wall tension allows greater shortening to occur at the LV mid-

wall than at the apex. For this reason, short-axis (circumferential) shortening contributes more to stroke volume than long-axis shortening.

Because of the regional differences in wall tension, when the LV dilates from a volume overload or thins as in a dilated cardiomyopathy, it tends to increase its dimension more in the short-axis direction rather than long axis. The result is that the LV becomes more spherical with either volume overload or in dilated cardiomyopathy. The opposite occurs in pathological pressure overload states, in which the LV walls thicken and there might be little change in the chamber diameter. In this setting, the wall tensions are low, and the LV might empty almost completely. The shape of the LV in pressure overload is ellipsoidal, with a narrower waist than

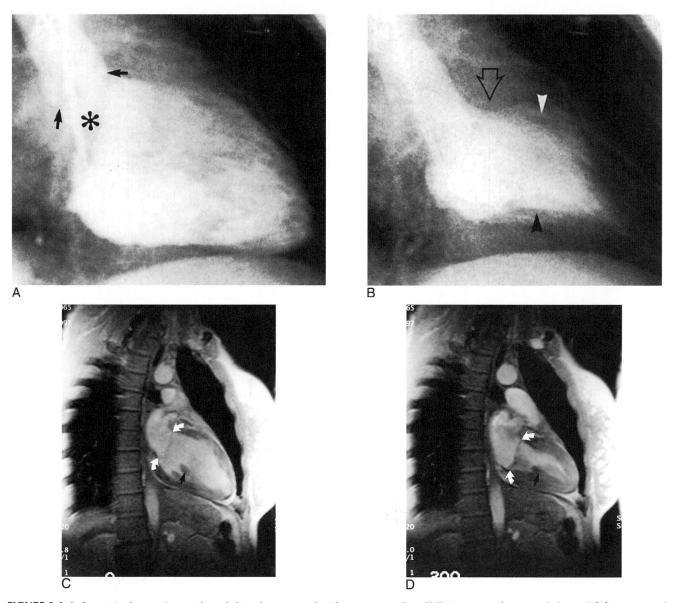

FIGURE 2-6. Left ventriculogram in systole and diastole compared with a corresponding CMR. Arrows at the upper left panel **(A)** represent the aortic valve plane on the RAO left ventriculogram. In the upper right panel **(B)**, the open arrow represents the location of the mitral valve and the closed arrows the papillary muscles. In the corresponding end-diastolic **(C)** and end-systolic **(D)** CMR images, the white arrows represent the mitral plane, and the dark arrows identify the papillary muscles. Note the relationship of the LV walls and papillary muscles to the LV contour. (From Hartnell GG, Raphael MJ. Cardiac anatomy and enlargement, in Grainger RG, Allison D, Adam A, Dixon AK (eds): *Diagnostic Radiology. A Textbook of Medical Imaging.* New York: Churchill Livingstone, 2001, p 679.)

normal. All these issues confound the development of appropriate mathematical models for LV volume determination and invalidate some of the quantitative wall motion analyses described later.

Frame-by-frame data from the LV volumes plotted over time (Figure 2-7) have been used to derive a number of systolic and diastolic parameters. Stroke volume is the difference between the LV end-diastolic and the LV end-systolic volumes. Ejection fraction is the most commonly used parameter derived from the volume curve data and is defined as LV stroke volume/LV end-diastolic volume. Ejection fraction can thus be obtained from knowledge of only two points on the volume-time curve.

These volume-time data can be matched with corresponding pressure from high-fidelity micromanometer pressure catheters to derive the entire pressure-volume relationship (Figure 2-8). The LV pressure-volume loop is counterclockwise with isovolumic contraction followed by systolic ejection, isovolumic relaxation, and diastolic filling, including the rapid filling phase and the passive filling phase. The area of the pressure-volume loop defines stroke work. By altering loading conditions, a series of pressure-volume loops is defined and can be used to calculate a variety of systolic and diastolic measures that are relatively load-independent assessments of contractile performance.[3] However, the complexity of such measures has limited

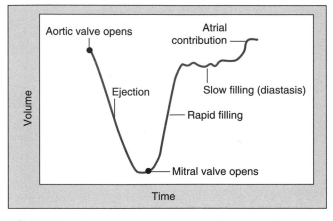

FIGURE 2-7. Schematic LV volume-time curve for a single beat.

their adoption into clinical practice, and, therefore, they will not be discussed in this chapter.

Right Ventricular Contraction and Function

After birth, the RV pumps into a pulmonary bed against low resistance. The RV is a thin-walled structure intended for volume and not pressure work. Although the RV shares the interventricular septum with the LV, the septum effectively functions as part of the LV. The curvature of the septum is toward the RV, and the RV pushes in a bellowslike manner against the septum to propel blood forward. RV contraction is complex, with several features occurring simultaneously. During systole, the RV trabeculae and papillary muscles pull the tricuspid valve toward the RV apex. At the same time, the RV free wall contracts and pushes the RV free wall toward the interventricular septum.

During LV contraction, the septum thickens and increases the septal curvature toward the RV. This tends to assist the RV in its bellows action. Right ventricular contraction pushes blood forward toward the pulmonary arteries, with the RV outflow tract contracting last. The pulmonary resistance is about 1/10th to 1/15th that of the systemic resistance. The result is that the RV pushes blood into a relaxed vas-

cular bed with blood flow continuing even after the onset of RV relaxation. This action results in the pulmonic valve closing later than the aortic valve, creating the normal splitting of the second heart sound. With inspiration, the reduced pleural pressure augments systemic venous return to the RV and reduces pulmonary venous return to the LV. Inspiration thus widens the splitting of the second heart sound.

When RV volume overload occurs, the chamber becomes more spherical, and the curvature of the interventricular septum may bow toward the LV during diastole. When the LV contracts in this situation, the septum seems to move "paradoxically" toward the RV during systole. During RV pressure overload, the normal bowing of the interventricular septum toward the RV during systole may be lost, and the septum appears flattened in both systole and diastole.

The pressure-volume relationship of the RV is similar to that of the LV, except that it varies greatly with respiration, and there is no true isovolumic relaxation slope. It is represented by a counterclockwise loop with isovolumic contraction followed by ejection, isovolumic relaxation, and finally filling of the RV.

GEOMETRIC MODELS OF VENTRICULAR VOLUMES

The volumes of the right and left ventricles can be determined by the different imaging techniques with variable degrees of accuracy. Each of the methods available makes assumptions regarding the shape of the ventricle on the basis of mathematical models. These models were derived from human heart casts and perform better when the LV and RV are of normal size and contractility. The models perform less well when disease states alter the basic architecture of the respective chambers. In addition, certain features of the imaging system, such as the inherent magnification created because of the divergence of X-rays used in contrast angiography or appropriate alignment of tomographic imaging planes using echocardiography, must be taken into account to estimate chamber volumes accurately for clinical purposes.

LV VOLUME MEASUREMENTS

The Area-Length Method

LV volumes are usually calculated in the cardiac catheterization laboratory using the area-length method applied to biplane LV angiograms (Figure 2-9). The basic assumption is that LV shape resembles an ellipse that has been rotated around its long axis. The concept capitalizes on the fact that the volume of an ellipsoid of revolution can be determined if the long axis (L) and the diameter of the ellipsoid in two short-axes (S and S' planes perpendicular to each other) are known.

The short axis can either be directly measured, or it can be calculated with knowledge of the long-axis dimension and the area of the ventricle in the long-axis view (hence the name area-length formula). The area of

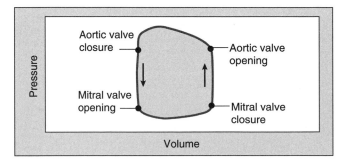

FIGURE 2-8. Schematic LV pressure-volume relationship for a single beat.

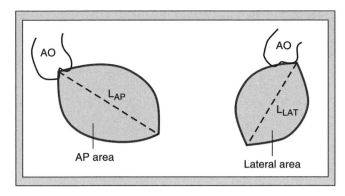

FIGURE 2-9. Modeling the cardiac chamber with an ellipsoid of revolution. The short-axis diameters are derived from the area. The only data needed, therefore, are the area and the length of the left ventricle. See text for formulas.

the chamber is planimetered. The formula for the volume of an ellipsoid is:

$$\text{Volume} = \frac{4\pi}{3} \times \frac{D}{2} \times \frac{D'}{2} \times \frac{L}{2}$$

where L is the long axis (longest chord that can be drawn) and D the short axis in one direction and D' the short axis in the other perpendicular direction.

From the planimetered area (A), the short-axis dimension can be derived by:

$$\text{Short axis } D = \frac{\text{Area}}{\pi L}$$

In biplane mode, D and D′ are each calculated from planimetered right anterior oblique (RAO) and left anterior oblique (LAO) views of the left ventricle. Thus, the formula becomes:

$$\text{Volume} = \frac{\pi L(D)(D')}{6} \text{ or } \frac{\pi L_{max}}{6} (4 A_{RAO}/\pi L_{RAO})(4 A_{LAO}/\pi L_{LAO})$$

Because the long axis in the LAO view is usually shorter than in the RAO view, the L_{max} cancels out of the equation, and the shorter of the two long axes (the LAO length) is used in the final formula:

$$\text{Area–Length Biplane Volume} = \frac{8}{3} \times \frac{A_{RAO} \times A_{LAO}}{\pi L_{min}}$$

The addition of the magnification correction factors (CF) completes the equation for calculating the volumes in a biplane mode. Note the correction factor is squared, because the formula uses an area determination in the numerator:

$$\text{Biplane volume} = \frac{8}{3} \times \frac{A_{RAO} \times A_{LAO}}{\pi L_{min}} \times \frac{(CF_{RAO})^2 \times (CF_{LAO})^2}{CF_{LAO}}$$

The area-length method can also be used for single-plane measurements, which assumes that the two short-axis diameters are equal. This assumption is only applicable when the LV is normal in size and function. Therefore, biplane determination is strongly recommended and should be considered the clinical "gold

standard." The area-length method can also be applied to other imaging modalities, such as echocardiography. The primary limitation of this model is that is assumes an elliptical geometry. In the case of spherical geometry (i.e., dilated cardiomyopathy) or distorted geometry (i.e., apical aneurysm), it is not as reliable.

Modified Simpson's Rule Method (Method of Disks)

Figure 2-10 outlines the use of Simpson's rule as applied to the LV. This method is based on the assumption that the cross-section of the LV can be defined as either circular or elliptical when sliced perpendicular to the long axis. As originally proposed, it required the measurement of corresponding horizontal axes at 1-mm intervals from the biplane cineangiogram. To obtain the best views of the ventricle for this purpose, biplane contrast angiography in the 25-degree RAO and 80-degree LAO projections are used. The volume (Vseg) of each segment is defined by the following: h = thickness of the each segment, A = the diameter of the segment in one view, and B = the diameter of the segment in the other view:

$$\text{Vseg} = \frac{\pi h (A \times B)}{4}$$

Total LV volume is calculated as the sum of the volumes of the individual segments. This requires the use of a computer, which is routine in the modern cardiac catheterization laboratory, but a major chore at the time this concept was developed. Biplane Simpson's rule is now the recommended method for calculating LV volumes by echocardiography. CMR is ideally suited to this model, because the slice thickness of each tomographic plane can be precisely known, and the volumes of a series of short-axis slices can be summed to obtain true LV volumes by Simpson's rule.

Three-Dimensional Imaging

By directly imaging the LV in three dimensions, reliance on geometric models is unnecessary. Several studies have

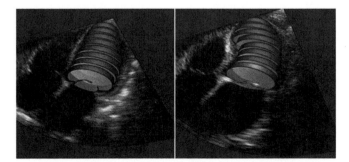

FIGURE 2-10. Simpson's rule method for determining LV volume. The volume of a series of disks from base to apex are summed to obtain LV volumes. The volume of each disk can be determined from its height and its major and minor axes. The latter is best determined from biplane measurements at cineangiography or echocardiography and may be directly measured by CMR. In this figure, a Simpson's rule measurement is illustrated for a normal LV (left) and an aneurysm of the LV apex (right). An area-length method would be inaccurate in the case of the aneurysm, because the geometric assumptions do not apply. As can be seen, Simpson's rule is still valid. (Courtesy of Brad Roberts, RDCS.)

used spatial three-dimensional (3D) reconstruction of echocardiographic images of the heart with good correlation of LV and RV volumes to in vitro and cineangiographic data. 3D reconstruction requires respiratory and ECG gating to orient images obtained in different planes at different times. Thus, a limitation of this technique is misregistration of images caused by cardiac motion, motion of the transducer, or changing cardiac cycle length. These problems should be eliminated by the recent development of real-time 3D image acquisition by echocardiography.[4]

Left Ventricular Mass

LV mass can be estimated by the area-length method by assuming a uniform shell of myocardium around the LV angiographic chamber (Figure 2-11). This requires an estimation of the LV wall thickness, which angiography does rather poorly compared with other techniques such as echocardiography and CMR. The wall thickness (h) on each side of the angiographic ellipsoid is added to each side of the ellipsoid. Thus, 2h is added to the long axis, and 2h is added to the calculated short axis to derive the epicardial shell of the ventricle. Each volume is then corrected by the appropriate regression equation. Subtraction of the angiographic shell from the calculated epicardial shell provides an estimate of total LV myocardial wall volume. Because the specific gravity of heart muscle is approximately 1.05, the total wall volume is multiplied by 1.05 to obtain the wall mass.

The calculations for biplane cineangiography are:

$$\text{Epicardial LV volume} = \frac{4}{3} \times \pi \times \frac{(L+2h)}{2} \times \frac{(S+2h)}{2} \times \frac{(S'+2h)}{2}$$

where L = the minimal long axis in the two views (usually the LAO) of chamber volume; S = short axis of chamber volume in RAO; and S' = short axis of chamber volume in LAO.

LV wall volume = Corrected LV epicardial volume – Corrected LV chamber volume
LV mass = 1.05 × LV wall volume

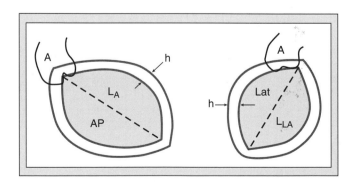

FIGURE 2-11. Schematic diagram for determining LV mass from biplane cineangiography. The width of the LV wall is added to the lengths and widths around the LV chamber to construct the LV volume that includes the wall thickness. Subtracting the LV chamber volume results in a shell representing the LV muscle volume. LV muscle volume (mL) × 1.05 mg/mL = LV mass. See text for details.

Given the difficulty in determining precise wall thickness by angiography, LV wall thickness might be better seen on the LAO view or might be directly measured by echocardiography, computed tomography, or CMR and added to the equation subsequently. Early echocardiographic estimates of LV mass were determined from single-dimensional M-mode measurements and corrected by a regression equation (Penn formula). Two-dimensional (2D) measurements have been validated, and it is reasonable to expect that 3D real-time measurements will be even more accurate. CMR has become the "gold standard" for quantifying LV mass because of its 3D spatial resolution.[5] By use of CMR, the volume of each of a series of short-axis slices is measured and Simpson's rule applied to calculate LV mass with a factor of 1.05 for the specific gravity of heart muscle.[5]

RV Volume Measurements

Given the complex shape and contraction pattern of the RV described previously, it is not surprising that there is no consensus regarding a model for determining RV volumes. The first attempt to measure RV volume applied Simpson's rule to the entire heart, then removed the left ventricle and interventricular septum. Other approaches have used the area-length method, a modified Simpson's rule, the parallelepiped method, a two-chamber model (an ellipsoid body and cylinder outflow), or assumed a prism shape or a three-sided pyramid. None of these models have achieved the level of acceptance required for incorporation into routine clinical practice. However, the advent of real-time 3D echocardiography and rapid CMR scanners now permits quantitation of RV volumes without geometric assumptions regarding RV shape.

CLINICAL ASSESSMENT OF VENTRICULAR VOLUMES AND GEOMETRY

Cardiac Catheterization/Contrast Angiography

The general shape of the LV is that of an ellipsoid of revolution as described previously. Figure 2-6 depicts the angiographic LV in the 30-degree RAO and compares it with a corresponding MR image to highlight the myocardium and papillary muscle locations. In modern cardiac catheterization laboratories, the RAO and LAO views are obtained on all patients. Failure to obtain the LAO view might result in inadequate description of septal and posterior wall motion. The cranial LAO view (hepatoclavicular view) can also be useful when the LV outflow tract needs to be well visualized, such as in localizing a ventricular septal defect or defining systolic anterior motion of the mitral valve, because this view best outlines the interventricular septum.

Early angiographic studies compared LV volumes with volumes of postmortem hearts filled with radiographic contrast material. It was observed that angiography tended to overestimate LV volumes because of the influence of papillary muscles and trabeculations.

Accordingly, specific regression equations were derived to correct angiographic volumes for this overestimation. These equations are shown in Table 2-1. Normal values for angiographic LV volumes in adults are shown in Table 2-2. Although normal values for angiographic LV mass were reported in these studies, angiography is unreliable for measuring LV mass, so that echocardiography or CMR should be used instead.

Biplane contrast angiography provides reasonable estimates of RV volume, although the unusual shape of the RV makes models of RV volume difficult to derive. Traditionally, the methods for determining RV volumes use the anteroposterior (AP) and lateral angiographic views. There have been numerous efforts to validate angiographic models to assess RV volumes, but there are difficulties inherent with all of these methods. These include a modification of the ellipsoid area-length method, the assumption that the RV can be converted to a parallelepiped, the assumption that the body of the RV resembles an ellipsoid and the outflow tract a cylinder (two-chamber model), the use of Simpson's rule, or the assumption that the RV shape is either a prism or a three-sided pyramid. In general, the difficulties inherent in these models have prevented angiography from being used in routine clinical practice to measure RV volumes.

Echocardiography

Echocardiography is the most widely used imaging modality in cardiology and is commonly used in clinical practice to measure ventricular size, mass, and geometry. Traditional echocardiographic measurements of LV size have used single-dimensional linear measurements, initially by M-mode and later by 2D echocardiography. A single linear dimension is inadequate to assess LV volumes. The American Society of Echocardiography has recommended the use of a biplane Simpson's rule method for calculating LV volumes from an apical four-chamber and apical two-chamber view. The values for 2D echocardiographic volumes in normal subjects are shown in Table 2-3. Echocardiography offers several advantages over angiography in calculating LV volumes.

■ ■ ■

TABLE 2-1 REGRESSION EQUATIONS CORRECTIONS FOR DETERMINING LV VOLUMES

Method	Regression equation	Author
Adults		
Biplane Dodge area-length RAO/LAO	$V_A = 0.989\, V_C - 8.1$	Wynne[*]
Biplane Dodge area-length AP/lateral	$V_A = 0.929\, V_C - 3.8$	Dodge[†]
Biplane Arcilla area-length AP/lateral	$V_A = 0.992\, Vc - 0.78$	Arcilla[‡]
Single-plane Dodge area-length RAO	$V_A = 0.938\, V_C - 5.7$	Wynne[*]
Single-plane Dodge area-length RAO	$V_A = 0.81\, V_C + 1.9$	Kennedy[§]
Single-plane Dodge area-length AP	$V_A = 0.951\, V_C - 3.0$	Sandler[‖]
Children		
Biplane Dodge area-length AP/lateral	$V_A = 0.733\, V_C$	Graham[¶]

V_A, Alveolar ventilation; V_C, pulmonary capillary blood volume.
[*]Wynne J, Green L, Mann T, Levin D, Grossman W. Estimation of left ventricular volumes in man from biplane cineangiograms filmed in oblique projections. *Am J Cardiol* 1978; 41:7226.
[†]Dodge HT, Sandler H, Ballew DW, Lord JDJ. The use of biplane angiocardiography for the measurement of left ventricular volume in man. *Am Heart J* 1960; 60:762.
[‡]Arcilla RA, Tsai P, Thilenius O, Ranniger K. Angiographic method for volume estimation of right and left ventricles. *Chest* 1971; 60(5):446.
[§]Kennedy JW, Trenholme SE, Kasser IS. Left ventricular volume and mass from single-plane cineangiocardiogram. A comparison of anteroposterior and right anterior oblique methods. *Am Heart J* 1970; 80:343.
[‖]Sandler H, Dodge HT. The use of single plane angiocardiograms for the calculation of left ventricular volume in man. *Am Heart J* 1968; 75:325.
[¶]Graham TP, Jr, Atwood GF, Faulkner SL, Nelson JH. Right atrial volume measurements from biplane cineangiocardiography. Methodology, normal values, and alterations with pressure or volume overload. *Circulation* 1974; 49(4):709-16.

It is noninvasive, relatively inexpensive, and has very good spatial and temporal resolution. On the other hand, high-quality images cannot be obtained in all patients with echocardiography caused by poor acoustic windows. Several studies have shown good correlation between LV volumes determined by biplane echocardiography and biplane LV angiography. However, compared with angiography, echocardiography tends to underestimate LV volumes. One important reason for this is foreshortening of the LV long axis because of failure of the

■ ■ ■

TABLE 2-2 REPRESENTATIVE NORMAL LV CHAMBER VOLUMES AND MASS IN ADULTS BY ANGIOGRAPHY

Method	EDV (mL)	ESV (mL)	EF (%)	LV mass (g)	Author
BP area-length	70 ± 20	24 ± 10	67 ± 8	92 ± 16	Kennedy[*]
BP area-length	72 ± 15	20 ± 8	72 ± 8		Wynne[†]
BP area-length	79 ± 4	28 ± 2	67 ± 3	93 ± 8	Hood[‡]
BP area-length	59 ± 4	14 ± 2	76 ± 2		Peterson[§]
BP area-length	57 ±18	14 ± 7	74 ±−11		Arvidsson[‖]
SP area-length	93 ± 18	27 ± 9	72 ± 6	93 ± 27	Rousseau[¶]
SP area-length	81 ± 15	−	70 ± 7	81 ± 18	Huber[**]

[*]Kennedy JW, Baxley WA, Figley MM, et al. Quantitative angiocardiography. I. The normal left ventricle in man. *Circulation* 1966; 34:272.
[†]Wynne J, Green L, Mann T, Levin D, Grossman W. Estimation of left ventricular volumes in man from biplane cineangiograms filmed in oblique projections. *Am J Cardiol* 1978; 41:7226.
[‡]Hood WPJ, Rackley CE, Rolett EL. Wall stress in the normal and hypertrophied heart. *Am J Cardiol* 1968; 22:550.
[§]Peterson KL, Skloven D, Ludbrook P, et al. Comparison of isovolumic and ejection phase indices of myocardial performance in man. *Circulation* 1974; 49:1088.
[‖]Arvidsson H. Angiocardiographic determination of left ventricular volume and its applications. *Radiology* 1967; 7:200.
[¶]Rousseau MF, Pouleur H, Charlier AA, Brasseur LA. Assessment of left ventricular relaxation in patients with valvular regurgitation. *Am J Cardiol* 1982; 50:1028.
[**]Huber D, Grimm J, Koch R, Krayenbuehl HP. Determinants of ejection performance in aortic stenosis. *Circulation* 1981; 64:126.

■ ■ ■

TABLE 2-3   NORMAL REFERENCE RANGES FOR 2D ECHOCARDIOGRAPHIC MEASUREMENTS OF LV VOLUMES AND MASS

Measurement	Reference range	
	Men	Women
LV end-diastolic volume (mL)	62-170	55-101
LV end-systolic volume (mL)	14-76	13-60
LV mass (g)	80-210	76-144
LV end-diastolic volume/mass ratio	0.49-1.17	0.62-1.21

Data from Wahr DW, Wang YS, Schiller NB. Left ventricular volumes determined by two-dimensional echocardiography in a normal population. *J Am Cardiol* 1983;1:863; and Byrd BF III, Wahr D, Wang YS, Bouchard A, Schiller NB. Left ventricular mass and volume/mass ratio determined by two-dimensional echocardiography in normal adults. *J Am Coll Cardiol* 1985; 6:1021.

■ ■ ■

TABLE 2-4   ABSOLUTE DIFFERENCE BETWEEN 2D ECHOCARDIOGRAPHIC AND CMR MEASUREMENTS OF LV VOLUMES AND EJECTION FRACTION

	Precontrast Echo–CMR	Postcontrast Echo–CMR	P value
LV end-diastolic volume (mL)	21 ± 13	15 ± 14	0.038
LV end-systolic volume (mL)	17 ± 13	12 ± 9	0.015
LVEF (%)	8 ± 6	5 ± 3	0.031

Modified from Hundley WG, Kizilbash AM, Afridi I, Franco F, Peshock RM, Grayburn PA. Administration of an intravenous contrast agent improves echocardiographic determination of left ventricular volumes and ejection fraction: a comparison with cine magnetic resonance imaging. *J Am Coll Cardiol* 1998; 32:1426.

transducer to overlie the true LV apex. This problem can be ameliorated by 3D reconstruction of multiple image planes or, more recently, by direct real-time 3D imaging. Lee et al[6] compared an early-generation real-time 3D echocardiography system with cine CMR for determination of LV volumes. An excellent correlation ($r = 0.99$ for both end-diastolic and end-systolic volumes) was observed. By Bland-Altman analysis, the 95% limits of agreement between the two techniques ranged from −24 mL to 24 mL for end-diastolic volume and −16 mL to 24 mL for end-systolic volume.

Other technical developments that improve the accuracy of echocardiography for determination of LV volumes are harmonic imaging and intravenous contrast agents (Figure 2-12). Signal dropout in the apical views often precludes accurate tracing of the endocardial borders. The use of a contrast agent virtually eliminates this problem and also allows salvage of a high percentage of technically difficult echocardiograms.[6] Recent studies have compared 2D echocardiography with and without contrast with cine CMR. The correlation coefficients between 2D echocardiography and CMR were excellent regardless of the use of a contrast agent; however, the absolute difference between echocardiographic and CMR measurements was significantly reduced by the addition of contrast (Table 2-4). Similar

findings were also reported by Thomsen et al[7] comparing LV volume measurements by harmonic contrast echocardiography, to electron-beam CT imaging. It is anticipated that the combination of real-time, harmonic 3D echocardiography and contrast agents will enable accurate measurements of LV volumes without the need for geometric assumptions about the shape of the ventricle.

In addition to measuring LV volumes, echocardiography is useful in the assessment of LV mass and geometry, which are important indices of LV remodeling in hypertension, valvular heart disease, cardiomyopathy, and after myocardial infarction. LV mass has been measured by M-mode echocardiography for many years and has been shown to predict cardiovascular mortality in large population studies. The formula for M-mode LV mass is based on the assumption of cuboid geometry and is calculated by the formula:

$$LVM = 1.04\ [(LVID + IVS + PW)^3 - (LVID)^3] - 13.6$$

where *LVID* is LV internal diameter, *IVS* is interventricular septal thickness, and *PW* is posterior wall thickness. The major limitation of M-mode measurements is that the 95% confidence intervals are very wide and interstudy reproducibility is poor. Thus, M-mode measurements of LV mass are not reliable for accurately detecting regression of hypertrophy within individual patients. Both 2D and 3D echocardiography are superior to M-mode for LV mass measurements. The American Society of Echocardiography recommends calculation of LV mass from 2D echocardiography by use of either the area-length method or truncated ellipsoid method that is shown in Figure 2-13.

Although LV end-diastolic volume is an important measure of LV remodeling, it does not convey specific information about LV shape. Accordingly, echocardiography is often used to measure the geometric change from an ellipsoidal LV to a more spherical LV. A practical method to calculate shape is to simply calculate the LV major-to-minor axis ratio from an apical four-chamber view (Figure 2-14). A normal end-diastolic major-to-minor axis ratio is 1.9 ± 0.2[8]; a decline in this value toward 1:1 indicates that the LV is assuming spherical geometry. A more sophisticated method is to define LV

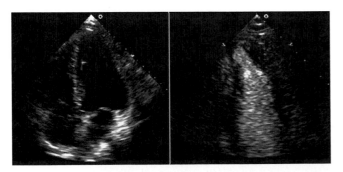

FIGURE 2-12. Echocardiograms obtained before (left) and after (right) administration of an intravenous contrast agent. Endocardial borders are more clearly seen, and a small apical aneurysm is only identified on the contrast-enhanced image. The image on the right is magnified. (Courtesy of Brad Roberts, RDCS.)

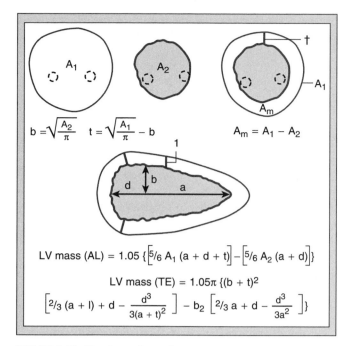

FIGURE 2-13. 2D echocardiographic measurements of LV mass. *Upper panel,* Schematic diagram of LV short-axis view at the papillary muscle tip level. Average myocardial thickness (t) and short-axis radius (b) are calculated from the traced epicardial (A_1) and endocardial (A_2) areas. *Bottom panel,* LV mass is calculated using the area-length (AL) or truncated ellipsoid (TE) formulas, where *a* = long-axis length from the widest minor axis radius to the apex, *b* = average short-axis radius, *t* = average short-axis wall thickness, and *d* = long-axis length from the widest minor axis radius to the mitral annulus plane. (Reprinted with permission from Schiller NB, Shah PM, Crawford M, DeMaria A, Devereux R, Feigenbaum H, Gutgesell H, Reichek N, Sahn D, Schnittger I. Recommendations for quantitation of the left ventricle by two-dimensional echocardiography. American Society of Echocardiography Committee on Standards, Subcommittee on Quantitation of Two-Dimensional Echocardiograms. *J Am Soc Echocardiogr* 1989;2:358.)

shape is to calculate the sphericity index, which is the LV end-diastolic volume determined by biplane Simpson's rule divided by the volume of a sphere whose diameter is equal to the length of the LV. An increase in the sphericity index toward 1.0 indicates spherical LV remodeling.

RV volume assessment by M-mode or 2D echocardiography is difficult because of the complex shape of the RV. Accordingly, RV volumes are not generally measured in clinical practice. However, the advent of 3D echocardiography promises to enable accurate measurements of RV volumes. Recently, real-time 3D echocardiography was evaluated in vitro and in vivo and found to be accurate in measuring RV volumes.[9] Importantly, the use of 3D imaging avoids the need for geometric assumptions about RV shape.

Cardiac Magnetic Resonance (CMR) Imaging

CMR is currently considered the "gold standard" for assessment of ventricular volumes and mass because of its high spatial resolution and the fact that it measures these parameters directly from a series of tomographic slices and does not require geometric assumptions. Figure 2-15 shows an example of calculation of LV volumes and mass by cine CMR with the gradient-echo technique. Current technology allows acquisition of a series of short-axis slices of known thickness (usually 8-10 mm) from base to apex during a single breath hold. The area of the cavity and myocardium is traced for each slice at end-diastole and end-systole and summed to determine LV volumes. Mass is determined by multiplying the summed myocardial volumes by 1.05 (specific gravity of tissue). The use of CMR to measure LV volumes and mass has been validated against human postmortem hearts. Subsequent clinical application has shown that interstudy[9] reproducibility of the measurements is superior to echocardiographic and nuclear techniques.[10,11] These factors render CMR superior to angiography or echocardiography for detecting small time-dependent changes in LV volumes or mass in individual patients.[12,13] Normal values for LV volumes and mass by CMR have been published and are similar to values obtained by LV angiography and echocardiography.[14]

Nuclear Imaging

Although nuclear methods are widely used to calculate LVEF (Figure 2-16) and to assess myocardial perfusion, their poor spatial resolution limits their accuracy for LV volumes or mass determination. Ioannidis published a

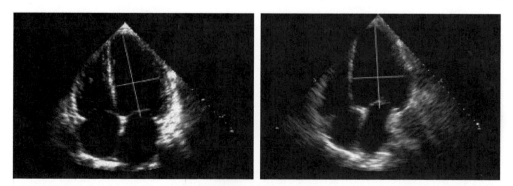

FIGURE 2-14. Major-to-minor axis ratio as a means of measuring LV shape changes associated with LV remodeling. At left is a normal LV with a major-to-minor axis ratio of 2.0. At right is a dilated LV with a major-to-minor axis ratio of 1.4. Sphericity index can be calculated as the volume of the LV (by biplane Simpson's rule) divided by the volume of a sphere whose diameter is equal to the major axis (length) of the LV. (Courtesy of Brad Roberts, RDCS.)

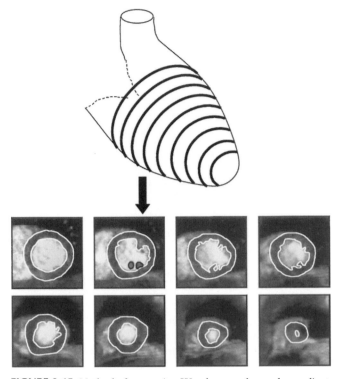

FIGURE 2-15. Method of measuring LV volume and mass by gradient-echo cine CMR. See text for details. (Reproduced from Myerson SG, Bellenger NG, Pennell DJ. Assessment of left ventricular mass by cardiovascular magnetic resonance. *Hypertension* 2002;39:750.)

meta-analysis of gated single photon emission computed tomography (SPECT) imaging compared with CMR for assessment of LV volumes.[11] Although good correlation coefficients were found between the two techniques, the rate of clinically significant misclassification of individual subjects was 37% for end-diastolic volume, 35% for end-systolic volume, and 23% for LVEF.

Computed Tomography

The development of spiral computed technology (CT) and electron-beam CT has enabled imaging of the heart within a single breath hold. An important feature of CT imaging is the excellent resolution of the endocardial and epicardial borders, resulting in accurate assessment of LV and RV volumes and LV mass.[15]

CLINICAL ASSESSMENT OF GLOBAL LV SYSTOLIC FUNCTION

LV Ejection Fraction

The left ventricular ejection fraction (LVEF) is the most commonly used measure of systolic function from a clinical and imaging standpoint. It was originally derived from angiographic LV volumes as the stroke volume (end-diastolic volume – end-systolic volume) divided by the LV end-diastolic volume. The normal

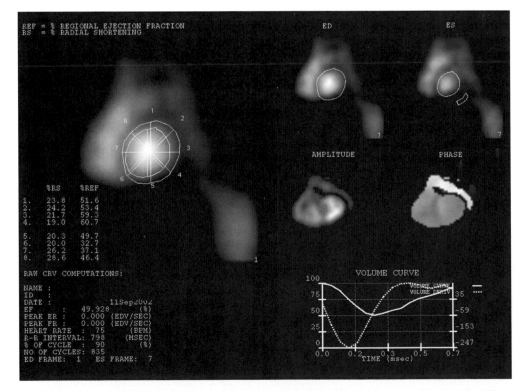

FIGURE 2-16. Radionuclide angiogram by MUGA technique. At the upper right, regions of interest are drawn around the left ventricle in a left anterior oblique projection at end-diastole (ED) and end-systole (ES). A volume-time curve showing radioactive counts during the cardiac cycle is shown at bottom right. The global LVEF is 50%. At upper left is a polar map showing percent radial shortening and percent ejection fraction in each of eight segments. (Courtesy of Michael Brophey, MD.) See also Color Insert.

LVEF is greater than 55%. LV angiography, echocardiography, cine CMR, and CT are commonly used to measure LVEF from LV volume data. The sources of error are related to technical issues in measuring volumes. For example, LV volumes and LVEF might be inaccurate by angiography in the setting of catheter-induced ectopy or if an inadequate amount of contrast is injected. Echocardiographic LVEF might suffer from endocardial "dropout" or poor acoustic windows. However, the use of echo contrast agents dramatically improves the accuracy of assessing LVEF.[7] CMR assessment of LVEF is accurate provided there are no motion artifacts or difficulties with ECG gating. Radionuclide angiography uses a count-based method in which radioactive counts at end-diastole and end-systole are used to calculate LVEF. This technique does not require calculation of LV volumes, is independent of LV shape, and has been widely used to measure LVEF in clinical trials. The advent of digital catheterization laboratories has enabled videodensitometry to calculate LVEF in a similar nongeometric method. Because X-rays are absorbed in an exponential manner, the X-ray signal must be logarithmically amplified to derive any linear relationship between the amount of contrast in the LV and the resultant video signal. Using a region of interest between the end-diastolic and end-systolic LV contours, an average background density can be derived and digital subtraction angiography used. The ejection fraction determined in this manner has correlated well with the area-length method ($r = 0.94$).

Although LVEF is a powerful prognostic tool in clinical cardiology, it has limitations that have stimulated a search for more fiducial measures of global LV systolic function. For example, LVEF is exquisitely dependent on afterload, preload, myocardial contractility, synchrony of the regional contractile pattern, and heart rate. These hemodynamic variables importantly affect what is considered the "normal" LVEF, for which reason there has been interest in further refining LVEF by dividing the change in stroke volume throughout systole into thirds. The percentage of stroke volume ejected during the first, second, and third portion of systole is then reported in an effort to further define the rate of LV ejection. Normal values have been reported to be $44 \pm 3\%$ for the first tercile, $33 \pm 2\%$ for the second tercile, and $21 \pm 3\%$ for the third tercile of systole. Another attempt to glean more information from the LV volume curve has been to assess the mean normalized systolic ejection rate. This is expressed as the LVEF/LV ejection time and results in an expression of end-diastolic volume per second, and as such represents an estimation of the rate of LV emptying. It has been proposed as a means to separate patients with normal LV function from those with depressed LV function with an apparently normal LVEF. However, these refinements have not proved useful clinically.

Still another attempt at defining LV performance relies on the determination of the rate of change of a midwall hoop around the equator of the LV ellipsoid. The rate of change of this hoop can be expressed in mean circumferences per second or the velocity of circumferential fiber shortening (Vcf). It is defined as:

$$Vcf = \frac{(M_{ed} - M_{es})}{ET \times M_{ed}}$$

where M_{ed} is the LV diameter at the minor equator in end-diastole, M_{es} is the LV diameter at the minor equator in end-systole, and ET is the LV ejection time. Although this is used sporadically clinically as a global index of contractile function, it is actually a measure of regional (minor equator) contractile performance with normal values of approximately 1.5 circumferences per second.

Correction of LVEF for Loading Conditions

Although widely used as a measure of global LV function, LVEF is more correctly a measure of chamber function rather than myocardial function. In the setting of abnormal loading conditions, such as valvular heart disease or hypertension, LVEF might reflect normal LV chamber function, even when intrinsic myocardial function is abnormal. Correcting LVEF for circumferential wall stress allows impaired myocardial function to be unmasked. This method has not been used widely in the clinical setting and is not as sensitive as the end-systolic pressure-volume relationship (see later) in detecting subtle decreases in contractility in aortic regurgitation. Figure 2-17 illustrates the relationship between LVEF and circumferential wall stress in normal subjects and in patients with aortic stenosis and dilated cardiomyopathy. Echocardiography has been used to plot LV fractional shortening or midwall shortening against end-systolic wall stress and shows a similar relationship to that seen in Figure 2-17.[16] Unfortunately, these echocardiographic techniques use single-dimensional M-mode measurements and are therefore dependent on the assumption that the myocardium is of uniform thickness and that the disease process is uniform. This can be overcome by the use of CMR, which can accurately measure wall stress and wall thickening in 3D space.[17]

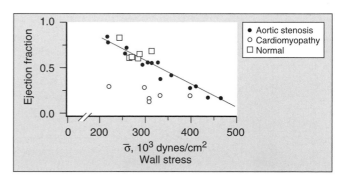

FIGURE 2-17. Relationship of LVEF to circumferential wall stress in normal patients, patients with aortic stenosis, and patients with dilated cardiomyopathy. Patients with aortic stenosis and normal controls fall along the normal LVEF-wall stress linear relation. Patients with cardiomyopathy have reduced LVEF for a given wall stress and fall below and to the left of the normal relation illustrated by the regression line. (Reproduced from Mirsky I, Tajimi T, Peterson KL. The development of the entire pressure-volume and ejection-afterload relations: a new concept of systolic myocardial stiffness. *Circulation* 1987; 76:343; with permission.)

End-Systolic Elastance

The optimal method of assessing myocardial contractility is to derive end-systolic elastance from a series of pressure-volume loops generated at different loading conditions (Figure 2-18). This is usually performed in the cardiac catheterization laboratory, where LV pressure is measured directly, preferably with a high-fidelity micromanometer-tipped catheter, and LV volumes are simultaneously measured using biplane cineangiography. Loading conditions are typically altered by infusion of vasoactive drugs to manipulate afterload or, alternately, by transient balloon occlusion of the inferior vena cava. The slope of the line connecting the end-systolic points on the pressure-volume loops is end-systolic elastance (Ees) and is a measure of contractility that is preload independent and incorporates afterload. Ees has been widely used to unmask myocardial contractile dysfunction in valvular heart disease, where abnormal loading conditions often result in normal LVEF. Unfortunately, the measurement of Ees is time-consuming and therefore rarely performed in clinical practice. Because measurement of Ees requires end-systolic LV pressure measurement, it is not usually obtained with noninvasive imaging techniques when end-systolic pressure is not measured directly.

Cardiac Output

Along with LVEF, cardiac output is one of the most widely used measurements of global LV performance. Invasive measurements of cardiac output using Fick, green dye, or thermodilution techniques actually measure RV cardiac output from catheters placed in the right side of the heart. However, imaging techniques can directly measure cardiac output from either ventricle as the difference between end-diastolic and end-systolic

volumes multiplied by the heart rate. The accuracy of such measurements is dependent on the accuracy of measurements of LV and RV volumes. As noted earlier, CMR is the most accurate and reproducible method of measuring LV volumes because of its high spatial resolution and the absence of geometric assumptions. Recently, CMR and 3D echocardiographic measurements of stroke volume have been validated against an electromagnetic flow probe in a sheep model.[17] Cardiac output can also be derived without using LV volumes. Both echocardiography and CMR can be used to measure aortic annulus velocity and cross-sectional area, the product of which is stroke volume. Figure 2-19 illustrates the Doppler method for calculation of cardiac output. The diameter of the LV outflow tract is measured, and the cross-sectional area of the LV tract is calculated assuming circular geometry. Pulsed-wave Doppler is used to obtain the velocity-time integral of blood flow in the LV outflow tract. The product of these two parameters is stroke volume; cardiac output is stroke volume multiplied by heart rate. Doppler LV outflow tract velocity-time integral is a measurement of stroke distance (the distance over which the heart would propel a red blood cell), which, unlike cardiac output, is independent of body surface area and therefore is a useful and simple measure of global LV function.[18] The normal stroke distance is 18 to 22 cm.

Isovolumic Phase Measurements of Global LV Function

LVEF is an ejection-phase index of global LV function. Isovolumic phase indices, such as first derivative of pressure measured over time (dp/dt), are usually measured from catheters placed in the LV rather than from imaging techniques. Some investigators have validated measuring dp/dt from the Doppler velocity spectrum of patients with mitral regurgitation. In mitral regurgitation, there is no true isovolumic period; however, the measured dp/dt correlates closely with that measured at catheterization. Another index is the Tei index, in which Doppler measurements are used to calculate the systolic ejection period, the isovolumic contraction period, and the isovolumic relaxation period. The Tei index has been proposed as a combined measure of systolic and diastolic LV function that is independent of heart rate and blood pressure. The Tei index is defined as the sum of isovolumic contraction time and isovolumic relaxation time divided by ejection time.

Global RV Function

As noted earlier, the complex shape of the RV makes it difficult to assess RV volumes by cineangiography or echocardiography, wherein assumptions regarding RV geometry are necessary. However, real-time 3D echocardiography and CMR can measure RV volumes without geometric assumptions, thereby resulting in accurate calculation of RVEF.[19] Likewise, radionuclide angiography yields RVEF on the basis of radioactivity counts, not on geometric assumptions. The latter technique has been used in clinical trials to assess RVEF.

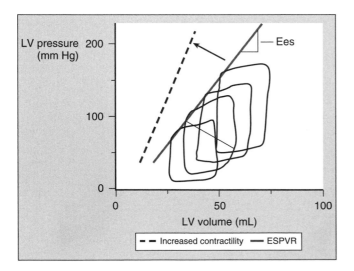

FIGURE 2-18. Schematic diagram of four pressure-volume loops generated at different levels of afterload. The end-systolic pressure-volume relation (ESPVR) is defined by the dark line, the slope of which is end-systolic elastance (Ees). A shift in the ESPVR to the left with an increase in Ees indicates increased contractility. A shift in the ESPVR to the right with a decrease in Ees (not shown) indicates decreased contractility.

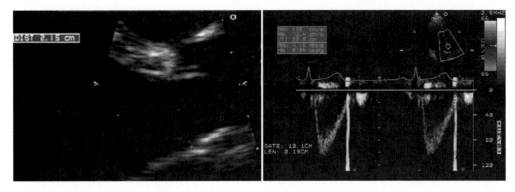

FIGURE 2-19. Doppler method of measuring cardiac output at the aortic annulus. *Left panel,* Parasternal long-axis view using zoom mode to magnify the measurement of the LV outflow tract diameter at the base of the aortic leaflets. *Right panel,* Pulsed Doppler velocity signal from the LV outflow tract. The modal velocity is traced to display the velocity-time integral in centimeters. This value is equal to the stroke distance or the distance that the heart would propel a single red blood cell. The product of stroke distance and LV outflow tract cross-sectional area is the stroke volume. (Courtesy of Brad Roberts, RDCS.) See also Color Insert.

CLINICAL ASSESSMENT OF REGIONAL WALL MOTION

Cardiac Catheterization/Cineangiography

Visual Grading of Wall Motion

Left ventricular regional wall motion is complex and is graded visually by comparing the contours of the angiogram from diastole to systole. Figure 2-20 reflects the terminology in general usage. Normal wall motion implies that the LV contour moves from its end-diastolic to end-systolic location vigorously and concentrically, reflecting normal ventricular wall thickening. Hypokinesia implies reduced end-diastolic to end-systolic wall motion and corresponds to reduced systolic wall thickening. Akinesia is lack of motion from end-diastole to end-systole caused by absent wall thickening. Dyskinesia is an outward movement of the LV contour during systole and corresponds to systolic ventricular wall bulging.

Visual estimates of the ejection fraction are more difficult than many appreciate. It has been our clinical experience that the larger the end-diastolic volume, the greater likelihood of underestimating true (calculated) ejection fraction by visual inspection of the cineangiogram.

Measurements of Regional Wall Motion

Regional wall motion abnormalities are particularly evident in patients with coronary artery disease. Although global measurements reflect the net performance of the LV chamber, quantitation of regional wall motion allows for greater sensitivity of regional wall motion abnormalities and assists with interpretation of global changes in the LVEF. Measurements of regional wall motion suffer from lack of a clearly defined "gold standard." Implantable metallic markers have been used to help validate some of the models described later, but these markers might underestimate the extent of endocardial shortening, because they do not completely account for LV wall thickening in the region of interest.

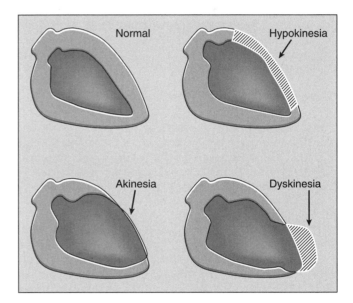

FIGURE 2-20. Visual grading of regional wall motion by cineangiography. See text for details.

The complex motion of the LV confounds efforts to quantify regional wall motion. For instance, to correct for the translational motion of the heart and the descent of the aortic and mitral valves, some of the methods that have been used have realigned the systolic and diastolic LV contours. The validity of this realignment has never been proven and might create artifactual wall motion measurements. Although regional wall-thickening measurements would obviate the concern regarding translational rotation of the heart, it easier to measure wall thickening by use of echocardiography or CMR tagging methods.

Wall motion analysis methods vary widely. All of the methods in current use are based on tracing the LV end-diastolic and LV end-systolic contours. These methods either realign the end-systolic and end-diastolic ventricular contours in some manner, such as aligning the coronary sinus or aortic valve planes or some central portion of the silhouette, or they make no effort to realign. The regional wall motion programs allow for measurement of regional wall motion changes using rectilinear systems, radial systems, area methods, or the centerline approach. The latter approach is the best and most commonly used.

Hemiaxial Rectilinear Method

In this system, the long axes of the diastolic and systolic contours are aligned, and perpendicular chords are drawn. The plane of the coronary sinus or the aortic valve may or may not be aligned, depending on the practices of individual laboratories. The assumption is that the endocardial surface moves toward the line defining the long axis of the LV during systole. To measure this change, the long axis of both the end-diastolic and end-systolic contours are divided into either four or five equal segments, and perpendicular hemiaxes to the long axis are drawn. The percent change of these hemiaxes defines the regional endocardial motion at each point along the LV contour (Figure 2-21). This change is usually normalized for the end-diastolic length and expressed as a fractional change:

$$\text{Fractional shortening} = \frac{\text{End-diastolic length} - \text{End-systolic length}}{\text{End-diastolic length}}$$

The use of the normalized shortening from both end-diastolic and end-systolic long axes is the preferable method. The area reduction of each of the segments outlined by the ventricular contour and the hemiaxes can also be plotted for each region (see Figure 2-21).

Hemiaxial Radial Methods

Radial methods assume the LV contracts toward a single point in the middle of the ventricle. That point is usually defined as the geometric center of gravity (centroid) or the midpoint of the long axis. The end-systolic silhouette center of gravity is then superimposed on the end-diastolic center of gravity, or the origins of both of the contours are aligned. Figure 2-22 displays the radial methods for quantitating region wall motion. Once the contours are aligned, radii are drawn from the center sweeping the LV outlines in a clockwise manner. The aortic valve region is usually excluded from the analysis. Anywhere from 8 to more than 100 radii can be drawn. The normalized change in the respective radii can then be plotted and compared with a set of normal values.

Area Reduction Methods

The hemiaxial and radial methods also lend themselves to analysis of the reduction in the areas subtended by the respectively drawn chords. Alternative approaches have even divided the LV into only three or four areas by bisecting the long axis of the LV. Comparisons of the hemiaxial, radial, and area reduction methods have yielded mixed results. The radial method was found to agree well with surgically implanted midwall myocardial markers.

Centerline Methods

Several inherent problems exist in the use of all the model systems described previously. First is the fact that the apex is a poorly visualized landmark with the highest degree of variability, and its use to define the length in earlier models is problematic. Second, the assumption that systolic wall motion proceeds toward the long axis or a centroid is unfounded. Third, the variable shape of the LV in differing views makes the use of the hemiaxial, radial, or area reduction methods impractical for the LAO

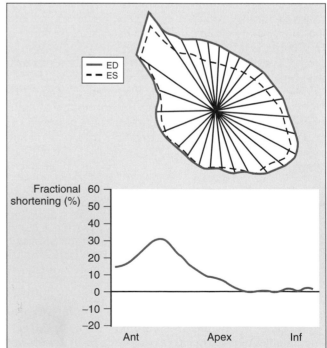

FIGURE 2-22. Radial methods for determining regional wall motion abnormalities. Either individual spokes of radii or the areas between them can be plotted to represent regional wall motion changes. ED = end-diastolic contour, ES = end-systolic contour.

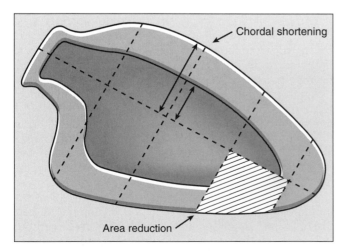

FIGURE 2-21. Hemiaxial methods for determining regional wall motion abnormalities.

ventriculogram or for the right ventricle. A different approach was adopted in which a centerline is drawn midway between the LV diastolic and systolic contours, and then 100 perpendiculars are constructed to this centerline. The degrees of movement of each of these perpendicular chords are then normalized by the LV end-diastolic contour and plotted. The data were compared with a normal population, and the results allow for the expression of regional motion in terms of standard deviations from the norm. The method is shown in Figure 2-23. The centerline method allows the wall motion abnormality to be identified, related to a given coronary artery distribution and defined statistically. However, clinicians might have difficulty understanding the output in terms of the variability in the standard deviation. The output display can be modified to relate to more familiar terms such as hypokinesia, akinesia, and dyskinesia, and the wall motion similarly compared with 100 normal controls. This modification is shown in Figure 2-24.

Echocardiography

Echocardiography is the most widely used imaging test for assessment of LV regional wall motion. Its advantages include cost, portability, high spatial and temporal resolution, and ability to image wall thickening in addition to endocardial excursion. Its primary limitation is the inability to acquire high-quality images in all patients. This latter problem can be overcome by the use of contrast agents (microbubbles) or transesophageal echocardiography. Both techniques have been shown to salvage technically difficult echocardiograms in the intensive care unit,[20-22] where ventilators and the inability to ideally position the patient might render transthoracic echocardiographic endocardial images technically nondiagnostic. Echocardiographic assessment of regional wall motion has proven to be valuable in numerous clinical conditions, including acute myocardial infarction, heart failure, hypertensive cardiovascular disease, cardiomyopathies, and valvular heart disease, and these clinical applications are reviewed in subsequent chapters.

Subjective Interpretation of Regional Wall Motion

The most widely used clinical method of analyzing regional wall motion by echocardiography is subjective visual grading. This is performed both during rest echocardiography and during exercise or pharmacological stress echocardiography. According to the American Society of Echocardiography, the LV should be divided into 16 segments according to the schematic diagram shown in Figure 2-25. Visual assessment of wall motion in each segment should be graded as 1 = normal or hyperkinetic, 2 = hypokinetic, 3 = akinetic, 4 = dyskinetic, or 5 = aneurysmal. A wall motion score index (WMSI) can be derived by summing the scores of each segment and dividing by 16. In the case of inadequate visualization of some segments, the WMSI can be derived by dividing the summed scores by the number of segments semiquantified. The echocardiographic WMSI has been shown to correlate with LVEF and to be

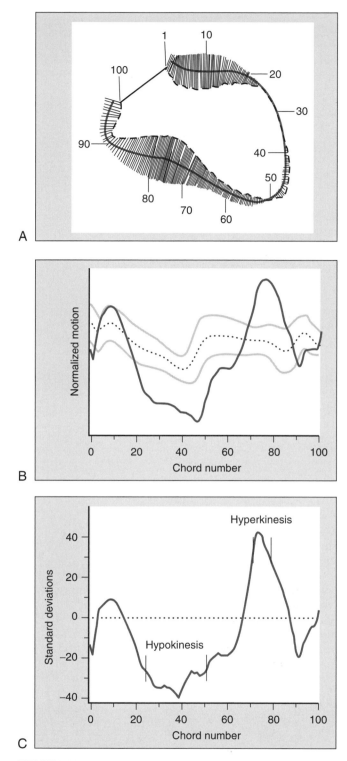

A

B

C

FIGURE 2-23. Centerline method for determining regional wall abnormalities. The outlines of the end-systolic and end-diastolic contours are drawn and a centerline constructed between them. Perpendiculars to this centerline are then drawn, normalized for the LV end-diastolic contour, and the degree of motion plotted versus a normal population. Data are expressed in standard deviations. **A,** Contours and the numbering scheme. **B,** Changes in the chords versus the normal control population. **C,** Outlines the 50% worse chords in the segments with hypokinesia and hyperkinesias. The mean standard deviation of these chords helps define the wall motion abnormality in a manner that aids in statistical analysis. (From Sheehan FH, Bolson EL, Dodge HT, et al. Advantages and applications of the centerline method for characterizing regional ventricular function. *Circulation* 1986; 74:293.)

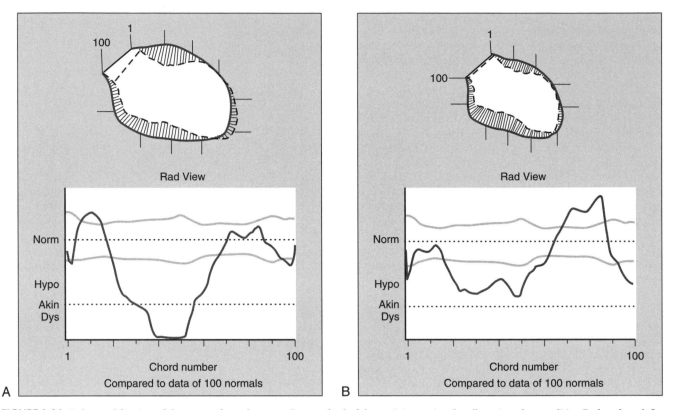

FIGURE 2-24. Duke modification of the output from the centerline method of determining regional wall motion abnormalities. Rather than define the wall motion changes in terms of standard deviations, the data are plotted relative to the severity of the wall motion change to include HYPO = hypokinesia, AKIN = akinesia, and DYS = dyskinesia. **A,** Patient with anterior dyskinesia during an acute myocardial infarction. **B,** Same patient during a follow-up angiogram in which there has been improvement in the anterior wall motion abnormality. (From Skelton TN. Angiographic techniques and data analysis, in Bashore TM (ed): *Invasive Cardiology.* Philadelphia: C.V. Mosby, 1990, p 216.)

an independent predictor of outcome in patients with ischemic heart disease.[23-25]

Visual grading of regional wall motion is the most complex and difficult aspect of echocardiography to teach or learn. It can be influenced by a variety of problems, including the effects of cardiac translational movement, bundle branch block, tachycardia, and improper alignment or foreshortening of the tomographic imaging planes. An important way to avoid these confounding influences is to incorporate a visual assessment of wall thickening into the grading scheme.[26] Wall thickening can be assessed in each segment and avoids the problem of translational motion. In addition, wall thickening and newer techniques using strain rate imaging are superior to endocardial wall motion in the presence of LV hypertrophy, where the latter might falsely indicate preserved regional LV function.[27,28] During stress echocardiography, where tachycardia and translational movement can easily confound the interpretation of regional wall motion, it is helpful to limit the display of LV function to systole only. This maneuver, which is easily achieved on current digital images, also facilitates interpretation of wall thickening in the patients with bundle branch block. Finally, careful attention to the orientation of the imaging planes is as important for assessment of regional wall motion as

it is for assessing LV volumes, mass, and ejection fraction. Foreshortening of the apex is a common problem, which can lead to overlooking apical wall motion abnormalities (see Figure 2-12). Often, there may be discrepancies between the wall motion in the same segment visualized in two different views. Usually this results because one of the views is improperly oriented (Figure 2-26). The short-axis views should be round; elliptical short-axis views suggest an oblique off-axis tomographic plane. A well-aligned short-axis view facilitates localization of the myocardial segments, because it identifies the anterior and posterior interventricular grooves, which in turn define the location of the left anterior descending and posterior descending coronary arteries. An apical four-chamber view should not show the anterolateral papillary muscle or the LV outflow tract. If the transducer is properly located on the true apex, rotation from a four-chamber to a two-chamber view will not result in movement of the LV apex from the apex of the echocardiographic sector. This enables LV foreshortening to be avoided.

The addition of contrast facilitates assessment of regional wall motion, because it provides a sharp distinction between the endocardial border and the LV cavity. Hundley et al[29] showed that contrast improved concordance between echocardiographic and CMR

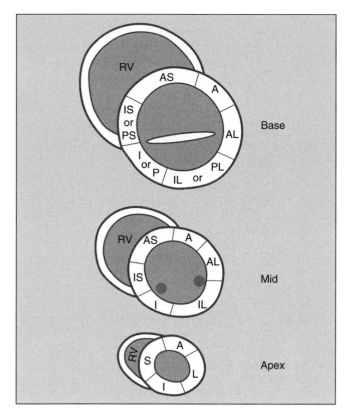

FIGURE 2-25. American Society of Echocardiography 16-segment model for assessment of regional wall motion. A = anterior, AL = anterolateral, PL or IL = posterolateral or inferolateral, I or P = inferior or posterior, IS or PS = inferoseptal or posteroseptal, AS = anteroseptal, L = lateral, S = septal. There are six segments at the base and mid-LV and four segments at the apex. (Reprinted from Schiller NB, Shah PM, Crawford M, DeMaria A, Devereux R, Feigenbaum H, Gutgesell H, Reichek N, Sahn D, Schnittger I. Recommendations for quantitation of the left ventricle by two-dimensional echocardiography. American Society of Echocardiography. Committee on Standards, Subcommittee on Quantitation of Two-Dimensional Echocardiograms. *J Am Soc Echocardiogr* 1989; 2:358.)

Quantitative Interpretation of Regional Wall Motion

A number of algorithms have been proposed to quantitate regional wall motion on the basis of the previously described angiographic models (Figures 2-21 to 2-24). Although these techniques are quantitative, they are somewhat cumbersome and therefore not widely used clinically. Furthermore, they have several inherent limitations. First, they usually quantify the motion of the endocardial border from end-diastole to end-systole and therefore are subject to translational motion of the heart. Second, they are subject to tethering. Third, methods that account for systolic wall thickening do so only in two dimensions and therefore do not account for the twisting motion of cardiac systolic contraction. Finally, these methods require off-line analysis of the images, which is impractical for routine clinical use.

Automatic Edge Detection

To avoid tedious off-line quantification of regional wall motion from echocardiographic images, automatic edge detection algorithms have been designed to track endocardial border excursion in real time from the acoustic backscatter signal. Measurements of global and regional LV function can be calculated automatically and displayed online by the imaging machine that has the theoretical advantage of reducing observer variability and providing a truly quantitative assessment of LV function. By color encoding the backscatter signal for each systolic frame, a graphical depiction of endocardial excursion, termed "color kinesis" can be displayed (Figure 2-27).[33] Unfortunately, automatic edge detection measures endocardial excursion rather than wall thickening and is still subject to translational artifacts, gain settings, and poor image quality. In our experience, the use of contrast markedly improves the image quality and reproducibility of color kinesis. Although it is a promising quantitative technique, it has not been adopted into routine clinical practice.

Tissue Doppler Imaging

A quantitative approach to measuring regional wall motion by echocardiography is the use of tissue Doppler imaging. The tissue Doppler signal reflects the high-amplitude, low-velocity motion of myocardial tissue while filtering out the low-amplitude, higher velocity signal from moving blood. Figure 2-28 depicts a 2D color tissue Doppler image and a pulsed-wave tissue Doppler image. There are two quantitative methods for analyzing regional wall motion by tissue Doppler: myocardial velocity gradient (MVG) and strain-rate imaging.[34] MVG represents the difference in velocity between the rapid movement of the endocardium and the much slower movement of the epicardium). It is calculated by the following equation:

$$MVG = (Vendo - Vepi)/L \cos \phi$$

where *Vendo* is the endocardial velocity, *Vepi* is the epicardial velocity, *L* is the thickness of the myocardium, and ø is the angle between the Doppler beam and the direction of tissue motion. In essence, the difference in

visual grading of regional wall motion from 76% to 91%, primarily because of salvage of inadequately visualized segments. Tissue harmonic imaging has also greatly improved the ability to detect endocardial borders by echocardiography. The combination of harmonic imaging and contrast has made the technically limited echocardiogram a rarity. This combination is widely used in stress echocardiography.[30,31] The use of harmonic contrast imaging has also improved interobserver and intraobserver variability in the interpretation of resting and stress regional wall motion.[29-31]

Other echocardiographic features are useful adjuncts to the assessment of ventricular function. For example, in the normal LV, descent of the base (mitral annulus) toward the apex is readily seen. Failure of the base to descend usually indicates severely depressed LV systolic function. Likewise, failure of the anterior mitral leaflet to fully open is an indicator of poor LV function. Wall thinning might occur after myocardial infarction caused by scarring and fibrosis. A thin (<0.6 cm), echogenic segment usually represents a transmural infarction without viability.[32]

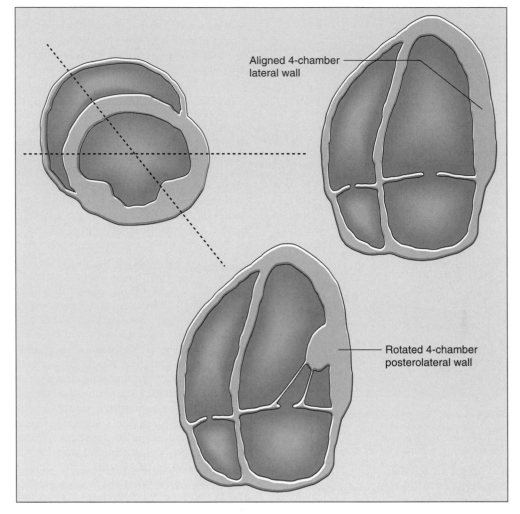

Aligned 4-chamber
lateral wall

Rotated 4-chamber
posterolateral wall

FIGURE 2-26. Examples of misalignment of echocardiographic planes resulting in apparent discrepancies in wall motion between two different views.

endocardial and epicardial velocities is a function of myocardial thickening and therefore is a promising quantitative measure of regional contraction. This method has the advantage of being independent of car-

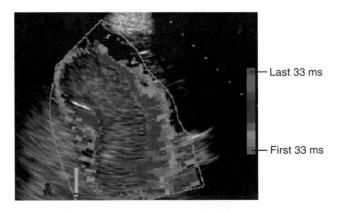

Last 33 ms

First 33 ms

FIGURE 2-27. Color kinesis images from a patient with apical akinesis *(arrows)*. Each color shown in the color bar represents endocardial motion during systole. Orange represents the first 33 ms and each subsequent 33-ms period is represented by a different color; bright blue represents the final 33 ms of systole (Courtesy of Brad Roberts, RDCS). See also Color Insert.

diac translation. Strain rate is the temporal rate of change of the spatial dimensions of a region of tissue or the rate of tissue deformation and, therefore, also reflects myocardial thickening. The concept of strain rate is more clearly understood if one considers the deformity of the biceps muscle during contraction. As the muscle contracts, its length is reduced (shortening), but its height and depth increase (thickening). Thus, there are three directional components to strain rate. In skeletal muscle, the fibers are arranged in parallel to the direction of shortening. In the heart, muscle fibers have a complex arrangement. Endocardial and epicardial fibers are arranged longitudinally from base to apex, but spiral in an opposite helical fashion such that the endocardial and epicardial fibers are nearly perpendicular to one another. The midmyocardial fibers are predominantly arranged in a circumferential pattern. This complex pattern has mechanical advantages for LV ejection. The three components of strain rate in the heart are longitudinal, radial, and circumferential. The relationship between strain rate in these three dimensions and myocardial fiber orientation in the different layers of myocardium has not been fully explored. The strain rate (SR) of a myocardial segment is determined from tissue Doppler velocities at two points within the segment according to the following formula (see Figure 2-29):

$$SR = \cos \emptyset \, (V_1 - V_2)/L$$

where V_1 is the velocity at one point, V_2 is the velocity at a second point, and L is the distance between the two points.[35] It is important to remember that this angle is 3D and is the primary source of error for tissue Doppler measurements.[36] Tissue Doppler cannot distinguish between longitudinal, radial, and circumferential strain and ideally measures strain rate along the path of the ultrasound beam, where $\cos \emptyset$ is 1. In apical views, longitudinal strain is predominantly measured, except for the actual apex, where SR is not reproducible because of the angle effect.[37] Conversely, in the short-axis view, the radial component of SR is predominantly measured in the anterior and posterior walls and the circumferential component is predominantly measured in the septal and lateral walls (Figure 2-29). Tissue Doppler SRs have been validated against tagged CMR, with good agreement observed for the short-axis and apical views.[38]

Applications of Newer Echocardiographic Techniques in Ischemic Heart Disease

Conventional stress echo methods have been shown to be reliable, easily obtained, and provide important prognostic data in large clinical studies.[39] Wall motion studies using tissue tracking techniques can characterize regional function and correlate well with CMR after myocardial infarction.[40] The assessment of myocardial perfusion by use of contrast echo methods has recently been validated in a multicenter trial and has demonstrated satisfactory performance compared with ^{99}Tc-methoxyisobutyl isonitrile (MIBI) nuclear techniques.[41] Contrast echocardiography (CE) has provided unique insights into the functional state of the microcirculation in evaluating viable myocardium after infarction.[42] CE allows differentiation between infarcted and borderzone myocardium before wall thinning occurs, which predicts the likelihood of functional recovery.[43] In addition, new real-time 3D echo permits assessment of mitral valve geometry in ischemic versus dilated cardiomyopathy and might suggest operative strategies for mitral valve repair.[44,45]

CMR

CMR can be used to grade regional wall motion in much the same way as cineangiography or echocardiography. Because of its excellent spatial resolution and image quality, CMR allows subjective assessment of wall thickening, as well as endocardial excursion. Semiquantitation of regional wall motion with CMR correlates well with cineangiography and echocardiography with a low interobserver variability. It can also be used with dobutamine or dipyridamole stress for diagnosis of coronary artery disease,[46,47] assessment of myocardial viability, and prediction of clinical outcome.[48]

CMR Tagging

Although subjective visual grading is clinically useful, regional wall motion can be quantified with CMR, primarily because its excellent spatial resolution provides unequivocal identification of endocardial and epicardial borders. The use of a centerline chord method for analyzing CMR wall motion has been proposed. However, the best quantitative methods use CMR tagging. CMR tagging, as discussed in Chapter 1, involves the labeling of a specific segment of myocardium by application of a radiofrequency pulse using a radial or "grid" (spatial modulation of magnetization [SPAMM]) technique. The tags move and deform with the myocardium throughout the cardiac cycle. Tags are placed perpendicular to the endocardial surface and appear as dark black lines, whose displacement can be tracked in 3D space (Figure 2-30). This method provides the capability to quantify transmural

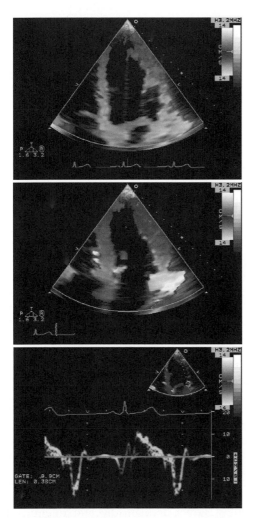

FIGURE 2-28. Tissue Doppler images. *Left panel,* 2D color tissue Doppler image in an apical four-chamber view. *Top panel,* Tissue Doppler image of myocardial velocities during systole in the apical four-chamber view. The red signal indicates diastolic tissue motion toward the transducer. *Middle panel,* Tissue Doppler image of myocardial velocities during diastole. The blue signal indicates diastolic tissue motion away from the transducer. *Bottom panel,* Spectral tissue Doppler display of velocities at the lateral mitral annulus. Systolic motion (S) is displayed above the baseline; early diastolic (E') and atrial contraction (A') velocities are below the baseline. (Courtesy of Brad Roberts, RDCS.) See also Color Insert.

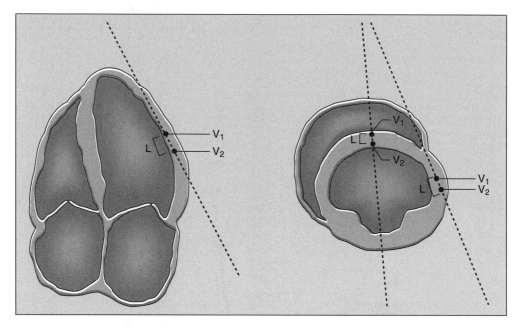

FIGURE 2-29. Schematic illustrating the measurement of strain rate by tissue Doppler in an apical four-chamber view *(left)* and a parasternal short-axis view *(right)*. The dashed lines represent ultrasound scan lines. V_1 is velocity at one point along the scan line, V_2 is the velocity at another point along the scan line, and L is the distance between the two points. In the apical view, the predominant directional component of strain rate is longitudinal along either the septum or lateral wall. In the short-axis view, the radial component of strain rate predominates in the anterior or posterior walls, whereas the circumferential component predominates in the lateral or septal walls (see text).

myocardial excursion, wall thickening, circumferential shortening, and longitudinal shortening simultaneously. Furthermore, all three spatial dimensions of regional myocardial strain or SR (see earlier), and the directions of those strains, can be accurately calculated using CMR tagging techniques.[37,49,50] Although not widely used clinically at present, CMR offers the optimal available method for quantifying regional wall motion by calculation of myocardial strains.

Nuclear Imaging

Equilibrium-gated radionuclide ventriculography is most often used clinically for its ability to accurately measure LVEF and RVEF. Gated SPECT imaging is primarily used for myocardial perfusion imaging. However, regional wall motion can be assessed by both techniques using either subjective visual grading or quantitative techniques. Although visual grading of radionuclide ventriculograms is most common, quantitative analysis of regional wall motion using radial or phase-analysis methods has been validated with contrast cineangiography. Visual grading of gated SPECT images has been shown to correlate favorably with visual grading by CMR.[51] Quantitative analysis of gated SPECT images has been performed, but this has not been rigorously validated against myocardial strain or SR by either tissue Doppler or CMR tagging. The primary strength of nuclear imaging for regional wall motion is that these studies are frequently performed for assessment of LVEF and/or myocardial perfusion. Simultaneous assessment of regional wall motion is convenient and clinically useful. The primary limitation of the technique is poor spatial resolution and the potential for errors caused by partial volume effects.

CLINICAL ASSESSMENT OF LV DIASTOLIC FUNCTION

Approximately 40% of patients with heart failure have normal LV systolic function and have symptoms caused by diastolic dysfunction. Accordingly, quantification of LV diastolic function is an important aspect of the evaluation of ventricular performance. To function effectively as a pump, the ventricles must fill with blood to eject blood. Diastolic filling involves a complex series of events that include isovolumic relaxation, rapid early filling, diastasis, and late atrial contraction. Disturbances in any of these phases of diastole can result in diastolic dysfunction.

Isovolumic relaxation occurs between aortic valve closure and mitral valve opening. It is an active adenosine triphosphate–dependent process in which calcium is transported from the cytosol back into the sarcoplasmic reticulum within the myocytes. In normal subjects, isovolumic relaxation occurs rapidly, and LV pressure falls well below LA pressure. As a result, when the mitral valve opens, LV filling occurs initially rapidly, such that about 70% of LV filling occurs during the rapid filling phase. As the pressures between the LA and LV equilibrate, filling slows dramatically and might even stop. This slow filling phase is often termed diastasis. Finally, LA contraction occurs, generating a new pressure gradient between the LA and LV that completes LV filling. Approximately 20% to 25% of LV filling occurs during atrial contraction. Loss of atrial contraction caused by atrial fibrillation can cause clinically significant impairment of LV filling, especially in patients with LV hypertrophy or restrictive cardiomyopathy.

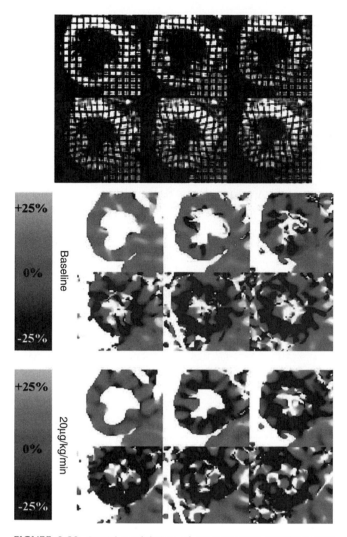

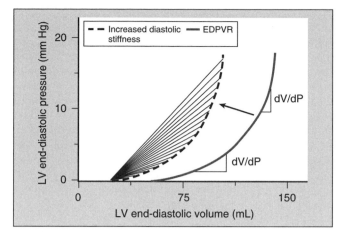

FIGURE 2-31. Schematic diagram of LV end-diastolic pressure-volume relation (EDPVR). Unlike the ESPVR, EDPVR is nonlinear. Therefore the slope of the EDPVR is different when measured at different end-diastolic volumes (see text). A shift in the EDPVR to the left indicates increased LV chamber stiffness.

diastolic pressure-volume relation. The slope of this relation represents chamber stiffness, but, as can be seen in Figure 2-31, this slope varies according to where it is measured on the pressure-volume relation. A potential solution to this problem is to use an exponential model to solve for chamber stiffness or to compare chamber stiffness at a common preload. Importantly, the pressure-volume relation allows measurement of LV chamber stiffness, not myocardial stiffness. The latter can be assessed by measurement of Langrangian stress-strain relations. In most clinical catheterization laboratories, neither chamber stiffness nor myocardial stiffness is usually measured, because the method is cumbersome and clinical and therapeutic usefulness are low.

Echocardiography

Echocardiography is by far the most commonly used method of assessing LV diastolic function. Earlier methods focused on the rate of change of LV wall movement during the rapid filling phase. These measurements are limited to assessment of rapid filling and are rarely used clinically. However, pulsed Doppler spectra of mitral inflow have become the clinical standard for assessment of LV diastolic function even though they are influenced by LV loading conditions. Mitral inflow velocities are measured with the Doppler sample volume located at the tips of the mitral leaflets. Because mitral inflow is normally directed toward the lateral wall, the transducer should be placed somewhat laterally to align the Doppler beam in parallel with the direction of flow. There are four distinct patterns of mitral inflow velocity associated with LV diastolic function: normal, impaired relaxation, pseudonormal, and restrictive. As shown in Figure 2-32, the normal signal has a rapid early filling peak (E wave) followed by a second peak at atrial contraction (A wave). The deceleration time is measured as the slope of the decay in velocity from the peak E wave velocity to its return to baseline. Even if the velocity does not actually reach baseline, the slope can be extrapolated

FIGURE 2-30. Spatial modulation of magnetization (SPAMM) CMR images illustrating the concept of tracking the motion of CMR tags, seen as dark lines overlying the images in the upper panel (see text). By measuring the spatial and temporal motion of the tags, 3D strain and strain rate can be determined accurately. The middle panel shows myocardial strain on a pixel-by-pixel basis at baseline; the bottom panel shows myocardial strain during dobutamine infusion. (Reprinted with permission from Garot J, Bluemke DA, Osman NF, et al. Fast determination of regional myocardial strain fields from tagged cardiac images using harmonic phase CMR. *Circulation* 2000; 101:981.) See also Color Insert.

Cardiac Catheterization/Cineangiography

During cardiac catheterization, isovolumic relaxation can be assessed from LV pressure tracings. The isovolumic relaxation time (IVRT) and peak negative dp/dt are highly dependent on aortic pressure, and other loading conditions. Tau represents the time constant of isovolumic relaxation, which is measured from the exponential decay of the LV pressure tracing from aortic valve closure to mitral valve opening. Because measurement of tau requires use of a high-fidelity micromanometer-tipped catheter and is load dependent, it is not widely measured in clinical practice.

LV pressure-volume loops can be generated to determine the passive filling characteristics of the LV during diastole. Figure 2-31 shows a schematic diagram of the LV

to the baseline to measure deceleration time. The normal pattern of mitral inflow has an E/A ratio of 1 or greater and a deceleration time of >140 ms.

The impaired relaxation pattern is associated with abnormal isovolumic relaxation, in which the fall in LV pressure is reduced in magnitude and prolonged in duration. As a result, the early diastolic pressure gradient between the LA and LV is reduced, and the E wave velocity is small with a prolonged acceleration time (Figure 2-32). There is increased LV filling during atrial contraction to compensate for the impaired early diastolic filling, and, therefore, the A wave signal is predominant. This pattern can also be seen in volume depletion, where

early diastolic filling is also reduced because of the low gradient between the LA and LV. An impaired relaxation pattern is common in elderly patients and those with LV hypertrophy. It is usually considered a sign of early diastolic dysfunction. Often these patients are asymptomatic and have normal LA pressure.

As LV diastolic function progresses, the impaired relaxation pattern might change to a pseudonormal pattern, in which the E/A ratio and deceleration times seem close to normal, despite significantly increased LA pressure and abnormal myocardial stiffness. This occurs because the increasing LA pressure increases the E wave velocity, whereas the A wave velocity decreases because of an ele-

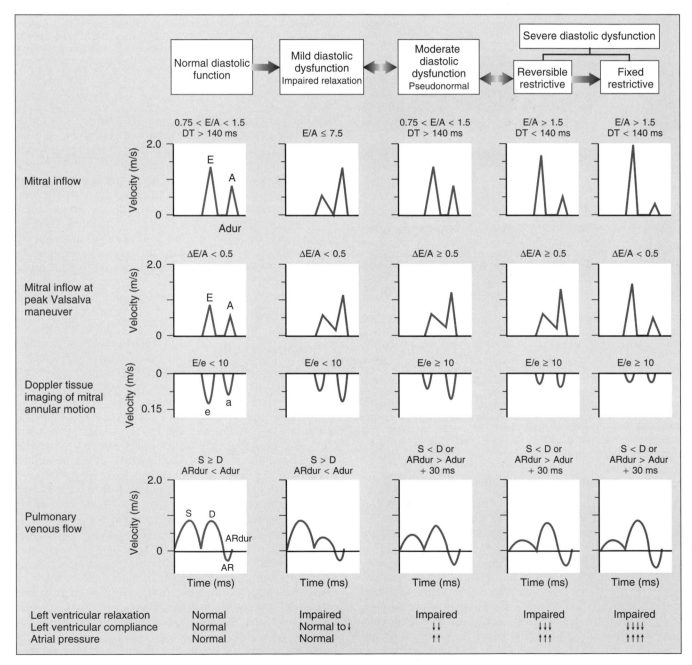

FIGURE 2-32. Doppler classification of LV diastolic function. (Reprinted from Redfield MM, Jacobsen SJ, Burnett JC, Maloney DW, Bailey KR, Rodenheffer RJ. Burden of systolic and diastolic ventricular function in the community: appreciating the scope of the heart failure epidemic. *JAMA* 2002; 289:194; with permission.)

vated LV end-diastolic pressure and/or decreased atrial systolic contractile function. During the Valsalva maneuver, a pseudonormal pattern typically reverts to an impaired relaxation pattern. Abnormal pulmonary venous flow velocities and tissue Doppler patterns also help unmask the pseudonormal pattern (see Chapter 10).

The restrictive pattern is characterized by a tall E wave, diminished A wave, and a deceleration time <140 ms. It is associated with increased LV stiffness because of severe hypertrophy, fibrosis, or infiltrative disorders, but it is also seen in constrictive pericarditis and severe mitral regurgitation. In patients with heart failure, a restrictive pattern is an independent predictor of adverse outcome. In patients with atrial fibrillation, a restrictive pattern can still be interpreted on the basis of an elevated E velocity and shortened deceleration time, even though there is no A wave.

The current approach to assessing diastolic function requires an integration of mitral inflow velocity patterns at rest and with Valsalva maneuver, tissue Doppler (Figure 2-32) at the mitral annulus, and pulmonary venous flow (see Chapter 10). This is important because of the known dependence of mitral inflow velocities on loading conditions and the fact that the pseudonormal pattern seems normal. Tissue Doppler measures the velocity of myocardial motion during diastole, which is less dependent on the pressure gradient between the LA and LV than Doppler velocities. Therefore, the tissue Doppler signal in pseudonormal patterns typically resembles the impaired relaxation pattern (Figure 2-32). Tissue Doppler can also be used to distinguish restrictive cardiomyopathy from constrictive

pericarditis.[52] In both conditions, the mitral inflow pattern will be restrictive. However, the tissue Doppler pattern indicates impaired relaxation in the former and restriction in the latter (Figure 2-33). Constrictive vs. restrictive physiology can also be ascertained by the respiratory variation in the mitral inflow velocity pattern. This is best determined with a nasal thermistor to record respiration while using a sweep speed of 25 mm/s. Restrictive physiology has little respiratory variation, whereas constrictive pericarditis is associated with a more than 25% drop in the peak E velocity after inspiration. Tricuspid inflow shows a 25% increase in E velocity after inspiration.

Tissue Doppler can also be used to assess strain rate during diastole, which is a measure of myocardial deformation[34,37,53] as previously described. As with systolic SR imaging, diastolic SR can only be measured in a single dimension, which is predominantly longitudinal, radial, or circumferential, depending on the imaging plane and myocardial location relative to the ultrasound beam (see Figure 2-29). It has also been reported that tissue Doppler can be used to estimate pulmonary artery wedge pressure. The normal tissue Doppler E wave (denoted E') measured at the mitral annulus is more than 10 cm/s. A value <8 cm/s is considered abnormal. The ratio of E/E' correlates well with pulmonary artery wedge pressure. An E/E' ratio >10 has been reported to predict a pulmonary artery wedge pressure >15 mmHg, with a sensitivity of 97% and specificity of 78%.

Another echocardiographic measurement of LV diastolic function is the color flow propagation velocity. This involves placement of an M-mode cursor parallel to mitral inflow and the use of color flow mapping to

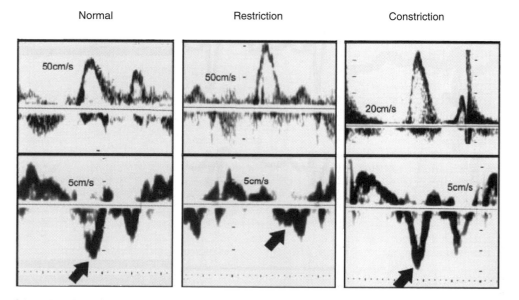

FIGURE 2-33. Use of tissue Doppler to help distinguish between restrictive cardiomyopathy and constrictive pericarditis. Mitral inflow pulsed Doppler flow velocities *(top panels)* and tissue Doppler spectral display of lateral mitral annulus velocities *(bottom panel). Left,* Normal mitral inflow and tissue velocities are seen with the E' signal shown by the arrow. In restriction and constriction, mitral inflow velocities show a characteristic restrictive filling pattern with a tall E wave and rapid deceleration. However, restriction is associated with a delayed onset of the E' tissue Doppler signal, which shows an impaired relaxation pattern. In contrast, myocardial constriction is associated with a restrictive pattern in both the mitral inflow and tissue Doppler spectra. (Modified and reprinted with permission from Garcia MJ, Thomas JD, Klein AL. New Doppler echocardiographic applications for the study of diastolic function. *J Am Coll Cardiol* 1998; 32:865.)

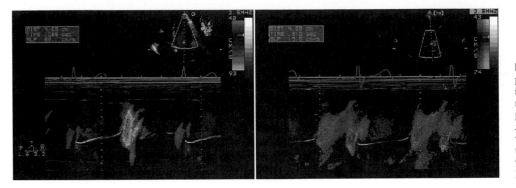

FIGURE 2-34. Color M-mode flow propagation as a measure of LV filling. *Left panel,* Tracing from a normal subject showing a flow propagation velocity of 62 cm/s. *Right panel,* Tracing from a patient with isolated LV diastolic dysfunction and a propagation velocity of 9 cm/s. (Courtesy of Brad Roberts, RDCS.) See also Color Insert.

image the temporal filling of the LV (Figure 2-34). The slope of the color flow propagation into the LV is termed Vp. The normal value for Vp is >55 cm/s in children and >45 cm/s in adults. A lower value indicates abnormal filling and might be useful in unmasking a pseudonormal pattern. The major limitation of this technique is that the slope is not always linear and can be difficult to define.

CMR

Cine-CMR provides highly accurate and reproducible measurements of LV volumes, as previously discussed. With modern scanners, frame rates are high enough to plot LV volumes throughout the diastolic filling period. This allows calculation of the peak filling rate of the LV.[54] Because the peak filling rate only evaluates the early fill-ing phase of diastole, it is not widely used clinically. By use of phase-contrast CMR, blood flow velocity across the mitral valve can be determined, providing a signal very similar to that of pulsed Doppler echocardiography (Figure 2-35). This technique can also be used to measure pulmonary vein flow velocities. The most promising use of cine-CMR for assessment of diastolic function is the use of tagging to calculate 3D strain within myocardial segments during diastole.[49,55] The primary disadvantage of CMR imaging is the long acquisition time. Even with newer faster scanners, a complete study encompassing quantitative measures of LV systolic and diastolic function, including gradient-echo, phase-encoded velocity measurements, and tagging, would take almost an hour. Additional time would be needed for off-line analysis. However, automated quantification algorithms will be developed to facilitate image analysis.

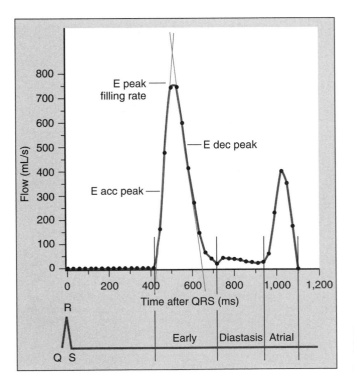

FIGURE 2-35. Phase-encoded cine-CMR display of mitral inflow velocity. (Reprinted with permission from Paelinck BP, Lamb HJ, Bax JJ, Van der Wall EE, de Roos A. Assessment of diastolic function by cardiovascular magnetic resonance. *Am Heart J* 2002; 144:198.)

Nuclear Imaging

Radionuclide angiography is capable of measuring peak early filling rate, time to peak filling, or filling fraction as indices of LV diastolic function. Peak early filling rate is often normalized to end-diastolic volume, stroke volume, body surface area, or peak ejection rate. Gated SPECT imaging can also measure peak filling rates[56] and their normalized values. Although these measurements have been shown to predict LV diastolic function, they are not widely used clinically, in part because they only reflect filling rates rather than intrinsic myocardial stiffness. Nuclear techniques do not have the spatial resolution required to measure myocardial strain or SR.

SUMMARY

Imaging methods for quantitation of ventricular function continue to evolve. The most commonly used techniques are echocardiography, cineangiography, and nuclear imaging techniques. CMR is less often used clinically but is the most accurate and reproducible method for quantification of ventricular function. With further advances in digital image processing, online edge detection algorithms, better contrast agents, and real-time 3D imaging, quantification of ventricular function is likely to be performed more routinely in clinical practice.

REFERENCES

1. Spotnitz HM. Macro design, structure, and mechanics of the left ventricle. *J Thorac Cardiovasc Surg* 2000; 119(5):1053.
2. Stuber M, Scheidegger MB, Fischer SE, Nagel E, Steinemann F, Hess OM, et al. Alterations in the local myocardial motion pattern in patients suffering from pressure overload because of aortic stenosis. *Circulation* 1999; 100(4):361.
3. Schmidt MA, Starling MR. Physiologic assessment of left ventricular systolic and diastolic performance. *Curr Prob Cardiol* 2000; 25:827.
4. Qin JX, Shiota T, Thomas JD. Determination of left ventricular volume, ejection fraction, and myocardial mass by real-time three-dimensional echocardiography. *Echocardiography* 2002; 17:781.
5. Myerson SG, Bellenger NG, Pennell DJ. Assessment of left ventricular mass by cardiovascular magnetic resonance. *Hypertension* 2002; 39:750.
6. Lee D, Fuisz AR, Fan P-H, et al. Real-time 3-dimensional echocardiographic evaluation of left ventricular volume: correlation with magnetic resonance imaging—a validation study. *J Am Soc Echocardiogr* 2001; 14:1001.
7. Thomson HL, Basmadjian AJ, Rainbird AJ, et al. Contrast echocardiography improves the accuracy and reproducibility of left ventricular remodeling measurements: a prospective, randomly assigned, blinded study. *J Am Coll Cardiol* 2001; 38:867.
8. Yiu SF, Enriquez-Sarano M, Tribouilloy C, Seward JB, Tajik AJ. Determinants of the degree of functional mitral regurgitation in patients with systolic left ventricular dysfunction: a quantitative clinical study. *Circulation* 2000; 102:1400.
9. Qin JJ, Jones M, Shiota T, et al. New digital measurement methods for left ventricular volume using real-time three-dimensional echocardiography: comparison with electromagnetic flow method and magnetic resonance imaging. *Eur J Echocardiogr* 2000; 1:84.
10. Grothues F, Smith GC, Moon JCC, et al. Comparison of interstudy reproducibility of cardiovascular magnetic resonance with two-dimensional echocardiography in normal subjects and in patients with heart failure or left ventricular hypertrophy. *Am J Cardiol* 2002; 90:29.
11. Ioannidis JPA, Trikalinos TA, Damas PG. Electrocardiogram-gated single-photon emission computed tomography versus cardiac magnetic resonance imaging for the assessment of left ventricular volumes and ejection fraction: a meta-analysis. *J Am Coll Cardiol* 2002; 39:2059.
12. Bellenger NG, Davies LC, Francis JM, Coats AJ, Pennell DJ. Reduction in sample size of remodeling in heart failure by the use of cardiovascular magnetic resonance. *J Cardiovasc Magn Reson* 2000; 2:271.
13. Myerson SG, Bellenger NG, Pennell DJ. Assessment of left ventricular mass by cardiovascular magnetic resonance. *Hypertension* 2002; 39:75.
14. Salton CJ, Chuang ML, O'Donnell CJ, et al. Gender differences and normal left ventricular anatomy in an adult population free of hypertension: a cardiovascular magnetic resonance study of the Framingham Heart Study Offspring Cohort. *J Am Coll Cardiol* 2002; 39:1055.
15. Roig E, Georgiou D, Chomka EV, et al. Reproducibility of left ventricular volume and mass measurement by ultrafast CT. *J Am Coll Cardiol* 1991; 18:99.
16. Wachtell K, Rokkedal J, Bella JN, et al. Effect of electrocardiographic left ventricular hypertrophy on left ventricular systolic function in systemic hypertension (The LIFE Study). *Am J Cardiol* 2002; 87:54.
17. Balzer P, Furber A, Delepine S, et al. Regional assessment of wall curvature and wall stress in the left ventricle with magnetic resonance imaging. *Am J Physiol* 1999; 277;H901.
18. Goldman JH, Schiller NB, Lim DC, Redberg RF, Foster E. Usefulness of stroke distance by echocardiography as a surrogate marker of cardiac output that is independent of gender and size in a normal population. *Am J Cardiol* 2001; 87:49.
19. Rominger MB, Bachmann GF, Pabst W, Rau WS. Right ventricular volumes and ejection fraction with fast cine MR imaging in breath-hold technique: applicability, normal values from 52 volunteers, and evaluation of 325 adult cardiac patients. *J Magn Reson Imaging* 1999; 10:908.
20. Yong Y, Wu D, Fernandes V, et al. Diagnostic accuracy and cost-effectiveness of contrast echocardiography on evaluation of cardiac function in technically very difficult patients in the intensive care unit. *Am J Cardiol* 2002; 89:711.
21. Reilly JP, Tunick PA, Timmermans RJ, et al. Contrast echocardiography clarifies uninterpretable wall motion in intensive care unit patients. *J Am Coll Cardiol* 2000; 35:485.
22. Grayburn PA, Mulvagh S, Crouse L. Left ventricular opacification at rest and during stress. *Am J Cardiol* 2002; 90(10 Suppl 1):21.
23. Galasko GI, Basu S, Lahiri A, Senior R. A prospective comparison of echocardiographic wall motion score index and radionuclide ejection fraction in predicting outcome following acute myocardial infarction. *Heart* 2001; 86:271.
24. Carluccio E, Tommasi S, Bentivoglio M, et al. Usefulness of the severity and extent of wall motion abnormalities as prognostic markers of an adverse outcome after a first myocardial infarction treated with thrombolytic therapy. *Am J Cardiol* 2000; 85:411.
25. Arruda-Olson AM, Juracan EM, Mahoney DW, et al. Prognostic value of exercise echocardiography in 5,798 patients: is there a gender difference? *J Am Coll Cardiol* 2002; 39:625.
26. Gibson RS, Bishop HL, Stamm RB, et al. Value of early two-dimensional echocardiography in patients with acute myocardial infarction. *Am J Cardiol* 1982; 49:1110.
27. Dong SJ, MacGregor JH, Crawley AP, et al. Left ventricular wall thickness and regional systolic function in patients with hypertrophic cardiomyopathy: a three-dimensional tagged magnetic resonance imaging study. *Circulation* 1994; 90:1200.
28. Yang H, Sun JP, Lever HM, Popovic ZB, Drinko JK, Greenberg NL, Shiota T, Thomas JD, Garcia MJ. Use of strain imaging in detecting segmental dysfunction in patients with hypertrophic cardiomyopathy. *J Am Soc Echocardiogr* 2003; 16(3):233.
29. Hundley WG, Kizilbash AM, Afridi I, Franco F, Peshock RM, Grayburn PA. Effect of contrast-enhancement on transthoracic echocardiographic assessment of left ventricular regional wall motion. *Am J Cardiol* 1999; 84:25.
30. Malhotra V, Nwogu J, Bondmass MD, et al. Is the technically difficult echocardiogram an endangered species? Endocardial border defi-

nition with native tissue harmonic imaging and Optison contrast: a review of 200 cases. *J Am Soc Echocardiogr* 2000; 18:771.

31. Rainbird AJ, Mulvagh SL, Oh JK, et al. Contrast dobutamine stress echocardiography: clinical practice assessment in 300 consecutive patients. *J Am Soc Echocardiogr* 2001; 14:378.

32. Sayad DE, Willett DL, Hundley WG, Grayburn PA, Peshock RM. Dobutamine magnetic resonance imaging with myocardial tagging quantitatively predicts improvement in regional function after revascularization. *Am J Cardiol* 1998; 82:1149.

33. Mor-Avi V, Spencer K, Gorcsan J, et al. Normal values of regional left ventricular endocardial motion: multicenter color kinesis study. *Am J Physiol* 2000; 279:H2464.

34. Trambaiolo P, Tonti G, Salustri A, Fedele F, Sutherland G. New insights into regional systolic and diastolic function with tissue Doppler echocardiography: From qualitative analysis to quantitative approach. *J Am Soc Echocardiogr* 2001; 14:85.

35. Heimdal A, Stoylen A, Torp H, et al. Real-time strain rate imaging of the left ventricle by ultrasound. *J Am Soc Echocardiogr* 1998; 11:1013.

36. Hashimoto I, Mori Y, Rusk RA, et al. Strain rate imaging: An in vitro "validation" study using a physiologic balloon model mimicking the left ventricle. *Echocardiography* 2002; 19:669.

37. Voigt JU, Lindenmeier G, Werner D, et al. Strain rate imaging for the assessment of preload-dependent changes in regional left ventricular diastolic longitudinal function. *J Am Soc Echocardiogr* 2002; 15:13.

38. Edvardsen T, Gerber BL, Garot J, et al. Quantitative assessment of intrinsic regional myocardial deformation by Doppler strain rate echocardiography in humans: validation against three-dimensional tagged magnetic resonance imaging. *Circulation* 2002; 106:50.

39. Sicari R, Pasanisi E, Venneri L, Landi P, Cortigiani L, Picano E. Echo Persantine International Cooperative (EPIC) Study Group. Echo Dobutamine International Cooperative (EDIC) Study Group. Stress echo results predict mortality: a large-scale multicenter prospective international study. *J Am Coll Cardiol* 2003; 41(4):589.

40. Borges AC, Kivelitz D, Walde T, Reibis RK, Grohmann A, Panda A, Wernecke KD, Rutsch W, Hamm B, Baumann G. Apical tissue tracking echocardiography for characterization of regional left ventricular function: comparison with magnetic resonance imaging in patients after myocardial infarction. *J Am Soc Echocardiogr* 2003; 16(3):254.

41. Wei K, Crouse L, Weiss J, Villanueva F, Schiller NB, Naqvi TZ, Siegel R, Monaghan M, Goldman J, Aggarwal P, Feigenbaum H, DeMaria A. Comparison of usefulness of dipyridamole stress myocardial contrast echocardiography to technetium-99m sestamibi single-photon emission computed tomography for detection of coronary artery disease (PB127 Multicenter Phase 2 Trial results). *Am J Cardiol* 2003; 91(11):1293.

42. Badano LP, Werren M, Di Chiara A, Fioretti PM. Contrast echocardiographic evaluation of early changes in myocardial perfusion after recanalization therapy in anterior wall acute myocardial infarction and their relation with early contractile recovery. *Am J Cardiol* 2003; 91(5):532.

43. Balcells E, Powers ER, Lepper W, Belcik T, Wei K, Ragosta M, Samady H, Lindner JR. Detection of myocardial viability by contrast echocardiography in acute infarction predicts recovery of resting function and contractile reserve. *J Am Coll Cardiol* 2003; 41(5):827.

44. Sitges M, Jones M, Shiota T, Qin JX, Tsujino H, Bauer F, Kim YJ, Agler DA, Cardon LA, Zetts AD, Panza JA, Thomas JD, Investigator: Thomas JD. Real-time three-dimensional color Doppler evaluation of the flow convergence zone for quantification of mitral regurgitation: validation experimental animal study and initial clinical experience. *J Am Soc Echocardiogr* 2003; 16(1):38.

45. Kwan J, Shiota T, Agler DA, Popovic ZB, Qin JX, Gillinov MA, Stewart WJ, Cosgrove DM, McCarthy PM, Thomas JD. Real-time three-dimensional echocardiography study. Investigator: Thomas JD. Geometric differences of the mitral apparatus between ischemic and dilated cardiomyopathy with significant mitral regurgitation: real-time three-dimensional echocardiography study. *Circulation* 2003; 107(8):1135.

46. Nagel E, Lehmkuhl HB, Bocksch W, et al. Noninvasive diagnosis of ischemia-induced wall motion abnormalities with the use of high-dose dobutamine stress CMR: comparison with dobutamine stress echocardiography. *Circulation* 1999; 99:763.

47. Hundley WG, Hamilton CA, Thomas MS, et al. Utility of fast cine magnetic resonance imaging and display for the detection of myocardial ischemia in patients not well suited for second harmonic stress echocardiography. *Circulation* 1999; 100:1697.

48. Hundley WG, Morgan TM, Neagle CM, et al. Magnetic resonance imaging determination of cardiac prognosis. *Circulation* 2002; 106:2328.

49. Garot J, Bluemke DA, Osman NF, et al. Fast determination of regional myocardial strain fields from tagged cardiac images using harmonic phase CMR. *Circulation* 2000; 101:981.

50. Gerber BL, Garot J, Bluemke DA, Wu KC, Lima JA. Accuracy of contrast-enhanced magnetic resonance imaging in predicting improvement of regional myocardial function in patients after acute myocardial infarction. *Circulation* 2002; 106:108.

51. Bax JJ, Lamb H, Dibbets P, et al. Comparison of gated single-photon emission computed tomography with magnetic resonance imaging for evaluation of left ventricular function in ischemic cardiomyopathy. *Am J Cardiol* 2000; 86:1299.

52. Rajagopalan N, Garcia MJ, Rodriguez L, et al. Comparison of new Doppler echocardiographic methods to differentiate constrictive pericardial heart disease and restrictive cardiomyopathy. *Am J Cardiol* 2001; 87:86.

53. Kukulski T, Jamal F, D'Hooge J, Bijnens B, De Scheerder I, Sutherland GR. Acute changes in systolic and diastolic events during clinical coronary angioplasty: a comparison of regional velocity, strain rate, and strain measurement. *J Am Soc Echocardiogr* 2002; 15:1.

54. Paelinck BP, Lamb HJ, Bax JJ, Van der Wall EE, de Roos A. Assessment of diastolic function by cardiovascular magnetic resonance. *Am Heart J* 2002; 144:198.

55. Fogel MA, Weinberg PM, Hubbard A, et al. Diastolic biomechanics in normal infants utilizing CMR tissue tagging. *Circulation* 2000; 102:218.

56. Kikkawa M, Nakamura T, Sakamoto K, et al. Assessment of left ventricular diastolic function from quantitative electrocardiographic-gated 99mTc-tetrofosmin myocardial SPECT. *Eur J Nucl Med* 2001; 28:593.

Quantitation of Myocardial Perfusion

C. Michael Gibson
Paul A. Grayburn
Marcelo F. Di Carli
Sharmila Dorbala
Debiao Li
Vibhas S. Deshpande
Norbert Wilke
Gilbert L. Raff
Prasad M. Panse
Steven R. Bergmann

ASSESSMENT OF CORONARY BLOOD FLOW AND MYOCARDIAL PERFUSION WITH THE CORONARY ARTERIOGRAM

Assessment of coronary blood flow on the coronary arteriogram has evolved in recent years. Traditionally, the TIMI (Thrombolysis In Myocardial Infarction) flow grade classification scheme has been used. The more objective TIMI frame count, in which the number of cine film frames are counted for dye to fill the artery, overcomes some of the limitations encountered with the use of the categorical and subjective TIMI flow grades.[1,2] More recently, there has been an emphasis on tissue level or microvascular perfusion. One angiographic method developed to assess tissue level perfusion is the TIMI myocardial perfusion grade (TMPG).[3]

The TIMI Flow Grade Classification Scheme

The TIMI flow grades were originally defined in the TIMI 1 study as follows:

Grade 0: No perfusion. No antegrade flow beyond the point of occlusion.
Grade 1: Penetration without perfusion. Contrast material passes beyond the area of obstruction but fails to opacify the entire coronary bed distal to the obstruction for the duration of the cineangiographic filming sequence.
Grade 2: Partial perfusion. Contrast material passes across the obstruction and opacifies the coronary artery distal to the obstruction. However, the rate of entry of contrast material into the vessel distal to the obstruction or its rate of clearance from the distal bed (or both) is perceptibly slower than its flow into or clearance from comparable areas not perfused by the previously occluded vessel.
Grade 3: Complete perfusion. Antegrade flow into the bed distal to the obstruction occurs as promptly as antegrade flow into the bed proximal to the obstruction, and clearance of contrast material from the involved bed is as rapid as clearance from an uninvolved bed in the same vessel or the opposite artery.

There has recently been "drift" in the way in which "TIMI grade 3 flow" is defined to include opacification of the coronary artery within three cardiac cycles. This revised definition has been applied in many of the recent intervention trials, and in particular in trials of primary coronary intervention for acute myocardial infarction. This departure from the original definition of TIMI grade 3 flow results in higher rates of TIMI grade 3 flow. For example, in recent thrombolytic trials, it requires just less than 1 second (26.8 ± 9.1 frames or 0.9 seconds, n = 693) or one cardiac cycle to traverse the length of the artery among patients with TIMI grade 3 flow. If the cutpoint for qualifying for TIMI grade 3 flow is increased from 1 to 3 cardiac cycles, then the newer "three cardiac cycle" definition of "TIMI 3" flow results in a 10% increase over the original definition of TIMI grade 3 flow. Thus, whereas rates of TIMI grade 3 flow of 95% are often reported in primary angioplasty trials, this number might be closer to 85% if the original definition had been applied.

There is interobserver variability in classifying the TIMI flow grades as well. Sometimes, TIMI grade 1 flow is misclassified as TIMI grade 2 flow. Strictly interpreted, to qualify as TIMI 2 flow, the dye must reach the apex during cinefilming. There is no confusion in classifying flow as TIMI grade 1 when dye barely penetrates the lesion. Confusion arises when dye penetrates the lesion, but the dye moves down the artery so slowly that the operator stops filming before it reaches the apex. In the TIMI angiographic laboratory, we would classify this second scenario as TIMI grade 1 flow. Operators at clinical sites often interpret this as TIMI grade 2 flow.

The rate of agreement between an angiographic core laboratory and clinical centers is higher if the question is whether the culprit artery is either open or closed (kappa value = 0.84 ± 0.05, which indicates good agreement). In contrast, when assessing the TIMI grade 3 flow, the rate of agreement is only moderate (kappa value = 0.55 ± 0.05) and is unfortunately poor in the assessment of TIMI grade 2 flow (kappa value = 0.38 ± 0.05).[2] Even between experienced angiographic core laboratories, there can be a frequent lack of concordance. In a recent study, the rate of agreement between two core laboratories in the assessment of TIMI grade 2 and 3 flows was only 83%, and three experienced angiographic core laboratories achieved complete agreement in only 71% of the cases. This high rate of discordance might be improved with the use of the TIMI frame count (see later section).

Although it is conceptually convenient to think of coronary blood flow as falling into different discrete categories, the fact is that coronary blood flow, like so many biological measures, is unimodally distributed as a continuous variable. Furthermore, coronary blood flow in the uninvolved nonculprit artery has been used as the "gold standard" for assessing TIMI grade flow in the infarct related artery. However, we have recently shown that flow in the uninvolved artery is often not normal and on average is slowed down by 40% in the acute myocardial infarction setting. As an ever-broader variety of reperfusion strategies achieve even higher rates of TIMI grade 3 flow, this categorical method might eventually yield limited statistical power and sensitivity in distinguishing the efficacy of different reperfusion strategies, because there are a range of velocities associated with TIMI grade 3 flow.[2]

The TIMI Frame Count

The corrected TIMI frame count (CTFC) overcomes many of the limitations of the categorical TIMI flow grade scheme.[4] In contrast to the conventional TIMI flow grade classification scheme, the CTFC is quantitative rather than qualitative, it is objective rather than subjective, it is a continuous rather than a categorical variable, and it is reproducible. Figure 3-1 shows the method used to determine the TIMI frame count. In the first frame included in the TIMI frame count, a column of dye touches both borders of the coronary artery and moves forward. In the last frame, dye begins to enter (but not necessarily fill) a standard distal landmark in the

artery. These landmarks are as follows: in the right coronary artery the first branch of the posterolateral artery; in the circumflex system the most distal branch of the obtuse marginal branch that includes the culprit lesion in the dye path; and in the left anterior descending (LAD) artery the distal bifurcation, which is also known as the "moustache," "pitch fork," or "whale's tail" (Figure 3-1). To correct for the longer length of the LAD, these frame counts are corrected for by dividing by 1.7 to arrive at the CTFC.[4]

In contrast to the TIMI flow grades, the CTFC is very reproducible. When angiograms are examined on two separate occasions 6 months apart, correlation of 0.97 in readings over time and a correlation of 0.99 between three different observers have been reported. Recently, the Cleveland Clinic Hospital and TIMI angiographic core laboratories analyzed the same set of films from a fibrinolytic trial. Although there were discrepancies in 21% of the TIMI flow grade readings (41 of 194, kappa = 0.76), excellent concordance was seen using the CTFC (overall median difference = 0 frames), with no significant difference in CTFCs being observed between the two experienced laboratories.

In the absence of acute myocardial infarction, we have demonstrated that normal blood flow in normal arteries requires 21 frames to traverse the artery, with the 95% confidence interval for normal flow extending from >14 frames to <28 frames. The impact of the force of injection on the CTFC has been studied by use of power injections performed at the 10th and 90th percentile of human injection rates, and this changed the CTFC by only two frames. Nitrate administration can significantly increase the CTFC. Dye injection at the beginning of diastole significantly decreases the CTFC from 30.1 to 24.4 frames ($P < 0.001$) for the left coronary artery and from 24.2 to 21.2 frames ($P < 0.001$) for the right coronary artery. Increasing heart rate significantly decreased the CTFC from 30.4 to 25.3 frames ($P < 0.001$). These confounders must, therefore, be considered in the design and interpretation of trials in which the CTFC is applied.

By use of the CTFC, coronary blood flow seems to be unimodally distributed as a continuous variable.[4] As a result, any division of flow into "normal" and "abnormal" categories is somewhat arbitrary. Although the TIMI Angiographic Core Laboratory does not use the CTFC to determine the TIMI flow grades, in a retrospective analysis, flow tended to be classified as TIMI grade 2 flow if the CTFC was >40 (~1.3 seconds).

Nonculprit Flow: A Flawed "Gold Standard" Against which to Gauge Flow in Acute Myocardial Infarction

Traditionally, it has been assumed that basal flow in nonculprit arteries in the setting of acute myocardial infarction after thrombolysis is "normal." However, in the setting of acute myocardial infarction, we have demonstrated that the mean CTFC at 90 minutes after thrombolysis in the nonculprit arteries (30.9 ± 15.0, n = 1817) was 45% higher than minimally diseased arteries with normal flow in the absence of acute myocardial infarc-

The TIMI Frame Count Method

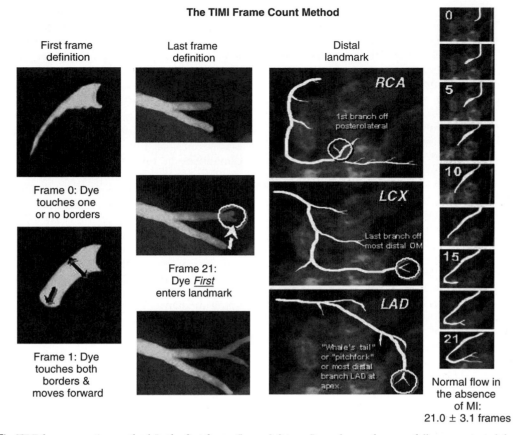

First frame definition

Frame 0: Dye touches one or no borders

Frame 1: Dye touches both borders & moves forward

Last frame definition

Frame 21: Dye *First* enters landmark

Distal landmark

RCA
1st branch off posterolateral

LCX
Last branch off most distal OM

LAD
"Whale's tail" or "pitchfork" or most distal branch LAD at apex

0
5
10
15
21

Normal flow in the absence of MI: 21.0 ± 3.1 frames

FIGURE 3-1. The TIMI frame counting method. In the first frame *(lower left panel)*, a column of near or fully concentrated dye touches both borders of the coronary artery and moves forward. In the last frame *(second column)*, dye begins to enter (but does not necessarily fill) a standard distal landmark in the artery. These standard distal landmarks are as follows: the first branch of the posterolateral artery in the right coronary artery *(upper panel, third column)*; in the circumflex system the most distal branch of the obtuse marginal branch, which includes the culprit lesion in the dye path *(mid panel, third column)*; and in the left anterior descending artery the distal bifurcation that is also known as the "moustache," "pitch fork," or "whale's tail" *(lower panel, third column)*.

tion (21.0 ± 3.1, $P < 0.001$). Not only is basal blood flow impaired in nonculprit arteries, but coronary flow reserve might also be impaired for several weeks after acute myocardial infarction. Thus, the conventional notion that flow in uninvolved arteries is "normal" might be erroneous and might lead to the misclassification of TIMI flow grades. This limitation is further compounded by the fact that in the RCA, no other "normal" artery is even present for comparison. Finally, the wide variety and subtle variation of current international cine-filming speeds (12.5, 15, 25, 30, 50, 60 frames/second) adds to the difficulties in assessing coronary blood flow. Abnormal flow in nonculprit arteries is not simply an angiographic aberrancy; abnormal flow in all three arteries is also related to adverse clinical outcomes just as is abnormal flow in the culprit artery.

A variety of mechanisms might mediate abnormal flow in the nonculprit artery. Slower flow in the nonculprit artery is associated with slower flow in the culprit artery, a longer length of culprit vessel distal to the stenosis (i.e., a larger infarct), a tighter stenosis in the nonculprit artery, and pulsatile flow in the culprit artery. The observation relating pulsatile culprit flow to delayed nonculprit flow provides some insight into the potential mechanism underlying abnormal flow in all three arter-

ies. A pulsatile pattern of flow with systolic flow reversal on the angiogram is analogous to systolic flow reversal observed during Doppler velocity wire studies, and this flow pattern reflects heightened downstream microvascular resistance. Thus, insofar as all three coronary arteries interdigitate downstream and insofar as they may share microvascular territories, it is not surprising that flow abnormalities in one artery might be linked to abnormal flow in the other arteries. To this end, we have recently demonstrated that percutaneous coronary intervention (PCI) of the culprit lesion is associated with an improvement in nonculprit artery flow after the intervention. Others have demonstrated that stent placement in the acute myocardial infarction setting improves both culprit and nonculprit flow, and by 15 minutes after stent placement in acute myocardial infarction, flow in the culprit and the nonculprit artery are both slower than at baseline. Likewise, fractional shortening of the left ventricle declines by 15 minutes after stent placement. Administration of an alpha-receptor blocker improves flow in both the culprit and the nonculprit territories and significantly improves wall motion. These data suggest that global flow abnormalities might be related to downstream "alpha-adrenergic storm." Along similar lines, we have recently demonstrated that stent placement after conventional percutaneous transluminal coronary angioplasty (PTCA) might be associated with a higher rate of staining of the myocardium, possibly secondary to downstream spasm or embolization.

Measurement of Coronary Velocity from the Angiogram

The length (cm) of arteries can be planimetered on the angiogram, and these data can be combined with the frame count (time) to calculate what is called the quantitative coronary angiography (QCA) velocity (cm/s). This method yields velocities that are nearly identical to that reported with Doppler velocity wires. The CTFC can also be used to calculate the coronary flow reserve. Essentially, if the time for dye to traverse the artery is cut in half (i.e., if the CTFC is cut in half), then the coronary flow reserve is 2.0 by definition. Coronary flow reserve (CFR) can be calculated by assessing the CTFC before and 15 seconds after intracoronary adenosine (24 to 36 µg in left anterior descending artery and left circumflex artery; 18 to 24 µg in right coronary artery). CFR can be calculated as the ratio of preadenosine CTFC ÷ postadenosine CTFC. This ratio has been validated in the literature as highly correlated with Doppler velocity wire–derived CFR ($r = 0.88, P < 0.0001$).

The PTCA guidewire velocity is another inexpensive method to assess coronary velocity. After PTCA, the guidewire tip is placed at the coronary landmark, and a Kelly clamp is placed on the guidewire where it exits the Y-adapter. The guidewire tip is then withdrawn to the catheter tip, and a second Kelly clamp is placed on the wire where it exits the Y-adapter. The distance between the two Kelly clamps outside the body is the distance between the catheter tip and the anatomical landmark inside the body. Velocity (cm/s) might be calculated as this distance (cm) divided by the time for dye to reach the landmark (CTFC divided by cinefilming speed yields time in seconds). By extension, flow (mL/s) may be calculated by multiplying this velocity (cm/s) and the mean cross-sectional lumen area (cm^2) along the length of the artery to the TIMI landmark.

The PTCA guidewire velocity technique demonstrates that TIMI grade 3 flow is actually rather heterogeneous. Among patients with TIMI grade 3 flow both before and after PTCA, the guidewire velocity actually increased 38% from 17.0 cm/s to 23.5 cm/s ($P = 0.01$). Likewise, flow increased 86% from 0.7 mL/s to 1.3 mL/s ($P = 0.001$).

The TIMI Myocardial Perfusion Grade (TMPG)

Myocardial contrast echocardiography has demonstrated that restoration of epicardial coronary blood flow does not necessarily imply tissue level or microvascular perfusion. Although myocardial contrast echo is an elegant tool to assess tissue level perfusion, difficulties in its day-to-day application currently limit its clinical usefulness. This led to the recent development of a new angiographic index of tissue level perfusion that is simple to apply called the TMPG.[5] Tissue level perfusion on the angiogram is graded as follows:

TMPG 3: Normal entry and exit of dye from the microvasculature. There is the ground-glass appearance ("blush") or opacification of the myocardium in the distribution of the culprit lesion that clears normally and is either gone or only mildly/moderately persistent at the end of the washout phase (i.e., dye is gone or is mildly/moderately persistent after three cardiac cycles of the washout phase and noticeably diminishes in intensity during the washout phase), similar to that in an uninvolved artery. Blush that is of only mild intensity throughout the washout phase but fades minimally is also classified as grade 3.

TMPG 2: Delayed entry and exit of dye from the microvasculature. There is the ground-glass appearance ("blush") or opacification of the myocardium in the distribution of the culprit lesion that is strongly persistent at the end of the washout phase (i.e., dye is strongly persistent after three cardiac cycles of the washout phase and either does not or only minimally diminishes in intensity during washout).

TMPG 1: Dye slowly enters but fails to exit the microvasculature. There is the ground-glass appearance ("blush") or opacification of the myocardium in the distribution of the culprit lesion that fails to clear from the microvasculature, and dye staining is present on the next injection (approximately 30 seconds between injections).

TMPG 0: Dye fails to enter the microvasculature. There is either minimal or no ground-glass appearance ("blush") or opacification of the myocardium in the distribution of the culprit artery indicating lack of tissue level perfusion.

To further quantitate the rate of dye entry into the myocardium, digital subtraction angiography (DSA) can be applied. To achieve good image alignment, DSA is consistently performed at end diastole by aligning cine-frame images before dye fills the myocardium with those at the peak of myocardial filling to subtract the spine, ribs, diaphragm, and the epicardial artery (Figure 3-2). A representative region of the myocardium is sampled that is free of overlap by epicardial arterial branches to determine the brightness of the myocardium when it first reaches its peak intensity. The size or circumference of the blush is then measured with a hand-held planimeter scaled to the size of the catheter. The number of frames required for the myocardium to first reach its peak brightness is converted into time (s). In this way the rate of rise in brightness (gray/s) and the rate of growth of blush (cm/s) can be estimated. Compared with normal patients, microvascular perfusion was reduced in patients with acute myocardial infarction on DSA as demonstrated by a reduction in peak gray (brightness) (10.9 vs. 7.8, $P < 0.0001$), the rate of rise in gray/s (2.8 vs. 2.1, $P < 0.0001$), the blush circumference (cm) (19.4 vs. 13.6, $P < 0.0001$), and the rate of growth in circumference (cm/s) (5.2 vs. 3.7, $P < 0.0001$). This technique has been successfully applied to evaluate drug efficacy in restoring tissue level perfusion.

Digital Subtraction to Quantitate Tissue Level Perfusion

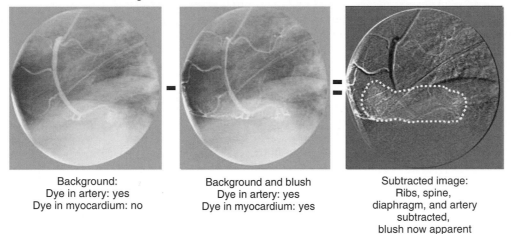

Background:
Dye in artery: yes
Dye in myocardium: no

Background and blush
Dye in artery: yes
Dye in myocardium: yes

Subtracted image:
Ribs, spine,
diaphragm, and artery
subtracted,
blush now apparent

FIGURE 3-2. Digital subtraction angiography (DSA) was used to quantitatively characterize the kinetics of dye entering the myocardium by use of the angiogram. DSA is performed at end-diastole by aligning cineframes images before dye fills the myocardium with those at the peak of myocardial filling to subtract spine, ribs, diaphragm, and the epicardial artery. A representative region of the myocardium is sampled that is free of overlap by epicardial arterial branches to determine the increase in the gray scale brightness of the myocardium when it first reached its peak intensity. The circumference of the myocardial blush is measured with a hand-held planimeter. The number of frames required for the myocardium to first reach its peak brightness is converted into time (s) by dividing the frame count by 30. In this way, the rate of rise in brightness (gray/s) and the rate of growth of blush (cm/s) can be calculated.

Relationship of Epicardial Coronary Blood Flow and Tissue Level Perfusion to Clinical Outcomes

There is a significant association between the 90-minute TIMI flow grade and mortality. Recently, we have demonstrated that the 60-minute TIMI flow grades are also similar to the 90-minute TIMI flow grades in the magnitude of their association with mortality. This is important insofar as many recent thrombolytic trials have now switched to the use of a 60-minute angiographic end point. One question that arises is whether injections at the earlier 60-minute time point alter patency at the later 90-minute end point. Recently, we demonstrated that early injections open about 10% of closed arteries, but given the low rate of vessel occlusion, the patency rate changes negligibly, by about 2%.

Another question that arises regarding the magnitude of mortality improvement, which could be anticipated on the basis of angiographic flow improvements. In GUSTO 1, an increase in the rate of TIMI grade 3 flow by 22 absolute percentage points (from 32% with streptokinase (SK) and intravenous [IV] heparin to 54% with front-loaded tissue plasminogen activator [tPA]) was associated with a mortality reduction of 1% (from 7.4% with SK and IV heparin to 6.3% with front-loaded tPA). Assuming a linear relationship between rates of TIMI grade 3 flow and mortality, current rates of TIMI grade 3 flow would need to improve from 60% to 80% to yield another 1% improvement in mortality. Although early trials of combination therapy for acute myocardial infarction hinted at a 20% improvement in TIMI grade 3 flow, pooled data from dose confirmation phases of various phase II angiographic studies of combination therapy demonstrate only an 8% improvement in TIMI grade

3 flow among patients treated with combination therapy (56% [n = 329] to 64% [n = 321]). If a 20% improvement is required to improve mortality by 1%, then an 8% improvement might be anticipated to improve mortality by 8/20 of 1% or by approximately 0.4%. This magnitude of mortality improvement is precisely what was demonstrated in the GUSTO V trial, consistent with the open artery hypothesis. To provide a more robust analysis of the relationship between TIMI flow grades at 90 minutes after thrombolysis and clinical outcome, a pooled analysis of 5498 patients enrolled in angiographic trials shows that the 30- to 42-day mortality rate was lowest (3.7%) among patients with TIMI grade 3 flow 90 minutes after thrombolysis. This was significantly lower than that in patients with TIMI grade 2 flow (6.1%, $P < 0.0001$) or TIMI grade 0/1 flow (9.3%, $P < 0.0001$) flow. Mortality differed significantly between patients with TIMI grades 2 and 0/1 flows ($P = 0.003$). Thus, TIMI grade 2 flow (partial perfusion) confers a significant survival advantage compared with TIMI 0/1 flow and therefore should not be regarded as a failure of reperfusion but rather as intermediate in benefit between TIMI grades 0/1 and 3 flows.

Assessment of TIMI grade 2 flow has, however, been limited by the interobserver variability. In addition, TIMI grade 2 flow encompasses a range of flow velocities from markedly delayed to near normal flows. Finally, most TIMI grade 2 flow is observed in the LAD artery (63%), whereas most TIMI grade 3 flow is observed in the right coronary artery (RCA) (approximately 75%). It is therefore possible that the poor outcomes observed among patients with TIMI grade 2 flow might be explained, at least in part, by the fact that this poor flow occurs more frequently in the LAD that subtends the anterior wall of the left ventricle.

The more objective CTFC is also related to clinical outcomes even when LAD location is corrected for. In the TIMI 4, 10A, and 10B trials, the flow in the infarct-related artery in survivors was significantly faster than in patients who died (CTFCs of 49.5 vs. 69.6, $P = 0.0003$). Mortality increased by 0.7% for every 10-frame rise in CTFC ($P < 0.001$). No patients with a CTFC <14 (hyperemic or TIMI grade 4 flow) died by 30 days. Likewise, in the broader population of the RESTORE trial (patients undergoing angioplasty for acute coronary syndromes including unstable angina and non-ST-elevation myocardial infarction), the CTFC after angioplasty was significantly faster in survivors than among those patients who died (CTFCs, 20.4 vs. 33.4, $P = 0.017$). Again, none of the 376 patients with a CTFC <14 after angioplasty died in this trial, underscoring the fact that within the subgroup of patients with "normal flow" there might be further subgroups with even better flow and even better outcomes.

The CTFC after PCI in this trial was also related to a lower rate of restenosis, even when postprocedure diameters were corrected for. Thus, not only is bigger better, but faster is also better. It has also been shown that the TIMI frame count/minimum lumen diameter predicts restenosis.

Independent of epicardial blood flow, tissue level perfusion using the TMPG is also associated with clinical outcomes.[5] The TMPG permits risk stratification even among patients with epicardial TIMI grade 3 flow. Despite normal TIMI grade 3 flow, those patients whose microvasculature fails to open (TIMI myocardial perfusion grade 0/1) have a persistently elevated mortality of 5.4%. This is in contrast to those patients with both TIMI grade 3 flow in the epicardial artery and TIMI myocardial perfusion grade 3, who have a mortality rate less than 1%. The TIMI flow grades and the TIMI myocardial perfusion grades can be used together to identify a group of patients at very low risk and alternatively very high risk for mortality. Those patients with both TIMI grade 3 flow and TIMI myocardial perfusion grade 3 flow had a mortality of 0.7%, whereas those patients with both TIMI grade 0/1 and TIMI myocardial perfusion grade 0/1 flow had a mortality rate of 10.9%.

Likewise, in the setting of unstable angina and non–ST-elevation myocardial infarction, we have demonstrated that TMPG 0/1 on diagnostic cardiac catheterization is independently associated with troponin elevation in a multivariate model, and if TMPG 0/1 persists after PCI, it is associated with a higher risk of death or myocardial infarction at 6 months. Finally, we have demonstrated that impaired tissue level perfusion after percutaneous coronary intervention in the unstable angina and non–ST-elevation myocardial infarction setting is associated with creatinine kinase-myocardial bound (CK-MB) elevations, as well as a higher risk of adverse clinical outcomes at 1 year. These data suggest a pathophysiological link between impaired tissue level perfusion, the release of cardiac markers, and adverse clinical outcomes in a variety of settings.

We have shown that both epicardial flow and tissue level perfusion are independently associated with improved 2-year survival after thrombolytic administration. In a multivariate model correcting for previously identified correlates of mortality (age, gender, pulse, LAD infarction, and any PCI during initial hospitalization), patency (TFG 2/3) (hazards ratio [HR] = 0.32, $P <$ 0.001), the CTFC ($P = 0.01$), and TMPG 2/3 (HR = 0.46, $P = 0.02$) all remained independently associated with reduced mortality. Although rescue PCI was associated with reduced long-term mortality in this study, improved microvascular perfusion (TMPG 2/3) before PCI was also related to improved long-term mortality independent of epicardial blood flow and the performance of rescue or adjunctive PCI.

These data suggest complementary mechanisms of improved long-term survival. It could be speculated that epicardial flow is related to long-term survival by virtue of its association with reocclusion, whereas tissue level perfusion might be more strongly related to infarct size. Indeed, we have recently demonstrated that abnormalities in perfusion are associated with larger infarcts, a pattern observed with different measures of both perfusion (TMPG and ST segment resolution) and infarct size (CK-MB and single photon emission computed tomography [SPECT]). Both angiographic and electrocardiographic measures of perfusion were independently associated with subsequent infarct size. This suggests a potential electromechanical dissociation between microvascular blood flow and myocyte function. It could be speculated that although the angiogram might reflect mechanical patency of the microvasculature and the integrity of the endothelium, the electrocardiogram may reflect the functional status of the supplied myocardium. These data indicate that angiographic and electrocardiographic measures are independent and complementary in their prognostic significance.

Finally, although perfusion and infarct size are associated with each other, the directionality of the causal relationship is unclear. It is unclear whether larger infarcts impair early microvascular flow or, conversely, whether early perfusion abnormalities lead to subsequent increases in infarct size. It is notable that after controlling for early left ventricular ejection fraction (a crude estimate of early infarct size), both TMPG and ST resolution seemed to provide additional prognostic information with respect to later SPECT infarct size.

QUANTITATION OF MYOCARDIAL PERFUSION: ECHO/DOPPLER METHODS

Myocardial perfusion imaging by echocardiography is a new technique that has been made possible by the development of microbubble contrast agents. Initially, myocardial contrast echocardiography (MCE) required intracoronary injection of microbubbles during echocardiographic imaging in the catheterization laboratory. However, recent technological advances have enabled MCE to be done at the bedside during IV infusion of microbubbles that are designed to traverse the pulmonary circulation to the left side of the heart. MCE offers several theoretical advantages over more traditional nuclear perfusion imaging. It avoids the use of radiation exposure, can be done at the bedside, and has much better spatial and temporal resolution. Potential clinical applications include assessment of reperfusion therapy for acute myocardial infarction, postmyocardial infarction risk area and infarct size, and myocardial viability. The addition of perfusion data to wall motion might augment the results of stress echocardiography. This section will describe the technological advances in contrast agents and related imaging technologies that enable myocardial perfusion to be assessed by echocardiography. In addition, clinical studies of myocardial perfusion by MCE will be reviewed.

Contrast Agents

The three most important properties of a microbubble are its size, gas, and shell composition. Myocardial perfusion after intracoronary injection of an ultrasound contrast agent was first described in 1980, but the large size of the bubbles used resulted in microcirculatory occlusion and death of the animals, and by 1983 the technique of sonication to produce smaller microbubbles was developed. The small size of such microbubbles allows them to pass through the capillary bed. The acoustic backscatter (brightness of the signal on echocardiography) of a bubble is related to the sixth power of its radius; therefore, even a small decrease in size can cause a large decrease in contrast effect. On the other hand, microbubbles that are too large might become lodged in the pulmonary capillaries, so that they do not cross the lungs and reach the left side of the heart. Thus, there is a delicate balance between the size of the microbubble and the size of the capillary. The ideal microbubble would be a large, compressible microbubble for a brighter ultrasound signal. However, most of the pulmonary capillaries are between 4 and 8 μm. Therefore, the ideal size of the microbubbles is probably about 4 μm, because larger microbubbles might become entrapped in the pulmonary microcirculation.

Early agents contained microbubbles of air in saline, indocyanine green, or sonicated dextrose. Air is highly diffusible and rapidly escapes from bubbles when mixed with blood. Accordingly, air-filled contrast agents generally do not opacify the left side of the heart after IV injection. Myocardial opacification with air-filled microbubbles could only be achieved by direct injection

of bubbles into the coronary system and was limited to the cardiac catheterization laboratory. Therefore, the development of microbubbles containing nondiffusible gases was undertaken to enable IV injection. The ideal gas would be insoluble in blood and slow to diffuse out of the bubbles. Perfluorocarbon gases meet this requirement and are also biologically inert and therefore safe. Microbubbles containing perfluorocarbon gases maintain excellent backscattering properties and are characterized by prolonged persistence and in vivo stability. Such agents have been demonstrated to opacify the left ventricular myocardium after intravenous injection.

Finally, shell composition is important. The gas in microbubbles is typically encapsulated in a shell composed of a protein, phospholipid, or polymer. Alternately, the microbubbles might exist as a free gas bubble in the circulation. The thickness and elasticity of the shell might influence diffusion of the gas out of the microbubble, potentially allowing greater persistence of the contrast effect. The shell composition might also increase compressibility of the microbubble (important for acoustic backscatter) or its resistance to ultrasound-mediated destruction.

Albunex and Levovist are often called first-generation contrast agents because they contained air (Table 3-1). Second-generation agents use primarily fluorocarbon gases and result in left ventricular opacification in most patients after venous injection. These agents provide prolonged and persistent opacification of the left ventricle, as well as more accurate and reproducible assessment of myocardial perfusion. Newer agents in development include polymer-coated microbubbles and anionically charged microbubbles.

Imaging Technologies

The optimal imaging method for contrast echocardiography is dependent on the physical characteristics of the particular microbubble used. A number of promising technologies are available. A major advance in MCE was the recognition that ultrasound energy at the high acoustic powers used for normal echocardiographic imaging destroys the microbubbles. A decrease in contrast reflectivity has been shown to correspond to a reduction in microbubble numbers. Microbubble destruction can be attenuated using intermittent

■ ■ ■

TABLE 3-1   CONTRAST AGENTS CURRENTLY AVAILABLE OR IN DEVELOPMENT

Agent	Shell composition	Gas	Mean diameter (μm)
Albunex (Molecular Biosystems, San Diego, CA)	Albumin	Air	4.3
Levovist (Schering, Berlin, Germany)	Galactose	Air	2-4
Optison (Molecular Biosystems, San Diego, CA)	Albumin	Perfluoropropane	3.9
Definity (Bristol-Myers Squibb, North Billerica, MA)	Phospholipid	Perfluoropropane	3-4
SonoVue (Braco Research, Geneva, Switzerland)	Phospholipid	Sulfur hexafluoride	2.5
AI-700 (Acusphere, Inc, Cambridge, MA)	Polymer	Perfluorocarbon	2.0
PB-127 (Point Biomedical, San Carlos, CA)	Polymer bilayer	Nitrogen	4.0
NC100100 (Nycomed AS, Oslo, Norway)	Unknown	Perfluorocarbon	3.5
PESDA (not commercial)	Albumin/dextrose	Perfluorocarbon	4.0
Imagent (Alliance Pharmaceutical Corp., San Diego, CA)	Buffered surfactant	Perfluorohexane/N2	3-4

imaging in which ultrasound pulses are limited to short electrocardiogram-gated pulses rather than continuous transmission at conventional 30-Hz frame rates. Reducing microbubble destruction improves myocardial opacification. Microbubble destruction can also be alleviated by reducing the ultrasound transmit power. This has the advantage of allowing real-time imaging.

Harmonic Imaging

Harmonic imaging is based on the fact that microbubbles undergo nonlinear oscillations when exposed to ultrasound. These oscillations give rise to backscatter signals at multiples of the original ultrasound frequency. By use of this principle, second harmonic imaging transmits ultrasound waves at one frequency and receives at twice that frequency. For example, the ultrasound signal may be sent at 1.3 MHz and received at 2.6 MHz. The harmonic signal is more likely to emanate from the microbubbles than from tissue. Not only does this make the image more vivid, it also requires less contrast than fundamental imaging. The combination of intermittent and harmonic imaging has been shown to be an improvement over conventional imaging for MCE. A number of clinical studies have shown that intermittent harmonic imaging is an improved technology for MCE, leading to both improved opacification of left ventricular cavities and assessment of myocardial perfusion.[6,7] A lower mechanical index (i.e., lower acoustic power) reduces microbubble destruction and therefore allows imaging to be done at frame rates high enough to interpret wall motion and perfusion simultaneously. This technique has been referred to as accelerated intermittent imaging. More recently, real-time perfusion imaging has been performed with very low acoustic power settings so as to cause microbubble resonance but not destruction.[8]

Power Doppler Harmonic Imaging

Power Doppler is an imaging modality that is very sensitive in the detection of ultrasound contrast agents.[9] Whereas conventional Doppler imaging processes the frequency shift of the received ultrasound signal to determine velocity, power mode Doppler analyzes the amplitude of the signal that is a marker of the number of ultrasound scatterers present (in this case, microbubbles). When performed at the harmonic frequency, this imaging mode is termed harmonic power Doppler imaging (HPDI). HPDI is more sensitive in detecting microbubbles than B-mode, largely because it transmits multiple bursts of ultrasound along each scan line. Two proposed mechanisms have been proposed for the ability to detect myocardial perfusion by HPDI. The first theory postulates that microbubble destruction produces an acoustic energy that results in an HPDI signal, termed "stimulated acoustic emissions." The second theory postulates that microbubble destruction results in a decrease in backscatter intensity and a change in phase between the sequential ultrasound bursts. HPDI interprets this change in phase as motion and therefore displays a signal. Regardless of which theory is correct,

microbubble destruction is necessary for HPDI to detect perfusion at high acoustic power. Recently, the use of low transmit power to avoid microbubble destruction and instead image the harmonic resonance of the microbubbles has enabled visualization of perfusion by HPDI in real time.

Physiology of Myocardial Contrast Echocardiography

Microbubbles have myocardial transit rates similar to red blood cells at the capillary level. Accordingly, MCE can provide a mechanism for quantifying myocardial blood flow with microbubbles by use of indicator dilution theory. Moreover, the microbubbles used in MCE remain entirely within the intravascular space. Because more than 90% of myocardial blood volume is located in the capillaries, MCE essentially provides an image of myocardial blood volume that is predominantly the amount of blood in the myocardial capillary bed. Moreover, because the velocity of blood flow in individual capillaries is very low (<1 mm/s), traditional Doppler velocity imaging cannot be used for MCE. As discussed previously, imaging the microbubbles within the myocardial capillary bed relies on either microbubble destruction techniques at high acoustic power or microbubble harmonic resonance at low acoustic power. MCE offers the possibility to evaluate perfusion of tissue at the capillary level and can provide pathophysiological insights into the myocardial microcirculation.[10]

As noted previously, because most microbubbles are intravascular tracers, MCE can be used to quantify myocardial blood volume by use of the indicator dilution theory. In dogs, myocardial perfusion can be quantified from time-intensity curves derived from direct injection of contrast into the left atrium and the background-subtracted peak video intensity that correlates closely with myocardial blood volume particularly during pharmacological hyperemia. Microbubbles are destroyed by ultrasound at high acoustic power, and Wei et al[11] took advantage of this fact to develop a novel method of quantifying myocardial perfusion. They administered microbubbles as a continuous infusion and then destroyed them within the myocardial capillary bed with triggered ultrasound. The hypothesis was that the reappearance rate of the microbubbles within the ultrasound beam would be a function of blood flow velocity and would depend on the time between ultrasound pulses (Figure 3-3). The peak microbubble concentration in the myocardium during steady state will reflect the myocardial blood volume. By determining both of these variables, it is possible to determine myocardial blood flow quantitatively as the product of the plateau videointensity and the rate of the replenishment curve.

Myocardial Perfusion Imaging by MCE

MCE has been shown to image myocardial perfusion after IV contrast injection in numerous animal models, as well as in humans. We studied perfluoropentane microbubbles in a canine model of acute coronary occlu-

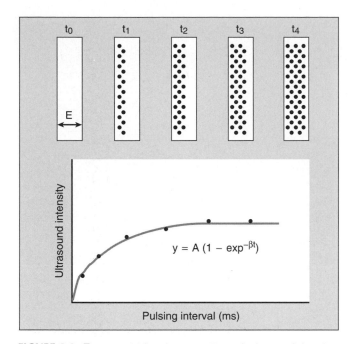

FIGURE 3-3. T*op panel,* The elevation (E) or thickness of the ultrasound beam is shown. At time 0 after a burst of ultrasound, there are no microbubbles present because of their destruction. On the first frame after a delay between ultrasound pulses (time 1), some microbubbles are seen to wash back into the beam. The longer the time delay, the more microbubbles replenish the beam until the beam is completely filled (time 4 in this schematic example). *Bottom panel,* Plotting the ultrasound signal intensity against the time delay between pulses yields a curve that fits the equation shown. The initial slope of the curve represents blood velocity, and the plateau represents myocardial blood volume. The product of A and B yields myocardial blood flow, which correlates closely with regional myocardial blood flow by radiolabeled microspheres in a dog model. (Adapted from Wei, et al. Quantification of myocardial blood flow with ultrasound-induced destruction of microbubbles administered as a constant venous infusion. *Circulation* 1998; 97:473.)

defect sizes during coronary occlusion correlate closely with postmortem risk area and infarct size.

These data have led to studies of the use of second-generation microbubbles to assess myocardial perfusion with coronary vasodilatation in a clinical setting.[13,14]

In a multicenter trial of patients who had a myocardial infarction in the prior year, the results of MCE were compared with SPECT imaging in 203 patients.[15] The MCE results were disappointing, because in segments with a diagnostic MCE, the segmental sensitivity ranged from 14% to 65%, and the specificity varied between 78% and 95% with SPECT scanning as the "gold standard." As expected, harmonic imaging was the more accurate imaging technique. The combined assessment of wall motion and perfusion by MCE yielded the highest sensitivity (46% to 55%) and specificity (82% to 83%). The study was criticized on the grounds that the echocardiographers who performed the study had little or no experience in MCE and did not receive specific training. SPECT was used as the "gold standard," and the low incidence of wall motion abnormalities in patients exhibiting SPECT defects calls into question the clinical significance of the SPECT findings.

A number of studies have shown the potential usefulness of MCE with harmonic power Doppler imaging. Heinle et al[16] performed MCE with harmonic power Doppler imaging with Optison in 123 patients who were referred for SPECT imaging for known or suspected coronary artery disease. MCE was performed during adenosine infusion (140 µg/kg/min) and was compared with sestamibi SPECT imaging. When MCE and SPECT were compared for agreement between normal perfusion vs. reversible defects vs. fixed defects, concordance was 82% for the LAD, 76% for the RCA, and 72% for the left circumflex artery (LCX). (Figure 3-4 shows an example of a patient with a fixed perfusion defect by both MCE and

sion and found that MCE accurately defined the extent of the area at risk and the infarct size, as determined by gross pathological specimen staining. Others have shown that MCE correctly detects the time course of changes in flow during occlusion-reperfusion, correlates significantly with regional blood flow, and accurately detects the progressive reduction in blood flow occurring within the postischemic microcirculation.

There have also been a number of studies looking at whether MCE can assess myocardial perfusion when there is a residual stenosis. With a canine model, Main et al performed MCE at baseline, during acute ischemia with residual flow, during physiological hyperemia, and during total coronary occlusion. They demonstrated that MCE can identify myocardial risk area in the setting of a severe coronary stenosis with residual antegrade flow.[12] A number of animal studies have shown that in the presence of coronary vasodilators, MCE can identify coronary stenoses with normal resting flow but impaired flow reserve. The magnitude of perfusion mismatch during hyperemia in the presence of a coronary stenosis correlates with the magnitude of a flow mismatch with radiolabeled microspheres and perfusion

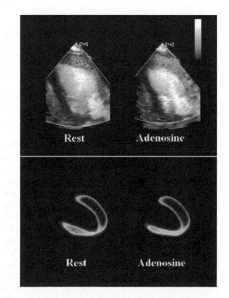

FIGURE 3-4. *Top panel,* Harmonic power Doppler images from an apical two-chamber view at rest *(left)* and during adenosine infusion *(right).* There is normal perfusion of the anterior wall but a fixed defect in the inferior wall. *Bottom panel,* SPECT sestamibi images confirm the fixed inferior defect in the same patient. See also Color Insert.

SPECT imaging.) The basal lateral wall tended to have a higher proportion of false-positive perfusion defects by MCE, largely because of acoustic shadowing and attenuation. Potential solutions to this problem include off-axis imaging and narrower transducer apertures with a more homogeneous beam profile.

MCE with harmonic power Doppler imaging has been shown to accurately predict the infarct-related artery after a Q-wave myocardial infarction and to identify stunned myocardium. Concordance between MCE and coronary angiography was excellent, and both MCE and SPECT imaging have comparable high sensitivity (93% and 94%, respectively) for detection of infarct artery patency as shown by coronary angiography. Main et al[12] have found that the combined assessment of microvascular integrity and contractile reserve improves differentiation of stunning and necrosis after acute anterior wall myocardial infarction.

To date, most studies of myocardial perfusion during stress have used vasodilators such as dipyridamole or adenosine. Despite the difficulty of increased heart rates complicating electrocardiographic gating, the technique of dobutamine stress echocardiography yields agreement with QCA of about 80% for perfusion compared with 70% for wall motion analysis. Shimoni et al[17] evaluated real-time perfusion MCE during supine bicycle exercise and treadmill exercise. Combining MCE and wall motion yielded a sensitivity of 86% and specificity of 88% compared with QCA. Agreement with SPECT was 76% for MCE perfusion.

Clinical Applications of MCE

In the setting of an acute myocardial infarction, MCE can be useful in assessing the area at risk, infarct size, and myocardial viability.[14] In addition, because MCE assesses myocardial perfusion, it can evaluate the no-reflow phenomenon. In patients with acute myocardial infarction studied before and after thrombolytic therapy with MCE, it has been shown that those patients who had a significant contrast enhancement within the risk area subsequently had an improvement in global left ventricular ejection fraction (LVEF) and regional left ventricular function. Some patients exhibited the no-reflow phenomenon characterized by TIMI grade 3 flow in the infarct-related artery but a residual perfusion defect, and they exhibited poor functional recovery of the post-ischemic myocardium. Patients with a high degree of microvascular damage and a large initial risk area have increased risk for subsequent cardiovascular events. Thus, coronary artery patency should not be thought to be synonymous with myocardial perfusion. The MCE assessment of microvascular integrity after reperfusion is a good predictor of the definitive infarct size and also provides useful estimates of myocardial viability. The development of myocardial perfusion imaging by IV MCE offers the potential to assess the no-reflow phenomenon at the bedside in patients with acute myocardial infarction. Because of its high spatial resolution, MCE offers the ability to identify subendocardial vs. Transmural perfusion abnormalities (Figure 3-5).

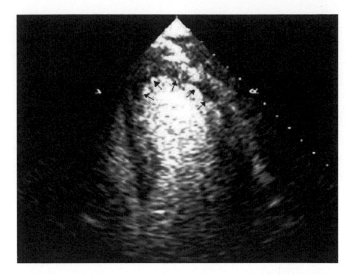

FIGURE 3-5. MCE study showing a subendocardial defect at the apex *(arrows)*. Unlike SPECT imaging, the high spatial resolution of echocardiography allows visualization of the transmural extent of perfusion defects.

Contrast agents can be beneficial in the assessment of coronary artery disease through improved visualization of left ventricular regional wall motion during stress echocardiography, when optimal endocardial visualization is essential. Improved visualization of the myocardium with contrast decreases interobserver and intraobserver variability, thus leading to more accurate and reliable stress echocardiograms. A high percentage of stress echocardiograms are difficult to interpret because of poor image quality, and contrast agents can improve the image quality dramatically. Another determinant of both infarct size and the amount of viable myocardium after acute coronary occlusion is the extent of collateral blood flow, and this can also be assessed by MCE.[18] The combination of MCE and dobutamine stress echocardiography provides information about contractile reserve and myocardial perfusion and seems to improve the diagnostic value of the individual tests.[19]

Future Directions

MCE is an emerging technology that might soon allow quantitative assessment of myocardial perfusion at the bedside. In the past 20 years, advances in both microbubble design and imaging technology have made it possible to study myocardial perfusion with MCE using IV agents. The use of high molecular weight gases has enabled consistent opacification of both the left ventricular cavity and myocardium. The use of intermittent harmonic imaging and harmonic power Doppler imaging has allowed assessment of myocardial perfusion and ventricular opacification, and real-time perfusion imaging, at low acoustic power, might offer the capability to assess perfusion and wall motion simultaneously and to take advantage of the high spatial and temporal resolution of echocardiography. Larger multicenter clinical trials are needed to demonstrate the applicability of these initial results to clinical practice. The low cost of MCE and its portability might eventually give it an advantage over current nuclear techniques.[13]

DETECTION AND EVALUATION OF CORONARY ARTERY DISEASE WITH MYOCARDIAL PERFUSION-GATED SPECT IMAGING

Perfusion Agents for Myocardial Perfusion SPECT Imaging

Regional myocardial blood flow can be assessed noninvasively by imaging the distribution of radiolabeled perfusion agents with SPECT.[20] (Table 3-2 summarizes the characteristics of perfusion tracers currently available for clinical use or undergoing clinical investigation.)

Thallium-201

Thallium is a metallic element in group III-A of the periodic table. Its principal photo peaks are at 135 and 167 keV, and it emits abundant X-rays of 69 to 83 keV (98%). The 69- to 83-keV X-rays allow imaging with high-resolution, low-energy collimators. After IV administration, the initial myocardial uptake of ^{201}Tl depends on myocardial blood flow and the extraction fraction. The cellular uptake of ^{201}Tl occurs by means of an active mechanism that depends on Na/K-ATPase. Under basal conditions, the extraction fraction is high and measured at 88%. During hyperemia, the extraction of ^{201}Tl falls once a flow rate of 2.5 mL/min/g is achieved. The myocardial extraction of ^{201}Tl is mildly decreased during hypoxia by 10% to 14% and is severely decreased in scarred myocardium that is unable to concentrate ^{201}Tl intracellularly.

After the initial extraction phase, the intracellular ^{201}Tl undergoes a continuous exchange with new ^{201}Tl from systemic recirculation in the myocardial capillaries. This influx and efflux of ^{201}Tl from the myocytes is known as *thallium redistribution,* which is defined as the total or partial resolution of initial defects over time after its IV administration. The process of ^{201}Tl redistribution begins soon after its IV administration and proceeds continuously until equilibrium is reached, which is determined by a net balance between myocardial ^{201}Tl influx and efflux. Redistribution results from a continuous exchange of ^{201}Tl between the myocardium and the extracardiac compartments. The presence of partial or complete ^{201}Tl redistribution over time (i.e., reversible defect) is characteristic of ischemia, whereas the lack of redistribution (i.e., fixed defect) denotes the presence of scarred myocardium.

^{99m}Tc-labeled Myocardial Perfusion Agents

Several ^{99m}Tc-labeled perfusion agents are currently available or under development for imaging regional myocardial blood flow and myocyte viability. The superior physical characteristics of ^{99m}Tc over ^{201}Tl make these perfusion agents ideal for myocardial perfusion imaging. First, the 140-keV photon energy peak of ^{99m}Tc is optimal for myocardial scintigraphy, resulting in higher quality images than those obtained with ^{201}Tl, owing to higher count statistics and decreased scatter. Second, the relatively short half-life of ^{99m}Tc (6 hours) results in more favorable patient dosimetry, and, thus, higher doses of the radiotracer (7 to 10 times larger than that of ^{201}Tl) can be administered, rendering better image quality with shorter acquisition time.

^{99m}Tc Sestamibi

^{99m}Tc sestamibi is a monovalent cation with a central Tc core surrounded by six identical lipophilic compounds coordinated through the isonitrile carbon. As with ^{201}Tl, the initial myocardial uptake of ^{99m}Tc sestamibi is linearly related to myocardial blood flow until a flow rate of approximately 2 mL/min/g is achieved, at which point a plateau is reached. Thus, ^{99m}Tc sestamibi underestimates myocardial blood flow at intermediate flow rates. Myocardial retention of ^{99m}Tc sestamibi is lower than that of ^{201}Tl at both intermediate and high flow levels, suggesting that the underestimation of flow is greater for ^{99m}Tc sestamibi than for ^{201}Tl.

The cellular uptake of ^{99m}Tc sestamibi involves passive diffusion across the sarcolemma and mitochondrial membranes. After reaching equilibrium, it is sequestered in the mitochondria. Moderate or severe ischemia decreases myocardial retention of ^{99m}Tc sestamibi. ^{99m}Tc sestamibi shows minimal redistribution after transient ischemia compared with what is seen

---

■ ■ ■

TABLE 3-2   COMPARATIVE CHARACTERISTICS OF RADIOLABELED PERFUSION IMAGING AGENTS

	^{201}Tl	^{99m}Tc-sestamibi	^{99m}Tc-teboroxime	^{99m}Tc-tetrofosmin	^{99m}Tc-NOET
Class	Metal	Isonitrile	BATO	Diphosphine	Nitrido
Charge	Cation	Cation	Neutral	Cation	Neutral
Myocyte uptake	Na-K-ATPase	Mitochondria	Passive diffusion	Mitochondria	Unknown
Redistribution	Yes	Minimal	Yes	No	Yes
Measure of peak MBF	Good	Adequate	Excellent	Adequate	Excellent
Injection to imaging	5-10 min	15-60 min	<2 min	15 min	10-15 min
Photopeak	68-80 keV	140 keV	140 keV	140 keV	140 keV
Physical half-life	73 h	6 h	6 h	6 h	6 h

MBF = Myocardial blood flow.

with [201]Tl. There is extensive and consistent evidence supporting the notion that the myocardial uptake of ^{99m}Tc sestamibi during a coronary occlusion correlates with occlusion flow (collateral dependent) and reflects the "area at risk." After reperfusion, the final defect size correlates with infarct size.

[99m]Tc Tetrofosmin

[99m]Tc tetrofosmin is a new diphospine, lipophilic, cationic complex of [99m]Tc. It shares similar myocardial uptake, retention, and blood clearance as ^{99m}Tc sestamibi. However, the clearance of ^{99m}Tc tetrofosmin from the liver and lungs is faster that that of ^{99m}Tc sestamibi. The initial myocardial uptake of ^{99m}Tc tetrofosmin is also linearly related to myocardial blood flow until a flow rate of approximately 1.5 to 2 mL/min/g is achieved, at which point a plateau is reached. As with other flow tracers, ^{99m}Tc tetrofosmin underestimates myocardial blood flow at intermediate flow rates. The cellular uptake of ^{99m}Tc tetrofosmin involves passive diffusion across the sarcolemma and mitochondrial membranes. Like ^{99m}Tc sestamibi, ^{99m}Tc tetrofosmin is also sequestered in the mitochondria.

Practical Implications

From the preceding, the difference in myocardial extraction among tracers suggests that ^{201}Tl might be more effective in detecting mild coronary stenoses, because it may be associated with better defect contrast between normal and abnormal zones than ^{99m}Tc-labeled sestamibi or tetrofosmin. On the other hand, the higher photon energy peak of ^{99m}Tc-labeled sestamibi or tetrofosmin results in consistently higher quality images than those obtained with [201]Tl. The higher count statistics with these imaging agents also result in less soft tissue attenuation and excellent gated images. In addition, the lack or minimal degree of redistribution over time of ^{99m}Tc-labeled sestamibi or tetrofosmin offers more flexibility than ^{201}Tl, because they do not require that imaging be performed soon after the radionuclide injection, particularly during stress. The latter is also an advantage for imaging in patients with acute ischemic syndromes, because imaging can be performed without interfering with patient management.

Stress Protocols for Myocardial Perfusion Imaging

Exercise stress is generally recommended for myocardial perfusion SPECT studies, because it is physiological, and it provides additional clinically important information (i.e., clinical and blood pressure responses, ST segment changes, exercise duration, and functional status). However, it is important to avoid submaximal stress that is associated with reduced sensitivity of the test. In these patients, pharmacological stress offers an adequate alternative to exercise stress testing. Pharmacological stress can be accomplished with coronary vasodilators such as adenosine and dipyridamole or beta_1-receptor agonists such as dobutamine.

Vasodilator Stress

Adenosine and dipyridamole are the most commonly used stressors in combination with myocardial perfusion imaging. The direct (adenosine) or indirect (dipyridamole) activation of A_2 receptors induces maximal coronary vasodilation, thereby increasing coronary blood flow. The hyperemic response to vasodilator stress is significantly greater than that achieved with exercise or dobutamine stress. Despite this differential flow response among stressors, however, the reported sensitivities and specificities of myocardial perfusion SPECT using pharmacological stress and exercise remain very similar. This is likely related to the fact that the relationship between myocardial radiotracer extraction and flow becomes nonlinear after reaching myocardial blood flows between 2 and 2.5 mL/min/g.

Dobutamine Stress

Dobutamine is a potent beta_1-receptor agonist that increases myocardial oxygen demand by augmenting contractility, heart rate, and blood pressure similar to exercise. It is generally used as an alternative to vasodilator stress in patients with chronic pulmonary disease. Peak doses of dobutamine used clinically (40 to 50 µg/kg/min) produce similar degrees of hyperemia than those achieved with exercise. The reported sensitivities and specificities for the detection of coronary artery disease with dobutamine myocardial perfusion imaging are similar to those reported with exercise and vasodilator stress. As with other stressors, sensitivity is significantly lower for detecting coronary stenoses of intermediate severity.

Myocardial Perfusion Imaging Protocols

A number of different protocols have been developed and tested for accuracy.[21,22] Imaging protocols must be tailored to individual patients on the basis of the clinical question, radiotracer used, and time constraints. ^{99m}Tc-labeled agents are now the most commonly used agents for myocardial perfusion imaging. Because ^{99m}Tc-labeled agents show minimal redistribution, two separate radiotracer injections are necessary for the rest and stress portions of the study to differentiate scar from ischemia. Ideally, two injections of 30 mCi each on separate days provide excellent quality perfusion and gated images, with no residual background activity. Because 2-day protocols are not convenient (especially for outpatients), single-day protocols have been developed. The commonly used imaging protocols for ^{99m}Tc agents or ^{201}Tl are described in the following.

Imaging Protocols for ^{99m}Tc-Labeled Perfusion Tracers

Single-day protocols are most widely used. The sequence of procedures can be rest-stress or stress-rest, with the former being the preferred. With any of these sequences, the initial study is always performed after IV injection of a low dose (8 to 12 mCi) while the subsequent study is acquired after administration of a higher dose (25 to 30 mCi) of the perfusion tracer.

Single-Day Rest-Stress Sequence

For optimal images, patients should be imaged approximately 60 minutes after the rest injection and 15 minutes after exercise. After pharmacological stress, acquisition of images should be delayed for approximately 60 minutes to allow for hepatic clearance of the perfusion tracer. Adjunctive exercise with vasodilator stress, especially with adenosine, helps to reduce the liver/heart ratio and shortens the test duration. ^{99m}Tc tetrofosmin clears faster from the liver; hence, it can be imaged approximately 15 minutes after the rest injection. Ideally, a 3-hour time interval is recommended between the two injections to reduce residual background counts.

Single-Day Stress-Rest Sequence

The advantage of this protocol is convenience and good image contrast for stress defects, because there is no background activity from a previous injection. This protocol allows for stress testing to be completed early in the morning, which might be preferable to many cardiologists. However, the potential limitations include a poorer quality stress image (which is the most important image for diagnosis) because of the low dose used, particularly in overweight patients. Second, this protocol has a reduced efficacy for defining reversible defects compared with the rest-stress sequence, because of "shine through" of the stress perfusion defect. Gated images are usually acquired after the rest injection (higher dose).

Two-Day Protocols

This protocol involves two separate injections of 20 to 30 mCi for the stress study (day 1) and for the rest study (day 2). Stress-rest imaging is the preferred sequence for 2-day protocols, because when stress images are normal, rest images can be safely avoided, especially if performed in conjunction with attenuation correction. Thus, imaging can be completed in a short time, which would be the significant advantage of this protocol as opposed to rest-stress 2-day protocols. This would be the ideal protocol for good-quality images and optimal image contrast. However, because of time constraints, in practice it is used only for obese patients (requiring two high-dose images).

Imaging Protocols for Thallium-201

The conventional thallium protocol for stress testing includes an injection of 3 to 4.5 mCi of ^{201}Tl at peak stress and imaging after 10 minutes. Delayed rest images are obtained at 3 to 4 hours. Thus, both stress and 3- to 4-hour delayed images can be obtained after a single injection because of redistribution of ^{201}Tl over time. Because of the better image quality with ^{99m}Tc tracers, it is estimated that only 30% of all stress tests are being performed using ^{201}Tl alone.

Imaging Protocols Combining ^{201}Tl and ^{99m}Tc-Labeled Agents

At present, ^{201}Tl is most often used in conjunction with ^{99m}Tc tracers; so-called dual-isotope protocols. Typically, a rest injection of 3 to 4.5 mCi of ^{201}Tl is followed by imaging 10 minutes after injection. Immediately after rest images are complete, stress testing is performed, and 25 to 30 mCi of ^{99m}Tc is injected at peak stress, followed by imaging starting 15 to 30 minutes after injection. There is minimal contribution of ^{201}Tl counts in the ^{99m}Tc energy window (2.9%), not necessitating any correction for cross-contamination between the two isotopes. The accuracy of defect reversibility with this protocol is similar to that of a single-day rest-stress ^{99m}Tc-labeled agents. The entire procedure can be completed in 1.5 to 2 hours for treadmill stress, which is the major advantage of this protocol. In addition, patients with fixed defects on the rest and stress images can be imaged at 24 hours for evaluation of myocardial viability.

Dual-isotope protocols have been modified to suit individual institutional needs. Inpatients can be injected with 3 to 4.5 mCi of ^{201}Tl in the evening and brought in for 12-hour delayed imaging the next morning, followed by stress testing and imaging with a ^{99m}Tc imaging agent. This protocol reduces the total duration of the procedure and allows evaluation of both hibernation and inducible ischemia. At our institution, we perform 3- to 4-hour redistribution imaging after a rest injection of 3 to 4.5 mCi of ^{201}Tl, followed by stress testing and imaging with 25 to 30 mCi of a ^{99m}Tc imaging agent. If defects remain fixed, we then proceed to ^{18}F-deoxyglucose imaging. This protocol is particularly well suited for patients with ischemic cardiomyopathy, in whom information about both viability and inducible ischemia are important in management decisions.

Despite the superiority of ^{201}Tl over ^{99m}Tc imaging agents for assessment of myocardial viability, the conventional 3- to 4-hour redistribution thallium images can occasionally underestimate detection of viable and ischemic myocardium. Reinjection of 1 to 2 mCi of ^{201}Tl after completion of stress or rest imaging with a pure thallium protocol or with a dual-isotope approach improves detection of viable but jeopardized myocardium.

Single-day simultaneous acquisition dual isotope protocols involve a rest injection of ^{201}Tl (with no rest imaging), followed by a stress test and injection of a ^{99m}Tc-labeled radiotracer. After stress, patients are imaged only once with two separate energy windows for rest thallium and stress ^{99m}Tc data. This protocol would significantly reduce the total test duration to less than 1 hour. However, this protocol is not recommended for clinical use until further validation of its accuracy.

Additional developments in the protocols for assessing myocardial viability include nitrate-enhanced SPECT and dobutamine-gated SPECT. Several studies have demonstrated that the administration of nitroglycerin during rest ^{99m}Tc-sestamibi imaging might enhance the detection of viable myocardium. There is growing and consistent evidence that in selected patients nitroglycerin reduces the magnitude of the resting perfusion defect, thereby enhancing the detection of viability. This reduction in resting defect size correlates with recovery of regional and global left ventricular function. It has been recently shown that low-dose dobutamine ^{99m}Tc SPECT provides better accuracy for functional recovery than rest SPECT alone.

Image Display and Interpretation

Interpretation of the rest and stress perfusion images should be performed initially without clinical information to minimize any bias in study interpretation. All relevant clinical data should be reviewed after a preliminary impression is formed.

Image Display

Display of SPECT images should follow the guidelines agreed to by committees of the American Heart Association, American College of Cardiology, and the Society of Nuclear Medicine.[23] Images from different acquisitions should be displayed aligned and adjacent to each other. Each set of images is generally normalized to the pixel with the highest count within the series, although they might be normalized to each individual slice.

Segmental Analysis of Perfusion and Functional Data

Before reviewing the reconstructed and processed data, the raw data (projection images) should be carefully reviewed for potential sources of artifact that may degrade image quality (e.g., patient motion, and excessive and/or differential soft tissue attenuation). In addition, the projection images should also be carefully examined for lung uptake of the tracer or uptake in organs other than the heart that might be of significance, because it might be associated with malignancy. Increased lung uptake of the radiotracer generally reflects increased pulmonary capillary pressure.

The interpreting physician must be aware of technical and clinical factors that can potentially lead to the creation of artifacts, which can significantly affect test specificity. The most common problems with SPECT imaging are related to patient motion and excessive soft tissue attenuation. Soft tissue attenuation artifacts (breast, diaphragm, lateral chest wall) appear as fixed perfusion defects and are commonly encountered in clinical practice. The implementation of routine attenuation correction, as it is used in PET imaging, will eventually resolve attenuation artifacts. Prone imaging is helpful for differentiating true inferior defects from diaphragmatic attenuation. The gated images are also helpful for differentiating fixed defects caused by myocardial scar (abnormal regional wall motion and thickening) from those caused by soft tissue attenuation (normal regional wall motion and thickening).

In addition to the qualitative assessment of perfusion defects, the reader should also apply semiquantitative approaches on the basis of a validated segmental scoring system. This approach standardizes the visual interpretation of scans, reduces the likelihood of overlooking clinically significant defects, and provides a semiquantitative index that is applicable to diagnostic and prognostic assessments. Perfusion images are evaluated visually and scored using a 17-segment model. In each segment, radiotracer uptake is generally scored with a 5-point grading system: 0 = normal, 1 = mildly reduced tracer uptake, 2 = moderately reduced tracer uptake, 3 = severely reduced tracer uptake, and 4 = absent tracer uptake. The use of a scoring system provides a reproducible semiquantitative assessment of defect severity and extent. A consistent approach to defining defect severity and extent is clinically important, because each of the two variables contains independent prognostic power. Furthermore, semiquantitative scoring can be used to more reproducibly and objectively designate each segment as normal or abnormal.

In addition to individual scores, calculation of summed or global scores either visually or using computer-based approaches is recommended. The summed stress score (SSS) equals the sum of the stress scores of all segments, and the summed rest score (SRS) equals the sum of the resting scores or redistribution scores of all segments. The summed difference score (SDS) equals the difference between the summed stress and the summed resting (redistribution) scores and is a measure of defect reversibility. In particular, the SSS and SDS seem to have significant prognostic power.

After reviewing the perfusion images, the gated SPECT study is then analyzed. Regional wall motion and wall thickening are usually scored in the same myocardial segments with a 6-point grading system for regional wall motion (0 = normal wall motion, 1 = mildly hypokinetic, 2 = moderately hypokinetic, 3 = severely hypokinetic, 4 = akinetic, and 5 = dyskinetic) and 4 grades for regional wall thickening (0 = normal, 1 = mild reduction in wall thickening, 2 = moderate to severe reduction in wall thickening, and 3 = absent wall thickening). Left ventricular volumes and global LVEF are then calculated automatically with validated computer-based programs. Subsequently, the patient's clinical history and stress data are reviewed, and the myocardial perfusion study can be reviewed again in light of the clinical information. The overall final reading is then rendered. To remain unbiased and objective, it is recommended that the interpretation change by no more than one grade in either direction (e.g., equivocal to probably normal for a low pretest likelihood of disease or probably abnormal for a high pretest likelihood of disease, but not to normal or abnormal).

Quantitative Image Analysis

Objective quantitative image analysis is a helpful tool for a more accurate estimation of defect size and severity, and it should be used in combination with the visual analysis. A variety of quantitative approaches have been developed, most of which compute the segmental radiotracer concentration and display this activity using a 2D or 3D polar map (Figure 3-6). Perfusion defect size, severity, and degree of reversibility are then defined by comparing the patient's polar map to reference polar maps derived from isotope- and gender-matched databases

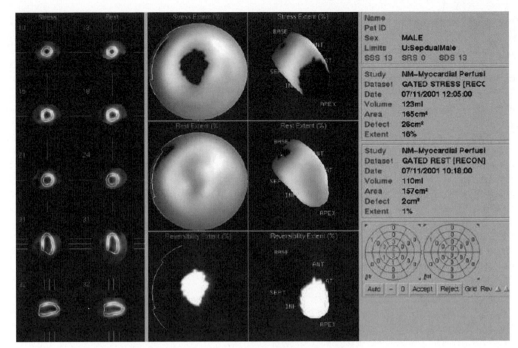

FIGURE 3-6. Display of quantitative results of a myocardial perfusion SPECT study. The left panel depicts the rest and stress myocardial slices used for quantitative analysis. The 2D *(middle panel)* and 3D *(right panel)* polar maps depict the relative quantitative tracer uptake during stress *(top)*, at rest *(middle)*, and their difference *(bottom)* reflecting the amount of defect reversibility. In the 2D polar maps, the left ventricular apex is represented at the center, the septum is to the left, the anterior wall is on the top, the lateral wall is to the right, and the inferior wall is at the bottom. The blackout regions in the polar maps reflect the extent of the perfusion abnormality, and the white color in the reversibility polar map reflects the amount of stress-induced ischemia. This example demonstrates a moderately large area of inducible ischemia in a patient with significant stenosis in the mid left anterior descending coronary artery. See also Color Insert.

established with patients with low probability of coronary artery disease (<5%). These quantitative approaches offer an objective interpretation that is inherently more reproducible than visual analysis. Quantitative measures of the defect size, severity, and degree of reversibility are particularly useful in describing changes in serial studies in the same patient. Quantitative analysis can also serve as a useful teaching aid for the less experienced observer who might be uncertain about normal variations in tracer uptake. Quantitative analysis should be used along with, and not as a substitute for, visual analysis.

Myocardial Perfusion for Detection of Coronary Artery Disease

Stress myocardial perfusion scintigraphy is an established method of diagnosing coronary artery disease. As with other tests applied for the detection of coronary artery disease, the diagnostic accuracy of myocardial perfusion imaging is also expressed as sensitivity and specificity.

Effect of Referral Bias on Sensitivity and Specificity

The reported sensitivity and specificity of noninvasive testing for detection of coronary artery disease might be confounded by referral bias. A flaw of having the angiogram serve as the "gold standard" to assess the diagnostic accuracy of noninvasive testing is the fact that

these patients are referred for cardiac catheterization, which in turn is markedly influenced by the amount of ischemia present on the myocardial perfusion study. This referral bias results in far more patients with positive scans being referred for coronary angiography. Thus, the measured sensitivity of the nuclear test (true positives/true positives + false negatives]) will be overestimated, because few false-negative patients will be referred for coronary angiography. Similarly, the measured specificity of the nuclear test (true negatives/[true negatives + false positives]) will be underestimated, because few true-negative patients will be referred for coronary angiography. Indeed, previous studies have reported a significant negative correlation between referral bias and test specificity. To address the impact of referral bias on specificity, the concept of "normalcy rate" was created and applied in many clinical studies. The normalcy rate is the observed rate of negative studies in a population of patients with a low pretest likelihood of coronary artery disease (<5%) on the basis of age, gender, symptoms, and the results of exercise electrocardiogram. This approach provides a surrogate for specificity that can be used when the referral bias is operational.

Diagnostic Accuracy of SPECT Imaging

The average reported sensitivity and specificity of SPECT imaging for detection of angiographically significant coronary artery disease are summarized (Table 3-3). The

■ ■ ■

TABLE 3-3 DIAGNOSTIC ACCURACY OF MYOCARDIAL PERFUSION SPECT IMAGING

	Sensitivity (%)	Specificity (%)	Normalcy rate (%)
[201]Tl	83	80	77
[99m]Tc sestamibi	90	93	100
[99m]Tc tetrofosmin	95	77	93

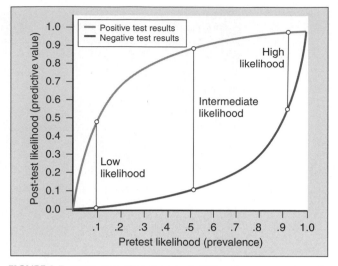

FIGURE 3-7. Estimation of posttest probability of coronary artery disease according to positive and negative stress nuclear testing results. (Adapted from Epstein SE. Implications of probability analysis on strategy used for noninvasive detection of coronary artery disease. *Am J Cardiol* 1980; 46:491.)

specificity of myocardial perfusion SPECT is slightly lower with ^{201}Tl than with ^{99m}Tc sestamibi or tetrofosmin. This is probably because ^{99m}Tc-labeled SPECT images are less affected by soft tissue attenuation and the use of gated SPECT. Despite the significant differences in extraction among the different perfusion-imaging agents, the reported sensitivities seem to be similar.

Likewise, the different perfusion-imaging agents seem to perform similarly in the evaluation of the extent of coronary artery disease. For example, the reported sensitivities for detecting single-vessel disease are 90% for both ^{201}Tl and ^{99m}Tc sestamibi. For detecting two-vessel disease, the sensitivities are 88% and 84% for ^{99m}Tc sestamibi and ^{201}Tl, respectively. For detecting three-vessel disease, the sensitivities are 98% and 96% for ^{99m}Tc sestamibi and ^{201}Tl, respectively.

Appropriateness of Stress Nuclear Testing

The basis for the diagnostic application of stress nuclear testing should be viewed in light of the concept of sequential Bayesian analysis of disease probability. This analysis requires knowledge of the prevalence of the disease in the population being tested (pretest probability), as well as the sensitivity and specificity of the test. The prevalence or pretest probability of coronary artery disease differs on the basis of age, gender, symptom classification, and coronary risk factors. With respect to symptoms, patients are classified into asymptomatic, nonanginal chest pain, atypical angina, and typical angina categories by use of three major characteristics of chest pain (i.e., substernal location, provocation by exercise, and relief gained from rest of nitroglycerin within 10 minutes). On the basis of the work of Diamond and Forrester, the prevalence or pretest probability of coronary artery disease might then be determined using the patient's age, gender, and symptoms. For practical purposes, one can consider that for 50-year-old men, the pretest probability of coronary artery disease is 5% for asymptomatic persons, 20% for those with nonanginal chest pain, 50% if atypical angina is present, and 90% for those with typical angina. For women, the same values apply but starting one decade later.

The posttest probability of coronary artery disease according to positive and negative stress nuclear testing results in patients with varying pretest probabilities of coronary artery disease (Figure 3-7). The line of identity (center line) represents a test with sensitivity and specificity of 50%. At any point along the centerline, the post-test probability of coronary artery disease is identi-

cal to the pretest likelihood of disease, indicating that such a test would have no diagnostic value. (The degree to which the lower and upper curves, reflecting normal and abnormal test results, deviate from the centerline represents the diagnostic value of the test.) It is evident from this graph that at both extremes of pretest probability of disease, the normal and abnormal test results, have almost no effect on the posttest probability of coronary artery disease. Thus, like any other imperfect test, stress nuclear testing has its maximum benefit when the pretest probability of coronary artery disease is intermediate (15% to 85%). For example, if a 60-year-old woman with nonanginal chest pain undergoes exercise electrocardiographic testing and the results are positive for ischemia, her postexercise probability of disease rises from 20% to approximately 50%. By use of sequential Bayesian analysis, the posttest results of the first test become the pretest probability of disease of the stress nuclear testing. Given the 90% sensitivity and specificity of myocardial perfusion scintigraphy, an abnormal result in a patient with a pretest probability of coronary artery disease of 50% would increase the probability of disease to 90%, whereas a normal test result would lower it to 10%.

Myocardial Perfusion for Risk Stratification

The power of myocardial perfusion SPECT for risk stratification is based on the fact that the major determinants of prognosis in patients with coronary artery disease are readily available from gated myocardial perfusion SPECT imaging. These include the amount of myocardial scar, the extent and severity of stress-induced ischemia, measurements of left ventricular size (i.e., volumes) and function, and other factors such as increased lung uptake of the radiotracer. The available evidence suggests that the prognostic power of myocardial perfusion imaging is independent of the perfusion imaging agent used, the type of stress or imaging protocol, the patients' age and gender, as well as the presence of documented coronary artery disease.

Chronic Coronary Artery Disease

For almost 20 years, the incremental value of myocardial perfusion imaging in providing prognostic information beyond clinical and historical variables, as well as the results of exercise electrocardiography, has been repeatedly demonstrated. Furthermore, it has been found that once SPECT information is known, cardiac catheterization data do not provide additional prognostic information. More recent data added to this body of literature by demonstrating that the incremental prognostic value of stress perfusion SPECT is applicable to patients with both normal and abnormal resting electrocardiograms. Similar findings have been reported in patients without known coronary artery disease, women, the elderly, and more recently in diabetes.

Because coronary artery disease represents a continuous spectrum of severity, it is important to assess the quantitative extent and severity of scan abnormalities (either visually or with the aid of computer-based programs) to maximize the prognostic power of these determinants and guide management decisions. The importance of the use of global scores (i.e., SSS, SRS, and SDS, see earlier) derived from the detailed segmental analysis of the perfusion images, rather than simply categorizing scan results as normal or abnormal, to assess clinical risk is supported by a wealth of clinical evidence. Indeed, it is well established that the extent and

severity of perfusion abnormalities, which reflects the magnitude of ischemia, are powerful and independent markers of prognosis. There is consistent evidence that a normal myocardial perfusion scan is generally associated with an excellent prognosis, with a cardiac event rate <1% per year of follow-up. Importantly, this consistently low event rate is unaffected by pre- or post-exercise tolerance test likelihood of coronary artery disease, patient symptoms, or gender. However, the "warranty" period of a normal scan seems to wane faster in patients with diabetes than in those without diabetes. Recent data from a large multiinstitutional study demonstrated a significant reduction in survival after 2 years of follow-up in patients with diabetes compared those without diabetes.

In risk-adjusted analyses, patients with mildly abnormal myocardial perfusion scans have a low risk for cardiac death or nonfatal myocardial infarction. Therefore, in a risk-based approach to management, patients with a normal or mildly abnormal myocardial perfusion scan would not require coronary angiography and subsequent revascularization, unless their symptoms are poorly controlled with medical therapy. On the other hand, patients with severely abnormal scans (e.g., multiple perfusion defects) are at high risk for death or myocardial infarction and, thus, require coronary angiography and prompt revascularization if appropriate (Figure 3-8). Patients with moderately abnormal scans have a low-intermediate risk of death or myocardial infarction, and the need for coronary angiography and revascularization in this group is uncertain.

This quantitative, risk-based approach to the analysis of stress perfusion imaging can also be applied to

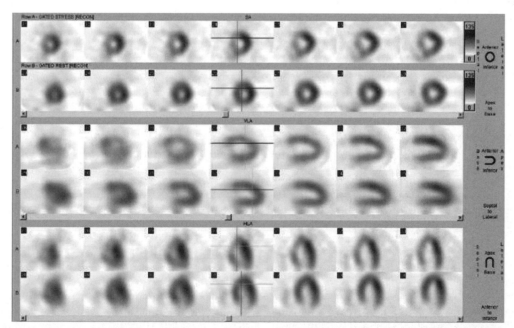

FIGURE 3-8. Example of a severely abnormal myocardial perfusion study (same-day rest-stress ^{99m}Tc) demonstrating a large, severe, and completely reversible perfusion defect throughout the mid and distal anterior and septal walls and the left ventricular apex. This is consistent with a large area of severe inducible ischemia throughout the left anterior descending coronary territory, which by quantitative analysis involved 23% of the left ventricle.

patients with known angiographic coronary stenoses, particularly those of intermediate severity. In these patients, stress nuclear testing can better define the physiological significance of these stenoses and the patient's clinical risk on the basis of the extent and magnitude of stress-induced ischemia. Indeed, the absence of ischemia on stress nuclear testing is generally associated with a relatively low risk for cardiac events, despite the presence of angiographic coronary artery disease.

In addition to the diagnostic and prognostic power of stress nuclear testing, this noninvasive approach to the evaluation of patients with known or suspected coronary artery disease also seems to be cost-effective. Shaw and colleagues[24] have demonstrated that for all levels of pretest clinical risk, the use of stress perfusion imaging plus selective coronary angiography results in a substantial cost reduction (30% to 50%) compared with a direct catheterization approach. More importantly, both strategies were associated with virtually identical rates of subsequent nonfatal myocardial infarction and cardiac death. However, the rate of subsequent revascularization (PCI and coronary artery bypass grafting) was substantially higher (50%) in the group of patients undergoing direct coronary angiography than among patients undergoing stress nuclear testing plus selective catheterization.

Acute Coronary Syndromes

There is growing and consistent evidence that the risk stratification concepts derived from the use of stress nuclear testing in patients with stable coronary artery disease can also be extended to patients with suspected or confirmed acute cardiac ischemia. Several studies have documented the value of rest perfusion SPECT imaging as a diagnostic and prognostic tool in patients with acute chest pain seen in the emergency department. The emerging concept from these clinical investigations is that a normal rest myocardial perfusion scan after radiotracer injection during or close to the resolution (approximately 1 hour) of chest pain has an extremely high negative predictive value (ranging from 95% to 100%) for excluding significant coronary artery disease or subsequent cardiac events. The positive predictive value of an abnormal scan for detecting acute cardiac ischemia is generally lower (12% to 90%) because of issues related to postscan "verification" bias, the specificity of the test, and the fact that perfusion defects could simply reflect chronic myocardial infarction. The effectiveness of this approach was tested in a large prospective multicenter randomized controlled clinical trial of perfusion imaging in the emergency department.[25] The ERASE Chest Pain (Emergency Room Assessment of Sestamibi for Evaluating Chest Pain) trial randomly assigned more than 2500 patients with symptoms suggestive of acute cardiac ischemia (but with a nondiagnostic test for acute ischemia or infarction) to one of two evaluation strategies. The control strategy was the usual emergency department strategy for evaluating such patients, which generally included enzyme analysis. The second strategy was the usual emergency department strategy supplemented by information from acute rest

SPECT sestamibi imaging. The investigators reported that among patients with an acute ischemic syndrome, both the scan and no scan randomization groups had a very high and appropriate admission rate to the hospital from the emergency department. Among patients who were ultimately ruled out for an acute ischemic syndrome, however, those initially randomly assigned to the scan strategy had a highly significant reduction in unnecessary hospitalizations. There was a 20% reduction in the relative risk of being hospitalized among those randomly assigned to the scan strategy who were ultimately found to be free of acute cardiac ischemia ($P < 0.001$). This reduction in the unnecessary hospitalization rate was seen in all age groups, in the presence or absence of risk factors, in men and in women, in hospitals with high or low volume emergency departments, and in hospitals with or without previous experience with imaging in this setting. In a multivariate analysis, the imaging data were among the most powerful factors associated with the decision to appropriately discharge the patient from the emergency department. Thus, the data were robust and potentially generalizable to a much wider setting.

The prognostic importance of the extent and severity of stress-induced ischemia is also applicable to patients after medically stabilized unstable angina or acute myocardial infarction. There is agreement that patients with prolonged ongoing rest angina, left ventricular dysfunction, dynamic ST segment changes, ischemic mitral regurgitation, or hypotension in the setting of ischemia should undergo emergent coronary angiography and revascularization. However, nuclear testing plays an important role in risk stratification of patients with unstable angina who fall in the low-intermediate risk category and who have been stabilized with medical therapy. In these patients, stress nuclear imaging performed after medical stabilization provides important information for management decisions, because it localizes the culprit vessel for subsequent revascularization and allows effective risk stratification. The absence of ischemia on stress nuclear imaging seems to be associated with a relatively low risk (2%) of subsequent cardiac events, whereas the presence of reversible perfusion defects identifies patients with a much higher risk of cardiac events (24%). This noninvasive approach is supported by the results of the TIMI IIIB trial demonstrating similar long-term outcomes in unstable angina patients who were stabilized on medical therapy and then randomly assigned to an invasive or a conservative, ischemia-guided strategy.

The quantitative measures of the extent and magnitude of infarcted and viable but jeopardized myocardium and the degree of left ventricular dysfunction derived from myocardial perfusion imaging are also powerful predictors of prognosis after myocardial infarction. There is a large body of literature supporting the value and accuracy of serial perfusion imaging for measuring myocardium at risk, infarct size, and the amount of salvaged myocardium after reperfusion therapy. These measurements of infarct size by predischarge SPECT perfusion imaging are also a useful marker of prognosis after myocardial infarction. With predischarge SPECT ^{99m}Tc sestamibi imaging, it has been reported that patients with infarcts involving >12% of the left ventricle had a significantly higher 2-year mortality than those with infarcts measuring <12% of the left ventricle. Assessment of prognosis after myocardial infarction might be further refined by considering the extent and severity of residual stress-induced ischemia and LVEF, which can be obtained with gated stress SPECT imaging. Quantitative information concerning the total amount of inducible ischemia or the amount of ischemia plus scar combined with measures of LVEF provides incremental prognostic information over baseline clinical data. In addition, recent data suggest that perfusion imaging with vasodilator stress can be safely performed on day 2 to 3 after myocardial infarction, thereby allowing early risk stratification. The effectiveness of stress perfusion imaging for risk stratification after myocardial infarction has also been confirmed in large clinical trials.

Preoperative Evaluation

There is extensive and consistent evidence demonstrating the effectiveness of stress nuclear testing for preoperative risk stratification.[26] There is general agreement that low-risk and high-risk patients can be identified clinically (i.e., age >70 years, Q waves on preoperative electrocardiograms, history of angina, history of ventricular ectopy requiring treatment, and diabetes; with = 3 variables defining high risk).[27] Stress nuclear testing seems most useful for risk stratification when applied to patients with intermediate clinical risk (i.e., one to two clinical variables). Indeed, a normal scan or the absence of reversible perfusion defects is associated with a low cardiac event rate (3.2%), whereas the presence of reversible defects is associated with a significantly higher event rate (29%).

Assessment of Myocardial Viability

Left ventricular function is a well-established and powerful predictor of outcome after myocardial infarction. Indeed, the occurrence of severe left ventricular systolic dysfunction (i.e., LVEF <35%) after myocardial infarction, especially if associated with heart failure, is associated with very poor survival. Despite the therapeutic advances, patients with coronary artery disease and severe left ventricular dysfunction have a poor prognosis when treated with medical therapy alone; however, in selected patients, surgical revascularization seems to afford a long-term survival benefit albeit with high surgical risk.

In some patients with coronary artery disease, left ventricular dysfunction results from myocardial infarction with attendant necrosis and scar formation. However, there is strong and consistent evidence that in many patients such myocardial dysfunction might be reversible with revascularization; this is otherwise referred to as hibernating and/or stunned myocardium. Consequently, the identification of ventricular dysfunction caused by fibrosis from that arising from viable but dysfunctional myocardium has important implications for patients with low ejection fraction in whom severe heart failure might be attributed to severe, widespread hibernation (or stunning or both) rather than to necrosis of a critical mass of myocardium. Failure to identify patients with these potentially reversible causes of heart failure might lead to progressive cellular damage, heart failure, and death.

Radionuclide Techniques for Assessing Viability with SPECT

Thallium-201 Imaging

The requirements for cellular viability include intact cell membrane function to maintain electrochemical gradients, preserved metabolic activity to generate high-energy phosphates, and residual myocardial blood flow to deliver substrates and remove the metabolites resulting from the metabolic processes. Because the retention of ^{201}Tl is an active, energy-requiring process that is a function of cell membrane activity and myocardial blood flow, myocardial uptake and retention of ^{201}Tl are very good markers of myocyte viability.

There are several approaches to the assessment of viability with ^{201}Tl scintigraphy (see "Imaging Protocols"). The selection of the approach should be tailored to the clinical question to be addressed in an individual patient. For example, rest-redistribution (either at 3 to 4 hours or at 24 hours) ^{201}Tl imaging might be appropriate for a patient in whom the question is the extent of viability of one or more dysfunctional myocardial territories, particularly when a perfusion defect is present at rest. On the other hand, stress-redistribution ^{201}Tl protocols might be more appropriate in a patient in whom the information of both stress-induced ischemia and viability are required. Alternately, protocols that combine ^{201}Tl (at rest) and ^{99m}Tc-labeled agents (stress; so-called dual-isotope) might provide similar information with the advantage of the superior gated images obtained with ^{99m}Tc tracers. The stress-redistribution ^{201}Tl or dual-isotope protocols are particularly well suited for patients with relatively preserved myocardial blood flow at rest, in whom left ventricular dysfunction might be caused by stunning rather than hibernation. With either protocol, the reinjection of ^{201}Tl facilitates the late uptake of thallium in regions with apparent irreversible thallium defects on redistribution imaging and thus helps to differentiate viable from nonviable myocardium.

^{99m}Tc-Labeled Agents

Like ^{201}Tl, the uptake and retention of ^{99m}Tc-labeled agents require intact cell membrane properties, suggesting that this approach should provide adequate information regarding tissue viability. However, in situations in which rest myocardial blood flow is reduced, ^{99m}Tc-labeled agents would also be expected to have inherent disadvantages compared with ^{201}Tl because of the lack of redistribution. Indeed, the uptake and retention of ^{99m}Tc sestamibi is very similar to that of ^{201}Tl, except in severe perfusion defects where it tends to underestimate the degree of viability.

Quantitative Analysis of Segmental Tracer Uptake

Objective quantitative assessment of regional tracer uptake has been shown to be an important tool in the assessment of tissue viability with nuclear imaging. The degree of regional tracer uptake correlates with the amount of myocyte viability by histological evaluation, with metabolic activity, and with recovery of regional function after revascularization.

18F-Deoxyglucose (FDG)

Under basal conditions, normal myocardium uses fatty acid oxidation as the primary source of high-energy phosphate. Fatty acid metabolism by means of β-oxidation in the mitochondria is highly dependent on oxygen availability and, thus, it declines sharply during myocardial ischemia. Under this condition, studies in animal experiments and in humans have shown that the uptake and subsequent metabolism of glucose by the ischemic myocardium is markedly increased. This shift to preferential glucose uptake plays a critical role in the survival of functionally compromised myocytes (i.e., stunned and hibernating), because glycolytically derived high-energy phosphates are critical for maintaining basic cellular functions. Consequently, noninvasive approaches that can assess the magnitude of exogenous glucose use, such as with FDG, play an important role in the evaluation of tissue viability in patients with myocardial dysfunction caused by coronary artery disease. With the FDG approach, areas of reduced blood flow but preserved FDG uptake (so-called perfusion-metabolism mismatch) identify viable myocardium, whereas areas of concordant reduction in blood flow and FDG uptake (so-called perfusion-metabolism match) identify areas of nonviable myocardium. Although originally the domain of dedicated PET scanners, FDG imaging can now be effectively performed with SPECT cameras (Figure 3-9).

Designing an Ideal Viability Protocol: A Pragmatic Approach

- Stress imaging provides important information for management decisions and should be part of the viability evaluation whenever possible.
- Thallium imaging or a dual-isotope approach that includes a thallium redistribution image should be the first diagnostic approach.
- FDG imaging provides incremental viability information over thallium SPECT, particularly in patients with severely reduced EF, and should be considered in patients with low EF and fixed perfusion defects

Relative Efficacy of Methods for Viability Assessment

Several approaches are currently available for the clinical evaluation of myocardial viability.[28] The data suggest that both SPECT and, especially, PET approaches are highly sensitive, with higher negative predictive value than dobutamine echocardiography, which in turn shows a higher specificity and positive predictive accuracy than the scintigraphic methods. Although the experience with contrast-enhanced cardiac magnetic resonance imaging (CMR) is more limited, recent results suggest that it offers similar predictive accuracies as those seen

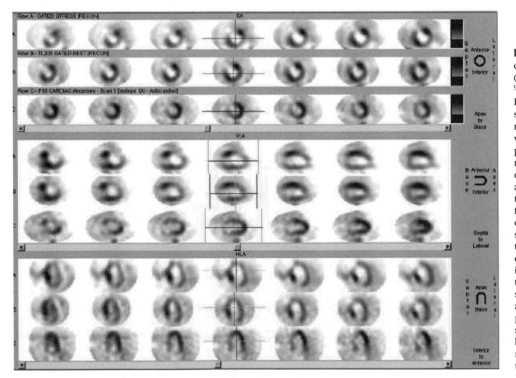

FIGURE 3-9. Example of a myocardial perfusion dual-isotope study (four redistribution [201]Tl[36] and stress ^{99m}Tc sestamibi *[upper row]*) and FDG metabolism *[lower row]* SPECT study in a patient with known coronary artery disease and severe left ventricular dysfunction. The stress perfusion images demonstrate a medium-sized and severe perfusion defect involving the mid and distal anterior and anteroseptal walls and the left ventricular apex, which is fixed. In addition, the stress images demonstrate a moderate-sized and severe perfusion defect throughout the inferolateral wall, showing near complete reversibility (reflecting ischemia in the left circumflex territory). The FDG images reveal preserved myocardial metabolism in the anteroapical wall and apex (so-called perfusion-metabolism mismatch), suggesting the presence of viable but hibernating myocardium in the mid left anterior descending territory.

with dobutamine echocardiography. However, such comparisons should be interpreted with caution, because these results are derived from isolated reports evaluating a single method, with only a few direct head-to-head comparisons between two or more of the available modalities.

Applying Viability Information in Management Decisions

A meta-analysis by Allman et al[29] pooled results from 24 viability imaging studies that reported long-term patient outcomes using stress echocardiography, SPECT ^{201}Tl, or FDG imaging. These reports were composed of a follow-up of 25 ± 10 months in 3088 patients (2228 men, 860 women) who had a mean ejection fraction 32 ± 8%. This meta-analysis found a strong association between revascularization and improved outcomes (cardiac death and nonfatal myocardial infarction) among patients with coronary artery disease and significant left ventricular dysfunction who had evidence of viable myocardium by noninvasive testing. The likelihood of improved outcome was greatest in the patients with demonstrated viability and the most severe left ventricular dysfunction. This association was seen only in revascularized patients with demonstrated viability. There was no detectable benefit associated with revascularization over medical therapy in the absence of demonstrated viability. Indeed, a trend toward higher death and nonfatal event rates was found under the latter conditions, possibly because of higher procedural risk for patients with severe left ventricular impairment associated with the revascularization itself in the absence of a balancing clinical benefit.

Multivariate modeling of the pooled study data in patients with viable myocardium demonstrated an inverse relationship between ejection fraction and the prognostic benefit associated with revascularization. That is, as the severity of left ventricular dysfunction increased, the potential benefit (reduction in risk of death and nonfatal events) associated with revascularization of patients with viable myocardium increased as well. This finding implies that despite an increasing risk of revascularization with worsening left ventricular dysfunction, noninvasive imaging evidence of preserved viability might provide information on clinical benefit to balance against that risk, informing clinical decision making.

Potential Role of Gated SPECT in Viability Assessment

Myocardial infarction, especially one that is large and transmural, can produce alterations in both the infarcted and noninfarcted regions that result in changes in left ventricular architecture known as left ventricular remodeling. In addition to the early thinning and elongation that occurs in the infarcted myocardium (infarct expansion), there are secondary changes in the noninfarcted zone characterized by a time-dependent associated increase in the end-diastolic length of viable myocytes that contribute to the overall process of left ventricular enlargement. Although this acute increase in cavity size tends to maintain pump function, this process usually leads to progressive ventricular dilation, heart failure, and decreased survival.

Increased left ventricular volumes and cavity size are also associated with poor outcomes in patients with ischemic cardiomyopathy undergoing coronary artery bypass graft (CABG) surgery, and left ventricular end-diastolic dimension >70 mm, as assessed by echocardiography, has also been shown to be a marker of poor outcome after revascularization. Likewise, others have shown that a preoperative left ventricular end-systolic volume index (LVESVI) >100 mL/m² , as assessed by contrast left ventriculography, was a predictor of mortality and postoperative heart failure and failure to improve regional and global left ventricular function after CABG. Importantly, these poor results in patients with severe left ventricular dilation were observed even in the patients with severe anginal symptoms, suggesting that progressive left ventricular remodeling after myocardial infarction might limit the benefits of revascularization on ventricular function and survival, even if there is evidence of viable (ischemic) myocardium.

CMR OF CORONARY ARTERIES

CMR is a promising screening technique for coronary artery disease, because it is noninvasive, does not require ionizing radiation or iodinated contrast media, can provide hemodynamic information in addition to vascular morphology, can provide 3D information, and might be significantly less expensive than conventional angiography. The CMR techniques for the evaluation of vascular anatomy, collectively known as magnetic resonance angiography (MRA), have advanced rapidly in the head and neck, lung, abdomen, and extremities. However, MRA of coronary arteries has been more difficult because of the challenges presented by both heart and respiratory motion, the close proximity of the coronary artery to cardiac chambers, and the small caliber and frequent tortuosity of coronary arteries. These require fast data acquisition to freeze the motion of coronary arteries during cardiac and respiratory cycles, techniques to eliminate or reduce motion effects, high-resolution volumetric coverage of the entire coronary artery tree, and optimal image processing and display methods.

Technical Considerations
Overcoming Cardiac Motion

To minimize the effects of cardiac motion, CMR data are usually collected during mid-diastole, when cardiac motion is minimized. This is done by acquiring the electrocardiographic signal of the patient and collecting CMR data after a certain delay from the R-wave. The electrocardiographic signal is usually acquired using three to four electrodes placed on the left anterior hemithorax. Data acquisition is limited to about 100 ms per cardiac cycle. To image coronary arteries using a 3D technique, the total acquisition time (TA) required is: TA = TR $\times$ $N_{line}\times$ N_{part}, where *TR* is the repetition time needed to collect one line of data, N_{line} is the number of lines per image, and N_{part} is the number of partitions for the imaging volume. For instance, for TR = 4.0 ms, N_{line} = 150 and N_{par} = 8, the total imaging time required will be 4.8 seconds, which will require 48 heartbeats to complete the measurement if the data acquisition window per heartbeat is 100 ms, during which 25 lines will be collected. Data collected from all heartbeats will be merged in K space and Fourier-transformed to form images. This scheme is called segmented data acquisition, in which part of the data space is collected in each heartbeat.

Overcoming Respiratory Motion

Two approaches have been used to eliminate the effect of respiratory motion. The first is breath hold, in which respiration is suspended during data acquisition. The advantages of breath-hold imaging include the fast speed to acquire a measurement and more complete elimination of respiration effects with cooperative patients. The data acquisition can be repeated if necessary. The short imaging time reduces the sensitivity to heartbeat irregularities that might occur over a long imaging time. The disadvantages of breath-hold imaging are the limited resolution, S/N ratio, and imaging volume per scan because of the constraint on imaging time. Another concern is that very sick patients have difficulty holding their breath for an adequate duration.

The second is respiratory gating, in which the displacement of the coronary artery caused by respiration is measured for the acquisition of each line of data; a decision is made to either accept or reject the data based on the displacement. In this method, a special navigator echo signal is collected corresponding to the acquisition of a segment of the K space within each cardiac cycle. This navigator echo is collected on a pencil beam along the liver-lung boundary in the superior-inferior direction. The displacement of the diaphragm during data acquisition is detected from the navigator echo and is used to determine whether the data are used for image reconstruction and whether slice correction is needed. The advantage of respiratory gating is that images are collected with free breathing, potentially allowing for relatively high resolution and S/N ratio. The disadvantages are the longer imaging time, sensitivity to irregular breathing patterns, and the variations in the relationship between diaphragmatic and cardiac motion between individuals.

Imaging Protocols and Procedures

There are many imaging protocols for coronary artery imaging. In this section, we will focus on two major approaches that have been clinically tested: volume-targeted breath-hold imaging; imaging with free breathing and navigator-echo–based motion correction.

Basic Imaging Scheme

The basic technique for coronary artery imaging is an electrocardiogram-triggered, segmented 3D gradient echo sequence. During each heartbeat, in phase encoding steps are acquired during mid-diastole. Data collected over several consecutive heartbeats is used to cover one plane of K space. This process is repeated until the entire 3D K space is covered. Data acquisition window per cardiac cycle is limited to less than 15% of the R-R interval to minimize the effect of cardiac motion. Before data acquisition during each heartbeat, there is a magnetization preparation stage to suppress the myocardial and epicardial fat signals. If a free-breathing approach is used, the navigator echo will be collected before data acquisition.

Volume-Target Breath-Hold Coronary Artery Imaging

With this protocol, a breath-hold scan is acquired to cover a major coronary artery branch. Repeated scans are collected to cover different parts of the coronary artery system, the left main artery (LM), LAD, left circumflex artery (LCX), and the RCA. Because of the limited volume coverage per breath-hold scan, it is critical to optimize the plane setup to maximize coverage of coronary arteries for each targeted scan. The first step in this process is localization of the heart. A single-shot true-fast imaging with steady-state precession (FISP) is used to acquire multislice 2D images in the three orthogonal planes (transverse, coronal, and sagittal). True-FISP is a new fast imaging technique that has found widespread applications in cardiac imaging in recent years.[30] The main advantages of this technique are the high S/N ratio and improved contrast between blood and myocardium compared with conventional gradient echo sequences such as fast low-angle shot (FLASH). Because each image is acquired in one cardiac cycle, the breath hold is relatively short, on the order of 6 to 9 seconds.

After the acquisition of the scout scans of the heart, an electrocardiogram-triggered, breath-hold, magnetization-prepared, segmented, 3D true-FISP sequence with a fat suppression prepulse is used to acquire a low-resolution 3D volume of the heart to find the orientations of the proximal and middle segments of coronary arteries. For LM and LAD localizations, the scan is oriented axially on the coronal scan, centered at the approximate origin of the LM, and rotated so that it follows the surface of the left ventricle. The imaging parameters are as follows: TR (repetition time)/TE (echo time) = 2.8/1.2 ms (asymmetric sampling of echo in the readout direction), flip angle = 70 degrees, readout bandwidth = 980 Hz/ pixel, FOV (field of view) = 200 × 300 mm^2, lines acquired per cardiac cycle = 41, in-plane matrix size = 82 × 256, number of partitions = 10 (interpolated to 20), slice thickness = 2 mm (after interpolation), total coverage = 40 mm. The duration of this scan is 20 cardiac cycles. A 3-point scan plan tool is then used to define the orientation of the LAD axis (Figure 3-10). To find the orientations for the RCA and LCX, another localizer 3D scan is run along the atrioventricular grove.

After the approximate orientations of the major coronary arteries are determined, high-resolution imaging of the coronary arteries can be collected by use of an electrocardiogram-triggered, breath-hold, magnetization-prepared, segmented, 3D true-FISP sequence. Typical

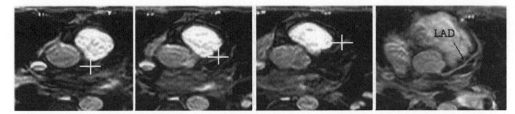

FIGURE 3-10. Procedure for finding the position and orientation of the left anterior descending (LAD) coronary artery using a 3-point graphic planning tool. Three images showing the proximal, middle, and distal segments of the LAD at different slice positions are seen in the three images on the left, respectively. When the points marked in the images are selected, the plane defined by those 3 points in space is determined. An image acquired by use of the orientation obtained by the preceding method *(on the right)* shows a clear delineation of the LAD.

imaging parameters are provided (Table 3-4). To visualize coronary arteries, the epicardial fat signal surrounding the coronary arteries needs to be suppressed. This is accomplished by the application of a frequency selective prepulse before data acquisition in each cardiac cycle. Contrast between blood and myocardium is created because the inherent T2/T1 weighting of the true-FISP signal (blood has a T2/T1 ratio of 0.21 and myocardium has a ratio of 0.06). A commercial two-element body phased-array coil on the Siemens imaging system is placed on patient's chest for signal reception. To avoid image wrap-around when using a small field of view (FOV), the coils built in the patient table are turned off.

Two major requirements for this method to be successful are consistent breath hold and uniform magnetic field. Although both inspiration and expiration breath holds have been used for coronary artery imaging, expiration breath hold tends to be more consistent, and inspiration breath hold tends to last longer. On the basis of our experience on the Siemens imaging system, default field setup is usually adequate in most patients. In some subjects, local field shimming or frequency shift might be required to improve the image quality.

Another data acquisition technique for 3D breath hold is contrast-enhanced FLASH. The advantage of this technique compared with true-FISP is the more complete suppression of the background tissue. The disadvantages are the need to determine the time delay of data acquisition after contrast injection and the limited number of scans per imaging session because of the Food and Drug Administration–mandated limit on how much con-

trast agent can be injected. Newly developed blood pool agents might alleviate this problem.

Coronary Artery Imaging with Free Breathing and Real-Time Slice Correction

The major problem with breath-hold coronary artery imaging is the limited resolution because of the constraint of imaging time. One method to alleviate this limitation is to acquire data during free breathing. The position shifts because of respiration during data acquisition of different parts of K space are corrected by changing the slice position in real-time such that the entire K space is acquired at the same slice position despite the motion of coronary arteries during respiration. To obtain a reference of position shifts of coronary arteries during data acquisition, navigator echoes are collected along the cranial-caudal direction at the dome of the diaphragm. The boundary between liver (high signal) and lung (low signal) is detected to track the motion of the diaphragm during breathing. The position shifts of the diaphragm are converted to coronary artery motion by use of a correction factor of 0.6 (Figure 3-11). The navigator echo can be collected with a pair of 90-degree and 180-degree pulses or a 2D excitation pulse.

Similar to the breath-hold approach, the first step is the localization of the coronary arteries. The localizing scan (approximately 1 minute) uses a multistack and multislice, segmented gradient echo sequence for localization of the heart and diaphragm in the three orthogonal planes. From the coronal data set, a navigator-gated

■ ▪ ■

TABLE 3-4 TYPICAL IMAGING PARAMETERS FOR THE BREATH-HOLD 3D TRUE-FISP AND FREE-BREATHING, MOTION-CORRECTED FLASH SEQUENCES

Type of acquisition	Breath-hold true-FISP	Free-breathing FLASH
TR/TE (ms)	3.5/1.4	7.7/2.2
Flip angle	70°	Variable
Lines/cardiac cycle	25-41	8
FOV (mm²) (phase × readout)	(160-175) × 380	360 × 360
Matrix size	(100-140) × 512	360 × 512
In-plane resolution (mm²)	(1.0-1.4) × 0.7	1.0 × 0.7
Number of partitions	6 (interpolated to 12)	10 (interpolated to 20)
Slice thickness (mm)	3 mm (interpolated to 1.5 mm)	3 mm (interpolated to 1.5 mm)
Coverage (mm)	18 mm	30 mm
Imaging time/scan	24-30 cardiac cycles	10-15 min

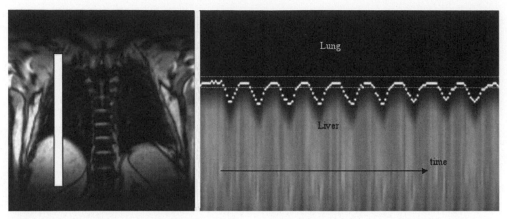

FIGURE 3-11. Tracking respiratory motion with navigator echoes. The coronal image of the chest on the left shows the column of tissue excited by the navigator echo. On the right is the resulting temporal display of multiple navigator echoes showing diaphragmatic motion. The boundary between the liver *(high signal in the lower portion of the image)* and the lung *(low signal in the upper portion of the image)* is marked with thick lines, and the range of motion accepted for image reconstruction is indicated by dotted lines.

3D segmented echo-planar localizer scan with 40 slices (approximately 2 minutes) is collected around the base of the heart to cover the region extending from the apex of the left ventricle to the pulmonary artery. This allows identification of the course of the major right and left coronary arteries. With the use of a 3-point plan scan tool, a plane through the major axis of the proximal and middle segments of the right coronary artery can be prescribed.

After localization of the coronary arteries, high-resolution scans are performed on a targeted volume. A navigator-gated 3D gradient echo scan is used to acquire the images. To delineate the coronary arteries better, a fat suppression prepulse and a T2 preparation are applied to suppress the signals from surrounding fat and myocardium, respectively. For the right coronary artery, a double-oblique 3D volume is imaged with use of the coordinates prescribed by the 3-point plan scan tool. For the LM, LAD, and LCX coronary arteries, a double-oblique transverse 3D volume with anterior-posterior and left-right angulations (5 degrees each) is imaged with the volume centered on the origin of the LM coronary artery as defined from the second localization scan. The navigator echo is collected on the right hemidiaphragm. The gating window used for the navigator is 5 mm at the end of expiration (Table 3-4). The time required for each scan is on the order of 10 to 15 minutes.

Image Analysis

One of the advantages of CMR imaging is the ability to acquire 3D data. It is thus desirable to display images in a 3D mode to enable viewing the arteries from different orientations. However, for both breath-hold and free-breathing approaches, the images do not have isotropic resolution. In addition, user interactions are required to remove background tissues. Therefore, for coronary artery MR image analysis, original source images are often displayed dynamically to the reviewer for disease diagnosis. Targeted maximum intensity

projection (MIP) has also been used to facilitate image presentation.

Preliminary Clinical Trials

A patient study using the breath-hold 3D true-FISP sequence (n = 30) was performed on the 1.5-T SONATA system (Siemens Medical Solutions, Erlangen, Germany) with a gradient subsystem of 40-mT/m maximum magnitude and 200-mT/m/ms maximum slew rate. The CMR images were analyzed by two reviewers blinded to the diagnosis of conventional angiography. They were compared with conventional angiography for the detection of clinically significant disease (at least 50% diameter stenosis). Images with poor quality (19%) were discarded without further analysis. The lengths of visualized coronary arteries were full length for LM, 6.4 (range, 2.9 to 10.3) cm for RCA, and 5.0 (range, 2.0 to 9.00) cm for LAD. The sensitivities of CMR to detect significant stenoses were overall, 88%; LM, 100%; LAD, 85%; RCA, 100%. The specificities were overall, 76%; LM, 91%; LAD, 60%; RCA, 69%. An example of coronary artery stenosis detection by use of this method is shown in Figure 3-12. CMR has also been used for identifying anomalous coronary arteries (Figure 3-13).

A multicenter study was conducted to evaluate the accuracy of free-breathing, motion-corrected coronary CMR among patients with suspected coronary artery disease.[31] The study was conducted on a 1.5-T system (Gyroscan ACS-NT, Phillips Medical Systems, Best, The Netherlands) equipped with Power-Trak 6000 gradients (23 mT/m, 219 (s rise time). One hundred nine patients were recruited in seven institutes. Seven coronary artery segments were evaluated: the LM artery and the proximal and middle segments of the LAD artery (0 to 2 cm and 2 to 4 cm), the LCX artery (0 to1.5 cm and 1.5 to 3.0 cm), and the RCA (0 to 2 cm and 2 to5 cm). Eighty-four percent of the coronary artery segments in CMR images had diagnostic image quality. The sensitivities of CMR to detect significant stenoses were LM, 67%; LAD, 88%; LCX, 53%; RCA, 93%. The specificities were LM, 90%;

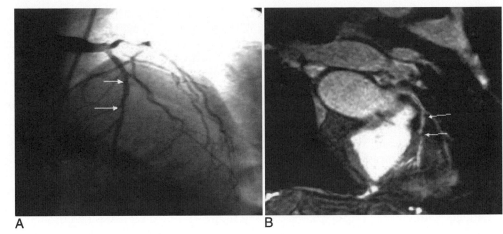

FIGURE 3-12. Coronary angiography in a 68-year-old patient with chest pain. The CMR coronary angiography **(A)** using the breath-hold 3D true-FISP sequence shows two high-grade stenoses in the proximal to middle segments of the LAD *(arrow)*. Conventional X-ray coronary angiography **(B)** confirms the presence of the stenoses *(arrow)*.

LAD, 52%; LCX, 70%; RCA, 72%. (Examples of coronary artery stenosis detection using this method are shown in Figure 3-14.)

Various other approaches have been developed for coronary artery CMR imaging in recent years. In addition to the two techniques introduced previously, other methods include multiple breath-hold 2D imaging, spiral imaging with breath-hold and diminished variance algorithm (DVA) with navigator-echo, multiple breath-hold imaging with a respiratory feedback monitor or real-time slice after, free breathing with retrospective respiratory gating or adaptive motion correction, hybrid ordered phase encoding for improved respiratory artifact reduction, real-time imaging, vessel tracking, black-blood imaging, echo-planar imaging, projection reconstruction, and

blood pool contrast agent–enhanced imaging. Although some of these techniques have been replaced by new methods, others continue to improve. With these techniques, it is now possible to consistently visualize proximal and middle portions of major coronary artery branches with a spatial resolution of 3 mm^3 in healthy volunteers and patients with coronary artery disease. CMR has a high negative predictive value and might be useful for ruling out clinically significant coronary artery

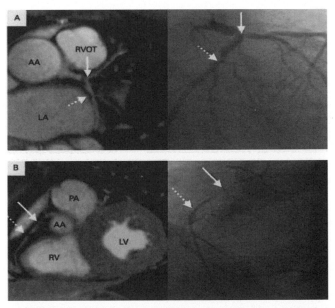

FIGURE 3-14. Coronary angiography in a 53-year-old man with exertional chest pain. A, Coronary magnetic resonance angiogram *(left)* and a corresponding X-ray coronary angiogram *(right)*, indicating a severe lesion at the bifurcation of the LAD and the LCX, involving the LM *(solid arrows)* and a more distal focal stenosis of the LCX *(broken arrows)*. B, Coronary magnetic resonance angiogram (left) and a corresponding X-ray image *(right)* indicating two stenoses of the proximal *(solid arrows)* and middle *(broken arrows)* RCA. AA = denotes ascending aorta, LA = left atrium, RVOT = right ventricular outflow tract, PA = pulmonary artery, RV = right ventricle, and LV = left ventricle. (Reproduced with permission from Kim, et al. Coronary magnetic resonance angiography for the detection of coronary stenoses. *N Engl J Med* 2001; 345:1863.)

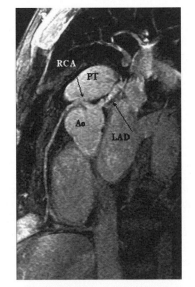

FIGURE 3-13. Coronary magnetic resonance angiography with breath-hold 3D true-FISP in a 51-year-old man demonstrates an anomalous RCA origin. The maximum intensity projection image shows the anomalous origin of RCA *(short arrow)* from the left sinus of Valsalva and the subsequent course between the pulmonary trunk (PT) and aortic root (Ao). The origin of the LAD coronary artery *(long arrow)* is normal.

disease in patients referred for conventional angiography. However, the sensitivity and specificity of detecting coronary artery disease with these techniques still need to be improved for general clinical applications. The major challenges are still to overcome the effects of respiratory motion and to improve spatial resolution. Both breath-hold and free-breathing approaches are likely to be useful in coronary artery imaging, but further refinements of the techniques are necessary. With improved CMR scanner hardware and software such as 3-T scanners, blood pool contrast agents, and fast, efficient imaging techniques such as true-FISP imaging with slice after and parallel imaging, CMR coronary artery imaging might play an important clinical role in the management of patients with coronary artery disease in the future.

QUANTITATIVE MYOCARDIAL PERFUSION BY MAGNETIC RESONANCE

Recent advances in myocardial perfusion imaging have been stimulated by an increased awareness of the role of microvascular function in coronary heart disease. Cardiac magnetic resonance imaging (CMR) has made substantial contributions to this field in the past 2 decades. Most recently, ultra-fast scanners have facilitated perfusion analysis by the magnetic resonance first-pass perfusion technique (MRFP). CMR relies on magnetic fields to reconstruct high-resolution images of myocardial structures. Its advantages include fine resolution of tissue structures (<2 mm), superior temporal resolution, ability to visualize tissue adjacent to the air-filled lungs, and lack of ionizing radiation. PET is the current clinical standard for myocardial blood flow assessment, but it is limited for clinical use by the need for an on-site cyclotron with consequent high expense and limited availability. SPECT is most commonly used, but its accuracy is lower, and both SPECT and PET are intrinsically limited to detecting transmural ischemia by their low resolution. First-pass CMR perfusion is capable of resolving subendocardial ischemia and with contrast agent kinetic modeling can also quantify myocardial blood flow and myocardial perfusion reserve.

CMR is unlike conventional cardiac imaging techniques in that it is not produced by shadowing or reflecting transmitted radiation. Hydrogen nuclei, or protons, are principal constituents of body chemistry, primarily in water molecules. Being ubiquitous, they constitute an ideal source of imaging information.

When magnetic objects like protons move, their magnetic field induces an electric current in metal coils in their field. The electric currents induced in detector coils placed on a patient's body are needed to produce the high-resolution MR images. Different tissues have different rates of relaxation; for example, free water molecules relax more freely than bound molecules, so tissues with more chemical free water can be differentiated this way. This forms the basis for the ability of CMR to image tissue contrast so well, even though the tissues may have similar X-ray densities.

The use of T1 MR contrast agents facilitates the use of these agents as sensitive blood flow indicators. Because they are mixed with blood, they increase the signal intensity in proportion to its concentration (mmol/kg), which allows in a broad sense the application of the indicator dilution principles with MR contrast agents as indicators for the quantification of myocardial blood flow.

Physiological Basis for First-Pass Myocardial Perfusion Analysis

Quantitative first-pass perfusion is an indicator dilution technique similar to densitometry or determination of cardiac output by dye dilution. It makes use of the physiology of myocardial flow to determine coronary stenoses and microvascular obstruction. Normal coronary flow resistance is determined by the distal arterioles and capillaries (diameter <300 μm), but when stenotic, the larger epicardial coronary arteries ("conduit vessels") can be flow limiting. Under normal conditions, a significant part of the myocardial capillary network is closed and represents excess capacity that is recruited during stress (myocardial perfusion reserve). This microcirculatory vasodilator reserve is fully recruited at rest in patients with severe coronary obstruction. When tested by a microcirculatory vasodilator challenge such as adenosine ("stress perfusion"), areas with adequate perfusion reserve can increase perfusion at least up to 500%, whereas in areas of abnormal perfusion reserve, flow might actually decrease (because of "coronary steal" as blood gets rerouted to less obstructed channels). Preferential flow to more normal vessels increases "flow heterogeneity," with ischemic zones remaining relatively hypoperfused. This effect can be visualized, as well as quantified by generating the myocardial segmental contrast agent signal-intensity versus time curves (SI-time curve).

With the spatial resolution of CMR, it is also possible to demonstrate other subtle early signs of ischemia. Blood flow is not uniform across the transmural extent of the myocardial wall but under normal circumstances favors the subendocardium. The blood flow ratio is normally 1.5:1 from endocardium to epicardium. As an early sign of coronary artery stenosis, flow is first diverted away from the subendocardium, with a ratio to subepicardium of <1.0, particularly with stress. These differences also can be visualized and measured with MRFP.

Image Acquisition: MRFP Perfusion Imaging

Perfusion studies are commonly performed after rest acquisition of MR cine function studies. Localizer images are used to establish the tomographic scan planes, which are most commonly through the short-axis of the left ventricle covering the left ventricular base, midventricle, and apex. Four-chamber views can also be easily acquired. Each image, including all slices, is acquired during a single pass of contrast agent and might be done with a single breath hold or alternately by free breathing with navigator gating. After a rapid IV bolus by means of either a central or large peripheral vein, the MR contrast agent (gadolinium [Gd]-diethylenetriaminepentaacetic acid [DTPA], 0.03 to 0.05 mmol/kg) will mix with the blood pool and will proportionally increase its signal while passing from the right ventricular chambers through the pulmonary circulation and into the left ventricular blood pool. Within 4 to 5 seconds, contrast will flush through the myocardial circulation and increase the signal intensity in proportion to the myocardial blood flow provided by the epicardial coronary arteries, medium-sized arterioles, and the capillary tree. A portion of the contrast will then recirculate, while another diffuses into the interstitium. Although contrast distributes Gd extracellularly at equilibrium, studies have shown that only 3% is extracellular during the first-pass circulation. The recommended rate of acquisition of images is generally one image per heartbeat with current ultrafast scanners, including multiple tomographic scans per heartbeat. In most cases, power injection is used to achieve a crisp bolus through an antecubital vein. For most patients, breath holding is used to reduce diaphragmatic motion, but navigator gating off the diaphragm can allow free breathing when necessary. ECG gating is used to time acquisitions in diastole to avoid systolic cardiac motion. Images are stored for postprocessing and are available immediately for visual, qualitative interpretation. The total dose of Gd-DTPA (<0.04 mmol/kg) is low enough to make repeat studies feasible.

Pharmacological Stress and Hyperemic Response

Repeat imaging is performed after a brief equilibration period of 3 to 5 minutes. The most common drugs for pharmacological stress are adenosine and dipyridamole, which are potent coronary vasodilators. A stepwise infusion MR protocol for adenosine up to a dose of 140 µg/kg/min over 6 minutes can be administered by an automatic infusion pump. An advantage of adenosine is its short half-life of 6 to 10 seconds after termination of infusion. Xanthine and caffeine block adenosine receptors, so patients should be instructed to abstain from coffee, caffeine-containing soda, and chocolate use for 12 hours before the procedure. Patients are continuously monitored for potential side effects or physiological responses such as increased heart rate, evidence of heart block caused by vagal stimulation of sinoatrial or atrioventricular nodes, or blood pressure response. Usually when vital sign changes necessitate discontinuing the infusion, successful imaging is still possible. Less significant side effects can be caused by vasodilation such as flushing, headache, chest pressure, and abdominal discomfort. Actual angina might be precipitated by coronary steal and can be treated by IV aminophylline if necessary. The effects of dipyridamole are more prolonged; thus it is more often necessary to administer 50 to 75 mg of aminophylline IV to eliminate side effects after the procedure. One dosage regimen for dipyridamole is 0.142 mg/kg/min over 4 minutes, with the maximal vasodilation occurring 4 minutes after infusion is completed. In patients for whom adenosine and dipyridamole are contraindicated, such as those with bronchospastic lung disease or patients who accidentally ingested caffeine, dobutamine is an alternative.

Perfusion Image Interpretation

Reconstructed perfusion images are customarily displayed in short-axis cine loop format. The rest perfusion cine loop should be examined for quality of the bolus and to find areas of lower signal intensity that represent hypoperfusion during the initial myocardial first pass. Images should be displayed about one per second. Images from the recirculation period should not be included in the analysis. Dark artifacts, called Gibb's rings, in the septal endocardial area are often due to magnetic susceptibility effects from the adjacent very bright myocardial blood pool. The distinction between artifact and perfusion defect can be made by noticing that the former tends to move every one or two frames, whereas the latter usually persists for at least three images. The characteristic form of the SI-time curve should also be examined (see Figure 3-15), comparing individual sectors against the wash-in curve of the left ventricular blood pool, looking for the upslope and delayed and reduced peak signal amplitude, either visually or numerically.

Quantitative Evaluation of Myocardial Perfusion

Quantitative perfusion analysis offers a number of advantages over visual analysis:

1. Better spatial resolution of segmental and transmural defects
2. Grading of lesion severity by measurement of myocardial perfusion reserve
3. Assessment of collateral-dependent flow to determine the regional absolute myocardial perfusion reserve

Visual assessment relies on differential signal enhancement of hypoperfused myocardium compared with normally perfused regions with higher signal intensities. Subtle changes below the visual threshold can be missed, such as might occur in regions supplied by collaterals with inadequate flow during stress. Adequate coronary flow reserve can only be assessed with quantification. After visual analysis, signal intensity vs. Time curves (SI-time) are generated by drawing regions of interest in six to eight sectors circumferentially around the short axis left ventricular wall and one within the left ventricular blood pool. Signal intensity is determined in each sector and slice during the passage of contrast and graphed against time (see Figure 3-15). By use of these data, there are two approaches to the quantification of MRFP.

The first is the analysis of perfusion indices derived from SI-time curves, such as the peak signal intensity or mean upslope of signal intensity vs. Time curves, time to peak intensity, amplitude of peak intensity, and determinations of relative myocardial perfusion index. These indices are used to relate resting to stress perfusion with the assumption that they are proportional to the flows involved.

The second approach uses contrast agent kinetic models to derive values for absolute myocardial flow and myocardial perfusion reserve. The input to the models are SI-time curves from myocardial sectors and left ventricular blood pool regions of interest and, in some cases,

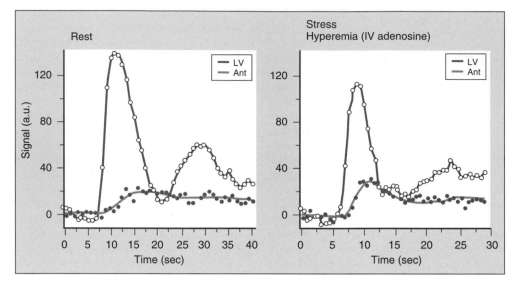

FIGURE 3-15. Typical example of regional signal intensity-time (SI) curves generated at rest and during stress. Shown is the left ventricular blood pool SI curve (LV) that serves as the input function for deconvolution of the tissue SI curves (ANT) of a representative normal anterior myocardial region of interest. The corresponding "fitted" myocardial curves are also demonstrated. The fitted curves revealed the myocardial blood flow. At rest, the SI curve slope is flat, and the peak SI amplitude is lower than at stress, which is induced by adenosine. The myocardial SI curve at stress has an increased slope and larger amplitude, reflecting a threefold increased myocardial blood flow. On the basis of rest and stress myocardial flow data derived from the fitted SI curves, the regional perfusion reserves can be derived as the ratio of stress over rest flows.

additional physiological parameters. These analyses reflect not only coronary flow but microcirculatory blood flow and endothelial function as well and have been extensively validated against standards such as radioactive microspheres, intracoronary Doppler flow probes, and PET scanning.

Studies have reported myocardial perfusion reserve values derived from the upslope of the CMR SI-time curve. Ibrahim and coworkers[32] found a mean value for myocardial flow reserve in normal individuals of 2.1 by CMR vs. 3.9 for PET. This study used parameters derived from CMR SI-time upslope and concluded that MRFP underestimates the values of normal myocardial perfusion reserve determined by PET and intracoronary flow Doppler.

Two studies that used contrast agent kinetic models have reported myocardial perfusion reserve measurements that were much more in agreement with invasive measurements and PET. Contrast agent kinetics models are probably more accurate than parametric measurement for determining myocardial perfusion reserve.

University of Minnesota: Requirements for Quantification

1. Contrast agent injection: Quantitative MRFP requires a very rapid bolus by power injector at an injection rate of approximately 5 to 10 mL/s. The entry of contrast into the myocardium is referred to as the "impulse" in contrast agent kinetics and ideally is a single sharp spike occurring in zero time. Recirculation, low ejection fraction, valvular regurgitation, and diffusion create error effects on the myocardial impulse signal that

are best corrected with a contrast agent kinetics model.

2. Scanner capability: Spatial resolutions should be less than 2.5 mm to resolve transmural variations in blood flow. The temporal resolution should be one to two images per heartbeat with T1-weighted ultrafast or real-time imaging.

3. CMR sequences: The choices are dictated by the trade-off between temporal resolution, spatial resolution, and acquisition time. The most common solutions at present are fast gradient echo sequences with T1 weighting. These typically have a preparatory inversion pulse followed by a TI delay chosen to null the myocardium just before contrast enhancement.

4. Multisided imaging: Simultaneous acquisition of multiple slices is attractive, because every slice has the same contrast agent input and is also much more time effective.

5. Contrast agent kinetic model: Models to interpret SI-time data have been developed to overcome the limitations from nonideal myocardial input because of dispersion of contrast in administration and transit into the myocardium. This correction of input function allows comparison of one study to another in the same patient at different times or between two patients.

The myocardial input function can be thought of as a train of impulses with heights determined by the height of the input function at each particular time point. By a mathematical process called "disconsolation," one can then infer the tissue response curve (an idealized curve) for a single impulse input. The height of the tissue residue impulse response is a measure of blood flow.

Microvasculature vs. Coronary Artery Obstruction

Studies of coronary reperfusion have shown that myocardial salvage is maximal if an occluded epicardial coronary artery is reperfused within 2 hours. Later infarct-related artery reperfusion has also been shown to improve long-term ventricular function and prognosis beyond the early period of myocardial salvage. Bridging collateral vessels on angiography can sustain myocardial viability in areas of coronary occlusion, and this might also be true with vessels too small to see. Testing this important issue in patients would rely on simultaneous assessment of viability and microvascular flow, a capability that CMR offers. Microembolization and loss of endothelial cell membrane integrity affect the microvascular bed. The "no-reflow" phenomenon occurs when the epicardial coronary artery is opened yet little or no flow occurs within the myocardium and the microcirculatory bed. Gd-DTPA tends to accumulate in infarct zones, leading to contrast hyperenhancement on delayed imaging. However, within the core of infarction, sequestration of neutrophils can lead to microvessel obstruction by erythrocytes, leukocytes, microemboli, and cellular debris. Consequently, this area might be inaccessible to reperfusion (and inflow of Gd contrast by CMR). This can be visualized as an area of low signal intensity depicted as a "hypoenhancement" on the perfusion images both visually and quantitatively.

Clinical Applications of CMR Myocardial Perfusion

Schwitter and colleagues[33] studied the accuracy of CMR first-pass perfusion compared with PET and coronary angiography in 48 patients undergoing cardiac catheterization for suspected coronary artery disease and in 18 healthy subjects. The method used was also analysis of the upslope of SI-time curves and visual analysis, with subendocardial and epicardial segments analyzed separately. Subendocardial upslope was found to be highly accurate in prediction of coronary artery disease by vessel compared with PET (sensitivity, 91%; specificity, 94%) and with quantitative angiography (87% and 85%, respectively). When transmural or subepicardial upslopes were used, the findings were less accurate.

In an assessment of myocardial viability by Lauerma et al before cardiac revascularization, PET scanning was compared with multimode dobutamine cine MR, adding either first-pass perfusion or Gd-DTPA late-enhancement as a second modality. A single Gd-DTPA perfusion scan was performed only during the dobutamine stress. The first part of the combination was the assessment of baseline wall motion. Cine wall motion was then measured at peak dobutamine, followed by a bolus injection of Gd for first-pass perfusion. The dobutamine/first-pass combination was the most accurate in predicting improvement in viable wall segments at a sensitivity of 97% and a specificity of 96%, compared with PET with 81% and 86%, respectively. Other protocols might be used to assess myocardial viability.[34] A combined approach using first-pass perfusion and delayed enhancement was reported by Rogers et al[35] in patients after first myocardial infarction. Regions of interest in reperfused infarcted regions were studied with resting first-pass perfusion and delayed enhancement done at 1 week and 7 weeks, and the functional recovery of these segments was measured. Abnormal segments were graded for decreased first-pass perfusion, abnormal delayed enhancement, or both. Regions designated as HYPO had only decreased first-pass wash-in rates, with a plateau of signal intensity at the same time as normal myocardium. HYPER regions had a continuous increase in signal intensity with time, beyond the plateau seen in normal myocardium during recirculation, and COMBO had both decreased early wash-in and delayed peaking. HYPO regions had both impaired regional wall motion compared with HYPER regions at week 1 and no significant improvement by week 7, whereas HYPER regions had marked improvement. COMBO regions were intermediate. They concluded that HYPO regions had more evidence of microvascular obstruction even with TIMI grade 3 flow on angiography. This study illustrates the combination of three different methods of CMR in each patient: cine function, delayed contrast enhancement, and first-pass myocardial perfusion.

CLINICAL APPLICATIONS OF PET IN THE HEART

PET is an advanced imaging technique that, although not widely available, provides sensitive and accurate assessment of myocardial perfusion and viability. This technology is extremely useful to clinicians in evaluating coronary artery disease and myocardial viability in their patients.

Background

PET is an outgrowth of the interest in imaging of the heart with radiotracers. The advantages of PET over SPECT include the fact that PET offers accurate and precise attenuation correction (unlike the current technology of SPECT). Two other physical characteristics make PET particularly attractive for studies of the heart. These include the fact that positron emission results in two photons of high energy (511 KeV compared with the more conventional single photon emission of ^{201}Tl, ~73 KeV; or Tc-99m, 140 KeV) and that when a positron annihilation occurs, the emission of the two simultaneous gamma photons with high energy occurs at 180 degrees. The high energy allows better penetration from the heart to the detector, and the emission of two photons at approximately 180 degrees permits more precise localization of the event source. All these factors result in superior heart imaging and more accurate localization with complete attenuation correction compared with SPECT imaging. However, this also makes PET cameras more complex, because the detector array needs to circumvent the body (leading to additional expense), and the crystals for capturing the higher energy emissions are more expensive.

The second issue related to PET that makes it more limited as a technology is the fact that positron-emitting radionuclides are not long-lived (Table 3-5). Most of the tracers that are used are made in a cyclotron, and those centers that use either oxygen-15–labeled water ($H_2^{15}O$) or carbon-11 (^{11}C) acetate for studies require an on-site cyclotron. Fluorine-18 has a sufficiently long half-life to enable transportation from remote sites for centers that do not have a cyclotron.

A tracer of special note, used for measuring myocardial perfusion, is rubidium-82 (^{82}Rb). This is the only Food and Drug Administration–approved tracer for measuring myocardial blood flow (MBF), and it is unique in that it is generator produced. That is, it needs on-site production, but this is performed in a generator system rather than by an on-site cyclotron. This is an extremely attractive approach, but the cost of the generator (approximately \$25,000/month) limits the ^{82}Rb generator to sites with reasonable patient loads and a dedicated PET camera.

Instrumentation

It is important that clinicians interested in using PET for cardiac applications understand the design characteristics, specifications, and limitations of PET. Commercially available systems are available for whole-body applications (oncology, neurology, and cardiac use), and this multipurpose application by nature results in a compromise. For example, some whole-body scanners have limited resolution needed for neurological applications, whereas high-resolution systems show reduced sensitivity for cardiac use. The requirements for cardiac PET have been described.

For imaging of the heart, the tomograph needs to have a field of use sufficiently large to obviate multiple data acquisitions. This is typically accomplished with a longitudinal field of view between 14 and 18 cm. This is the case for all commercially available cameras. The gantry opening must be sufficiently wide to fit the torso of large patients. This is easily accomplished on all commercially available PET systems.

■ ■ ■

TABLE 3-5   POSITRON-EMITTING TRACERS USED CLINICALLY FOR CARDIAC PET

Radionuclide (half-life)	Compound	Use
Cyclotron-produced		
Oxygen-15 (2.1 min)	H_2O	Blood flow
	CO	Blood volume
	CO_2	Blood flow
	O_2	Metabolism
Nitrogen-13 (10.0 min)	NH_3	Blood flow/ metabolism
Carbon-11 (20.4 min)	Palmitate	Metabolism
	Acetate	Metabolism
	Glucose	Metabolism
Fluorine-18 (110 min)	Fluorodeoxyglucose	Metabolism
Generator produced		
Rubidium-82 (76 sec)	RbCl	Blood flow/ cell viability

Because most cardiac studies are performed in the nongated mode (however, gated applications have been increasingly used [see later]), spatial resolution of cameras is usually not a limiting factor. However, it should be remembered that, because the average heart wall is approximately 1 cm, the spatial resolution of reconstructed images is typically not sufficient to interrogate transmural differences in blood flow or metabolism, because one needs to have approximately two times the full width at half maximum (FWHM) to resolve such differences. Although recent PET tomographs have spatial resolutions of 4 to 6 mm FWHM, heart motion with systole and diastole and with respiration limits reconstructed resolution. Although it is possible to acquire data with both cardiac and respiratory gating, the technique is not widely used because of the increased computer requirements for segregating data and the loss of count information.

The incomplete recovery of counts when the imaged object is less than two times FWHM results in a loss of tracer information that can be corrected for. For qualitative imaging, this is typically not performed. For quantitative information (i.e., measuring myocardial perfusion in mL/g/min or metabolism in μmol/g/min), correction for wall thickness needs to be performed. This is typically done within the mathematical model used to estimate perfusion or metabolism, but estimates of wall thickness can also be obtained with direct measurements of the wall with techniques such as echocardiography or CMR.

To measure myocardial perfusion and metabolism quantitatively, regions of interest in the blood (for the input function) and in heart tissue (for delineation of tissue time-activity curves) are required at data acquisition rates of between 5 and 10 seconds. This requires a computer with high time resolution that is available on all commercially available tomographs. For most qualitative cardiac applications, ungated "static" scans are acquired for 10 or 15 minutes without collecting dynamic data.

Radiotracers for Cardiac PET

One of the most attractive features for the use of cardiac PET is the ability to image sequentially heart perfusion, metabolism, and function with short half-life tracers. Although some tracers (Table 3-5) are used predominantly for research applications, those used clinically will be considered individually in the following.

It should be noted that in the United States in 2003, only two tracers are approved for clinical use. These are ^{82}Rb, which is used for the assessment of myocardial perfusion, and FDG, which is used for the assessment of myocardial viability. However, a number of other tracers have been used for clinical cardiac work, including $H_2^{15}O$ (for perfusion) and ^{11}C-acetate (for viability). Many insurance carriers will reimburse PET with these tracers when adequate expertise and experience have been demonstrated.

Clinical Use of Cardiac PET

Although one of the major strengths of cardiac PET is for research applications, for the practicing clinician, there are two primary roles for cardiac PET. These are (1) for the diagnosis of coronary artery disease and assessment of the efficacy of interventional strategies, and (2) for the assessment of myocardial viability.

Although PET is not typically used as a primary diagnostic tool for initial assessment of patients, it should be noted that there are some centers that use PET with ^{82}Rb specifically as an alternative for traditional SPECT stress myocardial perfusion imaging. This would be an appropriate strategy for centers that have patients whose body habitus often limits adequate evaluation with conventional SPECT tracers (i.e., women with large breasts or obese patients) and when the clinical volume is sufficient to justify the expense of a ^{82}Rb generator. However, it must be remembered that exercise cannot be performed in a PET gantry, and thus all evaluations of stress cardiac perfusion imaging are performed with pharmacological agents such as dipyridamole, adenosine, or dobutamine. For centers that do not have sufficient volume to justify the cost of an ^{82}Rb generator, most perfusion assessments are performed with nitrogen-13 ammonia (^{13}NH$_3$), a cyclotron-produced tracer. This is done predominantly for patients with equivocal studies from conventional SPECT perfusion imaging and in patients who do not want to undergo angiography.

For viability assessments, PET is an appropriate tool with a high sensitivity and specificity for delineation of patients who would benefit from revascularization procedures. Medicare requires an "equivocal" SPECT scan before PET for reimbursement to be made. As noted later, cardiac PET has been shown to identify significant myocardial viability in up to 60% of patients who have infarction by conventional SPECT studies and is thus an appropriate approach for delineating viable myocardium in patients who are revascularization candidates.

Assessment of MBF with PET

The delineation of blood flow is an essential noninvasive approach for the detection of macrovascular coronary artery disease and for evaluation of medical or interventional strategies to augment myocardial perfusion.

PET has been used for several decades for the delineation, both qualitative and quantitative, of MBF in patients with macrovascular coronary artery disease. Because PET allows quantification of myocardial perfusion on an absolute basis (i.e., mL/g/min), PET has also been used for the delineation of abnormal blood flow in the absence of macrovascular disease.

General Approach for Measurement of MBF with PET

A number of radiopharmaceuticals are suitable for the assessment of MBF with PET (Table 3-5). For clinical assessments of myocardial perfusion, two tracers, ^{13}NH$_3$ (cyclotron-produced) and ^{82}Rb-chloride (generator-produced), are used. The former requires an on-site cyclotron, whereas the latter requires an on-site generator system. H$_2^{15}$O is a cyclotron-produced tracer that has also been extensively used for the assessment of myocardial perfusion, but its use is limited to research applica-

tions, because the quality of H$_2^{15}$O images is not sufficiently high for clinical diagnosis (although the quantitative estimates with myocardial perfusion with H$_2^{15}$O are extremely accurate [see later]).

Both ^{13}NH$_3$ and ^{82}Rb-chloride are cationic tracers that are actively extracted by the myocardium as they pass through the coronary vasculature. The extraction of these tracers is high under resting conditions but decreases inversely and nonlinearly as blood flow increases. Because these tracers are highly extracted, they provide good to excellent quality images of myocardial perfusion and have been used extensively. The sensitivity and specificity for these tracers is high (Table 3-6). Image analysis is comparable to that performed with conventional SPECT tracers and will not be delineated here.

In addition to qualitative assessment of myocardial perfusion analogous to that which can be obtained using more conventional tracers such as ^{201}Tl or Tc-99m sestamibi or tetrofosmin, one of the advantages of PET is the ability to quantify blood flow in absolute terms, which is accomplished by performing dynamic acquisition (i.e., acquiring counts over time) and incorporating the input function (arterial time-activity curve) and tissue regions of interest into mathematical models. For most clinical applications, qualitative flow assessment is sufficient. However, the addition of quantitative measurements can be extremely useful to document absolute levels of flow in hearts with homogenous but abnormal perfusion such as seen in patients with chest pain but angiographically normal coronary arteries; in patients with cardiac transplants; or in patients with cardiomyopathy or balanced, multivessel coronary artery disease. In all these conditions, uptake of flow tracers might be homogeneous despite the presence of hypoperfusion on the basis of

■ ■ ■

TABLE 3-6 SELECTED STUDIES USING PET FOR DETECTION OF CORONARY ARTERY DISEASE

	Number of subjects	Sensitivity	Specificity
^{82}Rb			
Gould et al[*]	27	95	100
Stewart et al[†]	81	84	88
Simone et al[‡]	225	83	91
Go et al[§]	202	93	78
Williams et al[‖]	222	87	88
^{13}N ammonia			
Schelbert et al[¶]	45	97	100
Gould et al[*]	23	95	100
Yonekura et al[**]	60	97	99
Tamaki et al[††]	51	88	90

Data sources:
[*]Gould KL, et al. *J Am Coll Cardiol* 7:775-789, 1986.
[†]Stewart RE, et al. *Am J Cardiol* 67:1303-1310, 1991.
[‡]Simone GL, et al. *Am J Physiol Imaging* 7:203-209, 1992.
[§]Go RT, et al. *J Nucl Med* 31:1899-1905, 1990.
[‖]Williams BR, et al. *J Nucl Med* 35:1586-1592, 1994.
[¶]Schelbert HR, et al. *Am J Cardiol* 49:1197-1206, 1982. Yonekura Y, et al. *Am Heart J* 113:645-654, 1987.
[**]Yonekura Y, et al. *Am Heart J* 113:645-654, 1987.
[††]Tamaki N, et al. *J Nucl Med* 29:1181-1188, 1988.

absolute estimates of blood flow. Assessment of absolute blood flow can be made simply and requires no more than collecting data dynamically during the scan.

$^{13}NH_3$

$^{13}NH_3$ has been used extensively for assessment of myocardial perfusion with PET. This tracer exhibits high fractional extraction by the myocardium and has a relatively prolonged retention in the heart. Extremely high-quality images of the myocardium can be obtained, although intestinal uptake is frequently seen. Patients with severe congestive heart failure and smokers can have increased tracer uptake in the lungs, impairing assessment of the lateral wall.

Regional inhomogeneity of uptake of $^{13}NH_3$ has been described and can be problematic. This decreased uptake is seen predominantly in the inferolateral myocardium and is likely due to regional differences in metabolism of $^{13}NH_3$ rather than because of flow heterogeneity. This observation underscores one of the inherent difficulties in the use of all extractable tracers for estimating myocardial flow. Uptake and retention are inexorably linked with the specific metabolic pathways responsible for tracer uptake and retention. Nonetheless, as shown in Table 3-6, qualitative assessments of images obtained with $^{13}NH_3$ are quite sensitive and specific for assessment of coronary artery disease.

For delineation of blood flow with $^{13}NH_3$, approximately 20 mCi of tracer is injected IV, typically over 15 to 30 seconds with an infusion pump. For quantitative assessments, dynamic data are collected dynamically over the initial 2 to 3 minutes of tracer infusion. For image analysis, data from approximately 5 to 15 minutes are acquired in a "static" frame. These images readily delineate high myocardial to blood and lung contrast (Figure 3-16). For use for the diagnosis of coronary artery disease, after acquisition of rest images, imaging is repeated approximately 45 to 60 minutes later (allowing for the decay of radioactivity to background levels) after inducing vasodilatation with dipyridamole, adenosine, or dobutamine.

In addition to its use for assessment of coronary artery disease, $^{13}NH_3$ has been used in a number of extremely interesting research studies that show the importance of absolute flow determinations. For example, it has been documented that young patients with either familial or intrinsic hypercholesterolemia have reduced hyperemia in response to a coronary vasodilator, demonstrating that changes in nutritive perfusion can occur even in the absence of overt coronary artery disease. Interventions such as exercise or cholesterol lowering can improve flow reserve. These observations are important in recognizing factors that impair nutritive perfusion even in the absence of frank atherosclerotic coronary artery disease and in the development of interventions to improve perfusion.

^{82}Rb

^{82}Rb chloride is an attractive tracer for assessment of myocardial perfusion, because it is generator produced and commercially available. It should be of particular interest to sites without an on-site cyclotron and that perform a large volume of pharmacological coronary procedures or that perform studies in obese patients or others in which tissue attenuation can be problematic in the evaluation of the heart with SPECT. The extremely short physical half-life of ^{82}Rb (76 seconds) results in images that are of slightly lower quality than can be achieved with $^{13}NH_3$, although some of the problems seen with $^{13}NH_3$ such as increased lung uptake, regional inhomogeneity, or intestinal uptake have not been reported to date with ^{82}Rb. The short physical half-life also allows very rapid imaging protocols, because approximately 5 minutes after a rest scan, a stress scan can be performed (as opposed to the longer wait time needed for decay of radioisotope when using $^{13}NH_3$). A noted disadvantage of ^{82}Rb is the current high cost of the generator, which requires high clinical volume to make this approach cost-effective.

As is the case for all extractable tracers, ^{82}Rb uptake is related to metabolism (similar to potassium uptake). For human studies, typically 40 to 60 mCi is administered with an infusion system and after a 60- to 90-second delay, images are obtained for 6 to 10 minutes. For quantitative estimates of perfusion, images are obtained dynamically from the start of tracer administration. Reported studies of ^{82}Rb sensitivity and specificity are very high (Table 3-6). Although ^{82}Rb is approved for myocardial perfusion studies, the number of centers that routinely use this tracer with PET for cardiac studies is relatively limited, although fiscal considerations would argue that this approach is underused.

Quantification of myocardial perfusion can also be obtained using ^{82}Rb, although the short physical half-life of this tracer does induce some technical issues.

An additional feature of ^{82}Rb that has only been preliminarily explored is the concept that this tracer can also assess myocardial viability. Because ^{82}Rb has a similar biological fate as potassium, it was reasoned that the extrusion of extracted ^{82}Rb from the myocardium might be an index of myocardial viability. Gould et al demonstrated that decreased retention of ^{82}Rb correlated with uptake of FDG, suggesting that this tracer could potentially be used to delineate myocardial viability as well as perfusion. Larger studies with a more diverse patient population will be needed to corroborate this finding, but if proven, it would make this tracer very attractive for cardiac use.

$H_2^{15}O$

Although not used clinically because it does not provide diagnostically suitable images, $H_2^{15}O$ bears mentions, because it is the only tracer currently in wide use that allows assessment of myocardial perfusion in absolute terms for a tracer that is not affected by metabolism. $H_2^{15}O$ is considered freely diffusible in the myocardium, meaning that it enters and leaves the myocardium solely on the basis of flow. Qualitative estimates of perfusion with $H_2^{15}O$ have been demonstrated to be accurate over a very wide range.

Typically, 15 to 30 mCi is administered as a bolus, and dynamic acquisition is obtained for approximately 3 to 5

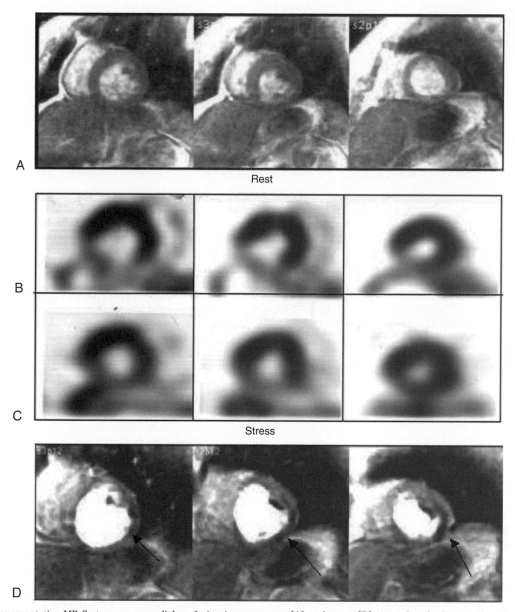

FIGURE 3-16. Representative MR first-pass myocardial perfusion images at rest (**A**) and stress (**D**) imaged at the base, mid, and apical level of the left ventricle *(from left to right)*. Shown are single-peak signal intensity images out of a series of 40 to 50 consecutive images after gadolinium-DTPA contrast injection of 0.04 mmol/kg. **A,** At rest, there is no qualitatively appreciated MR perfusion defect noted in the inferior septal and posterior segments. MRFP corresponded well with the coronary angiogram seen in Figure 3-17, with complete antegrade and retrograde collateral filling of a subtotal occluded right coronary artery. **B,** However, the SPECT (^{201}Tl/^{99m}Tc) study suggested a perfusion defect at rest (even so there was enough collateral blood flow supply as indicated by the collaterals in Figure 3-17). MRFP better depicted in this example the collateral dependent blood flow at rest. However, this could not be appreciated on the SPECT rest perfusion studies, which indicated some chronic infarction with significantly reduced rest flow. **C to D,** With stress (**D**) there is an area of inducible ischemia seen indicated by low signal intensity in the posterior and inferior septal segments (arrows in **D**) in good agreement with the stress SPECT study (**C**), indicating a "steal effect" in this area.

minutes. An alternative approach is to administer ^{15}O-labeled carbon dioxide ($C^{15}O_2$) by inhalation over 3 to 3.5 minutes and obtain images over 6 to 7 minutes. This approach relies on the rapid conversion of $C^{15}O_2$ to $H_2^{15}O$ in the lung by the enzyme, carbonic anhydrase. Because H_2^{15} has a short half-life, stress images can be obtained approximately 5 to 10 minutes after rest images.

Because $H_2^{15}O$ circulates in the vascular pool and the heart, images obtained must be corrected for vascular activity. This can be obtained using a separate tracer of the blood pool such as ^{15}O-labeled carbon monoxide;

with the initial 30 seconds of the $H_2^{15}O$ image to form an image of the vascular pool, or by factor analysis. Numerous studies have demonstrated that $H_2^{15}O$ accurately delineates perfusion and coronary artery disease. There is an inverse relationship between the severity of coronary stenosis and myocardial perfusion reserve in patients with single-vessel coronary artery disease. At rest, flow in patients is not different from age-matched controls, whereas after vasodilatation with dipyridamole, the hyperemic response is diminished distal to stenosis and correlates inversely with the degree of narrowing. In

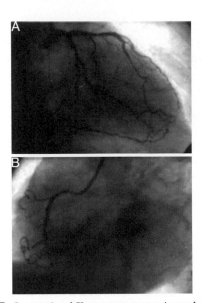

FIGURE 3-17. Conventional X-ray coronary angiography in the same patient as shown in Figure 3-16. Injection into the right coronary artery (B) demonstrated a total occlusion of the mid RCA with antegrade collateral supply of the left coronary artery. Injection into the left coronary artery (A) revealed complete retrograde collateral filling of the RCA. This suggested some preservation of blood flow in the territory of the RCA at rest as correctly depicted by the normal MRFP rest study but not the SPECT study. The quantitative regional myocardial perfusion reserve is a precise measurement of coronary artery severity and collateral dependent flow.

addition, this tracer has been used to show the efficacy of interventions such as angioplasty or thrombolytic therapy.

Similar to the case of ^{82}Rb, some investigators have demonstrated that a specific measure obtained with $H_2^{15}O$ can be used to delineate scar from viable tissue and therefore be used to predict recovery of function after either thrombolytic therapy or CABG. These studies suggest that $H_2^{15}O$ might be useful not only to assess perfusion but also myocardial viability. Although this observation has not been tested extensively, it provides an impetus for delineation of both perfusion and viability with a single tracer.

Assessment of Myocardial Viability

An extremely important role for cardiac PET is the delineation of myocardial viability. Although many diagnostic and therapeutic decisions can be made by use of conventional SPECT techniques with perfusion tracers such as ^{201}Tl or ^{99m}Tc sestamibi or tetrofosmin, these tracers underestimate viable tissue. Thus, although it has been shown that myocardium that has reversible defects with either ^{201}Tl or ^{99m}Tc-based flow, tracers will improve after revascularization; even with 24-hour delayed ^{201}Tl studies, up to 60% of segments that have scar by conventional SPECT imaging show evidence of viability by PET scanning, and these areas improve function after a revascularization procedure. Although some authors have suggested that there is equivalence between delineation of viability with SPECT techniques and PET, the preponderance of evidence is that PET is more sensitive

for delineation of viable, hibernating myocardium than conventional SPECT.

The delineation of viable to nonviable myocardium becomes particularly important in patients with markedly reduced EF. These patients are at most perioperative risk but also stand to derive the most benefit from revascularization procedures. Thus, it is in these patients that PET scanning offers the most critical diagnostic information.

Scheme of Myocardial Metabolism

To understand the basis for cardiac PET scanning for assessment of myocardial viability, a basic understanding of the metabolism of the heart is important. The heart is an intrinsically aerobic organ that requires sufficient oxygen and substrate to provide high-energy phosphates for profound ionic fluxes and myocardial contraction. Under fasting conditions, the heart predominantly uses fatty acids for energy, because these are abundant in blood but postprandially switches to carbohydrates because of the inhibitory effects of secreted insulin in response to ingested sugars on peripheral lipolysis. On the basis of an inverse relationship between myocardial fatty acid and glucose use, postprandially, glucose becomes a more important substrate for the production of adenosine triphosphate (ATP) compared with fatty acid. As insulin levels drop, plasma fatty acid increases, and the preponderance of fatty acid as a prime substrate recurs. This inverse relationship between myocardial fatty acid and glucose use (the Randle cycle) has important implications for imaging of the heart.

When oxygen is limited because of limited blood flow, cardiac metabolism is altered. Fatty acid oxidation is diminished, and glucose becomes more important, because it is well known that glucose can provide energy by means of anaerobic glycolysis. In addition, it has been shown that ischemia or hypoxia up-regulate glucose transporters, and the failing heart reverts to a more fetal-type of metabolism that is nearly exclusively glycolytic. With complete occlusion of the coronary artery such as might occur with acute myocardial infarction, upstream buildup of long-chain fatty acid intermediates might play a role in decreased myocardial contractility, as well as with increasing arrhythmogenesis. Although ATP can be made by anaerobic metabolism and this can partially compensate for the energy needs of the heart, experimental studies suggest that anaerobic glycolysis is insufficient to meet contractile function of the heart but might be sufficient for preservation of cellular viability, at least for a period of time. The conditions in human myocardium might be more complex. Down-regulation of function can reduce energy needs in areas distal to stenoses. These conditions might allow for the heart not only to alter its metabolic pathways but might also set up a condition whereby myocardial viability can be preserved for months or even years. Diminution of fatty acid metabolism and enhancement of glucose use is the metabolic signature of disordered myocardial metabolism, and the pattern of change that is key in the identification of ischemic myocardium with PET.

If blood flow is restored soon after acute coronary occlusion, the normal pattern of substrate metabolism is restored, although the recovery of the normal pattern of metabolism might be delayed for days to weeks. Restoration of the ability to oxidatively metabolize substrate is particularly important for the ultimate functional recovery of ischemic myocardium.

Specific Tracers of Myocardial Metabolism for Assessing Viability FDG

FDG is the most extensively used tracer in PET because of its use in studies of the brain, oncology, and for cardiac imaging. Because the physical half-life of FDG is 110 minutes, it can be shipped from remote locations and thus is available nationwide to centers that do not have cyclotrons.

FDG is not analogous to native glucose (i.e., it is an analog). Although the native substrate is available as ^{11}C-glucose, it has a more complex metabolism, requiring dynamic scanning, because it can undergo multiple metabolic fates, and the half-life of ^{11}C (20 minutes) requires an on-site cyclotron for production. In contrast, FDG has a unique metabolic fate. It crosses the sarcolemma similar to glucose, but once phosphorylated to FDG-6-phosphate, it is relatively impermeable for back-diffusion into the blood. In addition, FDG-6-phosphate is not a substrate for further metabolism. Although glucose uptake can be measured quantitatively by use of mathematical models, it has been demonstrated that the use of quantitative as opposed to qualitative estimates does not improve assessments of viability. Quantitative assessments of glucose uptake with FDG require the use of a "lumped constant" that corrects uptake of FDG for differences with glucose. The "lumped constant" can be influenced by plasma substrate concentration and levels of insulin.

For clinical use, there is some debate about whether patients should be studied under fasting conditions as opposed to after glucose loading or an insulin clamp. It might seem intuitive that ischemic myocardium might be best identified with the patient studied under fasting conditions (i.e., when normal myocardium is using fatty acid and ischemic myocardium is using glucose). However, under fasting conditions, uptake of glucose by the heart is so small that performing studies under fasted conditions results in an intolerably high level of uninterpretable scans because of poor FDG uptake. Thus, almost all centers performing viability scans use a glucose loading protocol. In addition, Gropler et al demonstrated regional heterogeneity of FDG uptake in healthy volunteers when studied under fasting conditions, whereas FDG uptake was nearly homogeneous under fed conditions. Signal in the septum during fasting conditions likely reflects regional heterogeneity in metabolism.

It is critical to follow a protocol to obtain diagnostically useful images of the heart with FDG. At our institution, when patients initially arrive at the laboratory they have a blood glucose level checked. They are then given an oral glucose load on the basis of their fasting glucose level. Nondiabetic patients with normal blood glucose will receive 50 g orally. Patients with higher baseline blood sugars receive less. Patients with diabetes may receive a small amount of oral glucose but then also are given insulin. Blood glucose levels are followed every 30 minutes and are used as a marker for insulin, which is anticipated to rise after oral glucose and then fall. As insulin levels rise, blood fatty acid levels are suppressed, and myocardial glucose uptake is maximal. As insulin levels fall, fatty acid levels will rise, and the heart will switch back to using predominantly fatty acids. We monitor blood glucose after the glucose load and after blood glucose rises and then is back toward baseline levels; then FDG is administered. Other laboratories use a euglycemic clamp instead of oral glucose loading. Eight to 10 mCi of FDG is then administered IV. For absolute quantification of regional myocardial glucose uptake, dynamic images are taken over 45 to 60 minutes. However, for most clinical assessments of viability, a single static image is usually obtained over 15 to 20 minutes starting 30 to 45 minutes after tracer administration. In our laboratory, we typically obtain a 1- or 2-minute "scout" scan to ensure adequate tracer uptake in the heart before performing the full diagnostic scan.

There is some controversy about the use of FDG early after acute myocardial infarction with or without reperfusion. Although glucose use is increased during acute ischemic states, the uptake of FDG during ischemia is typically reduced because of reduced perfusion. With reperfusion, although glucose uptake can be enhanced, FDG uptake can be variable, depending on levels of residual blood flow, arterial substrate concentrations, and time. In addition, inflammatory cells also can take up FDG. For this reason, it has been our practice, unsupported by data, not to perform viability scans for at least 3 weeks after acute myocardial infarction.

In chronic states, coupled with the use of a flow tracer (^{13}NH$_3$ or ^{82}Rb), discordances between myocardial perfusion and FDG uptake have been the mainstay for identification of hibernating myocardium from scar (Figure 3-18). Normal myocardium is characterized by normal function, normal perfusion, and matched, normal FDG uptake. Dysfunctional myocardium can show four different patterns (Figure 3-19). Infarcted myocardium has concordantly reduced perfusion and FDG uptake; hibernating myocardium has reduced perfusion, but FDG uptake is increased relative to perfusion; stunned myocardium has near normal flow, with a variable pattern of metabolism; and dysfunctional myocardium with relatively normal perfusion but reduced FDG uptake seems to represent viable tissue (Table 3-7).

■ ■ ■

TABLE 3-7 MYOCARDIUM AS DEFINED WITH PET

Classification	Function	Perfusion	FDG uptake relative to flow
Normal	Normal	Normal	Normal
Infarcted decrease	Decreased	Decreased	Matched
Hibernating	Decreased	Decreased	Increased
Stunned	Decreased	Normal	Variable
Viable but jeopardized	Decreased	Near Normal	Decreased

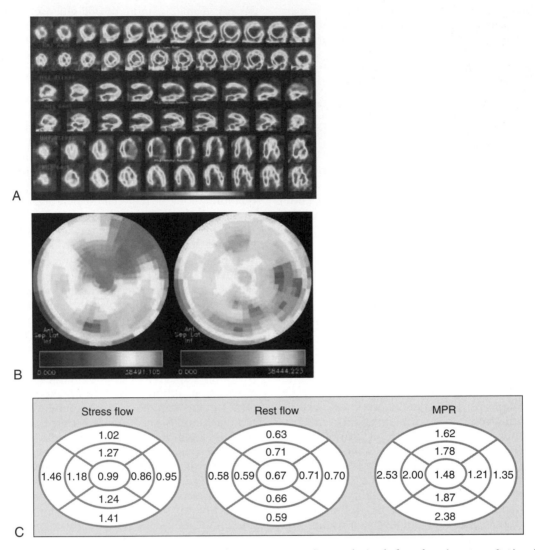

FIGURE 3-18. (A) Short- and long-axis images of a patient with coronary artery disease obtained after adenosine stress *(top)* and rest *(bottom)* using [13]NH[3]. There is a large anterolateral perfusion defect. **B,** Polar map of the stress perfusion image *(left)* and rest image *(right).* **C,** Quantitative estimates of myocardial perfusion based on mathematical modeling. Even in regions of apparently normal perfusion based on uptake of tracer, absolute quantification of flow indicates a blunted response to adenosine (i.e., these values are below the lower limits of normal). See also Color Insert.

We quantify perfusion in absolute terms (mL/g/min) in every patient. This is performed to assess absolute levels of myocardial perfusion to determine whether areas of apparent normal perfusion actually have decreased myocardial blood flow. However, absolute levels of myocardial perfusion cannot be used to distinguish viable from nonviable myocardium, because the overlap between regions is so large. FDG uptake is normalized to perfusion, with the region of most normal perfusion representing "100%" and FDG uptake in this region considered normal in the glucose-loaded state. Heart segments with FDG uptake greater than or less than 12% of perfusion in a region are considered to have enhanced or decreased FDG uptake. We divide the heart into nine contiguous regions (basal and distal anterior, inferior, lateral, and septal walls and apex) and consider these territories in conjunction with gated wall motion studies. For delineation of hibernating myocardium, based on the studies of Di Carli et al, 20% of contiguous myocardium

must be hibernating or viable for a recommendation that the territory would improve after revascularization.

Numerous studies that used FDG for delineation of viability have shown that up to 60% of regions with scar by traditional SPECT imaging have hibernating myocardium on the basis of PET. The finding of reduced function with reduced perfusion and decreased FDG uptake is specific for nonviable myocardium. In a meta-analysis by Bonow, based on 146 patients from six studies, the pattern of hibernating myocardium resulted in positive predictive accuracy of 82%, with a negative predictive accuracy of 83%. Those with the poorest function who are at the highest risk for perioperative morbidity or mortality had the greatest improvement after revascularization (Figure 3-20).

A recent study from our laboratory demonstrated that approximately 60% of patients with scar by ^{201}Tl SPECT imaging have evidence of significant viable myocardium by PET. In these patients, all with severely reduced EF

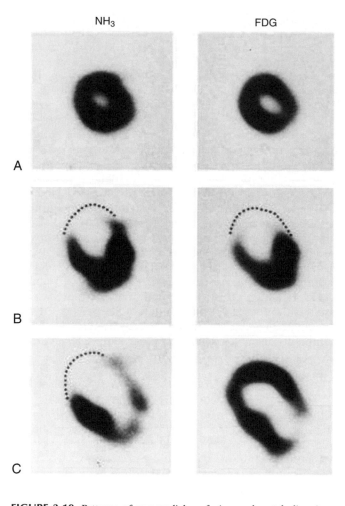

NH₃   FDG

A

B

C

FIGURE 3-19. Patterns of myocardial perfusion and metabolism in a normal volunteer (A), in a patient with myocardial infarction (B), and in a patient with hibernating myocardium (C). In the control subject, perfusion and FDG uptake is homogeneous, whereas in the patient with infarction, perfusion and metabolism are concordantly decreased. In the patient with hibernating myocardium, myocardial perfusion is markedly decreased, whereas glucose use is enhanced. This pattern is associated with recovery of function after revascularization. An additional pattern is sometimes observed consisting of normal perfusion and diminished FDG in dysfunctional regions. This latter pattern is associated and jeopardized by viable myocardium. Thus, assessment of the pattern of flow and metabolism is useful in delineating viable from nonviable myocardium and thus in predicting who will benefit from interventional procedures. (Reproduced with permission from Schelbert HR. Current status and prospects of new radionuclides and radiopharmaceuticals for cardiovascular nuclear medicine. *Semin Nucl Med* 1978; 17:145.)

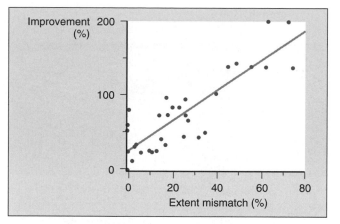

FIGURE 3-20. Relationship between the percent of a perfusion/metabolism mismatch defined by PET (as a percentage of the left ventricle involved) with the change in function status after coronary artery bypass grafting (expressed as a change from baseline symptoms). Thus, patients with the largest areas of viability have the highest perioperative morbidity and mortality; they are also the ones who derive the most functional benefit from revascularization. (Reproduced with permission from Di Carli, et al. Quantitative relation between myocardial viability and improvement in heart failure symptoms after revascularization in patients with ischemic cardiomyopathy. *Circulation* 1995; 92:3436.)

revascularization or not. This recent study corroborates previous studies in a very sick patient population. These studies suggest that patients with hibernating myocardium have an ischemic substrate that results in a high rate of sudden cardiac death, acute myocardial infarction, or worsening heart failure. On the basis of these data, our current algorithm for the delineation of

(average EF, 22%), the incidence of cardiac events was significantly higher in patients with hibernating myocardium who did not undergo revascularization as opposed to those who did, and EF improved significantly only in patients with hibernating myocardium who underwent revascularization. Similarly, survival was significantly better in a 2-year follow-up in patients with hibernating myocardium undergoing revascularization compared with those remaining on medical therapy. Patients with infarction by PET had no decrease in cardiac events or change in EF whether they underwent

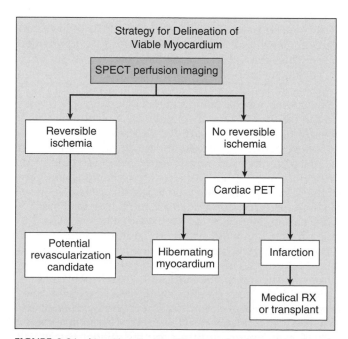

FIGURE 3-21. Algorithm for identification of viable myocardium in patients with myocardial dysfunction who may be candidates for revascularization therapy, as noted in text.

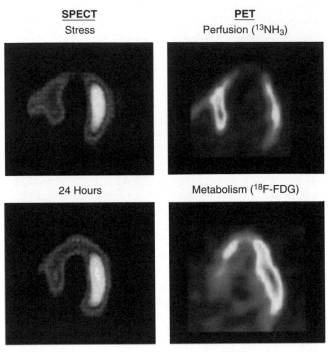

SPECT
Stress

PET
Perfusion (^{13}NH$_3$)

24 Hours

Metabolism (^{18}F-FDG)

FIGURE 3-22. Image taken from a patient showing discrepancies between perfusion obtained with SPECT and that obtained with PET. On the left are stress, 4-hour, and 24-hour redistribution images obtained after administration of ^{201}Tl. To the right are analogous images obtained after administration of ^{13}NH$_3$ and FDG. Areas of apparent decreased flow in the septum are actually caused by tissue attenuation in the SPECT scan, and analysis of a SPECT perfusion vs. PET FDG scan would result in a false-positive assessment of hibernating myocardium. Thus, caution must be used when performing interpretation obtained with SPECT and PET because of differences in tracer attenuation and attenuation correction. See also Color Insert.

myocardial viability in patients with heart failure is shown (Figure 3-21).

Centers that perform heart transplants in patients with severe heart failure often use PET imaging to determine patients in whom CABG can be performed rather than transplantation. It has been the experience of several centers that approximately 30% to 50% of patients referred for transplantation have significant hibernating myocardium that is amenable to bypass grafting rather than transplantation. Not only is this a less life-altering procedure for patients, but it also preserves scarce donor hearts for those who are most in need (patients with nonischemic cardiomyopathy or with ischemic cardiomyopathy but deemed to be inoperable). In a study from our laboratory, nearly 40% of patients referred for transplantation had evidence of hibernating myocardium. Of those who went on to bypass surgery, all did well with an improvement in EF. Thus, PET should be used for delineating viable from nonviable myocardium in patients with ischemic cardiomyopathy being referred to heart transplantation.

Because of the usefulness of FDG for delineating viable myocardium, a number of centers have evaluated whether this tracer can be used with conventional SPECT equipment outfitted for the higher energy of positron emitters that use improved columnization or coincidence detection. Although initial reports have been favorable, it should be cautioned that SPECT systems have worse resolution and sensitivity than the current generation of PET tomographs, and further studies are warranted. Another issue that is often raised is whether one can use a non–positron-emitting flow tracer with an FDG image in the PET camera for delineation of viability. In patients with dilated hearts, attenuation often occurs with conventional flow tracers, and thus one can obtain a false-positive signal of hibernating myocardium (decreased flow with enhanced FDG uptake) (Figure 3-22). Thus, extreme caution is warranted in comparing conventional SPECT tracers and images with true PET images. Use of gated wall motion analysis can be helpful, because regions of FDG uptake in dysfunctional myocardium typically represent viable myocardium. Although no study has been performed to compare the diagnostic accuracy of a hybrid SPECT perfusion/PET metabolism approach, with the advent of more SPECT cameras capable of imaging FDG, viability assessments with this tracer might become more widely used in the future. In addition, the wide use of FDG for oncologic imaging should provide an impetus for many centers to install a dedicated PET scanner even without an on-site cyclotron or generator.

^{11}C-Acetate

Although FDG has been extremely useful for delineating viable from nonviable myocardium, it has been shown both experimentally and clinically that the recovery of oxidative metabolism is critical for the recovery of myocardium after revascularization. ^{11}C-acetate is a tracer of overall oxidative metabolism, because it is metabolized nearly exclusively in mitochondria in the tricarboxylic acid cycle. Because this cycle is so tightly linked to oxidative phosphorylation, it provides an overall index of oxygen use. In addition, unlike glucose or FDG, the use of acetate is independent of the availability of alternative substrates.

For clinical imaging, approximately 20 mCi of acetate is administered IV, and dynamic acquisition is initiated from the time of tracer administration for 25 to 30 minutes. One disadvantage of the use of this tracer is that one needs to quantify kinetics of myocardial washout rather than simply looking at static images. Monoexponential or biexponential fitting of the washout from different myocardial regions is used for calculating the turnover rate constants, and images obtained from approximately 7 to 15 minutes after tracer administration are used to visualize the myocardium.

It has been shown that, in patients with acute myocardial infarction, profound decreases in uptake and clearance of ^{11}C-acetate are observed, and no change occurs over time. Patients treated with thrombolytic therapy recover oxidative metabolism, although it lags behind restoration of perfusion.

In patients with chronic coronary artery disease, viable myocardium has a regional oxidative metabolism similar to normal, whereas nonviable tissue has decreased regional oxidative metabolism. Acetate seems to be superior to FDG for delineating viable from nonviable myocardium on the basis of recovery of function after revascularization. Thus, use of ^{11}C-acetate is an alternative approach for delineating viable from nonviable myocardium, although it is not approved for reimbursement for this use and its imaging is somewhat more complicated by the need to perform dynamic data acquisition and analysis. Recent studies have demonstrated that quantitative flow can be obtained with ^{11}C-acetate that would further enhance the clinical capabilities of this tracer.

[11]C-Palmitate

Because fatty acid plays such a central role in myocardial metabolism, ^{11}C-palmitate has been extensively used in PET studies of the heart. Approximately 20 to 25 mCi of palmitate is administered IV, and dynamic scanning is initiated at the time of tracer administration for 25 to 30 minutes. Excellent quality images of the heart can be obtained when reconstructions from approximately 8 to 16 minutes are used.

Although the kinetics of ^{11}C-palmitate uptake and release are complex, they have been well characterized both experimentally and in clinical studies. A mathematical model has been developed and used for absolute quantification of myocardial fatty acid metabolism.

[11]C-palmitate can be used to define diminished long-chain fatty acid oxidation in children with specific defects of the β-oxidation fatty acid pathway. In addition, the cellular shunting of fatty acid from the cytosol to a slow-turnover pool, presumed to represent triglycerides, could be demonstrated. Whether this approach could be used for delineation of nonischemic cardiomyopathy or used for defining abnormalities in myocardial metabolism in adult patients with acquired cardiomyopathy remains to be defined.

Because of the paramount importance of myocardial fatty acids and the extensive PET literature showing the ability of fatty acids to image the heart, iodinated fatty acids have become of increasing interest and might provide an alternative approach for assessment of myocardial fatty acid metabolism using SPECT.

Functional Analysis

Although PET does not have sufficient resolution to serve as a primary diagnostic approach for measuring myocardial function, with tracers that are extracted and retained by the myocardium, gating of PET images to the cardiac cycle can provide estimates of regional wall motion at the same time that imaging is being performed for estimation of myocardial perfusion or metabolism. Images obtained with [13]NH$_3$ can be gated, and wall motion studies can be used to define regional wall motion at the time of perfusion or metabolic imaging and can help in delineating viable from nonviable myocardium. In addition, wall motion analysis aids in the identification of artifacts such as decreased uptake of [13]NH$_3$ in the inferolateral wall. With normal wall motion in this area, decreased tracer counts suggest uptake inhomogeneity rather than a perfusion defect. Although currently not routinely performed, the simultaneous assessment of function in patients undergoing cardiac PET studies should provide additional diagnostic and prognostic information and should be encouraged.

Miscellaneous Tracers

Because of the flexibility of incorporation of positron-emitting radioisotopes into the compounds and receptor and drug ligands, PET has been used in a number of research applications and has provided insight into a number of cardiac states such as the decrease in β-adrenergic receptor density in patients with dilated cardiomyopathy and the reinnervation of the transplanted heart. These approaches are not used clinically at present, although such agents should be able to define regional variations in adrenal receptor distribution that might be useful in both guiding antiadrenergic therapy in patients with heart failure and potentially in evaluating possible heterogeneity of adrenal receptor location or function leading to recurrent arrhythmias.

Radiolabeling of drugs with positron-emitting radiopharmaceuticals would enable improved drug development by allowing direct interrogation of the binding and residence time of the ligand with its target in the heart.

More recently, experimental studies have demonstrated the ability to incorporate receptor sites in transfer gene products that, when expressed, bind to PET radioligands. This strategy would undoubtedly allow evaluation of the distribution and expression of administered gene products and might become extremely useful in the future in the evaluation of therapies designed to increase blood vessels or cardiac myocytes to the heart.

Summary

PET of the heart enables precise, sequential measurement of regional myocardial perfusion and metabolism. Because of the accurate attenuation correction afforded by PET, the high energy of positron-emitting radionuclides, and the excellent localization based on the emission of two opposing annihilation photons, coupled with the radiotracers that can be labeled, PET has found a niche for the sensitive and specific diagnosis of coronary artery disease, especially in patients with equivocal studies from conventional SPECT imaging, and for the assessment of myocardial viability. Quantification of myocardial perfusion and metabolism is currently used for research studies but does have applications both to evaluate abnormal blood flow in patients with both macrovascular and microvascular disease and for evaluation of the efficacy of pharmacological, mechanical, and surgical interventions. Because of its limited availability, the use for diagnosis of coronary artery disease is most effective in patients with equivocal studies from conventional SPECT techniques. Quantitative assessment of perfusion should be considered in patients with triple-vessel disease, heart transplantation, and other clinical settings in which tracer uptake may be homogeneous but absolute flow in response to stress might be reduced.

Assessment of myocardial viability with PET is highly sensitive and specific for delineation of myocardium that will improve after revascularization and also identifies a subset of patients at high risk for cardiac events, those with significant amounts of hibernating myocardium. These patients should be revascularized, because the event rate is as high as 60% within 2 years, including a high incidence of sudden cardiac death. Although patients with severely reduced EFs are at the most perioperative risk, they will benefit most from revascularization and should be considered for a PET viability scan before revascularization if there is any question regarding the amount of viable myocardium at risk. Because conventional SPECT imaging underestimates viability, it is suggested that all patients with infarction by conventional SPECT imaging who are under consideration for revascularization undergo a PET viability scan.

PET is a unique imaging modality that enables characterization of the events that underlie myocardial dysfunction and provides an important diagnostic modality to optimize care for patients with cardiac disease.

REFERENCES

1. Gibson CM, Murphy SA, Rizzo MJ, et al. The relationship between the TIMI Frame Count and clinical outcomes after thrombolytic administration. *Circulation* 1999; 99:1945.
2. Barcin C, Denktas AE, Garratt KN, Higano ST, Holmes DR, Jr, Lerman A. Relation of Thrombolysis in Myocardial Infarction (TIMI) frame count to coronary flow parameters. *Am J Cardiol* 2003; 91:466.
3. Gibson CM, Cannon CP, Murphy SA, Marble SJ, Barron HV, Braunwald E. Relationship of the TIMI Myocardial perfusion grades, flow rates, frame count, and percutaneous coronary intervention to long-term outcomes after thrombolytic administration in acute myocardial infarction. *Circulation* 2002; 105:1909.
4. Gibson CM, Cannon CP, Daley WL, et al. The TIMI Frame Count: a quantitative method of assessing coronary artery flow. *Circulation* 1996; 93:879.
5. Gibson CM, Cannon CP, Murphy SA, et al. Relationship of TIMI perfusion grade to mortality after administration of thrombolytic drugs. Circulation 2000; 101:125.
6. Ronderos RE, Boskis M, Chung N, et al. Correlation between myocardial perfusion abnormalities detected with intermittent imaging using intravenous perfluorocarbon microbubbles and radioisotope imaging during high-dose dipyridamole stress echo. *Clin Cardiol* 2002; 25:103.
7. Petronio AS, Rovai D, Musumeci G, et al. Effects of abciximab on microvascular integrity and left ventricular functional recovery in patients with acute infarction treated by primary coronary angioplasty. *Eur Heart J* 2003; 24:67.
8. Porter TR, Xie F, Silver M, Kricsfeld D, Oleary E. Real-time perfusion imaging with low mechanical index pulse inversion Doppler imaging. *J Am Coll Cardiol* 2001; 37:748.
9. Muro T, Hozumi T, Watanabe H, et al. Assessment of myocardial perfusion abnormalities by intravenous myocardial contrast echocardiography with harmonic power Doppler imaging: comparison with positron emission tomography. *Heart* 2003; 89:145.
10. Shimoni S, Frangogiannis NG, Aggeli CJ, et al. Microvascular structural correlates of myocardial contrast echocardiography in patients with coronary artery disease and left ventricular dysfunction. *Circulation* 2002; 106:950.
11. Wei K, Jayaweera AR, Firoozan S, Linka A, Skyba DM, Kaul S. Quantification of myocardial blood flow with ultrasound-induced destruction of microbubbles administered as a constant venous infusion. *Circulation* 1998; 97:473.
12. Main ML, Magalski A, Morris BA, Coen MM, Skolnick DG, Good TH. Combined assessment of microvascular integrity and contractile reserve improves differentiation of stunning and necrosis after

acute anterior wall myocardial infarction. *J Am Coll Cardiol* 2002; 40:1079.
13. Rocchi G, Fallani F, Bracchetti G, et al. Non-invasive detection of coronary artery stenosis: a comparison among power-Doppler contrast echo, ^{99m}Tc-Sestamibi SPECT and echo wall-motion analysis. *Coron Artery Dis* 2003; 14:239.
14. Kontos MC, Hinchman D, Cunningham M, Miller JJ, Cherif J, Nixon JV. Comparison of contrast echocardiography with single-photon emission computed tomographic myocardial perfusion imaging in the evaluation of patients with possible acute coronary syndromes in the emergency department. *Am J Cardiol* 2003; 91:1099.
15. Marwick TH, Brunken R, Meland N, et al. Accuracy and feasibility of contrast echocardiography for detection of perfusion defects in routine practice: comparison with wall motion and technetium-99m sestamibi single-photon emission computed tomography. The Nycomed NC100100 Investigators. *J Am Coll Cardiol* 1998; 32:1260.
16. Heinle SK, Noblin J, Goree-Best P, et al. Assessment of myocardial perfusion by harmonic power Doppler imaging at rest and during adenosine stress: comparison with (99m)Tc-sestamibi SPECT imaging. *Circulation* 2000; 102:55.
17. Shimoni S, Zoghbi WA, Xie F, et al. Real-time assessment of myocardial perfusion and wall motion during bicycle and treadmill exercise echocardiography: comparison with single photon emission computed tomography. *J Am Coll Cardiol* 2001; 37:741.
18. Ha JW, Cho SY, Chung N, et al. Fate of collateral circulation after successful coronary angioplasty of total occlusion assessed by coronary angiography and myocardial contrast echocardiography. *J Am Soc Echocardiogr* 2002; 15:389.
19. Colonna P, Cadeddu C, Montisci R, et al. Post-infarction microvascular integrity predicts myocardial viability and left ventricular remodeling after primary coronary angioplasty. A study performed with intravenous myocardial contrast echocardiography. *Ital Heart J* 2002; 3:506.
20. Wagner A, Mahrholdt H, Holly TA, et al. Contrast-enhanced CMR and routine single photon emission computed tomography (SPECT) perfusion imaging for detection of subendocardial myocardial infarcts: an imaging study. *Lancet* 2003; 361:374.
21. Gibbons RJ, Balady GJ, Bricker JT, et al. ACC/AHA 2002 Guideline Update for Exercise Testing: Summary Article. A report of the American College of Cardiology/American Heart Association Task Force on Practice Guidelines (Committee to Update the 1997 Exercise Testing Guidelines). *J Am Coll Cardiol* 2002; 40:1531.
22. Ritchie JL, et al. Guidelines for clinical use of cardiac radionuclide imaging. *J Am Coll Cardiol* 1995; 25:521.
23. Updated imaging guidelines for nuclear cardiology procedures, part 1. *J Nucl Cardiol* 2001; 8:G5.
24. Shaw LJ, Hachamovitch R, Berman DS, et al. The economic consequences of available diagnostic and prognostic strategies for the evaluation of stable angina patients: an observational assessment of the value of precatheterization ischemia. Economics of Noninvasive Diagnosis (END) Multicenter Study Group. *J Am Coll Cardiol* 1999; 33:661.
25. Udelson JE, Beshansky JR, Ballin DS, et al. Myocardial perfusion imaging for evaluation and triage of patients with suspected acute cardiac ischemia. *JAMA* 2002; 288:2693.
26. Froehlich JB, Karavite D, Russman PL, et al. American College of Cardiology/American Heart Association preoperative assessment guidelines reduce resource utilization before aortic surgery. *J Vasc Surg* 2002; 36:758.
27. Eagle KA, Berger PB, Calkins H, et al. ACC/AHA guideline update for perioperative cardiovascular evaluation for noncardiac surgery? Executive summary: a report of the American College of Cardiology/American Heart Association Task Force on Practice Guidelines (Committee to Update the 1996 Guidelines on Perioperative Cardiovascular Evaluation for Noncardiac Surgery). *Circulation* 2002; 105:1257.
28. Shimoni S, Frangogiannis NG, Aggeli CJ, et al. Identification of hibernating myocardium with quantitative intravenous myocardial contrast echocardiography: comparison with dobutamine echocardiography and thallium-201 scintigraphy. *Circulation* 2003; 107:538.
29. Allman KC, Shaw LJ, Hachamovitch R, Udelson JE. Myocardial viability testing and impact of revascularization on prognosis in

patients with coronary artery disease and left ventricular dysfunction: a meta-analysis. *J Am Coll Cardiol* 2002; 39:1151.

30. Deshpande VS, Shea SM, Li D. Artifact reduction in true-FISP imaging of the coronary arteries by adjusting imaging frequency. *Magn Reson Med* 2003; 49:803.

31. Kim WY, Danias PG, Stuber M, et al. Coronary magnetic resonance angiography for the detection of coronary stenosis. *N Engl J Med* 2001; 345:1863.

32. Ibrahim T, Nekolla SG, Schreiber K, et al. Assessment of coronary flow reserve: comparison between contrast-enhanced magnetic resonance imaging and positron emission tomography. *J Am Coll Cardiol* 2002; 39:864.

33. Schwitter J, Nanz D, Kneifel S, et al. Assessment of myocardial perfusion in coronary artery disease by magnetic resonance: a comparison with positron emission tomography and coronary angiography. *Circulation* 2001; 103:2230.

34. Sandstede JW. Assessment of myocardial viability by MR imaging. *Eur Radiol* 2003; 13:52.

35. Rogers WJ Jr, Kramer CM, Geskin G, et al. Early contrast-enhanced CMR predicts late functional recovery after reperfused myocardial infarction. *Circulation* 1999; 99:744.

36. Senior R, Swinburn JM. Incremental value of myocardial contrast echocardiography for the prediction of recovery of function in dobutamine nonresponsive myocardium early after acute myocardial infarction. *Am J Cardiol* 2003; 91:397.

Imaging of Myocardial Antigens, Receptors, Hypoxia, Necrosis, Apoptosis, Metabolism, and Viability

Ignasi Carrio
Albert Flotats
Nagara Tamaki
Jagat Narula
Carina Mari
H. William Strauss

Measurements of myocardial receptor occupancy, utilization of metabolic substrates (mainly fatty acids and glucose), identification of focal zones of decreased oxygen tension (hypoxia), necrosis, and apoptosis may be useful in patients with a variety of cardiac diseases. Clinical decisions concerning the management of patients with heart failure, severe coronary disease (especially evaluating myocardial viability), acute infarction, myocarditis, transplant rejection, and vulnerable atherosclerotic plaques can be refined with data available from specific radionuclide studies. The information obtained can identify patients at risk for progression of heart failure, myocardial remodeling after infarction, rupture of vulnerable plaque, and sudden cardiac death. The following sections describe the imaging methods available to make these measurements and some clinical situations in which these data will be helpful (Table 4-1).

TARGETING MAJOR HISTOCOMPATIBILITY COMPLEX (MHC) CLASS II CARDIAC ANTIGENS

Cardiac transplant rejection is associated with upregulation of several adhesion receptors belonging to the immunoglobulin family including the MHC class II antigens. The increased expression of the MHC class II antigens during cardiac allograft transplant rejection is seen in the graft endothelium and on infiltrating mononuclear cells in endomyocardial biopsy samples. In a canine model that used radiolabeled monoclonal antibodies, it has been demonstrated that abnormal expression of MHC class II antigens can be detected noninvasively in rejecting allografts and that the uptake of radiolabeled antibody to class II antigen correlated with the histological severity of rejection using the International Society of Heart Transplantation (ISHT) gradations.[1] Despite statistically significant differences in uptake between these histological groups, there was overlap, especially with milder degrees of rejection.

Intercellular adhesion molecule-1 (ICAM-1, CD54) belongs to the immunoglobulin supergene family that interacts with the leukocyte β-2 integrins. Increased expression of ICAM-1 during acute allograft rejection has been shown in primate cardiac allografts. It has been demonstrated in rats that ICAM-1 induction can be assessed quantitatively by radioimmunoscintigraphy (by use of a ^{111}In-labeled anti-ICAM-1 monoclonal antibody).[2] Rejecting allografts showed increased uptake of radiotracer as early as 5 days after transplantation, and mildly rejecting allografts (mononuclear cell infiltration without significant myocyte necrosis) could be detected scintigraphically. The level of tracer uptake reflected the severity of rejection. In contrast, nonrejecting cardiac allografts and isografts did not show specific uptake. In distinction to anti-MHC class II imaging, the anti-ICAM-1 monoclonal antibody can be applied to the imaging of rejection irrespective of donor haplotype and seems to be more sensitive.

TARGETING PLATELET AGGREGATION

In acute coronary syndromes, potential targets for labeling include fibrin, platelets, and fibrinolytic molecules, but poor target/blood-pool ratios, low sensitivity, and technology limitations have slowed development. In an attempt to distinguish between stable and unstable coro-

TABLE 4-1   RADIOTRACERS TARGETING PATHOLOGICAL PROCESSES IN CARDIOVASCULAR DISEASES

Tracer group	Targeted pathology	Radiotracers	CV diseases
1. Agents that target sympathetic receptors	Myocardial innervation	MIBG-^{123}I, ^{11}C-epinephrine, hydroxyephedrine	CHF, myocardial ischemia
2. Agents that identify loss of sarcolemmal integrity	Necrosis	Antimyosin, glucaric acid	Acute MI, myocarditis, transplant rejection
3. Agents that target altered sarcolemmal composition	Myocyte apoptosis	Annexin V	Acute MI, myocarditis, transplant rejection, myocardial ischemia
4. Agents that target myocyte metabolic derangements	Myocardial viability	FDG, IPPA, BMIPP	Chronic myocardial ischemic disorders
5. Agents that target upregulation of accessory cardiocyte molecules or cytokine/humoral systems	Myocardial inflammation	HLA, ICAM, MCP1	Transplant rejection, endothelial derivative atherosclerosis
6. Agents used for supportive role in nuclear cardiology	Myocardial ischemia	Selective adenosine receptor analogs, hypoxia markers	Decreased intracellular Po_2
7. Atherosclerosis	Plaque	LDL, MCP-1, FDG, annexin	Vulnerable plaque

nary atherosclerotic plaques and to identify platelet-rich thrombus, a glycoprotein IIb/IIIa platelet inhibitor DMP-444, labeled with technetium (Tc)-99m, was tested in a canine model.[3] Varying amounts of coronary thrombus were achieved experimentally, and in animals with markedly positive nuclear images after the injection of ^{99m}Tc DMP-444, the presence of platelet-rich thrombus was confirmed post mortem by gross appearance, high nuclear counts, and abundant platelets on electron microscopy. The animals with negative images had lower counts, smaller thrombus weights, and fewer platelets by electron microscopy. Thus, activated platelets participating in acute thrombus formation were accurately detected by nuclear imaging with ^{99m}Tc DMP-444. In addition, ^{99m}Tc-labeled thrombospondin peptide receptor analogs TP-1201 and TP-1300 have favorable characteristics for imaging deep venous thrombosis and pulmonary embolism.[4]

Bacterial endocarditis is also characterized by aggregation of activated platelets, fibrin, and bacteria; in a canine model, there was clear focal accumulation of DMP-444 labeled with ^{99m}Tc in the aortic valve region when endocarditis was present, and 4 hours after injection the in vivo valve/blood-pool ratios were 1.9 in endocarditis and 1.0 in noninfected controls.[5] It was concluded that targeting activated platelets with the ^{99m}Tc-labeled GP IIb/IIIa antagonist DMP444 allowed a final diagnosis of experimental bacterial endocarditis within 4 hours because of high, specific, and fast in vivo uptake. Immunoscintigraphy in patients with subacute infective endocarditis provides valuable diagnostic information in equivocal echocardiographic findings and may be used to monitor antibiotic therapy.[6]

CARDIAC RECEPTORS

Adrenergic and Cholinergic Receptors

Imaging the regional myocardial distribution of adrenergic and cholinergic receptors in the heart[7] may be used to classify dysautonomias, to detect reduced adrenergic innervation in patients with heart failure (a sign of poor prognosis), to characterize arrhythmogenic cardiomyopathies, and to identify postinfarction patients who might be at high risk for arrhythmias.

Radiopharmaceuticals Used for Assessment of Adrenergic Innervation

Scintigraphic imaging of myocardial innervation uses radiolabeled forms or analogs of physiological neurotransmitters or false neurotransmitters (Figure 4-1).

Commonly used agents include:

1. Presynaptic: ^{18}F-fluorodopamine to assess norepinephrine synthesis[8] and ^{11}C-hydroxyephedrine, ^{11}C-epinephrine, ^{11}C-ephedrine, and ^{123}I-metaiodobenzylguanidine (MIBG) to assess presynaptic reuptake and storage.[9]

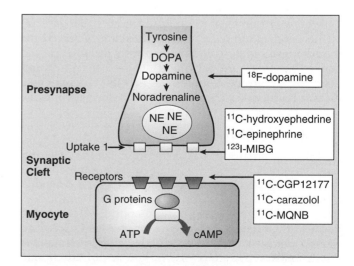

FIGURE 4-1. Most commonly used radioligands for assessment of cardiac presynaptic and postsynaptic processes.

2. Postsynaptic: beta-blockers such as the pindolol analog ^{11}C-CGP and ^{11}C-carazolol are used to assess β-adrenoceptor expression and density.[7]

Data can be recorded as static images to define the regional distribution of receptors or as dynamic images to calculate influx and efflux rate constants. Myocardial adrenoceptor density (B_{max}) can be measured by in vivo displacement assays.

Metaiodobenzylguanidine

Metaiodobenzylguanidine (MIBG) is a chemically modified form of guanethidine, the selective sympathetic blocking agent. This modification increases affinity for neuronal uptake sites and permits labeling with radioiodine to visualize sites of sympathetic innervation. Since 1980, when MIBG was first used for myocardial imaging, it has been shown MIBG and noradrenaline use the same uptake and storage mechanisms in the sympathetic nerve endings and that ^{123}I-MIBG, a catecholamine analog, is taken up into the neuron (by means of uptake-1) in a manner similar to that for norepinephrine, but it is not metabolized and therefore marks the location of functioning nerve terminals. Assessment of ^{123}I-MIBG uptake also allows unique characterization of alterations in regional sympathetic nerve function. This neuronal uptake of MIBG is characterized as a temperature-dependent, high-affinity (K_m (μmolar) of 1.22 ± 0.12 for MIBG and 1.4 ± 0.50 for noradrenaline, low-capacity system, and the kinetics of ^{123}I-MIBG mimic those of H-noradrenaline.

[18]F-Fluorodopamine

[18]F-fluorodopamine is concentrated by sympathetic nerve terminals and transported into axoplasmic vesicles, where it is converted and stored.[8] During sympathetic stimulation, ^{18}F-fluoronorepinephrine is released from sympathetic nerve terminals like norepinephrine. Cardiac ^{18}F-fluorodopamine images are analyzed by drawing regions of interest within the ventricular wall by use of a composite of the images for each plane. Time-activity curves are computed from the logarithm of the concentrations in the myocardium (adjusted for the administered dose and patient body weight) and the concentration in arterial blood. The mean concentration of ^{18}F-fluorodopamine in left ventricular myocardium peaks at 5 to 8 minutes in normal controls.

[11]C-Hydroxyephedrine and C-Epinephrine

[11]C-hydroxyephedrine, a false neurotransmitter, has the same neuronal uptake mechanism as norepinephrine (neuronal uptake-1). Hydroxyephedrine is not degraded by monoamine oxidase or catechol-methyl-transferase, the enzymes metabolizing norepinephrine in the heart. Because the storage and release properties differ from those of the physiological neurotransmitters, this agent is less useful for the study of the kinetics of adrenergic uptake. ^{11}C-epinephrine, on the other hand, is a more physiological tracer for the evaluation of presynaptic sympathetic nerve function and is useful to define uptake, vesicular storage, and metabolism. ^{11}C-epinephrine is rapidly transported into the presynaptic nerve terminal (by means of uptake-1) and is stored in the vesicles, like norepinephrine. After correction for the contribution of ^{11}C-labeled metabolites, the fraction of the intact molecule localized in the myocardium can be plotted as a function of time. The myocardial images can be analyzed by volumetric sampling procedures to assess the homogeneity of myocardial tracer distribution. The volume of distribution of ^{11}C-hydroxyephedrine in normal subjects is 71 ± 19 mL/100 g of tissue. Several other radio-labeled beta-receptor antagonists, including the pindolol analog CGP[10] and carazolol,[11] have been used for studies of the adrenergic system.

Radiopharmaceuticals for Assessment of Cholinergic Innervation

Methylquinuclidinyl benzilate (MQNB) is a highly specific antagonist of muscarinic receptors that can be labeled with C (C-MQNB) and iodine. The stimulation of local muscarinic receptors inhibits norepinephrine release from adrenergic nerve terminals. Although muscarinic receptors are present on sympathetic nerve endings in a prejunctional distribution, it is recognized that they play a role in neurotransmission within the intrinsic cardiac sympathetic nervous system. The labeling of MQNB with C provides an agent with specific radioactivities ranging from 12 to 90 GBq/μmol. Imaging of left ventricular receptors reveals a uniform distribution in the left ventricular myocardium of the normal heart.

Planar and Tomographic Imaging of the Heart with MIBG

Planar imaging has been used to determine cardiac MIBG uptake. Although myocardial uptake and distribution can be assessed visually, a semiquantitative measurement of myocardial MIBG uptake is often used to express myocardial innervation. Regions of interest are drawn over the left ventricular myocardium and the noncardiac portion of the mediastinum to produce a heart/mediastinum ratio. To eliminate superimposition of lung on the left ventricular myocardium, single photon emission computed tomography (SPECT) imaging has been proposed as a preferable approach. However, in heart failure or after myocardial infarction, conditions that markedly reduce myocardial MIBG uptake, the image quality may be reduced, making the data very difficult to interpret.

Positron Emission Tomography (PET) Imaging

PET imaging protocols vary according to the radiotracer characteristics and instrumentation. After acquisition, data sets are realigned according to standardized axes, and physiological parameters are calculated by use of tracer kinetic models. Region of interest analysis of the activity concentration inside the left ventricular cavity yields the time activity curve of arterial blood.

Examples of several protocols follow:

1. Continuous thoracic PET scanning is performed after F-fluorodopamine infusion for up to 3 hours. The total scanning time is divided into intervals of 5 to 30 minutes, and the tomographic results of each interval are assessed. Scan sequences may consist of five frames H 1 minute, five H 5 minutes, four H, 15 minutes, and three H 30 minutes.
2. PET scanning of ^{11}C-hydroxyephedrine and ^{11}C-epinephrine usually lasts for 60 minutes. Scan sequences may consist of 15 frames: six H 30 seconds, two H 60 seconds, two H 150 seconds, two H 300 seconds, two H 600 seconds, and one H 1200 seconds.
3. With ^{11}C-CGP continuous thoracic scanning, recording data in list mode is typically performed for 1 hour after infusion.
4. When ^{18}F-fluorocarazolol is used, acquisition protocols after infusion may consist of eight frames H 15 seconds, four H 30 seconds, four H 1 minute, four H 2 minutes, six H 4 minutes, and two H 10 minutes.
5. For ^{11}C-MQNB, recording of data is started with the first injection. Sixty sequential images may be acquired, by use of one of the cross-sections and reconstructing according to the specific protocol used. Scan sequences may consist of 24 time frames: eight H 15 seconds, four H 30 seconds, two H 60 seconds, eight H 150 seconds, after each infusion.

Primary Cardioneuropathies

Dysautonomias

Derangements of sympathetic and parasympathetic function are frequently encountered in patients with neurological and cardiac diseases. Three forms of primary dysautonomia can be distinguished: pure autonomic failure (defined as a sporadic, idiopathic cause of persistent orthostatic hypotension and other manifestations of autonomic failure that occur without other neurological features), Parkinson's disease with autonomic failure, and multiple system atrophy. The distinction between Parkinson's disease with autonomic failure from some forms of multiple-system atrophy is difficult, and unfortunately physiological and neurochemical tests often fail to properly separate the different forms of dysautonomia.

PET scanning with ^{18}F-fluorodopamine has been used to examine cardiac sympathetic innervation in patients with different types of dysautonomia and suggests that sympathetic neurocirculatory failure results from peripheral sympathetic denervation or reduced (or absent) sympathetic signal traffic. PET scanning correlates with signs of sympathetic neurocirculatory failure such as orthostatic hypotension and abnormal blood pressure responses associated with the Valsalva maneuver and with responsiveness to treatment with levodopa-carbidopa. Patients with pure autonomic failure or Parkinsonism and sympathetic neurocirculatory failure have no myocardial ^{18}F-fluorodopamine uptake or cardiac norepinephrine spillover, indicating loss of myocardial sympathetic nerve terminals. Patients with the Shy-Drager syndrome have increased levels of ^{18}F-fluorodopamine activity with intact nerve terminals and absent nerve traffic. Patients with dysautonomia without sympathetic neurocirculatory failure have normal levels of ^{18}F-fluorodopamine activity in the myocardium and normal rates of cardiac norepinephrine spillover. ^{18}F-fluorodopamine PET studies, in combination with neurochemical tests and clinical observations, support this new pathophysiological classification of dysautonomias, with enhanced diagnostic differentiation between multiple system atrophy, Shy-Drager syndrome, Parkinsonism with autonomic failure, and peripheral autonomic failure.

Heart Transplantation

During orthotopic heart transplantation, the recipient's diseased heart is excised except for the posterior atrial walls, to which the donor heart atria are anastomosed (Figure 4-2). During the process, the allograft becomes completely denervated, and lack of autonomic nerve supply is associated with major physiological limitations. Denervation of the sinus node might result in inadequate acceleration of heart rate during stress, hypovolemia, and reduced cardiac output. Furthermore, loss of vasomotor tone might adversely affect hemodynamic performance at rest and during exercise, during hemodynamic stresses, and result in decreased exercise capacity. The inability to perceive pain might reduce symptomatic recognition of coronary arterial stenosis caused by accelerated allograft vasculopathy. Scintigraphic uptake of ^{123}I-MIBG and ^{11}C-hydroxy-

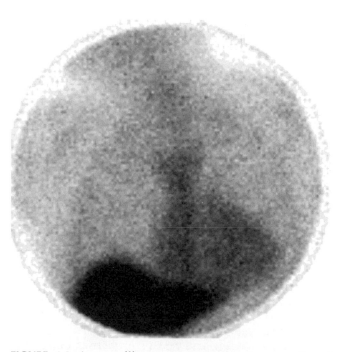

FIGURE 4-2. Anterior ^{111}In-antimyosin imaging from a patient 1 month after orthotopic heart transplantation, with diffuse uptake throughout the ventricle. Gradually decreasing activity in serial follow-up imaging at 3, 6, and 12 months provides useful information for risk stratification.

ephedrine suggests that there is spontaneous reinnervation after transplantation. Studies performed up to 5 years after heart transplantation suggest that cardiac reinnervation is a slow process, with some detectable reinnervation 1 year after transplantation, as reflected by an increase in the intensity of myocardial MIBG uptake in the anterior, anterolateral, and septal regions (Figure 4-3). Complete reinnervation of the transplanted heart is not seen, even 12 years after cardiac transplantation. Sympathetic reinnervation after cardiac transplantation is not simply a function of time but occurs earlier in young recipients, after fast and uncomplicated surgery, and in patients with less rejection.[10] Early vasculopathy may inhibit the process of sympathetic reinnervation of the transplanted heart. The relationship between reinnervation status and graft vasculopathy deserves further investigation and may help to differentiate subsets of transplant patients with different clinical outcomes.

Idiopathic Ventricular Tachycardia and Fibrillation

Malignant ventricular arrhythmias may be provoked by physical or mental stress or by catecholamine administration. By use of ^{123}I-MIBG, ^{11}C-hydroxyephedrine, and ^{11}C-CGP, it has been demonstrated that in patients with idiopathic right ventricular outflow tract tachycardia, both the presynaptic myocardial catecholamine reuptake and the postsynaptic myocardial β-adrenoceptors density are reduced despite normal blood catecholamine levels. The maximal binding capacity of the β-adrenoceptor antagonist is reduced in patients with right ventricular outflow tract tachycardia compared with controls (6.8 ± 1.2 vs. 10.2 ± 2.9 pmol/g). These scintigraphic findings suggest myocardial β-adrenoceptor downregulation in this clinical syndrome.

In a small study of patients with implantable cardioverter defibrillators (ICDs) those who had a history of ICD discharge had more abnormal MIBG imaging parameters (lower early MIBG heart/mediastinal ratio, higher MIBG defect scores, and more MIBG/^{99m}Tc sestamibi mismatching segments, reflecting denervation in areas of preserved viability) than patients without previous ICD discharge.[11] They also had reduced values for heart rate variability (suggesting abnormally increased sympathetic tone) compared with patients without a previous ICD discharge. These data suggest the possibility that noninvasive imaging data may eventually contribute to decisions concerning ICD implantation.

Secondary Cardioneuropathies

Dilated Cardiomyopathies

Persistent increased sympathetic activity might have deleterious effects on the cardiovascular system: the combination of vascular constriction and increased salt and water retention by the kidneys increase myocardial wall tension and hence energy requirements. Increased sympathetic cardiac adrenergic function might also cause arrhythmias, desensitization of postsynaptic β-adrenoceptors, and activation of other neurohumoral systems such as the renin-angiotensin system, which might also exert adverse effects and contribute to progression of myocardial dysfunction. Prolonged, elevated circulating levels of norepinephrine might contribute to cardiovascular disease progression by direct myocardial action and modification of cellular phenotype and ultimately cause myocyte death.

Alterations of cardiac sympathetic innervation might contribute to fatal outcomes in patients with heart failure. In patients with heart failure with impaired functional capacity and left ventricular ejection fractions less than 40%, multivariate analyses show that low MIBG uptake and reduced left ventricular ejection fraction are independent predictors of mortality. Impaired cardiac adrenergic innervation, as assessed by MIBG imaging, might be directly related to mortality (Figure 4-4). The heart/mediastinum ratio for both the early and delayed MIBG planar images and myocardial washout rate at 4 hours have been analyzed quantitatively in patients with dilated cardiomyopathy.[12] Multivariate analysis selected washout rate as the most powerful independent predictor of prognosis, and survival curves, with a threshold value of 52% for washout rate, were able to differentiate

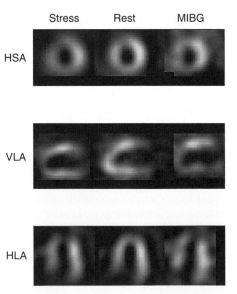

FIGURE 4-4. Myocardial exercise-rest perfusion (^{99m}Tc-tetrofosmin) and sympathetic innervation images (^{123}I-MIBG) in a patient with coronary artery disease. Myocardial perfusion study images anterior and apical ischemia. MIBG study shows decreased uptake in the same territories, suggesting persistent neuronal damage after repetitive myocardial ischemia. HSA = Horizontal short-axis, VLA = Verticle long axis, and HLA = Horizontal long-axis.

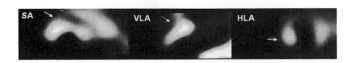

FIGURE 4-3. SPECT images of MIBG distribution in a patient initially seen with partial reinnervation after heart transplantation. Note the MIBG activity in the anterobasal segments of the myocardium (*arrows*). SA = short-axis; VLA = vertical long-axis; HLA = horizontal long-axis.

a negative outcome from survival. Patients with congestive cardiomyopathy typically have accelerated clearance (washout rates >25% from 15 to 85 minutes) compared with controls (<10%). In addition, MIBG parameters have been shown to correlate with other predictors of prognosis such as peak VO_2. Similarly, children with idiopathic dilated cardiomyopathy might have impaired cardiac adrenergic neuronal function. On the basis of a reduction of the heart/mediastinum count ratio, cardiac neuronal uptake of ^{123}I-MIBG was significantly decreased in children with dilated cardiomyopathy compared with cardiac uptake in control subjects.[9]

The concept that prolonged sympathetic hyperactivity is detrimental in chronic heart failure is supported by the trials demonstrating the beneficial effects of angiotensin-converting enzyme inhibitors and β-adrenoceptor antagonists. Thus, reduction of sympathetic activity is an important target for drug treatment of heart failure. Mechanisms that contribute to reduced β-adrenoceptor responsiveness in heart failure include downregulation of β-adrenoceptors, uncoupling of subtypes of β-adrenoceptors, upregulation of β-adrenoceptor kinase, increased activity of G protein, decreased activity of adenylyl cyclase, and increased nitric oxide. Noradrenaline can contribute to myocardial remodeling by direct stimulation of adrenoceptors on cardiac myocytes and fibroblasts. The hypertrophic effect of noradrenaline is associated with the re-expression of fetal genes and the downregulation of several adult genes.

Apoptosis occurs in the myocardium of patients with end-stage dilated cardiomyopathy.[13] The toxic effect of β-adrenoceptor stimulation is mediated in part by apoptosis, and in cultured myocytes, exposure to noradrenaline for 24 hours increases the frequency of apoptosis, which is inhibited by the β-blocker propranolol. In comparison, little is known about the effects of noradrenaline on the extracellular matrix, although noradrenaline stimulates the expression of transforming growth factors that regulate extracellular matrix proteins. Cardiac neurotransmission imaging might help to explain the mechanisms responsible for increased sympathetic activity in heart failure and how sympathetic overactivity exerts its deleterious actions.

Coronary Artery Disease

Sympathetic nervous tissue is affected by myocardial ischemia. There is reduced uptake of ^{123}I MIBG in areas of myocardial infarction, as well as in areas of acute and chronic ischemia. A decrease in MIBG uptake in ischemic tissue reflects the loss of integrity of postganglionic, presynaptic neurons, which are very slow to regenerate. Repetitive episodes of ischemia might result in permanent loss of sympathetic innervation (Figure 4-5). Early after infarction, sympathetic denervation in adjacent noninfarcted regions is frequently observed, and within 10 days of acute infarction, zones of reduced MIBG uptake, which are more extensive than the region of reduced perfusion, have been described. This possibly reflects a greater sensitivity of sympathetic nervous tissue to ischemia than myocytes. Such denervated zones

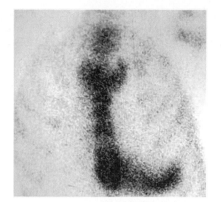

FIGURE 4-5. Anterior ^{99m}Tc-pyrophosphate imaging from a patient with acute inferior wall myocardial infarction with right ventricular involvement.

might be associated with increased susceptibility to ventricular tachyarrhythmias or spontaneous arrhythmias, because adrenergic denervation of viable myocardium results in denervation supersensitivity and an exaggerated response to sympathetic stimulation.

In patients with multivessel coronary artery disease without prior myocardial infarction, presynaptic sympathetic innervation has been studied by use of PET with N-ammonia and C-hydroxyephedrine.[14] Despite normal resting perfusion, significantly reduced C-hydroxyephedrine retention, indicating denervation, was found in most vascular territories, indicating that it can occur in the absence of myocardial infarction.[14] This is consistent with the hypothesis that sympathetic neurons are more susceptible than myocytes to ischemic damage.

Even after successful reperfusion after acute myocardial infarction, in reperfused acute myocardial infarction (AMI), the severity score of the MIBG abnormality, reflecting cardiac sympathetic nervous system abnormality, was a powerful predictor of ventricular dilation.[15] Transmyocardial laser revascularization improves perfusion but also causes denervation, evident at 3 months, which partially recovers by 12 months.[16] After myocardial infarction, reinnervation in peri-infarct regions has been demonstrated by the reappearance of MIBG uptake but often remains incomplete. The eventual concordance between the extent of decreased MIBG uptake at rest and the extent of the perfusion abnormality during exercise in patients with coronary artery disease suggests that mild degrees of ischemia injure myocardial sympathetic neurons. The correlation observed between the zone of decreased MIBG uptake and the area "at risk," defined by altered perfusion, supports the concept of neuronal damage in the ischemic territory.

Hypertrophic Cardiomyopathy

Autonomic dysfunction seems to play a role in the phenotypic expression of hypertrophic cardiomyopathy. Clinical features of hypertrophic cardiomyopathy suggest increased sympathetic outflow. The incidence of chest pain, myocardial hypercontractility, propensity to ventricular arrhythmias and sudden death, and the beneficial effect of β-blockers suggest increased delivery of norepinephrine to myocardial adrenoceptors. Cardiac presynaptic catecholamine reuptake is impaired in hypertrophic cardiomyopathy in association with reduced postsynaptic β-adrenoceptor density, suggesting an increased neurotransmitter concentration in the synaptic cleft. This can be shown by quantitative PET studies using ^{11}C-hydroxyephedrine and ^{11}C-CGP. The enhanced adrenergic stimulation is reflected in the increased washout (>25%) between initial and delayed images seen in this disease. The autonomic dysfunction in these patients is probably related to disease progression and ultimately heart failure.[17] In patients studied with ^{13}N-ammonia and ^{18}F-fluorodopamine, the ^{18}F/^{13}N ratio is lower in hypertrophied than in nonhypertrophied regions, indicating decreased neuronal uptake of catecholamines in hypertrophied myocardium of patients with hypertrophic cardiomyopathy.[17]

Arrhythmogenic Right Ventricular Cardiomyopathy

Fibrolipomatous degeneration of the right ventricular myocardium is the main structural abnormality in arrhythmogenic right ventricular cardiomyopathy. In these patients, who may exhibit provocable ventricular tachyarrhythmias and cardiac arrest during exercise or stress, involvement of the sympathetic nervous system in the pathogenesis of arrhythmias is strongly suggested.[18] Both MIBG-SPECT and ^{11}C-hydroxy-ephedrine PET demonstrate changes in the left ventricular myocardium, even though the left ventricle is not primarily involved. Patients with arrhythmogenic cardiomyopathy demonstrated a highly significant overall reduction in postsynaptic β-adrenergic receptor density compared with control subjects. There are no differences in myocardial blood flow, and plasma norepinephrine levels are within normal limits in patients and control subjects.[18] These findings suggest reduced activity of the noradrenaline transporter (uptake-1) with subsequent β-adrenoceptor downregulation.

Diabetes Mellitus

The sympathetic nervous system is activated during the early stages of diabetes, with elevated plasma catecholamine levels. Prolonged exposure to elevated catecholamines might lead to downregulation of adrenergic receptors and to alterations in adrenergic nervous fibers in the myocardium of patients with diabetes. Hyperglycemia and insulin deficiency might also contribute to the abnormalities in cardiac innervation in diabetes. Decreased cardiac ^{123}I-MIBG uptake in patients with diabetes with autonomic dysfunction has been correlated with increased mortality, and impairment of cardiac sympathetic innervation (demonstrated by MIBG studies) correlates with an abnormal response to exercise in patients with diabetes. In patients with reduced systolic function (left ventricular ejection fractions <50%), the presence of diabetes and early substantive loss of initial MIBG uptake were the most potent predic-

tors of subsequent cardiac mortality.[19] Patients with diabetes with scintigraphic evidence of denervation might exhibit increased sensitivity to dobutamine used in pharmacological stress tests.

Drug-Induced Cardiotoxicity

Anthracycline cardiotoxicity is associated with a persistent decrease in myocardial sympathetic innervation, and this is reflected by decreased myocardial MIBG uptake even in hearts with limited morphological damage and normal systolic function.[20] The decrease in myocardial MIBG accumulation parallels the decline of ejection fraction. At intermediate cumulative doses of anthracycline (240 to 300 mg/m^2), approximately 25% of patients exhibit some decrease in MIBG uptake, and at maximal cumulative doses, there is a significant decrease in MIBG uptake. These data suggest that the assessment of drug-induced sympathetic damage could possibly be used to select patients at risk of severe functional impairment who might benefit from either cardioprotective agents or changes in the treatment schedule or dosage of antineoplastic drugs.

Endothelin Receptors

The endothelin peptide family is composed of three isoforms (ET-1, ET-2, and ET-3), and endothelin-1 (ET-1) is produced by vascular smooth muscle cells and cardiac myocytes and is promitogenic and the most potent endogenous vasoconstrictor substance known. The diverse biological activities of ET-1 are mediated through two receptor subtypes (ETA and ETB) that are expressed in cardiac myocytes, vascular smooth muscle cells, and endothelium.[21] Labeling of the different endothelin system components has elucidated the anatomy, physiology, and pathology of the system.

Endothelin receptors have been quantitated in the human coronary artery and ventricular and atrial muscle by means of receptor autoradiography.[22] Specific binding was denser in atrium and coronary artery (especially in the media) than in ventricular muscle. In the human atherosclerotic aorta, the levels of endogenous ET and big ET-1 (the inactive precursor) detectable by radioimmunoassay were significantly higher than those in histologically normal tissue.[23] It seemed likely that this increase noted in atherosclerotic plaques came from endothelial cells and macrophages but not vascular smooth muscle cells. ETA receptors predominated in the media of both normal and diseased arteries, and ETB receptors, where present, were found on endothelial cells and macrophages. In atherosclerotic rabbit aortas, although the density and the ratio of endothelin receptor subtypes change, a lack of receptor-specific accumulation of ^{125}I-ET-1 in atherosclerotic areas suggests that endothelin receptor targeting is unsuitable for imaging of atherosclerosis.[24]

In humans with dilated cardiomyopathy and chronic heart failure, a persistent, approximately twofold, increase in immunoreactive ET-1 in the left ventricle has been described. In end-stage heart failure, there is decreased ETB receptor expression and increased ETA receptor density, but the ETA receptor signaling pathway seems to be desensitized. There is elevation of immunoreactive plasma ET-1 in heart failure (mainly the precursor "big" ET-1), and concentrations are significantly higher in patients with moderate and severe heart failure than in those with mild heart failure.[25] In end-stage heart failure, multivariate analysis reveals that elevation of plasma big ET-1 is strongly related to survival and seems to predict 1-year mortality better than other hemodynamic variables or levels of atrial natriuretic peptide.

HYPOXIA MARKERS

A marker of decreased intracellular oxygen tension (hypoxia) might be useful to identify dysfunctional tissue that is viable. The sensitivity of a radiopharmaceutical agent, or tracer, to detect hypoxic tissue will depend on a number of variables, including the amount delivered to the site of ischemia, the fraction that enters the tissue, the rapidity of clearance from normoxic cells, and the degree of retention in hypoxic cells. The specificity will depend on the contrast between the region of interest and background and between normal and hypoxic tissue and the oxygen concentration at which tracer trapping occurs.

The nitroimidazoles are a class of compounds that undergo different intracellular metabolism depending on oxygen availability. When a nitroimidazole enters a viable cell, the molecule undergoes a single electron reduction to form a potentially reactive species. In the presence of normal oxygen tension, the molecule is immediately reoxidized, and in the presence of hypoxia, further reduction ensues with the association of reduced nitroimidazole with various intracellular components. The agents clear from hypoxic tissue over time, and the oxygen tension at which they are retained may be reported as the *Km,* which is the oxygen tension at which retention or activity is 50% of the anoxic-normoxic value, and it is independent of the nitroimidazole concentration at imaging doses. The compounds used most frequently are the 2-nitroimidazoles (misonidazole or MISO). ^{99m}Tc-labeled nitroimidazoles preferentially bind to hypoxic tissue in the myocardium[26] and have considerable potential. Kinetics of a putative hypoxic tracer, ^{99m}Tc-HL91, in normoxic, hypoxic, ischemic, and stunned myocardium indicate that retention of ^{99m}Tc-HL91 correlates well with oxygen level and suggest that the agent might be a useful marker of the severity of myocardial hypoxia.[27] If successfully developed, these hypoxic imaging agents will provide insights into the pathophysiology of myocardial ischemia, cardiomyopathy, and angiogenesis.

MYOCARDIAL NECROSIS

The diagnosis of acute infarction can be problematic, even after evaluating the results of serial enzyme assays and electrocardiograms, because approximately 1% to 2% of patients with AMI are mistakenly discharged from emergency departments. Acute myocardial necrosis can be imaged with tracers that localize in necrotic tissue, resulting in a "hot spot" in the area of necrosis.[28] Two hot-spot imaging agents, ^{99m}Tc-pyrophosphate and ^{111}In-antimyosin, have been used in clinical studies of acute infarction, but both of these agents localize maximally in the area of myocardial damage several days after onset of necrosis rather than in the early hours of acute infarction, limiting their usefulness.

^{99m}Tc-Pyrophosphate

Increased sarcolemmal permeability in irreversibly damaged cells allows ^{99m}Tc-pyrophosphate access to the intracellular environment, where it binds to free calcium in the necrotic myocardium. Laboratory studies indicate that a minimum of several hours after the onset of necrosis is required for the cells to become sufficiently permeable for tracer localization. An additional problem is tracer delivery. In the case of an occluded vessel, only minimal tracer is delivered to the infarct site. In general, the infarct must be ≥12 hours old to get visualization if the vessel remains occluded. When the infarct-related artery is patent (e.g., because of reperfusion therapy with thrombolytic agents or angioplasty), the lesion can be seen earlier. Maximum infarct uptake occurs between 24 and 72 hours after infarction and usually lasts for 6 to 10 days. ^{99m}Tc-pyrophosphate concentration is maximal in areas with a moderate reduction of myocardial blood flow (20% to 40% of maximum) but is substantially reduced in regions of severely diminished perfusion. This might result in the so-called doughnut pattern associated with a large MI, where the maximal uptake occurs at the periphery of the infarct, with a probable overestimation of the necrotic tissue. ^{99m}Tc-pyrophosphate scintigraphy is 90% to 96% sensitive for Q wave infarctions and 38% to 92% for non-Q wave infarctions, with a specificity of 60% to 80%. False-positive results can occur in patients with secondary hyperparathyroidism, dystrophic cardiac calcification (e.g., valvular calcification), cardiac amyloidosis, myocarditis and myopericarditis, cardiac metastases, ventricular aneurysm, electrical cardioversion, and previous MI (up to 1 year after the acute event). If the test is performed <24 hours or >7 days after the onset of infarction, the false-negative rate increases. False-negative results might also occur with either small or non-Q wave MI. SPECT imaging allows the detection of smaller infarcts that might be missed by planar imaging and reduces the prevalence of persistent positive patterns. Patients manifesting extensive uptake (myocardial uptake in >50% of the cardiac area), a doughnut pattern, and persistence of myocardial uptake after the acute episode have a poor prognosis and a greater incidence of complications.

^{111}In-Antimyosin

An alternative to ^{99m}Tc-pyrophosphate scintigraphy uses ^{111}In-labeled murine monoclonal antimyosin Fab antibody fragments. ^{111}In-antimyosin targets the intracellular heavy chain of cardiac myosin, which becomes accessible to an extracellular tracer with sarcolemmal disruption. The small size of antimyosin Fab (65 H 35 Å) allows it to enter the membrane gaps created by complement membrane attack complexes or by inflammatory reactions that might subsequently result in myocyte necrosis.

Experimental and clinical evidence support the specific targeting of necrotic myocardial cells. Comparisons between ^{99m}Tc-pyrophosphate and ^{111}In-antimyosin imaging in MI detection have generally provided similar results: sensitivity of 87% to 98% for Q wave infarctions and 78% to 84% for non-Q wave infarctions, with antimyosin imaging being more specific (96%) than pyrophosphate (85%) in the diagnosis of acute MI. False-positive results might occur with imaging <24 hours after tracer injection because of residual activity in the blood pool. In contrast to ^{99m}Tc-pyrophosphate, ^{111}In-antimyosin is incorporated into the necrotic myocardium with an inverse relationship to regional flow, with maximum uptake in areas with severe flow impairment. This difference might be due to the longer circulating half-life of antimyosin-Fab (about 6 hours) compared with pyrophosphate (about 15 minutes). ^{111}In-antimyosin uptake is more intense in reperfused myocardium than in myocardium distal to persistent coronary occlusion. Focal ^{111}In-antimyosin uptake in infarcted myocardium has been demonstrated as long as 9 months after the acute event. This might be related to the persistence of the heavy chain of cardiac myosin at the sites of infarction because of its limited solubility. Therefore, it might be difficult to identify recurrent infarction with this imaging technique within 1 year of the original event. Other uses of ^{111}In-antimyosin have included the detection of allograft rejection in cardiac transplant recipients, doxorubicin-induced cardiotoxicity, myocarditis, and various cardiomyopathies.

Heart Transplant Rejection

Transplant rejection is associated with gradual, relentless immune-induced apoptotic and necrotic cell death of myocytes and vascular endothelial cells. Transplant patients with normal ^{111}In-antimyosin scans rarely experience histological evidence of rejection during long-term follow-up, whereas those with abnormal myocardial uptake usually will exhibit histological evidence of rejection. The intensity of antibody uptake correlates with the probability of detecting rejection in myocardial biopsy specimens and provides useful information for risk stratification.

Doxorubicin Cardiotoxicity

In addition to using MIBG as an indicator of doxorubicin cardiotoxicity, the myocyte oncosis caused by the drug can be detected by ^{111}In-antimyosin imaging. The antibody uptake intensity relates to the cumulative dose of doxorubicin, and its appearance precedes ejection fraction deterioration, making early identification of patients at risk feasible.

INFLAMMATION

Myocarditis

^{111}In-antimyosin scintigraphy might detect myocyte necrosis in patients with suspected acute myocarditis. A negative scan rules out the presence of myocardial necrosis (sensitivity >95%), which usually obviates the need for endomyocardial biopsy. ^{111}In-antimyosin scans have also been used successfully to alert clinicians to the possibility of myocarditis in patients who otherwise seem to have AMI or in patients who have unexplained ventricular tachyarrhythmias. In patients with dilated cardiomyopathies, there is a high prevalence (up to 70%) of ongoing myocyte necrosis, as demonstrated by myocardial uptake of the antibody. The scan provides prognostic data, because intense ^{111}In-antimyosin uptake is associated with increased mortality or the need for heart transplantation.

Similarly, in patients who abuse alcohol, uptake depends on alcohol consumption, and a reduction of antibody uptake has been observed with abstention accompanied by an increase in ejection fraction. ^{111}In-antimyosin imaging can also detect myocardial damage in HIV-myocarditis and in hypertrophic cardiomyopathy, particularly in the late dilated phases of the disease.

METABOLIC IMAGING AND MYOCARDIAL VIABILITY

Imaging the regional distribution of metabolic substrates used by the myocardium can provide significant information. The myocardium is omnivorous. The fully oxygenated healthy heart can consume fatty acids (with a marked preference for chain lengths between 14 and 18 carbons), lactate, and glucose. Under circumstances of ischemia, the metabolic choices are more restricted, and oxygen, required for β-oxidation of fatty acids, is present in very limited supply. The clearance of waste products is slowed, reducing intracellular pH. These circumstances markedly reduce catabolism of fatty acids, thus reducing myocyte contraction. In concert with the downregulation of contractile function, catabolism of glucose is increased to permit the cell to maintain vegetative functions. Glucose catabolism can provide at least two adenosine triphosphate (ATP) molecules without the requirement for oxygen. This level is insufficient to maintain contractile activity but sufficient to maintain cellular integrity. Imaging the regional distribution of perfusion and glucose use allows specific identification of areas of viable ischemic myocardium (Table 4-2).

Principles

Because perfusion and metabolism are tightly coupled in normal myocardium, the regional distribution of metabolic substrates (glucose, lactate, or fatty acids) should mirror that of perfusion. The specific substrate used by the myocytes depends on the hormonal milieu (primarily the insulin level), myocardial work, and the adequacy of perfusion. When insulin levels are elevated, myocytes

■ ■ ■

TABLE 4-2 PET AND SPECT TRACERS FOR ASSESSING MYOCARDIAL METABOLISM

Metabolism	PET tracers	SPECT tracers
Glucose	^{18}F FDG	None
Fatty acid	^{11}C palmitate	^{123}I-IPPA, ^{123}I-BMIPP
Oxidation	^{11}C acetate	None
	^{15}O oxygent	
Protein synthesis	^{11}C (^{13}N) amino acids	None

use glucose. When insulin levels are low, the heart uses lactate, ketone bodies, or fatty acids. Attempts have been made to develop a single photon agent that behaves like glucose, but they have been unsuccessful.

Glucose can be labeled by exchanging a stable carbon (^{12}C) with a radioisotope of carbon (^{11}C for positron studies, or ^{14}C for in vitro studies) or by substituting the radionuclide fluorine (^{18}F) for a hydroxyl group. When the fluorine is substituted for a hydroxyl group on the second carbon, the fluorinated molecule is a "deoxy" glucose because of the missing hydroxyl group, making the name for this substance 2-fluoro-2-deoxyglucose (FDG). FDG is recognized nearly as well as native glucose by the glucose transporters in the cell membrane. Once in the cell, FDG undergoes the same first step of metabolism as native glucose, phosphorylation to FDG-6-phosphate. The 6-phosphate form of glucose or FDG is impermeable to the cell membrane. The second step in glucose metabolism is conversion of glucose-1-phosphate to glucose-1,6-diphosphate. With FDG, the fluorine on the 2 position prevents this reaction from occurring, leaving intracellular FDG as FDG-6-phosphate. Some tissues, such as the liver, contain the enzyme glucose-6-phosphatase, which removes the phosphate from the molecule, allowing the molecule to diffuse out of the cell. This is the reason that the liver appears so faint on FDG images, even though the liver consumes large amounts of glucose. Myocardium, brain, skeletal muscle, and most tumors do not contain this phosphatase enzyme, which results in trapping of FDG that enters the cell by the glucose transporters.

Under circumstances of normal perfusion, the distribution of FDG in the insulin-stimulated heart is uniform and proportionate to perfusion in all regions. In the presence of ischemia, the zone of myocardium with decreased perfusion uses glucose to a greater degree than the decrease in perfusion, giving rise to the "perfusion metabolism mismatch," the hallmark of viable, ischemic myocardium. The relationship of perfusion to glucose use can be determined by imaging the distribution of perfusion with a flow tracer and that of glucose with FDG.

Patient Preparation

Myocardial glucose use increases in both normal and ischemic tissue. FDG uptake is similarly increased in both normal and ischemic areas, reducing the contrast between normal and ischemic tissue. However, for reasons that are not well understood, approximately 50% of patients without evidence of coronary disease have

a heterogeneous pattern of myocardial FDG uptake in the fasting state. In studies of normal volunteers, by use of the insulin clamp model, the myocardial response to increased glucose and insulin is nonuniform and accounts for the heterogeneity of FDG uptake. However, regardless of the etiology, the heterogeneity of uptake markedly reduces the specificity of the imaging study for the detection of viable myocardium. The heterogeneity of the FDG scan is reduced with glucose loading (for example, with a glucose clamp). Therefore, most myocardial studies are performed with glucose loading before FDG administration. Glucose loading increases insulin levels, causing increased myocardial glucose use.

Additional metabolic alterations occur with administration of drugs such as heparin or catecholamines. Heparin elevates plasma free fatty acid levels and suppresses glucose metabolism, as do high circulating catecholamine levels. These factors might limit evaluation of regional tissue viability with FDG-PET.

Clinical Applications

The perfusion studies required for comparison with FDG can be performed with positron-emitting perfusion agents, such as generator-produced rubidium-82 or cyclotron produced ^{13}N-ammonia, or with single photon–emitting perfusion agents. In either case, the perfusion data and metabolic data need to be combined into a "fusion" image, depicting the distribution of perfusion and metabolism (Figure 4-6). The combination of hypoperfusion and increased glucose use is identified by direct image inspection, creating a ratio image of perfusion/glucose metabolism or by generating a ratio "bulls-eye."

In patients with regional myocardial dysfunction, there are three distinct patterns:

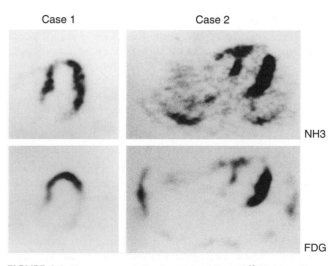

Case 1   Case 2

                                                    NH3

                                                    FDG

FIGURE 4-6. One representative transverse slice of ^{13}N-ammonia perfusion and FDG images in two cases with anterior myocardial infarction. **A,** Case 1 shows reduction of perfusion with increased FDG uptake in anterior region, indicating presence of myocardial ischemia. **B,** Case 2 shows reduction of both perfusion and FDG uptake, indicating myocardial scar.

1. Normal perfusion and metabolism.
2. Reduced perfusion, but glucose use is enhanced or at least greater than the perfusion (perfusion-metabolism mismatch).
3. Perfusion and metabolism are both reduced concordantly.

Combining the findings of decreased regional wall motion with the perfusion and metabolic findings results in the following three diagnostic categories:

1. Areas of normal perfusion and metabolism with abnormal regional wall motion represent *stunned myocardium*.
2. Zones of perfusion-metabolism mismatch represent *hibernating myocardium*.
3. Regions with a concordant decrease in perfusion and glucose metabolism represent *scar* (Figure 4-6).

FDG uptake in the presence of reduced blood flow has a high predictive value for recovery, whereas the absence of metabolic activity in segments with decreased perfusion is associated with a lack of recovery of contractile function. The magnitude of improvement in global left ventricular ejection fraction after revascularization can be predicted by the number of segments showing perfusion-metabolism mismatch. As a result, FDG-perfusion studies can help select the subset of high-risk patients with severe left ventricular dysfunction who have the highest likelihood of significant improvement in global function, heart failure symptoms, and quality of life after revascularization and thus a more acceptable surgical risk.

Oxidative metabolism

[11]C Acetate as a Marker of Oxidative Metabolism

Acetate is a major substrate of oxidative metabolism, because it enters the Krebs cycle and is rapidly catabolized to CO_2 and water with the production of ATP, reduced nicotinamide adenine dinucleotide (NADH), and reduced form of flavin adenine dinucleotide ($FADH_2$). A radiolabeled form of acetate, ^{11}C acetate is rapidly concentrated by the myocardium, converted to acetyl coenzyme A (CoA), and is oxidized by means of the tricarboxylic acid cycle in mitochondria to [11]CO_2 and water, reflecting overall oxidative metabolism.

Contractile function requires functioning oxidative metabolism. After an episode of ischemia, systolic function recovers in parallel with oxidative metabolism. After a short period of ischemia, both oxidative metabolism and systolic function are reduced, but both parameters increase in response to inotropic stimulation, a phenomenon known as "contractile reserve." This is a hallmark of stunned myocardium, in which myocytes have a reserve capacity to meet at least part of an increased sympathetic demand for increased function. When ischemia persists for 1 to 3 hours, oxidative metabolism might not return to baseline levels for at least 2 to 6 weeks, in parallel with systolic function.

Acetate clearance is relatively unaffected by insulin, allowing measurements to be made with the patient fed or fasting. ^{11}C-acetate is concentrated in proportion to perfusion. In normal myocardium, there is homogeneous uptake and clearance from the left ventricular myocardium, indicating homogeneous oxidative metabolism. A monoexponential or bi-exponential least square fit can be applied to the regional myocardial time activity curves to calculate the K mono or K1 values, which are useful as indices of regional myocardial oxidative metabolism. Cardiac efficiency can be calculated when myocardial oxygen consumption (calculated by ^{11}C acetate PET) is combined with measurements of left ventricular external work.

Clinical Studies of Oxidative Metabolism

[11]C acetate metabolism is reduced in zones of acute myocardial infarction. Markedly reduced oxidative metabolism occurs in the central zone of infarction with no recovery in the absence of reperfusion. When thrombolytic therapy is administered early after onset of infarction, function and metabolism can be restored in parallel. In patients with delayed successful thrombolysis, perfusion might be normalized within 24 hours, whereas impaired oxidative metabolism improves slowly, in parallel with improvement in regional systolic function. β-Blockers reduce oxidative metabolism in normal myocardium, suggesting a possible mechanism of myocardial protection. Oxidative metabolism is reduced in areas of perfusion-glucose metabolism mismatch in patients with recent myocardial infarction. In coronary patients with recurrent myocardial ischemia, who have not had a prior infarction, oxidative metabolism is preserved in areas with mature collaterals, but in areas with reduced collateral flow and abnormal wall motion, oxidative metabolism is reduced. Biopsy specimens obtained at the time of bypass surgery in these patients reveal cellular swelling, loss of myofibrillar content, and accumulation of glycogen.

Because of the importance of oxidative metabolism for the recovery of ventricular function after ischemia, ^{11}C acetate imaging has been used to detect viability. Concordant reduction of blood flow and oxidative metabolism suggests nonviable myocardium, and, thus, probable lack of long-term improvement in contractile function. In contrast, myocardium with a greater reduction of oxidative metabolism than blood flow might show improvement in contractile function. A threshold of regional perfusion (<0.5 ml/g/min) and oxidative metabolism (0.09 [k_2]) seems necessary for recovery, whereas myocardial areas beyond the threshold might be irreversibly injured. Other studies indicate that oxidative metabolism is generally reduced in proportion to myocardial blood flow and offers no additional information compared with measurements of perfusion and FDG.

Combining sequential ^{11}C acetate studies at rest and during dobutamine infusion offers the ability to assess oxidative metabolic reserve. Assessing oxidative reserve with low-dose dobutamine infusion might be a better marker of recovery of regional function than resting oxidative metabolism alone. [11]C acetate can also be used to assess patients with hypertrophic and dilated cardiomyopathy. In patients with dilated cardiomyopathy, heterogeneity of regional oxidative metabolism might be observed in proportion to heterogeneous ventricular dysfunction on echocardiography. The efficiency of contraction and external cardiac work is reduced in patients with dilated cardiomyopathy and myocardial hypertrophy.

Fatty Acid Imaging

Tracers for Assessing Fatty Acid Use

Long-chain fatty acids are the principal energy source for normally oxygenated myocardium and pass easily through the sarcolemmal membrane by a facilitated transport mechanism. In the cell, the fatty acid is activated by CoA to form acyl CoA and is transported into mitochondria by the acyl carnitine carrier system, where it is rapidly catabolized by β-oxidation. β-Oxidation reduces the chain length by two carbons for each turn through the system. Fatty acid catabolism is a rapid process, requiring only 1 to 2 minutes for the complete consumption of a 16- to 18-carbon fatty acid. The 2-carbon fragment is acetyl CoA, which enters the tricarboxylic acid cycle (mirrored by the ^{11}C acetate studies described previously) for further oxidation to become water and carbon dioxide.

A small fraction of the total fatty acid entering the myocyte is stored as either triglyceride or myocardial structural lipids and persists in the myocardium for a long time. In the fasting state, when insulin levels are relatively low, fatty acids are the major source of myocardial contractile energy. With myocardial ischemia, oxidation of long-chain fatty acid is suppressed, uptake of fatty acid is markedly reduced, and fatty acid that is taken up is stored in the cell. Under these circumstances, anaerobic glucose metabolism provides ATP to maintain sarcolemmal integrity.

Fatty acid metabolism has been evaluated with a fully metabolized fatty acid, such as ^{11}C palmitate, and a trapped fatty acid, such as ^{123}I BMIPP (Figure 4-7). ^{11}C palmitate is transported in the myocyte by facilitated diffusion, and most is esterified to palmitate-acyl-CoA and proceeds into mitochondria by way of the carnitine shuttle, where it undergoes repeated cycles of β-oxidation into 2-carbon fragments that are oxidized by means of the tricarboxylic acid (TCA) cycle to ^{11}C carbon dioxide and water. A minor fraction of palmitate-acyl-CoA enters the intracellular lipid pool, where it remains as either a triglyceride or phospholipid. Sequential images recorded after intracoronary or intravenous administration of ^{11}C palmitate demonstrate rapid uptake of the agent in pro-

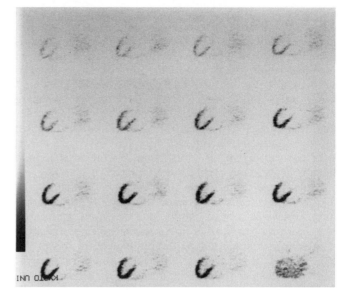

FIGURE 4-7. Serial dynamic images (2 minutes per frame) of the myocardium after administration of ^{11}C palmitate in a normal subject. Note a high myocardial uptake in the early stage with rapid washout from the myocardium.

portion to regional perfusion and a bi-exponential washout from the myocardium. The rapid clearance component that correlates with myocardial oxygen consumption corresponds to the fraction catabolized by β-oxidation, whereas the slow washout component reflects the turnover rate of the intracellular lipid pool.

Radioiodine, particularly ^{123}I, with its half-life of 13 hours and its gamma emission of 159 keV with no accompanying β-radiation, is an appropriate choice for labeling metabolic substrates. An even more compelling reason for the use of iodine is the wide availability of single photon imaging equipment. Thus, ^{123}I-labeled fatty acids have received great attention for assessing myocardial metabolism in vivo.

Two groups of iodinated fatty acids have been evaluated: straight-chain fatty acids and branched fatty acids (Table 4-3). The straight-chain fatty acids are metabolized by means of β-oxidation, and the radiolabel is released from the myocardium. The clearance of iodine from the myocardium, however, is not the same as $^{11}CO_2$ clearance, because there are back-diffusion components that must be considered. The uptake and regional retention of branched-chain fatty acids, which are retained in the myocardium, are easier to evaluate.

Branched-chain fatty acids provide excellent myocardial images within minutes of injection. The myocardial

■ ■ ■

TABLE 4-3 IODINATED FATTY ACIDS

Straight-chain fatty acids	Branched fatty acids
^{123}I-16-iodohexadecenoic acid	^{123}I-(p-iodophenyl)-3-(R,S)-methylpentadecanoic acid (BMIPP)
^{123}I-17-iodoheptadecanoic acid	^{123}I-(p-iodophenyl)-3,3-dimethylpentadecanoic acid (DMIPP)
^{123}I-iodophenylpentadecanoic acid	^{123}I-(p-iodophenyl)-9-(R,S)-methylpentadecanoic acid (9-Me-BMIPP)
	16-[^{123}I]-iodo-3-methylhexadecanoic acid
	13-p-[^{123}I]-3-(p-phenylene)-tridecanoic acid

localization of these agents is due to high myocardial extraction in areas that are normally oxygenated. Within the myocardium, branched-chain fatty acid clearance is related to the rate of α-oxidation and the turnover rate of the lipid pool, which is a very slow process compared with β-oxidation. To evaluate effectively the metabolic component of localization, it is necessary to measure both perfusion and fatty acid uptake. Such dual-tracer imaging is used to demonstrate perfusion-metabolism mismatch and to characterize fatty acid use. This is particularly important as the tissue becomes ischemic, because extraction changes with ischemia.

Under basal conditions, BMIPP has an extraction of 74% after intravenous injection and 65% after intracoronary injection, with only 9% washout from the myocardium. Coronary venous sampling might demonstrate the products of α-oxidation, back-diffusion of the fatty acid molecule, and a small component of β-oxidation metabolites. In the occlusion-reperfusion canine model, BMIPP uptake correlates with ATP levels, and equilibrium extraction is reduced in the presence of ischemia.

Clinical Applications of Straight-Chain Fatty Acids

In patients with coronary artery disease, a segmental or regional reduction of 15-(p[123I]-iodophenyl)-3,3-dimethylpentadecanoic acid (IPPA) correlates with reduced regional perfusion as determined by thallium imaging. The IPPA lesions are generally more prominent than thallium, probably because of reduced extraction of IPPA in ischemic tissue. These findings suggest that imaging the myocardial distribution of IPPA (with injections at rest) is useful for detecting coronary artery disease.

In ischemic territories, IPPA uptake is reduced, and clearance is delayed, whereas focal areas of decreased uptake are observed in infarcted myocardium. Therefore, a delayed washout with reversibility of the tracer uptake on the early and delayed scan is considered to be a key sign for identifying myocardial ischemia. A multicenter study showed the clinical value of rest IPPA SPECT imaging to assess viability and its ability to predict functional recovery after revascularization.[29] In patients with dilated cardiomyopathy, greater heterogeneity of IPPA uptake with faster washout is observed compared with normal subjects, indicating metabolic heterogeneity in this disease state. The unique ability to explore myocardial perfusion and fatty acid turnover with a single tracer is interesting, but the clinical niche of IPPA imaging is unclear.

15-(p[123I]-Iodophenyl)-3-Methylpentadecanoic Acid (BMIPP)

As with perfusion imaging agents, significant myocardial uptake of BMIPP occurs within 20 seconds of injection, reaches a plateau in 3 to 5 minutes, and remains essentially unchanged for about 60 minutes. There is minimal uptake in the liver and lung. Because BMIPP uptake is similar to that of perfusion imaging agents, both fatty acid uptake and perfusion should be determined to iden-

tify whether a regional decrease in tracer distribution represents an area of altered perfusion or fatty acid uptake. Less BMIPP uptake than perfusion (discordant BMIPP uptake) is often observed in ischemic myocardium, particularly in patients with acute infarction who have been reperfused and in patients with severe wall motion abnormalities. In patients with acute myocardial infarction, the reduced regions of fatty acid uptake identified by BMIPP images correlate with the area "at risk" assessed by perfusion imaging performed at the time of admission to the hospital. The relatively reduced BMIPP concentration in the myocardium might reflect preceding severe ischemia after successful reperfusion, so-called ischemic memory. These zones of ischemic memory seem to have a high likelihood of functional improvement on a follow-up study. These findings correlate with thallium reversibility or the perfusion-metabolism mismatch pattern seen with PET studies. In addition, areas of myocardium with contractile dysfunction associated with BMIPP-perfusion mismatch are more likely to exhibit contractile reserve than those areas with a matched pattern. They have minimal (<10%) fibrosis on histological examination and usually show improvement of regional function after successful revascularization.

BMIPP imaging at rest has been advocated to identify ischemic myocardium. A decrease in BMIPP uptake is associated with regional wall motion abnormalities in patients with no history of myocardial infarction (Figure 4-8). Unfortunately, the sensitivity of BMIPP imaging at rest is only 40% to 70% for detecting coronary artery lesions. However, in patients with vasospastic angina, reduced BMIPP uptake might be seen as a result of repetitive ischemic episodes. Because discordant BMIPP uptake might represent ischemic and jeopardized myocardium, studies of combined BMIPP and thallium imaging might have potential value for risk stratification in coronary patients. In follow-up studies of patients with acute myocardial infarction, among the various clinical, angiographic, and radionuclide prognostic indices, impairment of BMIPP uptake and perfusion-BMIPP mismatch patterns emerge as strong predictors of future fatal and nonfatal cardiac events. These data suggest that the BMIPP and thallium imaging might be useful for identifying high-risk subgroups among patients with coronary artery disease.

TARGETING MYOCARDIAL APOPTOSIS

Apoptosis is a complex, energy-requiring, genetically programmed process that has been evolutionarily conserved. Although it exists for the removal of unwanted cells and fulfills a physiological function, it is now recognized that exaggerated apoptosis might lead to degenerative disorders (such as congestive heart failure and Alzheimer's disease), and deficient apoptosis might be associated with excessive cellular proliferation (such as in neoplastic disorders or autoimmune diseases). Because apoptosis is a programmed process, it might be amenable to therapeutic manipulation. For such a management strategy to be successful, techniques must be

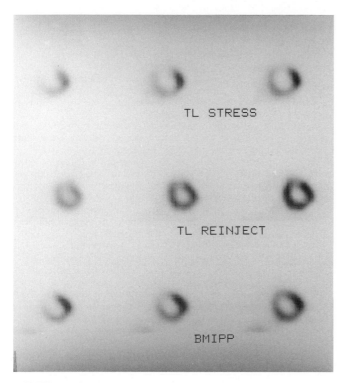

FIGURE 4-8. A series of short-axis slices of stress *(top)* and reinjection *(middle)* thallium SPECT and resting BMIPP SPECT *(bottom)* of a patient with unstable angina. Thallium study indicated stress-induced ischemia in anterior and septal regions. Reduction of BMIPP uptake is noted in the areas of thallium abnormality, indicating alteration of fatty acid metabolism in the ischemic myocardium.

developed to detect and monitor apoptosis and to assess the response to therapeutic interventions.

Apoptosis begins with a trigger, or initiation, phase followed by an execution phase of a common proteolytic cascade involving the family of cysteine proteases or caspases. Activation of caspases leads to proteolysis of cytoplasmic proteins and fragmentation of DNA. Necrosis, unlike apoptosis, is not part of normal homeostasis and is a result of a nonphysiological insult. The hallmark of necrotic cell death is the loss of membrane integrity, cell swelling, chromatin flocculation, and the uncontrolled spillage of intracellular contents leading to local inflammation. Examples of the nonphysiological noxious conditions that induce necrosis include severe hypoxia, ischemia, respiratory poisons, or inflammatory damage. Such insults destroy or permanently impair cellular integrity of a group of cells, adjacent healthy cells (tissues), and extracellular matrix, resulting in dysfunction, scar, and tissue deformity at the site of injury. With apoptosis, the cellular architecture remains intact, and the function of adjacent cells continues in uninterrupted fashion.[30]

Role of Apoptosis in Cardiovascular Diseases

Apoptosis might occur when a major insult results in cell injury but is not severe enough to induce cell death, and it has also been reported secondary to growth stimulation in which transcription factors and fetal genes are expressed in myocardium leading to cell hypertrophy

and preparing the cell to divide. However, because myocytes are terminally differentiated, they are unable to divide and die by apoptosis. Finally, if apoptosis does not occur normally during embryogenesis of the heart, various morphological anomalies can occur.

Noninvasive In Vivo Detection of Apoptosis

During apoptosis, the cell membrane develops protrusions and invaginations because of a disordered distribution of phospholipids in the lipid bilayer and cytoskeletal architectural alterations. Phosphatidylserine (PS), a component of the cell membrane that is normally maintained on the inner leaflet of the membrane, is expressed on the cell surface. The intracellular alterations of apoptosis often follow the exposure of PS on the cell surface. The caspases are activated and lead to proteolytic damage to the cytoskeleton (actin filaments) and nuclear matrix proteins (nuclear laminar proteins that rigidly support chromatin organization). Protein kinase C, an enzyme involved in the assembly of microfilaments needed to form membrane blebs and ultimately apoptotic bodies, is also activated. The apoptotic bodies are identified by PS receptors on macrophages, and the apoptotic cells are removed without spilling intracellular contents or inducing an inflammatory reaction.

The exposure of PS during apoptosis makes it an attractive target for radiopharmaceutical imaging.[28] Annexin V, an endogenous human protein with a molecular weight of 35 kDa, has a nanomolar affinity for exteriorized PS. The annexin V binds specifically to anionic phospholipids such as PS and phosphatidyl ethanolamine with essentially no binding to neutral or cationic phospholipids. Its affinity for PS is significantly higher than for phosphatidyl ethanolamine. The binding is Ca^{++} dependent, with rapid complete reversal after chelation. Annexin V labeled with fluorescein has been used in conjunction with flow cytometry for in vitro identification of apoptotic cells. It has been reasoned that in vivo imaging with radiolabeled annexin V could allow noninvasive detection of apoptotic cells.[31]

Annexin V, radiolabeled with ^{99m}Tc or iodine, has been used to detect PS expression in vivo in laboratory studies of apoptosis in tumor-bearing animals and several models of transplant rejection. Human studies in patients with tumors and heart transplant rejection have demonstrated the ability of radiolabeled annexin to localize at sites of apoptosis. A series of consecutive patients who had undergone heart transplantation had a scintigraphic study within 1 year using ^{99m}Tc-labeled annexin V. Analysis of SPECT images demonstrated no uptake of annexin V in 9 of 14 patients, their endomyocardial biopsies were unremarkable, and there was lack of immunohistochemical evidence of caspase-3 upregulation, confirming the absence of significant apoptosis. Five patients with a positive scan had histologically verified transplant rejection of grade 2/4 or higher. Caspase-3 upregulation in the patients with positive annexin-V scan confirmed the specificity of noninvasive detection of apoptotic process. Histological evidence of apoptosis was observed in both myocytes and nonmyocytic cells. Two of the five patients with positive annexin scans demonstrated diffuse global uptake of radiolabeled annexin V in the myocardium; their endomyocardial biopsy specimens revealed grade 3A/4 rejection and severe vascular rejection, respectively, and caspase-3 upregulation and activation was seen in myocytes and endothelial cells. Caspase-3 staining was particularly intense and was observed in most endothelial cells in the biopsy specimen of the patient with acute vascular rejection. Thus, all nine patients without histological evidence of rejection had a negative scan. As seen in these patients with rejection, ^{99m}Tc-annexin V imaging can identify cardiac apoptosis. Similarly, in acute myocarditis, annexin imaging identifies areas of acute myocardial damage.[32]

In patients with early, symptomatic postinfarction heart failure and evidence of persistent occlusion of the infarct-related artery (who died 10 days or more after acute myocardial infarction), the apoptotic rate was increased fourfold at the site of infarction.[33] In addition, both at the site of infarction and in unaffected regions, the apoptotic rate correlated significantly with parameters of progressive left ventricular remodeling, suggesting that apoptosis is strongly associated with and might be a major determinant of unfavorable left ventricular remodeling and early symptomatic postinfarction heart failure.

REFERENCES

1. McGhie AI, Radovancevic B, Capek P, et al. Major histocompatibility complex class II antigen expression in rejecting cardiac allografts: detection using in vivo imaging with radiolabeled monoclonal antibody. *Circulation* 1997; 96:1605.
2. Ohtani H, Strauss HW, Southern JF, et al. Intercellular adhesion molecule-1 induction: a sensitive and quantitative marker for cardiac allograft rejection. *J Am Coll Cardiol* 1995; 26:793.
3. Mitchel J, Waters D, Lai T, et al. Identification of coronary thrombus with a IIb/IIIa platelet inhibitor radiopharmaceutical, technetium-99m DMP-444: a canine model. *Circulation* 2000; 101:1643.
4. Pallela VR, Thakur ML, Consigny PM, Rao PS, Vasileva-Belnikolavska D, Shi R. Imaging thromboembolism with Tc-99m-labeled thrombospondin receptor analogs TP-1201 and TP-1300. *Thromb Res* 1999; 93:191.
5. Oyen WJ, Boerman OC, Corstens FH. Animal models of infection and inflammation and their role in experimental nuclear medicine. *J Microbiol Methods* 2001; 47:151.
6. Morguet AJ, Munz DL, Ivancevic V, et al. Immunoscintigraphy using technetium-99m-labeled anti-NCA-95 antigranulocyte antibodies as an adjunct to echocardiography in subacute infective endocarditis. *J Am Coll Cardiol* 1994; 23:1171.
7. Riemann B, Schafers M, Law MP, Wichter T, Schober O. Radioligands for imaging myocardial alpha- and beta-adrenoceptors. *Nuklearmedizin* 2003; 42:4.
8. Goldstein DS, Holmes C, Cannon RO 3rd, Eisenhofer G, Kopin IJ. Sympathetic cardioneuropathy in dysautonomias. *N Engl J Med* 1997; 336:696.
9. Maunoury C, Agostini D, Acar P, et al. Impairment of cardiac neuronal function in childhood dilated cardiomyopathy: An ^{123}I MIBG scintigraphic study. *J Nucl Med* 2000; 41:400.
10. Bengel FM, Ueberfuhr P, Hesse T, et al. Clinical determinants of ventricular sympathetic reinnervation after orthotopic heart transplantation. *Circulation* 2002; 106:831.
11. Arora R, Ferrick KJ, Nakata T, et al. ^{123}I MIBG imaging and heart rate variability analysis to predict the need for an implantable cardioverter defibrillator. *J Nucl Cardiol* 2003; 10:121.
12. Momose M, Kobayashi H, Iguchi N, et al. Comparison of parameters of ^{123}I-MIBG scintigraphy for predicting prognosis in patients with dilated cardiomyopathy. *Nucl Med Commun* 1999; 20:529.
13. Narula J, Haider N, Virmani R, et al. Apoptosis in myocytes in end-stage heart failure. *N Engl J Med* 1996; 335:1182.
14. Bulow HP, Stahl F, Lauer B, et al. Alterations of myocardial presynaptic sympathetic innervation in patients with multi-vessel coronary artery disease but without history of myocardial infarction. *Nucl Med Commun* 2003; 24:233.
15. Sakata K, Mochizuki M, Yoshida H, et al. Cardiac sympathetic dysfunction contributes to left ventricular remodeling after acute myocardial infarction. *Eur J Nucl* Med 2000; 27:1641.
16. Muxi A, Magrina J, Martin F, et al. Technetium 99m-labeled tetrofosmin and iodine 123-labeled metaiodobenzylguanidine scintigraphy in the assessment of transmyocardial laser revascularization. *J Thorac Cardiovasc Surg* 2003; 125:1493.
17. Li ST, Tack CJ, Fananapazir L, Goldstein DS. Myocardial perfusion and sympathetic innervation in patients with hypertrophic cardiomyopathy. *J Am Coll Cardiol* 2000; 35:1867.
18. Wichter T, Schafers M, Rhodes CG, et al. Abnormalities of cardiac sympathetic innervation in arrhythmogenic right ventricular cardiomyopathy: quantitative assessment of presynaptic norepinephrine reuptake and postsynaptic beta-adrenergic receptor density with positron emission tomography. *Circulation* 2000; 101:1552.
19. Nakata T, Wakabayashi T, Kyuma M, et al. Prognostic implications of an initial loss of cardiac metaiodobenzylguanidine uptake and diabetes mellitus in patients with left ventricular dysfunction. *J Card Fail* 2003; 9:113.
20. Nousiainen T, Vanninen E, Jantunen E, Remes J, Kuikka J, Hartikainen J. Anthracycline-induced cardiomyopathy: long-term effects on myocardial cell integrity, cardiac adrenergic innervation and fatty acid uptake. *Clin Physiol* 2001; 21:123.
21. Russell FD, Molenaar P. The human heart endothelin system: ET-1 synthesis, storage, release and effect. *Trends Pharmacol Sci* 2000; 21:353.
22. Bax WA, Bruinvels AT, van Suylen RJ, Saxena PR, Hoyer D. Endothelin receptors in the human coronary artery, ventricle and atrium. A quantitative autoradiographic analysis. *Naunyn Schmiedebergs Arch Pharmacol* 1993; 348:403.
23. Bacon CR, Cary NR, Davenport AP. Endothelin peptide and receptors in human atherosclerotic coronary artery and aorta. *Circ Res* 1996; 79:794.
24. Meding J, Dinkelborg LM, Grieshaber MK, Semmler W. Targeting of endothelin receptors for molecular imaging of atherosclerosis in rabbits. *J Nucl Med* 2002; 43:400.
25. Pacher R, Stanek B, Hulsmann M, et al. Prognostic impact of big endothelin-1 plasma concentrations compared with invasive hemodynamic evaluation in severe heart failure. *J Am Coll Cardiol* 1996; 27:633.
26. Sinusas AJ. The potential for myocardial imaging with hypoxia markers. *Semin Nucl Med* 1999; 29:330.
27. Imahashi K, Morishita K, Kusuoka H, et al. Kinetics of a putative hypoxic tracer, ^{99m}Tc-HL91, in normoxic, hypoxic, ischemic, and stunned myocardium. *J Nucl Med* 2000; 41:1102.
28. Leppo J. Imaging cell injury and death. *Curr Cardiol Rep* 2003; 5:40.
29. Verani MS, Taillefer R, Iskandrian AE, Mahmarian JJ, He ZX, Orlandi C. ^{123}I-IPPA SPECT for the prediction of enhanced left ventricular function after coronary bypass graft surgery. Multicenter IPPA Viability Trial Investigators. ^{123}I-iodophenylpentadecanoic acid. *J Nucl Med* 2000; 41:1299.
30. Kanduc D, Mittelman A, Serpico R, et al. Cell death: apoptosis versus necrosis [review]. *Int J Oncol* 2002; 21:165.
31. Flotats A, Carrio I. Non-invasive in vivo imaging of myocardial apoptosis and necrosis. *Eur J Nucl Med Mol Imaging* 2003; 30:615.
32. Tokita N, Hasegawa S, Maruyama K, et al. ^{99m}Tc-Hynic-annexin V imaging to evaluate inflammation and apoptosis in rats with autoimmune myocarditis. *Eur J Nucl Med Mol Imaging* 2003; 30:232.
33. Abbate A, Biondi-Zoccai GG, Bussani R, et al. Increased myocardial apoptosis in patients with unfavorable left ventricular remodeling and early symptomatic post-infarction heart failure. *J Am Coll Cardiol* 2003; 41:753.

chapter 5

Evidence-Based Medicine: A Guide to Cardiac Imaging

Raymond J. Gibbons

Rationale for Clinical Practice Guidelines
Overview of ACC-AHA Guideline Process
Evolution of the ACC-AHA Guidelines
Overview of Current Situation
Future Directions

Over the past 2 decades, there has been an explosion of scientific knowledge with respect to the diagnosis and treatment of cardiovascular disease. Before 1980, randomized trials in cardiovascular disease were infrequent. Currently, every new issue of a major cardiovascular journal reports the results of several such trials, which frequently involve thousands of patients. The application of this enormous base of new evidence to optimize cardiovascular practice is the underlying rationale for clinical practice guidelines, which are commonly defined as "systematically developed statements to assist practitioner and patient decisions about appropriate health care for specific clinical circumstances."[1,2] This chapter is intended to summarize the rationale for clinical practice guidelines, provide an overview of the American College of Cardiology–American Heart Association joint effort to develop practice guidelines, describe the ongoing evolution of these guidelines as well as their current status with respect to cardiac imaging, and offer some insights regarding potential important future developments.

RATIONALE FOR CLINICAL PRACTICE GUIDELINES

Unfortunately, the quality of medical care does not always meet ideal standards. The first important national recognition of suboptimal care occurred in the mid-1980s, when federal authorities recognized that permanent pacemakers were often implanted for inappropriate reasons. A retrospective analysis of a large number of pacemaker implantations[3] showed that there were definite appropriate indications for about 40% of implantations and possible indications in about 35% of implantations. However, the reasons for implantation in nearly 20% of cases seemed to be incorrect. This led to the initiation of the joint American College of Cardiology–American Heart Association (ACC/AHA) practice guidelines effort and formation of the first committee to develop

Practice Guidelines for the Implantation of Permanent Pacemakers.

Such early indications of suboptimal quality were not confined to cardiovascular disease. Comparisons of appropriate preventive care were performed for a number of different procedures in an attempt to show that managed care systems provided better preventive services than fee-for-service systems. One study examined the performance of every other year mammography in women older than the age of 50. Although there has been some controversy regarding the use of mammography before the age of 50,[4] or its use on an annual basis in older women, there has been no such controversy about the use of every other year mammography in women older than the age of 50. All authorities would agree that such imaging is appropriate. In one of the largest studies examining the performance of biannual mammography in women older than the age of 50, managed care systems had a higher rate of appropriate delivery of this service (about 50%) than fee-for-service systems (about 35%). However, it was not reassuring that the odds that such an important service was provided were no better than the flip of a coin.

Multiple studies have reported that therapies that are of unequivocal benefit in randomized trials are not provided consistently in practice. The Worcester Heart Study is a population-based, careful methodological effort to systematically collect data on cardiovascular care in Worcester, Massachusetts. The Worcester Heart Study has reported on the rate of use of aspirin and beta-blockers at the time of admission of patients with myocardial infarction, who had a definite history of a prior myocardial infarction. In the absence of definite contraindications, all these patients should have been taking both aspirin and beta-blockers because of their proven efficacy after myocardial infarction.[5] Although there was an increase in the percentage of patients taking beta-blockers between 1986 and 1995, the most recently published data from 1995 continued to show that only 45% of patients were actually taking beta-blockers. More surprising, although there was an increase in the use of aspirin between 1986 and 1995, only one half of the patients were taking aspirin, despite the wealth of randomized trial evidence showing the effectiveness of this inexpensive medication (Figure 5-1).

A variety of performance measures have been proposed as measures of the quality of care; these typically include not only appropriate medications but also appropriate diagnostic testing. A report from the Health Care

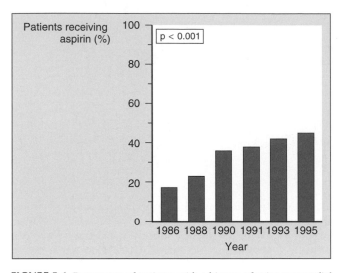

FIGURE 5-1. Percentage of patients with a history of prior myocardial infarction who were taking aspirin at the time of admission for a recurrent myocardial infarction. (From McCormick D, Gurwitz JH, Lessard D, Yarzebaki J, Gore JM, Goldberg RJ. Use of aspirin, beta-blockers, and lipid-lowering medications before recurrent acute myocardial infarction: missed opportunities for prevention? *Arch Intern Med* 1999; 159:561.)

Financing Administration[6] examined compliance with 24 appropriate performance measures for the treatment of six medical conditions by state. It demonstrated large regional differences in compliance (Figure 5-2). However, even those states in the upper quartile had rates of compliance that were generally less than 80%. One of the performance measures was the measurement of left ventricular ejection fraction during the initial evaluation of a patient with congestive heart failure. The best state in the country, New Hampshire, had a rate of compliance of 79%; the worse state in the country, Wyoming, had a rate of compliance of only 34%. There was a wide

spectrum of performance between these two extremes. A more recent review indicated that care for Medicare fee-for-service plan beneficiaries improved substantially between 1998 and 1999 and 2000 and 2001, but a large opportunity exists for further improvement.[7]

Wide geographical variations in the delivery of care have been documented and widely reported. The most widely cited compilation of such data is the Dartmouth Atlas of Cardiovascular Health Care.[8] The rates of angioplasty range from less than 3 to more than 20 per 1000 Medicare enrollees, approximately a 10-fold range, after adjustment for the basic demographics of the local population (Figure 5-3). Rates in New England, New York, Washington, and Oregon were distinctly lower than the national average. Rates in west Texas, Missouri, and the south were much higher. Although such variation may reflect legitimate variations in the practice of medicine, as well as patient preference in different locations, this degree of variability is very difficult to explain or understand.[9] It is certainly attractive to hypothesize that such variability might affect the quality of care, but it is difficult to define optimal use (i. e., the "right rate)."

The measured differences in quality of care, the wide variability in delivery of services, and general explosion of medical knowledge all support the need for the development of evidence-based clinical practice guidelines to improve the quality of care and possibly reduce inappropriate variation. The ACC and AHA have jointly supported the development of cardiovascular practice guidelines for more than 15 years.

OVERVIEW OF ACC-AHA GUIDELINE PROCESS

The ACC-AHA practice guideline effort is directed by the Task Force on Practice Guidelines, a distinguished group of senior physicians from both organizations who repre-

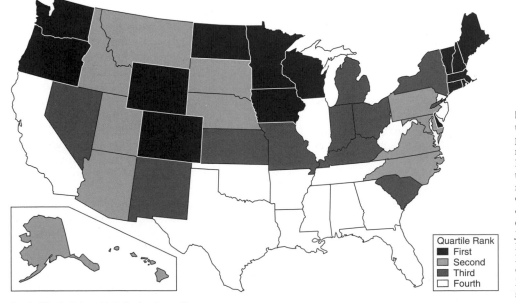

Puerto Rico (not shown) is in the fourth quartile

FIGURE 5-2. Ranking of individual states according to Medicare performance measures for six common conditions. States in New England, the northern Plains, and the Pacific Northwest generally ranked in the first quartile. California and states in the south constituted the fourth quartile. (Reproduced with permission from Jencks SF, Cuerdon T, Burwen DR, Fleming B, Houck PM, Kussmaul AE, Nilasena DS, Ordin DL, Arday DR. Quality of medical care delivered to Medicare beneficiaries: a profile at state and national levels. *JAMA* 2000; 284:1670.)

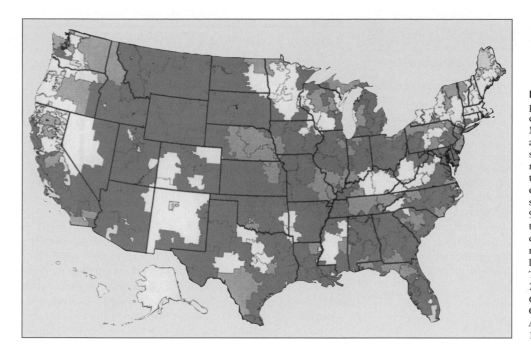

FIGURE 5-3. National map by hospital referral region of the rate of coronary angioplasty per 1000 Medicare enrollees, adjusted for age, gender, and ethnicity. Regions shown in the darkest color had rates that were several-fold higher than the regions shown in the lightest color. Key: in descending order, starting with darkest color: 1. 0 to 2. 97, 1.10 to <1.30, 0.90 to <1.10, 0.75 to <0.90, 0.35 to <0.75. Remaining color (see northwest Maine or northeast Minnesota) is "not populated." (From Wennberg JE, Bubolz TA, Fisher ES, Gittelsohn AM, et al. *The Dartmouth Atlas of Health Care in the United States*, in Cooper MM (ed): Chicago, IL: American Hospital Publishing, 1996:123.)

sent a spectrum of expertise and include many past officers of both organizations. This group is responsible for setting overall policy, identifying appropriate topics, and overseeing the selection of chairpersons and members of writing committees for these specific topics. Members of the writing committee are intentionally selected to represent a spectrum of expertise, different regions of the country, and, whenever possible, other specialties including general internal medicine and family medicine.

The writing committee follows a systematic step-by-step process (Box 5-1), including an exhaustive literature search, synthesis and interpretation of the available evidence, the writing of recommendations, and the classification of these recommendations with respect to both usefulness and strength of evidence. The classification of usefulness uses standardized definitions (Box 5-2). Levels of evidence are assigned to each recommendation on the basis of the strength of available evidence (Box 5-3). Implicit in this process is the recognition that many important clinical questions that are addressed in practice guidelines might not lend themselves to experimentation or may not yet have been addressed by high-quality investigations. Although randomized controlled trials might not be available, the clinical question may be so important that recommendations must be provided on the basis of expert consensus. Assigning a level of evidence of B or C is therefore not to be construed as implying that the recommendation is a "weak" one.

The writing committee typically meets on three or four occasions over the course of 12 to 18 months to complete its final draft. The task force then oversees an intensive review process, which includes at least three reviewers designated by each organization. There is a designated reviewer from the task force who examines the writing committee's responses to all of the reviews and provides appropriate oversight of the review

■ ■ ■

BOX 5-1   STEPS IN GUIDELINE CREATION

1. Determine the guideline scope and outline the document.
2. Define and conduct appropriate and comprehensive literature searches.
3. Sort and evaluate the evidence.
4. Synthesize and interpret the evidence (text and evidence tables).
5. Write recommendations on the basis of expert interpretation of the evidence.
6. Assign classification of recommendations and strength of evidence.
7. Create tables, diagrams, and mnemonics describing recommendations.

process. Once the designated task force reviewer and task force chair have approved the document, it is submitted to the leadership of both organizations for further review and official endorsement. The final guideline consists of both a full-length version (with complete refer-

■ ■ ■

BOX 5-2   CLASSIFICATION OF RECOMMENDATIONS

Class I: Conditions for which there is evidence and/or general agreement that a given procedure or treatment is useful and effective.

Class II: Conditions for which there is conflicting evidence and/or a divergence of opinion about the usefulness/efficacy of a procedure or treatment.

IIa: Weight of evidence/opinion is in favor of usefulness/efficacy.

IIb: Usefulness/efficacy is less well established by evidence/-opinion.

Class III: Conditions for which there is evidence and/or general agreement that a procedure/treatment is not useful/effective and in some cases might be harmful.

■ ■ ■

BOX 5-3   STRENGTH OF EVIDENCE

Level of evidence A: Data derived from multiple randomized clinical trials.
Level of evidence B: Data derived from a single randomized trial, or non-randomized studies.
Level of evidence C: Consensus opinion of experts.

■ ■ ■

TABLE 5-2   RADIONUCLIDE TESTING IN UNSTABLE ANGINA

Indication	Test	Class
Ischemia in distribution of "culprit"	Stress perfusion	I
LV function	RNA	I
Severity/extent in patients with ongoing ischemia	Rest perfusion	IIa
Severity/extent in patients who have been stabilized	Stress perfusion	IIa
Diagnosis when history/ECG unreliable	Rest perfusion	IIb

From *Circulation* 91:1278, 1995.

ences and between 25 and 100 printed pages of text) and an executive summary (with complete recommendations and limited text). In the past, the full-length and executive summary versions were published in *Circulation* and the *Journal of the American College of Cardiology*. More recently, the full-length version is only available on the Internet web page of both organizations. The executive summary is still published in a print version in these same journals.

EVOLUTION OF THE ACC-AHA GUIDELINES

Over the past few years, there have been several important developments in the evolution of the ACC-AHA guidelines process. The first development was a shift from procedure-specific guidelines such as echocardiography and radionuclide imaging to disease-specific guidelines, such as stable angina and unstable angina. Although procedure-specific guidelines are still useful and therefore produced and revised when necessary, they are now secondary in importance to disease-specific guidelines, because the latter provide more assistance to the practicing clinician within a more clinically useful context. In the past, procedure-specific guidelines might include recommendations for echocardiography and pericardial disease (Table 5-1) or radionuclide testing in unstable angina (Table 5-2). However, such recommendations would require a clinician to search through multiple guidelines to manage a patient with a particular problem and would demand that the clinician then understand how to use this information in the framework of clinical management. Flow diagrams began to appear in procedure-specific guidelines to address the issue of clinical context (Figure 5-4). However, such flow diagrams were generally unable to consider the "complete picture" of patient management. More recently, disease-specific

guidelines have provided such a complete picture in a series of flow charts (Figure 5-5).

The guidelines have also evolved to include shorter and briefer versions. Practicing clinicians are faced with an "information explosion" and little time to assimilate or prioritize all the information available to them. The most frequent complaint regarding the full-length versions of the ACC-AHA guidelines was that they were simply "too long and detailed." Although they provided complete background information and served the role of a "reference text," they did not allow the clinician rapid access to the specific information required. This led to the development of "pocket versions," which began with the *Perioperative Evaluation Guideline*. Such pocket versions were very popular and are now a standard part of all disease-specific guidelines, as well as selected procedure-specific guidelines. Pocket guidelines for stable angina, myocardial infarction, valvular heart disease, and unstable angina are already available. These pocket guides include laminated cards with brief, practical instructions facilitating application at the bedside. Several of them are now available in computerized versions for personal digital system devices such as the Palm Pilot computer. The guidelines process has also made an effort to develop simple mnemonics wherever possible, such as the ABCDE instructions for the management of all patients with stable angina (Box 5-4).

The guidelines process has recognized the need for much more frequent revisions because of the rapid development of new evidence in cardiovascular disease. Both the ACC and AHA maintain active Internet web pages on which the guidelines are available in searchable format. These Internet versions have facilitated the development of more rapid and timely "updates" whenever major new evidence appears on a given topic. The writing committees are asked to monitor the appearance of new evidence that might mandate a change in guideline recommendations. The first such update was issued for the *Myocardial Infarction Guideline* in 1999,[5] when the publication of the SHOCK trial[10] changed the recommendation for the use of primary angioplasty in patients with ST elevation or left bundle branch block, age <75, and the possibility of revascularization within 18 hours of the onset of chest pain to a class I recommendation from a class IIa recommendation (which had appeared in the 1996 release of the guideline). Updates have now been published for exercise testing,[11] periop-

■ ■ ■

TABLE 5-1   ECHOCARDIOGRAPHY IN PERICARDIAL DISEASE

Indication	Class
Suspected pericardial disease	I
Suspected bleeding in the pericardial space	I
Guidance/monitoring of pericardiocentesis	IIa
TEE for assessment of pericardial thickness	IIb
Routine follow-up of small effusion in stable patient	III

From *Circulation* 1997; 95:1686.

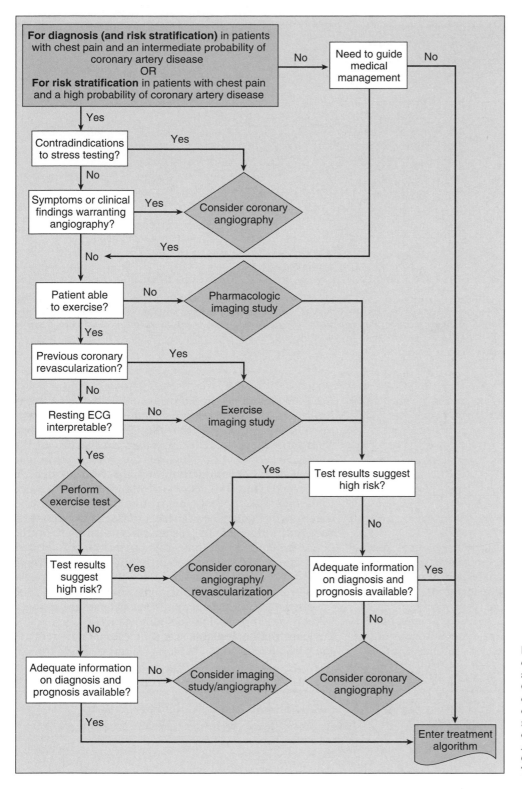

FIGURE 5-4. Overview of clinical decision making in the choice of an appropriate stress test. (From Gibbons RJ, Balady GJ, Beasley JW, et al. ACC/AHA guidelines for exercise testing: executive summary. A report of the American College of Cardiology/ American Heart Association Task Force on Practice Guidelines (Committee on Exercise Testing). *Circulation* 1997; 96:345.)

erative evaluation,[12] echocardiography,[13-15] stable angina,[16] and unstable angina.[17] This "ongoing, living" document process also requires ongoing change in the membership of the writing committee to ensure broad input and adequate representation. The task force has developed timelines for the stepwise replacement of the entire original committee by the time three such updates have been completed.

Finally, the guidelines have evolved to include full partnership with other interests and organizations. In the past, other organizations participated in a collaborative fashion by providing representatives on the writing committee and occasionally endorsing the final guideline. However, in recent years, the ACC-AHA task force has attempted to more formally involve other major organizations in a "full partner" role. This process began with

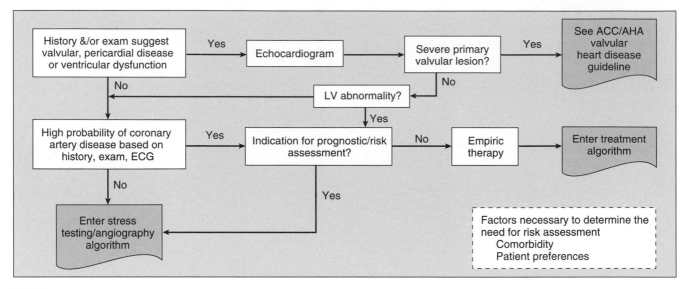

FIGURE 5-5. A portion of the clinical assessment of patients with stable angina, extracted from a larger flow diagram. (From Gibbons RJ, Chatterjee K, Daley J, Douglas JS, Fihn SD, Gardin JM, Grunwald MA, Levy D, Lytle BW, O'Rourke RA, Schafer WP, Williams SV. ACC/AHA/ACP-ASIM guidelines for the management of patients with chronic stable angina: a report of the American College of Cardiology/American Heart Association Task Force on Practice Guidelines (Committee on the Management of Patients with Chronic Stable Angina). *J Am Coll Cardiol* 1999; 33:2092.)

■ ■ ■

BOX 5-4   MNEMONIC FOR STABLE ANGINA

A = Aspirin and Antianginal therapy
B = Beta-blocker and Blood pressure
C = Cigarette smoking and Cholesterol
D = Diet and Diabetes
E = Education and Exercise

---

the *Stable Angina Guideline*. Because many such patients are managed by general internists, the American College of Physicians/American Society of Internal Medicine participated as a full partner in this effort, including the identification of one third of the membership of the writing committee, formal endorsement of the final guideline, and subsequent publication of a reformatted version for general internists in the *Annals of*

Internal Medicine. The European Society of Cardiology has served for the first time as a full partner on the development of the *Guideline for Atrial Fibrillation*.[18] Appropriate subspecialty organizations, such as the American Society of Nuclear Cardiology, American Society of Echocardiography, and the North American Society of Pacing and Electrophysiology have been asked to partner with the ACC and AHA on appropriate procedure-specific guidelines. These efforts have been well received and generally recognized to strengthen the entire process by avoiding the publication of overlapping, and potentially conflicting, guidelines. Although there was an initial concern about the ability of physicians from different perspectives to partner on such efforts, the efforts have generally proceeded in a collegial fashion by emphasizing the importance of basing the guideline on the available scientific evidence rather than the particular "opinions" of a given group.

■ ■ ■

TABLE 5-3   NONINVASIVE TESTS BEFORE AND AFTER ADJUSTMENT FOR REFERRAL BIAS

Modality	First author	Year	Total patients	SENSITIVITY		SPECIFICITY	
				Biased	Adjusted	Biased	Adjusted
Exercise ECG	Morise A	1995	Men: 508	0.56	0.40	0.81	0.96
			Women: 284	47	0.33	0.73	0.89
Exercise planar thallium	Schwartz RS	1993	Men: 845	0.67	0.45	0.9	0.78
Exercise planar thallium	Diamond G	1986	Overall: 2269	0.91	0.68	0.34	0.71
Exercise SPECT thallium	Cecil MP	1996	Overall: 2688	0.98	0.82	0.14	0.59
Exercise/ dipyridamole & SPECT sestamibi	Santana-Boado C	1998	Men: 100	0.93	0.88	0.89	0.96
			Women: 63	0.85	0.87	0.91	0.91
Exercise echo	Roger V	1997	Men: 244	0.78	0.42	0.37	0.83
			Women: 96	0.79	0.32	0.34	0.86

OVERVIEW OF CURRENT SITUATION

Both the procedure-specific and disease-specific guidelines that have already been mentioned provide important direction regarding the use of imaging procedures. It is beyond the scope of this chapter to provide all the details of that information. However, it is appropriate to highlight several general themes in existing guidelines and to cite some specific examples.

The guidelines often emphasize well-established scientific principles that have not been widely recognized in clinical practice. One example is the importance of posttest referral bias in the assessment of any diagnostic test. This is a well-established principle that has been emphasized in multiple previous publications. However, it continues to be ignored in many contemporary publications on diagnostic testing. The failure to recognize this principle often leads to inappropriate conclusions. This concept is emphasized in the *Stable Angina Guidelines,* which provides one of the few available tabulations of those published studies that have taken this principle into account with respect to the noninvasive diagnosis of coronary artery disease (Table 5-3). The guideline process will hopefully focus more attention on this important principle, which is a major limitation of recently published, and widely discussed, meta-analyses.[19,20]

Another example of how the guidelines process has attempted to focus clinicians on a more evidence-based approach is the issue of noninvasive risk stratification. A major meta-analysis of all the randomized trials comparing medical therapy and coronary artery bypass grafting[21] demonstrated that revascularization usually leads to an improved prognosis in patients with an annual mortality of greater than 3% per year and generally does not lead to an improved prognosis in patients with an annual mortality of less than 1% per year. Although well established by the published evidence, this concept has not generally been recognized. The *Stable Angina Guideline* has attempted to highlight its important by compiling specific examples of noninvasive test results that place the patient in low-, intermediate-, and high-risk categories.[16] These categories have clear implications for the potential to improve patient outcome and thereby help determine the need for early catheterization (Box 5-5).

The guidelines have attempted to provide an objective comparison of different imaging procedures that might potentially be used for the same purpose. The most visible example of this is the comparison of stress echocardiography and stress radionuclide perfusion imaging in the *Stable Angina Guideline.* The table that appeared in that guideline summarizing the available evidence and the strengths of each technique (Box 5-6), has now been widely reproduced. It attempts to place an objective, evidence-based overview on what is frequently a subjective, highly emotional issue. As part of this same process, the guidelines may highlight evidence that favors one imaging procedure over the other. The *Stable Angina Guideline* made recommendations that clearly favored vasodilator stress perfusion imaging for both diagnosis and risk stratification in patients with left bundle branch

block or ventricular paced rhythm. This procedure was recommended as class I for such patients compared with a class IIb recommendation for exercise echocardiography, dobutamine echocardiography, or exercise perfusion imaging for such patients.

■ ■ ■
BOX 5-5   NONINVASIVE RISK STRATIFICATION

High-risk (greater than 3% annual mortality rate)

1. Severe resting left ventricular dysfunction (LVEF <35%)
2. High-risk treadmill score (score, –11)
3. Severe exercise left ventricular dysfunction (exercise LVEF <35%)
4. Stress-induced large perfusion defect (particularly if anterior)
5. Stress-induced multiple perfusion defects of moderate size
6. Large, fixed perfusion defect with LV dilation or increased lung uptake (thallium-201)
7. Stress-induced moderate perfusion defect with LV dilation or increased lung uptake (thallium-201)
8. Echocardiographic wall motion abnormality (involving greater than two segments) developing at low dose of dobutamine (10 mg/kg/min) or at a low heart rate (<120 beats/min)
9. Stress echocardiographic evidence of extensive ischemia

Intermediate-risk (1% to 3% annual mortality rate)

1. Mild/moderate resting left ventricular dysfunction (LVEF, 35% to 49%)
2. Intermediate-risk treadmill score (–11<score<5)†
3. Stress-induced moderate perfusion defect without LV dilatation or increased lung uptake (thallium-201)
4. Limited stress echocardiographic ischemia with a wall motion abnormality only at higher doses of dobutamine involving two segments

Low-risk (less than 1% annual mortality rate)

1. Low-risk treadmill score (score, 5)
2. Normal or small myocardial perfusion defect at rest or with stress*
3. Normal stress echocardiographic wall motion or no change of limited resting wall motion abnormalities during stress*

*Although the published data are limited, patients with these findings will probably not be at low risk (LVEF <35%).
†Note on treadmill score: The Duke treadmill exercise score is calculated: [duration of exercise (in minutes) – [5 x maximal ST-segment deviation during or after exercise (in millimeters)] – [4 x treadmill angina index (0 = no angina, 1 = non limiting angina, 2 = exercise-limiting angina)]. A duke treadmill exercise score of 5 or greater is considered low risk; –10 to +4, intermediate risk; and less than – 10, high risk.

■ ■ ■
BOX 5-6   COMPARATIVE ADVANTAGES OF STRESS ECHOCARDIOGRAPHY AND STRESS RADIONUCLIDE PERFUSION IMAGING IN DIAGNOSIS OF CAD

Advantages of stress echocardiography

1. Higher specificity
2. Versatility more extensive evaluation of cardiac anatomy and function
3. Greater convenience/efficacy/availability
4. Lower cost

Advantages of stress perfusion imaging

1. Higher technical success rate
2. Higher sensitivity especially for single-vessel coronary disease involving the left circumflex
3. Better accuracy in evaluating possible ischemia when multiple resting LV wall motion abnormalities are present
4. More extensive published database especially in evaluation of prognosis

Evidence-based medicine may sometimes conclude that imaging procedures are unnecessary. For the initial noninvasive evaluation of patients with normal resting electrocardiograms, both the *Exercise Testing*[11] and *Stable Angina Guidelines*[16] have relied on the multiple published studies that have concluded that the incremental value of stress imaging compared with the exercise electrocardiogram is modest. As a result, treadmill exercise testing was given a class I indication for such patients in contrast to a class IIb indication for imaging. In contrast, the guidelines may sometimes strongly favor imaging. In the case of diagnostic testing for coronary artery disease, both the *Exercise Testing* and *Stable Angina Guidelines* strongly favored the use of stress imaging procedures rather than treadmill exercise testing for patients with marked resting ST depression, an inability to exercise, or previous coronary revascularization.

In some circumstances, the guidelines have highlighted the scarcity of data that are available to guide the proper clinical use of imaging procedures. This is particularly true with respect to the issue of patient follow-up. The available scientific evidence often focuses on the initial presentation of patients and does not reflect the clinical reality that most patients in clinical practice have been seen previously. There is surprisingly little published evidence to help clinicians in this regard. By highlighting this scarcity of data, the guidelines will hopefully help foster future studies. In the meantime, however, they help to provide an expert consensus about what is believed to be of "best clinical practice" on the basis of the scant data that are available. The *Valvular Heart Disease Guidelines*,[22] for example, provide clear direction with respect to the required interval of follow-up echocardiography in patients with valvular heart disease that does not yet warrant valvuloplasty or valve replacement. The *Stable Angina Guideline* provided information regarding the use of stress testing in patients who are otherwise clinically stable. The available process for rapid updates will hopefully permit the incorporation of new evidence about follow-up testing as it becomes available.

FUTURE DIRECTIONS

Given the growing interest in quality of care on a national level, there is every reason to believe that clinical practice guidelines, and evidence-based medicine, will be increasingly emphasized over both the short term and long term. Research has already identified multiple barriers to the implementation of practice guidelines and evidence-based medicine.[23,24] Reports are already beginning to appear in the scientific literature of a wide variety of efforts that are being tested to overcome these barriers. One of the largest such efforts is the ACC-sponsored Guidelines Applied in Practice (GAP) study, which is examining the effectiveness of a "tool kit" of eight different components on the quality of care after acute myocardial infarction in multiple hospitals in southeastern Michigan. The American Heart Association has initiated a national effort entitled "Get with the Guidelines," which is designed to assist hospitals and other health care facilities in the implementation of cardiovascular practice guidelines. These and other efforts are likely to expand greatly in the near future. The long-term efforts in this area will be determined by the success of these initial efforts.

The guidelines have often demonstrated the remarkable absence of evidence for important clinical decisions that are routinely part of current medical practice. They have helped to identify areas in which research is clearly warranted to develop better evidence. One early example of this phenomenon was the use of imaging studies after intermediate-risk treadmill exercise tests. The initial *AHCPR Unstable Angina Guideline* suggested that either coronary angiography or stress imaging procedures could probably be used in such patients, revealing the absence of evidence on this issue. As a result, a subsequent single-center study of myocardial perfusion imaging examined its potential incremental prognostic value in such patients.[25] A much larger, multicenter, longer term study was then undertaken with the support of the American Society of Nuclear Cardiology.[26] The results of that larger study demonstrated the value of a normal or near-normal perfusion image in the management of such patients (Figure 5-6).

Multiple other studies are under way to address other deficiencies in our knowledge. One example is the proper role of coronary revascularization in the management of patients with congestive heart failure. Although the potential etiological importance of coronary artery disease in such patients is widely recognized, clinicians struggle daily with the issue of how to evaluate and treat this possibility in the millions of

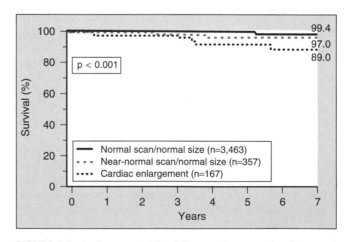

FIGURE 5-6. Cardiac survival for different subgroups of patients with intermediate-risk exercise electrocardiograms who did not have myocardial perfusion defects on radionuclide imaging. The patients with normal perfusion scans and normal heart size *(solid line)*, patients with near-normal scans and normal heart size *(dashed line)*, and patients with cardiac enlargement *(dotted line)* were significantly different from one another (*P* < 0.001). (From Gibbons RJ, Hodge DO, Berman DS, Akinboboye OO, Heo J, Hachamovitch R, Bailey KR, Iskandrian AE. Long-term outcome of patients with intermediate-risk exercise electrocardiograms who do not have myocardial perfusion defects on radionuclide imaging. *Circulation* 1999; 100:2140.)

Americans with congestive heart failure, because there is little current evidence on which to base this decision. The National Heart, Lung, and Blood Institute is currently considering a large multicenter trial to address this deficiency, which first became evident in the national *Congestive Heart Failure Guidelines* published by both the Agency for Health Care Policy and Research and the ACC-AHA.[27,28] A second example is the early emergency department triage of patients with acute chest pain syndromes. The deficiencies in our knowledge in this area with regard to the proper role of imaging procedures are readily apparent in any of the published unstable angina guidelines. A large, multicenter study that used myocardial perfusion imaging has already been completed.[29] Other studies with echocardiography are being reported.[30,31] It is hoped that publication of the scientific evidence from these endeavors will be incorporated in future guidelines and lead to improved patient care.

Clinical practice guidelines and evidence-based medicine are here to stay. Their role in medical practice is likely to expand rapidly over the next few years. There is a clear rationale for such an expansion. The ACC-AHA guideline effort is the dominant force in cardiovascular disease guidelines. It is hoped that this effort will continue to expand the involvement of other organizations. The current evolution toward disease problems, shorter versions, more rapid updates, and hand-held computer versions are all designed to facilitate the implementation of these guidelines. The major challenge for the health care system and for individual physicians is to apply these evidence-based principles in everyday practice in as many patients as possible in an effort to improve cardiovascular care. It is hoped that ongoing research will identify the best tools to assist physicians in this quality improvement effort.

REFERENCES

1. Gibbons RJ, Smith S, Antman E. American College of Cardiology/American Heart Association clinical practice guidelines. Part I. Where do they come from? *Circulation* 2003; 107:2979.
2. Gibbons RJ, Smith SC Jr, Antman E. American College of Cardiology/American Heart Association clinical practice guidelines. Part II. Evolutionary changes in a continuous quality improvement project. *Circulation* 2003; 107:310.
3. Greenspan AM, Kay HR, Berger BC, Greenberg RM, Greenspon AJ, Gaughan MJ. Incidence of unwarranted implantation of permanent cardiac pacemakers in a large medical population. *N Engl J Med* 1988; 318:158.
4. Josefson D. US issues new guidelines as mammography debate continues. *BMJ* 2002; 324:506.
5. Ryan TJ, Antman EM, Brooks NH, et al. 1999 update: ACC/AHA Guidelines for the Management of Patients With Acute Myocardial Infarction: Executive Summary and Recommendations: a report of the American College of Cardiology/American Heart Association Task Force on Practice Guidelines (Committee on Management of Acute Myocardial Infarction). *Circulation* 1999; 100:1016.
6. Jencks SF, Cuerdon T, Burwen DR, et al. Quality of medical care delivered to Medicare beneficiaries: a profile at state and national levels. *JAMA* 2000; 284:1670.
7. Jencks SF, Huff ED, Cuerdon T. Change in the quality of care delivered to Medicare beneficiaries, 1998-1999 to 2000-2001. *JAMA* 2003; 289:305.
8. Cooper MM. The Dartmouth Atlas of Health Care: what is it telling us? *Health Syst Rev* 1996; 29:44-5.
9. Beller GA. President's page: geographic variations in delivery of cardiovascular care: an issue of great importance to cardiovascular specialists. *J Am Coll Cardiol* 2000; 36:652.
10. Hochman JS, Sleeper LA, Webb JG, et al. Early revascularization in acute myocardial infarction complicated by cardiogenic shock. SHOCK Investigators. Should we emergently revascularize occluded coronaries for cardiogenic shock. *N Engl J Med* 1999; 341:625.
11. Gibbons RJ, Balady GJ, Bricker JT, et al. ACC/AHA 2002 guideline update for exercise testing: summary article: a report of the American College of Cardiology/American Heart Association Task Force on Practice Guidelines (Committee to Update the 1997 Exercise Testing Guidelines). *Circulation* 2002; 106:1883.
12. Eagle KA, Berger PB, Calkins H, et al. ACC/AHA guideline update for perioperative cardiovascular evaluation for noncardiac surgery: executive summary. A report of the American College of Cardiology/ American Heart Association Task Force on Practice Guidelines (Committee to Update the 1996 Guidelines on perioperative cardiovascular evaluation for noncardiac surgery). *Anesth Analg* 2002; 94:1052.
13. Cahalan MK, Stewart W, Pearlman A, et al. American Society of Echocardiography and Society of Cardiovascular Anesthesiologists task force guidelines for training in perioperative echocardiography. *J Am Soc Echocardiogr* 2002; 15:647.
14. Flachskampf FA, Decoodt P, Fraser AG, Daniel WG, Roelandt JR. Guidelines from the Working Group. Recommendations for performing transesophageal echocardiography. *Eur J Echocardiogr* 2001; 2:8.
15. Agricola E, Oppizzi M, De Bonis M, et al. Multiplane transesophageal echocardiography performed according to the guidelines of the American Society of Echocardiography in patients with mitral valve prolapse, flail, and endocarditis: diagnostic accuracy in the identification of mitral regurgitant defects by correlation with surgical findings. *J Am Soc Echocardiogr* 2003; 16:61.
16. Gibbons RJ, Abrams J, Chatterjee K, et al. ACC/AHA 2002 guideline update for the management of patients with chronic stable angina. Summary article: a report of the American College of Cardiology/American Heart Association Task Force on practice guidelines (Committee on the Management of Patients With Chronic Stable Angina). *J Am Coll Cardiol* 2003; 41:159.
17. Braunwald E, Antman EM, Beasley JW, et al. ACC/AHA 2002 guideline update for the management of patients with unstable angina and non-ST-segment elevation myocardial infarction. Summary article: a report of the American College of Cardiology/American Heart Association task force on practice guidelines (Committee on the Management of Patients With Unstable Angina). *J Am Coll Cardiol* 2002; 40:1366.
18. Fuster V, Ryden LE, Asinger RW, et al. ACC/AHA/ESC guidelines for the management of patients with atrial fibrillation. A report of the American College of Cardiology/American Heart Association Task Force on Practice Guidelines and the European Society of Cardiology Committee for Practice Guidelines and Policy Conferences (Committee to develop guidelines for the management of patients with atrial fibrillation) developed in collaboration with the North American Society of Pacing and Electrophysiology. *Eur Heart J* 2001; 22:1852.
19. Kwok Y, Kim C, Grady D, Segal M, Redberg R. Meta-analysis of exercise testing to detect coronary artery disease in women. *Am J Cardiol* 1999; 83:660.
20. Fleischmann KE, Hunink MG, Kuntz KM, Douglas PS. Exercise echocardiography or exercise SPECT imaging? A meta-analysis of diagnostic test performance. *JAMA* 1998; 280:913.
21. Yusuf S, Zucker D, Peduzzi P, et al. Effect of coronary artery bypass graft surgery on survival: overview of 10-year results from randomised trials by the Coronary Artery Bypass Graft Surgery Trialists Collaboration. *Lancet* 1994; 344:563.
22. Bonow RO, Carabello B, de Leon AC, et al. ACC/AHA Guidelines for the management of patients with valvular heart disease. Executive Summary. A report of the American College of Cardiology/ American Heart Association Task Force on Practice Guidelines (Committee on Management of Patients with Valvular Heart Disease). *J Heart Valve Dis* 1998; 7:672.
23. Borenstein J, Chiou CF, Henning JM, et al. Physician attitudes toward strategies to promote the adoption of medical evidence into clinical practice. *Am J Manag Care* 2003; 9:225.

24. Weingarten S. Critical pathways: what do you do when they do not seem to work? *Am J Med* 2001; 110:224.

25. Hachamovitch R, Berman DS, Kiat H, et al. Exercise myocardial perfusion SPECT in patients without known coronary artery disease: incremental prognostic value and use in risk stratification. *Circulation* 1996; 93:905.

26. Gibbons RJ, Hodge DO, Berman DS, et al. Long-term outcome of patients with intermediate-risk exercise electrocardiograms who do not have myocardial perfusion defects on radionuclide imaging. *Circulation* 1999; 100:2140.

27. Hunt SA, Baker DW, Chin MH, et al. ACC/AHA guidelines for the evaluation and management of chronic heart failure in the adult: executive summary. *J Heart Lung Transplant* 2002; 21:189.

28. Hunt SA, Baker DW, Chin MH, et al. ACC/AHA Guidelines for the Evaluation and Management of Chronic Heart Failure in the Adult: Executive Summary A Report of the American College of Cardiology/ American Heart Association Task Force on Practice Guidelines (Committee to Revise the 1995 Guidelines for the Evaluation and Management of Heart Failure): Developed in Collaboration With the International Society for Heart and Lung Transplantation; Endorsed by the Heart Failure Society of America. *Circulation* 2001; 104:2996.

29. Udelson JE, Beshansky JR, Ballin DS, et al. Myocardial perfusion imaging for Evaluation and Triage of Patients with Suspected Acute Cardiac Ischemia. *JAMA* 2002; 288:2693.

30. Kontos MC, Kurdziel K, McQueen R, et al. Comparison of 2-dimensional echocardiography and myocardial perfusion imaging for diagnosing myocardial infarction in emergency department patients. *Am Heart J* 2002; 143:659.

31. Mobasseri S, Hendel RC. Cardiac imaging in women: use of radionuclide myocardial perfusion imaging and echocardiography for acute chest pain. *Cardiol Rev* 2002; 10:149.

Diagnostic Decision Making

J. Sanford Schwartz

"Prediction is very difficult, especially about the future."

Niels Bohr

The goal of medical diagnosis is to improve patient outcomes through better selection of therapeutic interventions resulting from enhanced diagnostic accuracy. The base of medical knowledge is large, rapidly changing, and published in disparate sources. Decisions often represent high stakes and need to incorporate a range of patient, family, and provider perspectives, values, preferences, and needs. The rapid growth of a continually expanding array of ever more sophisticated diagnostic tests rather than simplifying the diagnostic task paradoxically has made clinical decision making increasingly complex and challenging while at the same time more effective and accurate.

Tests often are used for purposes other than diagnosis, for example, to assess disease severity, predict prognosis, or monitor disease status. Although this chapter will focus on the interpretation and use of diagnostic tests, these principles also guide assessment and use of tests for other clinical purposes.

Diagnostic tests are useful to the degree that they provide new information that will have a beneficial impact on subsequent diagnostic workup, clinical management, and health outcome. New information alone is of very limited benefit if it does not alter patient management and outcomes.

All clinical information has diagnostic value and can be considered as a diagnostic test. All diagnostic information is imperfect and subject to error. That which is available is frequently conflicting and of uncertain validity and reliability. Thus, all medical decisions are subject to some degree of uncertainty. Moreover, in addition to how well diagnostic tests discriminate between people with and without a disease, optimal selection, interpretation, and use of diagnostic tests also is a function of the clinical objective, effectiveness of therapy, physician selection of that therapy, patient adherence with the prescribed therapy, disease response to the therapy, and interactions with and confounding effects of coexisting disease.

For all clinical conditions the probability of disease in a given person varies between zero (definitely absent) and 1.0 (definitely present). For every clinical condition there is some probability (<1.0) above which the physician is sufficiently confident of the diagnosis to warrant therapeutic intervention, the "test-treatment threshold." Similarly, there is some probability (>0) below which one is confident enough that the condition is not present that the disease can be excluded and other diagnostic possibilities considered and pursued, the "test-no treatment threshold." The area between these two disease probabilities corresponding to when one is not sufficiently confident to either treat or not treat the patient is when diagnostic tests are potentially useful. The goal of such testing, singly or in combination, is to move one's estimate of disease probability either above the "test-treatment threshold" or below the "test-no treatment threshold" (see Figure 6-1).[1]

Treatment and testing thresholds are a function of the risks, costs, and benefits (mortality, morbidity, and quality of life) of treatment or lack thereof, as well as test performance characteristics (sensitivity and specificity). Greater diagnostic certainty is required before instituting therapy or testing (higher the treatment and testing thresholds) the riskier or more costly the test and the riskier and more costly or less effective the therapy. Less diagnostic certainty is required before instituting therapy or testing (lower the treatment and testing thresholds) the safer, more accurate, and less costly the test and the more effective, safer, and less costly the treatment. Reduced test risk and cost and improved test performance widen the probability range in which testing is appropriate, whereas increased test cost and risk and reduced sensitivity and specificity narrow the range for testing.

DIAGNOSTIC TEST PERFORMANCE

Precision and Accuracy

Diagnostic tests must be both precise (reliable) and valid. Precision and reliability refer to the ability of a diagnostic test to yield a consistent result; validity (accuracy) refers to the ability of a diagnostic test to yield a correct result. It is difficult to be accurate without being precise, but one can be precise without being accurate.

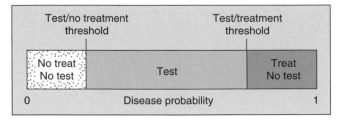

FIGURE 6-1. Threshold theory of decision making. (Adapted from Pauker SAG, Kassirer JP. The threshold approach to clinical decision making. *N Engl J Med* 1980; 302:1109.)

Discrimination of People with and Without Disease

The primary measure of diagnostic test performance is its ability to distinguish between the presence and absence of a specific disease. Ideally, a diagnostic test perfectly discriminates between those with disease (true positives [TP]) and without disease (true negatives [TN]) (Figure 6-2, *A*).[2] However, rather than directly detecting disease, diagnostic tests detect disease markers that are imperfectly correlated with the presence or absence of disease. Thus, some degree of misclassification exists for all diagnostic tests. In their simplest form, diagnostic tests are dichotomous (interpreted as either positive or negative). Two types of misclassification errors occur with dichotomous tests: people free of disease incorrectly classified as diseased (false positives [FP]) and people with the disease incorrectly classified as nondiseased (false negatives [FN]) (Figure 6-2, *B*).

Before ordering a diagnostic test, the physician needs to consider (1) the probability that the test will correctly identify people with and without the disease in question and (2) the probability that a positive test result correctly indicates the presence of disease and a negative test result correctly identifies those without disease.

Sensitivity measures the proportion of people with disease correctly identified by a diagnostic test. *Specificity* refers to the proportion of those without the disease correctly identified by the diagnostic test as nondiseased. Test sensitivity and specificity are not affected by disease prevalence or the estimated pretest probability of disease.

Optimal use of a diagnostic test requires the physician to estimate the probability of disease in a patient before performance of the test and then use of the information provided by the test to derive a revised posttest probability of disease. *Predictive value positive (PV+)* measures the posttest probability that a positive test correctly identifies people with the disease being assessed. *Predictive value negative (PV–)* measures the posttest probability that a negative test correctly identifies those without disease. Thus, sensitivity and specificity indicate the percent of diseased and nondiseased patients, respectively, correctly identified by a test, whereas PV+ and PV– indicate the percent of patients, respectively, testing positive or negative who have (PV+) or do not have (PV–) disease (see Table 6-1.)

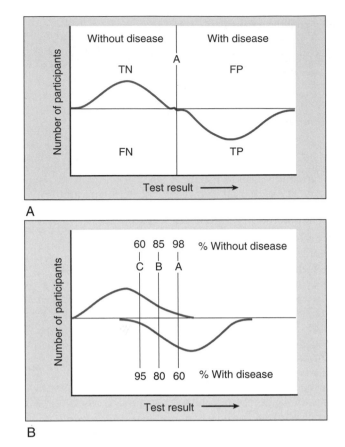

A

B

FIGURE 6-2. Diagnostic test discrimination between diseased and nondiseased subjects. Hypothetical distribution of results in an ideal test (**A**) and most tests (**B**) used in clinical medicine. TN = True-negative; FP = false-positive; FN = false-negative; TP = true-positive. (From Black ER, Panzer RJ, Mayewski RJ, Griner PF. Characteristics of diagnostic tests and principles for their use in quantitative decision making, in Black ER, Bordley DR, Tape TG, Panzer RJ (eds): *Diagnostic Strategies for Common Medical Problems*. ed 2. Philadelphia: American College of Physicians, 1999, p 7.)

Weiner et al[3] evaluated the diagnostic performance of the electrocardiographic stress test (EST) in 1465 men with exercise-induced chest pain. The EST was defined as positive if there was ≥1.0 mm of horizontal or downward sloping ST-segment depression compared with the resting baseline electrocardiogram (ECG) for at least 0.08 seconds (diagnostic criteria designed to be reasonably sensitive to detect ischemic coronary artery disease

■ ■ ■

TABLE 6-1   TEST PERFORMANCE CHARACTERISTICS

	Disease present	Disease absent	
Test positive	True positive (TP)	False positive (FP)	TP + FP
Test negative	False negative (FN)	True negative (TN)	FN + TN
	TP + FN	FP + TN	

Sensitivity = true positives/all patients with disease = TP/TP + FN; specificity = true negatives/all patients without disease = TN/TN + FP; PV+ = true positives/all patients with positive tests = TP/TP + FP; PV– = true negatives/all patients with negative tests = TN/TN + FN.

■ ■ ■

TABLE 6-2   ELECTROCARDIOGRAPHIC STRESS
TEST PERFORMANCE IN MEN UNDERGOING
CARDIAC CATHETERIZATION

	CHD present	CHD absent	
EST positive	815	115	930
EST negative	208	327	535
	1,023	442	

Sensitivity = 815/1023 = 0.80; specificity = 327/442 = 0.74; PV+ = 815/930 = 0.88; PV− = 327/442 = 0.61. Adapted from Weiner DA, Ryan TJ, McCabe CH, et al. Exercise stress testing: correlation among history of angina, ST-segment response and prevalence of coronary artery disease in the Coronary Artery Surgery Study (CASS). *N Engl J Med* 1979; 301:23.

■ ■ ■

TABLE 6-3   EFFECT OF PRIOR PROBABILITY
(PREVALENCE) ON PREDICTIVE VALUE OF
POSITIVE TEST RESULTS

Prior probability (Prevalence) (%)	Predictive value of positive test result(%)		
	Sensitivity 90% Specificity 90%	Sensitivity 95% Specificity 95%	Sensitivity 99% Specificity 99%
0.1	0.9	1.9	9.0
1	8.3	16.1	50.00
2	15.5	27.9	66.9
5	32.1	50	83.9
50	90	95	99.0

The predictive value of a positive test iss low when the disease prevalence is low. From Diagnostic tests, in Goroll AH, May L, Mulley AG (eds): *Primary Care Medicine*, ed 4. Philadelphia: Lippincott, 2000.

[CAD] while reducing false-positive results). The reference standard against which the EST was evaluated was the presence of ≥70% narrowing of one or more major coronary arteries as determined on cardiac catheterization. One thousand twenty-three of the tested men had evidence of ischemic coronary heart disease (CHD) on cardiac catheterization as defined previously, of whom 815 had a positive EST. Of the 442 men without CHD on cardiac catheterization, 115 had a positive EST. Sensitivity, specificity, positive predictive value (PV+), and negative predictive value (PV−) for the EST in these men with acute, exercise-induced chest pain undergoing coronary angiography are shown in Table 6-2.

In contrast to sensitivity and specificity, the predictive value of positive and negative diagnostic tests are strongly influenced by disease prevalence/pretest probability of disease.[4] A diagnostic test's positive predictive value is directly related to disease prevalence, increasing as the pretest probability of disease increases and decreasing as disease prevalence declines. Conversely, negative predictive value is inversely related to disease prevalence, declining as the pretest probability of disease increases and increasing as disease prevalence decreases. Thus, the higher the prevalence or pretest probability of disease, the more likely a positive test result is to represent a true-positive and the less likely a negative test result correctly identifies those without disease. If the probability of disease is very high, even a negative test will not exclude the disease. Conversely, the lower the prevalence or pretest probability of disease, the more likely a positive test result is a false positive and the more likely that a negative test result correctly identifies those without disease. If the pretest probability of disease is very low, a positive test likely represents a false-positive result (see Table 6-3).[5]

BIASES IN ASSESSING DIAGNOSTIC TEST PERFORMANCE

Much of the information about diagnostic test performance is obtained from the medical literature, the evaluation of which frequently is confounded by a number of potential problems and thereby suffers from several biases that tend to overstate diagnostic test perform-

ance. Thus, physicians must be able to evaluate the validity of published studies of diagnostic tests.

Reference (Gold) Standard Problems

Test performance is assessed in relation to a reference standard that establishes the presence or absence of a disease. However, true disease status is often difficult to establish. Ideally, diagnostic test performance is studied in populations with known true disease status. Thus, establishing true disease status requires an independent accurate "gold standard" test. However, true disease status often is difficult to establish because of safety, cost, ethics, and scientific limitations. Thus, frequently imperfect ("tarnished") "gold standards" must be used to establish disease status, with resulting misclassification. Imperfect reference standards distort estimates of test sensitivity and specificity. Although several methods have been developed to reduce the effects of biased reference standards, they only partially correct biased estimates of test performance.[6,7] For example, although coronary angiography is an appropriate reference standard for establishing a diagnosis of coronary vessel occlusion, it does not detect CAD patients at increased risk for a cardiac event with nonocclusive coronary lesions (e.g., potentially unstable, thin-walled coronary plaque).

Spectrum Bias

Estimates of diagnostic test performance are dependent on the spectrum of diseased and nondiseased subjects evaluated.[8] Ideally, diagnostic tests should be evaluated on a wide spectrum of diseased and nondiseased subjects large enough to estimate test performance in clinically relevant subgroups. The spectrum of patients for evaluating diagnostic tests should include healthy subjects with no disease and patients without the disease but with common comorbid conditions, with recent-onset asymptomatic disease, established asymptomatic disease, established symptomatic disease, advanced disease, end-stage disease, and other diseases affecting the same anatomical organs as the disease in question. Evaluation of diagnostic tests on an unrepresentative sample of diseased and nondiseased subjects usually results in overestimation of test sensitivity and specificity. For example, it has been estimated that EST sensitivity is 0.68 and specificity 0.77. However, diagnostic performance varies substantially, depending on the coronary vessel with CAD, with sensitivity highest in patients with left anterior descending (LAD) lesions, lower for right coronary lesions, and lowest for left circumflex lesions. Compared with those with single-vessel disease, among patients with multivessel CAD, EST sensitivity is higher (approximately 0.81) but specificity lower (approximately 0.66); these trends are further accentuated among patients with left main or three-vessel CAD (sensitivity 0.86; specificity 0.53).[9] Similarly, EST performance varies in relation to patient symptoms.[10]

Referral/Verification/Workup Bias

Referral bias occurs when the result of the test being evaluated is used to determine which subjects are further evaluated by the reference standard, resulting in unrepresentative application of the reference standard. Referral bias commonly occurs when the reference standard poses some risk, is expensive, or is uncomfortable and results in overestimation or underestimation of test sensitivity and specificity. Shortly after the widespread introduction of exercise radionuclide angiography into clinical practice, the test's specificity was noted to be lower than reported in initial published studies of test performance, a result of physicians using the test to select patients for further, more invasive evaluation by cardiac catheterization.[11] Although an appropriate use of the test, the apparent decline in test specificity indicates, in part, the degree to which using the results of a diagnostic test to select patients who receive the reference test can affect assessment of test performance. Because people testing positive on the test being evaluated generally are more likely to receive the reference test, workup bias often overstates the sensitivity but underestimates the specificity of the test being evaluated.[12]

Blinded Interpretation

Results of the test being evaluated should be interpreted without knowledge of the reference standard test result or the true diagnosis. When such blinded, independent test interpretation does not occur, test sensitivity and specificity may be overestimated.

As a result of these various biases, diagnostic test performance frequently is misestimated (and commonly overestimated) in the medical literature. The greater the discrepancy between study conditions and the setting in which the test will be used, the less applicable the study results are to clinical practice.

Uninterpretable Results

Uninterpretable results occur with varying frequency for diagnostic imaging tests as a result of limitations of technology, technician skill and experience, and patient physiology. For example, a patient's arthritis might limit the ability to exercise to the level of exertion required by a stress test. Technicians vary in their ability to obtain high-quality echocardiograms in obese patients or to avoid attenuation of the inferior wall on single photon emission computed tomography (SPECT). Uninterpretable test results might seriously impair estimates of diagnostic performance.[13] This is of particular importance when comparing alternative diagnostic tests, because the frequency of uninterpretable test results might vary significantly among tests. If, as commonly occurs, indeterminate results are not included in calculation of diagnostic test performance, test sensitivity and specificity will be overestimated. Inclusion of such results as either positive or negative will reduce test specificity and sensitivity, respectively. Assessing the performance of cardiac imaging tests, indeterminate results either most commonly are not included, are discarded, or are deleted.

SELECTION AND USE OF DIAGNOSTIC TESTS

The selection and use of diagnostic tests is a function of the test's performance characteristics (sensitivity and specificity) and the clinical situation in which it is used (e.g., severity of the disease being tested for and the safety and effectiveness of available therapies and other interventions). True-positive results help the physician select appropriate management, reducing patient morbidity and mortality and improving patient function. True-negative results provide reassurance and avoid unnecessarily risky, inconvenient, and costly tests and reduce anxiety. Conversely, false-positive results increase risk and costs from unnecessary and inappropriate tests and treatments and might increase anxiety and psychological harm, whereas false-negative results might result in missed diagnoses, adverse outcomes from untreated disease, or delayed treatment administered at an advanced stage, as well as subject patients to unnecessary additional tests and uncertainty and anxiety from diagnostic delay.

Tests with high sensitivity are preferred when the costs of missing a diagnosis are high (as in screening or when attempting to exclude a disease). Thus, a test with high sensitivity is desired when the intervention is effective; safe; inexpensive; false-positive results do not result in serious clinical, psychological, or economic harm; and when the goal is to minimize false-negative results. Tests with high specificity are required before instituting risky or expensive therapy. Thus, a test with high specificity is desired the lower the effectiveness and the greater the risk and expense of therapy, when false-positive results cause serious clinical, psychological, or economic harm, and when one seeks to minimize false-positive results.

In general, diagnosis is a multistage process, often beginning with screening or case finding, proceeding through excluding (ruling out) disease and culminating in confirming (ruling in) disease before initiating therapy or another intervention. The type and characteristics of appropriate diagnostic tests vary with the stage of the diagnostic process (see Table 6-4).

For example, a detailed history regarding the presence and character of chest discomfort is often used to screen for ischemic CHD. However, although a history of chest discomfort has modest sensitivity for clinically significant ischemic coronary heart disease, it is not specific (i.e., has a high false-positive rate). Thus, physicians commonly evaluate such patients with an imaging test (e.g., EST, stress echocardiography, nuclear stress test), which, although more expensive and complicated to perform, has high sensitivity. However, generally, tests with high specificity (e.g., coronary angiography) are required before definitive, expensive, or risky interventions are initiated.

The clinician can optimize sensitivity and specificity by careful selection among alternative tests with differing test performance characteristics, by altering the cutoff point of a test to emphasize *either* sensitivity *or* specificity (but not both simultaneously), or by the use of tests in combination (requiring a series of tests to be positive to consider the diagnosis present reduces sensitivity and increases specificity beyond that of any of the tests singly; considering the diagnosis to be present if any of a series of tests is positive increases sensitivity while reducing specificity beyond that of the individual tests).

SCREENING

Diagnostic tests commonly are used for screening, defined as detection of disease or elevated risk of disease in apparently well patients before the onset of symptoms. Selection of diagnostic tests for screening requires that one consider the disease burden, the test characteristics when used for screening, the characteristics of the follow-up tests that will be required if the screening test is positive, and the safety and effectiveness of early treatment. By definition, screening is conducted among patients and populations with low disease prevalence and among patients with a low pretest probability of disease. Thus, in most cases, screening is targeted toward identifiable populations at increased risk of disease (sometimes referred to as *case finding*).

Because of the low prevalence of disease among screening populations, tests used for screening purposes always produce a very high false-positive rate (low PV+). Unless screening is confined to a high-risk population (≥50%), even the very best screening tests will yield more false-positive than true-positive results. Furthermore, most people being screened will not benefit from the screening process, because only a small percentage of those being screened will actually have the condition of interest. Thus, screening is best confined to serious diseases for which a safe and effective treatment exists and for which it has been demonstrated that early detection and treatment significantly improve patient outcome. The screening test itself must have high sensitivity and specificity and be safe, inexpensive, convenient, and acceptable to the target screening population. In addition, because performance of the screening test will result in many false-positive results, appropriate follow-up tests with sufficiently high diagnostic performance, safety, and cost must be

TABLE 6-4 TEST PERFORMANCE CHARACTERISTICS DESIRED AT DIFFERENT STAGES OF DIAGNOSIS

Objective	Desire	Avoid	Risk	Cost
Screening/ case finding	High sensitivity	FN	Minimal	Low
Disease exclusion rule out disease moderate	High sensitivity	FN	Minimal-moderate	Low-moderate
Disease confirmation rule in disease	High specificity	FP	Minimal-high	Low-high

FN = False Negative, FP = False Positive.

available to identify and exclude those without the disease and to confirm the presence of disease in those affected. For this reason, generally, even the best screening tests are optimally confined to populations and patients at increased risk of disease as determined by known risk factors.

A screening test, as in Table 6-4, must have very high sensitivity, because the objective is to minimize false-negative results. This is perhaps counterintuitive to many physicians, who think that the objective of a screening test is to identify people with a disease. However, because of the low prevalence of disease in the screened population and the resulting high false-positive rate, patients testing positive on the screening test will need to undergo subsequent diagnostic testing to sort out those with the disease (TP) from those without the disease (false positive [FP]). In contrast, patients who are negative on the screening test will not undergo further evaluation. Thus, the primary goal is to minimize false-negative results, those people with the disease who falsely test negative.

The anticipated effectiveness and benefits of screening tests and screening testing programs are often overestimated because of biased assessment of screening tests and programs. In addition to the biases in test performance discussed earlier, screening tests are subject to *lead-time bias* and *length-time bias*.

Lead-Time Bias

A common pitfall in the evaluation of a screening program is to measure the time between disease detection and death as a measure of the success of the program. For the example in the second row of Figure 6-3,[14] one would incorrectly conclude that the screening program prolonged life, despite the fact that death did not occur any later than if it was not detected earlier by screening (i.e., the amount of time by which the disease diagnosis is accelerated by screening). This misinterpretation of the value of screening programs has been termed *lead-time bias. Lead time* is the time between disease detection by screening and time of usual symptomatic diagnosis and is a function of the rate of biological progression of the disease and screening test sensitivity. *Lead-time bias* refers to artifactual survival prolongation resulting from earlier disease detection in the absence of increased effectiveness of earlier intervention simply because the diagnosis is made earlier.

One of the questions to determine in deciding whether to screen for a disease is whether early diagnosis leads to increased or improved survival.[15] Consider the preceding diagram, which represents a hypothetical disease. The first row represents the natural history of the disease, with no screening and no treatment. In this row, the disease is diagnosed clinically, and the patient eventually succumbs to the disease. The second row represents the situation in which screening is possible, but where there is no effective intervention to prolong the length of survival (even if the diagnosis is made early through screening). The last row represents a disease in which early screening leads to earlier, more effective treatment. Here, the actual length of survival is improved, the goal of screening.

Nonexperimental (e.g., observational) studies and quasi-experimental (e.g., case control) studies often result in lead-time bias. Rigorous randomized clinical trials often are required to assess the true improved outcomes attributable to a screening test program.

Critical Point

The critical point in the natural history of a disease is the point beyond which there is no cure.

Depending on the disease, the critical point might occur at any point along the continuum in Figure 6-4. An effective screening test detects disease at A′ (between the points of biological onset [A] and usual clinical detection [B]) for a disease whose critical point is somewhere beyond (i.e., to the right of) A.′ The period from this detection point (A′) to the usual time of diagnosis (B) is the detectable preclinical phase. If the critical point is before the detectability of disease, screening is

not useful, because the only cases of disease detected will be those already progressed beyond cure.

Primary prevention occurs before biological onset (A) by eliminating causes of disease (e.g., prevention or delay of clinical CHD by improved more effective treatment of diabetes and hypertension, reduction of serum lipids, smoking cessation, exercise, or inhibition of platelet activation). Secondary prevention occurs between the "biological onset" (A) and "time of usual clinical detection" (B), as might occur with a true-positive EST or electron-beam computed tomography (EBCT) in an asymptomatic person. Tertiary prevention occurs subsequent to the "time of usual clinical detection" (B) but before either "severe illness develops" (C) or "death" (D), as occurs with management of CHD after its initial clinical manifestations of angina or acute myocardial infarction.

Length/Time Bias

Length/time bias refers to artifactually increased measured survival from selectively increased detection of less aggressive disease with better prognosis (Figures 6-5 and 6-6),[16] because patients with more aggressive disease are more likely to die between screening intervals.

Prevalence Bias

Prevalence bias is the unrepresentative impact of detection of prevalent cases in early screening cycles. The impact of incident cases increases with the number of subsequent screening cycles.

Adherence/Compliance Bias

Adherence/compliance bias is the overestimation of anticipated screening benefits as a result of enhanced participation by people more likely to adhere to recommended therapy. For example, the expected benefit from

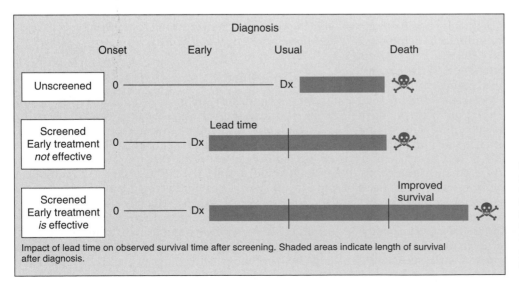

FIGURE 6-3. Lead time and lead time bias. Impact of lead time on observed survival time after screening. Shaded areas indicate length of survival after diagnosis (Dx). (Adapted from Fletcher RH, Fletcher SW, Wagner EH. *Clinical Epidemiology: The Essentials*, ed 2. Baltimore: Williams & Wilkins, 1982.)

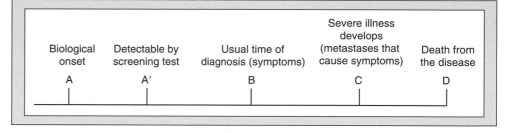

FIGURE 6-4. Continuum of disease natural history and critical point. (Adapted from Greenberg RS, Daniels SR, Flanders WD, Eley JW, Boring JR. Diagnostic testing, in *Medical Epidemiology*. Norwalk CT:Appleton & Lange, 1996, p 75.)

a screening program will be overestimated to the degree that adherence rates with screening tests in randomized trials exceed those observed in clinical practice.

All the preceding biases overestimate the perceived and estimated benefits of screening. Therefore, it is essential that promising screening tests and programs be rigorously evaluated by randomized clinical trials.

RECEIVER OPERATING CHARACTERISTIC (ROC) CURVES

An ROC curve is a plot of test sensitivity (TP rate) vs. 1–specificity (false-positive rate), because the criterion for a normal/abnormal test result (i.e., definition of positive test) is varied across the full range of clinically relevant values.[17-20] An ROC curve assesses the ability of the test–interpreter unit as opposed to the test itself, a particularly important distinction for cardiac imaging tests in which specifics of imaging agents, protocols, and technician and interpreter experience and skill exert considerable effect on test performance. Thus, comparison of diagnostic imaging performance across tests,

interpreters, and sites often is difficult and fraught with potential sources of bias.

Selection of a Test Cutoff Point

Diagnostic test sensitivity and specificity depend on the cutoff point chosen between a normal and abnormal test result.[13] Although for many tests a cutoff point may be selected such that no disease-free people are incorrectly categorized as diseased (specificity = 1.0), the same cutoff point erroneously classifies many people with disease as nondiseased, resulting in low test sensitivity. Conversely, a cutoff point selected so that all people with disease are correctly identified (sensitivity = 1.0) will misclassify disease-free people as diseased, resulting in low test specificity. An ROC curve is useful for identifying tradeoffs between true-positive and false-positive test results, thus identifying the optimal test cutoff point. Table 6-5 presents the tradeoffs between test sensitivity (TP rate), specificity (TN rate), and 1–specificity (false-positive rate) for alternative ST-segment positivity criteria for the EST (see reference 21 for additional information).

$$\frac{\text{Sensitivity}}{1 - \text{Specificity}} = \frac{\text{Net cost TN} - \text{Net cost FP}}{\text{Net cost TP} - \text{Net cost FN}} \times \frac{\text{Posttest probability no disease}}{\text{Pretest probability disease}}$$

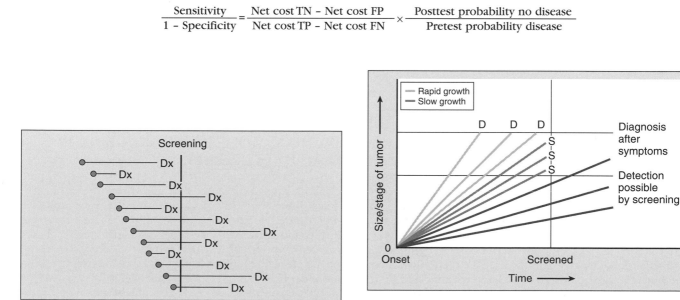

FIGURE 6-5. Length/time bias. Cases that progress rapidly from onset (●) to symptoms and diagnosis (Dx) are less likely to be detected during a screening examination. (From Fletcher RH, Fletcher WS, Wagner EH. *Clinical Epidemiology: The Essentials*. Baltimore: Williams & Wilkins, 1988, p 162.)

FIGURE 6-6. Length/time bias: rapidly growing tumors come to medical attention before screening, whereas more slowly growing tumors are detected by screening. D = Diagnosis after symptoms, S = diagnosis after screening. (From Fletcher RH, Fletcher WS, Wagner EH. *Clinical Epidemiology: The Essentials*. Baltimore: Williams & Wilkins, 1988, p 162.)

■ ■ ■

TABLE 6-5 RELATIONSHIP BETWEEN ST-SEGMENT DEPRESSION CRITERION AND EST SENSITIVITY AND SPECIFICITY

ST segment	Sensitivity	Specificity	1–Specificity
=0.5 mm	0.86	0.77	0.23
=1.0 mm	0.65	0.89	0.11
=1.5 mm	0.42	0.98	0.02
=2.0 mm	0.33	0.99	0.01
=2.5 mm	0.20	0.995	0.005

From Diamond GA, Forrester JS. Analysis of probability as an aid in the clinical diagnosis of coronary artery disease. *N Engl J Med* 1979; 300:1350.

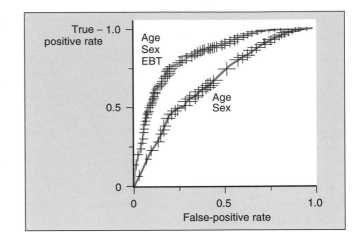

FIGURE 6-7. ROC curves for pretest model based on age and gender and for the combined model based on age, gender, and calcium scores. Vertical and horizontal bars represent 95% CIs for each plotted true-positive rate and false-positive rate derived from computed logistic probabilities. Addition of EBT increased the area under the ROC curve from 0.67 to 0.84 (*P* < 0.001). (From Budoff MJ, Diamond GA, Raggi P, Arad Y, Guerci AD, Callister TQ, Berman D. Continuous probabilistic prediction of angiographically significant coronary artery disease using electron beam tomography. *Circulation* 2002; 105:1791.)

Selection of the optimal diagnostic test cutoff point is a function of disease prevalence and estimated pretest probability of disease; test sensitivity and specificity; and the risks, costs, and benefits of correct and incorrect diagnoses (themselves a function of disease severity and the safety, effectiveness, and cost of therapeutic interventions).[13,22]

Published diagnostic test cutoff points generally are more subjectively determined and thus frequently may not be the most appropriate clinical value to use.

Comparison of Performance of Alternative Diagnostic Test Systems

The performance of alternative diagnostic tests must be compared over a range of cutoff points to avoid erroneous conclusions. An ROC curve demonstrates the inherent tradeoff between sensitivity and specificity, because the criteria for distinguishing between normal and abnormal results are varied over a range of cutoff points.[13] Thus, it is inappropriate and not informative to discuss either test sensitivity or specificity without consideration of the other, because test sensitivity always can be increased by adopting a more lenient positivity criteria, but only at the expense of decreased specificity.

When using ROC curves to compare diagnostic test performance, the diagnostic technology with the ROC curve highest and farthest to the left at a particular test result cutoff point is the preferred test (sensitivity is greater for any given level of specificity and vice versa). Over a range of cutoff points, the superior diagnostic technology is that with the greatest area under the ROC curve (or the greatest area under the clinically relevant range of the ROC curve).[23-25] Figure 6-7 shows the ROC curves for pretest model on the basis of age and gender and for the combined model on the basis of age, gender, and calcium scores. Of the three tests, the EBT exhibits the best diagnostic test performance, as indicated by its position up and to the left of the age and gender, indicating that for any level of sensitivity, the EBT has the highest specificity of the three tests and for any level of specificity, it has the highest test sensitivity. This is confirmed by the comparing the areas under the ROC curves (AUCs) for each of the three tests.

INFORMATION CONTENT

A diagnostic test's potential information content is a function of how much new additional information it provides to what is already known from the history, physical examination, and previously available diagnostic tests. A diagnostic test's incremental information is potentially greatest when one is most uncertain (intermediate prevalence or pretest probability) of the diagnosis being considered.[26] Even the best diagnostic test does not contribute new diagnostic information when one is certain that the disease either is present or absent. Conversely, diagnostic tests provide the greatest diagnostic information the more uncertain one is before testing. The information content of a diagnostic test is greater when one uses continuous criteria, such as when one considers the degree of positivity, than when using categorical (i.e., dichotomous test criteria) criteria.

DICHOTOMOUS VS. CONTINUOUSLY SCALED TEST RESULTS

Diagnostic tests commonly are interpreted as either positive or negative. However, dichotomous test results disregard valuable information, because a slightly abnormal test is more likely to be a false-positive result than a markedly abnormal test that is more likely to be a true-positive result. Similarly, a strongly negative test result is more likely to represent a TN than a slightly negative test result that is more likely to be a false-negative result. Borderline test results commonly are of limited diagnostic value. Most diagnostic test results can be continuously scaled or interpreted across a range of intervals. Thus, considering the degree of test abnormality provides more diagnostic information than a dichotomous ("positive" vs. "negative") result. For example, considering the extent of the electrocardiographic stress test positivity provides approximately one-third more diagnostic information than interpreting the test as either positive or negative (Figure 6-8).[27,28]

LIKELIHOOD RATIOS

The *likelihood ratio (LR)* of a test result provides the odds of the test result occurring in a person with disease compared with the test result occurring a person without disease. LRs provide a method to operationalize assessment of test performance over a range of test results, because they lend themselves to interpretation and use of interval-based (as opposed to dichotomous) diagnostic test results. LRs are not restricted to dichotomous outcomes but can be calculated for a range of test results, thereby facilitating use of continuous rather than dichotomous diagnostic test results in individual patients.

The LR of a positive test result (LR+) represents the TP/FP ratio for a test result and is obtained by calculating the probability of the positive test result among diseased subjects divided by probability of the same positive test result among nondiseased subjects.

$$LR = \frac{\text{Probability (result x)/disease}}{\text{Probability (result x)/Nondisease}}$$

An LR for a positive test >1 means that the test result increased the probability of disease (i.e., the posttest probability of disease is greater than that of the pretest probability of disease), with higher LR+ values indicating

a higher likelihood of disease. Conversely, a LR for a positive test <1 means that the test result lowered the probability of disease (i.e., the posttest probability of disease is lower than that of the pretest probability of disease). The higher a test's LR, the more likely the test result is to occur in a person with the disease as opposed to in a person who is free of the disease. The LR of a negative test (LR−) is the ratio of the likelihood of a negative test in all patients with disease to the likelihood of a negative test in all patients without disease, with greater LR− values indicating lower likelihood of disease.

By providing information for specific test results or ranges of test results, LRs maximize the information provided by diagnostic tests. For a given test result or interval:

$$LR+ = \frac{\text{Sensitivity}}{1-\text{Specificity}} = \frac{\text{Probability of T+/Disease}}{\text{Probability of T+/No disease}}$$

A literature-based pooled estimate of EST diagnostic performance for CHD in patients with chest pain syndromes for various magnitudes of exercise-induced horizontal or downward sloping ST-segment depression was developed by Diamond et al, with 50% diameter narrowing of at least one coronary artery as the reference standard.

By use of a dichotomous result criteria of ≥1.0 ST-segment depression as a positive test, the EST has a sensitivity = 0.65 and a specificity = 0.89. Use of interval LRs allows classification of results into multiple intervals (see Table 6-6).

Thus, by considering the *degree* of test positivity, the positive LR yields improved discrimination between those with and without disease.

Use of LRs in Clinical Practice

Although useful for evaluating diagnostic tests, sensitivity and specificity are difficult to use at the bedside because of the computational complexity of revising probabilities. Although odds and probabilities are interchangeable (Table 6-7 and Figure 6-3), likelihood ratios (which express test performance in terms of odds) are more use-

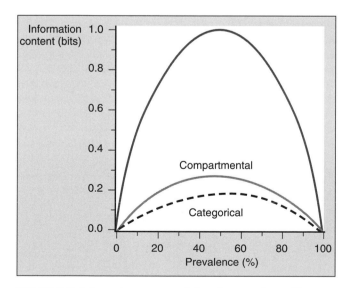

FIGURE 6-8. Information content of the electrocardiographic stress test: categorical vs. continuous diagnostic criteria. Improvement in information content by compartmental analysis. The area under the compartmental *(solid)* curve, average information content, is 41% greater than the area under the best categorical *(dashed)* curve (≥1.0). (From Diamond GA, Hirsch M, Forrester JS, Staniloff H, et al. Application of information theory to clinical diagnostic testing. *Circulation* 1981;63:915.)

■ ■ ■

TABLE 6-6   INTERVAL ELECTROCARDIOGRAPHIC STRESS TEST LIKELIHOOD RATIOS

EST positivity criteria (mm ST-segment depression)	Sensitivity (TP rate)	1–Specificity (FP rate)	Likelihood ratio (sensitivity/1–specificity)
0.0 ≤ ST <0.5	0.143	0.625	0.23
0.5 ≤ ST <1.0	0.208	0.227	0.92
1.0 ≤ ST <1.5	0.233	0.110	2.12
1.5 ≤ ST <2.0	0.088	0.021	4.19
2.0 ≤ ST <2.5	0.133	0.012	11.08
2.5 ≤ ST	0.195	0.005	39.0

Adapted from Diamond GA, Forrester JS. Analysis of probability as an aid in the clinical diagnosis of coronary-artery disease. *N Engl J Med* 1979; 300:1350.

TABLE 6-7 CONVERSION BETWEEN PROBABILITY AND ODDS

Odds	Probability
9:1	0.90
4:1	0.80
3:1	0.75
2:1	0.67
1:1	0.50
1:2	0.33
1:3	0.25
1:4	0.20
1:9	0.10

ful at the bedside, because odds ratios can be multiplied by each other and thus are easier to calculate at the bedside than revising probabilities. Thus, if the pretest odds of a disease being present are 1:3 and the LR of a positive test is 9:1, the posttest odds of disease are 3:1 (the product of the pretest odds and the test's LR). By providing information for specific test results or ranges of test results, LRs maximize the information provided by diagnostic tests.

$$\text{Pretest odds} \times \text{LR} = \text{Posttest odds}$$

where:

$$\text{Pretest odds} = \frac{\text{Pretest probability disease}}{1 - \text{Pretest probability disease}}$$

$$\text{Posttest odds} = \frac{\text{Posttest probability disease}}{1 - \text{Posttest probability disease}}$$

Thus, the posttest odds or probability of disease is a function of the pretest probability or odds and the LR of the test result (see Figure 6-9).

The relation between the posttest probability of CAD and the magnitude of EST ST-segment depression is illustrated in Figure 6-10 for a 45-year-old man and a 45-year-old woman with atypical angina.[14]

As likelihood ratios become more familiar to physicians and the number of tests for which likelihood ratio data availability increase, their use in clinical medicine will grow.

RELATIONSHIP OF ODDS AND PROBABILITY

LRs are odds ratios as opposed to probabilities. Odds and probabilities are related to each other by the formula:

$$\text{Odds} = \frac{\text{Probability}}{1 - \text{probability}}$$

and can be easily converted from one to the other, facilitating use of LRs in clinical practice.

A simple nomogram (Figure 6-11)[29] can be used to convert subjective estimated pretest probability of disease to calculated posttest disease probability for a given LR of a positive test (LR+).

THE USE OF TESTS IN COMBINATION

For most diagnostic problems, individual diagnostic tests are insufficient to guide clinical decisions. Therefore, multiple diagnostic tests are commonly used in combination to provide the diagnostic information required to cross patient management thresholds.

Multiple testing offers the advantages of increased information, improved diagnosis, speed of diagnosis, and convenience (patient, physician, laboratory), and, in some circumstances, reduced cost. However, multiple testing

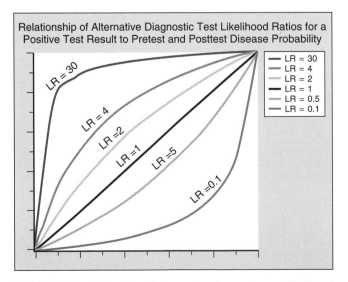

FIGURE 6-9. Relationship of alternative diagnostic test likelihood ratios for a positive test result to pretest and posttest disease probability. (Reference 29)

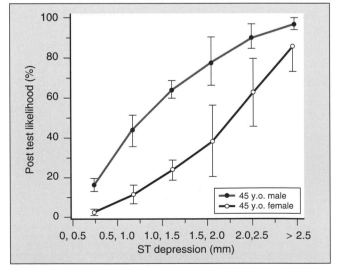

FIGURE 6-10. Posttest CAD probability for a 45-year-old man and a 45-year-old woman with atypical angina. (From Diamond GA, Forrester JS. Analysis of probability as an aid in the clinical diagnosis of coronary artery disease. *N Engl J Med* 1979; 300:1350.)

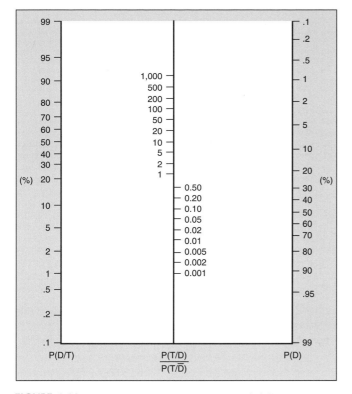

FIGURE 6-11. Nomogram to convert pretest probability to posttest probability using test likelihood ratios. (From Fagan RJ. Nomogram for Bayes's theorem [letter]. *N Engl J Med* 1975; 293:257.)

TABLE 6-8   COMBINATION TESTING: EST AND RNA

Test combination positivity criterion	Sensitivity	Specificity
EST	0.88	0.46
RNA	0.92	0.34
EST or RNA	0.96	0.29
EST & RNA	0.65	0.68

From Campos, et al. *Circulation* 1983; 67:1204. EST = electrocardiographic stress test, RNA = radionuclide angiograph.

the less additional information obtained from using tests in combination. Tests that measure different aspects of a suspected pathological condition or use different methods of diagnosis (e.g., serological tests and imaging tests) are more likely to provide independent information than test combinations that use similar methods.

Sequential vs. Concurrent Testing

When tests are used in combination, they can be performed either concurrently or sequentially, with performance of subsequent tests based on the results of previous tests. Concurrent test strategies result in faster diagnosis but involve performance of more tests than sequential testing. Thus, sequential testing is generally more appropriate when problem evolution is slow, when costs of slower diagnosis are lower such as in an outpatient setting, when test risk is high, and when the costs of delayed therapy are low. In contrast, concurrent testing is preferred when problem evolution is rapid, costs of delay are high such as in the inpatient setting, test risk is low, and costs of delayed treatment is high.

SUMMARY

Optimizing medical practice and health outcomes is dependent on accurate and efficient diagnosis. Diagnostic tests are useful to the degree they provide accurate, new information that will have a beneficial impact on subsequent diagnostic workup, clinical management, and health outcome. Thus, the goal of testing, singly or in combination, is to move one's estimate of disease probability either above the "test–treatment threshold" or below the "test–no treatment threshold."

All diagnostic tests are imperfect and subject to error. Thus, assessment and use of diagnostic tests must consider the ability of the test to discriminate between people with and without a disease and the clinical objective and safety, effectiveness, and cost of therapy. Test performance commonly is described in terms of the ability to correctly identify patients with disease (sensitivity) and without disease (specificity). Test sensitivity and specificity applied to pretest probability of disease provides an estimate of the probability that a positive test result accurately indicates disease and that a negative test result correctly indicates the absence of disease. The validity and reliability of test performance is undermined to the extent that test evaluation is biased by

also poses potential disadvantages. Some patients are exposed to the risks and costs of unnecessary additional tests and diagnostic and therapeutic delay. In addition, multiple testing is characterized by increased complexity of interpretation of discrepant test results (as the number of diagnostic tests performed increases, the opportunity for discrepancies among test results increases substantially). Although concordant test results increase confidence in a diagnosis, discordant results decrease confidence.

When multiple tests are performed, one must adopt criteria for interpreting discrepant test only combinations.[30,31] When conjunctive criteria are used, a test combination is interpreted as positive if *all* tests are positive. Conversely, disjunctive criteria interpret a test combination as positive if *any* of the tests performed are positive. Disjunctive criteria for interpreting test combinations increase sensitivity and decrease specificity relative to the individual tests, whereas conjunctive criteria decrease sensitivity but increase specificity relative to the individual tests (see Table 6-8).[31]

Thus, conjunctive criteria are preferred when false-positive results are undesirable and disjunctive testing when false-negative results are undesirable.

Test Correlation and Conditional Dependence[30,33,34]

Tests used in combination often are partially correlated with each other. The greater correlation among tests,

inappropriate selection of the spectrum of patients on whom the test is evaluated, selection of an inappropriate reference standard to establish the presence or absence of disease, and evaluation of diagnostic tests and biased referral of patients for the reference standard test. As a result of these various biases, diagnostic test performance frequently is misestimated (and commonly overestimated). The greater the discrepancy between study conditions and the setting in which the test will be used, the less applicable the study results are to clinical practice.

Tests with high sensitivity are preferred when the costs of missing a diagnosis are high (as in screening or when attempting to exclude a disease). Tests with high specificity are required before instituting risky or expensive therapy. Consideration of the degree of test abnormality (rather than interpreting tests as either positive or negative) increases the amount of diagnostic information obtained. When expressed in terms of a test's likelihood ratio it also facilitates estimation of the posttest probability (or odds) of disease.

Clinicians can optimize sensitivity and specificity either by careful selection among alternative tests with differing test performance characteristics, or by altering the cutoff point of a test to emphasize *either* sensitivity *or* specificity (but not both simultaneously). The use of tests in combination, requiring a series of tests to be positive to consider the diagnosis present, reduces sensitivity and increases specificity beyond that of any of the tests individually. In addition, considering the diagnosis to be present if any of a series of tests is positive increases sensitivity while reducing specificity beyond that of the individual tests. ROC curves facilitate identification of true-positive/false-positive tradeoffs, because one alters a test's cutoff point that is required to compare the diagnostic performance of alternative diagnostic tests.

REFERENCES

1. Pauker SAG, Kassirer JP. The threshold approach to clinical decision making. *N Engl J Med* 1980; 302:1109.
2. Black ER, Panzer RJ, Mayewski RJ, Griner PF. Characteristics of diagnostic tests and principles for their use in quantitative decision making, in Black ER, Bordley DR, Tape TG, Panzer RJ (eds): *Diagnostic Strategies For Common Medical Conditions*. Philadelphia: American College of Physicians, 1999; p 7.
3. Weiner DA, Ryan TJ, McCabe CH, et al. Exercise stress testing: correlation among history of angina, ST-segment response and prevalence of coronary artery disease in the Coronary Artery Surgery Study (CASS). *N Engl J Med* 1979; 301:230.
4. Galen RS, Gambino SR. *Beyond Normality: The Predictive Value and Efficiency of Medical Diagnosis*. New York, John Wiley & Sons, 1975.
5. Mulley AG. The selection and interpretation of diagnostic tests, in Goroll AH, May L, Mulley AG (eds): *Primary Care Medicine*. Philadelphia: Lippincott, 1987 p 7.
6. Begg CB, Greenes RA. Assessment of diagnostic tests when disease verification is subject to selection bias. *Biometrics* 1983; 39:207.
7. Gray R, Begg CB, Greenes RA. Construction of receiver operating characteristic curves when disease verification is subject to selection bias. *Med Decis Making* 1984; 4:151.
8. Ransohoff DF, Feinstein AR. Problems of spectrum and bias in evaluating the efficacy of diagnostic tests. *N Engl J Med* 1978; 299:929.
9. Froelicher VF, Myers J. *Exercise and the Heart*, ed 3. Philadelphia: WB Saunders, 1999.
10. Chaitman BR, Waters DD, Bourassa MG, Tubau JF, Wagniart P, Ferguson RJ. The importance of clinical subsets in interpreting maximal treadmill exercise test results: the role of multiple-lead ECG systems. *Circulation* 1979; 59:560.
11. Rozanski A, Diamond GA, Berman D, Forrester JS, Morris D, Swan HJ. The declining specificity of exercise radionuclide ventriculography. *N Engl J Med* 1983; 309:518.
12. Choi BC. Sensitivity and specificity of a single diagnostic test in the presence of work-up bias. *J Clin Epidemiol* 1992; 45:581.
13. Begg CB, Greenes RA, Iglewicz B. The influence of uninterpretability on the assessment of diagnostic tests. *J Chron Dis* 1986; 39:575.
14. Fletcher RH, Fletcher SW, Wagner EH. Prevention, in Fletcher RH, Fletcher SW, Wagner EH (eds): *Clinical Epidemiology: The Essentials*. Baltimore, Williams & Wilkins, 1988; p 161.
15. Greenberg RS, Daniels SR, Flanders WD, Eley JW, Boring JR. Diagnostic testing, in *Medical Epidemiology*. Norwalk, CT: Appleton & Lange, 1996, p 75.
16. Fletcher RH, Fletcher SW, Wagner EH. Prevention, in Fletcher RH, Fletcher SW, Wagner EH (eds): *Clinical Epidemiology: The Essentials*. Baltimore, Williams & Wilkins, 1988; p 162.
17. Green D, Swets J. *Signal Detection Theory and Psychophysics*. New York: John Wiley and Sons, 1966; p 45.
18. Lusted LB. Decision-making studies in patient management. *N Engl J Med* 1971; 284:416.
19. Goodenough DJ, Rossmann K, Lusted LB. Radiographic applications of receiver operating characteristic (ROC) curves. *Radiology* 1974; 110:89.
20. Swets JA, Pickett RM, Whitehead SF, et al. Assessment of diagnostic technologies. *Science* 1979; 205:753.
21. Diamond GA, Forrester JS. Analysis of probability as an aid in the clinical diagnosis of coronary-artery disease. *N Engl J Med* 1979; 300:1350.
22. McNeil BJ, Keeler E, Adelstein SJ. Primer on certain elements of medical decision making. *N Engl J Med* 1975; 293:211.
23. Hanley JA, McNeil BJ. The meaning and use of the area under a receiver operating characteristic (ROC) curve. *Radiology* 1982; 143:29.
24. Dorfman DD, Alf E. Maximum likelihood estimation of parameters of signal detection theory and determination of confidence intervals rating methods. *J Math Psych* 1969; 6:487.
25. Metz CE, Kronman HB. Statistical significance tests for binomial ROC curves. *J Math Psych* 1980; 22:218.
26. Shannon EC, Weaver W. T*he Mathematical Theory of Communication*. Urbana, IL: University of Illinois Press, 1949; p 125.
27. Diamond GA, Forrester JS, Hirsch M et al. Application of conditional probability analysis to the clinical diagnosis of coronary artery disease. *J Clin Invest* 1980; 65:1210.
28. Diamond GA, Hirsch M, Forrester JS, et al. Application of information theory to clinical diagnostic testing. The electrocardiographic stress test. *Circulation* 1981; 63:915.
29. Fagan TL. Nomogram for Bayes theorem. *N Engl J Med* 1975; 293:257.
30. Schwartz JS, Cebul RD. Strategies for using multiple tests, in *Teaching Medical Decision Making*. Philadelphia: Praeger Press, 1985.
31. Hershey JC, Cebul RD, Williams SV. Clinical guidelines for using two dichotomous tests. *Med Dec Making* 1986; 6:68.
32. Campos CT, Chul HW, D'Agostino HJ, Jones RH. Comparison of rest and exercise radionuclide angiography and exercise treadmill testing for the diagnosis of anatomically extensive coronary heart disease. *Circulation* 1983; 67:1204.
33. Schwartz JS, Kinosian B, Pierskalla W, Lee H. Strategies for screening blood for HIV virus antibody: use of a decision support system. *JAMA* 1990; 264:1704.
34. Schwartz JS, Dans PE, Kinosian BP. Human Immunodeficiency Virus test evaluation, performance, and use: proposals to make good tests better. *JAMA* 1988; 259:2574.

chapter 7

Cost-Effectiveness of Imaging Techniques in the Medical Marketplace

Kirsten E. Fleischmann

The availability of new, often expensive diagnostic and treatment modalities, as well as concern over the rising costs of health care, has led to increasing interest in cost-effectiveness analysis.[1-3] Once a tool of health policy and decision makers, cost-effectiveness analysis is now being used to weigh risks, benefits, and costs associated with various diagnostic and therapeutic strategies. Results of such analyses are used both by the individual clinician to help guide patient care and by policy makers concerned with the effective use of limited health care resources. Cost-effectiveness analysis can also help point out areas in which further research might be needed. As a first step to assessing the cost-effectiveness of imaging procedures in the medical marketplace, we will review some fundamental concepts of cost-effectiveness analysis. (See Box 7-1 for key terms.)

TYPES OF COST ANALYSES

Cost-effectiveness analysis seeks to balance costs, usually expressed in monetary terms, against effectiveness, generally couched in terms of medical benefits such as life-years saved, days of disease-free survival, or days of disability avoided[4-8] (Table 7-1). If the measure of effectiveness incorporates utility or quality of life, a cost/utility ratio is generated.[9] In contrast, cost/benefit analysis expresses both the costs and the benefits of treatment in monetary terms and often requires assigning a dollar value to the medical benefits described previously. Finally, cost-minimization analysis presumes that each of

the strategies considered is essentially equivalent from the standpoint of benefit and compares only costs among the various strategies. Of these, cost-effectiveness analysis with adjustment for quality-of-life considerations is most often used in medicine, and the subsequent discussion will focus on this type of analysis.

CLINICAL DECISION TREES

To analyze quantitatively the costs and benefits of various strategies, researchers often use a tool called a decision tree (Figure 7-1).[10] Such clinical decision trees explicitly outline the possible strategies and their outcomes. For example, for a patient seen with chest pain and electrocardiographic evidence of myocardial infarction, the clinical decision tree might include arms such as primary thrombolytic therapy, percutaneous transluminal coronary angiography, or conservative management without reperfusion therapy. Each arm is generally made up of a number of decision points known as nodes, which codify key decision-making points for the

■ ■ ■

BOX 7-1   KEY TERMS IN COST-EFFECTIVENESS ANALYSIS

Cost: Amount of resource required, usually expressed in monetary units

Effectiveness: Health benefit achieved, commonly expressed in units such as the number of lives saved, the days of disability avoided, the years of life saved, etc.

Clinical decision model: A model of the clinical problem, usually constructed in the form of a decision tree, in which various diagnostic or therapeutic options are outlined, and the possible clinical events and outcomes are enumerated and assigned probabilities and utilities. This can be used to analyze the cost or health benefit of various options.

Utility: The benefit associated with a specific outcome. By convention, perfect health is assigned a value of 1, whereas death is assigned a value of 0.

Sensitivity analysis: An analysis in which certain parameters in the clinical decision model are systematically varied over reasonable ranges, so as to determine whether the results of the model are significantly affected. This is especially important if there is significant uncertainty or variability in the values of certain parameters.

QALY: Quality-adjusted life-year.

Incremental cost-effectiveness: Additional cost-effectiveness of a new strategy compared with the baseline strategy.

From Key terms in cost-effectiveness analysis (modified from Wang S and Fleischmann KE, in Otto (ed): *Practice of Clinical Echocardiography*, Second Edition. Philadelphia: WB Saunders, 2002.)

■ ■ ■

TABLE 7-1   COST, EFFECTS, UTILITY, AND BENEFITS OF TREATING PATIENTS WITH DISEASE X WITH TWO ALTERNATE STRATEGIES, TREATMENT A AND TREATMENT B

Strategy	Treatment costs	Effectiveness (life expectancy)	Utility (Quality of life)	Utility (Quality-adjusted life expectancy)	Benefits
Treatment A	$20,000	4.5 y	0.80	3.6*	$4000
Treatment B	$10,000	3.5 y	0.90	3.15	$2000

$$\text{Incremental cost-effectiveness ratio} = \frac{\$20,000 - \$10,000}{4.5 \text{ years} - 3.5 \text{ years}} = \$10,000 \text{ per life-year gained}$$

$$\text{Incremental cost-utility ratio} = \frac{\$20,000 - \$10,000}{3.6 \text{ QALYs} - 3.15 \text{ QALYs}} = \$22,222 \text{ per QALY gained}$$

$$\text{Incremental cost/benefit ratio} = \frac{\$20,000 - \$10,000}{\$4000 - \$2,000} = 5$$

*QALYs = quality-adjusted life years.
From Detsky et al. Comparison of various types of cost analyses for patients undergoing one of 2 treatments, Treatment A and Treatment B. (Reproduced with permission from *Ann Intern Med* 1990; 113:147.)

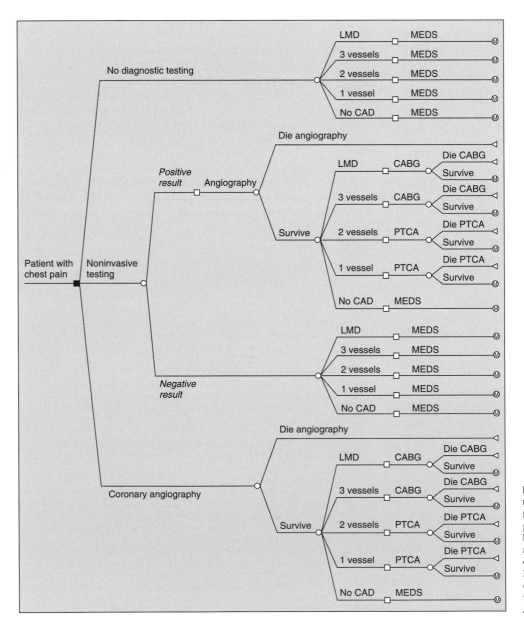

FIGURE 7-1. Example of a decision tree outlining diagnostic strategies for a patient initially seen with chest pain. CABG = coronary artery bypass grafting; CAD = coronary artery disease; LMD = left main disease; MEDS = medical therapy; PTCA = percutaneous transluminal coronary angioplasty. (Reproduced with permission from Kuntz et al. *Ann Intern Med* 1999; 130:709.)

clinician. Each arm is also assigned an outcome on the basis of risks and benefits of the strategy outlined. Such an estimate of the benefits of treatment is critically dependent on the assumptions made both in structuring the decision tree and in assigning estimates of the risks, benefits, and costs of certain actions. (See also the section on sensitivity analysis to follow.)

By calculating effectiveness for each strategy on the basis of its risk and benefit and a cost on the basis of its financial ramifications, cost-effectiveness analysis may be used to compare various strategies in terms of effectiveness and costs. Certain strategies might even be cost saving,[11,12] that is, they both save money and increase effectiveness compared with the baseline strategy. However, most interventions and strategies will obtain greater benefit or effectiveness at a cost. Therefore, the goal of most cost-effectiveness analyses is to find the lowest cost strategy that achieves a desired level of effectiveness or, conversely, to find a strategy that achieves the greatest effectiveness at a given cost. As is implicit from the prior discussion, cost-effectiveness analysis is generally conducted by comparing various strategies against a current or baseline strategy. In this case, the incremental benefit and cost over the baseline strategy is calculated (Table 7-1).

CALCULATION OF BENEFIT

The calculation of benefit assigned to a treatment strategy is generally derived from the medical literature. In its simplest form, survival data associated with each strategy may be used in their raw form. Often, however, an adjustment for patients' quality of life is added, leading to the metric of quality-adjusted life-year saved or "QALY."[13] Less commonly, other metrics of benefit are used, such as days of disability avoided.

Adjustment for quality of life seeks to quantify the reduction in the benefit of a diagnostic or treatment strategy when the health status of the patient is compromised by disability, pain, or other factors. QALY has been defined as "the number of years at full health that would be valued equivalently to the number of years of life as experienced" in less than perfect health. The degree of decrement associated with a given health state can be measured in a variety of ways. Commonly, utility of a given health state is measured by quantifying patients' perception of disease and their preferences for certain health outcomes. In its simplest form, utility can be measured on a linear scale, with death at one end and perfect health at the other.[14,15] Each patient or subject is then asked to mark where in that range a health state falls in terms of its desirability. A more complex means of measuring utility involves the "standard reference gamble."[16] In this method, the patient or subject is given a hypothetical between a compromised health state (for example, life with moderate angina) and a course of action that is likely to improve but in some cases might worsen the situation (for example, percutaneous transluminal coronary angioplasty). The patient is given a probability for a successful procedure and being restored to good health and the converse probability that a serious complication or death would be involved. The probabilities for favorable and unfavorable outcomes are varied, until a level of "indifference" is reached, which helps define the utility or value of the health state in which the patient lives with angina.

A common variation of the standard gamble approach is the time tradeoff.[17,18] In this situation, a patient or subject is asked whether he or she would prefer a given amount of time in perfect health or a longer period of time in a less than perfect health state. Returning to our angina example, a patient might be asked whether he preferred 10 years with mild angina or 9 years in perfect health. The time in perfect health is adjusted until the patient finds the two choices equivalent, which defines the utility of the health state. If, for example, the subject rated 10 years with angina as equivalent to 8 years in perfect health, the utility of the angina state would be 0.8. By convention, death is assigned a value of 0, whereas perfect health is scored as 1.0.

CALCULATION OF COSTS

Calculation of costs is also often based on the medical literature or on medical accounting systems. Costs may be of several types. For example, direct costs[19] might include such things as physician and staff salaries, whereas indirect costs may include such things as utilities, overhead, or time lost from work. In these analyses, costs should be distinguished from charges,[20,21] which are the set fee that third party-payers are charged to pay for a procedure or treatment. True costs may be derived from hospital accounting systems or other sources. Because they can be difficult to obtain, charges or charges adjusted for a ratio of costs to charges are often used as their surrogate.[22] However, charges, which are usually fixed for a given institution, may not reflect accurately the cost of a given procedure to the institution and often do not take into account the drop in cost that may be associated with increased volume. In addition, many analyses consider only direct costs rather than important nonmedical costs such as days of work missed, which might contribute importantly to the economic costs of a given strategy from society's perspective. Therefore, it is critical to define in each cost-effectiveness analysis the perspective from which the analysis is conducted, be it that of an individual clinician, an institution, a third-party payer, or society itself.

DISCOUNTING

In most analyses, costs and benefits that accrue early in a course of treatment are valued more highly than those that occur in the future.[23] For example, a 4-year strategy that costs $20,000 in the first year is considered more costly than one costing $5000 in year 1 and $5000 in each of the 3 successive years, because current money is generally valued more highly than money spent in future. Similarly, a strategy that saves 5 QALYs immediately is valued more highly than the one in which there is a downstream benefit of 5 QALYs after 10 years of treatment. After all, many things might happen in the intervening years of treatment that could keep a patient from realizing the full benefit of therapy. To account for this, most analyses use a convention known as "discounting." That is, future costs and benefits are discounted by a set amount, usually approximately 3% to 5% yearly, to reflect the effect of time on costs and benefits.

SENSITIVITY ANALYSIS

Because cost-effectiveness analysis is dependent on the estimates of the risks, benefits, and costs of each strategy, most cost-effectiveness analyses include a variety of sensitivity analyses for critical variables[10,24,25] (Figure 7-2). These analyses allow values for important variables to range within reasonable estimates and determine the effect on the conclusions of the analyses. For example, if mortality is one of the outcomes of interest, and meta-analysis of the published literature suggests an average all-cause mortality of 25%, one might use that value in a base-case analysis. However, if the literature suggests that the range of mortality may be as low as 10% and as high as 40%, a sensitivity analysis, which reruns the analysis within these ranges, would be conducted to ensure that the conclusions of the paper are robust within reasonable ranges. More than one variable can also be tested at one time, leading to so-called two-way or three-way sensitivity analyses that provide an idea of what the results of the analysis would be with various combinations of data (Figure 7-3).

MARKOV MODELS

One special type of analysis often seen in the literature is called a Markov or state transition model.[26,27] In the Markov model, a simulation is performed that allows a cohort of hypothetical patients to progress from one health state to another with time in proportion to their probability estimates. For example, in a cost-effectiveness analysis of stenting as a treatment for symptomatic single-vessel coronary disease,[28] a Markov model was designed to model long-term outcomes after the procedure. Patients could remain stable, have restenosis develop, have chronic angina develop, or die, in relation to the probabilities for each outcome. At the end of each time period or cycle, survivors could remain in the same state of health or could transition to another state of health. This Markov model allows estimate of the long-term prognosis after the procedure.

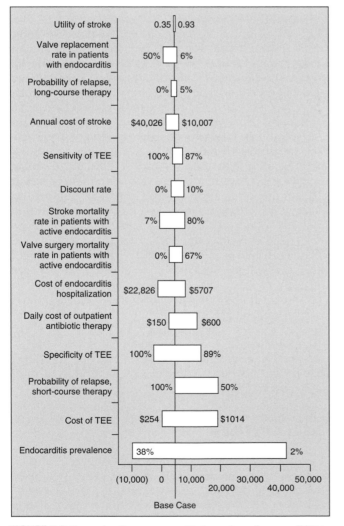

FIGURE 7-2. Example of one-way sensitivity analyses for use of TEE to guide antibiotic duration of therapy in catheter-associated *Staphylococcus aureus* bacteremia. The range of inputs for each variable is noted at the ends of each bar. (Reproduced with permission from Rosen et al. *Ann Intern Med* 1999; 130:810.)

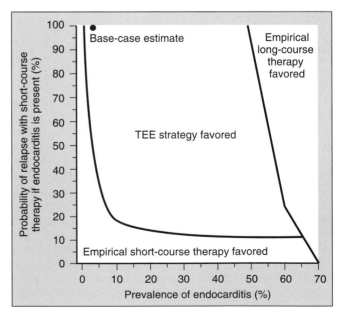

FIGURE 7-3. Graph of a two-way sensitivity analysis exploring the effect of the prevalence of endocarditis and probability of relapse on results of a TEE-guided strategy for determining duration of antibiotic therapy in catheter-associated *Staphylococcus aureus* bacteremia. (Reproduced with permission from Rosen et al. *Ann Intern Med* 1999; 130:810.)

DIAGNOSTIC TESTING AND THE BAYESIAN APPROACH

The cost-effectiveness of imaging techniques in the medical marketplace is also dependent on the setting in which the test is used.[29] In assessing a patient's symptoms, a clinician implicitly assesses a pretest probability of disease, an estimation of the clinical probability that a given disease is present. For example, in the patient with chest pain, a description of the quality of the discomfort, in conjunction with risk factors such as age and gender, may lead a physician to conclude that the patient's symptoms are most likely typical angina, or, conversely, an atypical angina or even noncardiac chest pain. This pretest likelihood of disease affects the physician's choice of diagnostic testing. A patient in whom angina and severe underlying coronary artery disease is suspected with a high degree of certainty may be referred directly to cardiac catheterization, whereas one in whom the diagnosis is less certain may first undergo noninvasive testing.

Combining the pretest probability of disease with the diagnostic accuracy of the test itself allows an estimate of the probability of disease after a given test result, or posttest probability of disease. The relationship between the pretest probability, the performance of the diagnostic test, and the posttest probability of disease is given by Bayes' theorem.[30] Applying this formula to our chest pain example, a 55-year-old man is seen with classical exertional chest pain at his physician's office (Figure 7-4). His physician diagnoses typical angina with roughly an 80% to 85% likelihood of underlying coronary artery disease. On the basis of the literature for exercise testing, this probability will rise to 95% after a positive exercise electrocardiogram and even higher, to approximately 99%, after a positive exercise scintigraphy. Conversely, a negative exercise test lowers the posttest probability of disease, but only to approximately 60%. Even with a negative scintigraphy, the residual estimated probability of disease, 30%, might still be high enough for the physician to choose to treat for angina or pursue further diagnostic testing. Therefore, a test is most useful from a diagnostic perspective when a negative or positive test result will change the probability of disease sufficiently to change management. Of course, diagnostic efficacy is not the only reason a diagnostic test may be ordered. Other valid reasons such as determination of severity of disease, expected prognosis, or the efficacy of treatment may also be helpful in caring for the patient.

Building on this theoretical foundation, the rest of the chapter will give several examples of the use of cost-effectiveness analysis of imaging techniques. These examples are not meant to be exhaustive but rather to illustrate common clinical problems that have been approached by cost-effectiveness analysis.

COST-EFFECTIVENESS OF IMAGING IN PATIENTS WITH CHEST PAIN

The cost-effectiveness of various strategies commonly used in the evaluation of chest pain was analyzed.[10] In this analysis, the published data to estimate the cost-effectiveness of five strategies for patients seen with chest pain without a history of myocardial infarction were used. It was assumed that patients were able to perform exercise stress testing. The five strategies included no testing, exercise electrocardiography, exercise echocardiography, or exercise single photon emission computed tomography (SPECT) as a first-line test, and coronary angiography alone (Figure 7-1). Direct coronary angiography compared favorably with a strategy of noninvasive testing (i.e., exercise echocardiography followed by angiography if the test is positive) when the probability of disease was high, for example, in a 55-year-old man with typical angina. In this situation, the incremental cost-effectiveness ratio for angiography was $36,400 per life-year saved, less than many well-accepted interventions. In patients with mild to moderate risk of coronary artery disease, noninvasive testing resulted in reasonable cost-effectiveness ratios. For example, in 55-year-old men with atypical chest pain, exercise echocardiography compared with standard exercise electrocardiography costs an additional $41,900 per QALY. In the event that exercise echocardiography was not available or not desired, exercise SPECT in these patients was associated with a cost-effectiveness ratio of $54,800 per QALY saved. Thus, noninvasive testing was preferred when the a priori, or pretest, probability of coronary artery disease was mild to moderate, whereas an invasive strategy was associated with favorable cost-effectiveness ratios for patients at high risk.

In a similar analysis of cost-effectiveness of alternate test strategies for the diagnosis of coronary disease by Garber and Solomon,[31] the effect of varying modeling strategies on analysis results is seen. Their analysis explored the relative cost-effectiveness of five noninvasive tests: exercise electrocardiography, planar scintigraphy, SPECT, stress echocardiography with a variety of stressors, and positron emission tomography (PET), all

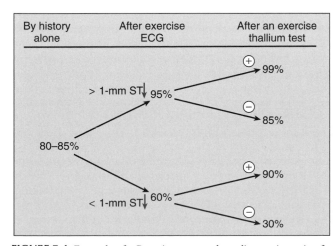

FIGURE 7-4. Example of a Bayesian approach to diagnostic testing for a patient with typical angina and a high probability of disease. The approximate posttest probability of coronary artery disease is given for each test result. (Reproduced with permission from Goldman L. Noninvasive tests in cardiology, in Branch WT (ed): *Office Practice of Medicine.* Philadelphia: WB Saunders, 1987.)

compared with a strategy of initial angiography. By use of this model, as well as slightly different estimates for the risks, benefits, and costs of various diagnostic tests, they found that stress echocardiography was cost-saving (that is, it improved outcomes and reduced costs) in many cases relative to stress electrocardiography and planar scintigraphy. The incremental cost-effectiveness ratio for SPECT relative to echocardiography was $75,000 per QALY and that of PET was $640,000 per QALY relative to SPECT. Immediate angiography in these patients with an intermediate pretest probability had an incremental cost-effectiveness ratio of $94,000 per QALY compared with SPECT. Thus, they concluded that noninvasive testing with stress echocardiography, or stress SPECT if local diagnostic accuracy and costs favor this approach, are appropriate diagnostic tests for patients at intermediate pretest risk of coronary disease. Immediate angiography may also be appropriate in some patients. An example of a cost-minimization approach to coronary artery disease management is given in the work of Shaw et al.[32] In this cohort study, researchers enrolled more than 11,000 patients with stable angina referred either for cardiac catheterization or for stress myocardial perfusion imaging. They matched a series of patients slated for each test by their clinical characteristics and pretest probability of coronary disease and then compared the costs of their care. Composite costs of care over 3 years for patients undergoing direct cardiac catheterization were compared with undergoing an initial stress scintigraphy test followed by selective catheterization for patients deemed at high risk. Because the rates of cardiac death or myocardial infarction were statistically similar, a cost-minimization analysis, presuming that benefits of the two strategies were similar, was pursued. In this observational study, the 3-year costs of care for direct cardiac catheterization patients ranged from $2878 to $4579 compared with $2387 to $3010 in patients undergoing initial stress perfusion testing. This difference was statistically significant. One potential explanation for these differences is found in the fact that coronary revascularization rates were higher for patients undergoing initial catheterization, even in patients at relatively low or intermediate risk of disease.

COST-EFFECTIVENESS OF TRANSESOPHAGEAL ECHOCARDIOGRAPHY (TEE) IN PATIENTS WITH SUSPECTED ENDOCARDITIS

As outlined earlier, what is considered "cost-effective" is often driven strongly by the pretest probability that disease is present. Another example of this comes from the work of Heidenreich et al,[33] who assessed the cost-effectiveness of TEE in the diagnosis of endocarditis. In this work, the authors constructed a decision tree and Markov model to simulate both costs and outcomes for patients undergoing evaluation for endocarditis. With a primary analysis of a 45-year-old man with a pretest probability of endocarditis of 20%, transesophageal imaging was cost saving compared with transthoracic echocardiography as a primary diagnostic test. That is,

TEE both improved quality-adjusted life expectancy and reduced costs. The strategy of transesophageal imaging without antecedent transthoracic imaging was optimal over a wide range of pretest probabilities ranging from 4% to 60%. Initial transthoracic imaging was the optimal strategy only over a very narrow range in patients with low probabilities of disease (i.e., 2% to 3%). These authors concluded that cost-effectiveness of transesophageal imaging was dependent on the a priori risk of disease but that transesophageal imaging was associated with favorable cost-effectiveness ratios over a wide range of pretest probabilities, well within the range seen in practice.

COST-EFFECTIVENESS OF TEE IN ASSESSING THE LENGTH OF TREATMENT FOR CATHETER-ASSOCIATED BACTEREMIA

Cost-effectiveness analysis is also useful in that immediate costs associated with one strategy can be weighed against downstream savings, either in terms of cost or improved outcomes. For example, Rosen et al[34] conducted a decision analysis and cost-effectiveness analysis to assess the cost-effectiveness of TEE for guiding the duration of therapy in catheter-related bacteremia with *Staphylococcus aureus*. The strategies compared an empiric short-course or prolonged course of intravenous antibiotics with a TEE-guided approach (with short-course therapy if the TEE was negative and longer duration therapy if the TEE was positive). In the base-case analysis, the TEE-guided strategy cost $4938 per QALY compared with empiric short-course therapy (Table 7-2). In contrast, an empiric 4-week course of antibiotic strategy was associated with cost-effectiveness ratios in excess of $1 million per QALY gained. A TEE-guided strategy was associated with reasonable cost-effectiveness ratios over a wide range of sensitivity analyses (Figures 7-2 and 7-3), suggesting that TEE to guide antibiotic duration is a cost-effective approach. In this case, addition of an extra diagnostic test (the TEE) is associated with additional costs. However, as the analysis showed, these costs were largely offset by potential cost savings in those patients who could be treated adequately with a shorter course of antibiotics.

COST-EFFECTIVENESS OF NEWER DIAGNOSTIC STRATEGIES

Assessment of cost and outcomes can also help guide development of newer diagnostic strategies. A technique called Challenge ROC (receiver operating characteristic) analysis has been used to estimate the diagnostic performance of imaging modalities such as echocardiography,[35] perfusion imaging,[36] magnetic resonance imaging,[37] or electron beam computed tomography[38] and the performance they must attain to be cost effective for the diagnosis of coronary artery disease.[39] It is estimated that newer techniques must be relatively inexpensive (i.e., less than $1000) and have excellent

■ ■ ■

TABLE 7-2   COST-EFFECTIVENESS OF TEE GUIDING DURATION OF ANTIBIOTIC THERAPY

Management strategy	Cost $	Effectiveness QALY	Cost $	Incremental effectiveness QALY	Cost-effectiveness ratio $/QALY
			TOTAL		
Discounted at 3% (base case)					
Short-course therapy	9830	5.424	—	—	—
TEE	10 051	5.469	219	0.0447	4938
Long-course therapy	14,136	5.471	4085	0.0024	1,667,971
Discounted at 5%					
Short-course therapy	9796	4.439	—	—	—
TEE	10 023	4.480	228	0.0411	5547
Long-course therapy	14 108	4.482	4085	0.0022	1,862,141
Undiscounted					
Short-course therapy	9895	8.418	—	—	—
TEE	10,103	8.470	208	0.0518	4013
Long-course therapy	14,187	8.473	4084	0.0031	1,335,863

TEE = transesophageal echocardiography; QALY = quality-adjusted life-year.
From Rosen et al. Results of a base case analysis of transesophageal echocardiography to guide duration of antibiotic treatment in catheter-associated *Staphylococcus aureus* bacteremia. *Ann Intern Med* 1999; 130:810.

sensitivity and specificity to compete effectively as a first-line technique for the diagnosis of coronary artery disease.

SUMMARY

These examples demonstrate that the tenets of cost-effectiveness analysis can help inform medical decision making, for individual patients and for the health care system and society at large. Although cost-effectiveness analysis, with its emphasis on both costs and benefits, is sometimes seen as being at odds with the priorities of a clinician treating an individual patient,[8] such analyses should be seen as contributing to the process of providing excellent care. Understanding the principles of cost-effectiveness analysis will allow physicians to optimize their choice of imaging modalities and lead to improved care both for the individual and for society at large.

REFERENCES

1. Fauchier L, Babuty D, Cosnay P, Fauchier JP. Cardiac resynchronization in chronic heart failure: some considerations about the cost-effectiveness. *Eur Heart J* 2003; 24:879.
2. Wilson K, Marriott J, Fuller S, Lacey L, Gillen D. A model to assess the cost effectiveness of statins in achieving the UK National Service Framework target cholesterol levels. *Pharmacoeconomics* 2003; 21(Suppl)1:1.
3. O'Hagan A, Stevens JW. Bayesian methods for design and analysis of cost-effectiveness trials in the evaluation of health care technologies. *Stat Methods Med Res* 2002; 11:469.
4. Weinstein MC, O'Brien B, Hornberger J, et al. Principles of good practice for decision analytic modeling in health-care evaluation: report of the ISPOR Task Force on Good Research Practices—Modeling Studies. *Value Health* 2003; 6:9.
5. Kupersmith J, Holmes-Rovner M, Hogan A, Rovner D, Gardiner J. Cost-effectiveness analysis in heart disease, Part I: General principles. *Prog Cardiovasc Dis* 1994; 37:161.
6. Kupersmith J, Holmes-Rovner M, Hogan A, Rovner D, Gardiner J. Cost-effectiveness analysis in heart disease, Part II: Preventive therapies. *Prog Cardiovasc Dis* 1995; 37:243-71.
7. Kupersmith J, Holmes-Rovner M, Hogan A, Rovner D, Gardiner J. Cost-effectiveness analysis in heart disease, Part III: Ischemia, congestive heart failure, and arrhythmias. *Prog Cardiovasc Dis* 1995; 37:307.
8. Detsky AS, Naglie IG. A clinician's guide to cost-effectiveness analysis. *Ann Intern Med* 1990; 113:147.
9. Capomolla S, Febo O, Ceresa M, et al. Cost/utility ratio in chronic heart failure: comparison between heart failure management program delivered by day-hospital and usual care. *J Am Coll Cardiol* 2002; 40:1259.
10. Kuntz KM, Fleischmann KE, Hunink MG, Douglas PS. Cost-effectiveness of diagnostic strategies for patients with chest pain. *Ann Intern Med* 1999; 130:709.
11. Goldman L, Weinstein MC, Goldman PA, Williams LW. Cost-effectiveness of HMG-CoA reductase inhibition for primary and secondary prevention of coronary heart disease. *JAMA* 1991; 265:1145.
12. Eisenberg JM. Clinical economics. A guide to the economic analysis of clinical practices. *JAMA* 1989; 262:2879.
13. Johannesson M, Pliskin JS, Weinstein MC. Are healthy-years equivalents an improvement over quality-adjusted life years? *Med Decis Making* 1993; 13:281.
14. Feeny D, Furlong W, Torrance GW, et al. Multiattribute and single-attribute utility functions for the health utilities index mark 3 system. *Med Care* 2002; 40:113.
15. Torrance GW. Looking back and looking forward: viewed through the eyes of George Torrance. *Med Decis Making* 2002; 22:178.
16. Morimoto T, Fukui T. Utilities measured by rating scale, time trade-off, and standard gamble: review and reference for health care professionals. *J Epidemiol* 2002; 12:160.
17. Melsop KA, Boothroyd DB, Hlatky MA. Quality of life and time trade-off utility measures in patients with coronary artery disease. *Am Heart J* 2003; 145:36.
18. Dolan P, Stalmeier P. The validity of time trade-off values in calculating QALYs: constant proportional time trade-off versus the proportional heuristic. *J Health Econ* 2003; 22:445.
19. Finkler SA. The distinction between cost and charges. *Ann Intern Med* 1982; 96:102.
20. Finkler SA. Allocating joint costs. *Hosp Cost Manag Account* 1992; 4:1.
21. Finkler SA. Total quality management: cost accounting specifics. Part 2. *Hosp Cost Manag Account* 1993; 5:1.
22. Mark DB, Hlatky MA, Califf RM, et al. Cost effectiveness of thrombolytic therapy with tissue plasminogen activator as compared with streptokinase for acute myocardial infarction. *N Engl J Med* 1995; 332:1418.
23. Durand-Zaleski I, Zaleski S. DEALE-ing and discounting: a simple way to compute the accrued costs of preventive strategies. *Med Decis Making* 1994; 14:98.

24. Sutton R, Bourgeois I. Cost benefit analysis of single and dual chamber pacing for sick sinus syndrome and atrioventricular block. An economic sensitivity analysis of the literature. *Eur Heart J* 1996; 17:574.

25. Laird NM, Weinstein MC, Stason WB. Sample-size estimation: a sensitivity analysis in the context of a clinical trial for treatment of mild hypertension. *Am J Epidemiol* 1979; 109:408.

26. Boll AP, Severens JL, Verbeek AL, van der Vliet JA. Mass screening on abdominal aortic aneurysm in men aged 60 to 65 years in The Netherlands. Impact on life expectancy and cost-effectiveness using a Markov model. *Eur J Vasc Endovasc Surg* 2003; 26:74.

27. Cooper NJ, Sutton AJ, Mugford M, Abrams KR. Use of Bayesian Markov chain Monte Carlo methods to model cost-of-illness data. *Med Decis Making* 2003; 23:38.

28. Cohen DJ, Breall JA, Ho KK, et al. Evaluating the potential cost-effectiveness of stenting as a treatment for symptomatic single-vessel coronary disease. Use of a decision-analytic model. *Circulation* 1994; 89:1859.

29. Spiegelhalter DJ, Myles JP, Jones DR, Abrams KR. Bayesian methods in health technology assessment: a review. *Health Technol Assess* 2000; 4:1.

30. Epstein SE. Implications of probabilty analysis on strategy used for noninvasive detection of coronary artery disease. *Am J Cardiol* 1980; 46:491.

31. Garber AM, Solomon NA. Cost-effectiveness of alternative test strategies for the diagnosis of coronary artery disease. *Ann Intern Med* 1999; 130:719.

32. Shaw LJ, Hachamovitch R, Berman DS, et al. The economic consequences of available diagnostic and prognostic strategies for the evaluation of stable angina patients: an observational assessment of the value of precatheterization ischemia. Economics of Noninvasive Diagnosis (END) Multicenter Study Group. *J Am Coll Cardiol* 1999; 33:661.

33. Heidenreich PA, Masoudi FA, Maini B, et al. Echocardiography in patients with suspected endocarditis: a cost-effectiveness analysis. *Am J Med* 1999; 107:198.

34. Rosen AB, Fowler VG Jr, Corey GR, et al. Cost-effectiveness of transesophageal echocardiography to determine the duration of therapy for intravascular catheter-associated *Staphylococcus aureus* bacteremia. *Ann Intern Med* 1999; 130:810.

35. Wagner RF, Wear KA, Perez JE, McGill JB, Schechtman KB, Miller JG. Quantitative assessment of myocardial ultrasound tissue characterization through receiver operating characteristic analysis of Bayesian classifiers. *J Am Coll Cardiol* 1995; 25:1706.

36. Fintel DJ, Links JM, Brinker JA, Frank TL, Parker M, Becker LC. Improved diagnostic performance of exercise thallium-201 single photon emission computed tomography over planar imaging in the diagnosis of coronary artery disease: a receiver operating characteristic analysis. *J Am Coll Cardiol* 1989; 13:600.

37. Kersting-Sommerhoff BA, Diethelm L, Teitel DF, et al. Magnetic resonance imaging of congenital heart disease: sensitivity and specificity using receiver operating characteristic curve analysis. *Am Heart J* 1989; 118:155.

38. O'Rourke RA, Brundage BH, Froelicher VF, et al. American College of Cardiology/American Heart Association Expert Consensus document on electron-beam computed tomography for the diagnosis and prognosis of coronary artery disease. *Circulation* 2000; 102:126.

39. Goldman L. Cost-effectiveness perspectives in coronary heart disease. *Am Heart J* 1990; 119:73; discussion 739.

Coronary Heart Disease—Acute Coronary Syndromes

John D. Rutherford
Alan C. Yeung
Sharon Coplen Reimold
DuWayne L. Willett
Bonnie L. Hiatt
David P. Lee
Joaquin E. Cigarroa
Ronald M. Peshock

Acute Myocardial Infarction with Electrocardiographic
   ST-Segment Elevations
Non ST-Segment Elevation AMI
Ischemic Ventricular Dysfunction
Stress Testing
Differential Diagnosis
Complications

The term *acute coronary syndrome* refers to symptoms compatible with acute myocardial ischemia and includes acute myocardial infarction (AMI) (ST-segment elevation and depression, Q wave and non-Q wave) and unstable angina.[1] The National Heart Attack Alert Program has developed guidelines for the rapid identification of such patients by emergency department registration clerks or triage nurses, which implies that they should be placed in an environment that allows continuous electrocardiographic monitoring, defibrillation capability, and that an electrocardiogram can be obtained and interpreted within 10 minutes. In some centers "chest pain units" or "short-stay units" are used to facilitate this activity. The most urgent early priority is to identify patients with AMI who qualify for immediate coronary reperfusion therapy and to recognize other serious medical conditions (e.g., aortic dissection, spontaneous pneumothorax, acute pericarditis, myocarditis, cholecystitis).

ACUTE MI WITH ELECTROCARDIOGRAPHIC ST-SEGMENT ELEVATIONS

Approximately 25% to 45% of patients with acute coronary syndromes are seen with prolonged chest pain within the previous 12 hours and 12-lead electrocardiograms with ST-segment elevations or a left bundle-branch block (LBBB) pattern and are ideally treated with fibrinolytic therapy or direct coronary revascularization usu-

ally by percutaneous transluminal coronary angioplasty (PTCA) or percutaneous coronary intervention (PCI). Guidelines produced by the American College of Cardiology and American Heart Association[1] provide general agreement, and evidence, that certain treatments or procedures are beneficial, useful, and effective in acute coronary syndromes. Fibrinolysis is indicated in patients with ST elevations >0.1 mV in two or more contiguous electrocardiographic leads in patients less than 75 years who had the onset of persistent, continuous chest discomfort within the previous 12 hours or who have a history suggesting AMI with bundle-branch block obscuring ST-segment analysis. Primary PTCA might be considered an alternative to fibrinolytic therapy in patients with AMI and ST-segment elevations or presumed new LBBB, who can undergo angioplasty of the infarct-related artery within 12 hours of the onset of symptoms or beyond 12 hours if symptoms persist. This latter procedure should be performed in a timely fashion by skilled personnel in centers that perform more than 200 PTCA procedures per year and have cardiac surgical capability. Most patients initially seen with AMI outside major cities, with tertiary health care centers, will be treated initially with fibrinolytic therapy because of the unavailability of primary PTCA.[2]

Noninvasive (Early)

Chest X-Ray

The first chest X-ray taken after admission to the hospital in patients with AMI provides prognostic information. In addition to age and a history of prior myocardial infarction, the presence or absence of cardiac enlargement or pulmonary congestion (or edema) is a determinant of outcome during initial hospitalization and 15-year follow-up. Those patients with cardiac enlargement and pulmonary congestion have a worse prognosis.

Echocardiography

Patients seen in the emergency department for evaluation of chest pain often have a differential diagnosis that includes cardiovascular, pulmonary, gastrointestinal, and musculoskeletal conditions. Usually clinical information including the patient's history, examination findings, and basic radiographic and laboratory data provide the diagnosis. In other situations, echocardiographic evaluation of the patient in the emergency department may confirm suspected diagnoses or identify unsuspected causes for chest discomfort.

In patients with chest pain and nondiagnostic electrocardiographic findings, transthoracic echocardiography may be used to distinguish between regional wall motion abnormalities associated with ischemia or myocardial infarction and normal myocardial contraction. Regional wall motion abnormalities develop if at least 20% to 25% of the myocardial wall thickness is infarcted or ischemic. Therefore, ischemia involving less than 20% to 25% of wall thickness will not be detectable with transthoracic imaging. From observations in the cardiac catheterization laboratory, it is clear that ventricular wall motion abnormalities develop within a few seconds of coronary artery occlusion (by balloon angioplasty catheters) and are more pronounced with greater reductions in coronary blood flow. Smaller degrees of ischemia will result in hypokinesis, and more significant degrees of ischemia will produce akinesis. Prompt identification of a regional wall motion abnormality of the ventricle corresponding to electrocardiographic ST elevations can support the decision to administer thrombolytic therapy or to perform primary coronary angioplasty. However, definitive treatment of ST-elevation myocardial infarction should not be delayed waiting for noninvasive imaging if the baseline electrocardiogram is consistent with this diagnosis. There are several limitations to using transthoracic echocardiography to identify myocardial infarction in the acute setting. Detection of regional wall motion abnormalities caused by acute ischemia, or infarction, may be difficult in patients with preexisting left ventricular dysfunction, prior extensive infarction, and in patients who have long pain-free intervals.

In patients with electrocardiographic ST-segment depressions, or nonspecific ST-segment changes, identification of a wall motion abnormality consistent with ongoing infarction might lead to a decision to perform emergent cardiac catheterization. Thrombolytic therapy in this situation is not warranted, because it has not been shown to be effective in non-ST-segment elevation syndromes. Patients with small myocardial infarctions might not have demonstrable regional wall motion abnormalities if less than 20% to 25% of the wall thickness is infarcted. The sensitivity of transthoracic echocardiography for the detection of regional wall motion abnormalities in patients seen in the emergency department with chest pain is 88% to 94% when regional wall motion abnormalities are used as the positive diagnostic criteria. In the same studies, specificity of regional wall motion abnormalities is 53% to 99%, presumably because of the inclusion of patients with global left ventricular dysfunction.

Echocardiography is also helpful in estimating infarct size and the location of the infarcted artery. The most widely used algorithm for quantitating myocardial infarction in based on a 16-segment model of the myocardium (Figure 8-1). Wall motion scoring is performed by assigning each myocardial segment a score: normal wall thickening, 1; hypokinesis, 2; akinesis, 3; dyskinesis, 4; aneurysmal, 5; akinesis with scar, 6; dyskinesis with scar, 7. (When calculating a wall motion index, "akinesis with scar" and "dyskinesis with scar" are assigned scores of 3 and 4, respectively.) All segments that can be evaluated are scored and an average score calculated. A mean score of 1 indicates no regional wall motion abnormalities and scores ≥2.0 are consistent with significant left ventricular dysfunction. AMI size estimated by echocardiography is frequently larger than pathological infarct size because of the detection by echocardiography of wall motion abnormalities at the infarct zone border.

The location of wall motion abnormalities might be used to predict the coronary artery involved. Each of the

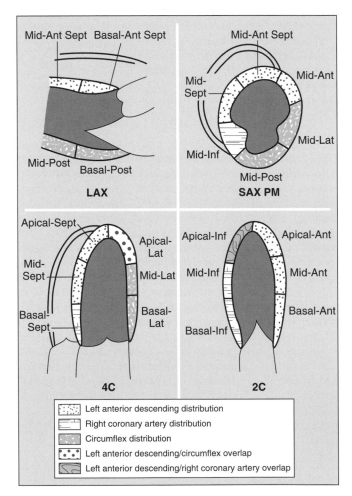

FIGURE 8-1. Diagram of the modified 16-segment model of wall motion abnormalities with areas of coronary artery distribution shown as areas of stippling or cross hatching. The overlap areas are represented as a combination of the graphics. LAX, long axis; SAX PM, short axis at the papillary muscle level; 4C, four chamber; 2C, 2 chamber; ANT, anterior; INF, inferior; LAT, lateral; LAX, long axis; POST, posterior; SEPT, septal. (Reproduced by permission from Segar DS, et al. *J Am Coll Cardiol* 1992; 19:1197.)

16 myocardial segments corresponds to one coronary artery distribution or an overlap zone (Figure 8-1). Two overlap zones exist. The apical lateral wall is supplied by either the left anterior descending artery or the left circumflex artery. The apical inferior wall is supplied by the right coronary artery or by the left anterior descending artery. The coronary artery supplying one of these zones may be deduced if adjacent nonoverlap zones are dysfunctional. For instance, if the apical septal and the apical inferior segments are dysfunctional, the apical inferior segment is likely supplied by the left anterior descending artery. Concordance of approximately 80% has been demonstrated between echocardiography and angiography in defining the culprit vessel in patients receiving thrombolytic therapy, with disagreement of infarct location occurring mainly in apical overlap zones.

In addition to the detection of regional wall motion abnormalities in the emergency department, underlying myocardial and valvular abnormalities have important prognostic significance. Detection of left ventricular dysfunction and/or significant mitral regurgitation in patients seen in the emergency department with chest discomfort is associated with increased 2-year mortality, even if an acute myocardial infarction is not evolving. Furthermore, if left ventricular systolic dysfunction is present on the initial echocardiogram, there is a 30% increase in significant arrhythmias, myocardial infarction, death, or the need for coronary revascularization.

Nuclear

The number of emergency department visits for chest pain in the United States exceeds 6 million annually or 5% of all visits, and the standard of care has become the admission of such patients to the coronary care units. However, only 10% to 30% of such patients will prove to have an acute coronary syndrome, and most will have no evidence of coronary artery disease after their evaluation is complete. There are approximately 2 to 3 million such "rule-out" admissions per year, at an estimated cost of $10 billion. Inevitably, third-party payers are restricting reimbursement to hospitals for the associated costs. Unfortunately, approximately 2% to 8% of patients with AMI are inappropriately sent out of emergency departments, and these cases are responsible for approximately 20% of all malpractice dollars paid out involving emergency department care. A need exists to safely reduce the number of persons admitted to the coronary care units with nonischemic chest pain, while simultaneously reducing the number of persons with acute infarction who are not admitted to the hospital. To attempt to achieve these goals, many hospitals have set up specifically targeted "chest pain centers" with evaluation algorithms and treatment protocols.

Exercise treadmill testing in the emergency department has been advocated for clinically stable patients without ongoing chest pain or electrocardiographic evidence of ischemia, either after serial enzymes exclude acute infarction, or, in the large group of clinically low-risk patients, even before serial enzymes are available. Exercise testing in chest pain centers has generally been reserved for the investigation of patients considered at low risk on the basis of history, physical examination, 12-lead electrocardiogram, and serum markers of myocardial damage.[3] In a large study of more than 1000 subjects, the specificity of exercise testing was 99% and the negative predictive value was 99% with respect to the diagnosis if admitted and during 30-day follow-up on all patients. The strategy has been safe in the relatively small number of patients studied to date who are low risk and in whom the prevalence of coronary artery disease is low. However, an estimated 10% to 40% of patients who might be candidates for this approach are either unable to exercise or have an abnormal resting electrocardiogram precluding a standard diagnostic exercise treadmill test. Last, the sensitivity of the standard electrocardiographic stress test for detection of coronary artery disease is modest (67%).[3]

Myocardial perfusion imaging can be performed with pharmacological stress in patients who cannot exercise and is a sensitive test in the presence of an abnormal resting electrocardiogram. Multiple studies have shown that there is a very low subsequent cardiac event rate after a normal stress myocardial perfusion study, generally about 1% per year. For these reasons, interest has developed in the use of radionuclide myocardial perfusion imaging in the emergency department evaluation of patients with chest pain and electrocardiograms that are either normal, or nondiagnostic, for an acute coronary syndrome.

[201]Tl is extracted by viable myocardial cells and after intravenous administration distributes in proportion to regional blood flow. Images of the heart show deficits in regions where blood flow is relatively reduced and in zones of nonviable myocardium (e.g., previous myocardial infarction). Over time, isotope "redistributes" from previously ischemic zones, so that ischemic myocardium normalizes or "fills in." Defects related to infarcted, or scarred, myocardium remain fixed and usually do not "redistribute" over time. Importantly, later imaging at 24 hours (or after reinjection of thallium-201) may show viable but hypoperfused segments not otherwise identified by an earlier standard redistribution study performed 3 to 4 hours after isotope injection.

By the use of [201]Tl Wackers et al performed pioneering studies evaluating rest images in acute coronary syndromes. Subsequently, rest imaging of patients with chest pain with ^{99m}Tc-based agents has been investigated and has been shown to be highly sensitive for detection of myocardial infarction and has a very high negative predictive value. The sensitivities of resting sestamibi imaging have been compared directly with serial measures of cardiac troponin I (cTnI) and the two are equivalent (92% vs. 90%), although the sensitivity of the initial cTnI level is low. Investigators at the Medical College of Virginia have demonstrated the effectiveness of a comprehensive strategy of risk identification and workup of chest pain in the emergency department using a 5 risk class scale and selective use of acute myocardial perfusion imaging. (A simple strategy for using rest and stress perfusion imaging selectively in evaluating patients with chest pain is shown in Figure 8-2.) Selection of a stress-testing modality in this situation is

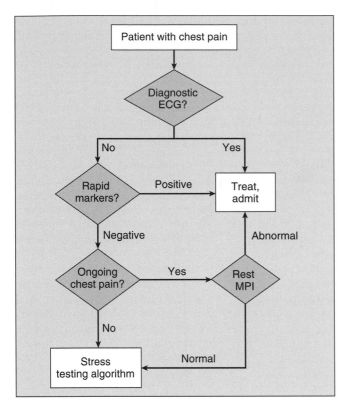

FIGURE 8-2. Flow chart of chest pain center activities. MPI, myocardial perfusion imaging. (Adapted from Tatum JL, Jesse RL. Emergency department triage and imaging of patients with acute chest pain. In: Zaret BL, Beller GA (eds): *Nuclear Cardiology: State of the Art and Future Directions.* St. Louis: Mosby, 1999.)

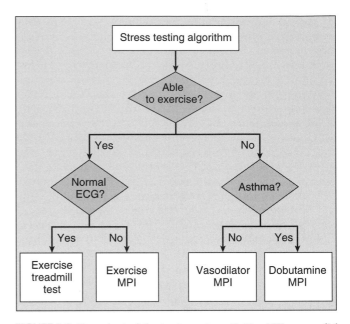

FIGURE 8-3. Flow chart of chest pain center activities. MPI, myocardial perfusion imaging. (Adapted from Tatum JL, Jesse RL. Emergency department triage and imaging of patients with acute chest pain. In: Zaret BL, Beller GA (eds): *Nuclear Cardiology: State of the Art and Future Directions.* St. Louis: Mosby, 1999.)

Invasive

Angiography

Coronary

The coronary artery atherosclerotic process in patients with symptoms of myocardial ischemia is usually diffuse, and severe, and nonquantitative coronary angiography measures the degree of narrowing by comparing severely narrowed arterial segments with less narrowed segments. Therefore, coronary angiograms may underestimate the amount of coronary artery luminal narrowing in symptomatic patients. In a comparison of cineangiographic and necropsy findings in patients with fatal coronary artery disease, underestimation of the degree of narrowing of moderate and severe coronary stenosis was common, and overestimation did not occur. In patients who die suddenly with acute coronary thrombosis, autopsy studies reveal layered thrombus, with successive deposits of different age and microemboli distal to thrombosed coronary arteries from peripheral embolization causing microinfarcts. Thus a process of dynamic thrombosis leads to infarction or sudden death. In 1962 Mason Sones, MD, first performed selective coronary angiography, and the structural and functional aspects have been subsequently described in detail (Figure 8-4).

The development of angulated views and multiple angiographic projections have reduced the problem of overlapping vessels, foreshortening of segments of coronary arteries, and the difficulty of assessing noncircular, eccentric coronary artery lesions. To profile the left main, proximal, and midleft anterior descending artery and its branches, the caudocranial left anterior oblique

analogous to selection in stable patients being evaluated for possible coronary artery disease (Figure 8-3).

In a prospective, multicenter study of patients presenting with symptoms suggestive of an acute coronary syndrome with normal, or nondiagnostic, electrocardiograms, patients were randomly assigned to a local standard clinical evaluation or resting ^{99m}Tc-sestamibi imaging interpreted promptly, so that physicians could incorporate the information into their clinical decisions.[4] Patients presenting at night, or with a history of prior myocardial infarction, were excluded. Use of resting myocardial perfusion imaging information reduced the rate of hospitalization for patients without acute myocardial ischemia from 52% to 42% without reducing appropriate admissions. The cost-effectiveness of this approach is still unclear. It should be noted that several limitations and obstacles need to be overcome to establish the capability for emergency department myocardial perfusion imaging, including immediate availability of radioisotope, 24-hour availability of a nuclear technologist to perform the scan and a nuclear cardiologist or radiologist to read the scan, access to a gamma camera in the emergency department, inability to distinguish a new from an old perfusion defect (unless the patient happens to have a prior scan at that institution), and defects related to attenuation artifacts in rest-only studies without a comparative stress perfusion image.

(half-axial) view is optimal and is achieved by moving the image intensifier left and angling it so that the X-ray beam passes in a caudocranial direction (cranial angulation) toward the head. A shallow left anterior oblique view (about 40 degrees left of sagittal) profiles the origin of the left main coronary artery but either superimposes the distal left main or proximal left anterior descending (on the proximal circumflex or intermediate coronary arteries) or views these vessels end-on. A deep inspiratory effort, which lowers the diaphragm, may reveal these branch origins, and if the X-ray beam is angled 30 to 40 degrees toward the head (40 degrees left anterior oblique with 30 to 40 degrees cranial tilt), these difficulties might be overcome. The "weeping willow" or craniocaudal left anterior oblique view (angled so that the X-ray beam passes in a craniocaudal direction toward the feet) profiles the left main, the origin and trunk of the proximal left anterior descending artery, and the origin and trunk of the proximal circumflex artery. The cranial right anterior oblique view might be useful to unmask disease in the midleft anterior descending coronary artery not seen in the standard right anterior oblique view, and the caudal right anterior oblique view

might be helpful to profile the circumflex marginal system. The proximal right coronary artery is usually well visualized with 50-degree left anterior oblique and 30-degree right anterior oblique views. Compared with standard left anterior oblique and lateral views of the right coronary artery, both the cranial right and left anterior oblique views may improve visualization of the distal right coronary artery and its branches.

Patients admitted with acute chest pain and an ST-segment elevation myocardial infarction or a new LBBB electrocardiographic pattern have a high prevalence of a coronary artery occlusion. DeWood and colleagues[5] described the angiographic findings in such patients. Within 4 hours of symptom onset, the artery was occluded in 87% and subtotally occluded 10% of patients. The occluded vessel often has an abrupt cutoff and may have a "beaked" appearance at the site of occlusion. Angiographic features consistent with thrombus were frequently found in patients admitted early after symptom onset (i.e., staining of the distal column of contrast was noted in 69%, dye retention in 20%, and intraluminal filling defects occurred in 10%), and patients who were seen later (within 12 to 24 hours of symptom

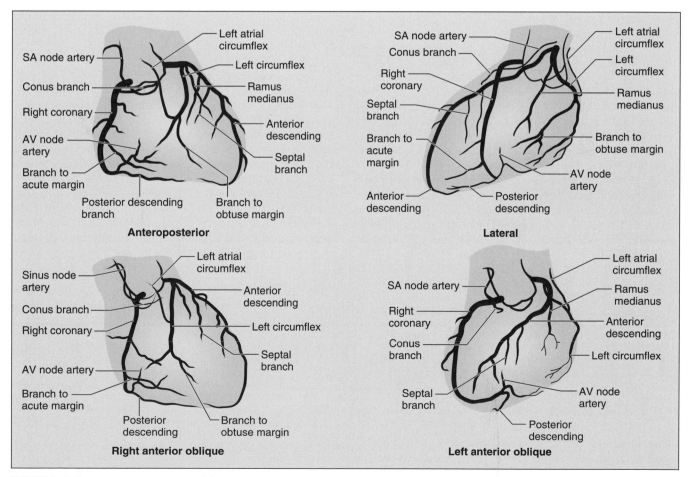

FIGURE 8-4. Anatomic representation of the coronary vessels as they are seen on a coronary angiogram. The combination of the left anterior oblique (LAO), lateral (LAT), and right anterior oblique (RAO) usually demonstrates all branches in profile, but cranial and caudal angulation may be needed to examine specific lesions or branches in detail. (Reproduced with permission from Abrams HL, Adams DF. The coronary arteriogram. Structural and functional aspects. *N Engl J Med* 1969; 281:1276.)

onset) had fewer total occlusions (65%) and more subtotal occlusions (16%). The increased coronary patency rates seen in the patients studied 12 to 24 hours after onset of symptoms and the fewer patients with angiographic features suggestive of thrombosis, demonstrate that 35% of patients admitted with ST-segment elevations will develop some antegrade flow because of endogenous thrombolysis but usually have a persistent, significant, residual epicardial stenosis. Angioscopy of the infarct-related artery provided additional insight into plaque morphology in patients with unstable angina or AMIs and demonstrated red thrombus in most patients with acute infarct and in only 25% of patients with unstable angina. These angioscopic findings demonstrate that fibrin-rich thrombus (responsive to thrombolytic therapy) is found in AMIs, whereas platelet-rich thrombus (responsive to antiplatelet therapy) is usually present in unstable angina.

The Thrombolysis in Myocardial Infarction Investigators demonstrated, in 1985, that intravenous tissue-type plasminogen activator was almost twice as effective as streptokinase in opening a totally occluded infarct-related coronary artery 90 minutes after the start of the drug infusion.[6] In this study, they introduced a new grading method of defining coronary artery patency, which is now called "TIMI flow" (Table 8-1). In this scheme TIMI grade 0 = no perfusion, TIMI grade 1 = penetration of contrast without perfusion, TIMI grade 2 = partial perfusion, and TIMI grade 3 = complete perfusion of the coronary artery bed distal to the obstruction. Subsequent studies examining the influence of thrombolytic therapy in acute myocardial infarction on infarct artery patency and subsequent prognosis have indicated that achieving TIMI grade 3 flow in epicardial coronary arteries (rather than TIMI grade 2 flow) achieves greater myocardial salvage, improves ventricular performance, and improves mortality. Similarly, improved epicardial coronary artery blood flow after thrombolytic therapy as assessed by TIMI frame counts[7] has been associated with reduced mortality. These methods have been further refined, and a simple, semiquantitative, classification scheme, the TIMI myocardial perfusion grade (TMP), allowing characterization of the filling and clearance of myocardial perfusion from a coronary angiogram, has been developed[8,9] (Table 8-2). The use of the TMP grade allows further stratification of patients, even among those with TIMI 3 flow. Patients with normal epicardial flow (TIMI grade 3 flow) and normal tissue-level perfusion (TMP grade 3) have a substantially lower mortality than those with slower myocardial perfusion (TMP grades 0 to 2).[8] Last, both improved epicardial flow (TIMI flow grades 2/3 and low corrected TIMI frame counts) and tissue-level perfusion (TIMI myocardial perfusion grades 2/3) at 90 minutes after thrombolytic administration are independently associated with improved 2-year survival.[10]

Guidelines have emphasized that percutaneous coronary intervention (PCI) is an effective method for reestablishing coronary perfusion in patients with ST-segment elevation AMI, and the reported rates of achieving TIMI 3 flow range from 70% to 90% are augmented by intracoronary stents. Stents decrease elastic recoil and remodeling and reduce restenosis. Furthermore, PCI reduces 6-month mortality in patients younger than 75 years with AMI complicated by cardiogenic shock.[11] In the PCI stent era, the classification of anatomical lesion risk has been modified (Box 8-1[12]).

Ventricular

The most important predictor of survival in patients with acute coronary syndromes or chronic stable angina is the cumulative amount of myocardial damage the patient has accrued, and the left ventricular ejection fraction consistently proves a key predictor of outcomes in studies of patients with myocardial infarction, even outweighing evidence of residual inducible ischemia. Left ventricular ejection fraction (LVEF) is also an important determinant for selection of patients with a survival benefit from surgical revascularization. The LVEF might be based on a visual estimate of contractile function or on semiquantitative methods such as the area/length method or Simpson's rule. Patients with ejection fractions of <40% are at increased risk of ventricular arrhythmias, worsening left ventricular dysfunction, and death in the 2 years after infarction. Patients with three-

■ ▨ ■

TABLE 8-1   DEFINITIONS OF TIMI FLOW

Grade 0 (no perfusion)	There is no antegrade flow beyond the point of occlusion.
Grade 1 (penetration without perfusion)	The contrast material passes beyond the area of obstruction but "hangs up" and fails to opacify the entire coronary bed distal to the obstruction for the duration of the cineangiogram filling sequence.
Grade 2 (partial perfusion)	The contrast material passes across the obstruction and opacifies the coronary bed distal to the obstruction. However, the rate of entry of the contrast material into the vessel distal to the obstruction or its rate of clearance from the distal bed (or both) is perceptibly slower than its entry into or clearance from the comparable areas not perfused by the previously occluded vessel (e.g., the opposite coronary artery or the coronary bed proximal to the obstruction).
Grade 3 (complete perfusion)	Antegrade flow into the bed distal to the obstruction occurs as promptly as antegrade flow into the bed proximal to the obstruction, and clearance of contrast material from the involved bed is as rapid as clearance from an uninvolved bed in the same vessel or the opposite artery.

Adapted from The TIMI Study Group. The thrombolysis in myocardial infarction trial. *N Engl J Med* 1985; 312:932.

■ ▪ ■

TABLE 8-2 TIMI MYOCARDIAL PERFUSION (TMP) GRADES

TMP grade 0	Failure of dye to enter the microvasculature. Either minimal or no ground-glass appearance ("blush") or opacification of the myocardium in the distribution of the culprit artery, indicating lack of tissue level perfusion.
TMP grade 1	Dye slowly enters but fails to exit the microvasculature. There is the ground-glass appearance ("blush") or opacification of the myocardium in the distribution of the culprit artery that fails to clear from the microvasculature, and the dye staining is present on the next injection (~30 s between injections).
TMP grade 2	Delayed entry and exit of dye from the microvasculature. There is the ground-glass appearance ("blush") or opacification of the myocardium in the distribution of the culprit artery that is strongly persistent at the end of the washout phase (i.e., dye is strongly persistent after three cardiac cycles of the washout phase and either does not or only minimally diminishes in intensity during washout).
TMP grade 3	Normal entry and exit of dye from the microvasculature. There is the ground-glass appearance ("blush") or opacification of the myocardium in the distribution of the culprit artery that clears normally and is either gone or only mildly/moderately persistent at the end of the washout phase (i.e., dye is gone or only mildly/moderately persistent after three cardiac cycles of the washout phase and noticeably diminishes in intensity during the washout phase), similar to that in an uninvolved artery. Blush that is only of mild intensity throughout the washout phase but fades minimally is also classified as grade 3.

Adapted from Gibson CM, Cannon CP, Murphy SA, et al. Relationship of TIMI perfusion grade to mortality after administration of thrombolytic drugs. *Circulation* 2000; 101:125.

vessel coronary artery disease have decreased 4-year survival if the ejection fraction is <35% compared with those patients with milder dysfunction (35% to 49%) and normal function (>49%), and patients with one-vessel coronary artery disease have increased mortality if their ejection fraction is <35%, but the survival difference between this group and patients with normal ejection fractions is less marked than in patients with multivessel coronary artery disease. In addition, assessment of ejection fraction has identified higher risk patients with low ejection fractions who will benefit from initiation of angiotensin-converting enzyme (ACE) therapy after myocardial infarction to attenuate adverse left ventricular remodeling and to improve survival. Even patients with mild dysfunction after myocardial infarction might benefit from ACE inhibitors. In an angiographic study of 605 patients with AMI, undergoing angiography within 1 to 2 months after infarction who were followed for more than 6 years, left ventricular end-systolic volume (calculated by an integration method from left ventriculography performed in the right anterior oblique position) was the primary predictor of survival and was superior to ejection fraction when ejection fraction was low (<50%) or if end-systolic volume was high.[13]

Ultrasound (Coronary)

Angiography, despite its significant limitations, has been the "gold standard" for diagnosis and treatment of coronary artery disease. When there are uncertainties regarding the etiology of a stenosis or the severity or length of a diseased segment, intravascular ultrasound can help guide the therapeutic strategy and can be influential in optimizing percutaneous coronary interventions. Intravascular ultrasound provides imaging of the coronary vessel wall, whereas angiography, as a silhouette technique, detects arterial disease that indents the luminal column of contrast. Therefore, intravascular ultrasound provides information about plaque characteristics, mural thrombus, intimal dissection, and microfractures, all of which are frequently missed by angiography alone.

There are two types of intravascular ultrasound catheters currently in use. The first is a mechanical catheter that consists of a rotating ultrasound crystal in the catheter tip. A motor outside the body drives the rotating core. The advantages to this system are its design

■ ▪ ■

BOX 8-1 ANATOMIC RISK GROUPS FOR PERCUTANEOUS INTERVENTION

Low risk

Discrete lesion (length <10 mm)
Concentric
Readily accessible
Nonangulated segment (<45°)
Smooth contour
Little or no calcification
Less than totally occlusive
Not ostial in location
No major side branch involvement
Absence of thrombus

Moderate risk

Tubular (length, 10-20 mm)
Eccentric
Moderate tortuosity of proximal segment
Moderately angulated segment (>45°, 90°)
Irregular contour
Moderate or heavy calcification
Total occlusions <3 months old
Ostial in location
Bifurcation lesions requiring double guidewires
Some thrombus present

High risk

Diffuse (length >20 mm)
Excessive tortuosity of proximal segment
Extremely angulated segments >90°
Total occlusions >3 months old
Inability to protect major side branches
Degenerated vein grafts with friable lesions

Adapted from Smith SC, Dove J, Jacobs AK, et al ACC/AHA guidelines for percutaneous coronary intervention: a report of the American College of Cardiology/ American Heart Association Task Force on Practice Guidelines (Committee to Revise the 1993 Guidelines for Percutaneous Transluminal Coronary Angioplasty). *J Am Coll Cardiol* 2001; 37:2239i.

simplicity, greater power output, and greater signal/noise ratio. One disadvantage is that the need for a central drive shaft precludes the use of a coaxial guidewire and the rapid-exchange guidewire that lies beside the imaging catheter and often appears in the displayed image. A second disadvantage is image distortion caused by variable rotation of the drive shaft (nonuniform rotational distortion), particularly when the catheter passes through a tortuous proximal vessel. The second type of intravascular ultrasound catheter is a solid-state catheter. This is a phased array or a dynamic-aperture array with 64 ultrasound crystals arranged around the circumference of the catheter tip, each activated sequentially to produce an electronically rotated ultrasound beam. This catheter is flexible and allows the use of a central lumen guidewire. The disadvantages with this imaging system are decreased power and a larger area adjacent to the catheter in which images cannot be obtained because of artifact (near field artifact). These catheters are as small as 2.6 F, and with imaging frequencies of 20 to 40 MHz, images of the component structures of the vascular wall can be obtained. These frequencies provide structural resolution from 150 to 175 μm.

The normal vessel consists of three echo layers as seen by intravascular ultrasound. The intima and internal elastic lamina form a single hyperechoic layer, with the hypoechogenic media directly external to the intimal layer. The adventitia is seen as an echodense zone beyond the medial layer because of its large amount of collagen. Plaque is by nature echogenic and is seen as increased echodensities and irregular thickness of the intimal layer extending into the lumen.

Intravascular ultrasound is used to detect mild coronary artery disease, to assess the indeterminate lesion, and to assess coronary stenoses before and after PCI. It can be particularly helpful in left main coronary artery lesions that are often difficult to quantitate with angiography because of overlapping branches, disease in the ostial segment, or diffuse disease.

In contrast to coronary angiography, intravascular ultrasound can also quantify atherosclerotic lesions without a normal proximal reference segment and eliminates underestimation of the amount of atherosclerosis when compensatory arterial enlargement occurs. However, intravascular ultrasound does not differentiate low echogenic thrombus and low echogenic soft plaques that contain high concentrations of lipids. By use of fiberoptic catheters to obtain optical coherence tomography images (by advancing them through the intravascular ultrasound core), a cross-sectional resolution of coronary vessels of approximately 10 μm is possible (fibrous caps are <65 μm). With this technique, it has been found that lipid-rich and fibrous plaques have distinct optical coherence tomography characteristics.[14] Intimal hyperplasia and echolucent regions, which may correspond to lipid pools, were identified more frequently by optical coherence tomography than by intravascular ultrasound.

Examination of plaque ruptures (comparing coronary angiographic lesion morphology and intravascular ultrasound) showed that plaque ruptures may be multiple, are eccentric, and are often not associated with lumen compromise but are close to a significant stenosis and to a side branch. If ultrasound identified a plaque cavity that communicated with the lumen with an overlying residual fibrous cap fragment, this strongly correlated with complex angiographic lesion morphology (ulceration in 81%, intimal flap in 40%, thrombus in 7%, and aneurysm in 7%).[15]

The most common complication associated with intracoronary ultrasound (which occurs in 2.9% of cases) is transient coronary spasm relieved with nitroglycerin. There is a less than 1% major complication rate, including acute occlusion, embolism, dissection, thrombus, and myocardial infarction possibly related to ultrasound imaging. These major complications usually occur in patients with acute coronary syndromes undergoing therapeutic intervention.

Intravascular Ultrasound and AMI

Intravascular ultrasound has been performed in patients within 6 hours of onset of AMI, and in approximately 90% of patients intravascular ultrasound was able to differentiate between scintillating, low-echogenic, intraluminal material suggestive of thrombus and the more highly echogenic atherosclerotic plaque. Low echogenic intraluminal material was found in approximately 75% of segments proximal to highly echogenic plaque and in two thirds of segments distal to it, suggesting prestenotic and poststenotic thrombus in acute myocardial infarction. The plaque was eccentric in approximately 75% of patients. The atherosclerotic lesions responsible for AMI were described as large, but minimally occlusive.

In studies comparing intravascular ultrasound imaging with atherectomy specimens within 1 week of presentation of patients with AMI, treated with intravenous thrombolytic therapy, mildly echogenic plaque identified by intravascular ultrasound and histological fibroatheromatous tissue was more frequently associated with thrombus than dense echogenic fibrocalcific tissue. All patients studied within 5 days of thrombolytic therapy had ultrasound evidence for intraluminal thrombus, frequently as an echogenic structure protruding into the central lumen. If studied longer than 5 days after thrombolytic therapy, an echogenic thrombus protruding into the lumen was rarely found. Instead, the thrombus appeared more linear, was adjacent to the wall, and its echogenic structure was more closely related to lose fibrous tissue. This variability of the echo density could predict the fibrin content and the degree of organization of the plaque. Identification of thrombus by intravascular ultrasound is easier if the structure is mobile within the lumen, and identification of older thrombus is more difficult, because the speckled appearance is often replaced by a more linear, mildly echogenic pattern. Thus, intravascular ultrasound is able to identify intraluminal thrombus and differentiate it from atherosclerotic plaque, which can be important before interventional procedures (Figure 8-5).

With AMI, reestablishing coronary blood flow is the most important goal. Although in most cases, reperfusion requires balloon angioplasty, reflow occasionally occurs with contrast injection into the arterial system or with manipulation of the coronary guidewire necessary

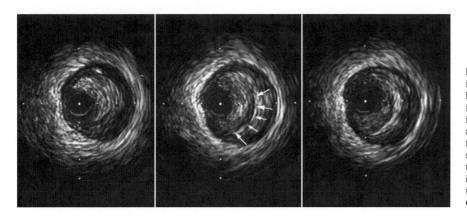

FIGURE 8-5. Coronary intravascular ultrasound images of a patient who presented with unstable angina. *Panel 1,* Intravascular ultrasound image proximal to an angiographic stenosis, illustrating an eccentric plaque with a fair amount of echogenicity. This is consistent with fibrofatty plaque. *Panel 2,* Intravascular ultrasound image of the stenosis. The arrows illustrate the interface between plaque and intraluminal thrombus. *Panel 3,* Intravascular ultrasound image of the distal lesion. See also Color Insert.

for PCI. Once flow is reestablished, intravascular ultrasound can be used to assess the degree of residual stenosis and to optimize the results of coronary intervention. Advantages to the use of intravascular ultrasound in the setting of acute myocardial infarction include the ability to visualize the intracoronary processes. Disadvantages of intravascular ultrasound include the additional time required for this procedure; although one study reported an intravascular ultrasound imaging time of 75 ± 22 s, which was a minimal proportion of the total duration of the invasive procedure (41 ± 15 min). The PCI guidelines indicate that intravascular ultrasound is not indicated routinely in all stent implantations but is useful in evaluating the results of high-risk procedures when the angiographic appearances are marginal, when there is poor TIMI flow or coronary flow reserve, or in patients with multiple stents.[12]

Angioscopy (Coronary)

Angioscopy is a percutaneous, catheter-based system designed to allow direct visual inspection of the endoluminal surface of the coronary arteries with a three-dimensional color image. This provides much more information than angiography alone, which is merely a "luminogram." Angioscopy better defines the nature of a luminal obstruction than angiography, especially for the detection and characterization of thrombus, ulceration, and calcification within the lesion. Because angiography displays only the silhouette of the luminal changes, it is inadequate to investigate the pathogenesis of acute coronary disorders, information that can be gained with angioscopy. Angioscopy is a forward-viewing technique revealing surface morphology, supplying different information than intravascular ultrasound, which provides a cross-sectional view of the arterial wall and data on plaque composition.

Angioscopy was initially performed intraoperatively while there was no coronary blood flow, and minimal flushing removed residual blood. This system often required no proximal occlusion of the coronary artery. Subsequently, percutaneous methods have been developed that require a balloon occluder proximal to the arterial segment being visualized, allowing for interruption and flushing of the blood to clear the field of view.

The current angioscopy imaging system consists of two elements that are both guided in a rapid exchange fashion over a single 0.014-inch angioplasty guidewire. The inner catheter contains an imaging bundle consisting of 3000 optical fibers. The inner catheter may be advanced or withdrawn independently of the outer catheter a distance of 6 cm, so that many segments of the vessel lumen can be examined. The outer catheter is 4.5 F in diameter, with a lumen for inflating and deflating the occlusion balloon at its distal tip. The occlusion balloon is compliant with a variable inflation diameter, depending on the volume of liquid introduced, maximum diameter 5.0 mm. Overinflation of the occlusion balloon is to be avoided, and the balloon should be inflated with just enough fluid to prevent forward injection of contrast medium to be visualized beyond the inflated balloon. The flush lumen, which exists between the two catheters, is connected to a power injector for infusion of warmed, lactated Ringer's at a rate of 0.5 to 1.0 mL/s. Each imaging sequence lasts approximately 30 to 45 seconds, after which the balloon is deflated and the flush discontinued.

The normal coronary artery intima has a smooth, glistening, white surface, whereas atherosclerotic plaque is frequently pigmented, from yellow to yellow-brown in color. Plaque in humans usually consists of lipid core with fibrous cap, intimal hyperplasia, fibrous tissue, calcification, and thrombus. Plaques that are white are likely to have a thick fibrous cap or to be fibrous. Comparing coronary angioscopy findings with integrated backscatter ultrasound findings, it was found that the surface color of plaques seen by angioscopy reflected the thickness of the fibrous cap but not the size of the lipid core.[16] Conversely, the size or thickness of the lipid core varied considerably among yellow, light yellow, and white plaques. Angioscopy provides lesion characterization on the basis of both plaque morphology and the presence and type of thrombus. Thrombus is characterized as either red (gelatinous material protruding into the lumen) or white (extending into the lumen from a disrupted intima). White thrombi are platelet rich, whereas red thrombi contain an abundance of fibrin mixed with erythrocytes and platelets.

Angioscopy is helpful in imaging the target vessel both before and after intervention including balloon and laser angioplasty, in guiding stent deployment, and in monitoring the results of thrombolytic therapy. The use of angioscopy is not without limitation. Despite improvements in size and flexibility from earlier angioscopes, it remains large (4.5 F) and therefore cannot be advanced into vessels less than 2.5 mm in diameter, and it tracks poorly around tortuous bends. The coronary artery that is being visualized is continuously flushed with Ringer's lactate to remove obscuring blood. This can result in ischemia in the territory of a diseased vessel. The requirement of a bloodless field also precludes imaging of the left main coronary and the ostia of the right coronary, left anterior descending, and circumflex arteries. Only the proximal to mid segments of relatively straight and large epicardial coronaries can be imaged. From 84% to 100% of target lesions are adequately visualized. An additional limitation to the use of angioscopy is that current systems are unable to easily extract absolute dimensional measurements from the collected images.

Angioscopy is associated with few complications. There have been reports of ventricular arrhythmia requiring defibrillation and transient atrioventricular block that had no clinical consequences. There is potential for developing ischemia on preimaging of interventional lesions and the development of dissection, acute closure, and/or thrombus on postimaging. There is also the potential for barotrauma to the vessel at the site of the occluding balloon, although at least one series failed to reveal any progression of disease at these sites.

Angioscopy in Acute Coronary Syndromes

Angioscopic imaging in patients with acute coronary syndromes demonstrates occlusive thrombi occurring more commonly in patients with AMI than in those with unstable angina, whereas mural (nonocclusive) thrombi are more common in those with unstable angina. Xanthomatous plaques are more common in patients with acute coronary disorders (50%) than in those with stable angina (15%) or old myocardial infarction (8%), whereas white and smooth plaques are seen in cases of stable angina and old myocardial infarction. These xanthomatous plaques have a distinctly yellow appearance and are likely to be cholesterol rich with a thin fibrous cap. White-appearing plaques are likely to have a thick fibrous cap or to be fibrous. This suggests that xanthomatous plaque probably predisposes to plaque rupture and that it might also be thrombogenic. It is also suggested that xanthomatous plaque might be thrombogenic, because there is a higher frequency of occlusive thrombi after PTCA at sites with greater lipid content.

In an angioscopic series of patients with AMI treated with thrombolytics followed by PTCA or directional coronary atherectomy (DCA), if reperfusion was incomplete, red and white thrombus, yellow plaque, and intimal flap was found in all patients evaluated before thrombolytic therapy. Others have reported the predominance of red thrombus in patients with AMI before reperfusion. After reperfusion, red thrombus was observed in only 30% of patients. This suggests that the fibrin-rich red thrombus is lysed, leaving platelet-rich thrombus at the disrupted yellow plaque. Angioscopic

follow-up has been performed at 20 to 30 days revealing white thrombus at the plaque site in 60% of patients, stressing the need for ongoing antiplatelet therapy.

Once coronary blood flow is reestablished, angioscopy can be used to assess the pathological process, the degree of residual stenosis, and to guide subsequent treatment. The data acquisition viewing time for angioscopy is approximately 30 to 60 seconds, with the average additional procedure time of approximately 12 to 15 minutes.

CMR

As described in an earlier chapter, magnetic resonance imaging (CMR) can provide information regarding cardiac structure, function, perfusion, coronary anatomy, and flow. Similar to other imaging techniques, CMR can be used to detect changes in wall thickness and wall thickening that occur in the setting of infarction. The imaging strategy is for the patient to hold their breath and to perform cine CMR with electrocardiographic gating to obtain images in each of the standard orientations: two chamber, four chamber, multiple short-axis sections spanning the entire left ventricle and long axis.[17] At present, conventional turbo field echo cine CMR requires an approximately 17-second (15 cardiac cycles) breath hold to obtain images with acceptable spatial and temporal resolution (approximately $2.5 \times 1.7 \times 6$ mm, 40 ms/frame). More recently, balanced field echo approaches (also termed fast imaging with steady-state precession [FISP] or steady-state free precession [SSFP]) have been developed, which can reduce the breath-hold time approximately by half. Grading of wall thickening is comparable to that used in echocardiography (Figure 8-6).

Early studies in animal models and patients demonstrated the ability of CMR to detect evidence of myocardial injury within hours of the onset of ischemia because of intrinsic changes in tissue relaxation times (particularly the spin-spin relaxation time T2) because of edema. However, this technique was not widely used because of lengthy imaging times and potential for artifacts. It was also noted at that time that extracellular CMR contrast agents, such as gadolinium diethylene triamine penta-acetic acid (DTPA), gadodiamide, or gadoteridol could be used to facilitate the detection of infarction and aspects of reperfusion. These contrast agents move rapidly from the vascular space into the interstitial space but do not enter myocardial cells. They are subsequently cleared from the bloodstream by the kidneys at a rate comparable to inulin. Thus, there is the opportunity to observe the initial appearance of the contrast agent in the myocardium and its subsequent clearance. It has been demonstrated that the initial appearance of the agent in tissue was dependent on myocardial blood flow and that its clearance was dependent on blood flow and the size of extracellular space. However, lengthy imaging times precluded the use of these techniques in patients.

With the recent development of faster CMR techniques, there has been considerable interest in the use of contrast-enhanced CMR (ceCMR) in the evaluation of

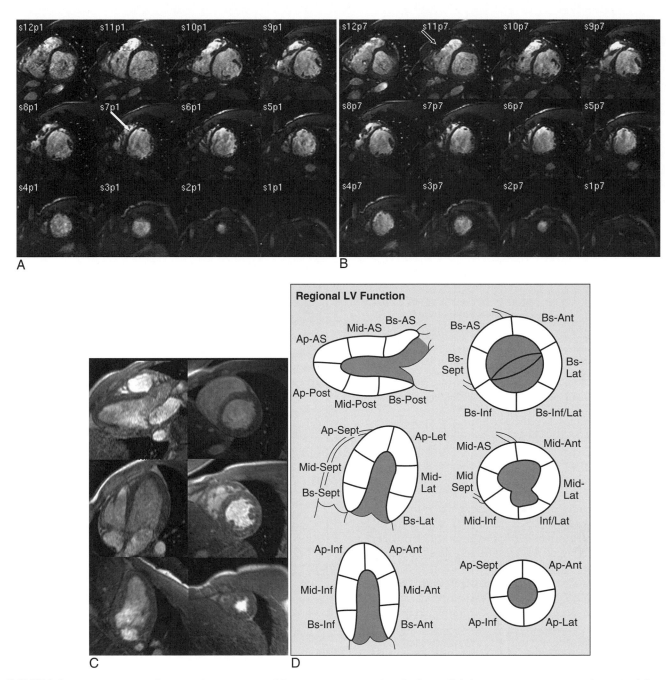

FIGURE 8-6. CMR assessment of ventricular structure and function. *Upper panel,* Multiple parallel short-axis views spanning the entire left ventricle obtained using a breath-hold cine CMR sequence. The end-diastolic images (left) and end-systolic images (right) demonstrate severe left ventricular dilation with marked thinning of the septum *(arrow).* Artifact from sternal wires from prior coronary artery bypass grafting is noted anteriorly *(open arrow). Lower panel,* Standard orientations obtained for the assessment of left ventricular structure and function. Images are interpreted using the same segments as used in echocardiography.

patients in the setting of acute ischemic syndromes. The basic approach involves the injection of the MR contrast agent in a peripheral vein. The recommended dose may vary, depending on the agent and the exact imaging sequence used. To look at the early distribution of contrast agent or to examine myocardial perfusion, the injection can be followed by immediate imaging. However, the critical delayed images are obtained 10 to 20 minutes after injection to examine at differences in clearance of the agent. To maximize efficiency, cine CMR to evaluate

function is frequently done between the initial images and the delayed images to evaluate function.

Immediate imaging during the first pass of the contrast agent through the myocardium can be used to detect differences in regional perfusion during stress and is discussed in detail in the section describing the evaluation of stable coronary artery disease. However, first-pass imaging at rest can demonstrate perfusion abnormalities at rest in the patient with an acute coronary syndrome. If imaging is performed early (in the first

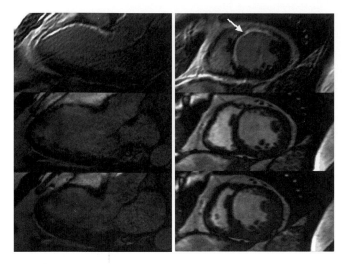

FIGURE 8-7. Contrast-enhanced magnetic resonance imaging used to assess myocardial viability. Long-axis *(left panel)* and short-axis images *(right panel)* from a contrast-enhanced CMR study for myocardial viability. Top image in each panel is obtained approximately 15 minutes after the administration of contrast agent and demonstrates delayed clearance of contrast agent from an extensive region involving the septum and anterior wall *(arrow)*. The middle image in each panel is the end-diastolic image from the cine CMR, whereas the bottom image in each panel is the end-systolic image from the same sequence. There is good correspondence between the region of enhancement and the region of wall thinning and decreased wall thickening on the cine sequence.

few minutes) after injection, regions of microvascular obstruction and no reflow will appear dark compared with the remainder of the myocardium.

The appearance on delayed imaging reflects three basic situations: (1) rapid wash-in and wash-out of the agent in regions of normal myocardium with normal perfusion, (2) relatively rapid wash-in and delayed wash-out in regions of perfusion but cellular injury, and (3) very delayed, if any, wash-in in regions of no reflow. Delayed imaging at 10 to 20 minutes permits wash-out of the contrast agent from the normal myocardium. The relatively slow wash-out in regions of injury then results in increased signal intensity in those regions relative to normal myocardium, permitting identification of regions of cellular injury (Figure 8-7).

The contrast agent concentration has recently been directly measured in animal studies by use of electron probe X-ray microanalysis. In acute infarction, it seems to be exclusively associated with regions of irreversible ischemic injury as defined by antimyoglobin antibody and increased sodium concentration. In chronically infarcted regions, the contrast agent concentration was also increased in areas of increased sodium concentration. The exact degree of contrast between the normal and injured myocardium depends on the exact imaging technique used, the time between the myocardial injury and the injection, and the time between the injection of contrast agent and delayed imaging. Thus, it is important to use a consistent protocol to obtain reproducible results.

This technique has been shown to be capable of detecting very small infarctions occurring in the setting

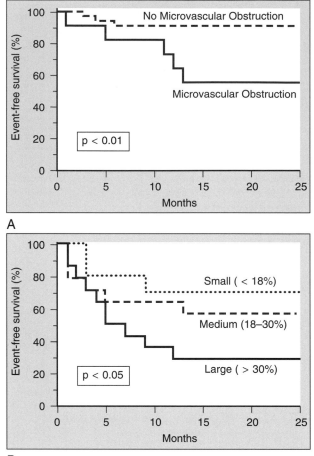

FIGURE 8-8. Event-free survival curves associated with magnetic resonance imaging evidence of microvascular occlusion and infarct size. **A,** Event-free survival (clinical course without cardiovascular death, reinfarction, congestive heart failure, or stroke) for patients with and without CMR microvascular obstruction. **B,** Event-free survival (clinical course without cardiovascular death, reinfarction, congestive heart failure, stroke, or unstable angina requiring hospitalization) for patients grouped by CMR infarct size. (From Wu KC, Zeerhouni EA, Judd RM, et al. The prognostic significance of microvascular obstruction by magnetic resonance imaging in patients with acute myocardial infarction. *Circulation* 1998; 97:765.)

of PCI.[18] Nine patients undergoing successful coronary stenting who had a mean myocardial-bound creatine kinase (CK-MB) elevation 2.3 times normal after the procedure demonstrated small regions of delayed enhancement in the perfusion territory of the target vessel. The average estimated mass of myocardial necrosis was 2 g. The extent of the hyperenhanced region appears to be predictive of future clinical events in patients with AMI (Figure 8-8). In patients followed over a year, the presence of microvascular obstruction by ceCMR predicted more frequent cardiovascular complications and was associated with fibrous scar and left ventricular modeling on follow-up scanning. The risk of adverse events increased with increased size of the region of hyperenhancement. Thus, there is increasing evidence that ceCMR can be used in the detection of AMI.

Noninvasive (Later After Onset of Symptoms)

Echocardiography

Echocardiography has become the most important, widely available, noninvasive technique to serially assess ventricular function in acute and chronic coronary syndromes. Quantitation of ejection fraction is possible by transthoracic echocardiography in most patients. However, in patients with technically difficult images, transesophageal echocardiography may be used to assess ejection fraction, as well as characterize valve structure and function and hemodynamic parameters. Radionuclide ventriculography provides a quantitative ejection fraction in patients in whom echocardiographic data are suboptimal.

Systolic and Diastolic Function

In the ischemic cascade, myocardial perfusion reductions temporally precede diastolic filling abnormalities, wall motion abnormalities, electrocardiographic changes, and finally chest discomfort. Doppler echocardiography can be used to evaluate left ventricular diastolic dysfunction. When pressures on the left side of the heart are normal, the mitral velocity in early diastole (E) exceeds that in the subsequent atrial systole (A). This relationship can change with normal aging, the presence of left ventricular hypertrophy, and myocardial ischemia. During acute ischemia, provoked by percutaneous balloon inflation during coronary angioplasty, the atrial systolic wave (A) becomes more prominent, consistent with abnormal diastolic filling secondary to abnormal cardiac relaxation and decreased early filling velocity into the left ventricle. Identification of such diastolic filling abnor-

malities of the ventricle is not useful as a diagnostic tool in AMI, or infarction, unless Doppler velocity recordings, taken before the acute ischemic episode, are available for comparison.

Hemodynamic Assessment

Two-dimensional and Doppler echocardiographic imaging may be used to estimate hemodynamics, including cardiac filling pressures. This application of echocardiography may be used in patients who are unstable or have hemodynamic abnormalities develop after myocardial infarction (Table 8-3). Stroke volume and cardiac output can be calculated from Doppler variables. Stroke distance is a surrogate for stroke volume and is equal to the velocity time integral (VTI) of aortic flow. In patients with a normal aortic valve, the normal stroke distance is 18 to 20 cm. Patients who have a hyperdynamic circulation have a stroke distance of >20 cm, whereas patients with severe left ventricular dysfunction have a stroke distance of <10 cm. Stroke volume can be calculated as the product of stroke distance and the cross-sectional area of the left ventricular outflow tract (assuming uniform shape of the outflow tract), and cardiac output may be calculated by multiplying stroke volume by heart rate. By knowing cardiac output, systemic blood pressure, and estimated central venous filling pressures, it might then be possible to estimate systemic vascular resistance.

Mitral inflow patterns and pulmonary venous flow patterns may be used to evaluate left ventricular filling pressures. Restrictive left ventricular filling patterns are defined as a prominent E wave with a smaller A wave (E > A) associated with shortened isovolumic relaxation and E wave deceleration times. The presence of an ejec-

■ ■ ■

TABLE 8-3 CLASSIFICATION OF HEMODYNAMIC STATES AFTER MYOCARDIAL INFARCTION USING ECHOCARDIOGRAPHY

Hemodynamic category	LVEF	RVEF	LVOT VTI	Mitral E/A	Pulmonary venous flow	PASP (TR velocity)	IVC
Normal	Normal	Normal	20 cm	A wave dominant	S > D	Normal	Normal
Hyperdynamic	Normal or increased	Normal	>20 cm	A wave dominant	S >D	Normal or increased	Normal
Hypovolemia	Variable	Normal	<20 cm	A wave dominant	S > D	Normal or decreased	Small, spontaneous collapse
LV failure:							
Mild	Mild decrease	Normal or decreased	Mild decrease	E wave dominant	S < D	Mild increase	Normal to plethoric
Severe	Moderate decrease	Normal or decreased	Moderate decrease	E wave dominant	S << D	Moderate increase	Normal to plethoric
Cardiogenic shock	Severe decrease	Normal or decreased	Severe decrease	E wave dominant	S << D	Moderate increase	Normal to plethoric
RV infarction	Variable	Decreased	Decrease	A wave dominant	S > D	Decreased	Severe plethora w/o collapse
MR	Normal to increased	Normal or decreased	Decreased	E wave dominant	SFR	Increased	Normal to plethoric
VSD	Normal to increased	Normal or decreased	Decreased	Variable	S < D	Increased	Normal to plethoric

LVEF, left ventricular ejection fraction; RVEF, right ventricular ejection fraction; LVOT VTI, left ventricular outflow tract velocity time integral; MR, mitral regurgitation; VSD, ventricular septal defect; TR, tricuspid regurgitation; PASP, pulmonary artery systolic pressure; S, systolic; D, diatolic; SFR, systolic flow reversal.

tion fraction of <35% and a mitral deceleration time <120 ms is correlated with a pulmonary capillary wedge pressure of >20 mmHg. Patients with elevated E/A ratios and decreased deceleration times in the presence of reduced systolic function (<40%) have an increased rate of adverse events during follow-up. Doppler tissue imaging detects the velocity of myocardial or annular movement over time. The ratio of peak transmitral velocity (E, cm/s) to the early mitral annular diastolic velocity (E′, cm/s) is predictive of elevated left atrial filling pressures.

Several groups have estimated left atrial pressure from pulmonary venous flow patterns. Quantitation of pulmonary venous flow patterns has demonstrated a relationship between the proportion of systolic fraction of flow and left atrial pressures. The velocity time integral of systolic and diastolic wave forms is integrated, and the proportion of total flow occurring in systole (systolic fraction) is calculated. In one study, the relationship between left atrial pressure and systolic fraction of pulmonary venous flow by transesophageal echocardiographic imaging was: Left atrial pressure = 0.35 to 0.39*(systolic fraction), (r = −.88; SEE = 3.5 mmHg).[19] Another study demonstrated a similar relationship by transthoracic echocardiography, with a technical success rate of >80% and found that a systolic fraction of <36% was consistent with a mean pulmonary capillary wedge pressure of ≥18 mmHg (sensitivity = 90%; specificity = 85%). The durations of the transmitral A wave and the pulmonary venous retrograde diastolic flow (occurring with atrial contraction) may be compared with estimated left ventricular end-diastolic pressure. Patients with a pulmonary venous retrograde duration greater than the transmitral A wave are likely to have an end-diastolic pressure of >15 mmHg (sensitivity = 85%; specificity = 79%).

Central venous filling pressures may be difficult to evaluate by physical examination, and measurement of inferior vena cava dimensions and their respirophasic variation yields noninvasive estimates of right atrial filling pressures. In patients with a low central venous filling pressure, the inferior vena cava is small (<1 cm in diameter) and collapses by >70% of its diameter with inspiration. Elevated filling pressures (>10 mmHg) are associated with inferior vena caval dilation (>2 cm in diameter) and a lack of respirophasic variation (plethora).

Pulmonary artery systolic pressure is most commonly estimated from the peak tricuspid regurgitant velocity using the modified Bernoulli equation (which states that the pressure gradient across a restrictive orifice = $4\,V^2$, where V is the peak instantaneous velocity of flow through the orifice [or in the acceleration zone]). Pulmonary artery pressure is estimated as right atrial pressure plus 4 times [tricuspid regurgitant peak velocity]^2. An empirical constant [5, 10, or 15 mmHg, depending on the size of the right atrium, severity of regurgitation, and appearance of the inferior vena cava] or floating constant [10% of the peak gradient] is usually assigned to right atrial pressure). This measurement is feasible in most patients with even a small amount of tricuspid regurgitation.

Echocardiography (High-Resolution Color and Contrast)

High-resolution color Doppler ultrasound has been successfully used in 61 consecutive patients with acute anterior myocardial infarction to image the left anterior descending coronary artery and perforators in the anteroapical wall. TIMI flow was also assessed by angiography.[20] The sensitivity, specificity, and diagnostic accuracy of color Doppler ultrasound in detecting left anterior descending patency were 86%, 98%, and 97%, respectively, on the basis of a recanalization score that was used. Futhermore, this recanalization score was a better discriminator of ventricular functional recovery than TIMI flow.

Detection of perfusion abnormalities by echocardiography is possible with myocardial contrast echocardiography. In this technique, a contrast agent (lipid/gas emulsion) is administered intravenously, crosses through the pulmonary vasculature, and is distributed to the myocardium by way of the coronary arteries. Myocardium with decreased blood flow will have absent, or diminished, distribution of the microbubbles with absent, or diminished, signal intensity. If either the "macro-" or "micro-" circulation of a region of myocardium is abnormal, this will be revealed by myocardial contrast echocardiography.

Intravenous myocardial contrast echocardiography and ultrasonic tissue characterization with integrated backscatter (IBS) shows some promise as a bedside technique to detect patency of the infarct-related artery. In the absence of any change in wall motion, there is recovery of cyclic IBS in the territories supplied by a patent infarct-related artery but not when the artery is occluded. By comparing peak-to-peak cyclic IBS in the infarct-artery territory with normal remote areas of myocardium in patients with AMI and using a 15% difference in cyclic IBS as a cutoff between infarcted and normal segments, the sensitivity, specificity, positive and negative predictive values were 92%, 75%, 81%, and 89%, respectively, for determining an occluded infarct-related artery. The cyclic IBS in the infarct-related artery territory was much lower when it was occluded.[21]

Nuclear

Assessing Ventricular Function

Radionuclide ventriculography (also commonly referred to as MUGA, for multigated acquisition) is an accurate and highly reproducible method for assessing LVEF. Interobserver and intraobserver variability are significantly less for radionuclide ventriculography than for echocardiography. The technique has probably been underused in the past in proportion to its proven value in assessing ventricular function after myocardial infarction. However, the advent of gated single proton emission computed tomography (SPECT) determinations of LVEF now allows determination of LV function at the time of myocardial perfusion imaging, and this reduces the need for a separate study to determine ventricular function.

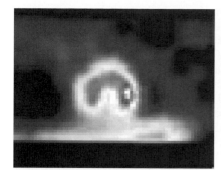

SAX - Apex

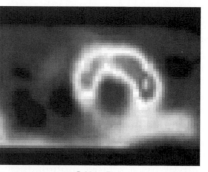

SAX - Base

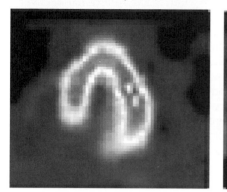

Horizontal LAX

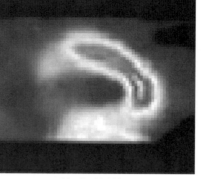

Vertical LAX

FIGURE 8-9. Sestamibi imaging of a patient with atypical chest pain. A 67-year-old woman was seen in the emergency room with atypical chest pain and an electrocardiogram with a left bundle-branch block pattern. A sestamibi scan revealed an inferior wall perfusion defect. Subsequent coronary angiography showed 99% stenosis of the proximal right coronary artery, which was successfully revascularized by percutaneous coronary intervention. SAX, short axis; LAX, long axis. See also Color Insert.

Detecting and Localizing AMI

The use of ^{201}Tl for acute rest imaging in myocardial infarction was originally reported by Wackers in 1975, and despite a subsequent publication showing the sensitivity of ^{201}Tl to be essentially 100% when done in the first 6 hours of infarction, the use of ^{201}Tl for acute infarct imaging never achieved widespread practice, in part because of logistical problems in obtaining the needed radiopharmaceutical in a timely manner. The development of the ^{99m}Tc-based agent sestamibi prompted a reexamination of myocardial perfusion imaging for the acute diagnosis of myocardial infarction because of several favorable tracer properties: (1) the ability to prepare the tracer agent locally from a "kit"; (2) the lack of significant sestamibi redistribution, allowing injection very early during medical stabilization of the patient, with subsequent imaging several hours later; (3) higher energy photons better suited for imaging with current gamma cameras, resulting in less attenuation artifacts; and (4) higher count densities, allowing suitable gated images to be performed in most patients and thus permitting simultaneous evaluation of myocardial perfusion and left ventricular systolic function. Several studies have shown that acute perfusion imaging with resting sestamibi or ^{99m}Tc-tetrofosmin injections can accurately provide early detection of myocardial infarction in patients with chest pain. The sensitivity of rest imaging with ^{99m}Tc-based agents is in excess of 90%, with a negative predictive value for AMI of 99%.

Infarct-Avid Imaging

Perfusion agents such as ^{201}Tl and ^{99m}Tc-sestamibi show an infarct as a "cold spot" or area of absent tracer uptake (Figure 8-9). An alternative approach is to use an agent that is preferentially taken up by an area of acute infarction. The original agent used for this purpose was ^{99m}Tc-pyrophosphate. The shortcomings of this included some difficulty distinguishing cardiac from thoracic cage uptake (especially on planar studies), and the agent is little used today. ^{99m}Tc-pyrophosphate can still play a role in evaluating patients seen late after a presumptive infarct (e.g., 72 hours), when biochemical markers may have returned to normal. If the test is performed outside this "time window" or when planar rather than SPECT imaging is used, false-negative results are frequent. However, pyrophosphate scans have no role in the acute determination of a fresh infarction. Indium-111–labeled antimyosin antibody is now available as an alternative infarct-avid agent; it is highly specific for myocardial necrosis, and thus avoids the problem with skeletal uptake. However, it is not suitable for rapid detection of a myocardial infarction, because blood pool uptake must be allowed to clear, and the optimal imaging time is 24 to 48 hours after injection. Additional agents are under evaluation but not yet clinically available, including ^{99m}Tc-glucarate, which can provide early imaging of infarct zones, and ^{99m}Tc-labeled annexin-V, a protein with high affinity for apoptotic cells.

Infarct Sizing

In addition to detecting and localizing myocardial infarctions, nuclear imaging techniques have proven accurate in measuring infarct size, both qualitatively and quantitatively. ^{99m}Tc-sestamibi with tomographic imaging can measure infarct size and correlates well with ejection fraction and wall motion score, and ^{201}Tl estimates of infarct size. Indeed, SPECT imaging with ^{99m}Tc-sestamibi might be the best available tool for measurement of infarct size.[22] Infarct size varies widely from subject to subject for a given site of coronary arterial occlusion, both in animal studies and in humans. Infarct size is a powerful predictor of late LVEF, left ventricular size, and long-term clinical outcome. Because of regions of stunned myocardium or regions of compensatory hyperkinesis, measures of LVEF during initial hospitalization for AMI may not correspond with eventual LVEF measured 6 weeks later.

Assessing Reperfusion

Reperfusion therapy for AMI is geared toward reestablishing patency of flow in the infarct-related artery, thereby salvaging ischemic but not yet permanently necrotic heart muscle tissue, with improvement in clinical outcomes. Thus, in addition to measuring final infarct size, it would be useful to have an accurate measure of the degree of myocardium at risk in patients with an acute transmural myocardial infarction. Because ^{99m}Tc-sestamibi does not undergo significant redistribution, myocardial perfusion imaging with sestamibi has developed into a useful technique for making these measurements, at least for clinical research.[22] Sestamibi may be injected early after patient presentation, even in the emergency department, with imaging delayed for several hours while other acute stabilization measures are being performed. The images then obtained provide a "snapshot" of what myocardial perfusion was like *at the time of initial tracer injection*. A repeat injection of sestamibi can be made 48, or more, hours later, with repeat imaging showing a more accurate representation of final infarct size. The difference in defect size between the two images represents the amount of myocardial salvage achieved. In a clinical research study, participants can then serve as their own "control" in studies of myocardial salvage. Because of this factor and the close relationship between infarct size and outcome, effective studies of treatments for myocardial infarction can be performed with significantly fewer subjects and at less cost than mortality studies. However, because of the need to reimage the patient 48 hours, or more, into the infarct period to assess myocardial salvage, this technique is clinically not helpful for evaluating infarct artery patency acutely (e.g., to help in making decisions regarding the need for "rescue" angioplasty after attempted thrombolytic therapy).

CMR Angiography

There has been considerable interest in the development of coronary artery magnetic resonance angiography (coronary MRA) as a means of performing noninvasive coronary angiography, because it does not use ionizing radiation and does not necessarily require the injection of a contrast agent. Initial reports suggested a moderate sensitivity and specificity for the detection of significant coronary stenosis. However, there are serious technical challenges in obtaining diagnostic images in many patients, including the complex three-dimensional course of the coronary arteries, respiratory and cardiac motion, and potential artifacts.[23] Despite these problems, significant progress has been made through the use of navigator echo techniques that correct for respiratory motion during free breathing by the patient (Figure 8-10).

In the first multicenter trial of coronary MRA,[24] free breathing coronary CMR was performed in 109 patients at seven centers before conventional contrast coronary angiography. The detection of lesions by MRA was compared with the presence of >50% reduction in diameter on X-ray angiography. Eighty-four percent of proximal and middle coronary artery segments could be analyzed, and 83% of clinically significant lesions were detected on coronary MRA. For left main or three-vessel disease, the sensitivity, specificity, and accuracy of coronary MRA were 100%, 85%, and 87%, respectively. The negative predictive value for any coronary artery disease was 81%, and for left main or three-vessel disease it was 100%. These results led the authors to conclude that noninvasive coronary MRA reliably identifies or excludes the presence of left main coronary or three-vessel coronary artery disease. Most patients with isolated distal coronary artery disease will be missed with this technique. In an accompanying editorial, concerns were raised regarding the average length of the examination (70 minutes) and that only 84% of proximal vessel segments could be analyzed. Recent studies indicate that CMR can be used to directly image the coronary wall and evaluate the progression of atherosclerotic process (Figure 8-11). However, at present, coronary wall imaging remains a research approach.

Thus, despite continuing improvement in technique, coronary MRA is not recommended in the general evaluation of patients. However, it can be used very effectively in the evaluation of patients with coronary artery anomalies, Kawasaki disease, and in the evaluation of coronary bypass graft patency. A complicating factor in coronary MRA is the extensive use of coronary artery stents. There is now considerable evidence that patients with coronary stents can be safely imaged with CMR; however, the stents do introduce an artifact in the image that prevents imaging in the region of the stent. A potential area of application of magnetic resonance spectroscopy is in the evaluation of patients with chest pain with normal coronary arteries. Another developing area is the measurement of coronary flow reserve in the epicardial coronary arteries with magnetic resonance flow-sensitive techniques. Studies in animals and man have demonstrated an excellent correlation between CMR assessments of coronary flow and flow reserve and invasive measures. This method has been applied to the evaluation of the functional significance of coronary stenosis and in the assessment of coronary artery restenosis.[25,26]

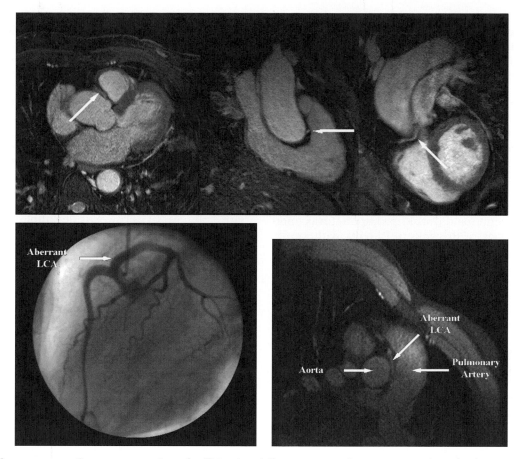

FIGURE 8-10. Coronary magnetic resonance angiography. *Upper panel,* Coronary magnetic resonance angiography demonstrating an aberrant right coronary artery *(arrow)* passing between the aorta and pulmonary artery/right ventricular outflow tract. The left image is in the axial plane, the center image demonstrates the vessel in cross section, and the right image is taken along the course of the vessel. *Lower left panel,* Contrast coronary angiography in a patient with an aberrant coronary artery. The left and right coronary arteries are seen to arise from a common anterior trunk. *Lower right panel,* MR coronary angiography demonstrating that the aberrant left coronary artery (LCA) courses between the aorta and pulmonary artery.

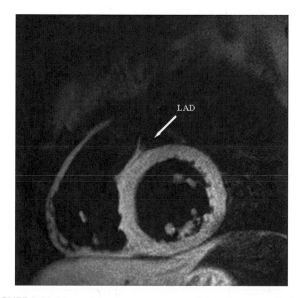

FIGURE 8-11. Magnetic resonance imaging of the coronary wall. Short-axis image of the proximal left anterior descending coronary artery (LAD). Fat suppression has been used to remove the signal from epicardial fat. The wall of the LAD is seen as a ring with a dark central lumen.

NON-ST-SEGMENT ELEVATION AMI

Patients with chest pain without ST elevations or patients who are seen >12 hours after symptom onset (about 50% to 70% of the population with acute coronary syndromes) have electrocardiographic findings such as T-wave inversions, ST depressions, or "nondiagnostic" findings and are part of a large, heterogeneous population with a wide range of risk for adverse outcomes. Some may be "low-risk" patients with noncardiac chest pain, and others may be "high-risk" patients with ventricular dysfunction and multivessel coronary artery disease. For the most part, these patients with unstable angina and non-ST-segment elevation AMI are more likely to have a history of diabetes, hypertension, heart failure, peripheral vascular disease, and prior myocardial infarction.

Noninvasive

Echocardiography

Another application of emergency department echocardiography is the triage of patients with chest pain and suspected acute myocardial ischemia. Patients with significant regional wall motion abnormalities of the ventricle may be admitted to the cardiac care unit, whereas patients without significant wall motion abnormalities may be admitted to a telemetry unit or to a "nonintensive care" chest pain unit for further evaluation. This strategy is safe, decreases the rate of hospitalization of such patients, and is cost-efficient. In patients with prolonged chest discomfort without diagnostic electrocardiographic changes, echocardiography may be used as a screening tool to identify unsuspected regional wall motion abnormalities, left ventricular dysfunction, or valvular dysfunction. The lack of regional wall motion abnormalities decreases the likelihood of significant myocardial infarction and should prompt an evaluation for other etiologies of discomfort. Patients with significant left ventricular dysfunction or mitral dysfunction remain at risk for the development of adverse cardiac outcomes. In addition to AMI, cardiac etiologies for prolonged chest discomfort and left ventricular dysfunction include myocarditis, myopericarditis, acute mitral valve dysfunction, and pericarditis.

In patients who do not have a suspected complication requiring early echocardiographic imaging, transthoracic imaging is typically performed on day 2 or 3 after myocardial infarction. Left ventricular systolic function, the extent of wall motion abnormalities, and associated valvular disease may be assessed with transthoracic echocardiography. This information is helpful for therapeutic purposes such as determining the need for anticoagulation after apical infarction or the initiation of ACE inhibitors. Echocardiographic data after myocardial infarction provide prognostic information as well. Patients with reduced ejection fraction are more likely to have complications, including arrhythmias and death. Patients with extensive wall motion abnormalities are more likely to have recurrent angina, heart failure, and death. Significant mitral regurgitation is a marker for adverse outcomes.

Nuclear

Myocardial perfusion imaging with ^{201}Tl or ^{99m}Tc-labeled tracers can be used in a similar fashion for patients with non-ST-segment elevation myocardial infarctions as with ST-segment elevation infarctions. Patients initially seen with chest discomfort without ST elevations usually have less extensive perfusion defects and higher ejection fractions than those with ST-elevation infarcts and have a more favorable in-hospital prognosis. However, patients with non-ST-elevation infarcts may have a larger amount of inducible ischemia (reversible defects) on predischarge exercise myocardial perfusion imaging. After hospital discharge, they have a larger number of reinfarctions and need readmission and revascularization, so that their cumulative long-term prognosis is effectively equal to those with initial ST-segment elevation myocardial infarctions. In the TIMI-IIIB study of patients with non-Q-wave myocardial infarction and unstable angina, those patients with increased lung thallium uptake on predischarge exercise or dipyridamole ^{201}Tl imaging had a higher subsequent cardiac event rate.

CMR

Contrast-enhanced (ce) CMR, as described previously, can be used to detect very small regions of cellular injury that do not result in ST elevation.[18] In addition, abnormalities associated with delayed clearance of contrast seem to persist for an extended time.[27] This might complicate determining whether new injury has taken place, but insufficient studies have been performed in patients to determine the sensitivity of ceCMR to detect new injury in the presence of preexisting abnormalities. Also, it is known that contrast enhancement occurs in the setting of other conditions such as cardiac sarcoidosis, which could mimic injury caused by coronary heart disease. CMR can be used to assess myocardial perfusion with the use of intravenously administered contrast agents. Similar to stress radionuclide perfusion studies, images are obtained at rest and with the administration of a vasodilator such as adenosine or dipyridamole. However, presently approved CMR contrast agents redistribute rapidly and require imaging during the first pass of the agent through the myocardium.

The MR contrast agent is typically injected through a peripheral vein with a power injector to obtain a reproducible bolus. The first pass of the contrast agent through the myocardium is observed at rest, and then the study is repeated after administration of the vasodilator in the same dose used in radionuclide or echocardiographic studies. Hypoperfused regions appear dark relative to normally perfused myocardium because of delayed wash-in of contrast agent and initially lower concentration of contrast agent during the first pass. Advantages include high spatial resolution and the ability to detect subendocardial ischemia. Disadvantages include the need to acquire images rapidly during the first pass of contrast agent through the heart.

Wash-in of contrast assessed by CMR has been compared with PET and coronary angiography in patients with suspected coronary artery disease referred for coronary angiography (Figure 8-12).[28] The best results for the detection of coronary disease by CMR involved assessing wash-in of contrast agent in the subendocardium and yielded a sensitivity of 91% and a specificity of 94% for CMR compared with reduced coronary flow reserve as defined by PET. In addition, the extent of abnormal myocardium as assessed by MR correlated closely with the PET measurement. The presence a >50% stenosis by quantitative coronary angiography was then compared with the presence of subendocardial MR perfusion abnormality. The sensitivity and specificity of MR in the detection of a >50% lesion was comparable for all three coronary arteries individually and for the number of involved vessels. A weakness of this study was the fact that patients with known prior infarction were excluded, so that sensitivity and specificity of the technique in those patients is unknown.

In another more recent study, flow reserve indices calculated from CMR perfusion studies were compared with quantitative coronary angiography and PET.[29] In healthy volunteers the flow reserve by CMR upslope analysis was lower at 2.1 ± 0.6 compared with PET at

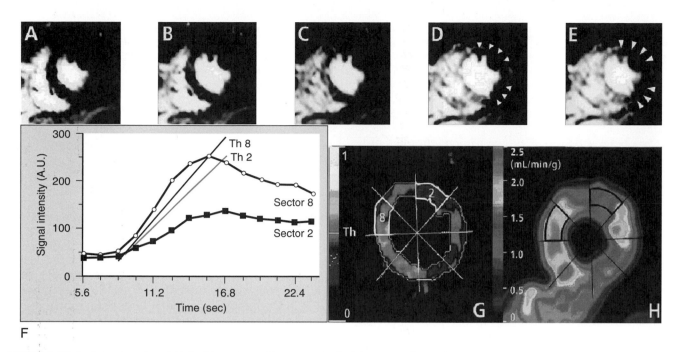

FIGURE 8-12. Perfusion imaging. **A-E,** In this patient with stenoses in the left anterior descending coronary artery and the right coronary artery, the transit of contrast material through the left ventricular myocardium during hyperemia demonstrates delayed wash-in in both the subendocardial and subepicardial layers of both arteries *(arrowheads)*. **F,** Representative signal intensity–time curves are shown for normal myocardium (sector 8) and hypoperfused myocardium (sector 2). On the parametric slope map **(G)**, pixels below/above the threshold (Th) are encoded in shades of blue/red, respectively. On the PET image **(H)**, reduced hyperemic flow is demonstrated in corresponding sectors. (Adapted from Schwitter J, Nanz D, Kneifel S, et al. Assessment of myocardial perfusion in coronary artery disease by magnetic resonance. A comparison with positron emission tomography and coronary angiography. *Circulation* 2001; 103:2230.) See also Color Insert.

3.9 ± 1.1 but correlated with PET flow reserve ($r = 0.70$). A CMR flow reserve of <1.2 predicted coronary artery narrowing (defined as >75% diameter stenosis) with a sensitivity of 69%, specificity of 89%, and a diagnostic accuracy of 79%. Thus, flow reserve by first-pass ceCMR underestimates flow reserve but seems to be capable of detecting significant stenosis in patients.

Invasive

Angiography

Routine coronary angiography after AMI seems to be cost-effective, especially in patients with a prior history of MI, postinfarction angina, or a positive exercise test. Coronary angiography, at the time of presentation of a non-ST elevation AMI, is more likely to reveal multivessel coronary artery disease without total occlusion of the culprit vessel.[1] In this cohort of patients, the ACC/AHA guidelines recommend early coronary angiography and/or interventional therapy in patients who, despite aggressive medical therapy, have persistent or recurrent episodes of symptomatic ischemia occurring spontaneously or induced by stress. In addition, those patients who have continuing hypotension, severe pulmonary congestion, or cardiogenic shock are all potential candidates for early coronary angiography and revascularization.[2]

Ultrasound

Coronary Pathology

Intravascular ultrasound has been used to evaluate the luminal differences between patients with unstable and stable angina. In patients undergoing elective balloon angioplasty, intravascular ultrasound reveals that most of the patients with unstable angina have soft plaques, composed of 80% thickened intimal echoes with homogeneous echodensity less than the adventitia. These soft lesions are likely to have a high content of thrombus, lipid, or fibromuscular components. Subintimal thickening corresponds to a concentric fibrous cap with variable degrees of fibromuscular or lipid deposition beneath. Echolucent zones, possibly corresponding with lipid pools, were documented more frequently in unstable lesions and were a more sensitive indicator of an unstable lesion. Patients with stable angina had more calcific and mixed plaques than did patients with unstable angina. Intravascular ultrasound, therefore, has the ability to identify potentially unstable lesions.

Low-echogenicity soft plaques are more frequently found in the angina-producing lesions of patients with unstable angina and also in younger patients with lesions located in the proximal arterial segments. There is a significantly higher frequency of echogenic (hard, fibrocalcific) plaques in older patients, those with stable angina, and those lesions located in the distal arterial segments. On the basis of these risk profiles, the symptom-producing lesions may be classified in groups likely to have either soft or hard plaque. Soft plaques with high cellular or thrombotic components, or both, may regress with appropriate treatment, whereas hard plaques with high dense fibrous or calcific components, or both, are unlikely to do so. Therefore, plaque regression therapy may be more appropriately directed toward patients likely to have soft plaques.

It has been shown that rupture-prone atherosclerotic lesions tend to be relatively soft and cholesterol rich with a thin fibrous cap overlying a lipid core and that plaque rupture is more common in eccentric plaques. This finding allows intravascular ultrasound to potentially identify lesions at risk for rupture and highlights the inability of angiography to identify vulnerable atheromas (Figure 8-13).

Additional investigation of the unstable lesion with intravascular ultrasound revealed a "layered" appearance within these lesions. This was thought to represent mural thrombus apposed to an underlying atheromatous plaque. Supporting this concept is that this appearance is seen in unstable lesions known to be thrombotic in nature, and the characteristics of the inner layer corresponded with published descriptions of experimentally induced intraarterial thrombus.

Recent studies have also demonstrated that the remodeling patterns are quite different in patients with unstable angina than patients with stable angina. Patients with unstable angina tend to have a larger vessel area/plaque area ratio, suggesting that these plaques have been undergoing recent expansion. Whether this remodeling process plays a role in the subsequent plaque rupture is unknown.

Mechanisms of Coronary Intervention

Intravascular ultrasound has also aided in determining the mechanism of PTCA. It has been shown that lumen enlargement with balloon dilatation results from a combination of dissection, arterial expansion, and axial plaque redistribution. It has also been shown that compared with stenoses without a disease-free wall, stenotic segments with a disease-free wall are associated with significantly lower lumen gains after balloon dilatation, and

this lumen enlargement is mainly obtained by wall stretch. This may increase restenosis because of late recoil, and therefore these lesions may be better treated with directional coronary atherectomy or stenting. The mechanism of angioplasty depends on the clinical situation. In most patients with unstable angina, angioplasty results in lesion remodeling, compression, or displacement of plaque material. In patients with stable angina, significant cross-sectional area reduction is less frequent, and vessel stretch is more frequently seen.

Assessing Residual Stenosis

In the setting of AMI, intravascular ultrasound may be an important clinical tool. The most important issue is to reestablish coronary flow. Although in most cases reperfusion requires balloon angioplasty, reflow occasionally occurs with contrast injection into the arterial system or with manipulation of the coronary guidewire necessary for PCI. Once flow is reestablished, intravascular ultrasound can be used to assess the degree of residual stenosis and to optimize the results of coronary intervention. Intravascular ultrasound characterization of the type of lesion present may also influence the therapeutic strategy for treatment of the lesion. Advantages to the use of intravascular ultrasound in the setting of AMI include the ability to visualize the intracoronary processes. Disadvantages include the additional time required for this procedure; however, one study reported an intravascular ultrasound imaging time of 75 ± 22 seconds, which was a minimal proportion of the total duration of the invasive procedure.

In patients with stable or unstable angina, intravascular ultrasound likewise has an important role. Intravascular ultrasound can be used to assess lesions of indeterminate severity and, similar to patients with acute myocardial infarction, can be used to optimize the results of percutaneous intervention. Advantages and disadvantages to intravascular ultrasound in this clinical situation are similar to those for patients with AMI; however, in this instance, the time disadvantage is even less critical because of the patient's relative stability.

Assessing the Indeterminate Lesion

Determining lesion severity in the cardiac catheterization laboratory is critical. Underestimation of disease severity leaves stenoses untreated, whereas overestimation of severity leads to unnecessary coronary interventions that might lead to the development of restenosis from vessel injury. Coronary angiography underestimates lesion severity within a vessel with diffuse atherosclerotic lesions and has other difficulties determining lesion severity, depending on lesion location, lesion morphology, and superimposition of arterial branches.

For example, evaluation for disease within the left main coronary artery is of the utmost importance. Unfortunately, measurements of the left main artery are the least accurate of any coronary segment analyzed by angiography. The difficulties arise from the lack of a reference segment and are caused by foreshortening or superimposition of other branches that often limit angio-

Vulnerable plaque

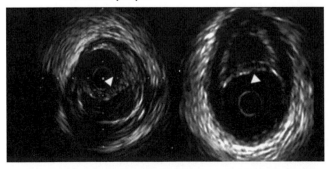

FIGURE 8-13. Intravascular ultrasound images of a highly remodeled coronary plaque with features of vulnerable plaque. There is an echolucent core and a thin fibrous cap (*arrows*). See also Color Insert.

graphic detection of disease within the left main coronary artery. In fact, a high percentage of patients with angiographically normal vessels have left main disease by intravascular ultrasound, including stenoses greater than 40%. Studies have been done to validate the use of intravascular ultrasound in the assessment of coronary artery stenosis severity. Nishioka et al, with stress myocardial perfusion imaging as the "gold standard," found several intravascular ultrasound-derived indices that quantitatively discriminated significant from nonsignificant coronary artery stenoses.[30] A lesion lumen area 4.0 mm^2 showed excellent diagnostic values of 88% sensitivity and 90% specificity. Overall vessel size or degree of coronary remodeling did not affect this measurement. The lesion percent area stenosis ((lesion external elastic lamina (EEL) area − lesion lumen area)/lesion EEL area) × 100), the luminal percent area stenosis ((mean reference lumen area − lesion lumen area)/mean reference lumen area} × 100), and corrected percent area stenosis ((mean reference EEL area − lesion lumen area)/mean reference EEL area) × 100) showed similar high sensitivities and specificities. Unlike other methods for indeterminate lesion assessment, including stress nuclear perfusion imaging, stress echocardiography, intracoronary Doppler flow measurement, and transtenotic pressure measurement, intravascular ultrasound is not affected by the microcirculation and is therefore a precise diagnostic imaging modality for independently assessing epicardial coronary stenosis severity.

Further study has been done to evaluate the left main coronary artery, given its importance and its notoriously difficult assessment by angiography. Critical left main coronary artery disease has been defined as a lumen area stenosis >80%, minimum lumen diameter <2.0 mm, and/or minimal lumen area <4.0 mm^2.

Guiding Therapy

Intravascular ultrasound not only assists in the assessment of an indeterminate coronary artery stenosis, it also guides the therapeutic strategy. Intravascular ultrasound allows the operator to base decisions not on lumenograms alone but also on assessment of the vessel wall. Intravascular ultrasound also accurately measures lumen size, plaque thickness, lesion length, and vessel wall size, enabling accurate sizing of interventional devices.

Intravascular ultrasound aids in optimal device selection such as whether to use rotoblators in calcified lesions or atherectomy devices in large plaques. Coronary artery calcification detected with intravascular ultrasound is predictive of a worse outcome with both PTCA, with larger and more frequent dissections, and DCA, with less tissue removed when superficial calcium is present. This might suggest rotablator as a therapeutic approach that preferentially removes atherosclerotic plaque composed of fibrous and calcific elements without extensive plaque disruption or arterial expansion.

Intravascular ultrasound demonstration of soft plaque juxtaposed to calcified plaque is the most important independent predictor of angiographic dissection after balloon angioplasty. Lesions with at least a 90-degree arc of superficial calcification identified by intravascular ultrasound have significantly greater residual plaque and smaller residual lumens than lesions with either less than a 90-degree arc of calcium or no calcium when treated with DCA. These lesions might be best treated with rotablator or stenting.

Intravascular ultrasound imaging identifies lesions with a disease-free wall. It has been shown that compared with stenoses without a disease-free wall, lesions with a disease-free wall are associated with significantly lower lumen gains after balloon dilatation and that this lumen enlargement is mainly obtained by wall stretch. This might increase restenosis, and therefore these lesions might be better treated with DCA or stenting. DCA might be more effective in cases of soft plaque and rotational atherectomy or laser angioplasty in cases of hard plaque.

Optimizing Coronary Intervention

After intravascular ultrasound has been used to assess the significance of an indeterminate lesion and guided the treatment strategy, it can be used to optimize the outcome of subsequent PCI. The need for PCI optimization is evidenced by angiographic results showing residual diameter stenosis of 15% to 25% after coronary intervention, whereas intravascular ultrasound assessment reveals plaque burden often to be >50% of the vessel's area. Intravascular ultrasound provides a more accurate assessment of lumen size after intervention, because angiography often overestimates the residual lumen size after balloon angioplasty. Fractures and dissections created with angioplasty can fill with contrast dye and "normalize" the angiographic silhouette even on orthogonal views. It is not uncommon to encounter a hazy lesion during angiography; this may represent thrombus, dissection, or calcium and often cannot be differentiated by angiography alone, requiring intravascular ultrasound to distinguish between these entities.

Not only does intravascular ultrasound provide helpful information regarding the diameter of a stenosis, it also helps delineate the length of the lesion. Through imaging of the vessel during catheter pullback, the lesion is visualized in its entirety. These data are helpful in choosing a stent length that will completely cover the diseased segment of the artery.

PTCA

It has been shown that the reference segment for a stenotic lesion often has a large plaque burden evident by intravascular ultrasound. The ultrasound appearance of the lesion after dilatation also demonstrates a large residual plaque burden despite acceptable post-PTCA angiography. The Clinical Outcomes with Ultrasound Trial (CLOUT), showed that intravascular ultrasound could be used to appropriately oversize PTCA balloons. In this study, after routine PTCA intravascular ultrasound imaging was performed, if atheromatous remodeling was present, PTCA was repeated with larger balloons. The demonstration of atheromatous remodeling by intravascular ultrasound permits the safe use of balloons that had

Red Clot and White Clot

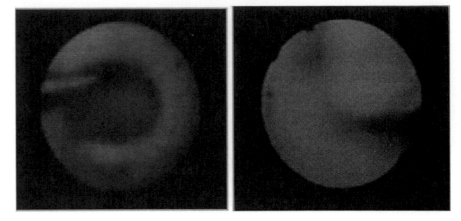

FIGURE 8-14. Angioscopy of two plaques in patients with a acute coronary syndrome. The left panel shows a plaque that is rich in red cells and probably fibrin. The right panel shows a plaque that is rich in platelets. (Reprinted from Abela et al. *Am J Cardiol* 1999; 83:94, with permission from Excerpta Medica Inc.) See also Color Insert.

been traditionally considered oversized, resulting in significantly improved luminal dimensions without increased rates of dissection or ischemic complications.

Coronary Stenting

Intravascular ultrasound is particularly helpful in optimizing coronary stent deployment and in detecting stent deployment abnormalities that are not detected with angiography, including incomplete stent expansion and apposition, articulation site prolapse, and inlet or outlet stenoses. In the CRUISE study, stent implantation was evaluated comparing intravascular ultrasound guidance to angiography guidance alone. In the intravascular ultrasound guidance group, 36% of patients required additional therapy because of incomplete apposition, edge dissection, and, most commonly, suboptimal minimal stent area (MSA). As a result, the MSA in this intravascular ultrasound subgroup increased from a mean of 7.06 mm^2 to 7.78 mm^2. At 9 months' follow-up, the intravascular ultrasound guidance group experienced a 44% relative reduction in target vessel revascularization (TVR), without a difference in death or myocardial infarction.[31]

High-pressure balloon inflation after stent deployment under angiographic guidance alone results in suboptimal stent expansion in >50% of cases, and further ultrasound-guided high-pressure dilatations can improve stent expansion. Optimal stent deployment is commonly defined as: (1) minimal lumen cross-sectional area >80% of the average reference segment area (proximal reference area minus distal reference area, or more than 100% distal reference area); (2) good apposition of struts against the vessel wall, so that no space separates the stent and vessel; (3) no dissection at the stent margins; and (4) circular or symmetric stent expansion.

Predicting Restenosis

Intravascular ultrasound has assisted in the discovery of factors that predict restenosis. After PTCA, luminal areas that are minimal seem to indicate restenosis, whereas morphological appearance is less predictive. Other factors that have been associated with restenosis are the absence of plaque fracture, the existence of a major dissection, and residual plaque burden >40% of vessel area. The postintervention intravascular ultrasound assessment of percent cross-sectional area narrowing, an index of plaque burden, is a powerful predictor of restenosis. This concept was supported by the results of the GUIDE trial, in which plaque burden was the most significant predictor of restenosis, whereas angiographic predictors were not significant. In the Restenosis after intravascular ultrasound Guided Stenting (RESIST) study, there was a 6% absolute reduction in the angiographic restenosis rate with intravascular ultrasound guidance, 23% vs. 29%. There was also a 20% increase in late lumen cross-sectional area in the intravascular ultrasound guidance group compared with angiography guidance alone. This highlights the importance of optimizing deployment at stent delivery.

Angioscopy

Unstable Angina vs. Stable Angina

Angioscopy has been used to study the pathophysiological differences within the artery among patients with unstable angina and stable angina (Figure 8-14). In a study of patients undergoing directional coronary atherectomy (DCA), Theime et al[32] evaluated angioscopic differences in patients with stable angina, postmyocardial infarction angina (defined as MI within 3 months), rest angina, crescendo angina, or primary angina. Lesion color was similarly distributed among patients with stable angina (57% yellow and 44% gray-white); however, lesions were predominantly yellow in patients with unstable angina and postmyocardial infarction angina (89% and 91%, respectively). Ruptured surfaces were found in 26% of patients with stable angina, 39% of patients with unstable angina, and 44% of patient after myocardial infarction. Histological analysis of the DCA specimen revealed that gray-white lesions represented fibrous plaque without degeneration in 64% and with degeneration in 36%, whereas gray-yellow lesions were associated predominantly with degenerated plaque (64%) and occasionally with fibrous plaque (21%) or atheroma (14%). Deep yellow or yellow-red lesions represented either atheroma (53%) or degenerated plaque (42%). The yellow color indicates the presence of a thin fibrous or mere endothelial layer covering free lipids. Subgroup analysis of the patients with yellow plaque explains the relative abundance of patients with stable angina. Forty percent of patients with stable angina and no prior MI were found to have yellow plaque, whereas yellow plaque was seen in 69% of patients with stable angina with MI >3 months and 91% with MI ≤3 months. Plaque color is a major indicator of instability and acute complications of coronary artery disease.

Several studies have assessed the angioscopic differences between patients with unstable and stable angina. Angioscopy performed during open-heart surgery revealed that none of the patients with stable angina had complex plaque or thrombus. All patients with accelerated angina had a complex plaque in the offending artery, but none had thrombus. All patients with rest angina had a thrombus in the offending artery, and one also had a complex plaque detected at another site in the offending artery.

When intracoronary angioscopy and intravascular ultrasound is performed in patients seen for elective coronary intervention, the presence of yellow plaque is similar in patients with stable and unstable angina, but angioscopy reveals thrombus more often in patients with unstable angina. Plaque rupture and thrombosis is present in approximately 17% of patients with stable angina, suggesting that this does not always lead to the clinical manifestation of an acute coronary syndrome.

Angioscopic characteristics of the different subtypes of angina have been defined. The crescendo type of unstable angina has been associated with white thrombi. Rest and postmyocardial infarction angina has been linked to red and pink thrombi. Most patients with stable angina have a smooth plaque surface without associated intracoronary thrombus. Most patients with recurrent ischemia after myocardial infarction still have red thrombus at the lesion site, and often this thrombus is occlusive, and it is this residual thrombus that is important in the development of recurrent ischemia after infarction. Restenotic lesions were all white, nondisrupted, and without thrombus.

Angioscopy may be helpful in patients with stable or unstable angina. It assists in assessment of the indeterminate lesion and, as in patients with acute myocardial infarction, can be used to optimize coronary intervention. The advantages and disadvantages to its use in this clinical situation are similar to those during AMI, with the time disadvantage less important because of the relative stability of the situation.

Assessment of the Indeterminate Lesion

As discussed, determination of the severity of a coronary lesion is critical, because underestimation leaves stenoses untreated, and overestimation leads to unnecessary procedures that might lead to the development of restenosis. The limitations of coronary angiography have been discussed, including its underestimation of lesion severity in diffusely diseased vessels and its diffi-culty determining lesion severity depending on its location, morphology, and superimposed branches.

Angioscopy more clearly defines the nature of the luminal obstruction than does angiography, especially for the detection and characterization of thrombus, ulceration, and calcification within the lesion. With angioscopy as the reference standard, angiography has a low sensitivity (approximately 20% to 66%) and a specificity of approximately 95% for the detection of thrombus. In patients with unstable angina, angioscopy is able to visualize disrupted plaques and intracoronary thrombi that frequently are angiographically silent. The detection of thrombus is important, because the presence of thrombus is a risk factor for both adverse outcome and restenosis.

Predicting Events

Information gained from angioscopic images can be used to predict future ischemic events. The ability of angioscopy, intracoronary ultrasound, and quantitative angiography to predict recurrent ischemia after interventional procedures has been compared, and two predictors, both of which were angioscopic, were identified plaque rupture on views taken before the procedure and thrombus visualized on imaging after the procedure. Therefore, angioscopic characteristics can identify patients who are at high risk.

In patients with unstable angina undergoing PTCA, angioscopy detects thrombus approximately 60% of the time (compared with detection by angiography in 20%), and its presence predicts an increased risk for major in-hospital complications (including death, recurrent ischemia, myocardial infarction, or emergency coronary bypass surgery).

Guiding Therapy

After angioscopy has assessed the culprit lesion, it can assist in guiding the particular therapeutic strategy. For example, angioscopy might be useful in selecting the specific therapy for abrupt occlusion, because it is superior to angiography for determining the etiology of abrupt occlusion. If angioscopy were to reveal thrombus, thrombolysis would be appropriate, whereas long balloon inflations or stents would be required for dissection.

In patients with unstable angina with the culprit lesion in a saphenous vein graft that was suitable for balloon angioplasty, angioscopy was more sensitive in detecting thrombus, dissection, and friable plaque than angiography. The information gained from angioscopy in this situation might indicate which patients would benefit from a distal protection device during percutaneous coronary intervention of a saphenous vein graft.

Optimizing Coronary Intervention

In addition to assessing the severity or etiology of a lesion seen angiographically and assisting in tailoring therapy to the specific cause, angioscopy can be used to optimize the results of a subsequent coronary intervention. Angioscopic pullback provides images along the length of a diseased segment. This information is helpful to accurately determine lesion length and to ensure that the entire lesion is adequately treated. Angioscopy provides a more accurate assessment of lumen size after angioplasty than angiography. Small fractures and dissections that occur after angioplasty can fill with contrast dye and "normalize" the angiographic silhouette despite imaging with orthogonal views. Angioscopy after intervention can identify dissections, intraluminal flap dissections, the adequacy of stent deployment, and residual thrombus.

PTCA

Angioscopy is helpful in assessing the result of PTCA. The neolumen that is created after coronary angioplasty often appears to be slitlike and much narrower by angioscopy than by angiography, suggesting that angiography underestimated the degree of residual stenosis after angioplasty. After balloon dilatation, angioscopy reveals that dissections are often present, and the lumen usually remains irregular with persistent narrowing. All coronary dissections visualized by angioscopy are generally abolished after stenting.

Angioscopy can be important in determining the cause of abrupt closure after PTCA, which is usually due to dissection, thrombosis, or spasm. Distinguishing between these entities is important, because the treatment varies for each condition.

Coronary Stenting

Angioscopy can be used to optimize the use of thrombolytic therapy and stent deployment. Thrombolytic therapy may be administered in cases in which thrombus is not suspected by angiography but in which it is seen on angioscopy, or it may be withheld when angiography suggests thrombus that is not confirmed by angioscopy. Angioscopy can be helpful in optimizing stent deployment, because patients may be treated with repeat angioplasty with a larger balloon if plaque is found to be bulging into the lumen at the stent articulation site. It also identifies patients who require additional stenting procedures either for significant disease proximal or distal to the stent or when a gap is present between two tandem stents. Investigators using angioscopy in this manner report a major improvement in the final luminal diameter and morphology when evaluated angioscopically.

Predicting Restenosis

Lesion characteristics by angioscopy assist in predicting the risk of restenosis after PTCA. It has been reported by some investigators that white plaque is a risk factor for restenosis, whereas others have found no correlation between plaque color and restenosis. Thrombus, especially protruding thrombus, has been described as a risk factor for restenosis.

Similar to intravascular ultrasound, intracoronary angioscopy provides additional information when angiography is ambiguous. Intravascular ultrasound sup-

plies a cross-sectional image, whereas angioscopy provides a topographical survey of the diseased artery. With experience, both assist in assessing stenosis severity and determining lesion length. They provide information that allows tailoring of the therapeutic strategy for the particular disease etiology, and assist in optimizing PCI. Currently, in the United States, intravascular ultrasound is more widely adapted because of its ease of use and its lower learning curve. Newer imaging modalities such as intravascular CMR and optical coherence tomography might provide even more detailed evaluation of the atherosclerotic process and guidance of the minimally invasive treatment techniques.

ISCHEMIC VENTRICULAR DYSFUNCTION

Types

Stunned Myocardium

The term "stunned myocardium" refers to prolonged, but temporary, postischemic ventricular dysfunction without irreversible myocyte damage. Its features include abnormal systolic and diastolic function, viable myocardium that exhibits contractile reserve, and absence of myocyte necrosis with routine microscopy.[33] Typically, a brief period of acute ischemia followed by restoration of coronary perfusion results in prolonged contractile dysfunction. This phenomenon has been observed after AMI with early reperfusion, unstable angina, coronary vasospasm, PTCA, exercise-induced ischemia, open-heart surgery, and after cardiac transplantation. Two clinical examples of myocardial stunning in the setting of acute myocardial infarction are illustrative of the phenomenon. In patients with AMI treated with fibrinolytic therapy within 6 hours of onset and successfully reperfused, it was found that both regional and overall left ventricular function (assessed by angiography) showed improvement 2 weeks after reperfusion, which was not observed within 24 hours. In the echocardiographic substudy of the Healing and Afterload Reducing Therapy Trial,[34] in which 352 patients with anterior myocardial infarctions were randomly assigned to ramipril or placebo, serial echocardiograms were obtained at 1 day, 14 days, and 90 days after myocardial infarction. Although ventricular dilation developed from day 1 to day 14, the degree of infarct zone akinesis, as measured by infarct perimeter, decreased consistent with recovery of function and resolution of stunned myocardium. Ventricular dilation was more prominent in the placebo-treated group, highlighting the benefit of ramipril in attenuating the early part of the remodeling process. Stunned myocardium may be identified by low-dose dobutamine echocardiography performed early after myocardial infarction. Stunned myocardium will develop improved wall thickening. These stunned areas might develop improved function over time.

Hibernating Myocardium

The term "hibernating" myocardium refers to severe, prolonged, cardiac dysfunction secondary to chronic ischemia with viable, although poorly contractile, myocardium.[33,35] As with "stunned" myocardium, the dysfunctional, but viable, myocardium exhibits contractile reserve and can be aroused by inotropic stimuli such as postextrasystolic potentiation or the infusion of a sympathomimetic amine. There is debate whether there is reduced flow or normal flow with reduced coronary vasodilator reserve. Patients with chronic left ventricular ischemic dysfunction might benefit from revascularization and show improvement in ventricular function. Regional myocardial function can be assessed during or after administration of nitroglycerin, after extrasystolic potentiation, catecholamine infusion (dobutamine) or exercise by echocardiography, nuclear imaging, or CMR. Myocardial perfusion, membrane integrity, and metabolism can be assessed by thallium scintigraphy, ^{99m}Tc-sestamibi, PET, and magnetic resonance spectroscopy.

Myocardial Viability/Contractile Reserve

Myocardial viability is an important determinant of left ventricular function and remodeling after myocardial infarction, as well as improvement in ventricular function after revascularization. Viability implies that the underlying myocardium is metabolically intact. Viable myocardium might exhibit normal contractile function or be hypokinetic or akinetic. Hypokinetic and akinetic segments have the capacity to develop improved contractile function if blood supply to that area is restored. Viable akinetic zones are often referred to as stunned or hibernating myocardium. The concept of contractile reserve refers to the capacity of the myocardium to develop improved or augmented contraction when exposed to stressors. Stressors can include exercise or pharmacological agents such as dobutamine.

Echocardiography

There has been interest in the use of low-level exercise to detect contractile reserve and viable myocardium. Because obtaining adequate serial echocardiographic images during treadmill exercise is technically difficult, this may be accomplished with supine bicycle exercise with serial echocardiographic imaging for the assessment of improvement in regional contractility with exercise.

Dobutamine echocardiography has been used to assess both viability and ischemia after myocardial infarction. The safety of administering dobutamine early after infarction in terms of provoking arrhythmias or mechanical complications has been a concern. The most common protocol early after infarction consists of serial infusion of dobutamine from 5, 10, to 20 µg/kg/min in 3- or 5-minute stages. The 20-µg/kg/min dose is the peak postinfarction dose and is the equivalent of a low-level stress test. Dobutamine echocardiography has been performed as early as 2 to 3 days after myocardial infarction in stable patients without a significant increase in adverse events. The normal response to dobutamine administration is for sequential increases in myocardial wall thickening. Normal, or hypokinetic, segments exhibit progressive attenuation or worsening of wall thickening consistent with an ischemic response. Segments may have increased contractility at low doses followed by decreased contractility at higher doses. This pattern constitutes the biphasic response and is consistent with myocardial viability and is predictive of recovery of regional myocardial function in the involved segments after successful revascularization. Myocardium that develops improved contractile function with low-dose dobutamine infusion (<20 µg/kg/min) is exhibiting contractile reserve and implies viable myocardium. Contractile reserve is associated with recovery of segmental motion over time (consistent with myocardial stunning) and improvement of regional function after revascularization (consistent with hibernation). Dobutamine echocardiography has increased specificity and accuracy compared with rest-redistribution thallium for the spontaneous return of regional left ventricular function after myocardial infarction. Prediction of nonviable tissue might be possible from transthoracic imaging. After transmural myocardial infarction, wall thinning and fibrosis occur. Akinetic zones that have a resting wall thickness of ≤6 mm on transthoracic imaging are unlikely to be viable as assessed by dobutamine echocardiography.

Myocardial contrast echocardiography provides a means of studying myocardial perfusion in patients with coronary artery disease and assessing microvascular integrity after AMI.[36] In a study comparing myocardial contrast echocardiography, with the use of intravenous contrast, and low-dose dobutamine echocardiography in predicting recovery of function in patients with recent AMI, contrast echocardiography compared favorably. When the two tests were concordant, the accuracy of prediction of recovery of segmental left ventricular function improved from approximately 75% to 85%.[37] Another study examined the histological correlates of myocardial contrast echocardiography parameters in humans with suspected myocardial hibernation and found that peak myocardial contrast intensity, an index of myocardial blood volume, correlates directly with microvascular density and capillary area and inversely with collagen content. When collagen content is high, and microvascular density is low, the contrast indices of myocardial blood velocity and flow are reduced, whereas they vary when microvasculature is preserved. Last, it was found that an intact microvasculature does not necessarily predict recovery of function and that parameters of blood velocity (the rate of increase of myocardial contrast intensity) and flow (peak myocardial contrast intensity × the rate of increase of myocardial contrast intensity) in these segments help differentiate hibernating from irreversibly damaged myocardium.

PET

PET tracers simultaneously emit two high-energy photons in opposite directions. Coincidence detection allows the PET scanner to detect these two simultaneously generated photons and to identify and localize true events and reject single (i.e., unpaired) photons as random, scattered photons. This improves spatial resolution compared with SPECT and allows correction for tissue photon attenuation. PET also has a high temporal resolution capability not available with SPECT. A number of tracers have been developed for clinical PET studies for the evaluation of regional myocardial blood flow, metabolic processes, oxygen consumption, receptor activity, and membrane function. The most frequently used agents to assess myocardial perfusion with PET are rubidium-82, nitrogen-13 (^{13}N) ammonia, and oxygen-15 (^{15}O) water. Carbon-11 (^{11}C)-labeled fatty acids and fluorine-18 (^{18}F) fluorodeoxyglucose are common metabolic tracers, and ^{11}C acetate is used as an agent to assess oxidative metabolism and oxygen consumption. These tracers require a local or on-site cyclotron for production, except for ^{18}F, which can be shipped for same-day use. PET scanners are more costly and less widely available than standard Anger cameras or SPECT systems. However, development of SPECT-like imaging systems for positron-emitting tracers (using annihilation coincidence circuits or high-energy photon collimators) may increase demand and lower cost for these radiopharmaceuticals.

In addition to the noninvasive detection of coronary artery disease and estimation of the severity of the disease, PET can assess myocardial viability in patients with coronary artery disease and left ventricular dysfunction[38]; it can also be used to evaluate left ventricular volumes, ejection fraction, and wall motion abnormalities.[39] The most common method is to determine whether metabolic activity is preserved in regions with reduced perfusion, with ^{18}F fluorodeoxyglucose as a marker of glucose use and thus tissue viability. Recently, plaque inflammation in the carotid artery was demonstrated by PET, and symptomatic, unstable plaques accumulated more ^{18}F fluorodeoxyglucose.[40] This method obviously opens up possibilities for atheromatous plaque imaging that reflects cellular pathology.

CMR

The detection of irreversibly injured myocardium by ceCMR can potentially be used to determine whether patients with severe left ventricular dysfunction will improve with revascularization. A study in patients with severe ischemic heart failure (mean ejection fraction 28%) compared ceCMR measurement of infarct or scar with reduced perfusion or glucose metabolism as assessed by PET.[41] The sensitivity and specificity of ceCMR for detecting scar tissue defined by PET were 0.96 and 1, respectively. CMR enhancement was present in 11% of segments defined as normal by PET. Of 34 segments with a mismatch on PET indicative of hibernating myocardium, CMR showed no enhancement in 23, nontransmural enhancement in 8, and transmural enhancement in 3. Thus, CMR can identify scar tissue more frequently than PET. Although these results are encouraging, the final role of ceCMR will require functional studies after revascularization to determine the significance of small regions of scar detected by CMR. The low interstudy variability of CMR assessments of chamber size and function permit studies of interventions in small groups of high-risk patients. Recently CMR has been used to demonstrate improvement in systolic wall thickening after laser myocardial revascularization in patients with medically refractory angina who were suboptimal candidates for conventional revascularization.[42]

STRESS TESTING

After admission to the hospital after onset of suspected non-ST-segment elevation MI or unstable angina, continuous risk assessment occurs starting with the initial clinical encounter and continues throughout hospitalization. Some patients are assessed as being at high risk of adverse events because of recurrent angina despite intensive medical therapy, hemodynamic instability, or severe left ventricular dysfunction and usually undergo invasive investigation with a view to revascularization. Other patients will be assessed as very low risk or have a noncardiac diagnosis and do not require risk stratification, because even an abnormal test finding would be unlikely to lead to revascularization therapy.[1] Patients who do not fall into either of these very high- or very low-risk categories constitute 35% to 60% of patients admitted with chest pain; these patients are usually candidates for risk stratification with noninvasive testing. In a meta-analysis of predischarge risk stratification evaluating exercise electrocardiography, myocardial perfusion imaging, and stress ventricular function, the markers of left ventricular dysfunction or heart failure (exercise duration, impaired systolic blood pressure response with exercise, and peak left ventricular ejection fraction) were more sensitive for identifying morbid and fatal outcomes than markers of ischemia (electrocardiographic ST-segment depression, angina, or a reversible perfusion defect).

Echocardiography

Postmyocardial infarction risk stratification includes an assessment for inducible ischemia in most patients. Patients with single-vessel coronary disease treated successfully with percutaneous coronary revascularization do not need an assessment for inducible ischemia before hospital discharge. Standard submaximal electrocardiographic exercise stress testing is appropriate to screen for low-level inducible ischemia if patients do not have resting electrocardiographic ST-segment abnormalities, left ventricular hypertrophy with strain, LBBB, paced rhythm, or digoxin therapy. Patients with these electrocardiographic abnormalities have reduced sensitivity and specificity on standard treadmill testing and benefit from addition of an imaging modality such as echocardiography or nuclear perfusion scanning.

With the availability of pharmacological therapy, including aspirin, clopidogrel, beta-blockers, glycoprotein IIb/IIIa inhibitors, thrombolytic agents, and use of interventional mechanical therapies such as PTCA and coronary artery stenting, the likelihood of developing a new complication of myocardial infarction beyond the fourth or fifth postinfarct day is low. This observation has led to the performance of exercise tests to risk stratify stable patients as early as 3 days after infarction. Low-dose dobutamine stress testing has been performed 2 to

5 days after uncomplicated infarctions without significantly increasing adverse side effects. Prompt risk stratification allows for early discharge of patients without significant ischemia and facilitates decision making regarding coronary catheterization and interventions in patients with evidence for inducible ischemia.

The addition of echocardiographic images to the standard electrocardiographic treadmill test increases the sensitivity and specificity for detection of ischemia, but relatively few studies have examined the usefulness of stress echocardiography early after myocardial infarction. Evidence of ischemia remote from the infarct zone was found to be a predictor of multivessel coronary artery disease and predicted a group of patients at high risk for reinfarction or recurrent angina in the first 3 months after infarction. Remote or adjacent myocardial asynergy on stress echocardiography is predictive of recurrent cardiac events during a follow-up of 6 to 10 months. Patients at high risk for recurrent cardiac events may be identified by presence of lower ejection fractions and by the extent of exercise-induced wall motion abnormality. Stress-induced echocardiographic wall motion abnormalities, ST-segment depressions detected during ambulatory electrocardiographic monitoring, and decreased heart rate variability have all been predictive of an increased risk of death over a 3-year period.

Stress echocardiography has been used to localize the area of ischemia and demonstrate resolution of ischemia in patients undergoing PCIs. In these studies, patients have had regional wall motion abnormalities on exercise echocardiographic imaging before angioplasty and have demonstrated resolution or improvement of these abnormalities after angioplasty. Stress echocardiography and ^{201}Tl SPECT have a concordance rate of approximately 80% before angioplasty and 90% after angioplasty, suggesting that either imaging modality can predict the results of interventions.

Stress echocardiography is typically performed by obtaining rest and peak exercise images. This is designed to detect ischemia as opposed to viability or contractile reserve; however, imaging at serial stages of exercise using supine, or upright bicycle, testing might yield information concerning viability and ischemia. In areas of akinesis, demonstration of increased regional contractility at low levels of exercise is suggestive of myocardial viability. If these areas become dysfunctional at higher workloads, myocardial ischemia is also present. Revascularization of these areas either percutaneously or by surgery might result in a decrease in ischemia and an improvement in overall myocardial function. This biphasic response might be the exercise equivalent to that seen with sequential dobutamine testing as described later.

Dipyridamole is a vasodilator used to induce cardiac ischemia. Dipyridamole echocardiography which is performed extensively in Europe has been used to predict the risk of subsequent cardiac events. The development of ischemia by electrocardiography or echocardiography and clinical symptoms predicts an increased risk of cardiac events and death. The most potent predictors of adverse events have been the detection of ischemia on echocardiography and the time to development of ischemia,

whereas the detection of an abnormal resting wall motion score index was only predictive of increased risk of death.

Dobutamine echocardiography has been used to risk stratify patients after AMI. When dobutamine echocardiography was performed in more than 200 patients early after myocardial infarction, the two multivariate predictors of subsequent morbid and fatal events were infarction zone nonviability and remote ischemia/infarction. Evidence for multivessel disease on dobutamine echocardiography was a more potent predictor of adverse outcome than angiographic multivessel disease. Dobutamine echocardiography has excellent specificity (97%) and moderate sensitivity (70%) for detecting ischemia remote from the infarct zone suggestive of multivessel coronary artery disease. In a large multicenter trial of dobutamine stress echocardiography after myocardial infarction, age and myocardial viability were predictive of future development of spontaneous cardiac events (death, recurrent ischemia or infarction), and when revascularization was also considered as an end point, older age, evidence of remote ischemia, and peak wall motion score index were predictive of adverse end points.

Standard-dose dobutamine echocardiography may be performed 4 to 6 weeks after infarction. By the use of full-dose dobutamine (40 μg/kg/min), the biphasic response to dobutamine administration has been noted. Hypokinetic and akinetic segments that develop improved wall thickening after low-dose dobutamine and a worsening of function at higher doses exhibit the biphasic response. These segments are the most likely to recover function if successful revascularization is performed. In addition, revascularized segments showing a biphasic response have increased augmentation to dobutamine after revascularization. Myocardial segments that have worsening of motion with increasing dobutamine infusion exhibit ischemic physiology. These segments may become nonischemic with revascularization but will not have an improvement in systolic function at rest; however, these segments might develop increased contractility with dobutamine infusion.

Myocardial contrast agents may be used as an adjunct to stress or dobutamine echocardiography, aiding in better identification of endocardium and endocardial motion.[43] These agents are injected through a peripheral vein and pass through the pulmonary circulation into the left side of the heart. When harmonic imaging is used, the contrast effect is seen in the left ventricle highlighting the endocardial border. Comparison of echocardiographic studies with standard imaging techniques and contrast/harmonics have demonstrated an increase in the number of segments that can be interpreted. The use of harmonics technology without contrast also increases endocardial resolution.

Nuclear

It has long been recognized that survivors of AMI are at increased risk of recurrent myocardial infarction and/or death, both during initial hospitalization and in the ensuing months. Predictors of posthospital discharge adverse events include LVEF and inducible ischemia. In the current era of revascularization and infarct size limitation, it is possible that inducible ischemia is relatively more important than previously. Traditionally, submaximal exercise treadmill testing has been advocated before hospital discharge, followed by a maximal exercise treadmill test 4 to 6 weeks later.

The 1999 update to the ACC/AHA Guidelines for Management of Acute Myocardial Infarction gives standard treadmill ECG testing a Class I indication ("conditions for which there is evidence for and/or general agreement that a given procedure or treatment is beneficial, useful, and effective"): (1) before discharge for prognostic assessment or functional capacity (submaximal at 4 to 6 days or symptom limited at 10 to 14 days); (2) early after discharge for prognostic assessment and functional capacity (14 to 21 days); and (3) late after discharge (3 to 6 weeks) for functional capacity and prognosis if early stress was submaximal.[2] Exercise or vasodilator stress perfusion imaging or exercise stress echocardiography are also given a Class I indication "when baseline abnormalities of the ECG compromise interpretation."

However, ST depression or angina on standard treadmill ECG testing have low sensitivity for identifying postinfarction patients who go on to experience adverse cardiac events. Studies examining risk stratification of postinfarction patients with myocardial perfusion imaging by use of either exercise or pharmacological stress have shown that the extent of inducible ischemia on stress perfusion imaging independently predicts risk after infarction. Ischemia detected in patients with myocardial infarction by sestamibi SPECT images is a better predictor of future cardiac events than electrocardiographic evidence of ischemia or exertional chest discomfort during the stress test. Investigators have begun looking at very early postinfarction risk stratification by use of vasodilator stress myocardial perfusion imaging, because some reinfarctions or deaths occur before exercise testing, particularly if not performed until 10 to 21 days after infarction. The current health care environment has made it desirable to identify as early as possible that group of post-MI patients who are at very low risk for recurrent events and can be safely discharged early from the hospital. This is an attractive method, because ischemia is uncommonly induced, and a markedly elevated rate-pressure product is avoided. Brown et al[44] reported on a multicenter trial comparing very early vasodilator myocardial perfusion imaging (2 to 4 days after infarct) with predischarge submaximal exercise stress perfusion imaging. Patients were randomly assigned to early vasodilator perfusion imaging and submaximal exercise perfusion imaging (N = 339) and to submaximal exercise perfusion imaging alone (N = 112). Clinicians were blinded to the results of the initial early vasodilator stress perfusion scan. Twenty-nine in-hospital events and 68 late cardiac events were subsequently noted. Importantly, the early vasodilator perfusion scan was more predictive of subsequent events than was the predischarge exercise SPECT study. No adverse effects from the early dipyridamole stress were seen.

Although the event rate is lower among acute infarction patients who are eligible for and receive throm-bolytic therapy, myocardial perfusion imaging remains a significant predictor of cardiac events in the thrombolytic era. Jain et al[45] have demonstrated that vasodilator perfusion imaging also remains valid in the elderly. In this study of 73 patients, aged 65 and older, with confirmed infarction, 33% had recurrent MI or death during 14-month follow-up. Multivariate analysis yielded four independent prognostic variables: nonuse of aspirin at hospital discharge, nonuse of beta-blocker at hospital discharge, depressed left ventricular systolic function, and evidence of reversible ischemia. Patients with ≥3 of these risk factors had an 83% chance of an adverse event compared with 6% in those with ≤1 risk factor. During follow-up (mean, 14 months), no patient with reversible defects who underwent revascularization died, whereas 37% (13 of 35) of those with reversible defects who were not revascularized died.[45] The finding of transient ischemic dilatation of the left ventricle at the time of stress perfusion imaging is a marker of severe and extensive coronary artery disease.

The use of technetium-based perfusion tracers such as sestamibi has allowed performance of gated SPECT measurements of LVEF along with the myocardial perfusion study. LVEF by gated SPECT has been shown to be accurate compared with first-pass radionuclide. Thus, two major determinants of postinfarction prognosis, LVEF and myocardial ischemia, can be obtained with a single test as early as 2 to 3 days after myocardial infarction.

The AHA Guidelines for uses of radionuclide imaging in acute myocardial infarction are summarized in Table 8-4, reproduced from the 1999 ACC/AHA Guidelines for the Management of Acute Myocardial Infarction.

CMR

Similar to other imaging techniques, CMR has been used in the setting of pharmacological stress for the detection of myocardial ischemia to risk stratify intermediate and low-risk patients.[25,26] The protocol for dobutamine infusion is the same as that used in stress echocardiography, including the use of atropine in patients who fail to achieve 85% of maximum predicted heart rate with dobutamine alone. An important concern with the use of dobutamine in association with CMR is that the magnetic field alters the appearance of the electrocardiogram because of the magnetohydrodynamic effect, so that the electrocardiogram during stress can be monitored for the presence of arrhythmias but not for the development of ST abnormalities. Therefore, images must be reviewed in real time for the development of wall motion abnormalities. Despite this concern, hundreds of patients have had stress CMR with dobutamine safely in multiple centers. The sensitivity and specificity for detecting >50% diameter narrowing are 83% and 87%, respectively. In studies comparing low-dose dobutamine (10 μg/kg/min) with ^{18}F-fluorodeoxy glucose PET (FDG-PET), there was a sensitivity of 81% and specificity of 100% for dobutamine CMR in detecting FDG-PET–defined myocardial viability. In patients referred for dobutamine/atropine stress CMR (because of poor left ventricular endocardial visualization with echocardiogra-

■ ▫ ■

TABLE 8-4   USES OF RADIONUCLIDE TESTING IN ACUTE MYOCARDIAL INFARCTION

DIAGNOSIS		RISK ASSESSMENT	
Indication	**Test**	**Indication**	**Test**
RV infarction	Rest radionuclide angiography ^{99m}Tc pyrophosphate	Residual ischemia	Stress thallium with redistribution Stress sestamibi with redistribution
Infarction not diagnosed by standard means; early presentation and successful reperfusion	Rest myocardial perfusion imaging ^{99m}Tc pyrophosphate	Myocardial infarct size	Tomographic thallium Tomographic sestamibi
Infarction not diagnosed by standard means; late presentation	^{99m}Tc pyrophosphate	Hibernating myocardium	Early, late thallium
Routine diagnosis	Any technique	Ventricular function	Radionuclide angiography

Adapted from ACC/AHA Guidelines. *J Am Coll Cardiol* 1995; 25:521.

phy), the presence of inducible ischemia (regional wall motion abnormalities) or a low LVEF is a predictor of future AMI or cardiac death during an average follow-up of 20 months.[46]

DIFFERENTIAL DIAGNOSIS

Aortic Dissection

Aortic dissection is a relatively rare, but important, cause of chest pain. Most patients are seen with severe, sharp chest pain and have a history of hypertension. Chest radiography frequently shows a widened mediastinum (type A, 66% of patients and type B, 55% of patients) and an abnormal aortic contour in 50% of patients. However, no chest X-ray abnormalities are found in approximately 10% of patients, and 31% of electrocardiograms are normal. The diagnosis of aortic dissection may be confirmed by several different imaging modalities, including transesophageal echocardiography, computed tomography, CMR, and aortography. They all have a relatively high sensitivity (88% to 100%), but their specificity is more variable (transesophageal echocardiography, 68% to 97%; CMR, 98% to 100%; computed tomography, 87% to 100%; aortography, 94%). If the diagnosis of aortic dissection is suspected, the imaging modality that can be performed most expediently should be obtained, because mortality increases at approximately 1% per hour after onset of symptoms. In an international registry, computed tomography was the initial imaging modality used in 61% of patients and is the most widely used noninvasive technique to diagnose thoracic aortic disease and define location, size, and extent of disease. However, CMR is emerging as the premier imaging method for the diagnosis of diseases of the thoracic aorta. Transthoracic echocardiography is a relatively insensitive method for detection of aortic aneurysm, which, if suspected, requires an additional imaging study. Because transesophageal echocardiography is the most portable of the preceding techniques, it is frequently used for bedside detection of aortic dissection.

However, transesophageal echocardiography may provide incomplete visualization of the aortic arch, which limits its diagnostic accuracy in this region. If questions concerning the presence or absence of aortic dissection persist after transesophageal echocardiography, then computed tomography, CMR, or aortography might be helpful.

Pericarditis and Pulmonary Embolism

Patients with pericarditis usually have chest pain and may have electrocardiographic abnormalities difficult to distinguish from those associated with acute coronary syndromes. In this situation, obtaining a transthoracic echocardiogram demonstrating normal endocardial wall motion decreases the likelihood of significant underlying infarction. In the subset of patients with chest pain caused by postinfarction pericarditis, usually echocardiographic evidence of a wall motion abnormality will exist.

Patients with pulmonary embolism may have discomfort that is difficult to distinguish from myocardial infarction. Echocardiography is normal in most patients after pulmonary embolism. Those patients with large pulmonary emboli may exhibit an electrocardiographic right ventricular strain pattern and echocardiographic evidence of right ventricular dilation with global and regional dysfunction.

Chest Trauma

In patients with chest trauma, both transthoracic and transesophageal echocardiography are used to evaluate the myocardium, pericardium, and aorta. The most common cardiac complication of trauma is cardiac contusion. These patients have a wide range of electrocardiographic abnormalities (ranging from nonspecific changes to findings compatible with infarction), and invariably cardiac enzymes are elevated. Transthoracic echocardiographic findings supporting the diagnosis of cardiac contusion include presence of a pericardial effusion, evidence of right ventricular dysfunction, and left ventricular regional wall motion abnormalities.

Disruption of the interventricular septum or cardiac valves caused by trauma may also be identified by transthoracic echocardiography. The use of transesophageal echocardiography in the evaluation of patients after trauma is helpful in evaluating descending aortic pathologic conditions, such as aortic transection, as well as in patients with technically difficult transthoracic images.

COMPLICATIONS

Mitral Regurgitation

Some degree of mitral regurgitation may be detected in up to 50% of patients after myocardial infarction by use of conventional transthoracic echocardiography. Mitral regurgitation present in the early hours of acute MI is usually clinically "silent," is more common with anterior MI, and is associated with an increased 1-year mortality. Moderately severe and severe mitral regurgitation complicating myocardial infarction can be associated with a 1-year mortality up to 50% and with increased mortality with coronary artery bypass surgery. Severe mitral regurgitation, resulting from papillary muscle rupture, usually is associated with an acute inferoposterior MI. In this latter situation, because mortality with medical therapy is approximately 90%, urgent cardiac repair is indicated, even though surgical mortality may approach 50%.

Echocardiography

Echocardiography may be ordered to evaluate a new murmur in the postinfarct patient. Echocardiographic imaging is 100% sensitive in distinguishing between ventricular septal defect and mitral regurgitation. Several physiological mechanisms exist for the development of mitral regurgitation after myocardial infarction. Disruption of the papillary muscle apparatus with the development of a flail mitral leaflet is the most devastating form of mitral regurgitation. More common mechanisms of mitral regurgitation in this setting include (1) mitral annular dilation caused by left ventricular enlargement and changes in wall stress and (2) contractile abnormalities of the papillary muscles or underlying myocardium. In those patients with systolic dysfunction, apical and posterior displacement of the papillary muscles may lead to mitral regurgitation. Structural abnormalities of the mitral leaflets, annulus, and adjacent myocardium are helpful in deducing the etiology of mitral regurgitation. Significant mitral regurgitation occurs equally after anterior and inferior myocardial infarction. Color Doppler techniques are used to map the extent of the systolic velocity disturbance of mitral regurgitation in the left atrium. Eccentric jets may be related to leaflet or papillary muscle dysfunction (i.e., posterior leaflet dysfunction results in an anteriorly directed jet of mitral regurgitation). Eccentric jets appear smaller than central jets for the same degree of regurgitation because of the interaction of the jet with the adjacent wall. Central jets may be due to bileaflet dysfunction or more likely to annular dilation. In acute mitral regurgitation, there may be a decreased pressure gradient between the left ventricle and left atrium caused by elevated left atrial pressures. Because of the lower driving pressure, this might result in a smaller color jet of mitral regurgitation than would be expected for the degree of regurgitation. Identification of systolic flow reversal in the pulmonary veins should heighten the suspicion for significant mitral regurgitation, even in the absence of a significant color jet of mitral regurgitation. The volume loading of the left atrium in mitral regurgitation results in an elevated early mitral inflow (E wave) velocities. Inflow velocities (E wave) greater than 1.2 m/s in the absence of mitral stenosis or prior repair are suggestive of significant mitral regurgitation. The echocardiographic interpretation should account for the jet characteristics and the patient presentation. Transesophageal echocardiographic imaging may be helpful in patients with limited, or nondiagnostic, transthoracic imaging. Transesophageal echocardiographic imaging does not provide different information but may provide better visualization of valve abnormalities and assessment of pulmonary venous wave patterns. Pulmonary venous flow patterns provide additional insight into the hemodynamic state of the patient. These waveforms are easier to obtain with transesophageal studies, but experienced sonographers should be able to record these spectra from transthoracic imaging in 70% to 80% of patients. The normal waveform consists of systolic forward flow (S) during atrial relaxation with a variable late systolic phase related to basal motion of the left ventricle, diastolic forward flow (D) during mitral valve opening, and retrograde flow occurring after atrial systole. In the normal individual, the systolic (S) wave is of greater magnitude than the diastolic component (D) (Figure 8-15). In patients with significant mitral regurgitation, there is reversal of the S wave with retrograde flow into the pulmonary veins. Blunting of the S wave may be associated with mitral regurgitation or elevation of left atrial filling pressures.

The most serious form of mitral regurgitation after myocardial infarction, papillary muscle rupture, is uncommon. Disruption may involve one or more heads of the papillary muscle. Complete rupture is associated with more significant left ventricular dysfunction and with increased mortality rates. The anterolateral papillary muscle has a dual blood supply, which serves as a protective mechanism against rupture. The posteromedial papillary muscle, which receives all of its blood supply from the posterior descending coronary artery, is more likely to rupture. Detection of papillary muscle rupture by echocardiography involves identification of either a flailing motion of the papillary muscle within the left ventricle or a flail mitral leaflet. The heads of the papillary muscle attached to the mitral leaflets may appear thickened and may be difficult to distinguish from vegetation. Most patients with suspected papillary muscle rupture are critically ill, with pulmonary edema. Transesophageal echocardiographic imaging is the preferred imaging technique for assessing mitral regurgitation in a critically ill patient, because it is portable and has high sensitivity and specificity for the diagnosis of significant mitral regurgitation.

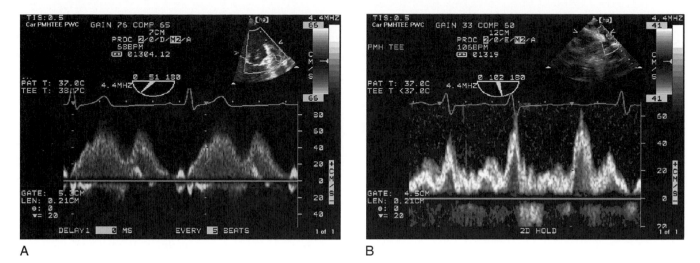

A   B

FIGURE 8-15. Pulmonary venous inflow patterns. **A,** Normal pulmonary venous flow depicted with antegrade flow in systole and diastole. Normally the systolic velocity and velocity time integral exceed the respective diastolic components. **B,** In the abnormal state, diastolic flow velocities exceed systolic flow velocities. This may be seen in individuals with low cardiac output, significant mitral regurgitation, or elevated left atrial filling pressures. See also Color Insert.

Echocardiographic signs of significant mitral regurgitation include an extensive left atrial color flow jet, systolic flow reversal in the pulmonary veins, elevated mitral inflow E wave velocities, and evidence for disruption of the mitral apparatus. Transesophageal echocardiography offers better images and more reliable information in patients with difficult transthoracic images and in those who are critically ill. In some instances, transesophageal images may be used to provide important confirmation of findings from a transthoracic study. Significant mitral regurgitation may be detected on left ventricular angiography, but echocardiography identifies the etiology of mitral regurgitation better than angiography (Table 8-5). In cases with eccentric color flow jets, echocardiography may underestimate the mitral regurgitant severity compared with left ventricular contrast angiography. In these cases, it is important to assess the impact of the regurgitation on left ventricular hemodynamics.

Ventriculography and Angiography

Left ventricular angiography performed in the right anterior oblique view provides an estimate of the severity of mitral regurgitation by grading the intensity of contrast that refluxes into the left atrium during ventricular systole. A semiquantitative scale is: no regurgitation = 0; regurgitation into the atrium that clears with each subsequent cardiac cycle = 1+; regurgitation with persistence of contrast in the atrium, which does not appear as dense as the ventricle = 2+; regurgitation with persistence of contrast in the atrium, which appears as dense as the ventricle = 3+; regurgitation with persistence of contrast in the atrium, which appears denser than the ventricle, or filling of the atrium in a single beat = 4+. Acute, severe, ischemic mitral regurgitation is usually associated with multivessel coronary artery disease and significant stenoses of the right and circumflex coronary arteries.

TABLE 8-5   IMAGING METHODS TO DETECT COMPLICATIONS OF MYOCARDIAL INFARCTION

	PA line	Transthoracic echocardiography	Transesophageal echocardiography	Nuclear imaging	CMR	Angiography
Mitral regurgitation	++	++	+++	0	++	+++
Ventricular septal defect	++	+++	++	+	+++	+++
Free wall rupture	0	+	+	0	0	0
Left ventricular aneurysm	0	+++	++	+	++	+++
Left ventricular pseudoaneurysm	0	+++	++	0	+++	+++
Right ventricular infarction	++	++	++	+	++	++
Thrombi	0	+++	+	0	++	+++
Pericardial effusion	0*	+++	+	0	+++	+

PA, Pulmonary arterial; CMR, cardiac magnetic resonance; +, may identify the suspected complication but not the preferred imaging technique; ++, frequently used technique for detecting complication; on occasion another technique may be needed to confirm the diagnosis; +++, best imaging method for detection of the underlying complication.
*May be useful if tamponade is present.

CMR

Disordered or "turbulent" flow results in the loss of signal intensity on cine CMR image permitting the qualitative detection of regurgitation similar to echocardiography. In addition, phase-contrast velocity mapping can be used to obtain quantitative measures of the amount of regurgitation that correlate well with invasive measures.

Ventricular Septal Defect

Rupture of the interventricular septum is an uncommon (1% or less)[47] but severe complication of myocardial infarction. In patients who have received thrombolytic therapy, there is a higher frequency of rupture that may occur earlier after the onset of infarction. The blood supply to the interventricular septum is derived from both the right coronary artery and the left anterior descending artery. Therefore, septal rupture can occur after anteroseptal or inferior myocardial infarction but is more common with anterior infarction. Ventricular septal defects develop at the perimeter of the infarcted septum and tend to be large. These defects are most commonly seen from 3 to 6 days after infarction as dyspnea, chest discomfort, or hemodynamic instability along with the development of a new, harsh, systolic murmur. Practice guidelines indicate that emergency surgical repair is now indicated for both hemodynamically stable patients and those with pulmonary edema and cardiogenic shock.[2] This is because the rupture site can abruptly expand and cause hemodynamic compromise even when left ventricular function is relatively unimpaired. Therefore, surgical referral and prompt insertion of an intraaortic balloon pump are recommended as soon as the diagnosis is made.[2] Indicators of poor prognosis include a low cardiac index, the presence of exten-

sive right ventricular and septal dysfunction on the two-dimensional echocardiogram, and early onset of rupture.

Echocardiography

Echocardiography is highly sensitive and specific for identifying ventricular septal defects and distinguishing these defects from mitral regurgitation. Ventricular septal defects occurring after anteroseptal myocardial infarctions typically develop in the apical third of the interventricular septum. These defects are best imaged from the apical four-chamber view. Slight angulation of the transducer may be required to optimize visualization of the defect. Posterior ventricular septal defects occur in the inferior septum and may be complex and difficult to visualize. Subcostal short-axis imaging at the base of the heart often provides the best imaging window for detection of tissue dropout in the inferior septum. Color flow Doppler imaging greatly enhances the ability to localize ventricular septal defects, identifying areas of turbulent flow across the septum. Two-dimensional imaging alone may detect 60% of defects; defect localization increases to 95% with color and pulsed Doppler techniques (Figure 8-16). As with mitral regurgitation, transesophageal echocardiography is often important in identifying defects in patients with difficult, or suboptimal, transthoracic imaging.

Important prognostic features of ventricular septal defects relate to the impact of the defect on right heart function. Right ventricular size and function may be assessed by echocardiography and by right atrial and inferior vena caval distention. Distention of the right heart is consistent with a significantly increased hemodynamic load because of increasing flow across the septal defect. Right ventricular dysfunction is predictive of increased mortality in patients with septal rupture. Development of pulmonary hypertension is consistent

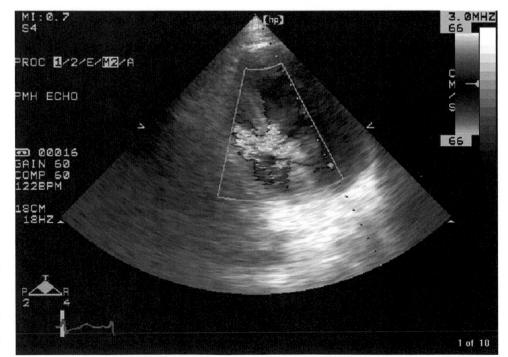

FIGURE 8-16. Echocardiographic imaging of a ventricular septal defect. A loud systolic murmur developed in this patient 4 days after an inferior myocardial infarction. **A,** A large defect is seen in the inferior septum from this modified apical projection. **B,** Color flow Doppler demonstrates left to right flow consistent with a postmyocardial infarction ventricular septal defect. See also Color Insert.

with a significant ventricular septal defect. Adverse risk factors for death after myocardial infarction complicated by a ventricular septal defect include inferior myocardial infarction, right ventricular and septal dysfunction identified by echocardiography, right atrial pressure >11 mmHg, cardiac shock/depressed cardiac index (cardiac index <1.76 L/m²/min), and rupture within the last week. Inferior ventricular septal defects are often difficult to repair surgically because of their location at the base of the heart and their complex, serpiginous, nature. Echocardiographic evidence of right atrial distention, bowing of the interatrial septum from right to left, and inferior vena caval distention are consistent with elevated right atrial pressure.

In general, transthoracic echocardiography provides the optimal imaging information when there is suspicion of a postinfarct ventricular septal defect. Apical defects may be difficult to visualize with transesophageal technology, but reports suggest excellent sensitivity and specificity with transesophageal studies. Assessment of the pulmonary/systemic flow ratios is helpful in quantitating defect size and suggests the possibility of shunting on the transthoracic study.

Role of Ventriculography and Angiography

If ventriculography is being used to image a ventricular septal defect, a left anterior oblique projection of 65 to 75 degrees allows tangential viewing of the interventricular septum, and if this is accompanied by 25 degrees of cranial angulation, foreshortening of the septum is reduced. Coronary angiography suggests that ventricular septal rupture is usually associated with total occlusion of the infarct-related artery and absence of collaterals; however, both single and multivessel coronary artery disease are associated with this complication.

CMR

Congenital ventricular septal defect has been demonstrated by CMR. However, echocardiography, because of its portability, is preferable for the evaluation of acute ventricular septal defect occurring in the setting of myocardial infarction.

Cardiogenic Shock

The incidence of cardiogenic shock has remained relatively constant over time, averaging approximately 7% to 10% of acute MI patients, with a hospital mortality of approximately 70% to 80%. In patients younger than 75 years with cardiogenic shock caused by acute MI with ST elevation, Q-waves or new LBBB treatment with emergency revascularization, compared with initial medical stabilization, does not alter 30-day mortality but reduces 6-month mortality (50% vs. 63%).[2,11]

Echocardiography and Left Ventricular Function Assessment

Transthoracic echocardiography can determine whether cardiogenic shock is due to myocardial dysfunction, unrecognized severe mitral regurgitation, ventricular septal defects, or right ventricular dysfunction. Transesophageal echocardiography augments this information in critically ill patients with suboptimal transthoracic imaging "windows." The presence of multivessel coronary artery disease and myocardial dysfunction in regions remote from the acute myocardial infarction are markers for the development of cardiogenic shock. In patients with large myocardial infarctions, and shock, all patients have hypokinesis of other regions of the heart.

Early echocardiographic imaging should be performed in patients with clinical evidence for large myocardial infarctions (ascertained by major electrocardiographic abnormalities and cardiac enzyme elevations), because the patients with extensive regional wall motion abnormalities involving both the infarct and noninfarct zones might benefit from aggressive mechanical and pharmacological support. Patients with cardiogenic shock are frequently supported by intraaortic balloon counterpulsation. Transthoracic echocardiography may be used to monitor the change in ventricular or valvular function over time and may be helpful in identifying additional complications of myocardial infarction, including pericardial fluid and intracavitary thrombi. Transesophageal echocardiography can be used to identify and localize the position of the balloon pump within the descending aorta. Left ventricular assist devices are used to support patients with cardiogenic shock after acute revascularization or as a bridge to cardiac transplantation. These patients typically have an open chest, and transthoracic imaging is often not feasible, but transesophageal echocardiography can be used to determine the position and function of the assist device conduit to diagnose the presence of pericardial fluid and valvular dysfunction and to assess left ventricular function and "unloading." In addition, transesophageal echocardiography may be used to help with weaning from the left ventricular assist device, noting the changes in left and right ventricular function, filling patterns, and atrioventricular valve regurgitation with decrease in assist device support.

Coronary Angiography

The index infarction of approximately 60% of patients with cardiogenic shock is anterior in location,[11] and primary revascularization is recommended (PTCA or coronary artery bypass grafting [CABG]) within 18 hours of the onset of shock and within 36 hours of the onset of acute ST-segment elevation or new LBBB acute MI, and who are younger than 75 years.[2] Occlusion of the infarct-related artery seems to be most strongly associated with mortality.

Acute Perfusion Imaging

Nuclear myocardial perfusion imaging (requiring transport of the patient outside the critical care area) therefore plays little, if any, role in this setting. Radionuclide ventriculography has been proposed as a test to evaluate the cause of cardiogenic shock: left and right ventricular function can be assessed, the presence of a pericardial effusion can frequently be inferred, and is possible to evaluate for large intracardiac shunts causing hemodynamic compromise. However echocardiography, and especially transesophageal echocardiography (1) can be performed acutely at the bedside and (2) provides more detailed information on possible causes of cardiogenic shock, and thus is almost always the preferred diagnostic test.

Ventricular Remodeling

Left ventricular remodeling occurs after myocardial infarction and results in progressive ventricular enlargement, with reduction in left ventricular systolic function. Large infarct size is the most highly associated clinical correlate to left ventricular remodeling. Patients with ejection fractions <40% form a high risk group more likely to have congestive heart failure or sudden death develop after myocardial infarction.

Echocardiography

In a serial echocardiographic study of patients with first AMI, thrombolytic therapy and patency of the infarct-related artery had independent and complementary effects on ventricular volume and function.[48] Thrombolysis had a beneficial effect on left ventricular size, even in patients with an occluded infarct-related artery 1 month after infarction (perhaps reflecting early reperfusion in some patients) compared with patients with occluded arteries who did not receive thrombolysis. However, the combination of thrombolysis and vessel patency was associated with higher ejection fractions and lower end-systolic volumes than in other patients. Interestingly, thrombolysis had its primary impact on initial ventricular volumes, whereas vessel patency related mainly to subsequent ventricular dilation.[48] Remodeling is more likely to occur in patients with large transmural myocardial infarctions and is attenuated by the administration of ACE inhibitors. The linkage between left ventricular enlargement and adverse clinical outcome was provided by the Echocardiographic substudy of the Survival and Ventricular Enlargement (SAVE) Trial of patients with acute MI and left ventricular ejection fractions of ≤40%, who were randomly assigned to placebo or captopril. Patients who had an adverse event at 1 year had more than a threefold increase in left ventricular cavity areas than those patients with an uncomplicated course. Attenuation of this enlargement with captopril was associated with a reduction in adverse events.[49]

Persistence or an increase in the number of negative T waves on standard electrocardiography is associated with progressive left ventricular dilation and worsening myocardial function. Viable myocardium seems to exert an important protective influence against adverse left ventricular remodeling. Univariate predictors of adverse remodeling and ventricular dilation included baseline ejection fraction, infarct size, age, and multivessel coronary disease. Infarct size is a predictor of ventricular dilation, and infarct-related viability is a negative predictor of dilation. Doppler echocardiography studies show that mitral deceleration times of ≤130 ms early after myocardial infarction are a strong predictor of ventricular dilation.

Segmental variation in contraction and filling can be assessed by tissue Doppler imaging. This technique allows display of myocardial velocities with high temporal resolution. Infarcted, or ischemic, zones have decreased myocardial velocities in systole compared with normal myocardium, and myocardial velocities may be color encoded and thus allow visual assessment of decreased myocardial thickening consistent with myocardial infarction. Echocardiographic harmonic imaging demonstrating abnormal videodensity has been shown to correlate with persistence of regional abnormalities in the infarct zone and with progressive left ventricular remodeling.

The concept of "no-reflow" has been propagated in the interventional cardiology literature. "No-reflow" implies significant myocardial damage that is not improved by reestablishing myocardial macroperfusion. The "no-reflow" concept has been investigated by use of intracoronary myocardial contrast echocardiography in patients after percutaneous reperfusion of myocardial infarction. Patients with "no reflow" are more likely to have pericardial effusions, develop early congestive heart failure, and progressive left ventricular dilation. Similar patients with normal myocardial contrast studies have a decrease in left ventricular chamber dimensions over time.

The incidence of left ventricular thrombi after myocardial infarction has decreased markedly in the past few decades, likely because of therapies to reduce infarct size (lytic agents) and decreased left ventricular remodeling (ACE inhibitors). The formation of left ventricular thrombus is most common after Q-wave anterior infarction, and although a severe depression of ejection fraction is not a prerequisite, an apical wall motion abnormality is almost always present. Embolic events tend to occur within the initial 4 to 6 months after AMI. Transthoracic two-dimensional echocardiography can usually identify thrombus, and thrombus that has a protruding configuration or is freely mobile is more likely to embolize. When adequate two-dimensional echocardiograms or contrast echocardiograms cannot be obtained, ^{111}In platelet scintigraphy seems to be highly specific and can detect thrombi that are actively incorporating platelets onto their surfaces. Those patients with thrombi have larger infarctions and are at risk for more extensive left ventricular remodeling.

CMR

CMR is intrinsically a three-dimensional technique that provides images in any orientation and is not limited by acoustic window or attenuation. Therefore, it provides a reproducible tool for the evaluation of ventricular size and remodeling, similar to echocardiography, and for assessing cardiac function.[50] In addition, the technique of myocardial tagging can be used to evaluate details of regional myocardial motion and regional myocardial strain. In studies in patients with first reperfused, transmural anterior myocardial infarction, CMR with myocardial tagging has demonstrated loss of regional ejection fraction and a significant reduction of longitudinal and circumferential stain in myocardium remote from the infarct. Studies combining ceCMR with tagging in animal models have shown that there is a relationship between the extent of microvascular obstruction by ceCMR and reduced local myocardial deformation in the infracted region and dysfunction of noninfarcted adjacent myocardium. These studies may help to explain the increased remodeling seen in patients with large regions of microvascular obstruction.

Ventricular Aneurysm

Left ventricular aneurysms develop over weeks to months after myocardial infarction. Early myocardial thinning associated with infarction represents infarct expansion.

Echocardiography

Aneurysmal expansion may be detected by echocardiography as early as 5 days after the infarct. Thrombolytic therapy has not been associated with a decrease in the incidence of aneurysms. Most commonly associated with anterior myocardial infarctions, aneurysms have thinned fibrotic myocardium that displays dyskinetic motion on echocardiography. Aneurysms have a thinned segment with dyskinesis in systole and maintain abnormal contour in diastole. Thrombi frequently form within aneurysms because of low-velocity flow within the aneurysm. Aneurysms are associated with the clinical development of heart failure, and arrhythmias and are associated with increased mortality. Detection of aneurysms is equally good with angiography and echocardiography. CMR may also identify and localize aneurysms. Surgical repair of aneurysms with good outcomes is possible in patients with at least 40% residual normal myocardium. Quantitation of the amount of residual myocardium is expected to be most accurate with three-dimensional techniques. The development of three-dimensional echocardiography and CMR may be optimal for assessing the extent of the aneurysm and residual normal myocardium. Currently, aneurysms are most commonly detected with transthoracic echocardiography. Because most aneurysms are apically located, transesophageal echocardiographic imaging may be suboptimal. Indications for surgical intervention include refractory heart failure, angina, or arrhythmias.

CMR

CMR can obtain images in any plane and is not limited by acoustic windows. A standard CMR study as described previously can readily be used to determine the size of a left ventricular aneurysm and to evaluate ventricular function.[50] CMR is presently considered the reference technique for the measurement of left ventricular volume in patients with ventricular aneurysms.

Right Ventricular Infarction

In up to 50% of patients with inferior or posterior myocardial infarction, the right ventricle is involved, especially in cases involving proximal occlusion of the right coronary artery, and in a smaller proportion this has adverse hemodynamic consequences. Clinical identification of right ventricular infarction includes the triad of elevated central venous pressures, hypotension, and absence of pulmonary congestion (provided left ventricular function is reasonable). This triad is specific but insensitive. ST-segment elevations in right precordial leads are sensitive and specific for right ventricular infarction. In patients with right ventricular infarction, complete reperfusion of the right coronary artery by PTCA within 12 hours of the onset of symptoms improves hemodynamics and outcome.

Echocardiography

Transthoracic echocardiography is useful for identifying and quantitating the degree of right heart dilation and global and regional dysfunction. Right atrial dilation may be seen because of atrial infarction or elevated right atrial pressures. Dilation of the inferior vena cava may represent elevated central venous pressures. Abnormal interventricular septal motion may be seen in severe right ventricular infarction. Tricuspid regurgitation may result from right ventricular dilation. Rarely, right atrial dilation leads to a stretched foramen and right-to-left shunting. Transesophageal echocardiography may be used to assess right ventricular function in patients without adequate transthoracic images. Because the right side of the heart is in the far field for the transesophageal probe, images may be difficult to evaluate.

CMR

Echocardiography has been used extensively in the detection of right ventricular infarction and has the advantages of portability and wide availability. CMR, however, can provide images of the right ventricular free wall without near-field artifact or limitations of acoustic window. For these reasons CMR has been shown to be highly accurate in the evaluation of right ventricular size and function. A third of patients with coronary disease have at least some mild depression of right ventricular function. Patients with left ventricular inferior wall motion abnormalities most frequently demonstrated reductions in right ventricular function; however, deterioration of right ventricular function is also noted in patients with left ventricular apical aneurysm.

Cardiac Rupture

Echocardiography

Rupture of the left ventricular free wall is usually a catastrophic complication of acute MI resulting in death and can occur both acutely, and subacutely (pseudoaneurysm). Left ventricular rupture occurs slightly more commonly than septal rupture (1%) and remains a major cause or contributor to death in hospitalized patients with infarction and outpatients with unrecognized infarction. Early reperfusion of myocardial infarction is associated with a decreased risk for myocardial rupture. Most patients with free wall rupture are seen abruptly with recurrent chest discomfort and hypotension progressing to cardiovascular death over seconds to minutes. Patients at highest risk for rupture are those with a thin infarct zone because of infarct expansion. A small proportion of patients will have a syndrome consisting of chest discomfort, nausea, and hemodynamic instability from impending or early rupture. These symptoms may lead to heightened suspicion for the diagnosis of myocardial rupture. Echocardiography in this setting may identify a pericardial effusion composed of echogenic material caused by hemopericardium. Impending rupture may also be identified by a localized area of hemorrhagic material in the pericardial space around the infarct zone. The actual site of myocardial rupture is rarely visualized. Identification of hemopericardium warrants emergent surgical therapy to decrease mortality. Mortality without intervention is essentially 100%. Surgical treatment of patients with impending rupture may decrease the mortality to 40%. If hemopericardium is suspected on the transthoracic echocardiogram in the absence of recent cardiac surgery, the two most likely etiologies are free wall rupture and aortic dissection into the pericardial sac. Both of these entities represent cardiac emergencies with surgical repair or appropriate treatment that can reduce mortality. Development of a false aneurysm or pseudoaneurysm of the left ventricle is a rare complication of myocardial infarction. Patients may be asymptomatic with a pseudoaneurysm, and it may be diagnosed incidentally by an echocardiogram performed for postmyocardial infarction assessment. A pseudoaneurysm results from subacute myocardial rupture that is contained by a localized area of pericardium. This pericardium is usually thickened and fibrosed, allowing for containment of the rupture. A pseudoaneurysm is distinguished from an aneurysm of the left ventricle by the appearance of a narrow neck with to-and-fro flow detected by pulsed Doppler imaging. The wall of the pseudoaneurysm is composed of pericardium and is thin and noncontractile as opposed to an aneurysm, which contains myocardium and is dyskinetic. The long-term risk of a pseudoaneurysm is related to its potential for late rupture. For this reason, most patients undergo surgical repair after identification of a pseudoaneurysm. From the surgical standpoint, anatomical localization of the defect and its relationship to the mitral valve and papillary muscles are important considerations. Transthoracic echocardiography is used to assess the anatomic location and extent of the pseudoaneurysm. Three-dimensional techniques such as CMR and real time three-dimensional echocardiography may offer more complete anatomical information.

CMR

CMR is accurate in detecting false aneurysm (subacute rupture or pseudoaneurysm), but 50% of these patients require further testing for definitive diagnosis.

Pericardial Effusion

Pericardial effusions develop in approximately 25% of patients after myocardial infarction and may be detected by standard two-dimensional echocardiography. The likelihood of a pericardial effusion developing increases with the size of the myocardial infarction detected by wall motion analysis or elevation of cardiac enzymes. These effusions may be asymptomatic or associated with typical pericardial discomfort but are rarely associated with the development of tamponade physiology. The development of tamponade physiology should raise the suspicion for occult left ventricular rupture. Blood in the pericardium may be a result of myocardial rupture and extravasation after transmural myocardial infarction treated with a lytic agent. Transthoracic echocardiographic is almost always sufficient to evaluate for pericardial effusion.

REFERENCES

1. Braunwald E, Antman EM, Beasley JW, et al. ACC/AHA guidelines for the management of patients with unstable angina and non-ST-segment elevation myocardial infarction: executive summary and recommendations. A report of the American College of Cardiology/American Heart Association task force on practice guidelines (Committee on the Management of Patients with Unstable Angina). *Circulation* 2000; 102:1193.
2. Ryan TJ, Antman EM, Brooks NH, et al. 1999 update: ACC/AHA Guidelines for the Management of Patients With Acute Myocardial Infarction: Executive Summary and Recommendations: A report of the American College of Cardiology/American Heart Association Task Force on Practice Guidelines (Committee on Management of Acute Myocardial Infarction). *Circulation* 1999; 100:1016.
3. Gibbons RJ, Balady GJ, Bricker JT, et al. ACC/AHA 2002 Guideline Update for Exercise Testing: Summary Article. A report of the American College of Cardiology/American Heart Association Task Force on Practice Guidelines (Committee to Update the 1997 Exercise Testing Guidelines). *J Am Coll Cardiol* 2002; 40:1531.
4. Udelson JE, Beshansky JR, Ballin DS, et al. Myocardial perfusion imaging for Evaluation and Triage of Patients with Suspected Acute Cardiac Ischemia. *JAMA* 2002; 288:2693.
5. DeWood M, Sores J, Notske R, et al. Prevalence of total coronary occlusion during the early hours of transmural myocardial infarction. *N Engl J Med* 1980; 303:897.
6. The TIMI Study Group. The Thrombolysis in Myocardial Infarction Trial. *N Engl J Med* 1985; 312:932.
7. Gibson CM, Murphy SA, Rizzo MJ, et al. The relationship between the TIMI Frame Count and clinical outcomes after thrombolytic administration. *Circulation* 1999; 99:1945.
8. Gibson CM, Cannon CP, Murphy SA, et al. Relationship of TIMI Perfusion Grade to Mortality after Administration of Thrombolytic Drugs. *Circulation* 2000; 101:125.
9. Barcin C, Denktas AE, Garratt KN, Higano ST, Holmes DR, Jr., Lerman A. Relation of Thrombolysis in Myocardial Infarction (TIMI) frame count to coronary flow parameters. *Am J Cardiol* 2003; 91:466.
10. Gibson CM, Cannon CP, Murphy SA, Marble SJ, Barron HV, Braunwald E. Relationship of the TIMI myocardial perfusion grades, flow rates, frame count, and percutaneous coronary intervention to long-term outcomes after thrombolytic administration in acute myocardial infarction. *Circulation* 2002; 105:1909.
11. Hochman JS, Sleeper LA, Webb JG, et al. Early revascularization in acute myocardial infarction complicated by cardiogenic shock. *N Engl J Med* 1999; 341:625.
12. Smith SC, Dove J, Jacobs AK, et al. ACC/AHA guidelines for percutaneous coronary intervention: a report of the American College of Cardiology/American Heart Association Task Force on Practice Guidelines (Committee to Revise the 1993 Guidelines for Percutaneous Transluminal Coronary Angioplasty). *J Am Coll Cardiol* 2001; 37:2239i.
13. White HD, Norris RM, Brown MA, Brandt PWT, Whitlock RML, Wild CJ. Left ventricular end-systolic volume as the major determinant of survival after recovery from myocardial infarction. *Circulation* 1987; 76:44.

14. Jang I-K, Bouma BE, Kang D-H, et al. Visualization of coronary atherosclerotic plaques in patients using optical coherence tomography: comparison with intravascular ultrasound. *J Am Coll Cardiol* 2002; 39:604.

15. Maehara A, Mintz GS, Bui AB, et al. Morphologic and angiographic features of coronary plaque rupture detected by intravascular ultrasound. *J Am Coll Cardiol* 2002; 40:904.

16. Kawasaki M, Takatsu H, Noda T, et al. In vivo quantitative tissue characterization of human coronary arterial plaques by use of integrated backscatter intravascular ultrasound and comparison with angioscopic findings. *Circulation* 2002; 105:2487.

17. Peshock RM, Franco F, Chwialkowski M, et al. Normal coronary anatomy, orientation and function. In: Manning WJ, Pennell DJ (eds): *Cardiovascular Magnetic Resonance*. New York: Churchill Livingstone; 2002.

18. Micciardi MJ, Wu E, Davidson CJ, et al. Visualization of discrete microinfarction after percutaneous coronary intervention associated with mild creatine kinase-MB elevation. *Circulation* 2001; 103:2780.

19. Channer S, Wilde P, Culling W, Jones J. Estimation of left ventricular end diastolic pressure by pulsed Doppler ultrasound. *Lancet* 1986; 3:1005.

20. Voci P, Mariano E, Pizzuto F, Puddu PE, Romeo F. Coronary recanalization in anterior myocardial infarction. The open perforator hypothesis. *J Am Coll Cardiol* 2002; 40:1205.

21. Hancock JE, Cooke JC, Chin DT, Monaghan MJ. Determination of successful reperfusion after thrombolysis for acute myocardial infarction. *Circulation* 2002; 105:157.

22. Gibbons RJ, Miller TD, Christian TF. Infarct size measured by single photon emission computed tomographic imaging with (99m)Tc-sestamibi: a measure of the efficacy of therapy in acute myocardial infarction. *Circulation* 2000; 101:101.

23. Fayad ZA, Fuster V, Nikolaou K, Becker C. Computed tomography and magnetic resonance imaging for noninvasive coronary angiography and plaque imaging. *Circulation* 2002; 106:2026.

24. Kim WY, Danias PG, Stuber M, et al. Coronary magnetic resonance angiography for the detection of coronary stenosis. *N Engl J Med* 2001; 345:1863.

25. Kraitchman DL, Sampath S, Castillo E, et al. Quantitative ischemia detection during cardiac magnetic resonance stress testing by use of FastHARP. *Circulation* 2003; 107:2025.

26. Kuijpers D, Ho KY, van Dijkman PR, Vliegenthart R, Oudkerk M. Dobutamine cardiovascular magnetic resonance for the detection of myocardial ischemia with the use of myocardial tagging. *Circulation* 2003; 107:1592.

27. Mahrholdt H, Wagner A, Honold M, Wedemeyer I, Sechtem U. Images in cardiovascular medicine. Magnetic resonance assessment of cardiac function, infarct scar distribution, and ventricular remodeling in the setting of ischemic cardiomyopathy. *Circulation* 2003; 107:e103.

28. Schwitter J, Nanz D, Kneifel S, et al. Assessment of myocardial perfusion in coronary artery disease by magnetic resonance. A comparison with positron emission tomography and coronary angiography. *Circulation* 2001; 103:2230.

29. Ibrahim T, Nekolla SG, Schreiber K, et al. Assessment of coronary flow reserve: comparison between contrast-enhanced magnetic resonance imaging and positron emission tomography. *J Am Coll Cardiol* 2002; 39:864.

30. Nishioka T, Amanullah AM. Clinical validation of intravascular ultrasound imaging for assessment of coronary stenosis severity. *J Am Coll Cardiol* 1999; 33:1870.

31. Fitzgerald PJ, Oshima A, Hayase M, et al. Final results of the can ultrasound influence stent expansion (CRUISE) study. *Circulation* 2000; 102:523.

32. Theime T, Wernecke KD, Meyer R, et al. Angioscopic evaluation of atherosclerotic plaques: validation by histomorphologic analysis and association with stable and unstable coronary syndromes. *J Am Coll Cardiol* 1996; 28:1.

33. Kloner RA, Bolli R, Marban E, Reinlib L, Braunwald E. Medical and cellular implications of stunning, hibernation, and preconditioning. An NHLBI Workshop. *Circulation* 1998; 97:1848.

34. Pfeffer M, Greaves S, Arnold J, et al. Early versus delayed angiotensin-converting enzyme inhibition therapy in acute myocardial infarction. The healing and early afterload reducing therapy trial. *Circulation* 1997; 95:2643.

35. Basso C, Valente M, Thiene G. "Hibernating" myocardium: not only a matter of semantics. *Circulation* 2003; 107:e10.

36. Shimoni S, Frangogiannis NG, Aggeli CJ, et al. Identification of hibernating myocardium with quantitative intravenous myocardial contrast echocardiography: comparison with dobutamine echocardiography and thallium-201 scintigraphy. *Circulation* 2003; 107:538.

37. Main ML, Magalski A, Morris BA, Coen MM, Skolnick DG, Good TH. Combined assessment of microvascular integrity and contractile reserve improves differentiation of stunning and necrosis after acute anterior wall myocardial infarction. *J Am Coll Cardiol* 2002; 40:1079.

38. Wiggers H, Botker HE, Sogaard P, et al. Electromechanical mapping versus positron emission tomography and single photon emission computed tomography for the detection of myocardial viability in patients with ischemic cardiomyopathy. *J Am Coll Cardiol* 2003; 41:843.

39. Schaefer WM, Lipke CS, Nowak B, et al. Validation of an evaluation routine for left ventricular volumes, ejection fraction and wall motion from gated cardiac FDG PET: a comparison with cardiac magnetic resonance imaging. *Eur J Nucl Med Mol Imaging* 2003; 30:545.

40. Rudd JHF, Warburton EA, Fryer TD, et al. Imaging atherosclerotic plaque inflammation with [^{18}F]-fluorodeoxyglucose positron emission tomography. *Circulation* 2002; 105:2708.

41. Klein C, Nekolla SG, Bengel FM, et al. Assessment of myocardial viability with contrast-enhanced magnetic resonance imaging. Comparison with positron emission tomography. *Circulation* 2002; 105:162.

42. Laham RJ, Simons M, Pearlman JD, et al. Magnetic resonance imaging demonstrates improved regional systolic wall thickening with myocardial perfusion of myocardial territories treated with laser myocardial revascularization. *J Am Coll Cardiol* 2002; 39:1.

43. Rocchi G, Fallani F, Bracchetti G, et al. Non-invasive detection of coronary artery stenosis: a comparison among power-Doppler contrast echo, 99Tc-sestamibi SPECT and echo wall-motion analysis. *Coron Artery Dis* 2003; 14:239.

44. Brown KA. Management of unstable angina: the role of noninvasive risk stratification. *J Nucl Cardiol* 1997; 4:S164.

45. Jain S, Baird JB, Fischer KC, Rich MW. Prognostic value of dipyridamole thallium imaging after acute myocardial infarction in older patients. *J Am Geriatr Soc* 1999; 47:295.

46. Hundley WG, Morgan TM, Neagle CM, Hamilton CA, Rerkpattanapipat P, Link KM. Magnetic resonance imaging determination of cardiac prognosis. *Circulation* 2002; 106:2328.

47. Birnbaum Y, Fishbein MC, Blanche C, Siegel RJ. Ventricular septal rupture after acute myocardial infarction. *N Engl J Med* 2002; 347:1426.

48. Popovic AD, Neskovic AN, Babic R, et al. Independent impact of thrombolytic therapy and vessel patency on left ventricular dilation after myocardial infarction. *Circulation* 1994; 90:800.

49. St John Sutton M, Pfeffer MA, Plappert T, et al. Quantitative two-dimensional echocardiographic measurements are major predictors of adverse cardiac events after acute myocardial infarction. *Circulation* 1994; 89:68.

50. Hundley WG, Hamilton CA, Rerkpattanapipat P. Magnetic resonance imaging assessment of cardiac function. *Curr Cardiol Rep* 2003; 5:69.

■ ■ ■ chapter 9

Chronic Coronary Heart Disease

Gary V. Heller
Georgios I. Papaioannou
Dudley J. Pennell
Gerard P. Aurigemma
Alan S. Pearlman
Jamshid Maddahi
John J. Mahmarian
Jeffrey A. Leppo

During myocardial ischemia, an imbalance occurs between myocardial oxygen supply and demand. Because the heart is an aerobic organ and relies almost exclusively on the oxidation of substrates for the generation of energy, it can develop only a small oxygen debt. The common clinical condition associated with anaerobic metabolism is an uncomfortable sensation in the chest, usually brought on by effort, called angina The underlying problem is usually disease of the coronary arteries or coronary atherosclerosis in which an abnormal narrowing of the coronary arteries decreases the blood supply to the myocardium to cause ischemia. Thus, the oxygen supply to the myocardial cells also falls, with anaerobic glycolysis and lactate production. Traditional objective methods used to determine the presence of ischemic heart disease include the measurement of metabolic products in the coronary venous drainage and contrast coronary angiography. Noncatheterization methods to detect ischemic heart disease depend on determinations of the consequences of altered regional coronary blood flow such as reduction in ventricular function or electrocardiographic changes from rest to stress (Figure 9-1). In addition to electrocardiograms acquired at rest and during stress, several cardiac imaging techniques are routinely used in clinical practice.

Because the objective demonstration of ischemia by electrocardiograms or cardiac imaging is associated with a significantly higher patient morbidity and mortality, the cellular basis of ischemia will be reviewed, and then the noninvasive techniques currently available for evaluating patients with possible ischemic heart disease will be outlined. The focus will be on the detection of ischemic heart disease and the determination of myocardial viability and prognosis.

MYOCARDIAL ISCHEMIA

In the heart, increased oxygen demands must be met almost entirely by increased coronary flow. The contractile function of myocardial cells becomes impaired during an ischemic insult lasting as little as 1 to 2 seconds, because anaerobic metabolism cannot adequately satisfy the metabolic demands of heart cells, and the heart cannot incur an oxygen debt. The detrimental effects of ischemia are usually reversible, but after periods of ischemia as short as 20 to 40 minutes, necrosis of myocardial tissue results. Most of the myocardial cell's energy use goes to maintain the contractile state. If energy is not constantly replenished by oxidative metabolism, energy stores will fall, metabolic by-products accumulate, and contractile activity declines. Although technically difficult, direct serial tissue measurements of myocardial energy stores (creatine phosphate and adenosine triphosphate) can provide a sensitive guide to the presence or absence of ischemia. Other less direct metabolic measures of ischemia include local Pco_2, lactate production, lactate/pyruvate ratio, potassium release, or phosphate release. However, most measurements that require myocardial sampling can only be used in experimental animals. Clinically, measurements of metabolites in coronary sinus blood require cardiac catheterization and can be altered by conditions other than ischemic heart disease, which makes direct evaluation of myocardial metabolism generally impractical in humans.

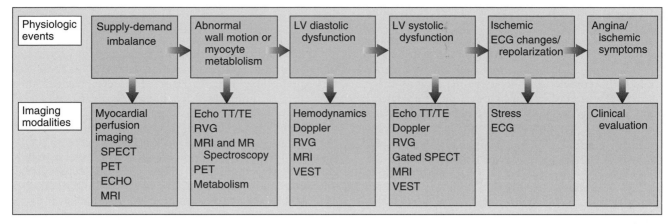

FIGURE 9-1. Schematic diagram of the cascade of physiological events during myocardial ischemia and the imaging correlates. Abn, abnormalities; ECG, electrocardiogram; LV, left ventricle; MRI: magnetic resonance imaging; RVG, radionuclide ventriculography; TT, transthoracic; TE, transesophageal; Vest, ambulatory radionuclide ejection fraction.

NONINVASIVE EVALUATION

Exercise Testing

Electrocardiogram

The pioneering work started by Master has led to an established role for the electrocardiogram-monitored exercise-stress test in the evaluation of ischemic heart disease. There are reports that question the usefulness of exercise testing, especially in populations in which ischemic heart disease would be expected to have a low prevalence. Nevertheless, dynamic exercise-stress testing supplies information useful for evaluating the predisposition to ischemia during normal daily activity. Most of the published reports in this field support the conclusion that ischemic heart disease is present when typical angina and reversible ST depression occur during a stress test.[1] In addition, a multifactor analysis of the entire stress test findings can improve the overall accuracy of an exercise evaluation and estimate prognosis.

The sensitivity of electrocardiographic testing for detecting coronary artery disease has in large part been based on the findings noted on coronary angiography. There are several potential problems with this analysis: (1) the presence of arterial stenoses does not necessarily imply that a region of myocardial tissue is ischemic, but rather that there is a potential for the attenuation of regional coronary reserve capacity; (2) electrochemical changes (ST depression) may not occur until the contractile state is already impaired, which suggests that a certain level of cellular ischemia must be reached before clinically apparent electrocardiographic changes; and (3) the effect of coronary collateral flow supply to the myocardium distal to a stenosis and the extent of small vessel disease is difficult to interpret. Therefore, one can conclude that in patients with angiographic coronary stenoses, the sensitivity of electrocardiographic evidence of ischemia ranges from 49% to 80%, and the specificity of this test is 41% to 95% (when 1 mm of ST depression was defined as a positive result).

Imaging

There are certain factors such as abnormal resting electrocardiogram, prior myocardial infarction, hyperventilation, neurasthenia changes, drug intake, and left ventricular hypertrophy that can make electrocardiographic interpretation difficult. It is in these more difficult cases and in patients with intermediate risk factors that noninvasive cardiac imaging can provide much greater diagnostic information.

The sequence of events occurring during the genesis of regional myocardial ischemia (Figure 9-1) emphasizes the concept that regional abnormalities in myocardial perfusion comprise a continuum from minor relative differences in flow without metabolic or regional functional consequences to the full expression of myocardial ischemia with systolic and diastolic dysfunction, electrocardiographic signs, and angina. Seminal studies of coronary blood flow in the early 1970s demonstrated that whereas a diameter stenosis of approximately 80% to 90% was necessary to induce a detectable regional coronary flow abnormality at rest, a stenosis on the order of approximately 50% diameter narrowing would result in regional flow disturbances during pharmacologically induced hyperemia. Radionuclide techniques evaluated myocardial perfusion and have been widely applied in the study of coronary blood flow in humans during stress. The concepts derived in animal models regarding the degree of stenosis required to induce a physiological flow abnormality during hyperemic stress were applied to radionuclide perfusion imaging studies, so that a 50% diameter stenosis on a coronary angiogram became the "gold standard" against which myocardial perfusion imaging was often tested. Other imaging modalities, including echocardiography and cardiac magnetic resonance imaging, are also being used to evaluate myocardial perfusion and with more widespread availability could reach the large population now being served with radionuclide techniques.

After perfusion imaging started, the ability to evaluate regional and global systolic ventricular myocardial function became available with the use of exercise radionu-clide angiography, echocardiography, and, more recently, magnetic resonance imaging. These techniques were also applied to the study of patients with known or suspected coronary disease to find a noninvasive diagnostic modality that would also be more efficacious than an exercise electrocardiogram. This is accomplished by measuring a physiological parameter that occurs earlier in the sequence of events after a regional supply/ demand imbalance than the ischemic ST depression detected by electrocardiography or by symptoms of angina.

Conceptually, on the basis of the cascade of myocardial cellular dysfunction, myocardial perfusion imaging should be the most sensitive technique to detect the presence of an epicardial coronary stenosis, with the study of stress regional wall motion abnormalities the next most sensitive, and exercise electrocardiograms the least sensitive. To some degree, this is reflected in numerous studies evaluating the sensitivities for detecting coronary artery disease and particularly the findings in several studies that myocardial perfusion imaging detects coronary disease more efficiently at lower workloads than functional imaging or exercise electrocardiography. Furthermore, positron emission tomographic (PET) techniques are likely to be the most sensitive, because absolute values of regional coronary flow reserve can be quantitated, presumably detecting more modest heterogeneities in regional flow during a hyperemic stress.

DETECTION OF CORONARY ARTERY DISEASE

Identification of traditional and newer risk factors for coronary artery disease is the first step in the evaluation of an individual's risk for having coronary artery disease. Those include advanced age and male gender, hypertension, hypercholesterolemia, family history of coronary artery disease in first-degree relatives younger than the age of 60, diabetes mellitus, smoking, obesity, sedentary lifestyle, and elevated homocysteine. Various clinical prediction models can be subsequently applied to further stratify patients into low, intermediate, and high risk for future cardiac events, including cardiac death and nonfatal myocardial infraction on the basis of these risk factors. A modified version of the Framingham risk score has been incorporated into the Third Report of the National Cholesterol Education Program (NCEP Guidelines) to estimate the 10-year risk for coronary artery disease developing.[2]

Although it is well recognized that sensitivity and specificity define the quality of a diagnostic test, the result cannot be satisfactory interpreted without additional knowledge of the prevalence of disease in a given population. Defining the pretest likelihood of coronary artery disease in a certain individual and determining the posttest probability after a positive or negative result is a key feature and is based on the concepts included in Bayes' theorem of conditional probability, and it is now well appreciated that cardiac imaging is of particular importance in patients at intermediate risk (those with

pretest probability between 20% and 80%), because a positive or a negative result influences further treatment decisions.

The decision to perform a stress test to obtain diagnostic and/or prognostic information in patients with chronic stable angina has been carefully reviewed in ACC/AHA guidelines.[3] There are also ACC/AHA Guidelines for exercise testing[1] and for the clinical use of radionuclide imaging[4] and prognostic risk indices developed for stress echocardiography.[5] There is also an expert consensus document concerning electron-beam computed tomography (EBCT) for the diagnosis and prognosis of coronary artery disease.[6] In general, these guidelines strongly recommend an imaging study as part of the evaluation in patients who are unable to exercise and in those with baseline electrocardiographic abnormalities (preexcitation, paced ventricular rhythm, >1 mm of resting ST-segment depression, complete left bundle branch block). The use of digoxin or the presence of left ventricular hypertrophy also decreases the specificity of exercise testing, whereas sensitivity may remain unaffected. Several other subsets of patients benefit incrementally with the use of cardiac imaging. Those groups involve patients with prior myocardial infarction, revascularization procedures (coronary artery bypass grafting [CABG] or percutaneous transluminal coronary angioplasty [PTCA]), known significant disease (for identification of the "culprit" lesion causing ischemia), diabetes, and patients with a previous positive imaging study (Box 9-1). At present, there are no specific guidelines for cardiovascular magnetic resonance (CMR) imaging, but information on this technique is included in this chapter for general information purposes and the expectation that this technique will play a more important role in routine clinical cardiology practice.

EBCT

The early detection of coronary atherosclerosis would seem desirable particularly among selected individuals

■ ■ ■

BOX 9-1 INDICATIONS FOR THE USE OF CARDIAC IMAGING RATHER THAN EXERCISE ELECTROCARDIOGRAPHY

- Complete left bundle-branch block
- Electronically paced ventricular rhythm
- Preexcitation (Wolff-Parkinson-White) syndrome or other, similar electrocardiographic abnormalities
- More than 1 mm of ST-segment depression at rest
- Inability to exercise to a level high enough to give meaningful results on routine stress electrocardiography*
- Angina and history of revascularization†

*Patients with this factor should be considered for pharmacological stress tests.
†In patients with angina and a history of revascularization, characterizing the ischemia, establishing the functional effect of lesions, and determining myocardial viability are important considerations.
Adapted from Gibbons RJ, Balady GJ, Timothy Bricker J, et al. ACC/AHA 2002 guideline update for exercise testing: summary article. A report of the American College of Cardiology/American Heart Association Task Force on Practice Guidelines (Committee to Update the 1997 Exercise Testing Guidelines). *J Am Coll Cardiol* 2002; 40:1531.

who are either at increased risk for the development of overt coronary artery disease on the basis of established clinical risk factor algorithms or have a strong genetic predisposition for premature coronary artery disease. The theoretical purpose behind screening is to (1) identify early atherosclerosis and potentially prevent its progression through intensive risk factor modification and (2) identify asymptomatic individuals with advanced atherosclerosis and silent myocardial ischemia who might benefit from antiischemic medical therapy and/or coronary revascularization.

EBCT is a simple, rapid, reproducible, and highly specific technique for the detection of early coronary atherosclerosis based on the presence and extent of coronary artery calcification.[7] Unlike spiral CT scanners, where image acquisition speed is limited by the mechanical rotation of the X-ray tube, EBCT uses electron beam technology with a <50-ms image acquisition time. Such rapid imaging allows a "freeze-frame" image of the myocardium and coronary arteries in end-diastole and literally eliminates distortion or blur from cardiac motion. Contrast angiography has also been successfully performed with EBCT to visualize both coronary artery bypass grafts and native coronary arteries.[8]

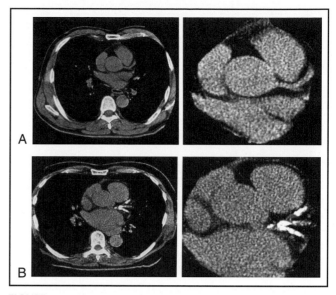

FIGURE 9-2. Single-level noncontrast EBCT scan of a normal subject *(top)* and an individual with severe coronary artery calcification *(bottom)*. Calcium is shown as intensely white areas within the coronary arteries.

Coronary Artery Calcification

The standard EBCT imaging protocol is to acquire 40 consecutive 3-mm-thick images at a rate of 100 ms/image from the base of the heart to just below the carina. Images are obtained at end-inspiration with electrocardiographic gating at end-diastole to accept beats within 80% of the predetermined RR interval. A calcified lesion is generally defined as either two or three adjacent pixels (0.68 to 1.02 mm² for a 512^2 reconstruction matrix and a camera field size of 30 cm) of >130 Hounsfield units (HU). The traditional Agatston scoring system multiplies each calcified lesion by a density factor as follows: 1 for lesions with a maximal density between 130 and 199 HU; 2 for lesions between 200 and 299 HU; 3 for lesions between 300 and 399 HU; and 4 for lesions >400 HU. The total coronary artery calcium score is calculated as the sum of each calcified lesion in the four main coronary arteries over all the consecutive tomographic slices (Figure 9-2).

The Agatston-derived coronary artery calcium score correlates extremely well with calcified areas found in individual coronary arteries as determined by histomorphometric measurements (Figure 9-3). Furthermore, excellent interobserver and intraobserver reproducibility is reported for recalculating the coronary artery calcium score on a single scan by use of the Agatston method. Temporal variability does exist when performing sequential imaging in the same patient, but this is primarily limited to patients with a very low initial coronary artery calcium score. Coronary artery calcium score variability has been demonstrated to be inversely related to the absolute value of the coronary artery calcium score and is greatest when the score is <10 (Figure 9-4).

A newer volumetric calcium scoring system calculates the volume of calcified plaque area rather than generating a coronary artery calcium score on the basis of an arbitrary plaque attenuation coefficient (i.e., Agatston method).[9] EBT shows promise in potentially tracking changes in calcified plaque.[10]

Calcium Score and Atherosclerotic Plaque Burden

The presence of coronary artery calcification indicates the presence of coronary atherosclerosis, and the coronary artery calcium score severity is directly related to the total atherosclerotic plaque burden present in the epicardial coronary arteries. Calcification is an active, organized, and regulated process occurring during atherosclerotic plaque development in which calcium phosphate in the form of hydroxyapatite precipitates in atherosclerotic coronary arteries in a similar fashion as observed in bone mineralization. Although lack of calcification does not categorically exclude the presence of atherosclerotic plaque, calcification occurs exclusively in atherosclerotic arteries and is not found in normal coronary arteries.

The presence and extent of histologically determined atherosclerotic plaque area has been compared with the total calcium area as assessed by EBCT in individual coronary arteries derived from autopsied hearts. A strong linear relation exists between the extent of total plaque area and coronary artery calcification in individual hearts and in individual coronary arteries. However, the total calcium area underestimates the total plaque area because of the presence of approximately five times as many noncalcified as calcified plaques. On the basis of current EBCT imaging protocols, small plaque areas of <5 mm² are generally not detected.

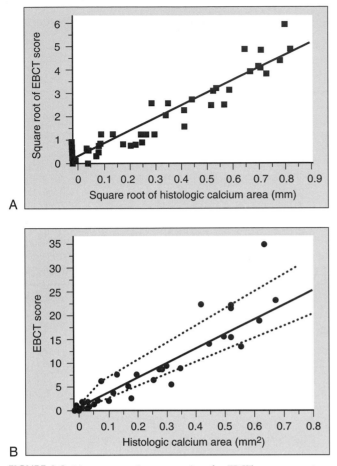

FIGURE 9-3. Linear regression comparing the EBCT coronary artery calcium score (square root transformation and actual data[2]) with the calcium area measured at histomorphometric examination. There is an apparent high-positive correlation between the EBCT calcium score and histomorphometric calcium area ($r^2 = .92$, $r = .96$; $P < 0.0001$). (From Mautner GC, Mautner SL, Froehlich J, Feuerstein IM, Proschan MA, Roberts WC, et al. Coronary artery calcification: assessment with electron beam CT and histomorphometric correlation. *Radiology* 1994; 192[3]:619.)

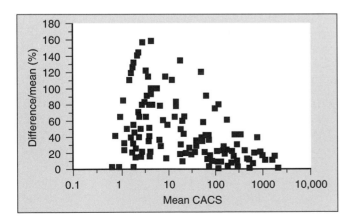

FIGURE 9-4. Graph depicts variability in sequential coronary artery calcium score results as a percentage of the mean coronary artery calcium score. Most variability in coronary artery calcium score is observed in subjects with an initial low score (<20). (From Bielak LF, Kaufmann RB, Moll PP, McCollough CH, Schwartz RS, Sheedy PF. Small lesions in the heart identified at electron beam CT: calcification or noise? *Radiology* 1994; 192[3]:631.)

Comparison of Coronary Artery Calcium Score and Angiography

Significant (>50%) coronary artery stenosis by angiography is almost universally associated with the presence of coronary artery calcium. However, stenosis severity is not directly related to the total coronary artery calcium score. A recent morphological study from autopsied hearts found a poor relationship between coronary stenosis severity and coronary artery calcium score, indicating the latter could not be used to estimate angiographic stenosis severity on a segment-by-segment basis. One explanation is that coronary artery diameter increases with increasing plaque burden, so as to maintain luminal patency. Although the extent of coronary calcification does not precisely predict stenosis severity, noncalcified plaques are almost universally associated with <50% diameter stenosis and typically <20% stenosis. Therefore, the lack of coronary calcification predicts a very low likelihood of obstructive coronary artery disease.

Clinical angiographic trials confirm the relationship between coronary artery calcium score severity and the presence of significant (≥50%) stenosis.[11] The likelihood of multivessel coronary artery disease increases with the calcium score in both men and women. A normal EBCT indicates a very low (<1%) risk of significant coronary artery disease. Although significant differences in coronary artery calcium score are noted among men and women, EBCT does predict significant coronary artery disease equally well in both genders on the basis of age-specific coronary artery calcium score thresholds (Figure 9-5). In the 15 largest studies evaluating EBCT and coronary angiography, the overall sensitivity and specificity for detecting obstructive (>50%) coronary artery disease were 97% and 39%, respectively (Table 9-1). The poor specificity of EBCT is not unexpected, because the presence of coronary calcification confirms the presence of atherosclerotic plaque that may not necessarily be obstructive in nature. Coronary artery calcium score severity may be a better barometer of obstructive coronary artery disease than the mere presence of calcium. Several reports in patients referred for coronary angiography have found that a coronary artery calcium score >100 best predicts obstructive coronary artery disease with an equally high sensitivity and specificity of 80%. There seems to be a threshold coronary artery calcium score above which most patients will have significant coronary artery stenosis. However, this may be gender-related and age-related (Figure 9-5). Despite the relationship between obstructive coronary artery disease and coronary artery calcium score severity, the latter is still too imprecise in itself to be used as a definitive criterion for proceeding directly to coronary angiography in asymptomatic persons.[12]

Coronary Artery Calcium Score and Stress Testing

Although patients with a normal EBCT are highly unlikely to have significant coronary artery disease and

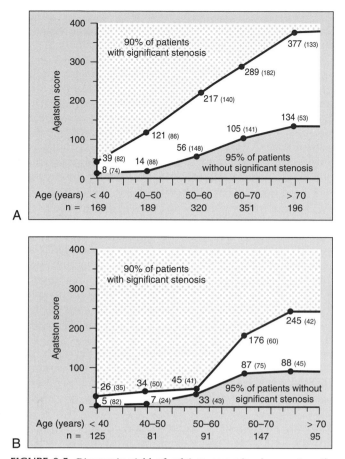

FIGURE 9-5. Diagnostic yield of calcium screening in symptomatic men (**A**) and women (**B**). The lower scores define the calcium score thresholds for the 95% of patients without significant stenoses. The higher scores give the calcium score thresholds for the 90% of patients with significant stenoses. Within the central area, the diagnosis is uncertain. The numbers in parentheses give the number of patients within the area. For example, a man at the age of 50 years is probably free of coronary stenosis if his score is <56. At score values >217, he bears a high risk of stenosis. (From Haberl R, Becker A, Leber A, Knez A, Becker C, Lang C, et al. Correlation of coronary calcification and angiographically documented stenoses in patients with suspected coronary artery disease: results of 1,764 patients. *J Am Coll Cardiol* 2001; 37[2]:451. Reproduced with permission.)

■ ■ ■

TABLE 9-1 ACCURACY OF EBCT CORONARY ARTERY CALCIFICATION IN DETECTING SIGNIFICANT (>50%) CORONARY ARTERY STENOSIS AS DEFINED BY ANGIOGRAPHY

Study author/year	N	Sensitivity (%)	Specificity (%)	Positive PA	Negative PA
Agatston 1990[a]	584	96	51	31	98
Breen 1992[b]	100	100	47	63	100
Bielak 1994[c]	160	96	45	57	93
Kaufman 1995[d]	160	93	67	81	86
Rumberger 1995[e]	139	98	39	59	97
Braun 1996[f]	102	93	73	93	73
Budoff 1996[g]	710	95	44	72	84
Detrano 1996[h]	491	95	31	51	89
Fallavollita 1996[i]	106	85	45	66	70
Baumgart 1997[j]	57	97	21	56	86
Kennedy 1998[k]	368	96	31	51	90
Schmermund 1997[l]	118	95	88	99	58
Haberl 2001[m]	1764	99	30	62	98
Bielak 2000[n]	213	99	39	64	98
Shavelle 2000[o]	97	96	47	80	82
Total	5169	97	39	61	92

PA, Predictive accuracy; [a]*J Am Coll Cardiol* 1990; 15:827; [b]*Radiology* 1992; 185:435; [c]*Radiology* 1994; 192:631; [d]*Mayo Clin Proc* 1995; 70:223; [e]*Circulation* 1996; 91:1363; [f]*Am J Kidney Dis* 1996; 27:394; [g]*Circulation* 1996; 93:898; [h]*J Am Coll Cardiol* 1996; 27:285; [i]*Circulation* 1994; 89:285; [j]*J Am Coll Cardiol* 1997;30:57; [k]*Am Heart J* 1998; 135:696; [l]*Circulation* 1997; 96:1461; [m]*J Am Coll Cardiol* 2001; 37:451; [n]*Circulation* 2000; 102:380; [o]*Am J Cardiol* 1995; 75:973.

require no further cardiac testing, an important clinical question is how best to proceed in patients with an abnormal EBCT who will have varying coronary artery calcium score severities. To proceed with invasive testing in this latter population is not warranted on the basis of the large degree of overlap between calcium scores and the presence of obstructive coronary artery disease. An alternative approach might be to perform noninvasive testing in selected patients at high risk for having myocardial ischemia on the basis of specific coronary artery calcium score thresholds. Stress myocardial perfusion imaging is one such well-established noninvasive technique for detecting the presence and determining the prognostic significance of coronary artery disease. Stress myocardial perfusion imaging can define high-risk and low-risk asymptomatic patients on the basis of the presence and extent of inducible myocardial ischemia. Although not recommended as a

screening test in asymptomatic patients because of the low prevalence of a positive test result (<5%), perfusion imaging might be used as a secondary test to identify myocardial ischemia once a certain threshold of atherosclerotic plaque burden had been identified by EBCT.

In a generally asymptomatic population who had risk factors for coronary artery disease development, the complimentary roles of EBCT and stress myocardial perfusion single photon emission computed tomography (SPECT) for identifying both preclinical coronary artery disease and silent myocardial ischemia were assessed.[13] The investigators attempted to identify patients with preclinical coronary artery disease who might benefit from aggressive risk factor modification and those at relatively higher short-term risk for cardiac events on the basis of the presence of silent myocardial ischemia. Among the 3895 subjects who had EBCT, 411 also underwent stress SPECT within a close temporal period (median, 17 days). Although only 22% of 374 subjects with an abnormal EBCT had an abnormal SPECT, the likelihood of an abnormal SPECT increased dramatically with the total coronary artery calcium score (Figure 9-6). Although only 1% of subjects with a total coronary artery calcium score <100 had an abnormal SPECT myocardial perfusion imaging (MPI), this was observed in 46% of those with scores ≥400. However, 10% of all 3895 subjects scanned with EBCT had a coronary artery calcium score ≥400. Large ischemic perfusion defects (i.e., ≥15% of the left ventricle) were virtually confined to subjects who had a coronary artery calcium score ≥400. Although a similar percentage of subjects had an abnormal SPECT (16%) or stress electrocardiogram (17%), only

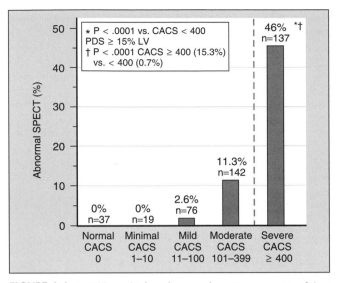

FIGURE 9-6. SPECT results based on total coronary artery calcium score (CACS). Few subjects with CACS <400 had abnormal SPECT (6.6%), and most (99.3%) had only small (<15%) perfusion defect size (PDS). LV indicates left ventricle. (From He ZX, Hedrick TD, Pratt CM, Verani MS, Aquino V, Roberts R, et al. Severity of coronary artery calcification by electron beam computed tomography predicts silent myocardial ischemia. *Circulation* 2000; 101[3]:244.)

the former was related to the total coronary artery calcium score, further illustrating the poor predictive accuracy of treadmill testing for detecting coronary artery disease in asymptomatic subjects.

The results of this study support the role of EBCT as an initial screening test for identifying subjects with varying degrees of coronary atherosclerosis. It also emphasizes the effectiveness of selectively combining SPECT with EBCT in the relatively small percentage of subjects who have a high (≥400) coronary artery calcium score to identify those with silent myocardial ischemia. This testing strategy may be optimal on the basis of the known prognostic value of SPECT and the apparent superior sensitivity of EBCT over SPECT for detecting preclinical coronary artery disease. Although the cost-effectiveness of the use of EBCT as a screening test demands further clinical investigation, it has been proposed that the coronary artery calcium score might be used to guide therapeutics and recommend the need for additional diagnostic testing.

Stress Myocardial Perfusion Imaging

Exercise Stress

Extensive data have demonstrated the high sensitivity of both ^{201}Tl planar and SPECT imaging for detecting coronary artery disease. With planar imaging incorporating visual assessment of myocardial scintigrams, sensitivity and specificity averaged 82% and 88%, respectively, in more than 4000 patients combined from multiple studies. Sensitivity varies with the extent of coronary artery disease. It approaches 79% for the detection of one-vessel disease (>50% stenosis), 88% for two-vessel disease, and 92% for three-vessel disease, with an average sensitivity of 86%. Application

of quantitative analysis increases the sensitivity (approximately 90%) with equal or occasionally slightly worse specificity.

With tomographic SPECT myocardial perfusion imaging technology, sensitivity averages 90% and specificity is approximately 70% in large series of patients. The lower specificity may be attributed to a referral bias in which patients with abnormal scans were more frequently referred for coronary angiography than patients with normal scans. This explanation is further supported by the high normalcy rate (89%) seen in a large series. In similar patients without a prior history of coronary artery disease, the overall sensitivity of ^{201}Tl SPECT imaging was 85%, with an average sensitivity of 83% for the detection of single-vessel disease, 93% for two-vessel disease, and 95% for three-vessel disease (Table 9-2).

Only a few comparative studies between planar and SPECT ^{201}Tl imaging are available. SPECT imaging seems superior, given the fact that it can detect an individual stenosis on the basis of localization of stress-induced perfusion defects. Sensitivity is enhanced in patients with known or extensive coronary artery disease, high-grade coronary stenosis, proximal location of stenosis, and the presence of wall motion abnormalities. Variables that diminish sensitivity for coronary artery disease detection are single-vessel disease, left circumflex coronary stenosis, branch vessel or distal stenosis, mild degree of stenosis (<50% luminal narrowing), inadequate heart rate response during exercise, and concurrent antianginal therapy. The low specificity with ^{201}Tl scintigraphy generally may be caused by a failure to recognize attenuation artifacts in the inferoapical and anteroseptal regions. The introduction of ^{99m}Tc-gated SPECT imaging permits the assessment of systolic wall thickening of end-diastole to end systole on multiple SPECT tomograms. Normal systolic thickening in an area of hypoperfusion in both stress and rest images represents an attenuation artifact rather than a myocardial scar that will be associated with reduced systolic thickening. Taillefer at al[14] compared the diagnostic accuracy of ^{201}Tl and ^{99m}Tc-sestamibi SPECT in 115 women (85 patients and 30 controls) in a prospective design. Women in the study underwent both perfusion (^{201}Tl and ^{99m}Tc-sestamibi) and electrocardiographic gated ^{99m}Tc-sestamibi SPECT imaging, and most of them had coronary angiography. The overall sensitivities for detecting ≥50% and ≥70% stenosis were 75% and 84%, respectively, for ^{201}Tl, and 72% and 80%, respectively, for ^{99m}Tc-sestamibi perfusion studies (both P = 0.48). The specificity for lesions ≥50% was 71% for ^{201}Tl, 86% for ^{99m}Tc-sestamibi perfusion (P = 0.05), and 94% for ^{99m}Tc-sestamibi gated SPECT (P = 0.002). For lesions ≥70%, the specificity was 67% for ^{201}Tl, 84% for ^{99m}Tc-sestamibi perfusion (P = 0.02), and 92% for ^{99m}Tc-sestamibi gated SPECT (P = 0.0004). In summary, the authors concluded that both ^{201}Tl and ^{99m}Tc-sestamibi had a similar sensitivity for the detection of coronary artery disease; however, ^{99m}Tc-sestamibi SPECT perfusion imaging showed a significantly better specificity, which was further enhanced by the use of electrocardiographic gating. This strongly suggests that all nuclear perfusion imaging should be performed with simultaneous gated wall motion.

TABLE 9-2   SENSITIVITY AND SPECIFICITY OF EXERCISE THALLIUM-201 SPECT

Study	MI	SENSITIVITY						Specificity	Normalcy rate
		Overall	MI	No MI	1VD	2VD	3VD		
Tamaki[a]	39%	98%	100%	96%	—	—	—	91%	—
(N = 104)		80/82	32/32	48/50				20/22	
DePasquale[b]	26%	95%	100%	92%	91%	99%	100%	74%	—
(N = 210)		170/179	47/47	123/134	85/93	72/73	13/13	23/31	
Iskandrian[c]	18%	82%	98%	78%	64%	87%	91%	60%	94%
(N = 461)		224/272	49/50	174/222	45/70	93/107	86/95	35/58	123/131
Maddahi[d]	47%	95%	100%	90%	83%	97%	98%	56%	86%
(N = 138)		87/92	43/43	44/49	15/18	32/33	40/41	10/18	24/28
Mahmarian[e]	33%	87%	99%	79%	84%	91%	100%	87%	—
(N = 360)		192/221	73/74	68/86	119/142	60/66	13/13	65/75	
VanTrain[f]	40%	94%	100%	90%	88%	96%	100%	43%	82%
(N = 318)		185/196	78/78	106/118	56/64	69/72	60/60	15/35	62/76
Total	31%	90%	99%*	85%	83%	93%†	95%†	70%	89%
		938/1042	322/324	563/659	320/387	326/351	212/222	168/239	209/235

*P = 0.0001 vs. no MI.
†P = 0.0001 vs. SVD.
1VD, single-vessel disease; 2VD, double-vessel disease; 3VD, triple-vessel disease; SPECT, single photon emission computed tomography; MI, myocardial Infarction.
[a]J Am Coll Cardiol 1984; 4:1213; [b]Circulation 1988; 77:316; [c]J Am Coll Cardiol 1989; 14:1477; [e]Am J Cardiol 1991; 67:1d; J Am Coll Cardiol 1990; 15:318; [d]J Am Coll Cardiol 1989; 14:1689; [f]J Nucl Med 1990; 31:1168.
Adapted from Mahmarian et al. Am J Cardiol 1991; 67:2D and J Am Coll Cardiol 1990; 15:318.

Several studies have addressed the diagnostic accuracy of ^{99m}Tc-sestamibi in comparison with ^{201}Tl imaging in the setting of suspected coronary artery disease. An analysis of studies that used exercise SPECT imaging yielded a 90% sensitivity for ^{99m}Tc-sestamibi and 83% for ^{201}Tl for the detection of coronary artery disease. Specificity for ^{99m}Tc-sestamibi was 93% compared with 80% for ^{201}Tl imaging, and the normalcy rate was 100% for ^{99m}Tc-sestamibi imaging and 77% for ^{201}Tl SPECT. ^{99m}Tc-sestamibi SPECT MPI had an excellent sensitivity for the detection of single-vessel coronary artery disease (90%), which was almost 20% higher than planar imaging.

To overcome some of the difficulties in distinguishing reversible from irreversible defects, a dual-isotope (rest ^{201}Tl/stress ^{99m}Tc-sestamibi SPECT imaging) protocol has been validated in patients with suspected coronary disease and prior myocardial infarction.[15] In this protocol 3 mCi of ^{201}Tl is injected at rest, with images acquired 10 minutes later. Subsequently, an exercise test is performed with 25 to 30 mCi of ^{99m}Tc-sestamibi injected at peak stress. Dual-isotope SPECT demonstrated high sensitivity for detecting patients with ≥50% coronary artery stenosis (approximately 90%) and with ≥70% stenosis (approximately 95%). Although high values for specificity were recorded in the study (75% for <50% stenosis, and 82% for <70% stenosis), the significance was uncertain, given the small number of patients with normal coronary angiograms. However, the normalcy rate was 95%, which is higher than ^{201}Tl and similar to ^{99m}Tc-sestamibi SPECT studies. Segmental agreement for defect type between ^{201}Tl and ^{99m}Tc-sestamibi studies was 97% in zones without previous myocardial infarction. In myocardial infarct zones, segmental agreement for defect type was 98%. The agreement for defect reversibility pattern (normal, reversible or irreversible) between first and second readings was 95%, and for the exact segmental score (range, 0 to 4) it was 86%.

The incremental benefit of dual-isotope SPECT over combined clinical information and the results of treadmill electrocardiographic stress tests in predicting adverse outcomes in 2200 patients with no prior known coronary disease referred for stress testing has been demonstrated.[16] The risk of either death or myocardial infarction over the next 18 months was 0.3% in individuals with normal scans, 4.7% in those with mild perfusion abnormalities, and 10% in those with severe abnormalities. Mild and severe perfusion scan abnormalities were found in individuals with a predicted risk of 0.9% to 2.5% by use of the Duke Treadmill Risk Score (which takes into account exercise time, electrocardiographic ST deviation, and the presence or absence of angina), and it was calculated that the perfusion imaging scans resulted in a fivefold increase in prognostic information. Thus, in a patient population at an overall low risk of 2% for "hard" events (cardiac death and myocardial infarction), myocardial perfusion SPECT imaging added incremental prognostic information and added to risk stratification provided by clinical and treadmill exercise test information. The dual-isotope approach also allows the use of ^{201}Tl for the evaluation of defect reversibility and detection of myocardial viability (greater redistribution of ^{201}Tl into areas of ischemic and viable myocardium).

Pharmacological Stress

Pharmacological stress myocardial perfusion imaging has become an important alternative noninvasive tool in the detection of coronary artery disease in patients who are unable to exercise. It has been reported that submaximal stress SPECT myocardial perfusion imaging is significantly less sensitive than maximal exercise in detecting coronary disease and may incorrectly identify patients with multivessel disease. Agents commonly used are dipyridamole, adenosine,[17] and dobutamine.[18] Both dipyridamole and adenosine induce a threefold to fivefold increase in myocardial blood flow with standard doses. Intravenous dobutamine is an alternative modality predominantly in patients with severe obstructive airway disease or high-grade atrioventricular block. Dobutamine infusion produces flow heterogeneity in the presence of significant coronary artery stenosis, because it increases myocardial oxygen demand by increasing heart rate, blood pressure, and contractility.

Multiple studies suggest a sensitivity of approximately 89% for dipyridamole, 90% for adenosine, and 82% for dobutamine myocardial perfusion imaging. Specificity is approximately 78%, 91%, and 73% for dipyridamole, adenosine, and dobutamine myocardial perfusion imaging, respectively. It seems that adenosine myocardial perfusion imaging has a slightly higher sensitivity and specificity compared with dipyridamole or dobutamine myocardial perfusion imaging, with a greater side effect profile. A recently published meta-analysis of 20 diagnostic studies that used dobutamine myocardial perfusion imaging for the detection of coronary artery disease confirmed a sensitivity of 88%, specificity of 74%, and diagnostic accuracy of 84%.[19] The combination of low-level exercise with intravenous adenosine infusions has been reported to be safe and reduces adverse reactions (especially related to bradycardia or first-degree atrioventricular block), improves image quality, and may provoke more episodes of myocardial ischemia.[20] This type of stress protocol may become a new preferred standard.

The diagnostic accuracy of myocardial perfusion studies in women is reduced by the high prevalence of single-vessel coronary disease, breast attenuation, and a smaller left ventricular chamber size than men.[21] With the use of gated SPECT the simultaneously derived information on perfusion and function helps differentiate attenuation artifact from myocardial infarction. Importantly, women are generally older when they are seen with coronary disease, and many are incapable of completing a symptom-limited exercise protocol and therefore those with an intermediate-to-high pretest likelihood of coronary artery disease should undergo pharmacological stress testing. There are insufficient data to firmly recommend a preference for a particular type of pharmacological stress test in women.[21] Finally, the ability of noninvasive tests to diagnose or localize coronary artery disease in patients with left bundle-branch block has been disappointing, although tomographic myocardial perfusion imaging with adenosine or dipyridamole stress provides important prognostic information in patients with left bundle-branch block.[22] Patients with left bundle-branch block and normal coronary arteries often have abnormal septal defects on exercise SPECT myocardial perfusion imaging. This false-positive rate of septal defects is significantly lower with dipyridamole or adenosine myocardial perfusion imaging. Current recommendations favor vasodilator stress imaging to determine the presence and prognostic significance of coronary artery disease in patients with left bundle-branch block.

PET

PET is increasingly being used for the noninvasive detection of coronary artery disease.[23] Most published literature and current clinical practice at PET centers rely on relative rather that absolute quantitation of myocardial blood flow (MBF) for detection of coronary artery disease, in a manner similar to the current practice with interpretation of myocardial perfusion SPECT studies (Table 9-3). Overall, the available literature suggests that for diagnosis of coronary artery disease, relative quantitation of myocardial perfusion is sufficient for routine clinical application and that absolute quantitation of MBF or coronary low reserve (CFR) by PET would not be required for this application.

Comparison Between PET and SPECT

PET has several theoretical advantages over SPECT imaging for detecting coronary artery disease. PET has higher spatial and contrast resolution. Furthermore, attenuation correction is well developed and is applied routinely in PET imaging, which improves specificity by eliminating attenuation artifacts. The pooled literature data for PET, ^{201}Tl SPECT, and ^{99m}Tc-sestamibi SPECT suggest that the sensitivities of the three methods are similar (94%, 91%, and 89%, respectively) for the detection of coronary artery disease. However, the specificity and normalcy rates of PET (83% and 96%) are higher than those of ^{201}Tl SPECT (70% and 89%) and ^{99m}Tc-sestamibi SPECT (36% and 81%). This is most likely related to a lower false-positive rate of PET, which is attained by routine application of attenuation correction. The difference between PET and SPECT, however, is likely to diminish with increasing application of gating and attenuation correction to SPECT studies, which are expected to improve identification of attenuation artifacts. Interestingly, no difference in patient management or cardiac event–free survival was demonstrated between management on the basis of ^{13}N-ammonia/[18]-fluoroprodeoxyglucose (FDG) PET and stress/rest ^{99m}Tc-sestamibi SPECT imaging.[24]

■ ■ ■

TABLE 9-3   PET FOR DETECTION OF CORONARY ARTERY DISEASE

Lead author	Patients	Sensitivity	Specificity	Normalcy
Schelbert[a]	45	97%	—	100%
Tamaki[b]	25	95%	—	100%
Demer[c]	193	83%	95%	—
Tamaki[d]	51	98%	100%	—
Yonekura[e]	50	97%	100%	100%
Go[f]	202	93%	79%	—
Stewart[g]	81	84%	—	88%
Khanna[h]	35	98%	—	96%
Simone[i]	225	82%	91%	—
Williams[j]	287	87%	88%	—

[a]Am J Cardiol 1982; 49:1197; [b]Eur J Nucl Med 1985; 11:246; [c]Circulation 1989; 79: 825; [d]J Nucl Med 1988; 29: 1181; [e]Am Heart J 1987; 113: 645; [f]J Nucl Med 1990; 31:1899; [g]Am J Cardiol 1991; 67:1303; [h]J Nucl Med 1993; 33:825; [i]Am J Physiol Imaging 1992; 7:203; [j]J Nucl Med 1994; 35:1586.

Echocardiography

Echocardiography, whether obtained with or without stress, is commonly used in patients with documented coronary artery disease. Standard, nonstress (resting) echocardiography is used for a variety of reasons: to evaluate systolic function (e.g., ejection fraction), to investigate the presence of focal wall motion abnormalities, to rule out superimposed acute ischemia, to diagnose complications of myocardial infarction, and to quantitate associated mitral regurgitation. Increasingly, exercise and pharmacological stress echocardiography are also used in patients with chronic coronary artery disease to investigate chest pain syndromes and to detect and evaluate the presence of coronary artery disease.

Resting Studies

The evaluation of ventricular systolic function is the most common indication for echocardiography, not only in patients with coronary artery disease but in general cardiology practice. In most institutions, two-dimensional (2D) echocardiography is the principal noninvasive method used for quantitating left ventricular volumes and assessing global and regional systolic function, with transesophageal echo being reserved for those situations when standard transthoracic imaging yields suboptimal images. Two-dimensional echocardiography, because of its superior spatial resolution, is used to guide appropriate positioning of the M-mode beam and is used for direct measurements of ventricular dimensions and for calculation of left ventricular volumes and ejection fraction. Such spatial resolution is especially important in patients with coronary heart disease, because shape distortions caused by myocardial infarction are common. In clinical practice, visual estimation of ejection fraction from 2D echocardiography is perhaps the most common method used, and, when performed by experienced readers, ejection fraction by visual estimation corresponds closely to that obtained by angiography or gated blood pool scanning. The administration of an echocardiographic contrast agent improves the delineation of the endocardial/left ventricular cavity interface and improves the accuracy of 2D echocardiographic estimates of ejection fraction. The use of second harmonic imaging, even without the administration of contrast agents, also improves the endocardial interface, thus facilitating identification of abnormal wall motion.

Besides quantitation of systolic function, echocardiography can diagnose mitral regurgitation resulting from a variety of mechanisms. Recent studies using three-dimensional (3D) echocardiography suggest that altered mitral valve geometry, occasioned by apical papillary muscle displacement, contributes importantly to mitral regurgitation in this setting. Color flow Doppler is used to provide an estimate of the severity of mitral regurgitation, assisting the cardiologist and cardiac surgeon in planning for corrective surgery. In patients with heart failure or significant ventricular arrhythmias, the presence or absence of ventricular aneurysm can be established, which also may be useful in planning surgery.

Stress Studies

Stress echocardiography, an alternative to stress nuclear perfusion imaging, has proven to have excellent diagnostic accuracy for detecting inducible ischemia in patients with intermediate to high pretest probability of coronary artery disease.[25] An obvious virtue of stress echocardiography compared with electrocardiographic stress testing is the ability to localize inducible myocardial ischemia. As expected, the sensitivity of this technique is greater in patients with multivessel disease than in those with single-vessel disease, and in those with >70% stenosis compared with those with less severe lesions.

The weighted mean sensitivity of exercise stress echocardiography is 86%, specificity 81%, and overall accuracy 85% (Table 9-4). The corresponding values for dobutamine stress echocardiography are 82%, 84%, and 83% (Table 9-5). Some limitations of the methods bear emphasis. Treadmill stress echocardiography may have lowered sensitivity if there is a significant delay from the end of the exercise to the acquisition of postexercise images. Sensitivity can also be diminished if all myocardial segments are not adequately visualized, and the diagnostic accuracy of stress echo can be improved in this setting with the use of contrast agents and second harmonic imaging.

Pharmacological stress echocardiography is used in situations in which exercise is not feasible, with the most common agents used being dobutamine and dipyridamole. Dobutamine, the most commonly used of the adrenergic stimulants, increases oxygen demand by increasing contractility, blood pressure, and heart rate. Dobutamine is most commonly administered in graded doses to titrate myocardial workload in a manner akin to standard exercise testing. Vasodilator agents, in contrast, cause heterogeneous myocardial perfusion without actually altering workload (or wall motion) directly. Comparative studies suggest a somewhat lower sensitivity for stress echocardiography with vasodilators compared with dobutamine. However, pharmacological stress echocardiography using vasodilator agents does seem to be useful in detecting inducible myocardial ischemia and particularly valuable in determining prognosis. Dobutamine stress has been used in conjunction with transesophageal echocardiographic imaging in patients with poor transthoracic windows. In an asymptomatic patient with prior infarction, stress echocardiography may be helpful in assessing risk and determining the need for cardiac catheterization, but it can be challenging to detect residual ischemia within an akinetic zone.

Comparison of Stress Echocardiography and Myocardial Perfusion Imaging (MPI)

Literature analyses comparing the diagnostic accuracy of myocardial perfusion imaging and stress echocardiography in patients with suspected or known coronary artery disease suggest that exercise SPECT scintigraphy has a sensitivity of approximately 90% and a specificity of approximately 70%, and exercise echocardiography a sensitivity of approximately 80% and specificity of approximately 90%. It seems that exercise SPECT is more

■■■

TABLE 9-4   DIAGNOSTIC ACCURACY OF EXERCISE ECHOCARDIOGRAPHY IN DETECTING ANGIOGRAPHICALLY PROVED CAD, SERIES PUBLISHED SINCE 1990

Year	Author	N	Sens (%)	Sens 1-VD	Sens MVD	Spec (%)	PPV (%)	NPV (%)	Acc (%)
1990	Sheikh[a]	34	74	74	—	91	94	63	79
1991	Pozzoli[b]	75	71	61	94	96	97	64	80
1991	Crouse[c]	228	97	92	100	64	90	87	89
1991	Galanti*[d]	53	93	93	92	96	96	93	94
1992	Marwick[e]	150	84	79	96	86	95	63	85
1992	Quinones[f]	112	74	59	89	88	96	51	78
1992	Salustri[g]	44	87	87	—	85	93	75	86
1992	Amanullah[h]	27	82	—	—	80	95	50	81
1993	Hecht[i]	180	93	84	100	86	95	79	91
1993	Ryan[j]	309	91	86	95	78	90	81	87
1993	Mertes[k]	79	84	87	89	85	91	75	85
1993	Hoffmann*[l]	66	80	79	81	88	95	58	82
1993	Cohen*[m]	86	88	82	91	80	89	77	85
1994	Marwick[n]	86	88	82	91	80	89	77	85

*Coronary stenosis >70%.

Sens, Sensitivity; 1VD, single-vessel disease; MVD, multivessel disease; Spec, specificity; PPV, positive predictive value; NPV, negative predictive value; Acc, accuracy.

[a]J Am Coll Cardiol 1990; 15:1043; [b]Am J Cardiol 1991; 67:350; [c]Am J Cardiol 1991; 67:1213; [d]Am Heart J 1991; 122:1609; [e]J Am Coll Cardiol 1992; 19:74; [f]Circulation 1992; 85:1026; [g]Am Heart J 1992; 124:75; [h]Clin Cardiol 1992; 15:585; [i]J Am Coll Cardiol 1993; 21:950; [j]J Am Soc Echocardiogr 1993; 6:186; [k]J Am Coll Cardiol 1993; 21:1087; [l]Am J Cardiol 1993; 72:555; [m]Am J Cardiol 1993; 72:1226; [n]Br Heart J 1994; 72:31.

sensitive compared with exercise echocardiography, with a trend toward higher specificity for the latter. Adenosine, dipyridamole, and dobutamine myocardial perfusion imaging studies provide similar diagnostic accuracy (sensitivity 89%, 90%, and 91%; specificity 83%, 78%, and 86%, respectively), and all are more accurate than dobutamine echocardiography (sensitivity 81%, specificity 83%).[26] Clinical specificity is similarly high with adenosine SPECT, dipyridamole echocardiography, and exercise echocardiography and lower with exercise SPECT. Normalcy rate is high for exercise SPECT (89%) and similar to clinical specificity for exercise echocardiography (90%). When the two major pharmacological stress imaging modalities were compared, adenosine

■■■

TABLE 9-5   DIAGNOSTIC ACCURACY OF DOBUTAMINE STRESS ECHOCARDIOGRAPHY IN DETECTING ANGIOGRAPHICALLY PROVEN CAD, SERIES PUBLISHED SINCE 1990

Author	Year	Protocol	N	Sens (%)	Sens 1-VD	Sens MVD	Spec (%)	PPV (%)	NPV (%)	Acc (%)
Sawada[a]	1991	DSE 2.5-30	55	89	81	100	85	91	81	74
Sawada[a]	1991	DSE 2.5-30	41	81	—	81	87	91	72	87
Previtali*[b]	1991	DSE 5-40	35	68	50	92	100	100	44	83
Cohen*[c]	1991	DSE 2.5-40	70	86	69	94	95	98	72	89
Martin[d]	1992	DSE 10-40	34	76	—	—	44	79	40	68
McNeill[e]	1992	DASE 10-40	28	71	—	—	—	—	-	71
Segar[f]	1992	DSE 5-30	88	95	—	—	82	94	86	92
Mazeika*[g]	1992	DSE5-20	50	78	50	92	93	97	62	82
Marcovitz[h]	1992	DSE 5-30	141	96	95	98	66	91	84	89
McNeill[e]	1992	DASE 10-40	80	70	—	—	88	89	67	78
Salustri[i]	1992	DSE 5-40	46	79	—	—	78	85	70	78
Marwick[j]	1993	DSE 5-4-	97	85	84	86	82	88	78	84
Forster[k]	1993	DASE 10-40	21	75	—	—	89	90	73	81
Günalp[l]	1993	DSE 5-30	27	83	78	89	89	94	73	85
Marwick[j]	1993	DSE 5-30	217	72	66	77	83	89	61	76
Hoffman*[m]	1993	DASE 5-40	64	79	78	81	81	93	57	80
Previtali[n]	1993	DSE 5-40	80	79	63	91	83	92	61	80
Takeuchi[o]	1993	DSE 5-30	120	85	73	97	93	95	80	88
Cohen*[p]	1993	DSE 2.5-40	52	86	75	95	87	94	72	87
Ostojic[q]	1994	DSE 5-40	150	75	74	81	79	96	31	75
Marwick[r]	1994	DSE 5-40	86	54	36	65	83	86	49	64
Beleslin[s]	1994	DSE 5-40	136	82	82	82	76	96	38	82

*Coronary stenosis >70%.

Sens, Sensitivity; 1VD, single-vessel disease; MVD, multivessel disease; Spec, specificity; PPV, positive predictive value; NPV, negative predictive value; Acc, accuracy.

[a]Circulation 1991; 83:1605; [b]Circulation 1991; 83:III27; [c]Am J Cardiol 1991; 67:1311; [d]Ann Intern Med 1992; 116:190; [e]Am J Cardiol 1992; 69:740; [f]J Am Coll Cardiol 1992; 19:1197; [g]J Am Coll Cardiol 1992; 19:1203; [h]Am J Cardiol 1992; 69:1269; [i]Eur Heart J 1992; 13:1356; [j]Circulation 1993; 87:345; [k]J Am Coll Cardiol 1993; 21:1591; [l]J Nucl Med 1993; 34:889; [m]Am J Cardiol 1993; 72:555; [n]Am J Cardiol 1993; 72:865; [o]J Am Soc Echocardiogr 1993; 6:593; [p]Am J Cardiol 1993; 72:1226; [q]J Am Coll Cardiol 1994; 23:1115; [r]Br Heart J 1994; 72:31; [s]Circulation 1994; 90:1168.

SPECT myocardial perfusion imaging had a significantly better sensitivity than dobutamine echocardiography (89% vs. 81%). Specificity for both modalities was 83%. In summary, both stress myocardial perfusion imaging and stress echocardiography have superior sensitivity and specificity compared with exercise electrocardiographic stress testing alone. Data from many studies confirm a higher sensitivity of SPECT myocardial perfusion imaging compared with stress echocardiography at the expense of specificity (Table 9-6). The addition of electrocardiographic-gated SPECT imaging with ^{99m}Tc-agents and the simultaneous evaluation of ventricular perfusion and function further improves the specificity and diagnostic accuracy of stress myocardial perfusion imaging.

CMR Imaging

CMR imaging is a new and rapidly evolving discipline. The clinical use of many CMR techniques is still being defined, and it is not yet in widespread clinical practice. The sequences and protocols described will probably change significantly in coming years, although the principles should remain constant. At this stage in its development, there is considerably more data on assessment of diagnosis in relatively limited populations rather than prognosis.

CMR Techniques for Assessing Regional Function

Cine CMR allows a qualitative assessment of regional cardiac function in the same way as echocardiography but with improved image quality and a lower loss of nonvisualized segments. CMR allows routine imaging in the true long and short axis of the heart, which assists in the comparison of regional wall motion between patients and as such does not suffer compromises that result from restricted angulation because of limited acoustic access.[27] Real-time CMR is now available, and comparisons with echo show superiority to echocardiography in patients with limited acoustic access.

In the assessment of resting ventricular function and mass, CMR has some fundamental advantages over other imaging techniques. CMR is both accurate and reproducible and does not require exposure to contrast agents or ionizing radiation. Early CMR techniques of assessing volumes and of the blood pool used the area-length

TABLE 9-6 SENSITIVITY AND SPECIFICITY OF NONINVASIVE TESTS FOR THE DETECTION OF CORONARY ARTERY DISEASE

Diagnostic test	Sensitivity (range)	Specificity (range)	Number of studies	Number of patients
Exercise ECG	68%	77%	132	24,074
Planar scintigraphy	79% (70%-94%)	73% (43%-97%)	6	510
SPECT MPI	88% (73%-98%)	77% (53%-96%)	8	628
Stress echo-cardiography	76% (40%-100%)	88% (80%-95%)	10	1174

Data on the ranges of sensitivity and specificity are from *Ann Intern Med* 1999; 130:719. Data on the sensitivity and specificity of exercise electrocardiography are from *Circulation* 1989; 80:87.

method with long-axis views, assuming that the left ventricle was a prolate ellipsoid of rotation. This was performed because the more complicated 3D coverage of the heart was too time-consuming. However, with faster scanners, this is no longer the case, and the area-length method has largely been abandoned, because the problems of geometric assumptions are manifestly incorrect in remodeled hearts. The 3D CMR approach (volumetry) is now in widespread use and is robust and practical. CMR offers the best current reference standard for the assessment of cardiac function and mass (Table 9-7), being both accurate and reproducible in normal and abnormal ventricles. Although much early CMR validation work was done with conventional non-breath-hold cines, the results using current breath-hold sequences show that the reproducibility of old and new techniques is similar. The most important clinical measure is that of interstudy reproducibility, because this describes the fidelity of a technique to determine changes in clinical parameters over time. This applies to individuals in whom a therapeutic response is being looked for or for research in which small changes between groups need to be identified and the sample size requirement is directly linked to the interstudy reproducibility.

A number of methods have been used to quantify cine CMR assessment of wall motion and wall thickening, but myocardial dynamics are more complicated than simple

TABLE 9-7 NORMAL CMR VALUES IN ADULTS FOR VOLUMES AND MASS OF THE LEFT VENTRICLE (LV)

PARAMETER	MALES		FEMALES	
	Absolute	Normalized to BSA	Absolute	Normalized to BSA
LVEDV	136±30 (77–195) mL	69±11 (47–92) mL/m²	96±23 (52–141) mL	61±10 (41–81) mL/m²
LVESV	45±14 (19–72) mL	23±5 (13-3) mL/m²	32±9 (13–51) mL	21±5 (11–31) mL/m²
LVSV	92±21 (51–133) mL	47±8 (32-2) mL/m²	65±16 (33–97) mL	41±8 (26–56) mL/m²
LVEF	67±5 (56–78) %	—	67±5 (56–78) %	—
LVM	178±31 (118–238) g	91±11 (70–113) g/m²	125±26 (75–75) g	79±8 (63–95) g/m²

BSA, Body surface area; EDV, end-diastolic volume; ESV, end-systolic volume; SV, stroke volume; EF, ejection fraction; M, mass including papillary muscles. Values are quoted as mean ± 1 standard deviation, with the 95% confidence interval for the normal range in brackets.
Data adapted from Lorenz et al. *J Cardiovasc Magn Reson* 1999; 1:71.

thickening and 2D motion because of a complex interaction of contraction, expansion, twisting, and through-plane motion. This can now be approached using CMR tagging, which has been validated against animal studies and which can provide a 3D solution.[28] Tagging CMR has revealed a fairly consistent pattern of normal regional variation in heart wall motion. Normal ventricular contraction is characterized by base to apex shortening, with little apical motion. Free wall contraction exceeds that of the septum, and endocardial thickening exceeds that of the epicardium. Although there is a fairly large regional variation in normal displacement, the regional deformation is more uniform, with the greatest systolic lengthening being approximately radially directed. There is also a normal torsional motion of the ventricle about its long axis, with a wringing action, with the base and with an apical myocardial infarction rotating in opposite directions. When tagging is performed in myocardial infarction in humans, the region of altered contraction often extends beyond the region of the infarct itself. This finding, which is considered important in remodeling, has been shown to respond to angiotensin-converting enzyme inhibition therapy. Studies such as these suggest that tagging CMR may find significant clinical and research application in the future, particularly once acquisition protocols are established and analysis tools are simpler to operate within shorter time frames.

Myocardial Ischemia

Myocardial ischemia can be investigated by CMR through the use of stress with either wall motion or perfusion analysis. The use of dobutamine wall motion is better established with CMR at present, and there are some reasonable clinical studies available. Other stress techniques have also been used in coronary disease. Finally, perfusion CMR is currently still in development, although significant progress has been made, and some small clinical studies have been reported.

Wall Motion Studies with Exercise

Supine dynamic exercise in the magnet is uncomfortable and leads to motion artifact, and therefore the reports of the use of dynamic exercise with CMR are limited to proof of concept studies, and there are none for the diagnosis of coronary artery disease. However, nonferromagnetic exercise devices are now commercially available for fitting to the magnet, and their use with real-time CMR techniques may in due course prove useful for exercise imaging. MR spectroscopy has used prone exercise and handgrip for stress to examine changes in high-energy phosphates, both in normal individuals and those with cardiovascular disease. During myocardial ischemia, a fall in the ratio of phosphocreatine (PCr) to adenosine triphosphate (ATP) has been demonstrated, and this change is abolished by successful revascularization. This early study suggests that metabolic CMR studies may prove useful in the future in understanding ischemia at the metabolic level and possibly contribute to clinical assessment.

Dipyridamole Wall Motion Studies

CMR has been used to detect the induction of regional wall motion abnormalities in coronary artery disease using dipyridamole (Figure 9-7).[29] The sensitivity of this method has been limited, with an inability to detect small areas of ischemia. Because of the disappointing results of dipyridamole CMR, it is not being actively used.

Dobutamine Wall Motion Studies

Dobutamine CMR in doses of up to 20 μg/kg/min seems to be a more sensitive pharmacological method of detecting wall motion abnormalities than dipyridamole.[28] Concordance has been seen in segments affected by perfusion and wall motion abnormalities, and the sensitivity of dobutamine CMR and MIBI SPECT is similar for the detection of disease (approximately 85%). Dobutamine CMR is valuable in patients whose echocardiographic image quality is poor, even with second harmonic imaging, with good results (sensitivity and specificity approximately 83%). The event-free survival rate was also been shown to be excellent in patients with normal dobutamine CMR.[28]

Dobutamine Global Ventricular Function Studies

CMR velocity mapping can also be used to assess global left ventricular function through changes in aortic flow during dobutamine stress, but further work is needed to evaluate the full value of assessing global ventricular function with CMR.

In summary, there are now a number of reports of the value of dobutamine stress CMR in patients with coronary artery disease, and the results are excellent, with good patient tolerance. The duration of the study is similar to echocardiography with the use of breath-hold CMR, and real-time CMR may also assist in improving patient throughput. Comparison with thallium imaging and stress echocardiography shows excellent correlation with the former and significant improvement over the latter. For the future, it may be that a combination of perfusion and wall motion in the same dobutamine CMR study may prove useful, and the possible role of quantification of myocardial contraction with tagging would be a great advance in improving the objectivity of the technique. Consensus statements on the performance of dobutamine CMR have been published.[30]

Use of CMR Imaging to Measure Myocardial Perfusion

Techniques and Validation

Techniques used to assess perfusion by CMR in humans have used extracellular gadolinium contrast agents. These agents shorten T1 relaxation times and increase signal on T1-weighted images. At the current stage of development, the technique relies on first-pass imaging of a gadolinium bolus with analysis of the myocardial signal changes that occur to determine parameters of

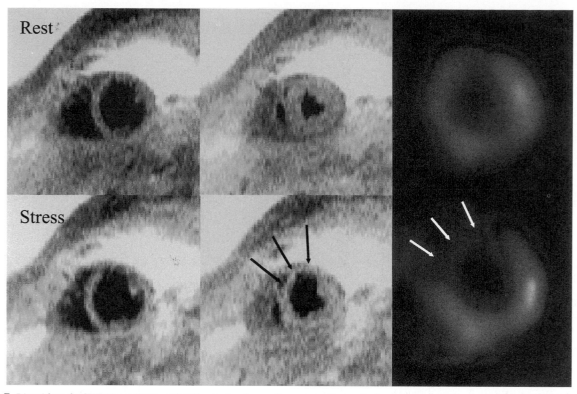

FIGURE 9-7. Dipyridamole CMR in a patient with left anterior descending artery disease. In the top row are short axis images before dipyridamole with postdipyridamole images in the lower row. End-diastole is in the left column, and end-systole is in the middle column. Left ventricular contraction is normal before vasodilatation but reduced in the anteroseptal region after dipyridamole *(black arrows)*. The stress-induced contraction abnormality is closely matched by the defect seen during dipyridamole thallium myocardial perfusion tomography *(white arrows on the color maps in the right column)*, which shows full reversibility. (Reproduced with permission from reference 29.) See also Color Insert.

perfusion. Ultrafast CMR techniques such as FLASH or hybrid echo-planar sequences provide the required temporal resolution to image the first pass through the myocardium with several short-axis–imaging planes per cardiac cycle, with good spatial resolution (2 to 3 mm). Pharmacological stress is used to provoke myocardial hyperemia, as is used with scintigraphic techniques, and has the advantage of limiting movement artifacts that would be created by exercise.

A good correlation has been demonstrated between inverse myocardial mean transit time and myocardial blood flow measured by microspheres. Different contrast enhancement has been shown in an occlusive rat model in perfused, and nonperfused, myocardium, and the technical feasibility of first-pass perfusion MR with gadolinium in humans has been demonstrated. Resting studies of patients with >90% coronary stenosis have found decreased peak signal intensity and a lower slope in distal perfused myocardium, and after revascularization the peak signal intensity returns to normal in most patients. The use of combined perfusion CMR with tagging reveals reduced regional deformation, and motion in myocardial areas with altered perfusion and a good correlation has been found between Doppler CFR and myocardial perfusion reserve in patients with nonsignificant coronary artery disease with multislice perfusion CMR.

Comparison of CMR with Thallium and MIBI SPECT Imaging

Gadolinium-enhanced snapshot MR imaging measuring first-pass signal intensity changes at several time points after bolus injection has generated circumferential profiles that were in close agreement with myocardial perfusion abnormalities detected by planar thallium scintigraphy in patients with coronary disease. A similar method has reported good correlations between CMR perfusion and results from planar or SPECT studies. In addition, Panting et al[31] reported the first clinical study of the use of a spin-echo, echo-planar MR technique at rest, and during adenosine stress, to assess perfusion in 26 patients with coronary disease and an abnormal thallium SPECT scan. For detecting abnormal coronary territories, this MR technique had a sensitivity and specificity compared with coronary angiography of 79% and 83%, which was similar to the results of thallium SPECT (Figure 9-8).

Comparison of CMR with PET and Coronary Angiography

Schwitter et al[32] reported the first comparison of multislice perfusion CMR with PET in 48 patients with coronary disease and 18 controls. A sensitivity and specificity of 87% and 85% vs. coronary angiography was

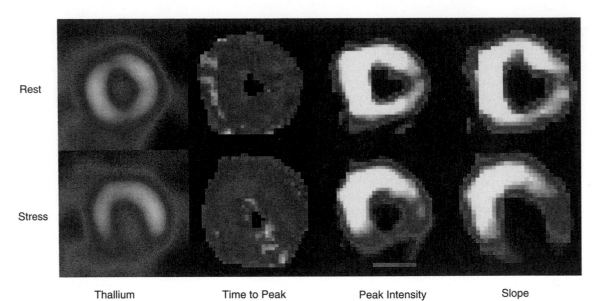

| | Thallium | Time to Peak | Peak Intensity | Slope |

Rest

Stress

FIGURE 9-8. Parametric map analysis for representation of perfusion CMR in a patient with an inferolateral reversible defect, with the corresponding thallium images *(first column)*. Columns 2 through 4 show the time to peak CMR myocardial signal intensity, the peak signal intensity, and the peak slope of the signal intensity vs. Time curves. There is good correlation between the CMR maps and the thallium scan. (Reproduced with permission from reference 31.) See also Color Insert.

found, which increased to 91% and 94% when compared with the PET findings for significant perfusion abnormality.

Two-dimensional breath-hold coronary CMR has problems with relatively low signal/noise, misregistration of images between different breath-holds, a significant requirement for high operator experience, and patients' intolerance of multiple breath holds. However, with this technique for the diagnosis of significant coronary artery stenosis, a sensitivity and specificity of 90% and 92%, respectively, have been described, with better results for the left main stem and left anterior descending arteries and worse results for the right coronary and left circumflex arteries. Three-dimensional and non-breath-hold techniques have been developed so that a volume slab containing many thin slices is acquired by typically using a segmented gradient echo sequence. These sequences have usually been acquired with respiratory gating (navigators) but with the newer ultrafast scanners the 3D slab can be acquired in a single breath hold (Figure 9-9).

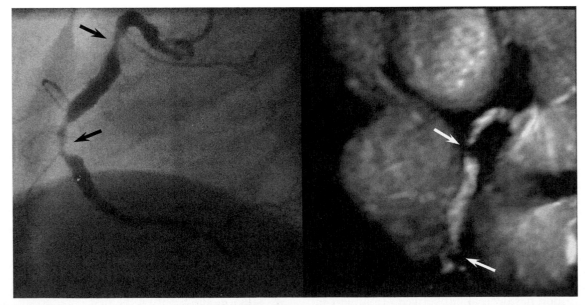

FIGURE 9-9. Comparison of x-ray invasive coronary angiography *(left)* in a patient with two tight stenoses of the right coronary artery *(black arrows)* with coronary CMR performed during a breath-hold showing similar appearances *(white arrows)*. (From van Geuns RJ, Wielopolski PA, de Bruin HG, Rensing BJ, Hulshoff M, van Ooijen PM, et al. MR coronary angiography with breath-hold targeted volumes: preliminary clinical results. *Radiology* 2000; 217[1]:270. Reproduced with permission.)

IMAGING TECHNIQUES USED TO ASSESS PROGNOSIS OF PATIENTS WITH CHRONIC CORONARY ARTERY DISEASE

Appropriate management of known coronary disease includes assessment of the individual risk of future cardiac events, including death and myocardial infarction. High-risk patients (e.g., those with left main disease and/or three-vessel disease with or without ventricular dysfunction) benefit from an aggressive approach with coronary angiography and revascularization. In contrast, most individuals with low annual risk for cardiac events can be managed conservatively.

Use of EBCT to Assess Coronary Artery Calcification

The likelihood of plaque rupture and the development of acute cardiovascular events are related to the total atherosclerotic plaque burden. Because there is a direct relationship between the coronary artery calcium score severity and the extent of atherosclerotic plaque, it would seem intuitive that the calcium score should predict risk for subsequent cardiovascular events among otherwise heterogeneous patient populations with cardiac risk factors.

Several recent trials have studied whether the extent of coronary artery calcification as assessed by EBCT can predict subsequent patient outcome. In an asymptomatic patient population referred for a screening EBCT and then followed for nearly 3 years, both the absolute coronary artery calcium score and the age-adjusted and gender-adjusted relative coronary artery calcium score percentiles predicted subsequent death and nonfatal myocardial infarction. Hard cardiac events occurred in only 0.3% of subjects with a normal EBCT, but this increased to 13% in those with a coronary artery calcium score ≥400.[33] In patients referred for coronary angiography, those with a coronary artery calcium score ≥100 had a 3.2-fold higher relative risk of death or myocardial infarction than those with a lower coronary artery calcium score during 7 years of follow-up.[34] A high coronary artery calcium score ≥1000 may portend a particularly high risk for death or myocardial infarction (i.e., 25%/year).[35]

The very low cardiac event rate in subjects with a coronary artery calcium score <100 is consistent with angiographic studies, indicating a comparably low likelihood of significant coronary artery disease and an extremely low incidence of stress-induced myocardial ischemia (1.5%) in such individuals. The increasing number of cardiac events with an ever-increasing coronary artery calcium score is also consistent with the dramatic increase in the incidence of stress-induced myocardial ischemia, particularly when scores are >400. All these data in asymptomatic patients indicate a potential novel role of EBCT in screening subjects for preclinical coronary artery disease on the basis of the presence and severity of coronary artery calcification.

Use of SPECT Imaging to Assess Prognosis

Combined myocardial perfusion and function results from stress MPI (^{201}Tl or ^{99m}Tc agents) have the ability to distinguish patients at high risk (greater than 3% annual mortality rate) from those at intermediate risk (1% to 3% annual mortality rate) or low risk (less than 1% annual mortality rate).[16,17,21,22,36] A normal ^{201}Tl or ^{99m}Tc-sestamibi scan is generally associated with low risk of future cardiac events. This low event rate approaches that of a normal age-matched population and also of patients with normal coronary angiograms. The same benign prognosis seems to persist even in patients with strongly positive electrocardiograms or angiographically significant disease. Studies demonstrating high-risk features (extensive ischemia of more than 20% of the left ventricle, defects in greater than one coronary vascular supply region, reversible ischemia in multiple segments, transient or persistent left ventricular cavity dilatation, increased ^{201}Tl lung uptake) predict an increase risk of cardiac events (Box 9-2; Figure 9-10).

Perhaps the most important feature of exercise or pharmacological stress perfusion imaging with ^{201}Tl or a ^{99m}Tc-labeled agent is its excellent negative predictive value for predicting low mortality and myocardial infarction rates (<1% per year) in patients with totally normal scans. The excellent prognostic value of ^{99m}Tc-sestamibi has been confirmed in a review of a large series of patients from 14 different prognostic studies.[37] A normal ^{99m}Tc-sestamibi image was associated with an average annual "hard" event rate of 0.6%, and patients with abnormal scans had a 12-fold higher event rate (7.4%).

The value of exercise MPI has been studied extensively in many large studies. The prognostic value of exercise testing with dual-isotope imaging (rest ^{201}Tl/stress ^{99m}Tc-sestamibi SPECT imaging) has been assessed on the basis of gender and race. In a large series of 4136 consecutive patients (2742 men and 1394 women), event rates for both men and women with normal results and increased clinical risk were similar (1.9% vs. 0.8%).[16] An abnormal study result, the presence of reversible perfusion defect, and summed scores reflecting the extent and severity of perfusion defects were associated with increased risk of cardiac death in both genders. However, the total mortality was greater in women with an abnormal study result than men (11% vs. 6%). On the basis of this finding, the investigators

■ ▪ ■

BOX 9-2 PREDICTORS OF STRESS-INDUCED ISCHEMIC EXTENT AND SEVERITY WITH MYOCARDIAL PERFUSION SPECT

- Number and/or location of reversible defections
- Magnitude (severity and extent) of stress defects
- Post stress pulmonary ^{201}Tl uptake*
- Transient ischemic left ventricle cavity dilatation after exercise*
- Delayed redistribution

*Best assessed by obtaining a 5-minute poststress and 4-hour redistribution or rest anterior planar scintigram before the initiation of SPECT imaging.
Adapted from *Prog Cardiovasc Dis* 2001; 43:281.

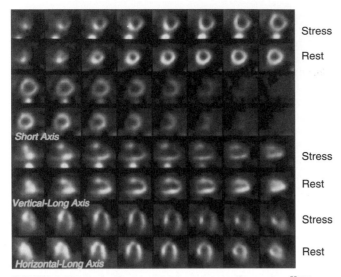

FIGURE 9-10. High-risk scan: Demonstration of exercise ^{99m}Tc-sestamibi myocardial perfusion imaging in multiple views (short-axis, vertical long-axis, horizontal long-axis; stress images on top of each row with test images on the bottom). Stress images demonstrate transient cavity dilation and extensive ischemia involving the anterior, anteroseptal, anterolateral, and anteroapical distribution. Rest images reveal normalization of the cavity size and elimination of the perfusion abnormalities. These findings predict a high risk for future cardiac events for the particular patient. See also Color Insert.

■ ■ ■

TABLE 9-8   RATES OF HARD EVENTS AND CARDIAC DEATH PER YEAR AND RATES OF REFERRAL TO EARLY CATHETERIZATION BY SCAN RESULT*

Summed stress score	Total	Normal (0-3)	Mildly abnormal (4-8)	Moderately abnormal (9-13)	Severely abnormal (>13)¶
Hard events (%/y)	4.9	1.6	3.5	5.7	10.6[†]¶
Cardiac death (%/y)	6.6	0.9	0.9	3.4	7.4[†]¶
Early catheterization (%)	14.1	3.8	9.7	23.1	27.2[†]¶

Hard events = cardiovascular death and myocardial infarction.
*The denominator for the hard event calculation is based on the censored population (n = 1079); the denominator for early catheterization is the entire population (N = 1159).
[†]Significantly different as a function of summed stress score.
Modified from Hachamovitch et al. Incremental prognostic value of adenosine stress myocardial perfusion single-photon emission computed tomography and impact on subsequent management in patients with or suspected of having myocardial ischemia. *Am J Cardiol* 1997; 80:426.

concluded that dual-isotope SPECT MPI is able to risk stratify women more effectively than men. In other studies MPI has provided similar prognostic information, regardless of racial difference.

Pharmacological stress imaging can also be used to assess prognosis in patients with chronic coronary artery disease who are unable to exercise and especially in patients who are scheduled to undergo major vascular surgery.[18,37] In these studies, a normal MPI is associated with a low annual event rate (cardiac death or nonfatal myocardial infarction) of less than 2% for men and women. In multivariable models, an abnormal MPI and/or a reversible defect are the strongest predictors for subsequent occurrence of cardiac death or nonfatal myocardial infarction. A normal MPI is usually associated with low cardiac event rate (<2%) compared with a 7% to 17% event rate for an abnormal study, a reversible perfusion defect, or a fixed defect, depending on the patient population under study. Both Cox proportional hazards and Kaplan-Meier analyses reveal that nuclear tests add incremental value after adjusting for known clinical and historical variables (Table 9-8).

In summary, the prognostic value of exercise and pharmacological tests with ^{201}Tl, ^{99m}Tc-sestamibi, and dual-isotope SPECT MPI in patients with stable coronary artery disease is comparable and provides valuable information. A normal study is generally associated with a low annual event rate of ≤2% for nonfatal myocardial infarction or death. Conversely, abnormal studies, particularly those with a reversible defect, are associated with significantly increased risk, with annual event rates from 7% to 17% for nonfatal myocardial infarction and death. Extent and severity of reversible defects and the presence of left

ventricular cavity dilation may provide additional prognostic information.

Prognostic Value of Stress Echocardiography

The presence or absence of inducible myocardial ischemia has prognostic value in both exercise and pharmacological stress echocardiography (Table 9-9). In general, a negative stress echocardiogram is associated with a low cardiovascular event rate. Specifically, in patients with an exercise electrocardiographic response suggestive of ischemia but no inducible wall motion abnormality detected by stress echo, there is a very low rate of adverse cardiovascular events during follow-up, but a higher rate than that seen in patients with no electrocardiographic evidence of ischemia. In patients with a positive wall motion abnormality provoked by stress echo, future cardiovascular events are more likely. Pooled results of studies involving approximately 6000 patients with chronic coronary artery disease indicate that the risk of future cardiac events can be stratified on the basis of the presence or absence of inducible ischemia on stress echocardiography testing.

ASSESSMENT OF MYOCARDIAL VIABILITY

Left ventricular function is a well-established powerful predictor of outcome after myocardial infarction. The occurrence of left ventricular dysfunction (LVEF <35%) after MI, especially if linked with symptoms of heart failure, is associated with poor survival. In selected patients with severe left ventricular dysfunction, revascularization seems to offer a long-term survival benefit. However, the selection of patients with low ejection fraction who would benefit the most from revascularization is critical because of the high operative mortality risk.

■ ■ ■

TABLE 9-9 PROGNOSTIC VALUE OF STRESS ECHOCARDIOGRAPHY IN VARIOUS PATIENT POPULATIONS

Author	Year	Total Pts	Stress	Follow-up (mos)	Events	% ANNUALIZED EVENT RATE		
						Ischemia	No Ischemia	Normal
Sawada[a]	1990	148	NL TSE	28	D, MI	—	—	0.6
Mazeika[b]	1993	51	DSE	51	D, MI, UA	16	3.8	—
Krivokapich[c]	1993	360	TSE	~12	D, MI	10.8	3.1	—
Afridi[d]	1994	77	DSE	10	D, MI	48	8.9	3
Poldermans[e]	1994	430	DSE	17	D, MI	6.6	3.4	—
Kamaran[f]	1995	210	DSE	8	D, MI	69	1	-
Williams[g]	1996	108	DSE	16	D, MI, Re	32.6	7.3	-
Anthopoulos[h]	1996	120	DSE*	14	D, MI	13.6	0	-
Marcovitz[i]	1996	291	DSE	15	D, MI	12.8	8.2	1.1
Heupler[j]	1997	508w	TSE	41	D, MI, Re	9.2	1.3	—
McCully[k]	1998	1325	NL TSE	23	D, MI	—	-	0.5
Chuah[l]	1998	860	DSE†	24	D, MI	6.9	6.3	1.9
Cortigiani[m]	1998	456w	DSE or DIP	32	D, MI	2.9	0.3	-
Davar[n]	1999	72w	NL DSE	13	D, MI	—	-	0

Prognostic value of inducible ischemia, detected with different forms of stress echocardiography.
*New wall motion abnormality considered "positive" for inducible ischemia.
†Any wall motion abnormality (at rest or with stress) considered "positive."
Adverse event rate = percentage of patients, per year, who had at least one adverse event develop during follow-up, depending on whether inducible ischemia was, or was not, demonstrated by stress echocardiography. The annualized event rate is also tabulated for those series describing patients who had normal resting and normal stress results (NL); CHF, development of severe congestive heart failure; D, death; DIP, dipyridamole stress echocardiography; DSE, dobutamine stress echocardiography; LD-DSE, low-dose dobutamine stress echocardiography; MI, nonfatal myocardial infarction, NL, series describing follow-up only in subjects with normal stress echo test results; Re, revascularization necessary; Stress, stress echocardiography protocol; TSE, treadmill stress echocardiography; Total pts, number of patients studied with stress echocardiography and subsequently followed for the development of adverse events (including death, nonfatal myocardial infarction, revascularization, or unstable angina; in posttransplant patients, development of severe congestive heart failure was also considered an adverse event); UA, unstable angina; w, patients in these series were all women.
[a]Am Heart J 1990; 120:49; [b]Am J Cardiol 1993; 71:33; [c]Am J Cardiol 1993; 71:646; [d]Am Heart J 1994; 127:1510; [e]Am J Med 1994; 97:119; [f]Am J Cardiol 1995; 76:887; [g]J Am Coll Cardiol 1996; 27:132; [h]J Am Coll Cardiol 1996; 28:52; [i]Am J Cardiol 1996; 78:404; [j]J Am Coll Cardiol 1997; 30:414; [k]J Am Coll Cardiol 1998; 31:144; [l]Circulation 1998; 97:1474; [m]J Am Coll Cardiol 1998; 32:1975; [n]Am J Cardiol 1999; 83:100-2,A8.

The assessment of myocardial viability by any imaging technique is extremely helpful in distinguishing hibernating from irreversibly injured myocardium in patients with ischemic cardiomyopathy who exhibit marked regional and/or global left ventricular dysfunction.[38] Thus, the accurate noninvasive determination of myocardial viability is critically important for clinical decision making with respect to revascularization. Although the assumption is that an improvement in left ventricular systolic function after revascularization may improve symptoms and prolong survival, this does not apply to all patients with low ejection fraction. It is also possible that additional benefits can be obtained from an improvement in blood flow to areas of stress-induced ischemia downstream from a severe coronary stenosis that are neither stunned nor hibernating. It is well documented that a revascularization strategy improves survival in patients with severe left ventricular dysfunction and anginal symptoms compared with medical therapy alone. However, this benefit has not been consistently associated with an improvement in resting left ventricular ejection fraction after revascularization. On the other hand, in patients with severe left ventricular dysfunction and predominant heart failure symptoms, revascularization of large areas of viable myocardium may lead to improved global left ventricular function, symptoms, and survival. In the same group of patients but with nonviable cardiac tissue, there is no difference in cardiac events after a medical treatment or revascularization strategy, and perioperative events at the time of revascularization are higher than in patients with viable myocardium. A meta-analysis of myocardial viability testing and the impact of revascularization in a total of 3088 patients (2228 men) with a mean left ventricular ejection fraction of 32% who were followed for 2 years has been reported.[39] In patients with myocardial viability, coronary revascularization was associated with a major reduction in annual mortality compared with medical treatment (16% vs. 3.2%). Patients without demonstrated myocardial viability had an intermediate mortality with revascularization vs. medical therapy (8% vs. 6%, P = NS) (Figure 9-11). Among patients with viable myocardium, there was a direct relationship between the severity of left ventricular dysfunction and the magnitude of benefit with revascularization. Therefore, viability assessment is less important in patients with low ejection fraction and severe angina with or without heart failure symptoms, because they seem to benefit from revascularization regardless of viability information. However, viability information is extremely helpful in most patients with left ventricular dysfunction, minimal or no anginal symptoms, and heart failure. Finally, in patients with recent myocardial infarction and jeopardized myocardium, in the infarct-related artery territory, the presence of residual viable myocardium that is not revascularized is an independent risk factor for future cardiac events.

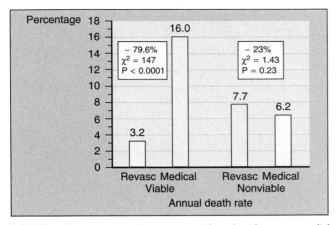

FIGURE 9-11. Death rates for patients with and without myocardial viability treated by revascularization or medical therapy. There is a 79.6% reduction in mortality for patients with viability treated by revascularization (16% vs. 3.2%, $\chi^2 = 147$, $P < 0.0001$). In patients without myocardial viability, there was no significant difference in mortality between the two strategies (7.7% vs. 6.2%, $\chi^2 = 1.43$, $P = 0.23$). (Reprinted and modified with permission from Allman KC, Shaw LJ, Hachamovitch R, Udelson JE. Myocardial viability testing and impact of revascularization on prognosis in patients with coronary artery disease and left ventricular dysfunction: a meta-analysis. *J Am Coll Cardiol* 2002; 39[7]:115.)

PET

PET imaging is considered by many to be the "gold standard" for noninvasive detection of viability with nuclear cardiology techniques.[24,32,40,41] Myocardial viability has been more extensively evaluated with the myocardial perfusion-FDG metabolism PET method than other protocols. With this protocol, regional myocardial perfusion is first evaluated with ^{13}N ammonia, ^{82}Rb, or ^{15}O water. Subsequently, FDG is used to assess regional myocardial glucose use. FDG is a glucose analog that crosses the capillary and sarcolemmal membrane at a rate proportionate to that of glucose. After myocardial uptake, FDG is phosphorylated to FDG-6-phosphate and is then trapped in the myocardium, because, unlike phosphorylated glucose, it is a poor substrate for glycogen synthesis, the fructose phosphate shunt, and glycolysis. Regional myocardial uptake of FDG, therefore, reflects relative distribution of regional rates of exogenous glucose use. In the fasting state, fatty acids are the preferred myocardial substrate for ATP production, and FDG is taken up minimally by the myocardium. In contrast, ischemic myocardial regions show substrate use shifts from fatty acid oxidation to glucose use. Hibernating myocardium, therefore, would demonstrate increased FDG uptake in the fasting state, unlike the surrounding normal myocardium. In the postprandial state, the normal myocardium shifts from fatty acid to glucose as the primary substrate for ATP production; thus hibernating and normal myocardium both would demonstrate FDG uptake. Therefore, preserved or even enhanced FDG uptake in dysfunctional myocardial regions represents presence of myocardial viability. Most clinical PET FDG studies are performed in the "postprandial" state to minimize heterogeneity in myocardial FDG uptake and to optimize image quality.

With the PET perfusion-metabolism protocol, when FDG is injected in the postprandial state, three different patterns of myocardial viability may be observed (Figure 9-12). Regional myocardial perfusion and FDG uptake may be concordantly reduced or absent, the so-called perfusion metabolism "match" pattern. On the basis of the severity of perfusion and FDG deficit, the "match" pattern may be categorized as transmural match (absent or markedly reduced perfusion and FDG uptake) or nontransmural match (mildly to moderately reduced perfusion and FDG uptake). These two terms were originally used to indicate that transmural match implies presence of transmural myocardial infarction, whereas nontransmural match suggests the presence of a mixture of viable and nonviable tissue in a given myocardial region and, thus, nontransmural myocardial necrosis. When regional myocardial FDG uptake is disproportionately enhanced compared with regional MBF, the pattern is termed perfusion-metabolism "mismatch." This PET pattern is thought to represent hibernating myocardium. Normal blood flow and normal, enhanced, or reduced glucose use may manifest regional dysfunction because of myocardial stunning.

Myocardial distribution of FDG may be evaluated by either coincidence imaging devices or by standard SPECT equipment and 511-keV collimators. To compare cardiac FDG uptake with perfusion, either ^{201}Tl or ^{99m}Tc-labeled tracers are used (Figure 9-13). The ^{99m}Tc-labeled tracers allow dual-isotope imaging, thereby avoiding misalignment between the FDG and the perfusion study. A number of studies have compared FDG PET with FDG

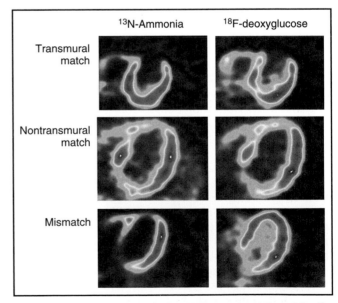

FIGURE 9-12. Regional myocardial perfusion (as evaluated by ^{13}N-ammonia) compared with ^{18}F-deoxyglucose (FDG) uptake in types of clinical situations. There may be concordant uptake of both tracers (the so-called perfusion metabolism "match" pattern), which may be categorized as transmural match (absent or markedly reduced perfusion and FDG uptake) or nontransmural match (mildly to moderately reduced perfusion and FDG uptake). The third pattern is "mismatch," which is typical for hibernating myocardium (reduced perfusion and uniform glucose uptake). See also Color Insert.

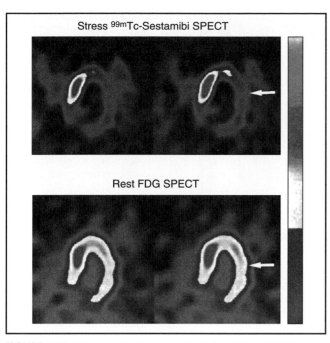

Stress 99mTc-Sestamibi SPECT

Rest FDG SPECT

FIGURE 9-13. Patient study demonstrating "mismatch" of FDG (glucose metabolism) and sestamibi (perfusion) performed on a SPECT imaging camera (not a dedicated PET camera). There is decreased perfusion in the posterior lateral wall, but glucose uptake is preserved (viable myocardium). See also Color Insert.

SPECT, showing a good agreement between PET and SPECT in the assessment of viable myocardium, ranging from 76% to 100%. The main shortcoming of these comparative studies is the lack of outcome data after revascularization.

Prediction of Recovery of Regional Left Ventricular Dysfunction After Revascularization

The mean positive predictive value is 71%, and the negative predictive value is 86% when FDG PET is used to detect improvement in regional contractile function after revascularization (Table 9-10). The criteria for viability were a mismatch pattern in 15 studies, normal perfusion in 5 studies, and a cutoff level of regional myocardial glucose use/percentage FDG uptake in 7 studies. Combined perfusion-FDG imaging seems to be superior to FDG imaging alone in predicting improvement in myocardial function after revascularization.

Prediction of Improvement in Left Ventricular Ejection Fraction (LVEF) After Revascularization

Literature reports on the value of PET for predicting improvement in LVEF are predominantly presented as comparison between prerevascularization and postrevascularization LVEFs in patients with and those without significant perfusion-FDG metabolism mismatch (i.e., PET evidence of myocardial viability) (Table 9-11). Usually the average LVEF (%) significantly increases from prerevascularization to postrevascularization in patients who have the PET pattern of myocardial viability. In the absence of the PET pattern

■ ▪ ■

TABLE 9-10   PET FOR PREDICTION OF RECOVERY OF REGIONAL LV DYSFUNCTION AFTER REVASCULARIZATION

Author/year	No. of patients	PPV (segments)	NPV (segments)
Tillisch, 1986[a]	17	85% (35/41)	92% (24/26)
Tamaki, 1989[b]	22	78% (18/23)	78% (18/23)
Tamaki, 1989[c]	11	80% (40/50)	38% (6/16)
Marwick, 1992[d]	16	68% (25/37)	79% (38/48)
Lucignani, 1992[e]	14	95% (37/39)	80% (12/15)
Carrel, 1992[f]	23	84% (16/19)	75% (3/4)
Gropler, 1993[g]	34	52% (38/73)	81% (35/43)
Paolini, 1994[h]	9	88% (23/26)	79% (11/14)
Vom Dahl, 1994[i]	37	48%-86% (NA)	84%-100% (NA)
Knuuti, 1994[j]	48	72% (23/32)	96% (50/52)
Tamaki, 1995[k]	43	76% (45/59)	92% (65/71)
Baer, 1996[l]	42	92% (24/26)	88% (14/16)
Gerber, 1996[m]	39	78% (18/23)	63% (10/16)
Vom Dahl, 1996[n]	52	68% (19/28)	93% (25/27)
Maes, 1997[o]	23	92% (10/11)	83% (10/12)
Wolpers, 1997[p]	30	90% (NA)	85% (NA)
Fath-Ordoubadi, 1998[q]	47	66% (190/286)	96% (48/50)
Pagano, 1998[r]	30	66% (190/286)	96% (48/50)
Kitsiou, 1999[s]	26	78% (NA)	82% (NA)
Weighted mean	563	71% (751/1059)	86% (417/483)

PPV, Positive predictive value; NPV, negative predictive value.
[a]N Engl J Med 1986; 314:884; [b]Am J Cardiol 1989; 64:860; [c]Am J Cardiol 1989; 64:86; [d]Circulation 1992; 85:1347; [e]Eur J Nucl Med 1992; 19:87; [f]Eur J Cardiothorac Surg 1992; 6:479; [g]J Am Coll Cardiol 1993; 22:1587; [h]Eur J Cardiothorac Surg 1994; 8:139; [i]Circulation 1994; 90:2356; [j]Am Heart J 1994; 127:785; [k]Circulation 1995; 91:1697; [l]J Am Coll Cardiol 1996; 28:60; [m]Circulation 1996; 94:651; [n]J Am Coll Cardiol 1996; 28:948; [o]J Am Coll Cardiol 1997; 29:62; [p]Circulation 1997; 95:1417; [q]Am J Cardiol 1998; 82:26; [r]Heart 1998; 79:281; [s]J Am Coll Cardiol 1999; 33:678.

of viability, LVEF remains unchanged or decreased after revascularization.

Prediction of Improvement in Heart Failure Symptoms After Revascularization

Because most patients with poor left ventricular function have heart failure symptoms, an important goal in assessing myocardial viability is to predict improvement

■ ▪ ■

TABLE 9-11   PET FOR PREDICTION OF IMPROVEMENTS IN LEFT VENTRICULAR EJECTION FRACTION (LVEF) AFTER REVASCULARIZATION

Author/year	No. of patients	Patients with mismatch LVEF (%)		Patients without mismatch LVEF (%)	
		Pre	Post	Pre	Post
Tillisch, 1986[a]	17	30 ± 11	45 ± 14	30 ± 11	31 ± 12
Lucignani, 1992[b]	14	38 ± 5	48 ± 4	—	—
Paolini, 1994[c]	17	28 ± 5	43 ± 8	—	—
Depre, 1995[d]	23	43 ± 18	52 ± 15	35 ± 9	24 ± 8

Pre and Post, Revascularization process.
[a]N Engl J Med 1986; 314:884; [b]Eur J Nucl Med 1992; 19:874; [c]Eur J Cardiothorac Surg 1994; 8:139; [d]Am J Physiol 1995; 268:H1265.

in heart failure symptoms after myocardial revascularization. This question has been addressed in three publications by use of myocardial perfusion-FDG metabolism PET imaging. Improvement in heart failure, by at least one class, seems to be related to the PET pattern (presence or absence of mismatch) and type of treatment (revascularization or medical therapy). More patients with the PET mismatch pattern who undergo revascularization have improvement in heart failure class than the other subgroups. Furthermore, the total extent of a PET mismatch before surgery seems to correlate linearly and significantly with a percent improvement in functional state after revascularization. Patients with large mismatches achieve a significantly higher functional state compared with those patients with minimal or no PET mismatch.

Thus, the PET pattern of myocardial viability predicts recovery of regional and global left ventricular dysfunction after myocardial revascularization and also identifies a subgroup of patients with poor left ventricular function and heart failure who are most likely to show relief of heart failure symptoms as a result of revascularization. Patients with large perfusion metabolism mismatches (i.e., greatest magnitude of ischemic viable myocardium by PET) exhibit the greatest clinical benefit after revascularization.

Prediction of Improved Survival After Revascularization

A major goal of noninvasive diagnostic procedures in the assessment of coronary artery disease is to evaluate prognosis and to assess the potential of survival benefit from a treatment plan. Because survival of patients with left ventricular dysfunction relates to the resting LVEF, it may be implied that perfusion-FDG metabolism PET imaging by predicting improvement in LVEF can also predict survival after myocardial revascularization. This hypothesis has been addressed in a few studies (Figure 9-14). The results indicate that in the subgroup of patients treated medically with viable myocardium as assessed by PET FDG imaging, the event rate (death or myocardial infarction) was approximately 50%. Importantly, in the patients with viable myocardium who underwent revascularization, the event rate was significantly lower at 13%. In patients without PET FDG evidence of myocardial viability, event rates were similar with medical therapy, and revascularization had similar event rates (15% vs. 13%, respectively). These data suggest that in patients with ischemic cardiomyopathy, revascularization should be recommended only in those with PET FDG evidence of myocardial viability.

Influence of PET FDG Metabolism Evaluation of Myocardial Viability on Clinical Decision Making and Patient Management

Cardiac transplantation has been the ultimate therapy for end-stage heart failure; however, because of the limited number of available donor hearts, the waiting period for a heart transplant by eligible recipients has been pro-

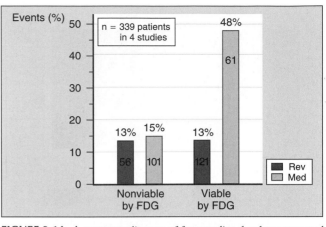

FIGURE 9-14. A summary diagram of four studies that have reported on cardiac events in patients after PET evaluations of myocardial viability. Patients are divided into two main groups (nonviable by FDG and viable by FDG) and then subdivided into those patients undergoing subsequent revascularization (Rev) or medical (Med) therapy. Events are highest in those patients who have viable myocardium and only get medical therapy.

longed and ranges from 8 months to 2 years. By detecting the presence of a sufficient amount of viable (hibernating) myocardium, potential candidates for myocardial revascularization may be identified. Such an approach not only lowers the number of patients who are waiting for a transplant but also reduces the overall cost of patient care by offering CABG to patients who would otherwise undergo more costly cardiac transplantation. Candidates for cardiac transplantation with ischemic cardiomyopathy may undergo PET perfusion-FDG metabolism imaging for assessment of the presence and extent of myocardial viability. If these patients have evidence of mismatch in at least two regions of the myocardium and suitable coronary targets for revascularization, consideration should be given to treatment with CABG, which is a more cost-effective therapy than cardiac transplantation with similar perioperative and long-term survival.

Use of SPECT Imaging to Assess Myocardial Viability

A number of radionuclide techniques can be used to assess myocardial viability in patients with ischemic heart disease.[15,39] Thallium-201 SPECT MPI is the most widely used and validated modality and continues to be the cornerstone of single photon radionuclide assessment of tissue viability. A delayed uptake of ^{201}Tl on rest-redistribution imaging is related to the presence of viable cells with intact cellular membrane. Several different protocols have been used to assess myocardial viability with ^{201}Tl SPECT MPI: rest-redistribution (either 4 or 24 hours), stress-redistribution, and the addition of ^{201}Tl re-injection techniques. Criteria to identify viability with ^{201}Tl have traditionally included the demonstration of redistribution and the uptake of the tracer >50% of normal uptake in an adjacent region on 4-hour redistribution imaging. However, this perfusion criteria cutoff to distinguish between viable and nonviable myocardium is actually more of a continuum. Several studies have shown an almost linear relationship between regional thallium activity and recovery of myocardium after revascularization. Myocardial segments with a low thallium uptake (<40%) are unlikely to improve after revascularization, and most myocardial segments with uptake greater than 80% will improve functionally after revascularization (Figure 9-15). The diagnostic accuracy of myocardial viability testing by use of ^{201}Tl rest-redistribution, ^{201}Tl stress-redistribution-reinjection, ^{99m}Tc-sestamibi MPI, ^{18}F-FDG PET, and low-dose dobutamine echocardiography in a pooled analysis suggests that the average sensitivity, specificity, and accuracy were 87%, 54%, and 70%, respectively, for ^{201}Tl techniques, but the specificity for both ^{201}Tl protocols was significantly lower than the other techniques. Although all techniques may accurately identify segments with improved contractile function after recovery, ^{201}Tl protocols may overestimate functional recovery. Low-dose dobutamine echocardiography appears to have a higher specificity and the highest predictive accuracy. However, because the differences in functional recovery generally involve small regions of myocardium, there is little or even no impact on late survival. This is supported by another prospective, randomized trial in which patients with ischemic cardiomyopathy were randomly assigned to clinical decisions for revascularization on the basis of ^{13}N-ammonia/^{18}F-FDG PET or ^{99m}Tc-sestamibi results.[24] There was no difference in patient management or cardiac event-free survival with either of the two techniques.

Although ^{99m}Tc-labeled agents (sestamibi, tetrofosmin) do not show significant redistribution over time, several studies have shown comparable accuracy for viability detection between these agents and [201]Tl. Analyses of the use of ^{99m}Tc agents to assess myocardial viability from multiple studies in patients with left ventricular dysfunction indicate an average sensitivity of 80%, a specificity of 60%, and diagnostic accuracy of 70%. The administration of nitrates (either sublingually or intravenously) before a resting injection of ^{201}Tl or ^{99m}Tc improves the sensitivity for the detection of viable myocardium.

Use of Echocardiography to Assess Myocardial Viability

A common clinical question is to decide whether dysfunctional myocardium is irreversibly damaged or "hibernating" (i.e., myocardium with a chronic reduction in perfusion sufficient to impair normal contractile function but preserve viability).[38] In patients with multivessel coronary artery disease and depressed left ventricular function, improvement in regional left ventricular function during dobutamine stress echocardiography indicates contractile reserve and is predictive of improved ventricular function after revascularization (Figure 9-16, A and B). The lack of contractile reserve during low-dose dobutamine infusion denotes a low likelihood of improvement after bypass surgery, and the presence or absence of contractile reserve by low-dose dobutamine stress echocardiography has positive and negative predictive values of approximately 80% (Tables 9-12 and 9-13).

In patients with heart failure caused by ischemic left ventricular dysfunction, evaluation of myocardial viability by dobutamine stress echocardiography can help determine the potential benefit of revascularization. The demonstration of significant regions of hibernating myocardium, which would suggest a high likelihood of improved function after successful revascularization, can help in deciding whether patients need coronary revascularization rather than heart transplantation.

COMPARISON BETWEEN DOBUTAMINE STRESS ECHOCARDIOGRAPHY AND FDG SPECT

Low-dose dobutamine echocardiography demonstrates contractile reserve in approximately 70% of viable segments detected by FDG SPECT (i.e., there is underestimation of viability by dobutamine echocardiography compared with FDG SPECT). In contrast, more than 90% of segments classified as nonviable by FDG SPECT have absence of contractile reserve during dobutamine echocardiography. Segments with contractile reserve and metabolic activity are likely to recover function after revascularization, but the functional fate after revascularization of the segments with preserved metabolic activity without contractile reserve has not been studied extensively. PET allows a quantitative assessment of MBF and metabolism and thus a more direct investigation of the mechanisms underlying ischemic left ventricular dysfunction than stress echocardiography.[26,39] Both techniques can identify viable myocardium and its potential recovery after revascularization with similar accuracy. The greater availability and the lower cost of dobutamine echocardiography may favor the use of this method in

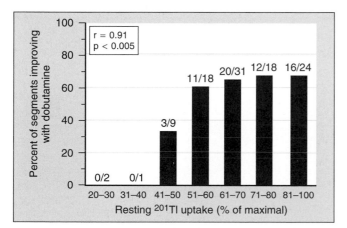

FIGURE 9-15. Demonstration of the linear relationship between the percentage of peak thallium activity on rest-redistribution imaging and the likelihood of segmental improvement after revascularization. Although various cutoff values have been proposed as thresholds, for viability, this figure indicates the continuous nature of this relation. (Reprinted with permission from Dilsizian V, Rocco TP, Freedman NM, Leon MB, Bonow RO. Enhanced detection of ischemic but viable myocardium by the reinjection of thallium after stress-redistribution imaging. *N Engl J Med* 1990; 323[3]:141.)

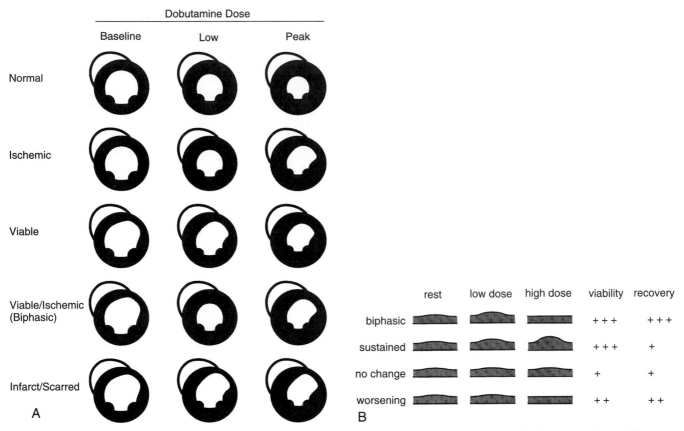

FIGURE 9-16. A, A short-axis view of the left ventricle at end-systole demonstrating various responses to a graded dobutamine infusion. The upper panel demonstrates a normal response. Subsequent panels show various abnormalities involving the anterolateral wall with a normal response in other ventricular segments. (From Orsinelli D, Daniels C. Pharmacologic stress echocardiography. *Cardiol Clin* 1999; 17:461. Reproduced with permission.) **B,** The different responses of dysfunctional myocardial segments to dobutamine at low dose and high dose and their relation to viability and recovery of contractile function after revascularization. (From Nagueh SF, Zoghbi WA. Stress echocardiography for the assessment of myocardial ischemia and viability. *Curr Prob Cardiol* 1996; 21:497. Reproduced with permission.)

■ ■ ■

TABLE 9-12   MYOCARDIAL VIABILITY: DETECTION OF STUNNED MYOCARDIUM BY DSE EARLY AFTER ACUTE MYOCARDIAL INFARCTION

Author	Year	Days after MI	Stress	N	Criteria	Sens (%)	Spec (%)	PPV (%)	NPV (%)	Acc (%)
Pierard[a]	1990	7 d	LD-DSE	17	impWM*	100	70	70	100	82
Barilla[b]	1991	4 d	LD-DSE	21	impWM*	95	—	—	—	95
Smart[c]	1993	2-7 d	LD-DSE	51	impWM*	86	90	86	90	88
Previtali[d]	1993	8 d	LD-DSE	42	impWM[†]	79	68	50	89	71
Watada[e]	1994	3 d	LD-DSE	21	impWM[†]	83	86	89	80	84
Poli[f]	1996	<10 d	LD-DSE	51	impWM[†]	72	68	50	85	69
Bolognese[g]	1996	3 d	LD-DSE	30	impWM[†]	89	91	86	93	90
Minardi[h]	1997	3-5 d	LD-DSE	50	impWM[†]	86	100	100	94	96
Smart[i]	1997	2-7 d	LD-DSE	115	impWM[†]	86	83	80	88	84

Acc, Overall accuracy; Criteria, findings on DSE considered as a "positive" indicator of viability; impWM, improved segmental wall motion seen on follow-up echocardiogram; d, days; LD-DSE, low-dose dobutamine stress echocardiography; MI, myocardial infarction; NPV, negative predictive value (likelihood of lack of subsequent improvement in patients without viability); PV, positive predictive value (likelihood of subsequent improvement in patients with evidence of viability; Sens, sensitivity for detecting viable myocardium; Spec, specificity for detecting viable myocardium; Stress, DSE protocol used for pharmacological stress.
Evaluation of myocardial viability with dobutamine stress echocardiography (DSE) early after acute myocardial infarction to detect stunned myocardium. The presence or absence of viability was established by follow-up resting transthoracic echocardiography.
N, Patients in this study were treated at admission with thrombolytic therapy.
*Wall motion analyzed by patient.
[†]Wall motion analyzed by segment.
[a]*J Am Coll Cardiol* 1990; 15:1021; [b]*Am Heart J* 1991; 122:1522; [c]*Circulation* 1993; 88:405; [d]*Am J Cardiol* 1993; 72:124G; [e]*J Am Coll Cardiol* 1994; 24:624; [f]*Heart* 1996; 75:240; [g]*J Am Coll Cardiol* 1996; 28:1677; [h]*Am J Cardiol* 1997; 80:847; [i]*Circulation* 1997; 95:1394.

■ ■ ■

TABLE 9-13 MYOCARDIAL VIABILITY: DETECTION OF HIBERNATING MYOCARDIUM BY DSE IN PATIENTS WITH CHRONIC CAD AND LV DYSFUNCTION

Author	Year	Stress	N	Criteria	Sens (%)	Spec (%)	PPV (%)	NPV (%)	Acc (%)
Marzullo[a]	1993	LD-DSE	14	Improve WM*	82	92	95	73	85
Cigarroa[b]	1993	LD-DSE	25	Improve WM†	82	86	82	86	84
Alfieri[c]	1993	LD-DSE	14	Improve WM*	91	78	92	76	88
LaCanna[d]	1994	LD-DSE	33	Improve WM*	87	82	90	77	85
Charney[e]	1994	DSE	17	Improve WM*	71	93	92	74	81
Afridi[f]	1995	DSE	20	Improve WM†	80	90	89	82	85
Senior[g]	1995	LD-DSE	22	Improve WM*	87	82	92	73	86
Haque[h]	1995′	LD-DSE	26	Improve WM*	94	80	94	80	91
Arnese[i]	1995	LD-DSE	38	Improve WM*	74	96	85	93	91
DeFilippi[j]	1995		23	Improve WM*	97	75	87	93	89
Iliceto[k]	1996	LD-DSE	16	Improve WM*	71	88	73	87	83
Varga[l]	1996	LD-DSE	19	Improve WM*	74	94	93	78	84
Baer[m]	1996	LD-DSE	42	Improve WM†•	92	88	92	88	90
Vanoverschelde[n]	1996	LD-DSE	73	Improve WM†	88	77	84	82	84
Gerber[o]	1996	LD-DSE	39	Improve WM*	71	87	89	65	77
Bax[p]	1996	LD-DSE	17	Improve WM*	85	63	49	91	70
Perrone-Filardi[q]	1996	LD-DSE	18	Improve WM*	79	83	92	65	81
Qureshi[r]	1997	LD-DSE	34	Improve WM*	86	68	51	92	73
Qureshi[r]	1997	DSE	34	Biphasic resp*	74	89	72	89	85
Nagueh[s]	1997	LD-DSE	18	Improve WM*	91	66	61	93	75
Nagueh[s]	1997	DSE	18	Biphasic resp*	68	83	70	82	77
Furukawa[t]	1997	LD-DSE	53	Improve WM*	79	72	76	75	76
Cornel[u]	1997	LD-DSE	30	Improve WM	89	82	74	93	85

Evaluation of myocardial viability with dobutamine stress echocardiography (DSE) in patients with chronic coronary artery disease (CAD) and impaired systolic left ventricular (LV) function to detect hibernating myocardium. In these patients, percutaneous or surgical revascularization was carried out after DSE testing. Those patients demonstrating improved wall motion on follow-up resting transthoracic echocardiography were considered to have had impaired LV function caused by hibernating myocardium, whereas those demonstrating no improvement despite revascularization were considered to have had impaired LV function caused by necrotic myocardium.

Acc, Overall accuracy; biphasic resp, biphasic response, defined as improvement in wall motion during low-dose dobutamine stress followed by worsening at high doses; Criteria, findings on DSE considered a "positive" indicator of viability; DSE, dobutamine stress echocardiography (dobutamine infused at both low and high doses); improvWM, improved wall motion during dobutamine stress in a previously asynergic segment; LD-DSE, low-dose dobutamine stress echocardiography; NPV, negative predictive value (likelihood that absence of viability by DSE is indicative of lack of functional recovery after revascularization); PPV, positive predictive value (likelihood that presence of viability by DSE is indicative of subsequent functional recovery after revascularization); Sens, sensitivity; Spec, specificity; Stress, DSE protocol used for pharmacological stress; N, number of patients with chronic CAD and LV dysfunction in whom DSE studies were analyzed.
*Wall motion analyzed by segment.
†Wall motion analyzed by patient.

[a]Am J Cardiol 1993; 71:166; [b]Circulation 1993; 88:430; [c]Eur J Cardiothorac Surg 1993; 7:325; [d]J Am Coll Cardiol 1994; 23:617; [e]Am Heart J 1994; 128:864; [f]Circulation 1995; 91:663; [g]Br Heart J 1995; 74:358; [h]Am Heart J 1995; 130:553; [i]Circulation 1995; 91:2748; [j]Circulation 1995; 92:2863; [k]Am J Cardiol 1996; 77:441; [l]Eur Heart J 1996; 17:629; [m]J Am Coll Cardiol 1996; 28:60; [n]J Am Coll Cardiol 1996; 28:432; [o]Circulation 1996; 94:651; [p]J Am Coll Cardiol 1996; 28:558; [q]Circulation 1996; 94:2712; [r]Circulation 1997; 95:626; [s]J Am Coll Cardiol 1997; 29:985; [t]Eur Heart J 1997; 18:798; [u]Eur Heart J 1997; 18:941.

most clinical settings. Finally, myocardial contrast echocardiography, which is a developing technique, has been proposed to identify viable myocardium in patients with both acute and chronic ischemic left ventricular dysfunction.[42] The availability of contrast agents that can be injected into a peripheral vein to measure myocardial perfusion seems to be an attractive alternative to nuclear studies.

Use of CMR Imaging to Assess Myocardial Viability

Scar Formation and Left Ventricular Wall Thickness

After transmural myocardial infarction, severe wall thinning may be present within several months of the acute event. In recent transmural infarcts, thinning is less marked, because local infarct remodeling is incomplete. Nontransmural infarcts may develop some wall thinning in proportion to the degree of myocardial damage. Therefore, the finding of preserved diastolic myocardial wall thickness in the territory of a known chronic infarct is likely to represent nontransmural infarction with a substantial overlying rim of viable myocardium. CMR is well suited for defining regional wall thickness because of its resolution and ability to image in any plane without limitation. Using a cutoff of 5.5 mm for left ventricular wall thickness, which is similar to that defined in pathological studies of transmural MI, it has been shown that akinetic regions of myocardium that exhibit end-diastolic thinning have significantly reduced FDG uptake. In most patients, the viability assessments based on FDG-PET and CMR are identical.

Contractile Reserve of Viable Myocardium

The predictive value of preserved end-diastolic wall thickness in determining recovery of myocardial function after revascularization is low. However, if contractile reserve can be demonstrated in dyssynergic segments, recovery of function is common after revascularization, and CMR is capable of providing such images.

Low-dose dobutamine CMR has been used to determine viability compared with FDG-PET and has shown a sensitivity of approximately 80% with a specificity of 95%.[29] Dobutamine CMR has also been used to predict postrevascularization functional recovery (sensitivity and specificity approximately 90%), and the use of FDG PET for comparison seems more sensitive than transesophageal echocardiography in detecting viable myocardium (81% vs. 77%) with similar sensitivity.

Late Gadolinium Hyperenhancement in Myocardial Infarction

Gadolinium contrast agents are used in CMR to decrease T1, which leads to an increased signal with appropriate imaging sequences.[32] Commercially available gadolinium agents distribute in the extracellular space, which is limited in the heart, and therefore there is rather little myocardial enhancement. During acute myocardial infarction, myocyte rupture occurs, which expands the extracellular space and increases effective voxel concentration of gadolinium. In addition, infarct tissue kinetics for the passage of gadolinium are slow compared with normal myocardium. Both of these effects lead to significant signal enhancement within the infarct.[43] The recent implementation of inversion recovery sequences, which null signal from normal myocardium, has allowed dramatic increases in contrast between infarcted and normal myocardium. The optimal time for imaging infarction after injection of a gadolinium bolus is when blood pool activity is falling, and this occurs about 10 minutes after injection. Therefore, this technique is referred to as "late enhancement." The technique has now been extensively validated in animal experiments, with the area of late gadolinium contrast enhancement correlating closely with areas of infarction, and, for the first time in vivo, high-quality imaging of the transmural distribution of scar is possible (Figure 9-17). Late enhancement of infarction also occurs in chronic infarcts because of a continuing increase in partition coefficient for gadolinium and delayed contrast agent kinetics. The technique has obvious implications for the assessment of viability, and a significant relationship exists between the transmural extent of gadolinium hyperenhancement within a segment and its potential for postrevascularization functional recovery in both animals and humans. With transmural enhancement of 25% or less, recovery is usual, but with enhancement of greater than 50%, there is little likelihood for recovery. When borderline (25% to 50%) hyperenhancement is demonstrated, recovery of myocardial function with revascularization is unpredictable.

Clinical Applications for Quantitation of Absolute MBF and Flow Reserve

Quantitative PET has been used to study MBF in response to interventions and in a variety of cardiac diseases such as syndrome X, hypertrophy cardiomyopathy, and cardiac transplantation vasculopathy. In these conditions, MBF is affected fairly uniformly (i.e., no significant regional differences in MBF are detectable). Therefore, absolute quantitation of MBF and flow reserve rather than relative quantitation of MBF are helpful in evaluating these conditions.

Syndrome X

Patients with syndrome X typically exhibit subjective (chest pain) or objective (ST-segment depression) evidence of myocardial ischemia despite absence of angiographically detectable coronary artery disease. In syndrome X patients, compared with normal volunteers, no significant differences in resting and hyperemic MBF or CFR are noted. However, some syndrome X patients have a reduced flow reserve that may be a result of significantly higher resting blood flow and consequently lower relative hyperemic MBF. Others have demonstrated a more heterogeneous distribution of blood flow at rest and during pharmacological hyperemia in syndrome X patients. Overall, quantitative flow measurements with PET have not yet suggested a uniform coronary flow mechanism in patients with syndrome X.

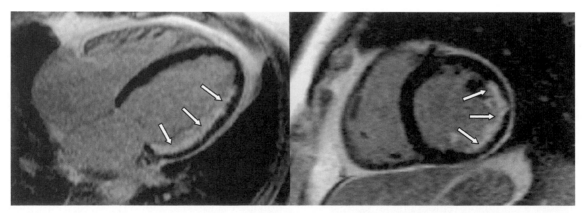

FIGURE 9-17. CMR using late gadolinium enhancement in a patient with an occluded left circumflex artery and lateral wall infarction *(arrows)*. *Left,* horizontal long axis; *right,* short axis. The infarction is nontransmural except for one small area seen on the short axis. Myocardial infarctions caused by ischemia invariably involve the subendocardium, but the transmural extent depends on the time to reperfusion and the presence of any collaterals.

Use of CMR Imaging to Evaluate Transmural Perfusion

The high spatial resolution of perfusion CMR facilitates the study of in vivo transmural variations in myocardial perfusion. Areas of myocardium perfused by a stenotic coronary artery have decreased subendocardial enhancement and lower enhancement in subendocardium compared with subepicardium.

Evaluation of Coronary Flaw Reserve (CFR)

In addition to homeostatic functions, the normal vascular endothelium may regulate vascular tone, and blood flow, by production of vasodilators (e.g., nitric oxide) and vasoconstrictors (e.g., endothelin-1), and because endothelium can be damaged by atherosclerosis, endothelial dysfunction may ensue. By use of CMR, acute cigarette smoking has been shown to be associated with an increased resting MBF and a reduced hyperemic myocardial flow. By use of dynamic ^{13}N-ammonia PET imaging in conjunction with intravenous adenosine, an abnormal vasodilatory response has been detected in male patients with a family history of coronary artery disease and high-risk lipid profiles, and CFR may also be decreased in anatomically normal coronary arteries of hypercholesterolemic patients. Improved cardiovascular conditioning alone, or in association with a low-fat diet, may improve coronary vasodilator capacity.

PREOPERATIVE CARDIAC RISK EVALUATION FOR NONCARDIAC SURGERY

Ischemic heart disease is a major cause of morbidity and mortality among patients undergoing elective noncardiac surgery and accounts for approximately one half of all perioperative deaths. Fortunately, most patients with known coronary artery disease can safely undergo major noncardiac surgery. The physiological importance of the coronary lesion(s) rather than the coronary anatomy per se has been established as the standard for evaluating cardiac risk in patients with coronary artery disease undergoing elective noncardiac surgery.

The major question is which subpopulations benefit from preoperative cardiac risk stratification. Recently, the ACC/AHA Task Force on Practice Guidelines has published an update on the recommendations for perioperative cardiovascular evaluation for noncardiac surgery.[44] These guidelines suggest that noninvasive cardiac testing should be used in patients with intermediate cardiac risk factors (mild angina, prior myocardial infarction, compensated or prior heart failure symptoms, or diabetes mellitus) who have either low functional capacity (<4 METs) or high-risk surgery (especially vascular). Patients with minor risk predictors do not need noninvasive risk stratification unless both their functional capacity is poor (<4 METs) and they are undergoing a high-risk surgical procedure. The results of noninvasive

testing (typically exercise testing or stress MPI or echocardiography) can be used to determine further preoperative management, such as cardiac catheterization and/or coronary revascularization, intensive medical therapy, or delay and/or cancellation of an elective noncardiac operation.

It is well appreciated that clinical indices alone (such as the Goldman index) have insufficient sensitivity or specificity for predicting perioperative cardiac events in patients with known coronary artery disease. Reviews of pharmacological stress MPI or echocardiography have shown that both techniques are useful in the risk stratification of these types of patients. In addition, MPI studies have demonstrated significant prognostic value in the later follow-up period and the perioperative period. Reports on the use of dobutamine echocardiography also support its utility in cardiac risk assessment in the perioperative period.[45] A number of investigators that used dipyridamole perfusion imaging to risk stratify patients with transient perfusion defects have shown a cardiac event rate of 1% to 2% in patients with normal scans and a gradient of risk of events from 8% to 50% as more coronary vessel perfusion defects are noted. Echocardiography also reveals a prognostic gradient of wall motion abnormalities that can predict increasing vulnerability to adverse short-term outcomes.

Preoperative risk stratification allows the clinician to predict the short-term risk for a particular patient but also to estimate a late cardiac event. In patients having dipyridamole ^{201}Tl MPI before elective vascular surgery, the best predictor of late cardiac events was the presence of moderate to large-sized fixed defects reflecting abnormalities in systolic ventricular function.

Finally, although myocardial SPECT imaging can successfully identify patients at high risk for perioperative and long-term cardiac events, the validity of a strategy of routine coronary revascularization before noncardiac surgery remains unclear.

In summary, stress MPI and echocardiography in conjunction with clinical predictors of risk, functional capacity, and surgery specific risk can accurately assess the perioperative cardiac risk among selected patients (intermediate-risk group) undergoing noncardiac surgery. A normal study has a high negative predictive value, whereas a positive study predicts a higher event rate that seems to increase in proportion to the magnitude of jeopardized myocardium or ventricular dysfunction.

RISK ASSESSMENT IN WOMEN

The selection of the appropriate noninvasive prognostic test in women requires careful consideration. Several factors play an important role in this decision. First, the risk profile in women differs compared with men. Second, epidemiological data suggest that women tend to present with their first anginal symptoms 10 years later and sustain their first myocardial infarction 20 years later than their male counterparts. Nonrandomized trials and observational studies attribute this partially to the cardioprotective role of estrogen. Third, several studies

■ ▣ ■

TABLE 9-14   DIAGNOSTIC ACCURACY OF STRESS ECHOCARDIOGRAPHY IN DETECTING ANGIOGRAPHICALLY PROVEN CAD IN WOMEN

Author	Year	Protocol	Signif CAD	Total Pts	Sens (%)	Sens 1VD	Sens MVD	Spec (%)	PPV (%)	NPV (%)	Acc (%)
Masini[a]	1988	DIP	≥70%	83	79	—	—	93	91	84	87
Sawada[b]	1989	TSE or UBE	≥50%	57	86	88	82	86	86	86	86
Severi[c]	1994	DIP	≥75%	122	68	—	—	96	90	86	87
Williams[d]	1994	UBE	≥50%	70	88	89	86	84	83	89	86
Marwick[e]	1995	TSE or UBE	≥50%	161	80	75	85	81	71	87	81
Takeuchi[f]	1996	DASE	≥50%	70	75	78	73	92	79	90	87
Roger[g]	1997	TSE or UBE	≥50%	96	79	—	—	37	66	54	63
Dionisopoulos[h]	1997	DASE	≥50%	101	90	79	94	79	90	79	86
Laurienzo[i]	1997	DS-TEE	≥70%	84	82	—	—	100	100	94	95
Elhendy[j]	1997	DASE	≥50%	96	76	64	92	94	96	68	82
Ho[k]	1998	DSE	≥50%	51	93	89	95	82	87	90	88

Diagnostic accuracy of stress echocardiography, using either exercise or pharmacological stress, in detecting angiographically proved coronary artery disease (CAD) in women. A new or worsening regional wall motion abnormality induced by stress generally was considered a "positive" result.
1 VD, test results positive in patients with single-vessel CAD; Acc, overall accuracy; CAD, coronary artery disease; DASE, dobutamine/atropine stress echocardiography; DIP, dipyridamole stress echocardiography; DSE, dobutamine stress echocardiography; DS-TEE, dobutamine stress transesophageal echocardiography; MVD, test results positive in patients with multivessel CAD; NPV, negative predictive value (likelihood of absence of angiographically significant CAD in patients without inducible wall motion abnormalities by stress echocardiography); PPV, positive predictive value (likelihood of angiographically significant CAD in patients with inducible wall motion abnormalities by stress echocardiography); Protocol, exercise or pharmacological protocol used in conjunction with transthoracic echo imaging; Pts, patients; Sens, sensitivity; Signif CAD, % coronary luminal diameter narrowing, documented by selective coronary angiography, considered to represent "significant" CAD; Spec, specificity; TSE, treadmill stress echocardiography; Total Pts, number of women in each series undergoing selective coronary angiography in whom stress echo studies were also carried out and wall motion analysis performed; UBE, upright bicycle stress echocardiography.
[a]*J Am Coll Cardiol* 1988; 12:682; [b]*J Am Coll Cardiol* 1989; 14:1440; [c]*Circulation* 1994; 89:1160; [d]*Am J Cardiol* 1994; 74:435; [e]*J Am Coll Cardiol* 1995; 26:335; [f]*Cor Art Dis* 1996; 7:831; [g]*Circulation* 1997; 95:405; [h]*J Am Soc Echocardiogr* 1997; 10:811; [i]*Am J Cardiol* 1997; 80:1402; [j]*Am J Cardiol* 1997; 80:1414; [k]*Am Heart J* 1998; 135:655.

have detailed the lack of diagnostic value of exercise testing in women. In those studies, sensitivity for the detection of significant coronary artery disease (≥50% or ≥70% angiographic stenosis) was similar in men and women (60% to 80% in women and 65% to 87% in men); however, specificity was significantly lower in women (63% to 68%) than men (74% to 89%).

Use of Stress MPI in Women

Stress MPI shows improved sensitivity and specificity in the detection of coronary artery disease in women.[14,16,21] Planar ^{201}Tl imaging has a sensitivity of 71% to 75% and a specificity of 91% to 97% in women with no prior history of coronary artery disease, and exercise SPECT MPI has been found to be more sensitive than planar imaging. Similar results can be obtained with pharmacological radionuclide imaging. By use of adenosine SPECT MPI with dual-isotope (rest ^{201}Tl/stress ^{99m}Tc-sestamibi for the detection of coronary stenosis of ≥70%) the sensitivity, specificity, and diagnostic accuracy was 95%, 66%, and 85%, respectively, with 93% normalcy rate. These results are similar for all women, regardless of the presenting symptoms, a history of myocardial infarction, or the pretest probability of coronary artery disease. The role of ^{99m}Tc agents and the addition of electrocardiographic-gated SPECT imaging further improve the specificity compared with ^{201}Tl imaging. In fact, stress MPI with either ^{99m}Tc or ^{201}Tl should be gated in all patients, not just women.

Thus, taking all data together, both exercise and pharmacological SPECT MPI provide significant independent and incremental prognostic information to clinical, physiological, and coronary angiographic data in women.

Use of Stress Echocardiography for Diagnosis of Coronary Artery Disease in Women

It has been established that the accuracy of exercise testing is lower in women than in men, owing in part to the higher prevalence of coronary disease in men. In studies of nearly 1000 women with suspected coronary artery disease where the presenting complaint was usually chest pain (Table 9-14), the diagnostic accuracy of stress echocardiography, with coronary arteriography as the reference standard, is good. The weighted mean sensitivity is 81% (89% in women with multivessel disease), specificity of 86%, and overall accuracy is 84%. Stress echocardiography clearly has a higher diagnostic accuracy than conventional treadmill exercise testing and may be a cost-effective diagnostic strategy in women with an intermediate pretest probability of coronary artery disease.

In summary, although a negative exercise stress test is extremely helpful in women with suspected coronary artery disease, a positive result may be misleading, especially in combination with atypical symptoms. Stress MPI improves the sensitivity and the specificity in the diagnosis of coronary artery disease and gives important prognostic information. The use of ^{99m}Tc agents with simultaneous assessment of perfusion and function further enhance the diagnostic accuracy of MPI in women.

REFERENCES

1. Gibbons RJ, Balady GJ, Timothy Bricker J, et al. ACC/AHA 2002 guideline update for exercise testing: summary article. A report of the American College of Cardiology/American Heart Association Task Force on Practice Guidelines (Committee to Update the 1997 Exercise Testing Guidelines). *J Am Coll Cardiol* 2002; 40:1531.

2. Third Report of the National Cholesterol Education Program (NCEP) Expert Panel on Detection, Evaluation, and Treatment of High Blood Cholesterol in Adults (Adult Treatment Panel III) final report. *Circulation* 2002; 106:3143.

3. Gibbons RJ, Abrams J, Chatterjee K, et al. ACC/AHA 2002 guideline update for the management of patients with chronic stable angina—summary article: a report of the American College of Cardiology/American Heart Association Task Force on Practice Guidelines (Committee on the Management of Patients With Chronic Stable Angina). *Circulation* 2003; 107:149.

4. Ritchie JL, Bateman TM, Bonow RO, et al. Guidelines for clinical use of cardiac radionuclide imaging: A report of the American College of Cardiology/American Heart Association Task Force on assessment of diagnostic and therapeutic cardiovascular procedures (Committee on Radionuclide Imaging)—developed in collaboration with the American Society of Nuclear Cardiology. *J Nucl Cardiol* 1995; 2:172.

5. Mazur W, Rivera JM, Khoury AF, et al. Prognostic value of exercise echocardiography: validation of a new risk index combining echocardiographic, treadmill, and exercise electrocardiographic parameters. *J Am Soc Echocardiogr* 2003; 16:318.

6. O'Rourke RA, Brundage BH, Froelicher VF, et al. American College of Cardiology/American Heart Association Expert Consensus document on electron-beam computed tomography for the diagnosis and prognosis of coronary artery disease. *Circulation* 2000; 102:126.

7. SoRelle R. Incremental benefits seen for electron-beam tomography. *Circulation* 2003; 107:e9045.

8. Gerber TC, Kuzo RS, Karstaedt N, et al. Current results and new developments of coronary angiography with use of contrast-enhanced computed tomography of the heart. *Mayo Clin Proc* 2002; 77:55.

9. Callister TQ, Cooil B, Raya SP, Lippolis NJ, Russo DJ, Raggi P. Coronary artery disease: improved reproducibility of calcium scoring with an electron-beam CT volumetric method. *Radiology* 1998; 208:807.

10. Budoff MJ, Diamond GA, Raggi P, et al. Continuous probabilistic prediction of angiographically significant coronary artery disease using electron beam tomography. *Circulation* 2002; 105:1791

11. Nallamothu BK, Saint S, Bielak LF, et al. Electron-beam computed tomography in the diagnosis of coronary artery disease: a meta-analysis. *Arch Intern Med* 2001; 161:833

12. Rumberger JA, Brundage BH, Rader DJ, Kondos G. Electron beam computed tomographic coronary calcium scanning: a review and guidelines for use in asymptomatic persons. *Mayo Clin Proc* 1999; 74:243.

13. He ZX, Hedrick TD, Pratt CM, et al. Severity of coronary artery calcification by electron beam computed tomography predicts silent myocardial ischemia. *Circulation* 2000; 101:244.

14. Taillefer R, DePuey EG, Udelson JE, Beller GA, Latour Y, Reeves F. Comparative diagnostic accuracy of ^{201}Tl and Tc-99m sestamibi SPECT imaging (perfusion and ECG-gated SPECT) in detecting coronary artery disease in women. *J Am Coll Cardiol* 1997; 29:69.

15. Berman DS, Kiat H, Friedman JD, et al. Separate acquisition rest thallium-201/stress technetium-99m sestamibi dual-isotope myocardial perfusion single-photon emission computed tomography: a clinical validation study. *J Am Coll Cardiol* 1993; 22:1455.

16. Hachamovitch R, Berman DS, Kiat H, et al. Effective risk stratification using exercise myocardial perfusion SPECT in women: gender-related differences in prognostic nuclear testing. *J Am Coll Cardiol* 1996; 28:34.

17. Shaw LJ, Hendel R, Borges-Neto S, et al. Prognostic value of normal exercise and adenosine (99m)Tc-tetrofosmin SPECT imaging: results from the multicenter registry of 4,728 patients. *J Nucl Med* 2003; 44:134.

18. Navare SM, Kapetanopoulos A, Heller GV. Pharmacologic radionuclide myocardial perfusion imaging. *Curr Cardiol Rep* 2003; 5:16.

19. Geleijnse ML, Elhendy A, Fioretti PM, Roelandt JR. Dobutamine stress myocardial perfusion imaging. *J Am Coll Cardiol* 2000; 36:2017.

20. Samady H, Wackers FJ, Joska TM, Zaret BL, Jain D. Pharmacologic stress perfusion imaging with adenosine: role of simultaneous low-level treadmill exercise. *J Nucl Cardiol* 2002; 9:188.

21. American Society of Nuclear Cardiology consensus statement: Task Force on Women and Coronary Artery Disease. The role of myocardial perfusion imaging in the clinical evaluation of coronary artery disease in women. *J Nucl Cardiol* 2003; 10:218.

22. Wagdy HM, Hodge D, Christian TF, Miller TD, Gibbons RJ. Prognostic value of vasodilator myocardial perfusion imaging in patients with left bundle-branch block. *Circulation* 1998; 97:1563.

23. Simone GL, Mullani NA, Page DA, Anderson BA Sr. Utilization statistics and diagnostic accuracy of a nonhospital-based positron emission tomography center for the detection of coronary artery disease using rubidium-82. *Am J Physiol Imaging* 1992; 7:203.

24. Siebelink HM, Blanksma PK, Crijns HJ, et al. No difference in cardiac event-free survival between positron emission tomography-guided and single-photon emission computed tomography-guided patient management: a prospective, randomized comparison of patients with suspicion of jeopardized myocardium. *J Am Coll Cardiol* 2001; 37:81.

25. Marwick TH. Stress echocardiography. *Heart* 2003; 89:113.

26. O'Keefe JH Jr., Barnhart CS, Bateman TM. Comparison of stress echocardiography and stress myocardial perfusion scintigraphy for diagnosing coronary artery disease and assessing its severity. *Am J Cardiol* 1995; 75:25D.

27. Ichikawa Y, Sakuma H, Kitagawa K, et al. Evaluation of left ventricular volumes and ejection fraction using fast steady-state cine MR imaging: comparison with left ventricular angiography. *J Cardiovasc Magn Reson* 2003; 5:333.

28. Kuijpers D, Ho KY, van Dijkman PR, Vliegenthart R, Oudkerk M. Dobutamine cardiovascular magnetic resonance for the detection of myocardial ischemia with the use of myocardial tagging. *Circulation* 2003; 107:1592.

29. Baer FM, Crnac J, Schmidt M, et al. Magnetic resonance pharmacological stress for detecting coronary disease. Comparison with echocardiography. *Herz* 2000; 25:400.

30. Nagel E, Lorenz C, Baer F, et al. Stress cardiovascular magnetic resonance: consensus panel report. *J Cardiovasc Magn Reson* 2001; 3:267.

31. Panting JR, Gatehouse PD, Yang GZ, et al. Echo-planar magnetic resonance myocardial perfusion imaging: parametric map analysis and comparison with thallium SPECT. *J Magn Reson Imaging* 2001; 13:192.

32. Schwitter J, Nanz D, Kneifel S, et al. Assessment of myocardial perfusion in coronary artery disease by magnetic resonance: a comparison with positron emission tomography and coronary angiography. *Circulation* 2001; 103:2230.

33. Raggi P, Callister TQ, Cooil B, et al. Identification of patients at increased risk of first unheralded acute myocardial infarction by electron-beam computed tomography. *Circulation* 2000; 101:850.

34. Keelan PC, Bielak LF, Ashai K, et al. Long-term prognostic value of coronary calcification detected by electron-beam computed tomography in patients undergoing coronary angiography. *Circulation* 2001; 104:412.

35. Wayhs R, Zelinger A, Raggi P. High coronary artery calcium scores pose an extremely elevated risk for hard events. *J Am Coll Cardiol* 2002; 39:225.

36. Elhendy A, Bax JJ, Poldermans D. Dobutamine stress myocardial perfusion imaging in coronary artery disease. *J Nucl Med* 2002; 43:1634.

37. Iskander S, Iskandrian AE. Risk assessment using single-photon emission computed tomographic technetium-99m sestamibi imaging. *J Am Coll Cardiol* 1998; 32:57.

38. Kloner RA, Bolli R, Marban E, Reinlib L, Braunwald E. Medical and cellular implications of stunning, hibernation, and preconditioning: an NHLBI workshop. *Circulation* 1998; 97:1848.

39. Allman KC, Shaw LJ, Hachamovitch R, Udelson JE. Myocardial viability testing and impact of revascularization on prognosis in patients with coronary artery disease and left ventricular dysfunction: a meta-analysis. *J Am Coll Cardiol* 2002; 39:1151.

40. Schelbert HR. PET contributions to understanding normal and abnormal cardiac perfusion and metabolism. *Ann Biomed Eng* 2000; 28:922.

41. Koskenvuo JW, Sakuma H, Niemi P, et al. Global myocardial blood flow and global flow reserve measurements by CMR and PET are comparable. *J Magn Reson Imaging* 2001; 13:361.

42. Senior R, Swinburn JM. Incremental value of myocardial contrast echocardiography for the prediction of recovery of function in dobutamine nonresponsive myocardium early after acute myocardial infarction. *Am J Cardiol* 2003; 91:397.

43. Messroghli DR, Niendorf T, Schulz-Menger J, Dietz R, Friedrich MG. T1 mapping in patients with acute myocardial infarction. *J Cardiovasc Magn Reson* 2003; 5:353.

44. Eagle KA, Berger PB, Calkins H, et al. ACC/AHA Guideline Update for Perioperative Cardiovascular Evaluation for Noncardiac Surgery—Executive Summary. A report of the American College of Cardiology/ American Heart Association Task Force on Practice Guidelines (Committee to Update the 1996 Guidelines on Perioperative Cardiovascular Evaluation for Noncardiac Surgery). *Anesth Analg* 2002; 94:1052.

45. Boersma E, Poldermans D, Bax JJ, et al. Predictors of cardiac events after major vascular surgery: role of clinical characteristics, dobutamine echocardiography, and beta-blocker therapy. *JAMA* 2001; 285:1865.

chapter 10

Heart Failure

Martin G. Keane

Jorge R. Kizer

Eric D. Popjes

Lee R. Goldberg

Evan Loh

The normal heart adapts to meet the metabolic needs of the peripheral tissues. Clinical heart failure results when cardiac dysfunction leads to elevated filling pressures and inadequate cardiac output. In the United States alone, 4.6 million people are treated for heart failure, and 550,000 new diagnoses are made each year. Prevalence doubles with each decade after age 45 and approaches 10% for persons aged 75 and older. The condition is the primary indication for approximately 3 million office visits, 870,000 hospitalizations, and 45,000 deaths per year, with estimated treatment costs of $38 billion annually.[1]

Both systolic and diastolic dysfunction cause heart failure. Diminished systolic contractile function and impaired left ventricular emptying cause elevated left ventricular end-diastolic volume. Increasing myocyte fiber length optimizes myosin-actin interaction and enhances myocardial contraction, but this compensation is limited by a progressively steep rise in left ventricular end-diastolic pressure at high end-diastolic volume. Impaired left ventricular diastolic passive or active relaxation results in a left-shifted pressure-volume relationship, with abnormally elevated end-diastolic pressures at normal end-diastolic volume. The resulting pulmonary venous hypertension and retrograde elevation of right ventricular and systemic venous pressure cause congestion of the pulmonary and systemic venous circulations, regardless of the underlying etiology. Progressive physical incapacity, damage to dependent organ systems, ventricular arrhythmias, and thromboembolic complications all contribute to high morbidity and mortality.

Although clinical presentation is similar, long-term prognosis and therapy for systolic and diastolic heart failure differ.[2] Thus, distinguishing systolic from diastolic dysfunction is important for the accurate management of congestive heart failure.

SYSTOLIC HEART FAILURE

Decreased systolic contractile function can result from ischemic heart disease, cardiomyopathy, chronic valvular disease, hypertension, and infiltrative syndromes (Table 10-1). Coronary artery disease is the most common cause of heart failure in developed countries today. Myocardial infarction results in loss of myocytes and decreased systolic contractile function and subsequent ventricular remodeling may progress to heart failure.[3] Postinfarction ventricular dilation augments ventricular wall stress and stimulates compensatory myocyte hypertrophy. Volume overload results in cavity dilation, distortion of ventricular geometry, and progressive heart failure.[3] Ischemic papillary muscle damage causes tethering of the affected leaflet and malcoaptation with mitral regurgitation (Figure 10-1), resulting in additional volume load, further affecting cavity enlargement and progressive systolic failure. Impaired contractility without myocardial necrosis can occur from transient interruption of myocardial perfusion ("stunning") or prolonged low-grade coronary insufficiency (hibernation).

The second most common etiology of left ventricular systolic dysfunction is primary cardiomyopathy.[4] The World Health Organization/International Society and Federation of Cardiology (WHO/ISFC) recognizes five categories of myocardial disease: dilated, hypertrophic, restrictive, arrhythmogenic right ventricular cardiomyopathy, and unclassified cardiomyopathy (Table 10-1). Dilated cardiomyopathy is characterized by left ventricular dilation and global systolic dysfunction (Figure 10-2) and may result from hereditary and acquired disorders or from autoimmune processes stimulated by myocarditis or cytotoxic agents (Box 10-1). In most cases, however, the cause of dilated cardiomyopathy is unknown.[4] Right-ventricular dilation resulting from the myopathic process or from pulmonary hypertension is also common.

Chronic volume and pressure overload from valvular disease and hypertension frequently lead to progressive left ventricular dilation and systolic failure. Historically, hypertension and valvular disease were the primary causes of heart failure, but their importance relative to coronary artery disease has decreased significantly over the past two decades. A rare form of dilated cardiomy-

■ ■ ■

TABLE 10-1   CLASSIFICATION OF THE CARDIOMYOPATHIES

SYSTOLIC DYSFUNCTION

Disorder	Description
Dilated cardiomyopathy	Dilation and impaired contraction caused by familial/genetic, viral and/or immune, alcoholic/toxic, or unknown factors
Ischemic cardiomyopathy	Depressed ventricular function secondary to ischemic damage (sometimes out of proportion to coronary artery disease)
Valvular cardiomyopathy	Ventricular dysfunction from abnormal loading conditions produced by the valvular stenosis and/or regurgitation
Inflammatory cardiomyopathy	Cardiac dysfunction as a consequence of myocarditis
Muscular dystrophies	Duchenne, Becker-type, and myotonic dystrophies
Neuromuscular disorders	Friedreich's ataxia, Noonan's syndrome, and lentiginosis
Sensitivity/toxic reactions	Alcohol, catecholamines, anthracyclines, irradiation, and miscellaneous
Peripartum cardiomyopathy	Heterogeneous disorders that first manifest in the peripartum period
Arrhythmogenic right ventricular cardiomyopathy	Fibrofatty replacement of the right ventricular myocardium, with occasional involvement of the left ventricle
Unclassified cardiomyopathy	Diseases that do not fit readily into any one category

DIASTOLIC DYSFUNCTION

Disorder	Description
Hypertrophic cardiomyopathy	Left and/or right ventricular hypertrophy, often asymmetrical, involving the interventricular septum
Restrictive cardiomyopathy	Restricted filling and reduced diastolic size of either or both ventricles with normal or near-normal systolic function
	Idiopathic or associated with infiltrative disease (amyloid, hemochromatosis, endomyocardial disease)
Hypertensive cardiomyopathy	Left ventricular hypertrophy with cardiac failure from predominant diastolic dysfunction (late-stage systolic failure)
General systemic disease	Includes connective tissue disorders, infiltrations, and granulomas

From Richardson P, McKenna W, Bristow M, et al. Report of the 1995 World Health Organization/International Society and Federation of Cardiology Task Force on the Definition and Classification of Cardiomyopathies. Copyright 1995, American Heart Association.

opathy is arrhythmogenic right ventricular dysplasia (ARVD), characterized by progressive, diffuse, or segmental myocardial atrophy of the right ventricular wall and replacement by fibrofatty tissue (Figure 10-3).[5] ARVD commonly presents with ventricular arrhythmias, which account for 20% of sudden cardiac death in young people and athletes.[5] Involvement of the left ventricle may result in biventricular failure, which is clinically indistinguishable from dilated cardiomyopathy.

DIASTOLIC HEART FAILURE

The normal aging process of the heart is the most common cause of intrinsic, isolated diastolic dysfunction (Table 10-1).[6] Myocyte attrition and progressive myocardial fibrosis contribute to increased passive stiffness of the ventricle in the elderly. Hypertrophy of remaining myocytes in response to systolic hypertension and age-related abnormalities of calcium handling add to abnor-

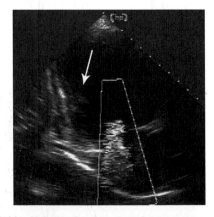

FIGURE 10-1. Apical two-chamber view demonstrates eccentric, posteriorly directed mitral regurgitation. The inferior wall and posteromedial papillary muscle (arrow) are scarred from prior myocardial infarction. Restricted systolic motion of the posterior mitral valve leaflet results in an overriding anterior mitral leaflet and eccentric regurgitation. See also Color Insert.

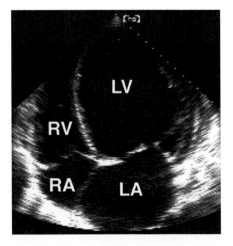

FIGURE 10-2. Apical four-chamber view of idiopathic dilated cardiomyopathy. There is dilatation of all chambers. There is increased echogenicity of the left atrial and left ventricular cavities, known as spontaneous echo contrast ("smoke"). This is consistent with sluggish intracavitary blood flow and low cardiac output.

■ ■ ■
BOX 10-1   KNOWN CAUSES OF DILATED CARDIOMYOPATHY

Toxins
Ethanol*
Chemotherapeutic agents (doxorubicin, bleomycin)
Cobalt*
Antiretroviral agents (zidovudine,* didanosine,* zalcitabine*)
Phenothiazines*
Carbon monoxide*
Lead*
Cocaine*
Mercury*

Metabolic abnormalities
Nutritional deficiencies (thiamine,* selenium,* carnitine*)
Endocrinologic disorders (hypothyroidism,* acromegaly,* thyrotoxicosis,* Cushing's disease, pheochromocytoma,* diabetes mellitus)
Electrolyte disturbances (hypocalcemia,* hypophosphatemia*)

Inflammatory or infectious causes
Infectious

Viral (coxsackievirus, cytomegalovirus,* human immunodeficiency virus)
Rickettsial
Bacterial (diphtheria*)
Mycobacterial
Fungal
Parasitic (toxoplasmosis,* trichinosis, Chagas' disease)

Noninfectious

Collagen vascular disorders (scleroderma, lupus erythematosus, dermatomyositis)
Hypersensitivity myocarditis*
Sarcoidosis*
Peripartum dysfunction*

Neuromuscular causes
Duchenne's muscular dystrophy
Facioscapulohumeral muscular dystrophy
Erb's limb-girdle dystrophy
Myotonic dystrophy
Friedreich's ataxia

Familial cardiomyopathy

*Potentially reversible, either spontaneously or with treatment, according to case reports.
From Dec WG, Fuster V. Idiopathic dilated cardiomyopathy. *N Engl J Med* 1994; 331:1564. Copyright 1994, Massachusetts Medical Society.

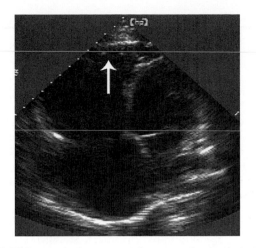

FIGURE 10-3. In arrhythmogenic right ventricular dysplasia (ARVD), the right ventricle is markedly dilated, and the free wall demonstrates evidence of fibrofatty replacement *(arrow)*.

mined and not attributable to increased afterload.[8] Myocardial hypertrophy is typically asymmetrical, predominantly involving the interventricular septum (Figure 10-4). One quarter of cases have left ventricular outflow tract obstruction resulting from systolic anterior

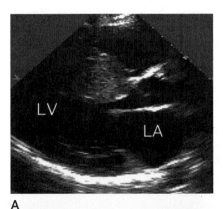

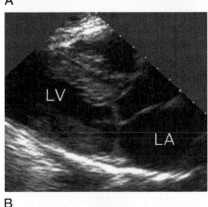

FIGURE 10-4. **A,** Parasternal long-axis view of hypertrophic obstructive cardiomyopathy (HOCM) at end-diastole. The asymmetrical septal hypertrophy (ASH) is evident in this view, where the upper interventricular measures 2.7 cm. **B,** Parasternal long-axis view of HOCM at end-systole shows characteristic anterior motion of the mitral valve apparatus (SAM), which obstructs the left ventricular outflow tract. This, in combination with ASH, is responsible for the dynamic outflow tract obstruction of the disease.

mal active and passive relaxation.[6] Superimposed valvular disease, hypertension, and atrial dysrhythmias might exacerbate diastolic heart failure.

Hypertensive heart disease is the second most common cause of isolated diastolic dysfunction. Ventricular hypertrophy initially normalizes increased myocardial wall stress caused by volume and pressure overload, preserving normal systolic function. The process becomes maladaptive as abnormal forms of myocardial components accumulate, including fetal myoglobin, alpha troponin, abnormal mitochondria, and impaired function of the sarcoplasmic reticulum.[7] Abnormal diastolic function occurs early in the hypertrophic process, whereas systolic dysfunction develops much later.

Ventricular diastolic abnormalities also occur in hypertrophic cardiomyopathy, in both obstructive and nonobstructive forms. Hypertrophic cardiomyopathy is characterized by a thickened, nondilated left ventricle, in which the degree of hypertrophy is genetically deter-

motion of the mitral leaflets into a subaortic area that is narrowed by the asymmetric septal hypertrophy. Systolic function is usually normal or supranormal. Diastolic dysfunction is due to abnormal cellular structure, functional impairment from myocyte hypertrophy, disorganization of muscle bundle alignment, and excess interstitial fibrosis.[8]

Less common etiologies of diastolic dysfunction include infiltrative diseases such as amyloid and hemochromatosis. Infiltration of the interstitial connective tissue by abnormal proteins increases myocardial stiffness and abnormalities of passive and active relaxation. Myocardial restrictive physiology is present in advanced stages of these diseases, with markedly reduced diastolic filling. Restrictive cardiomyopathy may be idiopathic or result from noninfiltrative disorders, storage diseases, or endomyocardial fibrosis. Heart failure symptoms result from diastolic dysfunction, when systolic function is still normal.

ASSESSMENT OF HEART FAILURE

Although the history, physical examination, electrocardiogram, and chest X-ray establish the clinical diagnosis of heart failure, cardiac imaging is essential for determining pathology and prognosis. Differentiation of systolic from diastolic failure is the key initial step. Determination of ventricular size, geometry, and performance provides prognostic information and is crucial in appropriate patient management and monitoring therapy.

SYSTOLIC HEART FAILURE

Early differentiation of ischemic from nonischemic causes of systolic ventricular failure is crucial. Prognosis is worse for ischemic left ventricular systolic dysfunction, and patients with left ventricular dysfunction from coronary artery disease might benefit from coronary bypass surgery. A history of angina pectoris, myocardial infarction, and the presence of atherosclerosis risk factors indicate an ischemic etiology of systolic dysfunction. Conversely, a history of familial cardiomyopathy, heavy alcohol use, postpartum status, or features of myocarditis are associated with a nonischemic etiology.

Noninvasive modalities can distinguish ischemic from nonischemic causes of left ventricular dysfunction. The presence of regional wall motion abnormalities, wall thinning, and scarring on two-dimensional echocardiography is strongly suggestive of prior myocardial infarction or chronic ischemia. Fixed or reversible perfusion defects on myocardial perfusion scintigraphy also indicate an ischemic etiology, although defects on ^{201}Tl imaging or ^{13}N-ammonia positron emission tomography might occasionally occur in patients with non-ischemic ventricular regional abnormalities and heart failure.[9] Stress-induced regional abnormalities in left ventricular contraction patterns on dobutamine echocardiography and exercise ^{99m}Tc-sestamibi assessment of perfusion and function allow further differentiation between ischemic and nonischemic etiologies.[9] Cardiac catheterization is the definitive test for coronary artery disease if the noninvasive workup is equivocal.

Nonischemic Heart Failure

Cardiac imaging can determine the diagnosis of underlying etiology of nonischemic ventricular dysfunction and identify structural and functional abnormalities of the left ventricle that predict prognosis and response to therapy.

Imaging for Etiology

Valvular vs. Nonvalvular

Differentiating primary, nonvalvular left ventricular dysfunction from heart failure secondary to chronic volume overload of valvular regurgitation may be difficult. In nonvalvular systolic dysfunction, mitral regurgitation typically occurs in the absence of structural leaflet or chordal abnormalities. Ventricular dilation and increased sphericity lead to posterior, mediolateral, and apical displacement of the papillary muscles, whereas chordae tendinae length remains fixed.[10] Increased distance between the coaptation point and the mitral annulus results in malcoaptation and mitral insufficiency (Figure 10-5).[10] Enlargement of the mitral annulus from chamber dilation and inadequate dynamic reduction of annular diameter because of impaired contractility cause further malcoaptation, worsening mitral regurgitation, and ongoing left ventricular dilation.

Evidence of intrinsic structural valve disease by two-dimensional echocardiographic images, including rheumatic, myxomatous, or calcific degeneration, suggests a valvular cause for ventricular systolic dysfunction. Annular dilation caused by cavity enlargement with central malcoaptation is more consistent with a nonalvular etiology. Color Doppler provides additional information as to the cause of the mitral regurgitation. In dilated cardiomyopathy of nonvalvular origin, the jet is typically central, reflecting symmetrical displacement

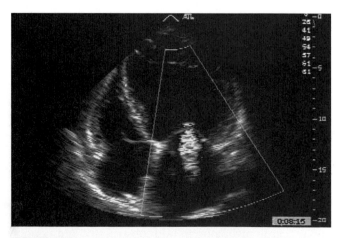

FIGURE 10-5. Atrial and ventricular cavity enlargement result in uniform dilation of the mitral annulus, with central malcoaptation of the mitral valve leaflets. This results in centrally oriented mitral regurgitation. See also Color Insert.

of the papillary muscles, whereas structural mitral disease is typically associated with an eccentric mitral regurgitation jet.

Valvular repair or replacement might prevent worsening of mild-to-moderate ventricular dysfunction from progressive volume or pressure overload.[11] In the case of mitral regurgitation, ventricular ejection into the low-pressure atrium masks the impaired left ventricular performance in patients with mitral regurgitation and is an important consideration before valvular repair or replacement. Morbidity and mortality of surgical correction of valve disease might be prohibitively high with severe ventricular dysfunction and heart failure.

Infiltrative vs. Noninfiltrative

Infiltrative disorders such as amyloidosis and hemochromatosis can be detected by two-dimensional echocardiography and usually have increased left and right ventricular wall thickness and normal ventricular size (Figure 10-6). In cardiac amyloid, the valves are diffusely thickened, and the interatrial septum is usually thicker than normal. Cardiac amyloidosis is also characterized by a "sparkling" appearance of the thickened myocardium because of the altered acoustic impedance of the amyloid deposition (Figure 10-6). The myocardium has more diffusely increased echogenicity in hemochromatosis, which is seen best with tissue Doppler techniques.[12] In early stages of both diseases, systolic function is typically preserved, but diastolic function is restrictive. Systolic contractile dysfunction and heart failure predominate in later stages of the disease.

Nuclear imaging demonstrates abnormally increased uptake of technetium in amyloidosis in <20% of patients. Assessment of myocardial tissue density abnormalities by cardiac magnetic resonance imaging (CMR) has demonstrated benefit for detection of both amyloid and hemochromatosis and can differentiate these from other noninfiltrative cardiomyopathies.[13]

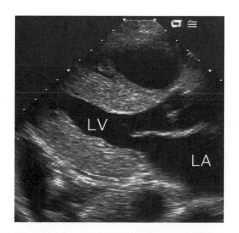

FIGURE 10-6. Uniform ventricular hypertrophy is characteristic of cardiac amyloid because of deposition of amyloid protein. This is a focal process and results in a "sparkling" appearance as a result of focally hyperrefractile echo densities seen here throughout the myocardium.

Diagnosing Myocarditis

Acute ventricular systolic dysfunction and heart failure may suggest myocarditis. Echocardiographic findings are nonspecific and must be interpreted in combination with other diagnostic tests. Global left ventricular dysfunction is common, but contractile dysfunction may be focal and lead to an erroneous diagnosis of coronary disease. Patients with fulminant or early myocarditis may have normal left ventricular size despite severe diffuse hypocontractility, whereas those who have subacute myocarditis typically have dilated chambers. Other echocardiographic findings include abnormal diastolic filling patterns, left ventricular thrombi, and increased wall thickness (consistent with interstitial hemorrhage or edema), especially in fulminant myocarditis. Left ventricular apical aneurysm is suggestive of Chagas' disease.

It is important to rule out valvular heart disease, congenital heart disease, and infiltrative myopathies as the cause of left ventricular systolic dysfunction. Ischemia or prior myocardial infarction must be ruled out when nonspecific electrocardiographic changes, chest pain, and elevated cardiac enzymes are present. Nuclear perfusion images are usually normal in myocarditis, although scarring that does not correspond to coronary distribution that might be present. Coronary angiography is occasionally performed when noninvasive testing is equivocal.

Radionucleotide-labeled antibody techniques may facilitate the diagnosis of acute myocarditis. Antimyosin scanning uses ^{111}In-labeled monoclonal antimyosin antibody, injected intravenously with imaging performed 48 hours later.[14] Antimyosin antibodies attach to the myosin heavy-chain component of disrupted myocytes and can be quantitated (Figure 10-7). The sensitivity of an antimyosin scan for detecting myocarditis has been reported to be 83% to 100%.[14] Antimyosin scans also have prognostic value, with improved left ventricular function over time primarily in those with positive scans.

Right ventricular endomyocardial biopsy–obtained histological examination remains the diagnostic "gold standard," with a specificity of approximately 50% and a negative predictive value of 90% to 92%. Fluoroscopy or echocardiography can localize the bioptome in the right ventricle, reducing the risk of ventricular perforation or damage to the tricuspid valve (Figure 10-8). For patients with acute heart failure, an initial antimyosin scan might help determine who should proceed to endomyocardial biopsy. Less than 10% of patients with a negative scan have a positive biopsy, but the positive predictive value of an antimyosin scan is only 33%.[14] The diagnostic schema for myocarditis incorporates antimyosin scanning and right ventricular endomyocardial biopsy (Figure 10-9).

Imaging for Prognosis and Therapy Direction

In addition to establishing diagnosis, a comprehensive imaging approach for nonischemic cardiomyopathy includes assessment of ventricular size and evaluation of indices of systolic performance. Cavity size and geometry establish the acuity of myocardial dysfunction and

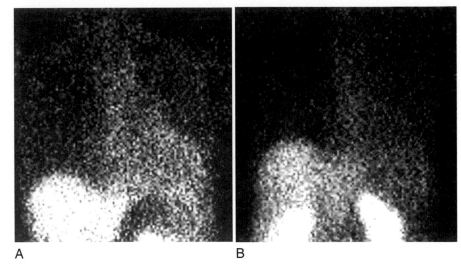

FIGURE 10-7. A, Initial antimyosin scan (indium-111) in a patient with acute onset of heart failure reveals diffuse antimyosin antibody uptake, suggesting myocarditis. Endomyocardial biopsy confirmed presence of myocarditis. **B,** After treatment with azathioprine and prednisone, follow-up scan shows significant resolution of antimyosin uptake. Biopsy also indicated healing myocarditis. The patient's left ventricular ejection fraction increased from 27% to 44%.

provide important prognostic information. Left ventricular size is used in the optimal timing of operative intervention in valvular heart disease.[11] Assessment of ventricular systolic function provides further prognostic information in heart failure.

Cavity Size and Volume

Noninvasive cardiac imaging techniques provide an accurate assessment of left ventricular cavity size and volume. Systolic and diastolic internal diameters measured at the tip of the mitral valve leaflets are clinically relevant, but calculation of ventricular volumes with two-dimensional echo is a more accurate measurement of ventricular cavity size. Geometric formulations of left ventricular volume are accurate when ventricular size is near normal but are inaccurate when cavity dilation is severe or regional, as in the presence of ventricular aneurysm (Figure 10-10). Simpson's method divides the ventricle along its major axis into multiple disks of equal

thickness, and the volumes of the disks are added to obtain overall cavity volume (Figure 10-11). The method allows calculation of systolic and diastolic volumes independent of shape or function.

Angiographic contrast and radionuclide ^{99m}Tc measurements permit nongeometric determination of ventricular volume but are less commonly used. Three-dimensional echocardiography and cardiac magnetic resonance imaging also provide accurate assessment of ventricular volume but require precise acquisition and are time-consuming. A real-time three-dimensional technique can accurately quantify ventricular volumes, even in the presence of aneurysms.[15]

In nonischemic cardiomyopathy, increased cavity size or volume predicts increased cardiovascular mortality. The prognostic importance of left ventricular size is further supported by the favorable effect of ventricular volume reduction by angiotensin-converting enzyme (ACE) inhibition, biventricular pacing, and surgery on cardiovascular morbidity and mortality.[16] Increase in chamber dimensions precedes development of systolic failure in valvular cardiomyopathies and is a key guide for the timing of surgical intervention.[11]

Ventricular Shape

Left ventricular enlargement in cardiomyopathy is characterized by a disproportionate increase in the diameter of the minor ventricular axis relative to the diameter of the major ventricular axis. As the minor axis approaches the major axis dimension, the normally ellipsoid left ventricle becomes more spherical (Figure 10-12). Sphericity of the ventricle correlates with prognosis in dilated cardiomyopathy and chronic volume overload states.[17] The mechanical disadvantage of spherical geometry may precipitate heart failure and is associated with development of mitral regurgitation.

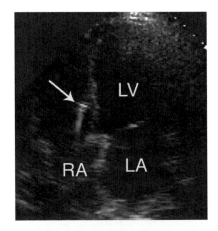

FIGURE 10-8. The echogenic tip of the bioptome is seen in the right ventricle on this apical four-chamber view *(arrow)* in proper position for biopsy of the mid-interventricular septum. There is bulging of the interventricular septum toward the left ventricle as pressure is applied for biopsy.

Ventricular Mass

Left ventricular mass can be measured noninvasively by echocardiography or CMR as the difference of endocar-

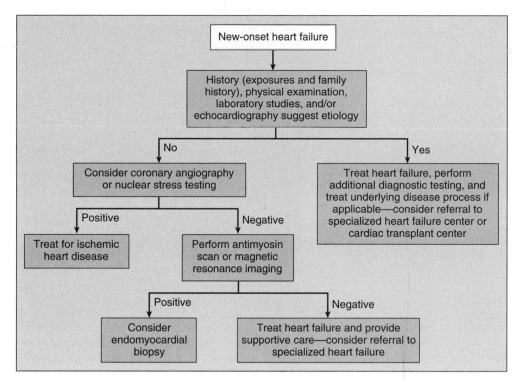

FIGURE 10-9. Imaging approach to the diagnosis of acute myocarditis.

dial and epicardial ventricular volume (myocardial volume) converted to mass by adjusting for myocardial density (1.04 g/mL). The ventricular walls thicken in response to increases in wall stress caused by volume or pressure overload, as described by the Laplace relationship (Figure 10-13). Ventricular hypertrophy normalizes increased wall stress due to cavity dilation and pressure overload and reduces myocardial oxygen consumption. Dilated, nonischemic cardiomyopathies are associated with hypertrophy because of enlarged cavity size. The ratio of wall thickness to cavity radius (relative wall thickness) remains normal. Prominent wall thickening and conserved ventricular cavity size are more commonly associated with pressure overload or hyper-

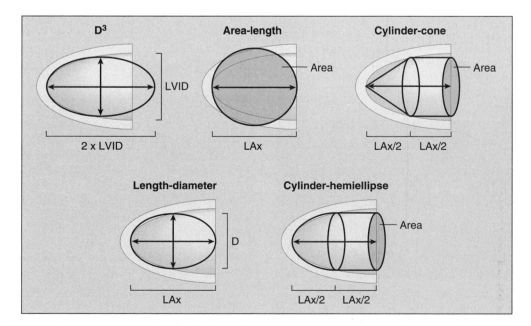

FIGURE 10-10. Some of the numerous geometric approximations of left ventricular volume are shown. LAx, long axis; LVID, left ventricular internal dimension.

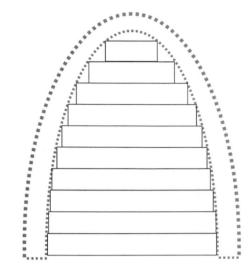

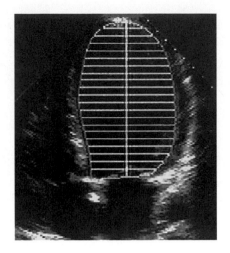

FIGURE 10-11. Simpson's method is applied by use of the apical four-chamber view of the left ventricle. Simplified diagram of the Simpson's method. Volume of each disk is calculated as $\pi R^2 h$ (h, disk height; R, disk radius). The ventricular endocardium has been digitized off line, and a computer algo0rithm is used to generate disks of equal height. The volumes of the disks are summed to obtain a ventricular volume.

trophic cardiomyopathy. Left ventricular hypertrophy predicts a two- to four-times increased incidence of adverse cardiovascular events and mortality.[18] In clinical practice, measurement of left ventricular wall thickness from two-dimensional or M-mode echocardiography is used to provide an estimate of the severity of hypertrophy.

CMR acquires data in a more spatially unambiguous manner than echo, with three-dimensional relationships of one image plane to another that are easily ascertained. Calculation of left ventricular (LV) mass by CMR methods has been demonstrated to be accurate and reproducible in both normal and myopathic hearts and is the "gold standard" for estimating LV mass. Newer acquisition techniques that reduce costs and scan time might make CMR more practical as a general prognostic tool.

Ejection Fraction

Noninvasive assessment of ventricular systolic function in nonischemic cardiomyopathy provides further prognostic information. The most commonly used clinical index of ventricular systolic performance is ejection fraction (EF), which is a key determinant of prognosis in heart failure. It is calculated from diastolic and systolic volumes measured with echocardiography, CMR, or cine ventriculography. Fractional shortening on M-mode or fractional area change of the ventricular cavity by use of endocardial border–detection techniques are surrogate measures of ejection performance but are unreliable in ventricles with regional variation in contractile function. Ejection fraction can be estimated by nuclear ventriculography, with the proportionality between ^{99m}Tc counts and blood volume to calculate the change in volume between systole and diastole, and has the advantage of being independent of asymmetry or regional variation in function.

Severely decreased ejection fraction (<20%) is associated with high morbidity and mortality in both nonis-

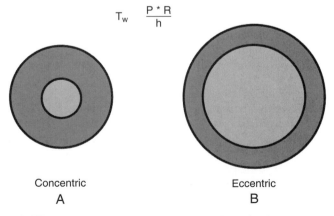

$$T_w \quad \frac{P * R}{h}$$

Concentric
A

Eccentric
B

FIGURE 10-13. Laplace's law expresses the relationship between ventricular pressure, radius, and wall stress (T_w, wall stress; P, intracavitary pressure; R, cavity radius; h, wall thickness). **A,** Ventricular hypertrophy in response to primary pressure overload results in compensatory increase in wall thickness without significant change in cavity radius. This "concentric" hypertrophy is represented in this short-axis diagram. **B,** Ventricular hypertrophy in response to primary volume overload results in a compensatory increase in wall thickness that matches increases in cavity radius. This results in "eccentric" hypertrophy geometry.

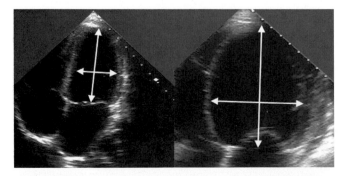

FIGURE 10-12. A, In the normal ventricle, the long-axis dimension (LAx) is significantly larger than the short-axis dimension (SAx). **B,** In dilated cardiomyopathy, the length of the short-axis dimension (SAx) becomes similar to that of the long axis (LAx). The ventricle has become more spherical in shape.

chemic and ischemic cardiomyopathy. In patients with heart failure, ejection fraction <35% predicts decreased survival and more frequent hospitalization, independent of the prognostic value of elevated ventricular mass.[19] There is little relationship between ejection fraction and other important prognostic indicators such as exercise tolerance or peak Vo_2, and the risk conferred by severely lowered EF must be assessed in conjunction with these other factors.

Stroke volume and cardiac output can be measured with Doppler echo or radionuclide techniques. Although without long-term prognostic significance, these measures of systolic performance can guide therapy during acute, decompensated heart failure. More commonly, invasive right heart catheterization is used for continuous monitoring of intracavitary pressures, pulmonary capillary wedge pressure, and cardiac output, allowing rapid adjustment of vasodilator, inotropic, and diuretic therapy.

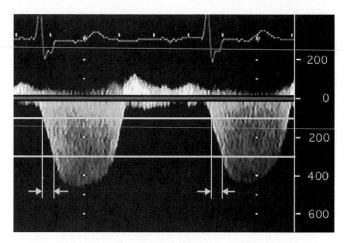

FIGURE 10-14. Spectral display of continuous-wave Doppler of mitral regurgitation taken from the atrial window. The time interval between the velocity of 1 m/s and 3 m/s is proportional to the dP/dt of the ventricle and is an index of systolic function.

Ejection Phase Indices

The principal determinants of systolic function are preload, afterload, and contractility. The interrelationships among these factors and their influence on systolic performance have been extensively studied with invasive hemodynamic measurements.[20] Ventricular loading conditions can be determined by calculation of ventricular wall stress in systole (afterload) and diastole (preload). Systolic pressure-volume and wall stress-length relationships reflect myocardial contractility, independently of loading conditions.[20] Measurement of wall stress by echocardiography or CMR allows systolic performance indices to be assessed noninvasively. Related ejection-phase indices (fractional shortening, fractional area shortening, velocity of circumferential fiber shortening, or V_{cf}) have limited prognostic significance in nonischemic cardiomyopathy but are useful measures of ventricular contractile improvement in therapeutic intervention trials.[21]

Isovolumic contraction and relaxation phase indices (change in pressure per unit time or dP/dT) can be measured from continuous-wave Doppler tracings of mitral regurgitation velocity (Figure 10-14). These represent reasonably load-independent measures of contractility and diastolic relaxation, respectively. In patients with severe chronic systolic heart failure, lower contractile dP/dt (<600 mmHg/s) and lower relaxation dP/dt (<450 mmHg/s) are both associated with poor short-term prognosis.[22] Measured invasively from pressure-volume loops, these isovolumic indices are reliable predictors of 10-year survival in patients with systolic dysfunction and heart failure.[23]

Pulmonary Hypertension

The degree and reversibility of pulmonary hypertension have profound impact on prognosis and management of nonischemic dilated cardiomyopathy. Morbidity and mortality are elevated in patients with moderate or severe pulmonary hypertension, particularly those with a history of myocarditis.[24] Increased left ventricular end-diastolic pressure, compounded by mitral regurgitation, causes pulmonary venous hypertension. Pulmonary artery pressure increases out of proportion to elevated pulmonary venous pressure because of pulmonary vasoconstriction and increased pulmonary vascular resistance. Early vascular endothelial dysfunction is reversible, but progressive intimal fibrosis and medial hypertrophy of the pulmonary arterioles lead to fixed pulmonary hypertension. Fixed, severe pulmonary hypertension worsens the surgical outcome of coronary bypass or valvular surgery and constitutes a contraindication to cardiac transplantation.[25] The donor right ventricle acutely fails in such circumstances because of inordinate elevation in pulmonary vascular resistance and afterload.

Tricuspid regurgitation is observed in three quarters of patients with pulmonary hypertension and practically all patients with pulmonary artery systolic pressure greater than 50 mmHg. Echocardiographic evaluation of pulmonary hypertension by use of the peak velocity of the tricuspid regurgitation jet and the modified Bernoulli equation ($P = 4V^2$) correlates well with manometry during cardiac catheterization. Right heart catheterization is invasive but allows measurement of pulmonary vascular resistance in addition to pulmonary artery pressures. Pulmonary vascular resistance of >2.5 Wood units predicts poor outcome after cardiac transplantation, although reduction of pulmonary vascular resistance by intravenous or inhaled vasodilators predicts an improved outcome with perioperative vasodilators.[26]

Chronic pulmonary hypertension increases right ventricular afterload, leading to right ventricular hypertrophy, enlargement, and systolic failure. The dilated right ventricle becomes apex forming, and the moderator band appears at a more perpendicular angle to the interventricular septum (Figure 10-15). Diminished contractile function is present, with reduced right ventricular wall thickening and minimal change in chamber area from systole to diastole. Ventricular enlargement produces dilation and distortion of the tricuspid annulus, increasing tricuspid regurgita-

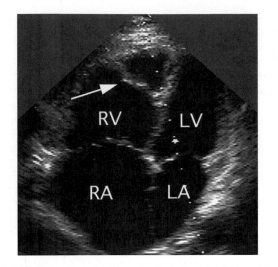

FIGURE 10-15. In the apical four-chamber view, the failing right ventricle (RV) enlarges and becomes the apex-forming ventricle. The moderator band *(arrow)* becomes prominent.

tion and exacerbating right ventricular dysfunction and enlargement. The extent of right ventricular dilation and the severity of right ventricular contractile dysfunction are predictors of poor long-term survival in dilated cardiomyopathy.[27]

Ischemic Cardiomyopathies

Similar to nonischemic cardiomyopathy, larger left ventricular size, increased ventricular sphericity, lower EF, and the present of significant pulmonary hypertension or right ventricular dysfunction also predict increased cardiovascular morbidity and mortality in ischemic cardiomyopathy.[24,28] Additional considerations to be addressed by the imaging evaluation of ischemic cardiomyopathy include characterization of the location and extent of ischemic damage, assessment for suitability of revascularization, and evaluation of secondary mitral regurgitation.

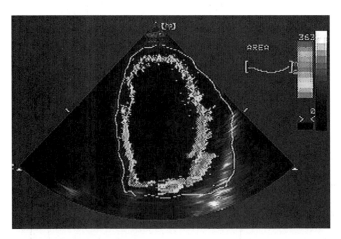

FIGURE 10-16. Color kinesis display of the left ventricular long axis. See also Color Insert.

Imaging for Etiology

Regional Systolic Function

Echocardiography, CMR, and radionuclide perfusion studies may all be used to evaluate regional wall motion abnormalities. Assessment of thickening and excursion of 16 individual left ventricular myocardial segments on transthoracic echocardiography allows clinical semiquantitative assessment of regional function. Echocardiographic border detection and color-coded display of endocardial motion may improve quantitation of regional wall function (Figure 10-16). Regional contraction and relaxation can also be measured by tissue Doppler, in which myocardial velocities correlate with the degree of fibrosis and β-adrenergic receptor density in ischemic ventricular dysfunction.[29] In addition, color tissue Doppler imaging permits resolution of the subendocardium from the subepicardium. Higher systolic velocity of the subendocardium in normal ventricles results in a myocardial velocity gradient, which is abolished or attenuated in the setting of ischemia and stunning.[29]

CMR techniques can precisely identify the location and severity of regional wall motion in three-dimensional space and assess regional wall stress and myocardial strain.

Acuity and Remodeling

Evaluation of left ventricular size and estimation of the acuity of the ischemic process are also important. Compensatory ventricular dilation and hypertrophy are important components of the remodeling that accompanies virtually all cases of myocardial infarction.[3] Monitoring ventricular chamber size thus permits assessment of this remodeling process and evaluation of the effectiveness of therapy with afterload reducing agents. Attenuation of the progressive ventricular dilation process after acute myocardial infarction has important, positive prognostic significance.[3]

Imaging for Prognosis and Therapy Direction

Myocardial Viability

In addition to the effects of impaired systolic function, ongoing ischemic damage has an adverse impact on long-term prognosis in ischemic cardiomyopathy. Evaluation of the extent of inducible and rest ischemia is required to determine the amount of myocardium that is salvageable by revascularization. Coronary bypass surgery is of greatest benefit with three-vessel disease and moderate LV dysfunction (EF, 35% to 50%). Surgical intervention for patients with demonstrable myocardial viability results in improved survival. Patients with ischemia or viability treated medically have a poor prognosis.

Positron emission tomography (PET) is the traditional "gold standard" for viability assessment but is restricted by expense and limited availability.[30] A perfusion tracer (^{13}N-ammonia) is used in conjunction with a metabolic marker (^{18}F-fluorodeoxyglucose) to highlight discrepancies between myocardial blood flow and metabolism.

Ischemic myocardium shifts to glucose as the principal energy substrate, and ^{18}F-fluorodeoxyglucose accumulates preferentially in hypoperfused but metabolically active and "viable" myocytes. ^{13}N-ammonia uptake is proportional to myocardial blood flow, and perfusion-metabolism "mismatch" detects segments of hibernating myocardium (Figure 10-17). Such flow-metabolism discordance accurately predicts functional recovery in hypocontractile areas and is reliable for predicting outcome of surgical revascularization.

Planar and single photon emission computed tomography (SPECT) imaging techniques are more widely available alternatives for detection of ischemia and viability. Intravenous ^{201}Tl initially distributes to the myocardium proportional to regional blood flow, followed 2.5 to 4 hours later by redistribution into jeopardized myocardial segments (rest-redistribution). Exercise-redistribution imaging allows evaluation of stress-induced ischemia. Another option is ^{99m}Tc-sestamibi, whose accumulation in the myocardium relies on preserved mitochondrial transmembrane electrochemical gradients. Reinjection is required, because ^{99m}Tc-sestamibi does not redistribute. For both ^{201}Tl and ^{99m}Tc agents, myocardial activity is inversely proportional to the extent of fibrotic replacement of the myocardial segment(s) of interest. Demonstration of ischemia, and not just viability, enhances predictive accuracy for functional recovery.[31]

Stunned or hibernating myocardium increases contractile function in response to low levels of inotropic stimulation with dobutamine. Echocardiographic detection of this contractile reserve predicts functional recovery after revascularization and improved survival in patients with ischemic left ventricular dysfunction.[32] The most specific response for predicting recovery of function after revascularization is the "biphasic" pattern, characterized by enhanced systolic function at low dobutamine doses, which disappears at higher doses.[33] A biphasic response predicts a high probability of functional recovery after revascularization in patients with ischemic left ventricular dysfunction.[33] Worsening of segmental motion at low doses predicts an intermediate chance of recovery, whereas segments with no change in contractility have the lowest likelihood of functional recovery. In addition, echocardiographic left ventricular wall thickness <6 mm indicates extensive transmural fibrotic replacement and nonviable myocardium (Figure 10-18), without potential for functional recovery.[34]

Contrast echocardiography and CMR are newer viability techniques. Echocardiographic contrast can evaluate perfusion at the microcirculatory level, with graded opacification of myocardium in proportion to the extent of blood flow.[35] Nonviable regions do not opacify with contrast because of destruction of the coronary microcirculation. Opacification of regions with preserved microvascular integrity occurs even when perfusion is markedly reduced and indicates viability.[35] Opacification with contrast predicts functional recovery of hypokinetic segments, but predictive accuracy is lower for akinetic regions. This reflects a distinction between microvascular integrity and contractile reserve as measures of myocardial viability. Use of contrast in dobutamine echocardiography may allow simultaneous assessment of both parameters.

CMR can assess coronary perfusion, contractile reserve, and cellular metabolism. Spin-echo or ultrafast CMR is used to measure perfusion, whereas cine CMR measures systolic wall thickening. Metabolic integrity is determined by magnetic resonance spectroscopy. Newer contrast-enhancement techniques can identify necrotic or fibrotic myocardium.[36] Hyperenhancement of nonviable myocardium with gadolinium quantitates and differentiates subendocardial from transmural fibrosis. CMR viability techniques have better prognostic reliability for functional recovery of akinetic and dyskinetic segments than nuclear scintigraphy and dobutamine echocardiography.[36]

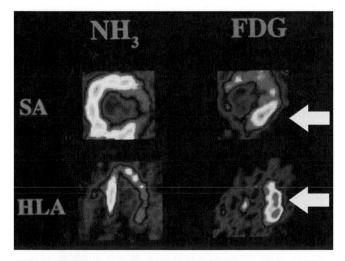

FIGURE 10-17. PET scan from a patient with angina and heart failure. Echocardiogram demonstrated LV ejection fraction of 30% with lateral akinesis. ^{18}F-fluorodeoxyglucose scan shows significant metabolic activity in the lateral wall *(arrow)*, but ^{13}N-ammonia uptake is minimal in this region. This perfusion-metabolism mismatch is consistent with hibernating myocardium. After redo bypass of the circumflex, LV ejection fraction increased to 65%, with return of lateral wall function (SA, short axis; HLA, horizontal long axis). (Courtesy of Luis Aruago, University of Pennsylvania.) See also Color Insert.

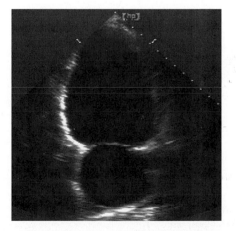

FIGURE 10-18. The inferior wall is significantly thinned (<6 mm) and echogenic on this apical two-chamber view *(arrow)*. This finding is consistent with scarred, nonviable myocardium.

Ischemic Mitral Regurgitation

Mitral regurgitation is common in ischemic cardiomyopathy. Papillary muscle rupture accounts for a minor proportion of mitral regurgitation but causes severe regurgitation that requires emergent surgical intervention (Figure 10-19). More typically, myocardial dysfunction of a papillary muscle results in leaflet tethering and malcoaptation. Posteromedial papillary dysfunction is most common because of its single coronary supply. Decreased posterior leaflet mobility results in an eccentric jet directed posteriorly into the atrium (Figure 10-1). Systolic dysfunction and cavity dilatation can result in functional mitral insufficiency similar to nonischemic heart failure.

Significant mitral regurgitation worsens prognosis in patients with ischemic cardiomyopathy. Postinfarction mitral regurgitation can be improved if LV enlargement and remodeling is attenuated by ACE inhibition.[37] In cases of established ischemic ventricular dilation and mitral regurgitation, valvular repair or replacement decreases volume overload, retards progression of ventricular dysfunction, and improves prognosis.[11] Transthoracic or transesophageal echocardiography can characterize the determinants of mitral regurgitation and assist in the choice of appropriate surgical strategy. Patients undergoing coronary bypass revascularization should be assessed for mitral repair or replacement. Interpapillary ventricular resection, infarct plication, chordal elongation, and annuloplasty may improve outcomes in these patients.

LV Thrombus

Intracavitary thrombi frequently complicate ischemic and nonischemic cardiomyopathies but are most common in akinetic or aneurysmal regions (Figure 10-20). Thrombi are a potential cardiac source of embolus and increase morbidity and mortality. On two-dimensional transthoracic echo, thrombus frequently appears hypoechoic compared with adjacent myocardium and may appear as a sessile mass or as a laminated crescent. Endocardial muscular trabeculations in the apical region may appear similar to thrombus (Figure 10-21). Systematic scanning of the apex and akinetic or aneurysmal regions is performed with a high-frequency, short-focus transducer, and diagnosis is based on thrombus visualization in orthogonal views. Frequently, spontaneous echocardiographic contrast is noted in the left ventricle or atrium. This accompanies severe reduction in cardiac output and increases the risk for future thrombus formation. The morphological appearance and mobility of the thrombus correlate with the likelihood of thromboembolism.

The left atrial appendage is also a site of thrombus formation, particularly in the context of atrial flutter or fibrillation. Transesophageal echocardiography is the

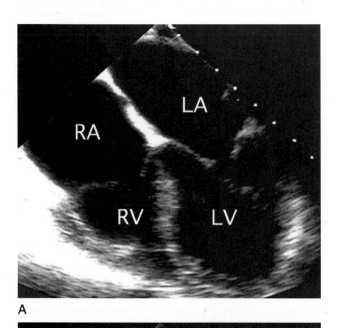

A

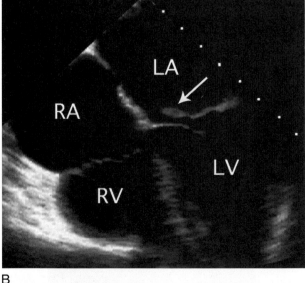

B

FIGURE 10-19. Four-chamber transesophageal views demonstrate the appearance of a ruptured posterior papillary muscle in diastole (**A**) and systole (**B**). The papillary muscle tip can be seen in the left atrium (*arrow*) during systole. This is typically associated with severe mitral regurgitation and represents a surgical emergency.

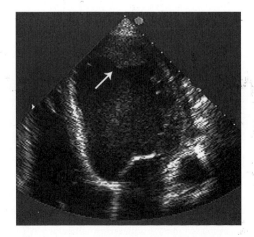

FIGURE 10-20. Sessile thrombus (*arrow*) is visualized in an area of akinesis and scarring in this chronic ischemic cardiomyopathy.

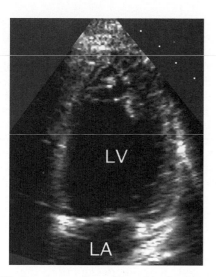

FIGURE 10-21. Prominent echocardiographic densities are noted in the apex of this ventricle and are consistent with LV apical myocardial trabeculations. In contrast to thrombus, these are more echodense and are present in a region of normal contractility.

modality of choice for exclusion of appendage-associated thrombus.

DIASTOLIC HEART FAILURE

Clinical findings of heart failure in the presence of normal LV systolic function mimic those of systolic failure. Morbidity from diastolic heart failure is similar to that seen in systolic failure.[2] Although mortality from diastolic heart failure has traditionally been considered lower than that from systolic failure, recently published 5-year mortality rates range from 24% to 40%. Diastolic heart failure is the most common reason for admission in patients older than the age of 65, with more deaths caused by diastolic heart failure in this group.[38]

Diagnostic Strategy

Identification of populations with diastolic heart failure has been difficult, and formal diagnostic criteria have only recently been proposed.[39,40] Confirmation of clinical congestive heart failure is the first priority (Table 10-2), because signs and symptoms are not specific.

■ ■ ■

TABLE 10-2 DIAGNOSTIC STRATEGIES FOR DIASTOLIC HEART FAILURE

RULE OUT OBVIOUS NONCARDIAC ETIOLOGIES OF SYMPTOMS

	Vasan & Levy[40]	European Society of Cardiology[39]
Symptoms and signs	Confirmed heart failure	Confirmed heart failure
Normal systolic function	EF ≥50%	EF ≥45%
Abnormal diastolic function	Hemodynamic	Hemodynamic Echocardiographic

Symptoms of noncardiac diseases (chronic obstructive pulmonary disease, obesity, and chronic venous insufficiency) might be mistaken for diastolic heart failure when LVEF is normal. In addition, valvular or ischemic heart disease might be present with congestive heart failure (CHF) and normal baseline systolic function. Pericardial diseases present with heart failure symptoms because of extrinsic diastolic constriction and should not be mistaken for intrinsic diastolic abnormality.

Once heart failure has been diagnosed, confirmation of normal left ventricular systolic function by angiographic ventriculography, echocardiography, or radionuclide blood pool scans is essential. Echocardiography is typically most helpful, because valve disease, ischemia, and pericardial disease can be ruled out simultaneously. Evaluation of heart failure at presentation is important to detect transient wall motion abnormalities or ischemic mitral regurgitation, which might be mistakenly attributed to diastolic dysfunction once resolved.[41]

Imaging of Diastolic Function

Accurate assessment of diastolic function is crucial because of the clinical impact of diastolic heart failure and the prevalence of clinically silent diastolic dysfunction. Despite underlying impaired myocardial relaxation, diastolic filling can be acutely altered by fluctuation of intravascular volume status, left atrial pressure, atrial compliance, and heart rate.

Cardiac Catheterization

Measurement of intracardiac hemodynamics during cardiac catheterization is the most reliable diagnostic assessment of diastolic function.[40] Plotting left ventricular pressure against simultaneous ventricular volume during the cardiac cycle allows precise demonstration of the abnormal features of the ventricular pressure-volume relationship. However, routine cardiac catheterization in the large population of elderly or hypertensive patients with suspected diastolic heart failure is neither cost-effective nor advisable.[40] Thus, in most cases, diastolic function is assessed noninvasively. Invasive hemodynamic assessment might be necessary in specific cases in the absence of obvious risk factors or clear noninvasive documentation of diastolic dysfunction. When appropriate, simultaneous coronary angiography may be useful to assess potential ischemic etiology of heart failure.

Echocardiography

Assessment of diastolic function by echocardiography has traditionally relied on Doppler measurements of LV inflow through the mitral valve (Figure 10-22).

Mitral Inflow Doppler

Several pulsed-wave Doppler parameters are useful for diastolic assessment. In normal cardiac physiology, the peak early filling velocity (E wave) is typically higher than the late peak filling velocity (A wave) (Figure 10-22).[42] Peak E and A-wave velocities are often expressed

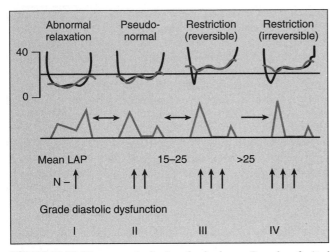

FIGURE 10-22. Diagrammatic display of pulsed-wave Doppler of mitral inflow patterns from the apical position. Normal diastolic filling is characterized by a velocity of the early filling wave of 0.8 to 1.0 cm/s, which is higher than the atrial wave velocity. **I,** Diastolic dysfunction pattern. The early filling wave velocity is lower than the A wave, and the deceleration time of the E wave has increased compared with normal **II,** Pseudonormalized pattern. Increased left atrial pressure results in increased early driving force for transmitral flow. The E wave again becomes prominent, despite impaired relaxation. **III,** and **IV,** Restrictive patterns. The E wave demonstrates a rapid deceleration time because of restrictive disease. The A wave is diminutive in this case because of atrial systolic failure. (Adapted from Tajik.) See also Color Insert.

as a ratio (E/A ratio), which is >1 in normal diastolic filling. The time required for early filling to terminate is measured from the peak of the E wave to its termination (deceleration time, DT) and ranges between 150 and 220 ms with normal ventricular relaxation.[43] Isovolumic relaxation time (IVRT) can be measured from the Doppler tracing as the time interval between cessation of LVOT outflow and the onset of the E wave and is 60 to 90 ms in normal subjects.[42] Although these parameters reflect underlying ventricular myocardial compliance, they are also dependent on afterload, preload, and heart rate.

In early stages of diastolic dysfunction, the volume of blood flow across the mitral inlet during early passive filling diminishes as a result of impaired ventricular relaxation, and a greater volume of blood crosses during atrial contraction. The E-wave Doppler velocity decreases, and A-wave velocity increases (Figure 10-22). This reversal of peak velocity between early and late filling stages (E/A ratio <1) is an echocardiographic hallmark of diastolic dysfunction. Impaired LV relaxation also results in prolonged isovolumic relaxation time of >100 ms.[42] This is typically an early indicator of diastolic dysfunction and precedes changes in E/A ratio. In addition, the deceleration time of the E wave becomes prolonged to >220 ms in early diastolic dysfunction.

Mitral diastolic peak inflow velocities and the E/A velocity ratio are sensitive to loading conditions, heart rate, and left atrial pressure. Progressive left atrial volume overload, dilation, and dysfunction result in left atrial pressure surpassing elevated ventricular diastolic pressure. Elevated atrial pressure provides enhanced driving force for early diastolic filling, with re-emergence of a higher velocity E wave and the E/A ratio returns to >1 (Figure 10-22). Increased atrial driving force also results in earlier onset of mitral inflow and shortening of IVRT to the "normal" range. The E-wave deceleration time also normalizes to <220 ms. Because of these changes, Doppler measurements of diastolic transmitral flow velocity can appear normal (pseudonormalization), despite the presence of advanced diastolic abnormalities of the left ventricle. The Valsalva maneuver can differentiate pseudonormalization of Doppler inflow from normal filling.[42] The first phase of the Valsalva maneuver diminishes left atrial preload, partially removing the atrial driving force. In patients with normal filling, the Doppler inflow pattern remains normal. In those with diastolic dysfunction, the pseudonormalized pattern reverts to a E/A <1 during Valsalva.

In advanced diastolic dysfunction, compliance and relaxation of the left ventricle are so diminished that minimal diastolic filling results in a marked rise in intracardiac pressures. Left atrial pressures are significantly increased in this circumstance, resulting in a high-velocity E wave. Duration of early filling is curtailed because of the rapid equilibration of atrial pressure and LV end-diastolic pressure (EDP). The E-wave deceleration time is typically very short, measuring <150 ms. Atrial contraction results in minimal increase in driving force, and flow during atrial systole is diminished. This "restrictive" inflow pattern is characterized by a high-velocity E wave and a relatively diminutive A wave (Figure 10-22). The IVRT is also very short, usually <60 ms.[42] Such restrictive filling is typically observed in amyloid and other infiltrative diseases but can also be present in end-stage hypertensive heart disease and hypertrophic cardiomyopathy.

Pulmonary Vein Flow Doppler

Pulmonary venous flow patterns complement mitral inflow pulse wave analysis and can help to distinguish between truly normal and pseudonormalized patterns. Pulmonary vein flow velocity is measured in the apical four-chamber view with pulse Doppler recording (Figure 10-23). Normal vein flow consists of prominent forward systolic flow, with two component waves (S_1,

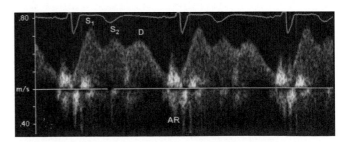

FIGURE 10-23. Normal pulmonary vein Doppler flow demonstrates two prominent systolic waves of forward flow (S_1, S_2) and a less prominent diastolic wave of forward flow (D). Reversal of flow occurs during atrial systole (AR). (Adapted from Tabata T, Thomas JD, Klein AL. Pulmonary venous flow by Doppler echocardiography: revisited 12 years later. *J Am Coll Cardiol* 2003; 41:1243.)

S_2) followed by a lower velocity diastolic forward flow (D), and subsequently a small degree of flow reversal back into the vein during atrial systole (AR) (Figure 10-23).[44] With normal ventricular systolic and diastolic function and normal left atrial (LA) pressure, the ratio of $S_{1,2}$/D is >1. When LA pressure is elevated, there is decreased filling of the left atrium from the pulmonary veins during ventricular systole, and the systolic velocity is reduced. A pattern resembling the E/A wave reversal in the mitral Doppler measurement occurs, the $S_{1,2}$/D ratio becomes <1, and the retrograde atrial component (AR) becomes more prominent and prolonged. Measured AR of > 35 cm/s is useful to distinguish pseudonormal mitral inflow.[44] Similar to the mitral valve (MV) inflow measurement, pulmonary venous flow is also load dependent, and the flow pattern may be altered by changes in heart rate, respiration, or with severe mitral regurgitation.

Tissue Doppler Imaging

Motion of the atrioventricular/annular plane toward and away from the apex of the heart during the cardiac cycle reflects myocardial fiber contraction and relaxation, respectively. Echocardiographic tissue Doppler imaging (TDI) measures the velocity of mitral annular motion (Figure 10-24). The early diastolic annular velocity (E') is measured in the apical four-chamber view with pulsed TDI of either the lateral or medial aspect of the mitral annulus. Because annular motion occurs away from the apex (and Doppler transducer), the direction of E' is opposite that of the E wave of the mitral inflow pattern. Normal velocity measurements of the medial annulus are 10 to 15 cm/s and 15 to 20 cm/s in the lateral annulus. Although measurement of medial mitral annular velocity is more accurate and reproducible, lateral mitral annular velocities are higher and easier to measure.[29]

Abnormally low velocity of annular motion is a reliable and reproducible indicator of intrinsic myocardial diastolic dysfunction, which is independent of loading conditions or left atrial pressure.[29] Annular velocities can differentiate normal from pseudonormal transmitral diastolic filling velocity patterns. Despite normalization of the E wave of mitral inflow with LA pressure elevation (and return of E/A to >1), the E' velocity remains low, reflecting persistently impaired myocardial relaxation underlying the pseudonormal mitral inflow pattern. The ratio of E-wave peak velocity to mitral annular early velocity (E/E') is typically <8 with normal diastolic function. The ratio remains unchanged in early diastolic dysfunction, because velocities of both E and E' decrease simultaneously. With superimposed atrial pressure overload and pseudonormalization of mitral inflow, E/E' typically exceeds 15.[29] The ratio increases further with advanced diastolic dysfunction and the onset of a restrictive filling pattern.

Abnormal TDI is a sensitive and clinically useful indicator of primary myocardial diastolic dysfunction, able to discriminate between physiological hypertrophy and pathological pressure overload hypertrophy and to identify individuals with preclinical hypertrophic cardiomyopathy.[45]

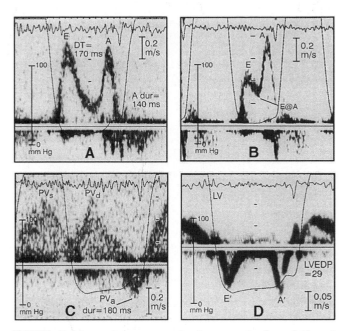

FIGURE 10-24. Simultaneous mitral inflow Doppler (**A** and **B**), pulmonary venous Doppler (**C**), and mitral annular tissue Doppler (**D**) from a patient with diastolic dysfunction and pseudonormalization of mitral inflow. Despite normal velocity of early filling and E/A ratio (*A*), the velocity of mitral annular early excursion (*E'*) is reduced (<8 cm/s). Valsalva maneuver results in abnormal mitral inflow (**B**), consistent with pseudonormalization. (Adapted from Ommen SR, Nishimura RA, Appleton CP, Miller FA, Oh JK, Redfield MM, Tajik AJ. Clinical utility of Doppler echocardiography and tissue Doppler imaging in the estimation of left ventricular filling pressures: a comparative simultaneous Doppler-catheterization study. (From *Circulation* 2000; 102:1788.)

Color Doppler M-Mode

During diastole, blood flow propagates along the long axis of the left ventricle toward the apex. Early diastolic inflow is first measurable at the mitral annulus and progresses distally in the ventricle. In the presence of impaired diastolic function, the propagation of this velocity wave through the ventricle is prolonged. Color Doppler displays a velocity map throughout the ventricular cavity from the base to the apex. Visualization of the color Doppler signal by M-mode tracing adds a temporal component, allowing precise velocity measurements over time.

Color Doppler of the diastolic inflow is assessed in the apical four-chamber view during M-mode recording (Figure 10-25). The Doppler/M-mode cursor is placed parallel to the central axis of ventricular diastolic flow as detected on two-dimensional color Doppler images. The slope of the first aliasing velocity (early filling) is measured from the mitral valve plane to a point approximately 4 cm distal in the left ventricular cavity. This slope of early diastolic flow is the diastolic "propagation velocity" (Vp, Figure 10-25), a measure of the propagation of the wave front of flow from the mitral leaflets to the left ventricular apex. In individuals with normal diastolic function, Vp is typically >45 cm/s. In the presence of early and advanced diastolic dysfunction, Vp becomes <45 cm/s and is a reliable indicator of underlying impaired myocardial relaxation.[46] The time delay (TD,

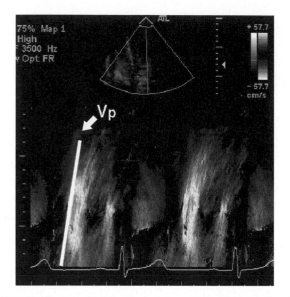

FIGURE 10-25. Color Doppler M-mode recording of mitral inflow. The normal early filling wave propagates rapidly toward the apex. The slope of the color signal demonstrated by the straight line on the second filling pattern is the velocity of propagation of early filling. Note that the velocity of the early wave is higher than the A wave and reaches farther into the LV cavity. See also Color Insert.

Figure 10-25) between the appearance of maximal early velocity at the mitral valve plane and at the apex represents an alternative measurement to Vp and is prolonged in cases of diastolic dysfunction.

Propagation velocity correlates with the LV relaxation time constant (τ, tau) in numerous disease states. Similar to tissue Doppler, the propagation velocity is load independent and is a useful adjunct to the load-dependent pulsed mitral inflow velocities. Although preload-independent, the propagation velocity can vary with differences in systolic function and end-systolic volume index.[47] Thus, propagation velocity must not be interpreted in isolation.

Alternative Imaging Techniques

In routine clinical cardiology practice, echocardiographic techniques provide some insight into underlying diastolic abnormalities. Synthesis of the data from two or more techniques may enhance the accuracy of diastolic assessment. Radionucleotide blood pool scans may also be used to assess diastolic filling, IVRT, and to determine the contribution of early rapid filling relative to diastolic filling as a whole. The radionuclide technique is limited in its inability to discern the LA-LV pressure gradient or to evaluate changes in LV pressure and volume during the diastolic phase.[48]

CMR offers numerous advantages to echocardiographic and other noninvasive modalities. Myocardial tagging allows detailed assessment of the complex diastolic untwisting motions (torsion) of myocardial relaxation. Longitudinal and radial elongation rates and wall thinning rates are reduced in the presence of diastolic myocardial abnormalities, independent of ventricular loading conditions.[49] Another advantage of CMR is the

ability to assess *regional* diastolic myocardial abnormalities, particularly useful in hypertrophic cardiomyopathy and ischemic heart disease.[49] Phase-contrast CMR measures blood flow velocity and pressure gradients between chambers. Volume flow for both mitral inflow and pulmonary veins can be measured accurately and correlates with analogous Doppler flow measurements in normal and abnormal diastolic function. Although determination of mitral and pulmonary venous flows is more accurate with CMR, assessment of diastole by means of CMR velocity/volume flow analysis is limited by the same preload dependence that affects echocardiographic Doppler assessments.

CARDIOVASCULAR IMAGING AFTER CARDIAC TRANSPLANTATION

Success of heart transplantation has improved over the past 20 years because of advances in immunosuppression and the early recognition and treatment of the long-term complications. Noninvasive and invasive imaging techniques have played important roles in improving outcomes for transplant patients. Echocardiography is vital for management, providing accurate assessment of graft function, evaluation of coronary artery disease, and rejection. Angiography has been the principal method for evaluating transplant-related coronary vasculopathy, but intravascular ultrasound (IVUS) continues to grow in use and has improved understanding of transplant-related vasculopathy. Newer nuclear and CMR technology offers promise to add to our knowledge of transplant biology and complement the technology available today. Because early and late postoperative periods have unique findings, imaging assessment of the transplanted heart varies during posttransplant phases.

Imaging in the Early Postoperative Period

Echocardiography

Early in the postoperative period, the left ventricle has increased mass and wall thickness and decreased cavity size, secondary to myocardial edema from reperfusion ischemic injury during organ preservation. Decreased cavity volume results from decreased vascular volume and preload and decreased ventricular compliance caused by reperfusion ischemic injury. LV wall motion is generally normal after transplantation, with the exception of the interventricular septum. Septal motion is paradoxical, with a rightward shift during systole, which may improve over time. The cause of abnormal septal motion is unclear, but it may be related to the anchoring of the heart to the thorax, pericardial disease or nonclosure, and conduction disturbances. Significant LV systolic dysfunction in this period is rare and should prompt the consideration of ischemic injury (secondary to poor preservation) or acute humoral rejection, which may require immediate and aggressive treatment.

Diastolic function in the early postoperative period is rarely normal. IVRT, the mitral valve pressure half time (MVP), and early mitral filling velocity have been used as measures of diastolic function. An initially restrictive filling pattern (Figure 10-22) is present, which evolves into a nonrestrictive pattern over the course of 6 weeks after operation. This reflects a decrease in filling pressures, decreased myocardial edema and stiffness, and improvement of diastolic function in the weeks after transplantation. Marked or persistent diastolic dysfunction correlates with a suboptimal clinical outcome and decreased long-term survival.[50]

The right ventricle (RV) is typically enlarged postoperatively but has normal function. RV hypertrophy may also be present. Dilation of the RV is primarily caused by preoperative pulmonary hypertension and elevated pulmonary vascular resistance, but ischemia and rejection may play a role in early RV dysfunction. Maximum RV enlargement occurs in the first month postoperatively and may take months to years to resolve, despite a return to normal pulmonary artery pressures and pulmonary resistance within several weeks. This may in part be explained by volume overload secondary to chronic tricuspid regurgitation. Substantial tricuspid regurgitation (TR) may be one explanation that RV function seems preserved despite elevated RV afterload. Significant RV systolic dysfunction after transplantation should raise suspicion of rejection, inadequate organ preservation, or prolonged warm ischemic times.

In patients with direct anastomosis of native and donor atria (the biatrial technique), the atria are enlarged and have an hourglass appearance (Figure 10-26). The suture lines appear as midchamber prominences or thickening and can be mistaken for an intracardiac mass. Turbulent flow may be seen across the anastomosis site, but frank obstruction is rare. In patients who have undergone a bicaval anastomosis, the right atrium is usually normal in appearance and dimension. There is little change in atrial anatomy over time. Case reports of spontaneous echo contrast or "smoke," a finding consistent with abnormal flow, have been reported, but the significance of this is unknown.[50]

TR is the major valvular lesion in transplant patients and seems to correlate with RV size. The degree of TR is typically more severe than mitral regurgitation and does not seem to be related to gender, endomyocardial biopsy (EMB) grade, hemodynamics, or time from transplant. Although the severity of regurgitation of all valves in the early transplant period is increased compared with that of donor age-matched controls, only TR causes symptoms. In some patients, TR may be related to distortion of the TV annulus from the surgical anastomosis and is worse in patients who have undergone biatrial anastomoses compared with those with the bicaval technique.[51] Mitral regurgitation is much less common than TR and usually not of hemodynamic significance. When it is present, distortion of the MV annulus secondary to the left atrial anastomosis or a primary abnormality of the valve should be considered. Aortic and pulmonic regurgitation are generally mild in nature and decrease with time.

A pericardial effusion is present in up to 50% of posttransplant patients but usually resolves spontaneously. On rare occasions, cardiac tamponade develops, and drainage is required. Effusions may be related to myocardial rejec-

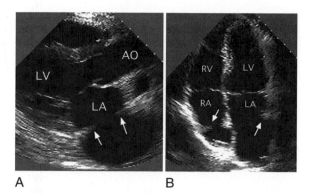

FIGURE 10-26. A, Parasternal long axis view showing the left ventricle (LV), aorta (AO), left atrium (LA), and mitral valve (star). The arrows indicate the LA anastomosis site. Note that the size of the recipient LA is larger than that of the donor. B, Apical four chamber view showing marked biatrial (LA, RA) enlargement and mild right ventricular (RV) enlargement. The arrows mark the sites of atrial anastomosis.

tion but more typically are secondary to postoperative bleeding or mismatches between donor heart size and recipient pericardial size.

In the early posttransplant period, imaging through the thorax is sometimes severely limited by poststernotomy changes, hyperinflation of the lungs, chest tubes, and other limitations to imaging. In these cases, transesophageal echocardiography provides valuable imaging information for assessment of posttransplant structure and function, especially when transthoracic echocardiography is technically limited.

Imaging in the Late Postoperative Period
Echocardiography

Data on long-term echocardiographic follow-up of transplant patients is limited and inconsistent, with little information on survivors of cardiac transplantation beyond 5 to 10 years. Persistent increase in LV mass is present in many transplant patients, correlating with postoperative blood pressure and cyclosporine levels.[50] Adjustment for body surface area, obesity, and donor-recipient size mismatch normalizes increase in LV mass in many patients. Systolic function usually remains normal long after transplant, and abnormalities raise concern for rejection or the development of transplant-related coronary artery disease (CAD) and ischemia. The RV remains dilated in 50% of patients for an extended time after transplantation. Wall thickness is also increased by approximately 50%. Despite these dimensional changes, fractional area change and function are comparable to normal individuals.

Tricuspid regurgitation tends to decrease over time as early postoperative intracardiac and pulmonary vascular hemodynamics return toward normal. However, the severity of TR can increase with time, especially when chronic, severe RV dysfunction develops. Iatrogenic TR is caused by damage to the tricuspid leaflets, chordal apparatus, and papillary muscles at the time of EMB (Figure 10-27). The degree of regurgitation can be hemodynamically significant and clinically evident and may require replacement or repair of the valve.

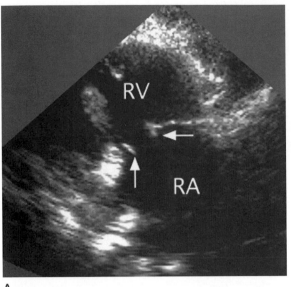

A

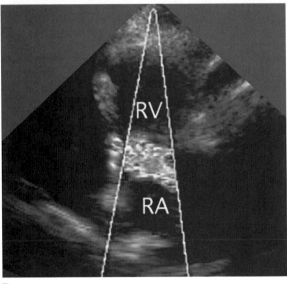

B

FIGURE 10-27. A, Parasternal right ventricular inflow view demonstrates a perforation in the septal leaflet of the tricuspid valve in a heart transplant recipient *(arrows)*. This was likely the result of injury during attempted right ventricular endomyocardial biopsy **(B).** The perforation results in a wide-based color Doppler jet of tricuspid regurgitation. See also Color Insert.

Angiography

The most vexing and difficult long-term complication of cardiac transplantation is accelerated coronary arteriopathy. Moderate to severe proximal or midvessel disease by angiography predicts a mortality of up to 50% in 2 years. Transplant-related CAD is multifactorial, including risk factors of donor age, time from transplant, donor undersize, donor smoking history, white race, rejection, cytomegalovirus infection, and triglyceride levels.

Angiography has been the "gold standard" for the detection of coronary disease in both transplant and nontransplant patients. Although angiography is the test of choice for epicardial vessel flow-limiting stenoses, transplant-related CAD is not a focal epicardial disease. It is typically a diffuse process of intimal thickening that does not initially affect luminal diameter at the epicardial vessel level. Rather, flow is limited in vessels not seen on angiography, which may be undetected for prolonged periods of time, delaying its diagnosis and treatment. Clinically significant CAD can occur suddenly and progress rapidly, leading to infarcts in major epicardial vessels or ischemia in the microcirculation.

With the advent of IVUS, angiography is no longer the "gold standard" for the detection of CAD in transplant patients. The sensitivity and specificity of angiography in the detection of moderate to severe intimal thickening may be at best 64% and 81%, respectively.[52] Luminal irregularities reported as noncritical or insignificant on angiography may represent severe transplant vasculopathy characterized by intimal thickening that is only appreciated on IVUS examination. Although detection of epicardial CAD is correlated with decreased survival, a normal angiogram does not indicate lack of CAD.

IVUS

IVUS provides important information for the understanding of CAD in the post-transplant population, with high-resolution images of the arterial wall and lumen that help to characterize plaque size and content (Figures 10-28 and 10-29). What was previously seen only at autopsy or organ explantation can now be directly visualized in the catheterization laboratory. The risks of IVUS are similar to that of angiography with bleeding (anticoagulation is usually administered for the procedure), coronary dissection, and coronary spasm.

IVUS is more sensitive than angiography and has been an integral part of the evaluation of the extent and natural history of CAD in heart transplant recipients. In one study, IVUS of the left anterior descending artery demonstrated negligible intimal proliferation within 1 month of transplant.[53] At 1 year after transplantation, all patients had at least mild intimal thickening (28% moderate, 35% severe), yet 72% had normal angiograms.[53] Most patients 1 year after orthotopic heart transplantation (OHT) have evidence of intimal thickening, and luminal narrowing can occur with the first year.

The detection of intimal smooth muscle cell proliferation by IVUS predicts future angiographically evident CAD.[52] Serial IVUS studies show progression of intimal thickness over time in some patients, with calcification of plaques after several years. Studies early in the transplant course reveal an eccentric plaque morphology indicative of preexisting atherosclerosis, whereas later studies (more than 1 year after transplantation) show a more diffuse concentric intimal thickening and homogeneous distribution of plaque, suggesting a combination of preexisting disease and transplant-related process.

The degree of intimal thickening also seems to have a strong effect on outcome. An intimal thickness of greater than 0.3 mm correlates with suboptimal clinical outcome, regardless of the angiographic findings, and this is independent of time from transplant or prevalence of rejection episodes. The presence of severe intimal thickening increases the risk of severe vasculopathy developing fourfold, whereas a normal IVUS predicts freedom from angiographic disease.[52]

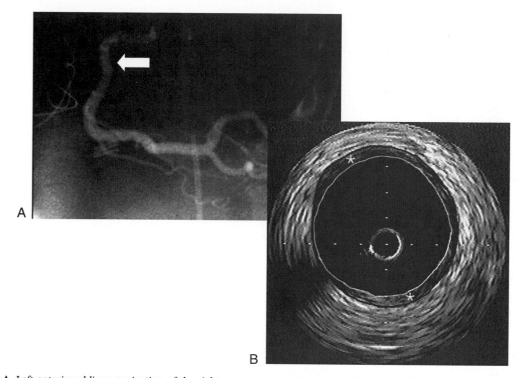

FIGURE 10-28. A, Left anterior oblique projection of the right coronary artery in a patient 1 year after heart transplant. The arrow indicates the area of the IVUS image of Figure. There is no significant lesion seen throughout the vessel's course, despite the IVUS abnormalities seen. **B,** IVUS image of the right coronary artery seen in A. There is moderate intimal thickening and proliferation (borders outlined by circular lines and marked by asterisks), despite a nearly normal angiographic appearance. The maximal intimal dimension is 0.4 mm. (Courtesy of Robert Wilensky, University of Pennsylvania.)

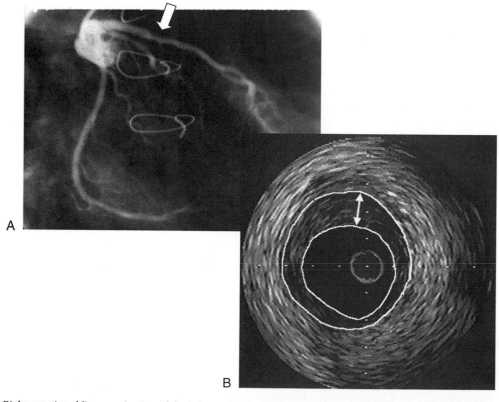

FIGURE 10-29. A, Right anterior oblique projection of the left anterior descending and left circumflex vessels. The arrow indicates the area of the IVUS image B. Note the diffuse luminal narrowing of the LAD and the small caliber and paucity of branch vessels. **B,** IVUS of the left anterior descending artery seen in A, showing marked intimal thickening and proliferation, the borders of which are outlined by the circular lines. The maximal thickness *(at the arrow)* is 1.5 mm. Each calibration mark measures 1 mm. (Courtesy of Robert Wilensky, University of Pennsylvania.)

Stress Echocardiography

Noninvasive detection of accelerated transplant-related coronary arteriopathy is of great interest, given the severe, delayed impact on the posttransplant patient. Exercise echocardiography has low sensitivity but good specificity compared with angiography that uses simultaneous IVUS.[54] There is a high false-negative rate for those with moderate disease (40% to 69% stenosis). False-positive echocardiograms in patients without a critical stenosis may correlate with the presence of mild-to-moderate intimal proliferation. The angiogram underestimates the extent of disease and is unable to detect small-vessel disease that could cause an abnormal stress test (secondary to impaired endothelial function and coronary flow reserve).

In many institutions, the primary noninvasive tool for coronary disease in transplant patients is the dobutamine stress echocardiogram (DSE). Similar to exercise echo, it may overestimate the presence of angiographically evident CAD. Sensitivity and specificity range from 72% to 86% and 80% to 91%, respectively.[54] A positive DSE study, characterized by a new reversible wall motion abnormality with stress, LV cavity dilation, marked diastolic dysfunction, or increased mitral regurgitation, predicts death or graft failure. Patients with persistent wall motion abnormalities during stress have a significantly increased risk of adverse cardiovascular events. A negative DSE is associated with a low cardiac event rate and predicts excellent intermediate-length survival.[54] Stress echocardiography can be positive without angiographically apparent CAD but with evidence of intimal thickening on IVUS imaging.

Nuclear Imaging

Nuclear imaging techniques have played a limited role in the clinical imaging of transplanted hearts, but perfusion studies may be useful for evaluation of ischemia and transplant-related CAD. Thallium scintigraphy has been shown to have a specificity of up to 100% and sensitivity of approximately 70% to 80% in the detection of lesions with a $\geq$50% luminal stenosis, and patients with a negative study have an excellent intermediate event-free survival. Lower observed specificity of 33% in one study was ascribed to factors such as rejection, myocardial edema, and inflammation creating false-positive results.[55] Thallium scintigraphy does not correlate with intimal thickening, because this diffuse process creates small-vessel ischemia and balanced perfusion on imaging.

On the basis of clinical signs and symptoms of ischemia that long-term survivors develop, it has long been presumed that the nerves innervating native heart, severed at the time of transplant, grow to reinnervate the transplanted heart. Nuclear techniques have provided important proof of reinnervation of the posttransplant heart. Studies using ^{123}I-metaiodobenzylguanidine (^{123}I-MIBG), a norepinephrine analog that is taken up by myocardial sympathetic nerves, have provided proof of sympathetic reinnervation.[56] Reinnervation begins within the first year or two after transplantation, precedes functional recovery of the nerve itself, takes greater than one decade to complete, and may occur less frequently in patients with a history of idiopathic dilated cardiomyopathy.

CMR

CMR is a useful tool in evaluating transplanted heart function, hypertrophy, and pericardial disease. Transplanted hearts demonstrate increases in LV mass with decreases in LV wall stress and wall stress/volume ratios on CMR, indicating a reduced contractile state in transplanted hearts after transplantation. CMR studies on atria have shown lower stroke volumes, volume changes, and filling rates in hearts with biatrial anastamoses.[57] Last, CMR angiography has revolutionized peripheral vascular disease imaging, but its application to evaluate CAD in transplant patients has been limited by low sensitivity, specificity, and negative and positive predictive values for certain vessels (i.e., LAD and LCx) and the inability to detect distal lesions in most vessels.

Imaging Techniques to Detect Myocardial Rejection

Rejection is an omnipresent complication of heart transplantation, and most patients will have at least one episode of rejection requiring treatment during the course of their graft survival. Surveillance for rejection is a major part of the patient's postoperative care. The "gold standard" for the detection of rejection is histopathological examination of tissue obtained by EMB. This procedure is performed frequently in the early (first year) postoperative period, but, in the absence of rejection, the frequency decreases significantly over time. A histological grading scale for cellular rejection takes into account the extent of lymphocytic infiltrate (focal or diffuse), the intensity of infiltration, and the presence or absence of myocyte necrosis, edema, and hemorrhage (Table 10-3). EMB is expensive, invasive, and carries the risks of vascular damage, tricuspid valve trauma, and right ventricular perforation. It is subject to sampling errors and may

■ ■ ■

TABLE 10-3 INTERNATIONAL SOCIETY OF HEART AND LUNG TRANSPLANTATION ENDOMYOCARDIAL BIOPSY GRADING SCHEME

Grade	Histological findings
0	Normal myocardium
1A	Focal lymphocytic infiltrate without necrosis
1B	Diffuse but sparse lymphocytic infiltrate without necrosis
2	One focus only of aggressive lymphocytic infiltrate and/or focal myocyte necrosis
3A	Multiple areas of aggressive infiltration and/or myocyte necrosis
3B	Diffuse lymphocytic infiltration with necrosis
4	Diffuse, aggressive, and polymorphous infiltration with necrosis (edema, hemorrhage, or vasculitis may be present)

From The International Society of Heart Transplantation. A working formulation for the standardization of nomenclature in the diagnosis of heart and lung rejection: Heart Rejection Group. *J Heart Transplant* 1990; 9(6): 587.

not detect focal rejection or rejection in areas outside the interventricular septum. The ideal mechanism for the detection of rejection would be a test of high specificity and sensitivity, ease of use, low cost, accessibility, and noninvasive design.

Echocardiography

Changes in LV systolic function, LV mass, and indices of diastolic function are all potentially useful noninvasive markers of rejection. Ventricular systolic function usually remains normal with mild to moderate rejection, and LV systolic dysfunction is consistent with severe rejection.[50] For this reason, echocardiographic assessment of systolic function cannot be used to detect or rule out most episodes of rejection. Ventricular mass and wall thickness also increase during rejection episodes and resolve with treatment.[50] Chronic cyclosporine therapy minimizes changes in mass and thickness, which have become less sensitive markers of rejection.

Changes in diastolic parameters are more useful echocardiographic parameters for detection of rejection. Late appearance of a restrictive filling pattern (Figure 10-22, C) is associated with a high incidence of rejection.[50] Abnormally short IVRT or low Vp and abnormally high early E-wave velocity occur with rejection. These measurements are more difficult to interpret when baseline diastolic function is abnormal without rejection. Significant decreases in IVRT and Vp followed serially occur with rejection, but individual changes are often within range of spontaneous variation observed in the absence of rejection. The filling pattern in an individual patient should be documented in the absence of rejection, and a subsequent intrapatient comparison made to detect abnormalities. Overall, the sensitivity of these Doppler findings is poor to fair, and their specificity is at best 80%. By use of a decrease of 15% in IVRT as a marker of grade 3 rejection, sensitivity and specificity are 22% and 73%, respectively. Using intrapatient changes in Vp and peak E-wave velocity, sensitivity and specificity are 59% and 74% for Vp and 47% and 83% for E-wave velocity.[58]

It remains to be seen whether newer echocardiographic techniques, including tissue Doppler, acoustic quantification, and automatic border detection, will offer any additional benefit for the noninvasive assessment of rejection.

Nuclear Imaging

Nuclear imaging for the detection of rejection has focused primarily on the use of ^{111}In-labeled antimyosin antibody (Figure 10-7). Extracellular myosin after transplantation is a marker of cell damage secondary to rejection.[14] Indium-labeled antimyosin scanning has a negative predictive value of 98% and a positive predictive value of 16%. The high negative predictive value and specificity indicate the potential clinical usefulness of a negative antimyosin scan in avoiding the need for repeated biopsies. The lack of technical expertise in the use of the antibody and skill in the interpretation of this technique has limited its wider application.

CMR

Investigation of CMR for detection of myocardial rejection has been limited to animal studies, focusing on LV structure, increased myocardial enhancement, prolonged relaxation times, and myocardial phosphate content. As seen on echocardiography, increases in LV mass and wall thickness can be detected on CMR during episodes of rejection. Increase in mass correlates with the histological grade of rejection. Ventricular wall thickness is greater in patients with evidence of rejection on EMB compared with normal volunteers, nonrejecting patients, and those with resolving rejection. Increased myocardial enhancement in transplanted animal hearts with biopsy-documented rejection has been shown by several investigators.[59] In human subjects, there is less enhancement in those without rejection but no significant difference in enhancement between those with mild, moderate, or severe rejection. The limited data that are available suggest that CMR is a highly sensitive technique for the detection of rejection, but this may be at the expense of specificity. Myocardial relaxation can be evaluated with T2-weighted scanning. Few small studies have shown prolonged relaxation in patients with rejection and little or no difference between those without rejection and normal controls, but this aspect of imaging in transplant patients remains unclear.

Magnetic resonant spectroscopy (MRS) is an area of CMR technology that has been applied to detect myocardial rejection, but, like other aspects of transplant CMR, the available data are limited. It relies on the detection of high-energy phosphates (adenosine triphosphate, phosphocreatinine) that are critical to tissue metabolism. A decrease in these organic phosphates and an increase in inorganic phosphates suggest cellular damage. In animal studies, phosphate MRS correlates with EMB results and may differentiate between ischemic injury and rejection.[60]

REFERENCES

1. Kannel WB. Vital epidemiologic clues in heart failure. *J Clin Epidemiol* 2000; 53:229.
2. Kitzman DW, Little WC, Brubaker PH, Anderson RT, Hundley WG, Marburger CT, Morgan TM, Stewart KP. Pathophysiological characterization of isolated diastolic heart failure in comparison to systolic heart failure. *JAMA* 2002; 288:2144.
3. St John Sutton M, Sharpe N. Left ventricular remodeling after myocardial infarction: pathophysiology and therapy. *Circulation* 2000; 101:2981.
4. Wynne J, Braunwald E. The cardiomyopathies and myocarditides, in Braunwald E, Zipes DP, Libby P (eds): *Heart Disease*, ed 6, Philadelphia: W.B. Saunders, 2001, p 1751.
5. Corrado D, Basso C, Thiene G. Arrhythmogenic right ventricular cardiomyopathy: diagnosis, prognosis, and treatment. *Heart* 2000; 83:588.
6. Kitzman DW, Gardin JM, Gottdeiner JS, Arnold A, Boineau R, Aurigemma G, Marino EK, Lyles M, Cushman M, Enright PL. Importance of heart failure with preserved systolic function in patients >65 years of age. *Am J Cardiol* 2001; 87:413.
7. Varagic J, Susic D, Frohlich E. Heart, aging, and hypertension. *Curr Opin Cardiol* 2001; 16:336.
8. Maron BJ. Hypertrophic cardiomyopathy. *Lancet* 1997; 350:127.
9. Danias PG, Ahlberg AW, III BAC. Combined assessment of myocardial perfusion and left ventricular function with exercise tech-

netium-99m sestamibi gated single-photon emission computed tomography can differentiate between ischemic and nonischemic dilated cardiomyopathy. *Am J Cardiol* 1998; 82:1253.

10. Yiu SF, Enriquez-Sarano M, Tribouilloy C, Seward JB, Tajik AJ. Determinants of the degree of functional mitral regurgitation in patients with systolic left ventricular dysfunction: a quantitative clinical study. *Circulation* 2000; 102:1400.

11. Enriquez-Sarano M. Timing of mitral valve surgery. *Heart* 2002; 87:79.

12. Palka P, Macdonald G, Lange A, Burstow DJ. The role of Doppler left ventricular filling indexes and Doppler tissue echocardiography in the assessment of cardiac involvement in hereditary hemochromatosis. *J Am Soc Echocardiogr* 2002; 15:884.

13. Fattori R, Rocchi G, Celletti F, Bertaccini P, Rapezzi C, Gavelli G. Contribution of magnetic resonance imaging in the differential diagnosis of cardiac amyloidosis and symmetric hypertrophic cardiomyopathy. *Am Heart J* 1998; 136:824.

14. Yasuda T. Detection of disruption of sarcolemmal membrane by indium-111 labeled antimyosin antibody scan, in Figulla et al eds): *Idiopathic Dilated Cardiomyopathy.* New York, Springer-Verlag, 1993.

15. Qin JX, Jones M, Shiota T, et al. Validation of real-time three-dimensional echocardiography for quantifying left ventricular volumes in the presence of a left ventricular aneurysm: in vitro and in vivo studies. *J Am Coll Cardiol* 2000; 36:900.

16. St John Sutton M, Plappert T, Abraham W, Smith A, DeLurgio D, Leon A, Loh E, Kocovic D, Fisher W, Ellestad M, Messenger J, Kruger K, Hilpisch K, Hill M. Effect of cardiac resynchronization therapy on left ventricular size and function in chronic heart failure. *Circulation* 2003; 107:1985.

17. Koilpillai C, Quinones MA, Greenberg B, Limacher MC, Schindler D, Pratt CM, Benedict CR, Kopelen H, Shelton B. Relation of ventricular size and function to heart failure status and ventricular dysrhythmia in patients with severe left ventricular dysfunction. *Am J Cardiol* 1996; 77:606.

18. Benjamin EJ, Levy D. Why is left ventricular hypertrophy so predictive of morbidity and mortality? *Am J Med Sci* 1999; 317:168.

19. Quinones MA, Greenberg BH, Kopelen HA, et al. Echocardiographic predictors of clinical outcome in patients with left ventricular dysfunction enrolled in the SOLVD registry and trials: significance of left ventricular hypertrophy. *J Am Coll Cardiol* 2000; 35:1237.

20. Grossman W. Evaluation of systolic and diastolic function of the ventricles and myocardium, in Baim DS, Grossman W (eds): *Grossman's Cardiac Catheterization, Angiography, and Intervention,* ed 6, Philadelphia, Lippincott Williams & Wilkins, 2000, p 367.

21. Leotta E, Patejunas G, Murphy G, JSzokol, McGregor L, Carbray J, Hamawy A, Winchester D, Hackett N, Crystal R, Rosengart T. Gene therapy with adenovirus-mediated myocardial transfer of vascular endothelial growth factor 121 improves cardiac performance in a pacing model of congestive heart failure. *J Thorac Cardiovasc Surg* 2002; 123:1101.

22. Kolias TJ, Aaronson KD, Armstrong WF. Doppler-derived dP/dt and -dP/dt predict survival in congestive heart failure. *J Am Coll Cardiol* 2000; 36:1594.

23. Kim IS, Izawa H, Sobue T, Ishihara H, Somura F, Nishizawa T, Nagata K, Iwase M, Yokota M. Prognostic value of mechanical efficiency in ambulatory patients with idiopathic dilated cardiomyopathy in sinus rhythm. *J Am Coll Cardiol* 2002; 39:1264.

24. Cappola TP, Felker GM, Kao WHL, Hare JM, Baughman KL, Kasper EK. Pulmonary hypertension and risk of death in cardiomyopathy: patients with myocarditis are at higher risk. *Circulation* 2002; 105:1663.

25. Tenderich G, Koerner M, Stuettgen B, Mirow N, Arusoglu L, Morshuis M, Bairaktaris A, Minami K, Koerfer R. Pre-existing elevated pulmonary vascular resistance: long-term hemodynamic follow-up and outcome of recipients after orthotopic heart transplantation. *J Cardiovasc Surg* 2000; 41:215.

26. Lindelow B, Andersson B, Waagstein F, Bergh CH. High and low pulmonary vascular resistance in heart transplant candidates. A 5-year follow-up after heart transplantation shows continuous reduction in resistance and no difference in complication rate. *Eur Heart J* 1999; 20:148.

27. Ghio S, Gavazzi A, Campana C, Inserra C, Klersy C, Sebastiani R, Arbustini E, Recusani F, Tavazzi L. Independent and additive prognostic value of right ventricular systolic function and pulmonary artery pressure in patients with chronic renal failure. *J Am Coll Cardiol* 2001; 37:183.

28. Zornoff LAM, Skali H, Pfeffer MA, Sutton MSJ, Rouleau JL, Lamas GA, Plappert T, Rouleau JR, Moye LA, Lewis SJ, Braunwald E, Solomon SD. Right ventricular dysfunction and risk of heart failure and mortality after myocardial infarction. *J Am Coll Cardiol* 2002; 39:1450.

29. Waggoner AD, Bierig SM. Tissue Doppler imaging: a useful echocardiographic method to assess systolic and diastolic ventricular function. *J Am Soc Echocardiogr* 2001; 14:1143.

30. Wiggers H, Botker H, Sogaard P, Kaltoft A, Hermansen F, Kim W, Krusell L, Thuesen L. Electromechanical mapping versus positron emission tomography and single photon emission computed tomography for the detection of myocardial viability in patients with ischemic cardiomyopathy. *J Am Coll Cardiol* 2003; 41:843.

31. Kitsiou AN, Srinivasan G, Quyyumi AA, Summers RM, Bacharach SL, Dilsizian V. Stress-induced reversible and mild-moderate irreversible thallium defects: are they equally accurate for predicting recovery of regional left ventricular function after revascularization? *Circulation* 1998; 98:501.

32. Chaudhry FA, Tauke JT, Alessandrini RS, Vardi G, Parker MA. Prognostic implications of myocardial contractile reserve in patients with coronary artery disease and left ventricular dysfunction. *J Am Coll Cardiol* 1999; 34:730.

33. Afridi I, Kleiman NS, Raizner AE, Zoghbi WA. Dobutamine echocardiography in myocardial hibernation. Optimal dose and accuracy in predicting recovery of ventricular function after coronary angioplasty. *Circulation* 1995; 91:663.

34. Cwajg JM, Cwajg E, Nagueh SF, He ZX, Qureshi U, et al. End-diastolic wall thickness as a predictor of recovery of function in myocardial hibernation. *J Am Coll Cardiol* 2000; 35:1152.

35. Colonna P, Cadeddu C, Chen L, Iliceto S. Clinical applications of contrast echocardiography. *Am Heart J* 2001; 141:S36.

36. Poon M, Fuster V, Fayad Z. Cardiac magnetic resonance imaging: a "one-stop-shop" evaluation of myocardial dysfunction. *Curr Opin Cardiol* 2002; 17:663.

37. Otsuji Y, Handschumacher MD, Liel-Cohen N, Tanabe H, Jiang L, et al. Mechanism of ischemic mitral regurgitation with segmental left ventricular dysfunction: three-dimensional echocardiographic studies in models of acute and chronic progressive regurgitation. *J Am Coll Cardiol* 2001; 37:641.

38. Gottdiener JS, McClelland RL, Marshall R, Shemanski L, Furberg CD, Kitzman DW, Chusman M, Polak J, Gardin JM, Gersh BJ, Aurigemma GP, Manolio TA. Outcome of congestive heart failure in elderly persons: influence of left ventricular systolic function. *Ann Intern Med* 2002; 137:631.

39. Remme WJ, Swedberg K. Guidelines for the diagnosis and treatment of chronic heart failure: task force for the diagnosis and treatment of chronic heart failure, European Society of Cardiology. *Eur Heart J* 2001; 22:1527.

40. Vasan RS, Levy D. Defining diastolic heart failure: a call for standardized diagnostic criteria. *Circulation* 2000; 101:2118.

41. Gandhi SK, Powers JC, Nomeir AM, Fowle K, Kitzman DW, Rankin KM, Little WC. The pathogenesis of acute pulmonary edema associated with hypertension. *N Engl J Med* 2001; 344:17.

42. Ommen SR. Echocardiographic assessment of diastolic function. *Curr Opin Cardiol* 2001; 16:240.

43. Appleton CP, Hatle LK, Popp RL. Relation of transmitral flow velocity patterns to left ventricular diastolic function: new insights from a combined hemodynamic and Doppler echocardiographic study. *J Am Coll Cardiol* 1988; 12:426.

44. Tabata T, Thomas J, Klein A. Pulmonary venous flow by Doppler echocardiography; revisited 12 years later. *J Am Coll Cardiol* 2003; 41:1243.

45. Ho CY, Sweitzer NK, McDonough B, Maron BJ, Casey SA, Seidman JG, Seidman CE, Solomon SD. Assessment of diastolic function with Doppler tissue imaging to predict genotype in preclinical hypertrophic cardiomyopathy. *Circulation* 2002; 105:2992.

46. Garcia MJ, Thomas JD, Klein AL. New Doppler echocardiographic applications for the study of diastolic function. *J Am Coll Cardiol* 1998; 32:865.

47. Barbier P, Grimaldi A, Alimento M, Berna G, Guazzi MD. Echocardiographic determinants of mitral early flow propagation velocity. *Am J Cardiol* 2002; 90:613.

48. Mandinov L, Eberli FR, Seiler C, Hess OM. Diastolic heart failure. *Cardiovasc Res* 2000; 45:813.

49. Paelinck B, Lamb H, Bax J, VanderWall E, deRoos A. Assessment of diastolic function by cardiovascular magnetic resonance. *Am Heart J* 2002; 144:198.

50. Burgess M, Bhattacharyya A, SG R. Echocardiography after cardiac transplantation. *J Am Soc Echocardiogr* 2002; 15:917.

51. Kavarana MN, Sinha P, Williams MR, Barbone A, Malhotra SM, Naka Y, Mancini DM, Edwards NM. Bicaval or biatrial technique for orthotopic heart transplant. *Circulation* 2000; 102:489.

52. Young J. Perspectives on cardiac allograft vasculopathy. *Curr Atheroscler Rep* 2000; 2:259.

53. St. Goar FG, et al. Intracoronary ultrasound in cardiac transplant recipients. In vivo evidence of "angiographically silent" intimal thickening. *Circulation* 1992; 85:979.

54. Konig A, Spes C, Schiele T, Rieber J, Stempfle H, Meiser B, Theisen K, Mudra H, Reichart B, Klauss V. Coronary Doppler measurements do not predict progression of cardiac allograft vasculopathy: analysis by serial intracoronary Doppler, dobutamine stress echocardiography and intracoronary ultrasound. *J Heart Lung Transplant* 2002; 21:902.

55. Howarth DM, et al. Evaluation of 201 Tl SPECT myocardial perfusion imaging in the detection of coronary artery disease after orthotopic heart transplantation. *Nucl Med Commun* 1996; 17:105.

56. Estorch M, et al. Sympathetic reinnervation of cardiac allografts evaluated by 123-I-MIBG imaging. *J Nucl Med* 1999; 40:911.

57. Laurema K, et al. Assessment of right and left atrial function in patients with transplanted hearts with the use of magnetic resonance imaging. *J Heart Lung Transplant* 1996; 15:360.

58. Holzmann G, et al. Usefulness of left ventricular infow Doppler in predicting rejection in pediatric cardiac transplant recipients. *Am J Cardiol* 1994; 73:205.

59. Johansson L, Johansson C, Penno E, Bjornerud A, Ahlstrom H. Acute cardiac transplant rejection: detection and grading with MR imaging with a blood pool contrast agent: experimental study in the rat. *Radiology* 2002; 225:97.

60. Buchthal S, Noureuil T, denHollander J, Bourge R, Kirklin J, Katholi C, Caulfeld J, Prohost G, Evanochko W. 31P-magnetic resonance spectroscopy study of cardiac transplant patients at rest. *J Cardiovasc Magn Reson* 2000; 2:51.

chapter 11

Valvular Heart Disease

Susan E. Wiegers
Howard C. Herrmann
Ted Plappert
Martin G. St. John Sutton

The prevalence of valvular heart disease varies geographically and socioeconomically. Rheumatic valvular heart disease has diminished in the United States and Western Europe over the past two decades but remains a major cause of cardiovascular mortality and morbidity in developing countries. Degenerative valve diseases involving the aortic and mitral valves, including senile calcific aortic stenosis, mitral valve prolapse, and ischemic mitral regurgitation, have increased proportionately as the average life expectancy has increased. Recent advances in imaging technology have facilitated earlier diagnosis of valvular heart disease in asymptomatic patients and have characterized the changes associated with transition from asymptomatic to symptomatic valvular heart disease. Noninvasive imaging and invasive imaging have not replaced the need for careful clinical examination of the cardiovascular system but provide methods for unequivocal diagnosis of valve disease. A wide spectrum of indications for noninvasive imaging are now recognized, extending from excluding valvular heart disease in asymptomatic patients with cardiac murmurs to assessing the severity of valve disease and directing medical and surgical therapy. Recently, portable ultrasonoscopes or "pocket-sized ultrasound stethoscopes" with full Doppler hemodynamic capabilities have been introduced that may revolutionize the cardiac physical examination. The purpose of this chapter is to describe the optimal and appropriate use of the complete range of cardiac imaging techniques in the diagnosis and management of patients with valvular heart disease in contemporary clinical cardiology practice.

Valvular heart disease may be suspected on the basis of symptoms of dyspnea, chest discomfort, or syncope related to the severity of disease or may be detected serendipitously by auscultation of a cardiac murmur in an asymptomatic patient at routine physical examination. Symptomatic patients with valvular heart disease require accurate diagnosis and warrant further evaluation to assess the hemodynamic severity of the valve disease and its effects on cardiac geometry and function, which may be pivotal in determining optimal treatment. Asymptomatic subjects with grade 3 or greater systolic murmur or with any diastolic murmur should undergo echocardiography with Doppler evaluation. This recommendation extends to asymptomatic patients with grade 1 or 2 systolic murmurs and abnormalities on electrocardiograms or chest X-ray. However, a large proportion of asymptomatic and especially young patients with grade 1 and 2+ ejection systolic murmurs with a normally splitting second heart sound, no associated abnormal findings on physical examination, normal electrocardiogram and chest X-ray can be managed clinically and do not require cardiac imaging.

This chapter addresses the diagnostic approach to suspected or known valvular disease with current imaging techniques. Echocardiography is currently the most frequently used method for anatomical and hemodynamic evaluation of valvular heart disease. Valvular anatomy and imaging of the four heart valves will be described, followed by discussion of the assessment of various disease states. Optimal assessment and management of patients with valve disease depends on determining (1) the pathoetiology of the valve malfunction; (2) the extent of involvement of the valve components; (3) the severity of the valve disease in terms of its impact on intracardiac hemodynamics and ventricular function; and (4) the ideal treatment strategy for individual patients that most favorably influences clinical outcome, which includes pharmacological treatment of heart failure therapy, catheter-based procedures, and surgical valve repair or replacement.

MITRAL VALVE DISEASE

Anatomical Evaluation

The function of the normal mitral valve is to open after isovolumic relaxation and allow blood flow from the left atrium into the left ventricle throughout diastole without resistance. Left atrial systolic contraction augments left ventricular filling, after which the mitral valve closes for the duration of ventricular systole preventing regurgitation of blood into the left atrium. The mitral valve apparatus consists of four components: the annulus, two leaflets, chordae tendineae (subvalve tensor apparatus), and the papillary muscles, all of which function as an integrated unit. Disease processes may involve changes in one or more of these subunits with different clinical consequences.

The anterior and posterior mitral leaflets are fine, mobile structures that coapt after atrial contraction and seal the mitral orifice, preventing regurgitation. The mitral valve annulus, part of the cardiac fibrous skeleton, forms the atrioventricular junction of the left side of the heart and provides electrical insulation of atrial from ventricular myocardium. The mitral subvalve tensor apparatus consists of the chordae tendineae that take origin from the papillary muscles and insert into the free margins of the ventricular surface of both mitral leaflets. The chordae from the anterolateral papillary muscle attach to the lateral half of both leaflets, whereas those from the posteromedial papillary muscle attach to the medial half of both leaflets. Each mitral leaflet is divided into three scallops: the posterior scallop P1 extends from the anterolateral commissure, scallop P3 extends from the posterior medial mitral commissure, and P2 is between P1 and P3. The anterior leaflet has three scallops: A1, A2, and A3, which coapt during systole with their corresponding posterior leaflet scallops.

Echocardiography

Transthoracic and transesophageal Doppler echocardiography enable complete and detailed characterization of the mitral valve and subvalve apparatus with simultaneous assessment of intracardiac hemodynamics.

In transthoracic echocardiographic studies, the mitral valve leaflets are best visualized from the parasternal long- and short-axis views (Figure 11-1). The thickness of the leaflets can be measured by M-mode or two-dimensional echocardiographic images and is normally <2 mm. Harmonic imaging may cause the appearance of thickening in normal valves and should not be used during the assessment of valve thickness.[1] The motion of the leaflets during the cardiac cycle is also best assessed in parasternal long- and short-axis and the four-chamber views. Restricted diastolic opening may be caused by thickening and calcification of the leaflets or by fusion of the commissures or chordal shortening caused by the rheumatic process. Systolic prolapse of the valve is usually best demonstrated in parasternal long axis. The parasternal short axis of the mitral valve orifice allows direct inspection of the commissures, assessment of valve opening, mitral orifice area, and assessment of

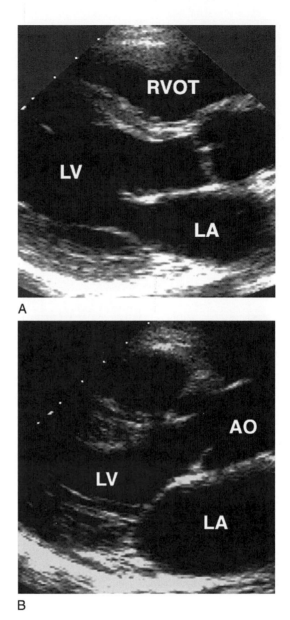

A

B

FIGURE 11-1. A, Parasternal long-axis view in diastole. The mitral valve leaflets are open in diastole, and the aortic valve is closed, with the coaptation point in the center of the aortic root. The sinotubular junction is represented by the point at that the sinus of Valsalva terminates and the diameter of the ascending aorta narrows. B, Parasternal long-axis view in diastole. The chordal attachments to the mitral leaflets are visualized. The aortic valve leaflets have not fully opened in this early systolic image. The right coronary cusp is imaged anteriorly and the noncoronary cusp is seen posteriorly. RVOT, right ventricular outflow tract; LA, left atrium; LV, left ventricle; AO, ascending aorta.

the three anterior and posterior leaflet scallops (Figure 11-2). The mitral annulus is usually not visualized as a distinct structure, except in the presence of calcification or thickening because of extension of endocarditis to the annulus per se. The apical views are optimal for demonstrating the chordal attachments to the valve leaflets. Redundant chords with excessive motion or thickened and retracted chords may be identified. The motion of the valve leaflets should be evaluated in these views. Conditions that interfere with complete closure

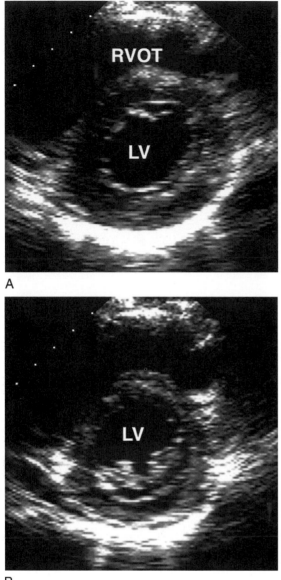

A

B

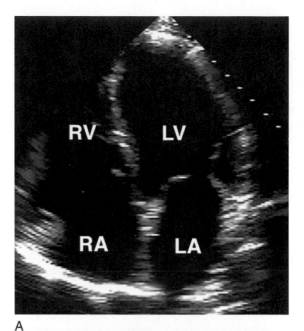

A

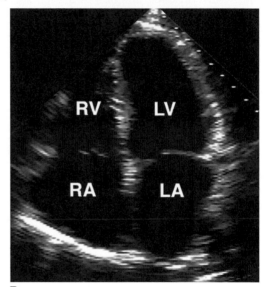

B

FIGURE 11-2. A, Parasternal short-axis view in diastole at the level of the mitral valve orifice. The mitral valve leaflets are fully opened. **B,** Systolic frame of the parasternal short-axis view. The mitral valve leaflets coapt completely. The medial commissure is visible to the left of the image and the lateral commissure to the right. The right ventricle appears enlarged. RVOT, right ventricular outflow tract; LV, left ventricle.

FIGURE 11-3. A, Apical four-chamber view in diastole. The mitral and tricuspid valves are opened in diastole. The lateral wall and the posterior septum are imaged in this view. The anterior mitral valve leaflet is seen to the left of the image and the posterior leaflet to the right. The septal attachment of the tricuspid valve is more apical than the mitral valve annulus. The septal and anterior tricuspid leaflets are imaged in this view. **B,** Apical four-chamber view in systole. Normal closing of the mitral and tricuspid valves is demonstrated. The tips of the leaflets are coplanar with the bodies of the leaflets.

Continued

of the valve can also be assessed in the apical views (Figure 11-3).

The positions of the two papillary muscles within the left ventricle are almost constant. They are well seen in the parasternal short axis at the level of the papillary muscle tips and may also be seen in the apical views. The papillary muscles are an integral part of the left ventricular myocardium, which, in conjunction with the mitral tensor apparatus, maintain the normal left ventricular chamber architecture and mitral valve competence. Diseases that disrupt the integrated function of the components of the mitral valve or alter the nor-

mal ventricular cavity geometry may result in mitral regurgitation.

Doppler evaluation of the mitral valve by both pulsed-wave and color Doppler imaging should be carried out in all views. The jet of mitral regurgitation may be markedly eccentric, making complete assessment in all views mandatory. The mitral valve inflow jet is normally parallel to the ultrasound beam only in the apical views

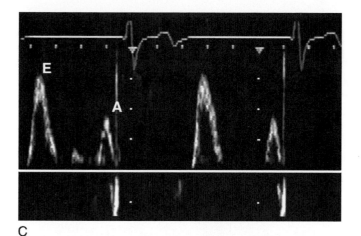

C

FIGURE 11-3, cont'd C, Spectral display of pulsed-wave Doppler across the mitral valve. The transducer is in the apical position, and the sample volume has been placed at the level of the tips of the mitral valve leaflets. The left ventricular diastolic filling is toward the transducer and so displayed above the baseline. This normal filling pattern demonstrates a "E" wave, with a peak velocity of approximately 0.6 m/s, and a smaller "A" wave, with a peak velocity of 0.4 m/s (calibration marks 0.2 m/s).

and should be used to measure diastolic gradients (Figure 11-3, *C*).

Transesophageal imaging of the mitral valve has been a dramatic advance in our ability to diagnose the structural basis for valvular dysfunction. The mitral valve leaflets are seen from the midesophagus in the transverse plane (imaging angle, 0 degrees). Omniplane examination allows a systematic assessment of the valve from multiple views, and the individual three scallops of the anterior and the posterior leaflets can be evaluated and their motion pattern assessed (Figure 11-4). Transesophageal imaging in the five-chamber view from the midesophagus at 0 degrees visualizes mitral scallops A1, A2, and P2. Advancement of the probe to obtain the four-chamber view visualizing the crux of the heart having excluded the aorta at 0 degrees brings into view mitral scallops A2 and P2. Rotation of the imaging plane to between 40 degrees and 60 degrees visualizes anterior mitral scallops A2 and A3 and the posterior scallop P3. Further rotation of the imaging plane to between 75 degrees and 90 degrees brings into view the entire left atrial appendage, in which plane from the lateral left atrial appendage to the medial left atrial junction the sequence of mitral scallops is P1, A2, and P3. At the same rotation, more anterior angulation visualizes the scallops P2, A3, and A2. By contrast, posteriorly directed imaging visualizes all three posterior scallops: P1, P2, and P3. Between 120 degrees and 140 degrees in the long-axis plane of the left ventricle, the mitral scallops visualized are P2 and A2. Advancing the probe into the stomach enables all of the mitral scallops A1 through A3 and P1 through P3 to be visualized in the short axis. The long-axis view in the transgastric position 90 degrees demonstrates mitral scallops P3, A2, and P1.[2,3] Detailed anatomy of the chordae can be imaged in the transgastric long-axis view of the left ventricle by transesophageal echocardiography. The mechanism of mitral regurgitation can usually be clarified by transesophageal echocardiography. This assessment is vitally important in planning the surgical approach to mitral valve repair.

MITRAL STENOSIS

Pathophysiology and Hemodynamics

The mitral valve may become stenotic because of abnormalities of any of its components. In rheumatic mitral disease, the most common cause, commissural fusion between the leaflets, has long been considered a pathological hallmark. However, leaflet thickening, fibrosis, and calcification, as well as shortening, thickening, and fusion of the chordae, are frequently present. The net result is a funnel-shaped structure with a fishmouth appearance of its base. Some degree of coexisting mitral regurgitation is common, and the rheumatic process may affect the aortic and tricuspid valves as well. The most prevalent cause of nonrheumatic stenosis of the mitral valve orifice is severe mitral annular calcification that extends apically and impedes the normal opening of the leaflets. The leaflets may also become involved in the calcification process, leaving only the leaflet tips uninvolved and producing moderate and occasionally severe stenosis. Mitral stenosis may also result as a congenital deformity of the mitral valve apparatus. Congenital mitral stenosis may occur as an isolated defect, but it is more frequently associated with other abnormalities, including defects in the atrial and ventricular septum, aortic stenosis, and coarctation. The cusps, commissures, or chordae tendineae may be abnormal or attached to a single papillary muscle that is known as a parachute mitral valve. The signs, symptoms, and hemodynamic effects of mitral stenosis are all secondary to the obstruction of blood flow by the mitral valve. The restricted left ventricular diastolic filling leads to an elevation of left atrial pressure, which is transmitted to the pulmonary venous circulation. As the left atrial pressure progressively increases, the left atrium enlarges, increasing the likelihood of atrial fibrillation, blood stasis, and thrombus formation. The pulmonary venous pressure elevation leads to pulmonary congestion and the eventual development of secondary pulmonary artery hypertension. Long-standing pulmonary hypertension can become fixed because of intimal and medial hyperplasia and fibrosis of the pulmonary arterial wall as it remodels in response to chronic pressure elevation. The right ventricle hypertrophies as a result of the pressure overload caused by the pulmonary hypertension. As the pulmonary arterial pressure rises, the right ventricle enlarges and in so doing alters the geometry of the tricuspid valve apparatus, causing secondary tricuspid regurgitation and further right ventricular dilation, which in combination culminate in the signs and symptoms of right heart failure.

The chest X-ray in patients with mitral stenosis may show changes in the border of the cardiac silhouette and in the lung fields. Straightening of the left heart border in the posteroanterior view indicates left atrial enlargement. A giant left atrium is usually indicative of

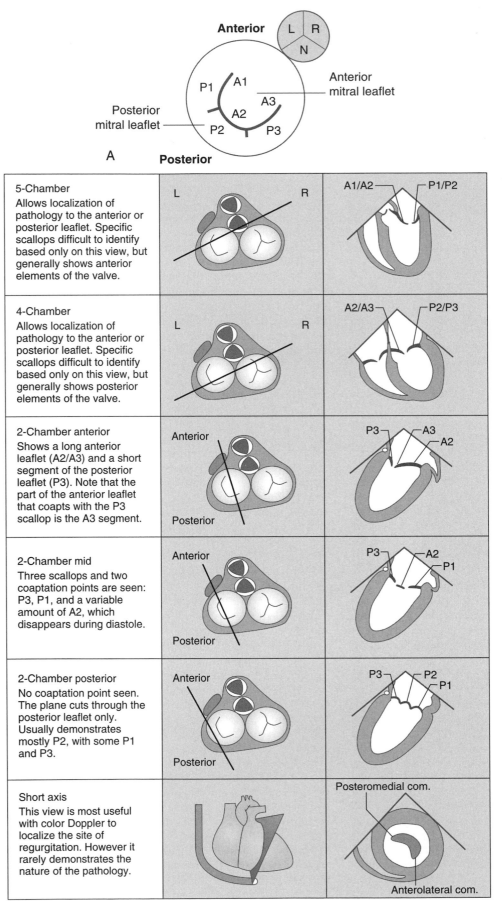

FIGURE 11-4. A, Carpentier nomenclature of the mitral valve scallops. The mitral valve is seen from the left atrium (surgeon's perspective). (Reprinted with permission from Lambert A, et al. *Anesth Analg* 1999; 88:1205.) B, Summary of a systematic mitral valve examination. The middle column shows the planes of the different cross-sections, and the right column demonstrates the leaflet segments visualized in each view. (Reprinted with permission from Lambert A, et al. *Anesth Analg* 1999; 88:1205.)

concomitant severe mitral regurgitation or associated atrial fibrillation. Rarely, the left atrium may be calcified. In the presence of pulmonary hypertension, the pulmonary artery and right ventricle may be enlarged. Finally, pulmonary venous distention in the upper lung fields, interstitial edema, or frank pulmonary edema may be detected. The findings of pulmonary congestion may be masked by tricuspid regurgitation (either rheumatic or functional secondary to pulmonary hypertension), which may decompress the pulmonary vasculature at the expense of reduced cardiac output.

The normal mitral valve orifice is between 4 and 5 cm^2 and may vary throughout diastole by as much as 20% to 40%. The signs and symptoms of mitral stenosis, dyspnea and fatigue, do not usually occur until the valve area is between 1.5 and 2.0 cm^2. Many patients remain well compensated and relatively free of symptoms with minimal treatment until the valve area is close to 1.0 cm^2. In this regard, it is noteworthy that many prosthetic mitral valves have effective orifice areas of only 2.0 cm^2. The transdiastolic gradient across the mitral valve rises with a decrease in diastolic filling time or with an increase in flow. Many patients with mild or moderate stenosis who are asymptomatic at low levels of exercise have heart failure develop with tachycardia or increases in cardiac output. The onset of atrial fibrillation with a rapid ventricular response, pregnancy, or severe exertion may first produce symptoms of mitral stenosis.

Anatomical Evaluation

Echocardiography

Two-dimensional transthoracic echocardiography (TTE) is the single most useful imaging modality in this disease. It provides direct visualization of the valve apparatus to determine etiology, allows quantification of the mitral valve area, and can detect complications of the disease, including left atrial thrombi, pulmonary hypertension, and mitral regurgitation.

Visualization of the valve apparatus allows estimation of the opening excursion, degree of leaflet thickening, calcification, mobility, and involvement of the subvalvular structures. Stenosis of the mitral valve, which is not due to commissural thickening, produces decreased leaflet mobility but not diastolic doming characteristic of rheumatic involvement. Subvalvular involvement by the rheumatic process is most clearly demonstrated in the apical four-chamber or apical long-axis views. Rheumatic involvement of the valve may be assessed by an echo score, which has proven useful in predicting both the short-term and long-term results of percutaneous balloon valvuloplasty (Figure 11-5). The most widely used echocardiographic scoring system (the Massachusetts General Hospital [MGH] score) assigns a value of 1 to 4 for each of four individual factors to create a sum between 4 and 16. The variables include leaflet mobility, thickening and calcification of the leaflet, and subvalvular involvement. The higher the score, the more severe the rheumatic involvement. Optimal results are obtained in patients with pliable valves and a minimum of leaflet thickening, immobility, calcification, and subvalvular

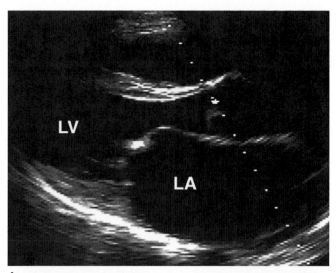

A

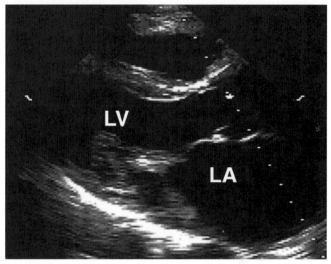

B

FIGURE 11-5. A, Parasternal long-axis view in diastole. The mitral valve leaflets dome and are thickened at the tips. The opening is restricted compared with the normal valve. The left atrium is enlarged but the left ventricle is normal. **B,** Similar view in systole. The subvalvular involvement is evident, with thickened and mildly calcified chords extending from the papillary muscle to the leaflets. The aortic valve is mildly thickened.

involvement. The ideal candidate for percutaneous balloon valvuloplasty is a patient with a total score of ≤8 and little mitral regurgitation. This mitral valve score was initially derived in patients undergoing double-balloon procedures but has proven applicable to newer mitral valvuloplasty techniques. Other echocardiographic scoring systems with greater emphasis on the presence or absence of commissural calcification may be particularly useful for predicting the severity of mitral regurgitation after the procedure.

The angiographic assessment of mitral valve stenosis usually does not add much information to noninvasive imaging techniques. Fluoroscopic valve calcification is an important predictor of both acute and chronic outcomes of percutaneous balloon valvuloplasty. Left ventriculography can be used to assess systolic function and mitral regurgitation but has limitations. The mitral leaflets may be visible with this negative contrast and their degree of immobility or prolapse assessed. The size of the left atrium may be determined by dye opacification secondary to associated mitral regurgitation or by the late phase of a pulmonary artery injection.

Quantification of Severity of Stenosis

Echocardiography

The valve area in mitral stenosis can be measured echocardiographically by planimetry of the mitral valve orifice area in the parasternal short-axis view (Figure 11-6) and correlates well with the valve area determined by cardiac catheterization. The accuracy of this technique requires careful measurement in a true perpendicular axis and may not take into account the contribution of the subvalvular apparatus to the severity of stenosis. The method tends to underestimate the area when the valve is heavily calcified and may be unreliable after surgery or valvuloplasty, because the complete mitral valve orifice may no longer be visualized in a single plane as a result of deformity of the valve. The true orifice of the valve is often not parallel to the short-axis view, and off-axis views are necessary. Up to 10% of patients have inadequate images to attempt planimetry.

The spectral Doppler time velocity envelope across the stenotic mitral valve demonstrates an elevated peak velocity and a delayed fall in velocity because of the persistent diastolic gradient (Figure 11-6, *C*).

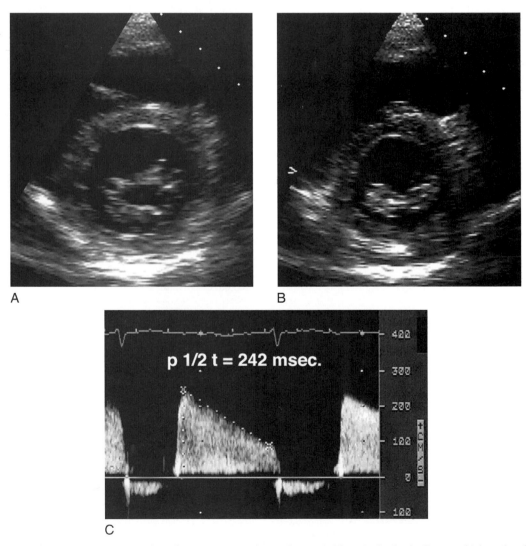

FIGURE 11-6. A, Parasternal short-axis view in diastole in a patient with mitral stenosis. The mitral valve leaflets are thickened and mildly calcified. There is marked restriction of diastolic opening compared with the image of the normal valve. The commissures are partially fused. The area of the diastolic orifice may be planimetered to yield the mitral valve area. **B,** Similar view in systole. The thickening of the leaflets is again appreciated. **C,** Spectral display of mitral valve inflow velocity measured by continuous-wave Doppler in a patient with mitral stenosis. The peak velocity is 2.5 m/s, which is consistent with a peak gradient of 25 mmHg across the valve. The mean gradient may be obtained by integrating the spectral envelope over time. The pressure half time (½ t) is marked on this figure. A pressure half time of 242 ms predicts a mitral valve orifice area of 0.9 cm².

The peak pressure gradient is calculated with the simplified Bernoulli equation:

$$\text{Peak pressure gradient} = 4\ v^2 \qquad \text{(Equation 1)}$$

where v is the peak velocity measured by continuous-wave Doppler. The mean pressure gradient is obtained by integrating the velocity envelope over time, which is equivalent to the area under the curve. An important observation was that the mitral valve area could be calculated from the pressure half time of the mitral valve velocity envelope. The pressure half time refers to the time, measured in milliseconds, required for the initial maximum pressure gradient to fall to half its value. The pressure half time can be automatically calculated online by most ultrasound machines. The longer the pressure half time, the more severe the stenosis. The mitral valve area is given by the equation:

$$\text{MVA} = 220/\tau \qquad \text{(Equation 2)}$$

where *MVA* is the mitral valve area in cm^2 and τ is the pressure half time given in milliseconds. This measurement is reproducible and independent of cardiac output, mitral regurgitation, and atrial fibrillation. If the spectral Doppler envelope does not have a linear slope, it is more accurate to use the middiastolic slope rather than the initial one. However, the valve area calculated from the pressure half-time measurement may be overestimated in the presence of aortic regurgitation and is also affected by acute changes in atrial or ventricular compliance, which occur immediately after balloon valvuloplasty. Similarly, the presence of a significant atrial septal defect with flow from the left atrium to the right atrium will result in underestimation of the severity of the obstruction. The peak pulmonary artery pressure is calculated by application of the modified Bernoulli equation to the tricuspid regurgitation jet.

Color Doppler examination has become an essential part of the evaluation of mitral stenosis. The detection of the proximal isovelocity surface area allows calculation of the mitral valve area.[4] The flow accelerates in isovelocity hemispheres as it approaches the stenotic valve. The color Doppler baseline is adjusted so that the radius from the valve orifice to the level of the first aliasing of the color Doppler jet proximal to the valve is easily measured. The peak velocity across the valve is measured by continuous-wave Doppler. Assuming a circular geometry of the orifice, the continuity equation allows calculation of the mitral valve area by the equation:

$$\text{MVA} = 2\pi\ R^2 \times V_{NYQUIST}/V_{PEAK} \qquad \text{(Equation 3)}$$

where *MVA* is the mitral valve area, *R* is the radius to the first aliasing surface, $V_{NYQUIST}$ is the velocity at the Nyquist limit, and V_{PEAK} is the peak velocity across the valve, measured with continuous-wave Doppler. The mitral valve area obtained with this method correlates closely with invasive methods of determining mitral valve area by use of the Gorlin hydraulic formula (Equation 4) and surgically measured anatomical areas.[5] Color Doppler velocity mapping is also important in detecting associated abnormalities, particularly mitral regurgitation. Three-dimensional echocardiographic analysis of the stenotic valve orifice with real-time volumetric assessment of flow may prove in the future to be a clinically reliable tool.[6]

Transesophageal echocardiography (TEE) is recommended to evaluate hemodynamics when TTE is suboptimal and to assess the presence of left atrial thrombus in patients before percutaneous mitral valvuloplasty or cardioversion[7] (Figure 11-7). The superior visualization of the valve may also provide additional clinically important morphological information, including the severity of subvalvular disease, chordal rupture, and a more accurate estimate of the degree of mitral regurgitation. The mitral diastolic flow is parallel to the ultrasound beam in the four-chamber view at the midesophageal level (imaging angle, 0 degrees). Analysis of the spectral envelope and measurement of the mitral valve area with the proximal isovelocity surface area (PISA) method is easily accomplished with this technique. However, short-axis imaging of the mitral orifice for planimetry is usually not feasible. TEE has become an invaluable imaging tool in the management of patients with mitral stenosis before, during, and after balloon valvuloplasty.

Cardiac Catheterization

Nowadays, mitral stenosis is rarely an unsuspected diagnosis in a patient undergoing cardiac catheterization. Its role is therefore usually confirmatory.

The hemodynamic assessment of mitral stenosis requires an understanding of both the pathophysiology

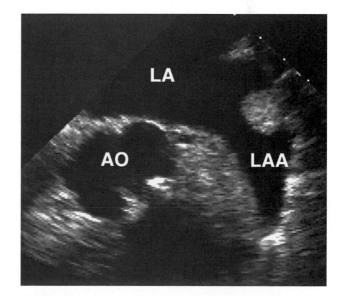

FIGURE 11-7. Transesophageal echocardiogram in the transverse plane (imaging angle 0 degrees) from the high esophagus. The left atrial appendage is visualized as an outpouching of the left atrium. There is an echodense mass at the mouth of the appendage (LAA), which is a thrombus attached to the left atrial wall and protruding into the appendage.

of this disease and the limitations of the catheterization techniques used in its assessment. The mitral valve area is calculated using the modified Gorlin formula, which is derived from standard fluid dynamic principles:

$$\text{MVA (cm}^2) = \frac{\text{Cardiac output (mL/min)/diastolic filling period (s)}}{37.9 \ \sqrt{\text{mean diastolic gradient (mmHg)}}}$$

(Equation 4)

The cardiac output determination is critical and can be obtained by the thermodilution technique in the absence of significant tricuspid regurgitation or by use of the Fick principle in the patient with multivalvular disease. To use the Fick principle, the patient's oxygen consumption must be measured. The use of an estimated value for oxygen consumption introduces additional variability. The mean transmitral diastolic gradient is derived from simultaneous measurements of left atrial and left ventricular pressures. Usually, the more easily obtained pulmonary capillary wedge pressure is substituted for direct left atrial pressure measurement. This substitution is a frequent potential source of error in the mitral valve area calculation because of attenuation of the pressure wave peaks in the wedge tracing and the need to correct the measurement for time delay. When a satisfactory wedge recording cannot be obtained or when the recorded pressure is discrepant with other assessments of the expected pressure, direct left atrial pressure recording is warranted by transseptal left heart catheterization.

The mitral valve area can be calculated by the Gorlin formula, and the pulmonary artery and pulmonary capillary wedge pressure can be directly measured, which may be useful in assessing the need and risk of surgery or valvuloplasty (Figure 11-8). These pressures may also provide important data on other potential causes of dyspnea. Left ventriculography may be performed to assess the degree of coexistent mitral regurgitation and other aortic and/or tricuspid valvular lesions. Finally, coronary angiography is necessary in selected patients before percutaneous therapeutic interventions or surgery.

Clinical Evaluation

The patient discovered to have any degree of mitral stenosis should undergo complete evaluation, including TTE with assessment of mitral valve gradients, mitral valve area by more than one method if possible, and estimation of the peak pulmonary artery pressure. TEE and cardiac catheterization are rarely needed in the initial evaluation. In the asymptomatic patient, annual clinical evaluation is usual, but repeat echocardiography is necessary only for a change in clinical status.[7] The rate of progression of mitral stenosis is not predicted by initial valve area, and right heart disease may progress without significant change in mitral valve area. Some patients may have atypical symptoms that are difficult to attribute to mild or moderate mitral stenosis. Exercise testing with treadmill or dobutamine stress may reveal a significant rise in pulmonary pressures or transmitral gradient that justifies intervention. The transmitral gradients obtained with echocardiography may be more reliable than those obtained in the catheterization laboratory, particularly when the pulmonary capillary wedge pressure is substituted for the left atrial pressure. Cardiac catheterization is indicated in cases in which significant mitral stenosis is suspected and the echocardiogram is technically limited or to clarify discrepant echocardiographic findings. Cardiac angiography is indicated in older patients or those with significant risk factors for atherosclerosis, but routine catheterization before surgery is not recommended.[7]

Medical treatment of mitral stenosis is usually effective for the patient with mild symptoms. Diuretics reduce pulmonary congestion. β-Blockers prolong diastolic filling time and thereby reduce the transmitral gra-

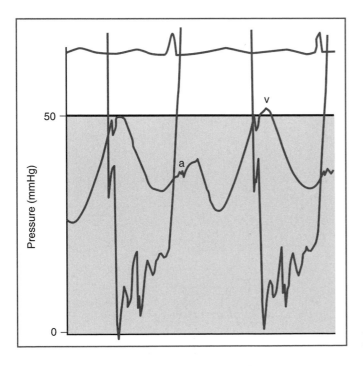

FIGURE 11-8. Simultaneous left ventricular pressure and pulmonary capillary wedge recordings in a patient with a mean transmitral gradient of 19 mmHg and a calculated mitral valve area of 1.0 cm².

dient. In patients with atrial fibrillation, β-blockers and digoxin may be helpful in controlling the ventricular rate and improving left atrial emptying. Patients with mitral stenosis and atrial fibrillation have a particularly high risk of systemic embolism (20% to 25%/year) in the absence of anticoagulation and should receive warfarin with a target international normalized ratio (INR) of 2.5 to 3.5. Finally, patients younger than 25 years of age and those with recurrent rheumatic fever should receive long-term penicillin therapy. All patients with mitral stenosis are advised to take antibiotic prophylaxis against endocarditis.

Treatment

For patients with symptoms despite medical therapy or with pulmonary hypertension (pulmonary artery systolic pressure >50 mmHg), mechanical relief of the obstructed valve is indicated. In some developing countries, closed commissurotomy is still the most frequent procedure performed for mitral stenosis. Open commissurotomy has become the preferred surgical procedure with amputation of the left atrial appendage. However, percutaneous balloon valvuloplasty has largely supplanted commissurotomy, because studies have demonstrated equivalent or better results with the less invasive procedure. In patients with heavily calcified degenerative mitral valve disease or with associated moderate regurgitation not suitable for surgical commissurotomy or balloon valvuloplasty, mitral valve replacement should be performed.

Percutaneous balloon valvuloplasty was first described by Inoue in 1984 and popularized in the United States by Lock. Single- and double-balloon techniques were first used but subsequently supplanted by Inoue's device. The balloon(s) catheters are introduced across the mitral valve by way of an antegrade transseptal approach (Figure 11-9). The major mechanism of successful balloon valvuloplasty requires splitting of fused commissures, analogous to surgical commissurotomy. Typical hemodynamic results achieved include a >50% reduction in mean transmitral gradient and an approximate doubling of the baseline mitral valve orifice area. Randomized comparisons of different techniques, as well as between percutaneous and surgical commissurotomy, have failed to document important short- or long-term differences in hemodynamic effects, prevalence of restenosis, or functional status. In long-term follow-up, the absence of need for mitral valve replacement or repeat valvuloplasty is the most objective measure of a successful procedure and is approximately 50% at 5 years. Higher event-free survivals up to 90% at 5 to 10 years have been reported in selected patients with lower echocardiographic morphological scores.[8]

Percutaneous balloon valvuloplasty dramatically improves dyspnea and functional capacity. Most patients report clinical improvement with documented changes of one to two functional classes and greater exercise capacity. Complications of valvuloplasty include a small incidence (0.5% to 3%) of death, usually related to perforation and cardiac tamponade. This complication has virtually disappeared with the use of the Inoue balloon and trans-

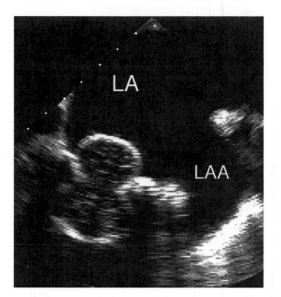

FIGURE 11-9. Transesophageal echocardiogram in the transverse plane (imaging angle 0 degrees) in the midesophagus at the level of the mitral valve. A valvuloplasty balloon has been placed across the stenotic valve and inflated. The waist in the balloon represents the level of the stenosis.

esophageal or intracardiac echocardiographic guidance of the transseptal puncture. Other reported complications include systemic embolism (1% to 4%), arrhythmias, vascular injury, persistent atrial septal defects, and mitral regurgitation. The incidence of systemic embolism is greatly reduced by the exclusion of patients with left atrial thrombus identified by preprocedure TEE imaging. Minor increases in the grade of mitral regurgitation are common after balloon valvuloplasty, occurring in up to 50% of patients; however, moderate and severe regurgitation are uncommon (5% to 10%).

Echocardiography is an indispensable part of the preprocedure, periprocedure, and postprocedure evaluation of balloon valvuloplasty patients. Preprocedure TTE is valuable to assess specific features of valvular morphology, to confirm the severity of both mitral stenosis and regurgitation, and to assess the patient for other valvular abnormalities. TEE should be routinely performed before the procedure to identify patients with thrombus in the left atrium or appendage, which is a contraindication to balloon valvuloplasty. During the procedure, transesophageal monitoring has been advocated to guide the transseptal puncture and to assess the result of each balloon inflation on both valve opening and on development of regurgitation. TEE can be used to guide the transseptal puncture and to assess the hemodynamic changes (peak and mean diastolic gradients and mitral valve orifice areas) and the degree of regurgitation after each balloon inflation. An alternative approach is to use intracardiac echocardiography to guide the transseptal puncture and transthoracic studies after each balloon inflation. The recent availability of intracardiac probes with full Doppler capabilities has also proved useful in assessing patients undergoing balloon valvuloplasty. Currently available high-quality, low-frequency directional devices with

Doppler capability will likely prove useful during therapeutic procedures.[9]

Echocardiographic imaging after balloon valvuloplasty can determine the presence and mechanism of complications, including mitral regurgitation and persistent atrial septal shunts, at the transseptal site. In one series of patients undergoing Inoue balloon valvuloplasty, the incidence of severe regurgitation was 7.5%, most often (45%) caused by rupture of the chordae tendineae to the anterior or posterior mitral leaflet. Other causes of acute procedure-related mitral regurgitation identified by echocardiography included leaflet tears and wide commissural splitting with a central regurgitant jet. At follow-up, approximately 80% of selected patients obtain long-term improvement after balloon valvuloplasty. Clinical and echocardiographic follow-up for evidence of recurrent symptomatic mitral stenosis and/or worsening regurgitation is essential. Significant left-to-right shunting across the interatrial septum is uncommon on long-term follow-up.

MITRAL REGURGITATION

Pathophysiology and Hemodynamics

The pathoetiology of mitral regurgitation (MR) can be considered in terms of diseases that affect the function of the individual components of the mitral valve unit. The severity of MR is dependent on the interaction of a number of factors, important among which are the size of the effective regurgitant orifice area, left ventricular loading conditions, the pressure difference between the left atrium and left ventricle during ejection, heart rate, and the compliance of the left atrium. MR may be acute or chronic, and the left ventricular geometry, contractile function, and the compensatory mechanisms activated during remodeling are markedly different. Acute severe MR caused by the abrupt onset of severe volume overload is characterized by a nearly normal sized or only slightly dilated left ventricle, with increased stroke volume but without compensatory hypertrophy or significant enlargement of the left atrium. Sinus tachycardia, hypotension, pulmonary congestion, and acute heart failure ensue. Chronic MR is characterized by a dilated, eccentrically hypertrophied left ventricle, left atrial enlargement, and stable hemodynamics (normotension and normal heart rate) that develop over months or years. These two distinct clinical syndromes of acute and chronic MR must be distinguished, because their respective prognoses and treatments are different. Although the hemodynamic severity of MR and its impact on left ventricular size and function can be assessed by a variety of techniques (cardiac catheterization, radionuclide angiography, and magnetic resonance imaging), the exquisitely detailed anatomical structure and function of the entire mitral valve apparatus unique to transthoracic and transesophageal Doppler echocardiography renders it the optimal technique for diagnosis and clinical decision making.

Chronic MR in its mildest form is common, usually asymptomatic, and may not result in left ventricular dilation or change in left ventricular function. MR of greater than mild severity initiates a series of compensatory changes in left ventricular geometry and function. Chronic MR is a volume overload state in which to maintain normal cardiac output the left ventricle must eject a larger than normal stroke volume that includes both the forward volume flow into the systemic circulation and the regurgitant or backward volume flow into the left atrium. Chronic volume overload causes the left ventricle to dilate initially in diastole by increasing myocyte length over a prolonged period of time. This increase in diastolic volume increases diastolic wall stress by Laplace's law. Increased wall stress is a powerful stimulus for hypertrophy, which alters the architecture of the ventricle to an eccentric pattern of hypertrophy. Early compensatory eccentric hypertrophy with increase in the number of sarcomeres arranged in series conserves the normal relationship between left ventricular mass and cavity volume and is the mechanism by which left ventricular loading conditions are normalized and contractile function preserved. Although left ventricular diastolic volume increases initially, systolic volume remains unchanged. Ejection-phase indices of contractile function may be normal or supranormal, because the left ventricle empties more completely into the low-pressure left atrium. Chronic MR of mild-to-moderate severity may remain symptomatically stable for many years, with no measurable difference in left ventricular volumes or contractile function and no progressive left atrial dilation over time. However, prolonged exposure to severe volume overload from MR eventually results in progressive left ventricular dilation initially in diastolic and subsequently systolic volumes with distortion of ventricular shape. When the increase in left ventricular systolic volume is no longer accompanied by adequate compensatory hypertrophy, systolic wall stress increases, and ejection-phase indices of contractile function deteriorate, since they vary inversely with wall stress. Changes in left ventricular architecture include cavity dilation, inadequate hypertrophy, and development of a more spherical cavity shape caused by a disproportionately greater increase in cavity diameter than cavity length. Left ventricular dilation results in stretching of the mitral annulus, enlargement of the mitral annular area, further disruption of the geometry of the mitral subvalve apparatus, and escalation in the severity of MR. Thus, chronic mitral regurgitation in altering left ventricular architecture facilitates further development of MR and so contributes to the increase in left ventricular loading conditions, further deterioration in contractile function, and onset of congestive heart failure. The transition in left ventricular topography and function from normality to end-stage heart failure resulting from chronic MR can be characterized by TTE.

Left ventricular size and function in chronic moderate-to-severe MR vary with changes in preload and afterload induced either pharmacologically or with exercise. Because MR is so exquisitely sensitive to perturbations in left ventricular load, it may be difficult to dissociate deterioration in ventricular function caused by myocyte dysfunction from changes in loading conditions. Progression of chronic MR is also dependent on the etiology of the mitral valve disease process, is difficult to anticipate in individual patients. Regular surveillance of left ventricular size and function is important to avoid irreversible contractile dysfunction. The trigger for ventricular decompensation and development of heart failure usually cannot be identified by any imaging modality, but this transition phase is signaled by a number of important changes in left ventricular architecture and function that are detectable by noninvasive imaging and accompanied by worsening symptoms of dyspnea, fatigue, and exercise intolerance.

Acute severe MR differs from chronic mitral regurgitation in its etiology, timing, and changes in left ventricular size and function. Acute MR is usually due to ischemia, papillary muscle dysfunction, degenerative mitral valve disease with flail leaflet, chordal rupture, or vegetative endocarditis. Acute severe MR is not associated with the same magnitude of derangements in left ventricular architecture as chronic MR. The stigmata associated with chronic MR, such as left ventricular dilation, left atrial dilation, and left ventricular hypertrophy, are not present in acute severe MR. The left ventricle has little or no opportunity to dilate or develop compensatory hypertrophy to offset the sudden increase in volume load. The left ventricle is usually hyperdynamic with reduced systolic volume, only mildly increased diastolic cavity volume, and resting sinus tachycardia. Sinus tachycardia results, because modulation of stroke volume is diminished, so that tachycardia is the only means of maintaining resting cardiac output. The hyperdynamic left ventricular function may make detection of regional wall motion abnormalities difficult. The diagnosis of acute severe MR is often suggested by the discrepant clinical symptoms of severe dyspnea and the hyperdynamic left ventricular function. Acute severe MR requires urgent and definitive diagnosis, because timely restoration of mitral competence is mandatory and necessitates surgical valve repair or replacement with or without myocardial revascularization rather than temporizing with afterload reduction.

Anatomical Evaluation

Echocardiography

The pathoetiology and mechanism of MR can be ascertained by TTE in >90% of all patients and in 99% by TEE. TEE is significantly better for detecting mitral valve vegetations, leaflet prolapse, flail segments, and ruptured chordae. Definition of the pathoanatomy of the mitral valve apparatus is critically important in clinical decision making, and echocardiography is unique for determining whether repair of the mitral leaflets and restoration of mitral competence is feasible, whether additional chordal lengthening/shortening procedures are indicated, and when the mitral valve is irreparably damaged by degenerative changes and necessitates prosthetic valve replacement.

Abnormalities of the Mitral Valve Leaflets

MR may result from alteration in the material properties of the valve leaflets, causing restrictive or excessive leaflet motion that impairs adequate leaflet coaptation and valve competence. A frequent cause of increased mitral leaflet thickness is rheumatic heart disease, which results in slowly progressive fibrosis, calcification, and deformity of the leaflets characterized by leaflet rigidity, restricted leaflet motion, and chordal shortening that impairs valve opening and closure. The pathognomonic feature of rheumatic mitral valve disease is fusion of the valve commissures, which is often associated with MR from inadequate leaflet coaptation. Progressive deformity of the valve leaflets may be accompanied by more hemodynamically significant MR than mitral stenosis. MR may also result after percutaneous balloon mitral valvuloplasty caused by tears in the valve leaflets during balloon inflation, causing acute increase in the severity of MR that can be localized to the site of the leaflet tear by TTE or TEE. Mitral leaflet thickness and motion in rheumatic MR can be evaluated by transthoracic Doppler echo in the parasternal long- and short-axis views, as well as the apical two-, four-, and long-axis views or in similar apical views by TEE.

Mitral valve prolapse occurs in 2% to 4% of the population and is associated with increased leaflet thickness and excessive motion of the mitral valve leaflets, which interrupts the normal leaflet coaptation, resulting in MR. Mitral valve prolapse is the most common cause of isolated MR in adults. The diagnosis of mitral valve prolapse is established by echocardiographic evidence of thickened mitral valve leaflets (≥5 mm) and billowing of one or both mitral leaflets 2 mm or more beyond the plane of the mitral valve annulus in the parasternal long-axis view (Figure 11-10). The associated MR is detected by color flow Doppler. Because the mitral valve annulus is saddle-shaped rather than monoplanar, the diagnosis of mitral leaflet prolapse should be established echocardiographically in the parasternal or apical long-axis views of the left ventricle and not in the apical four-chamber view

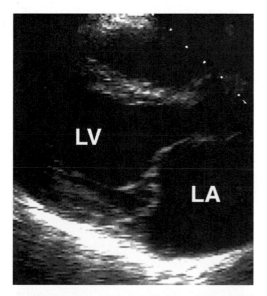

FIGURE 11-10. Parasternal long axis in systole from a patient with mitral valve prolapse. Both mitral leaflets are thickened and moderately myxomatous. The posterior leaflet prolapses into the left atrium and crosses the mitral annular plane by more than 5 mm.

alone.[10] Three-dimensional echocardiography may allow further definition of mitral anatomy (Figure 11-11).

Mitral valve prolapse may involve one or both leaflets, but when only one leaflet is involved, it is more commonly the posterior leaflet than the anterior leaflet, and the MR may be holosystolic or late systolic. There is a wide spectrum of alterations in the mitral valve leaflets and subvalve components evident on echocardiographic examination that varies from near-normal leaflets to the thickened, myxomatous floppy leaflets and a dilated mitral annulus as occurs in connective tissue disorders such as Ehlers-Danlos and Marfan's syndrome. Identification of the individual scallop or scallops that are prolapsing may demonstrate the mechanism of MR and should be attempted in all cases, especially when there is sufficient regurgitation to warrant surgical intervention. Transitory mitral valve prolapse may occur during tachycardia, ventricular ectopy, intravascular volume depletion, and in the presence of large pericardial effusions despite the valve and subvalve apparatus being intrinsically normal. In these circumstances, mitral valve prolapse usually disappears with restoration of normal hemodynamics. Initial descriptions of the natural history of mitral valve prolapse reported widely varying prevalence of prolapse-related adverse cardiovascular events and resulted from the original criteria used for the diagnosis. Recent community-based cohorts that used strict criteria of >2 mm of scallop displacement and leaflet thickness of >5 mm have shown that most patients with mild mitral valve prolapse and hemodynamically insignificant MR remain stable over many years without adverse cardiovascular events. However, in a minority of subjects, mitral prolapse is characterized by slowly progressive degenerative mitral valve disease punctuated by rupture of minor chordae, leading to partial or completely flail leaflets with increased severity of MR, left atrial dilation, and progressive contractile dysfunction necessitating valve repair or replacement.[11] Associated complications of mitral valve prolapse include recurrent arrhythmias, conduction disease, endocarditis, and thromboembolic stroke. Studies that used TTE have identified age, mitral leaflet thickness, MR, increased left atrial and left ventricular size, low ejection fraction, and atrial fibrillation to be associated with adverse prognosis, which are useful for risk stratification.

There are important additional reasons for establishing the diagnosis of mitral valve prolapse. First, to detect associated MR, which, if present, necessitates antibiotic prophylaxis for dental therapy, lower intestinal endoscopy, and to reduce the risk of endocarditis. Second, to assess the severity of MR, its impact on left ventricular function, and to identify subjects at high risk for adverse outcome by serial two-dimensional echocardiography over time. When MR is of a severity to warrant surgical intervention, preoperative TEE should be performed to plan the details of the surgical procedure. TEE (Figures 11-4, B and 11-12) provides precise pathoanatomical details of each of the three anterior (A1, A2, A3) and three posterior scallops (P1, P2, P3) of the mitral leaflets and of the subvalve apparatus.[2,3] This information is invaluable in assessing whether the prolapsing anterior and/or posterior leaflet scallops can be repaired, whether quadrangular leaflet resection or additional chordal shortening procedures are required, and whether the mitral annular diameter requires reduction.[12] Similarly, after operative mitral valve repair or replacement, intraoperative TEE after bypass is mandatory to assess the integrity of the mitral repair procedure and ascertain whether valve competence is maintained with resting hemodynamics and during challenges with increased ventricular afterload. When there is significant residual regurgitation after repair at intraoperative TEE, further repair or replacement can be performed by reinstituting cardiopulmonary bypass. No other imaging techniques provide the anatomical detail or are sufficiently portable to guide the surgical mitral valve repair intraoperatively and confirm competence of the valve after repair.

Acute bacterial endocarditis may be associated with changes in the mitral leaflets, which range from nonspecific inflammatory thickening to discrete vegetations from 2 to ≥15 mm in diameter, with excessive leaflet motion, leaflet perforation, or destruction causing from mild to severe MR. In approximately two thirds of patients with acute vegetative endocarditis, the vegetations can be detected by TTE. By contrast, vegetations are detected in >95% of patients with documented infective endocarditis by TEE. Therefore, in patients with thickened mitral valve leaflets and a clinical suspicion for endocarditis, TEE is mandatory to establish the diagnosis. Vegetations can be visualized in exquisite detail, and the attachment of mitral valve vegetations, described originally only of postmortem, can be demonstrated taking origin from the atrial surface of the mitral leaflets by TEE.

Congenital anomalies of the mitral valve leaflets presenting in adults are rare, but cleft mitral valve leaflets or duplication of the mitral valve orifice, may be associated with MR. Congenital cleft mitral valve may occur as an isolated anomaly or more commonly in association with partial or complete atrioventricular canal defects (see

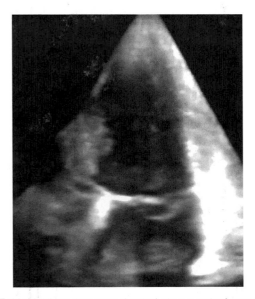

FIGURE 11-11. Three-dimensional apical view acquired as a full volume and cropped to demonstrate prolapse of the posterior leaflet. A partial flail is demonstrated in this view.

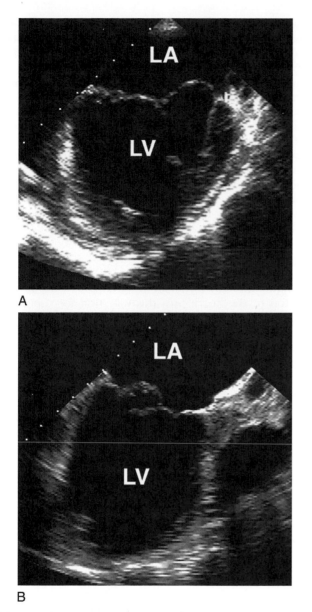

A

B

FIGURE 11-12. A, Transesophageal image of the four-chamber view in the transverse plane (imaging angle 0 degrees) from the midesophageal level. The P2 scallop of the posterior leaflet prolapses into the left atrium. **B,** Same patient in the longitudinal plane (imaging angle 130 degrees) two-chamber view. The posterior leaflet prolapses (scallop P2), whereas the anterior mitral valve leaflet appears normal.

Chapter 14). The congenitally cleft anterior mitral valve leaflet usually appears thickened in the parasternal long-axis view of the left ventricle by two-dimensional echocardiography. However, the cleft in the anterior leaflet can be optimally visualized in the parasternal short-axis view of the left ventricle, in which the altered systolic coaptation can be seen to be the cause of the MR that may vary from mild to severe. The mitral regurgitant jet can be precisely localized by color flow Doppler to occur through the defect in the anterior leaflet.

Acquired nonspecific mitral leaflet thickening with reduced leaflet mobility causing MR may be caused by exuberant mitral annular calcification (MAC) extending into the posterior mitral valve leaflet. MAC is prevalent in

end-stage renal disease and is associated with aging and senile calcific aortic stenosis and hypertrophic cardiomyopathy. Systemic lupus erythematosus, cardiac amyloidosis, and prolonged exposure (>6 months) to an anorexigen use may also cause thickening of the leaflets with restricted motion. These less common causes of mitral leaflet thickening and MR can usually be diagnosed by the presence of associated echocardiographic abnormalities and the accompanying medical history and physical examination.

Abnormalities of the Chordae Tendineae

Disorders of the tensor apparatus associated with MR include shortening and scarring, elongation, and rupture of the chordae tendineae. Rheumatic mitral valve disease involves the leaflets and subvalve tensor apparatus and results in fibrosis, scarring, shortening, and even calcification of the chordae tendineae, causing leaflet retraction, inadequate valve closure, and MR.

Myxomatous degeneration of the mitral valve leaflets is often accompanied by elongated and redundant chordae that not only allow systolic prolapse but also permit overriding of the mitral leaflets and failure of adequate coaptation. The excessive leaflet motion in mitral leaflet prolapse applies increased traction to the chordae that lengthen and occasionally rupture with worsening MR. Ruptured chordae can usually be visualized by TTE as mobile threadlike structures within the left ventricular cavity attached either to the mitral leaflet or to the papillary muscle tip. Mitral chordal rupture with severe MR may also develop in acute, vegetative bacterial endocarditis either from excessive traction on the chordae by large extremely mobile vegetations or by necrosis of the chordal/leaflet junction by destructive microorganisms such as *Staphylococcus aureus*. Chordal rupture can be defined anatomically and must be distinguished from a mobile vegetation or tumor mass by TEE.

Acute MR secondary to chordal rupture may occur after inferior myocardial infarction usually involving the posteromedial papillary muscle. Separation of chordae from the tip of the necrotic papillary muscle characteristically occurs from 2 to 7 days after acute infarction. Acute chordal separation is usually associated with sudden severe hemodynamic decompensation and a new murmur caused by severe acute MR, which, if not diagnosed and corrected rapidly, usually leads to deterioration in left ventricular function, pulmonary edema, and congestive heart failure. The diagnosis is rarely made with TTE and should be established by emergent transesophageal Doppler echocardiography, which demonstrates the flail-like motion of chordae attached to the separated tip of the papillary muscle, severe MR by color flow Doppler, and segmental left ventricular wall motion abnormality (Figure 11-13).

Abnormalities of Papillary Muscles and Left Ventricular Myocardium

After myocardial infarction, papillary muscle rupture (as discussed previously) may be the cause of acute severe

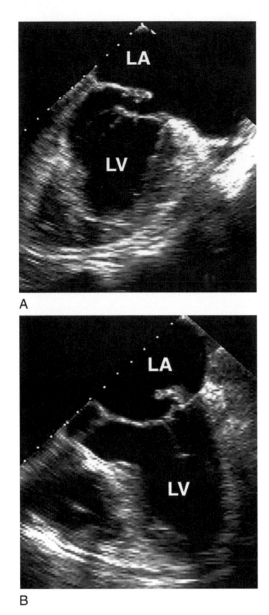

A

B

FIGURE 11-13. A, Transesophageal image in the longitudinal plane (imaging angle 120 degrees) in systole in a patient with acute severe mitral regurgitation. The posterior leaflet is flail, whereas the anterior leaflet maintains a normal position. The tip of the posterior leaflet is thickened. This may represent an intrinsic abnormality of the leaflet or the tip of the papillary muscle. The systolic bulging of the inferior wall at the base is evident in this image. The patient had sustained an inferior myocardial infarction several days earlier. **B,** Transesophageal image in the transverse plane (imaging angle 0 degrees) in the modified five-chamber view from the same patient. The tip of the posterior papillary muscle is prolapsed into the left atrium in this systolic frame.

MR requiring emergency surgery. Transient "ischemic MR" occurs in approximately one third of patients after myocardial infarction because of loss of the normal coordinated contraction of the ventricular walls from ischemia and to alteration in systolic position and direction of contraction of the papillary muscles. Concomitant enlargement of the mitral valve annulus also contributes to development of MR. Early MR after myocardial infarction usually resolves or lessens in severity as the left ven-

tricle stabilizes rather than remodels. Left ventricular remodeling and development of ischemic MR has been characterized by serial quantitative two-dimensional TTE and portends a poor long-term prognosis.[13]

In patients with advanced, obstructive coronary artery disease, intermittent acute episodic myocardial ischemia may cause papillary muscle dysfunction or acute cavity dilation and result in "flash" pulmonary edema because of acute severe or worsening of chronic MR without any anatomical disruption of the papillary muscle. Detection of severe evanescent MR from global ischemia or from regional myocardial ischemia with or without papillary muscle dysfunction is important, because it may be reversed by myocardial revascularization (see Ischemic MR later).

Abnormalities of the Mitral Valve Annulus

The mitral annulus forms an integral part of the fibrous skeleton of the heart, provides insertion for the mitral valve leaflets, and provides electrical insulation between the left atrium and ventricle. Normal mitral annular dimensions in adults vary over a narrow range. The annular area index is 3.9 ± 0.7 cm^2/m^2. The mitral annular dimension can be measured in orthogonal planes from the apex of the left ventricle by TTE and exhibit a direct relationship with the long axis of the left ventricle. Left ventricular dilation and concomitant changes in ventricular shape to a more spherical configuration as occurs in idiopathic dilated cardiomyopathy is frequently accompanied by MR of varying severity (Figure 11-14). Alteration in ventricular shape disrupts the normal geometry of the mitral valve apparatus, separating the papillary muscles and increasing the angle the chordal tendineae subtend to the mitral valve annulus, as well as causing mitral annular dilation. Normal mitral valve closure cannot occur, even though the leaflets and subvalve apparatus are normal, resulting in mild to severe MR. Progressive left ventricular dilation and cavity distortion begets MR, which in turn begets further left ventricular dilation and escalation in the severity of MR and deterioration in ventricular function. The mechanism of this functional MR is due in part to "tenting" of the mitral valve leaflets, which limits leaflet coaptation to the leaflet tips such that systolic displacement of the leaflet bodies toward the annulus is restricted.[14] The major determinant of mitral tenting is apical and posterior displacement of the papillary muscle consequent on left ventricular dilation and dysfunction. The impaired leaflet coaptation caused by tenting is exacerbated by mitral annular dilation and loss of systolic annular function.[15] Mitral leaflet tenting relates directly to effective mitral regurgitant orifice area. Recently, epicardial restraint devices have been used to reduce left ventricular dilation and MR to prevent progressive deterioration in left ventricular function. Splinting of the posteroinferior left ventricular wall, reduction in mitral leaflet tenting, and restoration of near-normal mitral valve geometry have been shown to decrease the severity of MR.[16]

Intraoperative transesophageal measurements of the mitral annular diameter are useful for "sizing" mitral prostheses before valve replacement surgery. The annu-

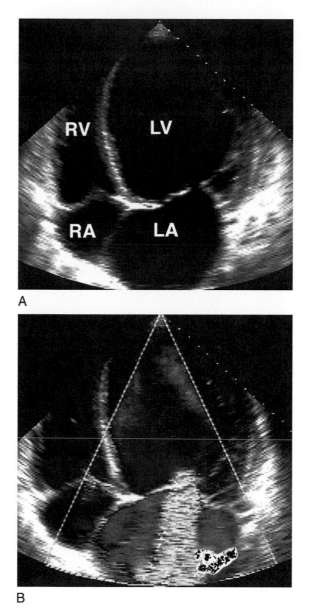

A

B

FIGURE 11-14. **A,** Four-chamber apical systolic image from a patient with idiopathic dilated cardiomyopathy. The left ventricle (LV) is severely dilated, and the systolic function is markedly decreased. In systole, the mitral valve leaflets fail to coapt completely, and the tips of the leaflets are tented, pointing toward the left ventricular apex. The left atrium (LA) is also dilated. The right ventricle (RV) is enlarged and systolic function is mildly decreased. **B,** Similar view in the same patient with color Doppler flow imaging in systole. A large color jet of mitral regurgitation extends to the posterior wall of the left atrium. The mitral regurgitation begins in the left ventricle at the level of the mitral leaflet tips, more apically displaced than is normal. A jet of tricuspid regurgitation is incompletely visualized in the right atrium (RA). See also Color Insert.

lus is usually measured in the transverse plane in the modified four-chamber view. Mitral annular diameter increases progressively with left ventricular dilation. Increase in mitral annular area alters the geometry of the mitral subvalve apparatus and interrupts the normal coaptation of the mitral leaflets, resulting in MR. Reversal of left ventricular dilation by intravascular volume depletion with intravenous diuretic therapy or afterload reduction with vasodilators decreases mitral

annular area and the severity of MR. Similarly, surgical mitral valve repair by mitral annuloplasty ring achieves mitral competence, primarily by reducing mitral annular area and secondarily by restoring toward normal the geometry of the mitral subvalve apparatus. Intraoperative transesophageal monitoring of mitral geometry and assessment of residual MR by Doppler color flow mapping after mitral valve annuloplasty repair is now standard surgical practice.

Disease processes involving the mitral annulus that cause MR usually do so indirectly by annular dilation. However, bacterial endocarditis involving the mitral valve leaflets may extend into the annulus and adjacent myocardium, resulting in abscess formation with destruction of the valve support structures and worsening MR. Recognition of mitral annular abscess is of critical importance, because medical therapy with intravenous antibiotics is not curative, and urgent surgical evacuation of the abscess and valve replacement offers the only potential cure. Mitral annular abscess can only be reliably diagnosed by TEE, and the extent of myocardial involvement and proximity to vital adjacent structures such as the left circumflex coronary artery must be clearly defined preoperatively.

Quantification of Severity of Regurgitation

Evaluation of MR should include quantitation of left ventricular size or volume, regurgitant fraction, regurgitant volume, or regurgitant orifice area, and contractile function, which in aggregate but not in isolation, describe the severity of the MR. Accurate assessment of left ventricular volumes and ejection fraction is important prognostically in chronic severe MR, because these measurements predict postoperative survival in patients undergoing valve surgery. The pathoetiology of MR should be determined, because this provides insight into the likely temporal course of the disease, for example, the clinical outcome in ischemic MR is poorer than with nonischemic MR.[13]

Echocardiography

Doppler echocardiography is the imaging technology most frequently used for the diagnosis of MR, assessment of the severity of acute and chronic MR, and quantitation of its effects on left ventricular function. Doppler color flow mapping unequivocally establishes the presence of MR. Continuous-wave and color flow Doppler enable estimation of the hemodynamics and quantitative assessment of the severity of MR. Doppler echocardiography can be repeated and is thus ideal for long-term surveillance of patients with MR to detect worsening regurgitation, progressive left ventricular dilation, and deterioration in left ventricular function. A number of Doppler echocardiography measurements are used to assess the severity of MR, none of which individually represents the "Rosetta stone." Integration of the selected measurements described in the following sections enable accurate assessment of the severity of MR and differentiation of clinically mild from moderate and moderate from severe MR.

Left Ventricular Dimensions, Volumes, and Ejection Fraction

Echocardiographic measurements of left ventricular size, volume, and ejection fraction indicate the severity of chronic MR, predict survival, and for this reason drive the clinical algorithm that determines treatment strategy.[7] Measurement of left ventricular end-systolic and end-diastolic dimensions by transthoracic two-dimensionally directed M-mode echocardiography can be obtained in most patients from parasternal long-axis images of the left ventricle. These M-mode measurements are reliable in left ventricles with uniform wall thickness that contract concentrically, but need to be interpreted with caution in left ventricles with regional wall motion abnormalities and nonuniform wall thickness from coexistent coronary artery disease. In addition, left ventricular dimensions vary with changes in left ventricular loading conditions. However, in the management of chronic severe MR, a left ventricular end-systolic diameter of >45 mm is recommended as a cut-point to stratify treatment of patients in New York Heart Association (NYHA) symptom classes I and II.[7]

Quantitation of left ventricular end-systolic and end-diastolic volumes is preferable to measurements of single dimensions, because the volume computational algorithms recommended by the American Society of Echocardiography make no assumptions about fixed left ventricular shape. Furthermore, the entire left ventricle is sampled from the base to the apex for volume calculations and is more representative of the adaptive changes in cavity shape as the heart remodels in response to chronic MR. Left ventricular volumes are ideally computed from biplane, near-orthogonal apical images of the long axis of the left ventricle by use of the modified Simpson's method or the method of disks. Volumes are usually obtained by manual digitization of the endocardial boundaries of left ventricular silhouettes, although automated edge detection algorithms for estimating volume by use of acoustic quantitation are now commercially available. Left ventricular volumes computed from single-plane apical images approximate closely biplane values but differ systematically with increasing ventricular volumes and distortion in cavity shape. A small study that used three-dimensional estimation of left ventricular volumes also correlated closely with biplane values, but their variance was less than with biplane volume estimates. Assessment of left ventricular end-systolic volume is important in chronic severe MR, because it is a powerful predictor of survival after mitral valve surgery.

Estimation of left ventricular cavity volumes allows calculation of ejection fraction, which is also a strong predictor of survival in patients with severe chronic MR undergoing valve surgery. Left ventricular ejection fraction of 60% and end-systolic dimension of 45 mm are used as cut-points in combination with NYHA functional class (I through IV) to provide objective measures that comprise the framework for current ACC/AHA recommendations for the management of patients with chronic severe MR.[7]

Regurgitant Volume and Regurgitant Fraction

Although left ventricular volumes are important in assessment of chronic MR, quantitation of the regurgitant volume or regurgitant fraction more directly addresses the severity of the hemodynamic burden. Mitral regurgitant volume (MRV) is the difference between the volume of blood entering the left ventricle through the mitral valve (mitral stroke volume, MSV) and the volume of blood ejected through the aortic valve (left ventricular stroke volume, LVSV) in each cardiac cycle:

$$MRV = MSV - LVSV \qquad \text{(Equation 5)}$$

There are two echocardiographic methods for quantifying MSV. The first method quantifies the difference between left ventricular end-diastolic (EDV) and end-systolic (ESV) volumes from biplane apical echocardiographic images:

$$LVSV = EDV - ESV \qquad \text{(Equation 6)}$$

The second method uses the Doppler principle that blood volume flow can be estimated as the product of the area under the velocity time curve (the velocity time integral [VTI]) and the cross-sectional area (CSA) of the flow stream. Thus, MSV is calculated as the product of transmitral Doppler velocity time integral (VTI_{mitral}) and the cross-sectional area of the mitral annulus (CSA_{mitral}), which is assumed to be circular and calculated from measurement of the annular diameter in the apical four-chamber view.

$$MSV = VTI_{mitral} \times CSA_{mitral} \qquad \text{(Equation 7)}$$

LVSV is quantified as the product of the left ventricular outflow tract Doppler velocity time integral (VTI_{LVOT}) obtained in the apical five-chamber view and the CSA of the left ventricular outflow tract calculated (πr^2) from the diameter of the LVOT in the left parasternal long-axis view, again assuming a circular cross-section. MRV is calculated as described in Equation 5.

Regurgitant fraction (RF) provides a quantitative estimate of the severity of MR and is defined as the percentage of the forward blood flow volume (MSV) that is regurgitated, and is calculated as the ratio of regurgitant volume and total antegrade flow across the mitral valve.

$$\text{Regurgitant fraction} = MRV/MSV \times 100\% \qquad \text{(Equation 8)}$$

Regurgitant volumes and RFs calculated using these two methods correlate closely. The severity of MR can be reliably estimated in terms of regurgitant volume and RF by quantitative TTE in 70% to 80% of patients in whom apical biplane left ventricular images are obtained compared with almost all patients using Doppler VTIs. Because of this shortfall and the labor intensity of manual or automated digitization of biplane apical left ventricular images to obtain volumes, the Doppler VTI method is more practical for routine clinical use. There is good agreement in RF between the two methods. An RF of <30% defines mild MR and corresponds to (1+) MR by contrast angiographic grade. RF between 30% and 50% corresponds to 2+ to 3+ MR by angiographic grade, and

RF >50% indicates severe MR in 4+ MR by angiographic grade.[3]

Doppler Color Flow Mapping

Doppler color flow mapping was initially believed to provide a means of evaluating the severity of MR. The length, width, and area of the MR jet were correlated with the severity of MR but did not reliably separate individual patients with mild from those with moderate or severe MR. Subsequently, regurgitant mitral jet area measured in three planes expressed as a ratio of left atrial area was shown to approximate with contrast angiographic grade of severity of MR. Although this more rigorous method did distinguish between population group means, considerable overlap remained between groups and rendered management of individual patients with MR problematic. The reason Doppler velocity color flow mapping seems ambiguous in assessing the severity of chronic MR relates to a number of factors that impact either directly or indirectly on the distribution of the color-encoded velocity jet in the left atrium. The area of the Doppler velocity color flow jet is affected by gain settings of the recording instrument, the initial MR jet velocity, the size and compliance of the left atrium, left ventricular loading conditions, and whether the regurgitant jet collides with the left atrial wall or septum, loses its momentum, and fails to propagate into the left atrium and pulmonary veins. Color flow Doppler tends to overestimate central regurgitant jets and underestimate eccentric jets, especially wall jets. Although, color flow Doppler mapping of the distribution of the MR jet does not provide quantitative information or direct individual patient management per se, when integrated with clinical history and examination findings, it is often helpful in guiding therapy. Caution should be used when assessing MR by TEE, especially in patients under general anesthesia. The alteration in loading conditions may cause underestimation of the degree of regurgitation. Three-dimensional reconstructions of the regurgitant jet may add additional insight into the severity of the regurgitation.[17]

Pulmonary Venous Blood Flow Velocity

Pulmonary venous blood flow velocity profiles can be sampled with pulsed-wave Doppler echocardiography by the transesophageal and transthoracic routes and may provide useful information relating to the severity of MR (Figure 11-15). TEE allows high-fidelity recording of pulmonary venous blood flow velocity patterns, which may be useful in the intraoperative assessment of MR before and after mitral valve repair. The pulmonary veins can be sampled by TTE in the apical views in most patients.

In normal subjects, pulmonary venous velocity signals show reversed blood flow during atrial systole, because there are no venous valves to prevent reflux of blood into the pulmonary venous system when the atrium contracts. This is followed by antegrade pulmonary venous flow in ventricular systole (systolic wave) as intrapericardial pressure falls, which is followed by increased forward flow during ventricular diastolic filling (diastolic

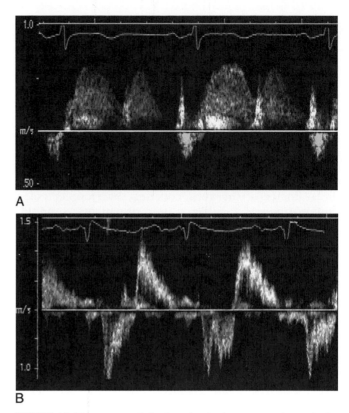

FIGURE 11-15. A, Spectral display of pulsed-wave Doppler with the sample volume placed in the ostia of the right superior pulmonary vein. The transducer is in the apical position. There is normal systolic filling and a slightly lower velocity wave in early diastole. Brief reversal of flow occurs with atrial contraction. **B,** Spectral display of pulsed-wave Doppler from a transesophageal study with the sample volume placed approximately 1 cm into the left superior vein. The patient had severe MR caused by a flail mitral valve scallop with an anteriorly directed jet. There is reversal of flow into the pulmonary vein in systole, with filling occurring only during diastole.

wave). Severe MR results in attenuation or reversal of flow during left ventricular systole, with loss or decrease in the systolic velocity wave, especially if the regurgitant blood flow jet is directed into the pulmonary vein in which the Doppler sample volume is located. When the regurgitant mitral jet is directed away from the pulmonary vein in which the pulsed-wave Doppler recordings are obtained, a normal pulmonary venous velocity spectra may be obtained, which may spuriously underestimate the severity of MR. Thus, a normal pulmonary venous velocity pattern does not reliably exclude severe MR. However, a ratio of systolic velocity/diastolic velocity >1.0 effectively excludes severe MR.

Vena Contracta Measurement

Although Doppler color flow mapping of regurgitant jet morphology provides only a semiquantitative assessment of the severity of MR, quantitative information can be extracted from color flow Doppler velocity signals that correlate with severity of MR. These Doppler color flow techniques involve measurements of the vena contracta or the radius of the proximal flow convergence zone.

The vena contracta is the term applied to the narrowest central flow region of a jet and approximates to or slightly underestimates effective regurgitant orifice area (EROA). The jet orifice area in MR can be measured by Doppler color flow imaging (Figure 11-16). Initial studies using transthoracic and multiplane transesophageal echocardiographic imaging demonstrated close agreement with angiographic assessment of MR and to measurements of regurgitant volume. These early clinical observations were confirmed in an animal model, and correlations between vena contracta width and severity of MR extended to regurgitant fraction. Measurement of the diameter of the vena contracta by Doppler color flow mapping is possible in >90% of patients, is simple, and allows differentiation of mild from severe MR. These measurements of the vena contracta can only be made from high-quality images. Measurements are optimally made using high-resolution mode or zoom function or better still with high-quality TEE images. Vena contracta width measurements of <0.3 cm correspond to mild MR, a vena contracta diameter from 0.3 to 0.5 cm corresponds to moderate MR, and >0.5 cm corresponds to severe MR. Although regurgitant orifice area calculated from biplane measurements of vena contracta diameter correlates with regurgitant volume, it systematically underestimates volumetric regurgitant orifice. The diameter of the vena contracta has subsequently been demonstrated to vary unpredictably with changes in left ventricular loading conditions and does not reliably determine whether the regurgitant orifice is fixed or dynamic. The role of vena contracta width in ascertaining the severity of mitral regurgitation remains to be clarified. In clinical practice, when visual assessment of Doppler color flow in chronic MR is integrated with left ventricular size, function, and symptomatic presentation, the vena contracta diameter provides additional insight that enables mild, moderate, and severe disease to be differentiated in most patients and correlates with EROA, RF and angiographic grading from 1+ to 4+. The ability of multiplane TEE to obtain orthogonal views, specifically oriented to assessing the vena contracta width, is superior to single-plane studies in evaluating the severity of mitral regurgitation.

Proximal Isovelocity Surface Area (PISA)

PISA as an echocardiographic estimate of MR relies on the flow convergence or proximal isovelocity surface area method to calculate the effective regurgitant orifice area. This method is based on the principle of conservation of mass and assumes that blood flow in the convergence region enters the regurgitant orifice region exclusively. Blood flow velocity increases as it approaches and enters the regurgitant orifice, producing a continuous series of hemispherical "shells" proximal to the orifice. The shells that converge around the regurgitant orifice are known as isovelocity surfaces, with increasing velocity and decreasing surface area. The velocity at any point on the surface of each shell is constant. Regurgitant flow is equal to the product of the area of the shell and the velocity at that same shell surface, assuming that the shape of the proximal isovelocity surface is hemispherical (Figure 11-17). The isovelocity surface in the convergence zone is made visible by shifting the baseline of the Doppler color flow velocity scale such that the radius to the first aliasing velocity is easily seen. The radius of the isovelocity shell is measured in the centerline of the outermost convergence zone of the ultrasound beam. Thus, regurgitant flow can be quantitated as:

$$\text{Regurgitant flow rate} = 2\pi r^2 \times V_N \qquad \text{(Equation 9)}$$

where V_N = velocity of the shell (the Nyquist limit), and r = radius of the shell. By the principle of the continuity equation, the flow at each isovelocity surface is equal to the flow at the regurgitant orifice. From the regurgitant flow rate, the EROA can be calculated as:

$$\text{EROA} = \frac{\text{Regurgitant flow rate}}{\text{Peak regurgitant velocity}} \qquad \text{(Equation 10)}$$

where peak regurgitant velocity is measured by continuous wave Doppler.

Finally, the regurgitant volume is equal to the velocity integral of the MR jet multiplied by the effective regurgitant orifice.

$$RV = 2\pi r^2 \times V_N (VTI_{MR})/V_P \qquad \text{(Equation 11)}$$

where RV is the regurgitant volume, r is the radius to the isovelocity surface area, VTI_{MR} is the velocity time integral of the MR jet measured by continuous-wave Doppler, V_P is the peak velocity of that jet, and V_N is the Nyquist velocity.

Although hemispheric geometry is applicable to unconstrained flow convergence zones, when the flow convergence zone is constrained, hemispherical geome-

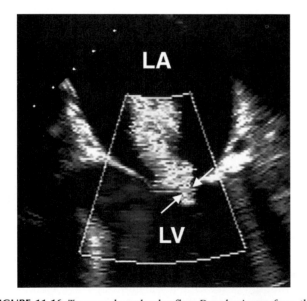

FIGURE 11-16. Transesophageal color flow Doppler image from the transverse plane in a patient with moderate mitral regurgitation. The vena contracta *(indicated by arrows)* is the narrowest area of the jet as it passes just beyond the mitral valve leaflets. The vena contracta in this patient is approximately 0.4 mm, consistent with moderate mitral regurgitation. See also Color Insert.

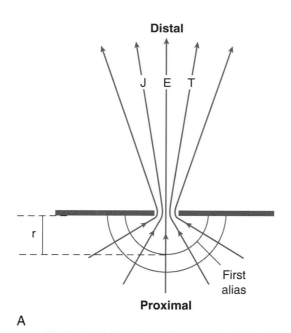

Distal

J E T

r

First alias

Proximal

A

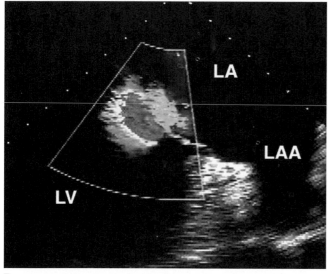

LA

LAA

LV

B

FIGURE 11-17. A, Schematic diagram of the proximal flow convergence region for a circular orifice. The streamlines of flow are shown approaching the orifice. The points at which flow has the same velocity form concentric hemispheric isovelocity contours. These can be visualized as the accelerating jet aliases as the velocity increases. The first aliasing velocity is the Nyquist limit, which can be read from the ultrasound machine display. (Reprinted with permission from Rodriquez et al. *Circulation* 1993; 88:1157.) **B,** Demonstration of PISA phenomenon in a patient with severe mitral regurgitation caused by a flail anterior leaflet. The jet is very eccentric, and its course cannot be visualized in the left atrium in this plane (LAA, left atrial appendage). See also Color Insert.

try may not be met, and in such cases EROA can be adjusted by measurement of the arc angle "α" of the constrained flow convergence zone by a factor of $\alpha/180$. Peak regurgitant velocity is measured by continuous-wave Doppler in the center line of the convergence beam. In the early use of the PISA flow convergence method, technical difficulties were encountered with regard to stability of the Doppler color flow signal, and this diminished enthusiasm for this method. However, the

stability and reproducibility of this method has been subsequently definitively established. PISA technique has been validated in vitro across a range of driving pressures and regurgitant orifice shapes and sizes and also validated clinically in large numbers of patients undergoing simultaneous cardiac catheterization and quantitative echocardiograms. Calculated EROA correlates closely with stroke volume assessed by two-dimensional echocardiography and with contrast angiographic grading of MR. Optimal flow convergence Doppler signals are obtainable in most patients (92% to 98%), are therefore practical for assessing the severity of MR, and only rarely overestimate the severity of MR, except when the flow convergence signal is suboptimal, typically in mitral prolapse.

The severity of MR can be graded by effective regurgitant orifice area calculated by the PISA method. An EROA <20 mm² is consistent with mild regurgitation (1+ by angiographic grade), EROA 20 to 40 mm² is moderate MR (2+ to 3+ angiographic grade), and EROA >40 mm² indicates severe MR (4+ angiograde grade).[18] The time-dependent progression of the severity of MR can be quantified in terms of regurgitant volume, RF and effective regurgitant orifice area, and the impact of therapeutic modulation of left ventricular afterload assessed. Recently, a semiquantitative index of the severity MR has been proposed, which is a composite of six echocardiographic variables: jet penetration, PISA, continuous-wave Doppler characteristics of the regurgitant jet, pulmonary artery pressure, pulmonary venous flow pattern, and left atrial size.[19] Each variable is scored on a scale of 0 to 3. This index correlates with RF and effective regurgitant orifice area but requires further clinical validation.

Cardiac Catheterization

Traditionally, assessment of chronic MR has been performed in the cardiac catheterization laboratory by measurement of right and left heart hemodynamics and left ventricular contrast angiography, which often provides insight into the pathoetiology of the mitral valve disease. Hemodynamic measurements in moderate to severe chronic MR demonstrate increased pulmonary capillary wedge pressure because of the presence of a large "v" wave, which may exceed mean pulmonary capillary wedge or left atrial pressure by twofold to threefold. Occasionally, resting hemodynamic measurements in chronic severe MR are only mildly abnormal and seem to exclude significant MR. In such circumstances, hemodynamic measurements should be repeated with exercise or with increased left ventricular loading induced by pharmacological stress to unmask severe MR, particularly in patients with ischemic MR. The impact of chronic severe MR on left ventricular contractile function can be underestimated, because ejection occurs into a low-pressure sink (left atrium), and left ventricular emptying appears vigorous and nearly complete. However, deviation from the normal pressure-volume relationship can be assessed during perturbations in left ventricular loading conditions by administration of intravascular volume or pharmacological agents that either increase or decrease preload and/or afterload. The slope of the left ventricular end-systolic pressure-volume relationship over a series of load perturbations enables characterization of intrinsic myocardial contractility independent of load.

Quantitative left ventricular contrast angiography enables accurate and reproducible assessments of left ventricular EDVs and ESVs, stroke volume, and ejection fraction from biplane or single-plane left ventricular angiographic silhouettes. Estimation of cardiac output either by thermodilution or Fick together with stroke volume allows quantitation of regurgitant volume from which RF can be calculated. Ventricular volumes have important prognostic information in patients undergoing mitral valve surgery. Left ventricular volumes are not quantitated routinely in most clinical catheterization laboratories, even in patients with valvular heart disease. The severity of MR may be semiquantitated in patients in sinus rhythm by visual estimation are made of the extent and timing of opacification of the left atrium after contrast left ventricular angiography. Similar qualitative visual estimation are made of left ventricular end-diastolic volume and ejection fraction. Angiographically mild (1+) MR is graded when left ventricular injection of contrast does not opacify the entire left atrium and clears in one cardiac cycle. Moderate (2+) MR is designated when the left atrium is opacified, but contrast does not clear after one cardiac cycle. Moderately severe (3+) MR is when the left atrium is completely opacified such that the density of contrast in the left atrium is equal to that in the left ventricle. Severe (4+) MR is when the entire left atrium is opacified within one cardiac cycle after left ventriculography, intensifies with each cycle, and refluxes into the pulmonary veins in systole.

These angiographic grades of severity of MR from mild (1+) through severe (4+) correspond to regurgitant fractions of less than 20%, 20% to 40%, 40% to 60%, and greater than 60%, respectively. Assessment of the severity of MR by contrast angiography is influenced by a number of factors, important among which are the size and compliance of the left atrium, left ventricular loading conditions, left ventricular function, and presence of ventricular ectopy during contrast injection into the left ventricle. Thus, contrast angiographic grading of MR is an approximation and cannot be regarded as a true "gold standard" for comparison with other techniques.

Cardiac catheterization remains an important means of assessing the severity of MR and should not be restricted to patients in whom TTE and/or TEE are inconclusive or technically limited. Cardiac catheterization is indicated, especially when there is discrepancy between the severity of MR assessed by Doppler echocardiography and clinical symptoms and in ischemic MR when the coronary artery disease can be evaluated and revascularization by coronary intervention performed. Patients older than 35 years of age or with more than one risk factor for coronary artery disease and MR of sufficient severity to warrant surgical intervention require preoperative coronary arteriography to evaluate coexistent, asymptomatic obstructive coronary artery disease.[7] Catheterization is also indicated in patients in whom the etiology of the MR is ischemia. Cardiac catheterization may be safely confined to assessment of coronary anatomy in patients in whom the history, physical examination, left ventricular geometry, and severity of MR by Doppler echocardiography are concordant.[7]

Radionuclide Angiography

Radionuclide angiography was formerly used in patients with MR for two discrete purposes: First, to assess left ventricular volumes and RF from the ratio of right ventricular and left ventricular stroke volumes, and second, to estimate left ventricular function and functional reserve as the change in ejection fraction from rest to exercise, respectively. Failure to increase ejection fraction or a decrease in left ventricular ejection fraction with exercise, is indicative of impaired left ventricular function. However, radionuclide techniques are now rarely used to assess patients with isolated MR but may be of value in the assessment of concomitant coronary artery disease.

Cardiac Magnetic Resonance (CMR)

CMR is acknowledged as the "gold standard" for quantitation of left ventricular volumes, mass, chamber topography, and ejection fraction, all of which are important in assessment of the severity of MR. Regurgitant volume and the velocity of the mitral regurgitant jet can also be quantitated by CMR. However, characterization of the pathologic changes in the rapidly moving mitral valve leaflets and subvalve apparatus remains limited by the low temporal resolution of conventional CMR pulse sequences. Despite recent improvements in temporal resolution and signal/noise ratio, current CMR spatial resolution is unsatisfactory to resolve leaflet pathology, and CMR is not routinely used clinically in assessing patients with mitral valve disease. Furthermore, image acquisition may be problematic because of electrocardiographic gating in patients with mitral valve disease in atrial fibrillation and with elevated heart rates. Further limiting its clinical application are the nonportability of the CMR scanner and the difficulty imaging patients with retained metallic fragments and permanent pacemakers or implantable defibrillators.

MR can be diagnosed by CMR, because the regurgitant jet causes turbulent flow, which leads to signal loss detectable on cine gradient echo images. The size of the signal void permits semiquantitative assessment of the severity of MR and correlates well with color Doppler techniques, although the mitral regurgitant jet signal void tends to be smaller than the total color jet area. Potential advantages of CMR techniques in quantitating the severity of mitral regurgitation relate to the greater sampling of the three-dimensional jet volume, and therefore a more accurate assessment of total jet area. Recent studies evaluating CMR techniques in quantifying the degree of MR described agreements of >90% with conventional measures and an interobserver reproducibility of 93%.[20] New, fast spiral phase-contrast sequences permit real-time color mapping of jets, similar to color Doppler mapping techniques.[21] The current inability of CMR to resolve mitral leaflet and subvalve pathology combined with the fact that CMR technology capabilities are limited to tertiary referral centers are reasons that restrict its use in the routine assessment of MR.

Clinical Evaluation

The diagnosis of MR can usually be made on physical examination, and this clinical diagnostic information should not be usurped by "routine" use of imaging technology. The clinical diagnosis of MR is based on the presence of an apical holosystolic murmur that characteristically radiates to the axilla. A number of recent studies have demonstrated a poor correlation between the severity of MR assessed clinically and quantitative echocardiography. However, usually an approximation of the severity of chronic MR can be determined by the location and character of the apical impulse that provides information about left ventricular size and global function. The presence of a third heart sound usually indicates that the MR is at least moderate. Displacement of the apical impulse indicates that the left ventricle is enlarged. Inability to localize the apical impulse in patients with normal body habitus suggests impaired left ventricular contractile function. However, in subjects with abnormal chest geometry because of chronic obstructive pulmonary disease, kyphoscoliosis, or truncal obesity, the apical impulse may not be localized. The presence of pulmonary hypertension secondary to MR is indicated by augmentation of the pulmonary component of the second heart sound and evidence of right ventricular prominence. Left ventricular decompensation and related congestive heart failure is suggested by the presence of a gallop rhythm with third and fourth heart sounds, and pulmonary congestion is indicated by the presence of rales bilaterally. Insight into the possible etiology of chronic MR may be available from clinical history, including mitral prolapse, vegetative endocarditis, acute myocardial infarction, long-standing coronary artery disease, familial hypertrophic or dilated cardiomyopathy, or previous valvular surgery. In summary, although the history and clinical examination may provide important diagnostic information, this is insufficient for accurate assessment of severity in a proportion of patients and underscores the importance of the parallel use of noninvasive Doppler echocardiographic imaging for optimizing management.

The electrocardiogram in patients with chronic moderate to severe MR is nonspecific but includes left atrial and left ventricular enlargement, left ventricular hypertrophy, and in the minority of patients with associated severe pulmonary hypertension, right-axis deviation with right ventricular hypertrophy may be present. Chest radiographs in chronic MR of moderate severity demonstrate enlargement of the left atrium and left ventricle and dilation of the pulmonary trunk in those with associated pulmonary arterial hypertension. The radiographic appearance of lung fields provides information regarding pulmonary venous and pulmonary arterial hypertension. Cephalization of pulmonary venous blood flow indicates increased pulmonary venous pressure, whereas interstitial pulmonary edema and pleural effusions denote the presence of congestive heart failure.

Optimal management of chronic MR is initially thorough clinical assessment and appropriate use of diagnostic tests to establish the severity and etiology of the regurgitation and its impact on left ventricular geometry and function. The appropriate use of diagnostic techniques allows differentiation of patients with left ventricular dysfunction caused primarily by MR from those with primary left ventricular dysfunction and MR secondary to left ventricular remodeling. Patients who have significant MR caused by dilated cardiomyopathy or postinfarction remodeling may demonstrate reduced regurgitation after diuresis and optimization of afterload reduction. However, there is no indication for afterload reduction in patients with preserved left ventricular function who do not have systemic hypertension. Annual or semiannual echocardiographic studies are indicated to follow asymptomatic patients with chronic severe MR.

Special consideration should be given to ischemic MR. This term refers to MR caused by myocardial infarction or myocardial ischemia from occlusive coronary artery disease and must be distinguished from degenerative mitral valve disease associated with but not causally related to coronary disease. Between one third and one half of all patients with acute myocardial infarction have early detectable MR develop either clinically or by Doppler echocardiography. In patients with acute myocardial infarction undergoing cardiac catheterization within 6 hours of the onset of symptoms, 18% had ischemic MR. In most postinfarction patients, the MR is mild and resolves early after infarction. These observations indicate that ischemic MR is common and clinically important, because even mild MR is associated with a significantly increased 1-year mortality.[13] MR occurring early after acute myocardial infarction before the left ventricle has dilated significantly may result from dysfunction of the papillary muscle because of reduced perfusion, causing loss of systolic myocardial shortening, which prevents central coaptation of the mitral leaflets. When the papillary muscles are not directly involved in the infarction, extensive regional wall motion abnormalities may result in left ventricular dyssynchrony, incoordinate contraction, and mitral insufficiency, all of which may be ameliorated by revascularization by either percutaneous catheter intervention or coronary bypass surgery and by angiotensin receptor-blocking agents.

In approximately one third of patients who survive acute myocardial infarction, the left ventricle remodels to offset the acute loss of contractile elements. MR facilitates further left ventricular dilation; thus MR begets MR and is associated with a time-dependent deterioration in left ventricular function and development of congestive heart failure.[13] Patients with ischemic MR can be further risk stratified for survival by estimating regurgitant volume and effective regurgitant orifice area[13] (Figure 11-18). Patients undergoing cardiac catheterization for symptomatic coronary artery disease with even mild chronic MR had a 1-year mortality of almost 17%. Mild (1+) MR was associated with a 1-year mortality of 10% compared with 6% in those without MR, whereas moderate (3+) to severe (4+) MR had a mortality of almost 40%. These mortality statistics underscore the impor-

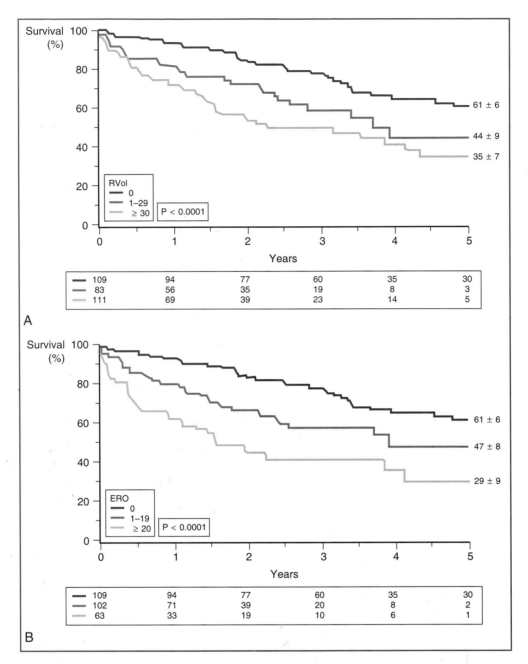

FIGURE 11-18. A, Survival after diagnosis according to degree of ischemic MR as graded by regurgitant volume (RVol) ≥30 mL/beat or <30 mL/beat. Numbers at the bottom indicate patients at risk for each interval. **B,** Survival after diagnosis according to degree of MR graded by effective regurgitant orifice (ERO) area ≥20 mm² or <20 mm². Numbers at the bottom indicate patients at risk for each interval. (Reprinted with permission from Grigioni et al. *Circulation* 2001; 103:1759.)

tance of recognition of ischemic MR and institution of appropriate treatment, including afterload reduction with angiotensin-converting enzyme inhibitors and β-receptor blockers early after infarction to prevent left ventricular remodeling.

Ischemic MR may be associated with recurrent episodes of flash pulmonary edema with systemic hypotension, and it is important to recognize, because it is usually reversible by revascularization with percutaneous catheter intervention or coronary bypass surgery. Chronic ischemic MR, resulting in a progressive increase in symptoms or heart failure, may become refractory to conventional therapy, and there is accumu-

lating evidence that revascularization and mitral valve repair offers survival benefit over continuing medical therapy. Two-dimensional echocardiography has been used to characterize the changes in left ventricular geometry, function, and leaflet coaptation during the early postinfarction period and also through late follow-up to 5 years.[13] Assessment of interval changes in the severity of ischemic MR quantitated by Doppler echocardiography with the proximal flow convergence method to estimate regurgitant volume and effective regurgitant orifice area are powerful predictors of survival at 5-year follow-up. In addition, the severity of ischemic MR is related to the extent of regional wall motion abnormalities at rest and with exercise stress or pharmacological-induced stress.

A small minority of patients with MR cannot be adequately assessed by TTE or less often by TEE because of technical difficulties, so that the optimal management strategy cannot be determined. In such patients, and in patients in whom there is discordance between the clinical and echocardiographic assessment of severity of MR, clarification of these problems can be resolved by hemodynamic measurements and contrast ventriculography at cardiac catheterization. Contrast ventriculography has limitations in quantitating the severity of mitral regurgitation, and these have been described previously, but when performed with care in patients in sinus rhythm, they usually provide sufficiently accurate information for making decisions regarding treatment. Coronary angiography is recommended for all patients in whom mitral valve repair or replacement is contemplated who are older than 35 years of age, in those with risk factors for coronary heart disease, and/or when the etiology of the MR is thought to be ischemic.[7]

Surgical Intervention in Native Valve MR

The prerequisite for the optimal timing of surgical intervention in patients with MR is availability of a noninvasive yardstick that reliably detects time-dependent changes in left ventricular topography and function, and this should be the combination of left ventricular volumes, ejection fraction, regurgitant volume, and effective regurgitant orifice area. There is currently no single invasive or noninvasive measurement that reliably stratifies patients in terms of hemodynamic severity and predicts long-term clinical outcome in all patients. Elective preoperative stratification of patients who would benefit from valve repair versus valve replacement can be achieved by rigorous assessment of the functional anatomy of the MR by TEE. In addition, the timing of operative intervention before the onset of irreversible left ventricular dysfunction is critical to avoid postoperative left ventricular remodeling and progressive deterioration in ventricular function.[22]

Quantitative Doppler echocardiographic assessment of left ventricular size, hemodynamics, and function in conjunction with clinical history and physical examination provides indications and guidelines for timing for surgical intervention. A number of prospective and retrospective studies of patients with chronic MR have demonstrated that preoperative left ventricular size, geometry, and contractile function are major predictors of postoperative clinical outcome. Clinical algorithms have been formulated by the ACC/AHA task force for management of valvular heart disease for optimal treatment strategies in patients with chronic MR from the combination of echocardiographic assessment of left ventricular size, ejection fraction, and NYHA functional class (Figure 11-19). Echocardiographic cut-points of left ventricular end-systolic size $\geq$45 mm and ejection fraction $\leq$60% have proved useful in differentiating good

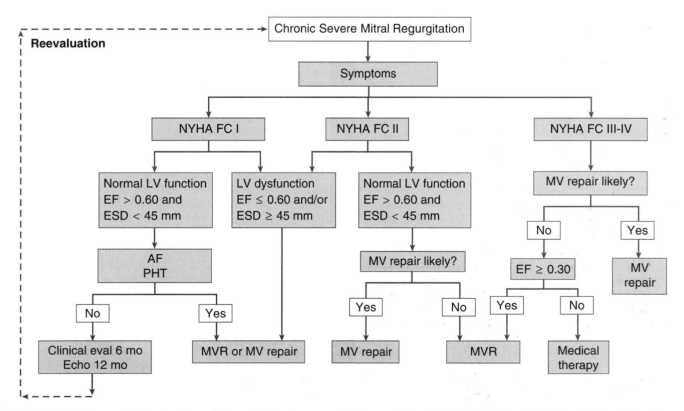

FIGURE 11-19. Management strategy for patients with chronic severe mitral regurgitation. (AF, atrial fibrillation; EF, ejection fraction; ESD, end-systolic diameter; FC, functional class; MV, mitral valve; NYHA, New York Heart Association; PHT, pulmonary hypertension.) (Reprinted with permission from Bonow et al. *J Am Coll Cardiol* 1998; 32:1486.)

from poor postoperative outcome and are used for recommending surgical intervention in patients with chronic MR.[7]

There are two types of surgical correction for chronic MR, of which repair and reconstruction of the native valve with restitution of mitral competence is the preferred technique. Echocardiography plays a primary role in determining whether a mitral valve is reparable or needs replacement. Complete detailed assessment of the leaflet scallops, commissures, the integrity and length of the chordae, and the degree of dilation of the mitral valve annulus should be undertaken preoperatively by TEE in almost every case in which the technical quality of the TTE is not ideal. Intraoperative prebypass and postbypass TEE is mandatory for mitral valve repair, and the competence of the repaired valve should be tested with volume or pressure loading before complete separation from cardiopulmonary bypass if there is any residual MR (Figure 11-20). A decision must be made intraoperatively as to whether the surgeon should reinstitute cardiopulmonary bypass and attempt further repair or replace the valve with a biological or mechanical prosthesis. Occasionally, after mitral valve repair, cardiac output may be low despite vigorous left ventricular contraction, which should suggest the possibility of dynamic left ventricular outflow tract obstruction, resulting from anterior mitral leaflet tissue escaping from the sewing ring and causing systolic anterior motion (SAM) of the mitral valve into the left ventricular outflow tract. SAM is readily detected on intraoperative TEE images of the excessively mobile mitral chordal or leaflet tissue partially obstructing systolic ejection and causing premature aortic valve closure. Mitral valve repair is technically more challenging than valve replacement, requires longer bypass time, and when sinus rhythm is present does not need long-term anticoagulation. The success of mitral valve repair is dependent on the anatomy of the entire mitral valve unit and on the surgical expertise at the point of care. However, improved surgical outcome is associated with repair. When mitral valve replacement is contemplated, preoperative echocardiographic imaging is useful for accurately estimating the appropriate size of the prosthesis so as to avoid prosthesis-patient mismatch and postoperatively to determine that the valve is well seated and competent. Valve replacement should include chordal sparing, which has salutary effects on left ventricular architecture and postoperative ejection performance.[23]

Postoperative assessment of left ventricular function is imperative not only to characterize remodeling but also to identify those patients with left ventricular dysfunction who are at high risk for heart failure developing and in whom appropriate afterload reduction therapy with angiotensin-converting enzyme inhibitors or angiotensin receptor blockade should be instituted.

NORMAL AND ABNORMAL FUNCTION IN PROSTHETIC HEART VALVES

Mitral valve prostheses have considerably smaller orifice areas than the normal mitral annular area. These valves

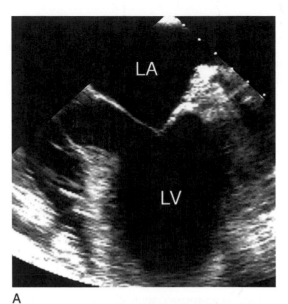

A

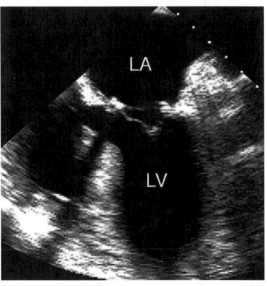

B

FIGURE 11-20. A, Transesophageal echocardiogram in the transverse plane at the level of the midesophagus in a patient with dilated cardiomyopathy. The left atrium (LA) and left ventricle (LV) are moderately dilated, and the mitral annulus is enlarged. In this systolic frame, mitral leaflets coapt more apically than normally, which results in significant mitral regurgitation. **B,** Similar view from the same patient after undergoing mitral repair with the placement of an annuloplasty ring. The mitral annular dimension has been reduced. The chambers are still enlarged, but there was no residual mitral regurgitation.

consist of either central occluders consisting of either a ball and cage or one or two tilting disks or biological leaflets mounted on a frame. Each valve prosthetic design has its individual idiosyncratic Doppler velocity profiles and range of transvalve gradients that can and have been determined with the modified Bernoulli equation and tend to decrease in amplitude with increase in valve size (Table 11-1).[24]

Prosthetic valves have finite durability. Biological mitral valve replacements, especially when placed in young patients (<60 years), have a significant primary failure rate from early calcification and leaflet fracture or

TABLE 11-1   NORMAL DOPPLER VALUES FOR MITRAL PROSTHESES

Mitral prostheses	Peak velocity(m/s)	Mean gradient (mmHg)	Area mean (cm²)	Area range (cm²)
Starr-Edwards	1.8 ± 0.4	4.6 ± 2.4	2.1	1.2-2.5
Bjork-Shiley	1.6 ± 0.3	5.0 ± 2.0	2.4	1.6-3.7
St. Jude Medical	1.6 ± 0.3	5.0 ± 2.0	2.9	1.8-3.9
Medtronic Hall	1.7 ± 0.3	3.1 ± 0.9	2.4	1.5-3.9
Omniscience	1.8 ± 0.3	3.3 ± 0.9	1.9	1.6-3.1
Hancock	1.5 ± 0.3	4.3 ± 2.1	1.7	1.3-2.7
Carpentier-Edwards	1.8 ± 0.2	6.5 ± 2.1	2.5	1.6-3.5

From Zabalgoitia M, Oraby M. Evaluation of prosthetic heart valves, in Pohost G (ed): *Imaging in Cardiovascular Disease,* Philadelphia, Lippincott, Williams & Wilkins, 2000, p 617.

stenosis, which can be detected either as a progressive increase in peak and mean transvalve gradients denoting partial obstruction. Alternatively regurgitation may occur, which is detected by Doppler color flow velocity mapping. Similarly, mitral valve repair procedures that develop either early or late failure can be accurately diagnosed. When TTE does not clearly identify the site and/or mechanism of malfunction of either a biological prosthesis or mitral repair, TEE is essential for diagnosis. Assessment of mechanical prosthetic malfunction is more difficult with TTE, because the non-biological components of the mitral valve "interfere" with the Doppler ultrasound, and if mechanical prosthetic malfunction is suspected, urgent TEE should be performed, especially if obstruction of the tilting leaflets is anticipated. Prosthetic obstruction to mechanical prostheses may occur because of valve thrombosis from inadequate oral anticoagulation, tissue ingrowth in long-standing prostheses over time, and endocarditis. TEE demonstrates the mechanism of obstruction for example as failure of the tilting disk to open (Figure 11-21). TEE imaging of the mitral prosthesis enables direct inspection of the biological or mechanical valve leaflets, which should be imaged throughout repetitive cardiac cycles to determine normal and equal leaflet excursion during opening and closure. Partial obstruction of a mechanical prosthesis is usually associated with an abnormal degree of prosthetic regurgitation. Prosthetic valve regurgitation may be difficult to detect, because the position of the prosthesis may preclude reliable Doppler velocity signals, particularly color flow Doppler signals from the apical views. However, continuous-wave Doppler velocities across the prosthetic valve are usually technically adequate. In mechanical prostheses, peak early diastolic velocity is a

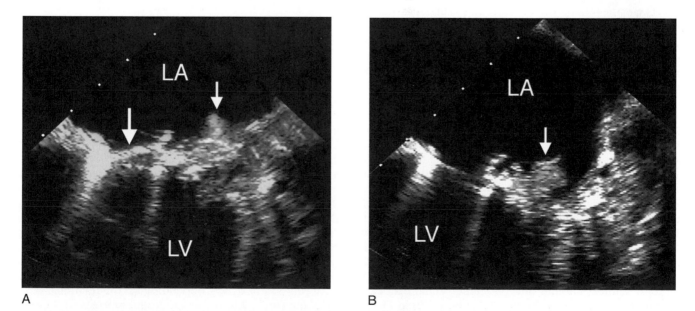

A   B

FIGURE 11-21. A, Transesophageal echocardiogram from a patient with a bileaflet mechanical mitral valve prosthesis. The imaging angle is approximately 30 degrees, and the transducer is in the midesophagus. The left atrium (LA) is enlarged. One of the mechanical leaflets is clearly seen to the left of the image *(arrow).* There is shadowing of the left ventricle (LV) by the artifact produced by the mechanical valve. The other leaflet is obscured by an indistinct mass that appears attached to the lateral annulus *(smaller arrow).* This is a thrombus that was interfering with valve function. **B,** Similar view in diastole. The medial leaflet is opened and projects into the ventricle. The thrombus *(arrow)* is attached to the more lateral leaflet and is preventing complete opening of this leaflet.

more reliable index of valve function than pressure half time.[25] Transmitral Doppler flow velocities should be recorded and fall within the normal published range of velocities for each type of prosthesis. A low threshold for proceeding to transesophageal Doppler echocardiographic interrogation of the prosthesis must be maintained.

TEE is ideally suited to examine the detailed anatomy of the mitral annulus, and the sewing ring of the prosthesis, the tilting disk motion, and the color flow Doppler signals that enable perivalvar regurgitation and dehiscence to be distinguished from mechanical failure of the prosthesis. In summary, the principles involved in prosthetic malfunction can be simply divided into those with predominant obstruction in which the Doppler mean and peak gradients are usually severely increased and those with predominant regurgitation in which transmitral flow velocities are usually normal or only minimally increased. Important prosthetic MR after valve repair, biological, or mechanical prostheses is optimally diagnosed by transesophageal Doppler echocardiography.

INFECTIVE ENDOCARDITIS OF THE MITRAL VALVE

Infective endocarditis is an inflammation of the endovascular surface of the cardiac valves or chambers and has an overall mortality of 10%. Infective endocarditis was formerly a clinical diagnosis established on basis of auscultatory findings, hemodynamics, and peripheral stigmata that was confirmed by identification of a causative microorganism. Nowadays, the diagnosis is made earlier, and most of the classic cutaneous stigmata that occur late in the course of the disease are rare and of interest as clinical curiosities that corroborate the diagnosis. Most patients with native valve infective endocarditis are initially seen with nonspecific symptoms of fevers, weight loss, and a heart murmur and are found to have persistent bacteremia that triggers a request for a transthoracic or more often a transesophageal two-dimensional echocardiogram, which demonstrates valvular vegetations. The clinical presentation may follow a more fulminant course, with rapid valve destruction, thromboembolism, septicemia, and symptomatic heart failure resulting from a virulent strain of *S. aureus* in which TEE may reveal avulsion of the mitral valve, florid valvular vegetations, mitral ring abscess, and hemodynamically severe regurgitation. Almost three quarters of patients with native valve endocarditis have anatomical or physiological abnormalities of the valve that predispose to infective endocarditis. Because of the wide variety of symptoms and signs that occur in infective endocarditis, a number of major and minor criteria (Duke criteria) have been proposed that combine clinical findings and two-dimensional echocardiographic features that facilitate diagnosis (Box 11-1). Definitive diagnosis of infective endocarditis is established by the presence of two major, one major and three minor, or five minor criteria. A possible diagnosis of infective endocarditis is suggested by the presence of minor criteria that are not sufficient to meet the requirements

---

■ ■ ■

BOX 11-1   DEFINITION OF TERMS USED IN THE DUKE CRITERIA FOR THE DIAGNOSIS OF IE

Major criteria
1. Positive blood culture for IE
   A. Typical microorganism consistent with IE from 2 separate blood cultures as noted below:
      (i) viridans streptococci,* *Streptococcus bovis*, or HACEX group, or
      (ii) community-acquired *Staphylococcus aureus* or enterococci, in the absence of a primary focus, or
   B. Microorganisms consistent with IE from persistently positive blood cultures defined as
      (i) ≥2 positive cultures of blood samples drawn >12 hours apart or
      (ii) all of 3 or a majority of ≥4 separate cultures of blood (with first and last sample drawn ≥1 hour apart)
2. Evidence of endocardial involvement
   A. Positive echocardiogram for IE defined as
      (i) oscillating intracardiac mass on valve or supporting structures, in the path of regurgitant jets, or on implanted material in the absence of an alternative anatomic explanation, or
      (ii) abscess, or
      (iii) new partial dehiscence of prosthetic valve, or
   B. New valvular regurgitation (worsening or changing of preexisting murmur not sufficient)

Minor criteria
1. Predisposition: predisposing heart condition or intravenous drug use
2. Fever: temperature ≥38.0°C
3. Vascular phenomena: major arterial emboli, septic pulmonary infarcts, mycotic aneurysm, intracranial hemorrhage, conjunctival hemorrhages, and Janeway lesions
4. Immunologic phenomena: glomerulonephritis, Osler's nodes, Roth spots, and rheumatoid factor
5. Microbiological evidence: positive blood culture but does not meet a major criterion as noted above† or serological evidence of active infection with organism consistent with IE
6. Echocardiographic findings: consistent with IE but do not meet a major criterion as noted above

Reprinted from Durack et al,[5] *American Journal of Medicine*, with permission from Excerpta Medica Inc.
*Includes nutritionally variant strains (*Abiotrophia* species).
†Excludes single positive cultures for coagulase-negative staphylococci and organisms that do not cause endocarditis.

---

for definitive diagnosis. The diagnosis can also be confidently excluded with these criteria. Two-dimensional echocardiography and especially TEE is the diagnostic imaging modality of choice for infective endocarditis in contemporary cardiology practice and contributes both major and minor diagnostic criteria. The echocardiographic evidence for infective endocarditis is established primarily by identification of valvular vegetations that usually appear as a mobile irregular mass attached to a valve leaflet (Figure 11-22). Rarely, vegetations may be attached to the endocardial surface of a cardiac chamber.

The sensitivity of TTE for detecting vegetations in proven native valve endocarditis is reported to vary between 60% and 70%, depending on the technical quality of the study; the size, location, and mobility of the vegetation; and the experience of the echocardiographic interpreter. The specificity of transthoracic two-dimensional echocardiography for detecting vegetative endocarditis is approximately 90%, because nonspecific thickening or myxomatous thickening of the mitral valve

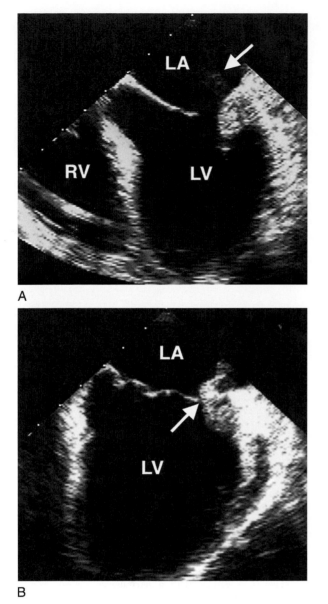

A

B

FIGURE 11-22. A, Transesophageal echocardiogram in the transverse plane (imaging angle 0 degrees) at the level of the midesophagus. There is a large vegetation *(arrow)* in the left atrium (LA) attached to the posterior annulus. The vegetation, which protruded into the left atrium, exhibited high-frequency chaotic motion. The posterior leaflet is severely thickened at the base and is involved by the mitral annular abscess associated with the vegetation in this patient with *Staphylococcus aureus* endocarditis. **B,** Transesophageal image in the two-chamber posterior view. The posterior abscess is visualized adjacent to P1 (posterior scallop1). The continuity of the annular abscess *(arrow)* and the vegetation is more evident in this systolic view. RV, right ventricle; LV, left ventricle.

leaflets, minor chordal rupture, mitral prolapse, and mitral fibroelastomas may be incorrectly interpreted as valvular vegetations. Small linear valvular excrescences have been reported in some transesophageal studies with a frequency of up to 38% of healthy volunteers and should not be mistaken for vegetations. Multiple, large, comparative studies have reported the greater sensitivity and specificity of transesophageal vs. transthoracic echocardiography for the detection of vegetations. The

sensitivity and specificity of TEE for vegetative endocarditis varies between 94% and 98% and 95% and 97%, respectively. Thus, the diagnosis of infective endocarditis cannot be excluded by TTE alone, and if the diagnosis is deemed clinically likely, TEE should be performed to exclude or confirm the presence of vegetative endocarditis.

In addition to the high sensitivity and specificity in the diagnosis of native valve vegetative endocarditis, echocardiographic assessment of the size and morphological characteristics of vegetations provides incremental prognostic information that is predictive of adverse cardiovascular complications, especially embolization. Mitral valve vegetations >10 mm in diameter, mobile, and/or pedunculated are more frequently associated with embolization, and thus large size alone has been suggested as a criterion for surgical intervention. A time-dependent increase in vegetation size is also associated with greater prevalence of embolization, abscess formation, and the need for valve replacement. Mobility and size of vegetations defined by TEE are predictive of embolization. Furthermore, mobile vegetations >15 mm are suggested as an indication for surgery, regardless of the presence of valve destruction or regurgitation.[26] The risk of embolization decreases with the institution of antibiotic therapy. Vegetations on the mitral valve have a higher risk of embolization compared with aortic vegetations.

Two-dimensional echocardiography plays a central role in diagnosis, prognosis, and recognition of the complications of infective endocarditis that influence decision making and optimal management of individual patients. Perforation or avulsion of the mitral valve leaflets and ruptured chordae are all associated with an acute increase in severity of mitral regurgitation and deterioration in left ventricular function, which can be readily recognized by Doppler echocardiography as described previously. Myocardial abscess and mitral ring abscesses are best detected by TEE and, when present, are indications for emergent valve replacement, because continued nonsurgical treatment is associated with a worse clinical outcome. Before the introduction of widespread use of TEE, the diagnosis of myocardial abscess was made serendipitously at operation or at necropsy, because no other imaging technique was diagnostic. Vegetations of the mitral valve may extend from the free edges of the anterior leaflet to the junction with the aortic valve leaflets, and mobile mitral valve vegetations may inoculate the aortic valve leaflets directly by contact and disrupt the fibrous cardiac skeleton of the heart. Direct extension of infection from the mitral valve leaflets to the myocardium, pericardium, mitral annulus, and aortic valve can only be reliably detected by two-dimensional transthoracic or optimally by TEE. This anatomical information is vitally important to ascertain before valve replacement surgery.

Prosthetic valve endocarditis makes up between 10% and 15% of all cases of infective endocarditis and has a prevalence of 1% to 1.5% per patient year, affecting mechanical and biological prosthetic valves with similar frequency. The diagnosis of prosthetic mitral valve endocarditis is established by the presence of the usual clinical criteria for native valve endocarditis. However, there may be difficulties detecting vegetations attached to mechanical valves by TTE because of multiple reflections from the nonbiological components of the prosthetic valve. Vegetations may be detected more easily by TTE on mitral bioprostheses than on mechanical prostheses, because their low profile sewing ring and stents allows the ultrasound beam to interrogate the valve and assess leaflet thickness, motion, and competence. Vegetations may also be detected by TTE on mechanical prosthetic valves before they disrupt valve opening or closure. However, vegetations taking origin from the sewing ring or leaflets per se interfere with valve leaflet opening and or closure, resulting in abrupt alteration in circulatory hemodynamics. When mechanical mitral valve prostheses become partially obstructed by vegetations growing into the moving components of the valve preventing adequate leaflet opening, the transmitral Doppler velocity profile will enable estimation of the increased pressure gradients and corroborate the presence of prosthetic obstruction. Similarly, vegetative material may extend into the mechanical mitral prosthesis, preventing normal coaptation of the leaflets resulting in mild through severe MR. Mitral prosthetic regurgitation is recognized as high-velocity turbulent systolic regurgitant flow into the left atrium by color flow Doppler mapping. Before transesophageal echocardiography was used routinely, obstruction of the poppet in ball-and-cage prostheses and obstruction of disk motion in unileaflet and bileaflet mechanical prostheses were studied by fluoroscopy. In a proportion of patients with mechanical or biological mitral prosthetic valves, infective endocarditis may present with symptoms of dyspnea and reduction in exercise capacity associated with acute MR. MR may result from perivalvular regurgitation because of localized destruction of the mitral annular tissue into which the prosthesis is seated, with partial dehiscence of the valve sewing ring, mitral ring abscess, or formation of a fistulous track adjacent to the sewing ring. All these complications are more common in prosthetic than in native valve infective endocarditis.[27]

TEE plays an especially important role in prosthetic valve endocarditis, both in diagnosis and in excluding the diagnosis, and is much superior to TTE (Figure 11-23). Systematic Doppler color flow velocity mapping of biological and mechanical prostheses in suspected infective endocarditis should be performed to identify mechanical failure and perivalvular regurgitation for which TEE is exquisitely sensitive. Transesophageal Doppler color flow mapping is essential for the detection of abnormal blood flow into fistulous tracks in the paravalvular tissues, myocardial and mitral ring abscesses, which, if present, require urgent surgical intervention. When infective endocarditis involves either a native or a prosthetic mitral valve, the aortic valve that is contiguous with it must be very carefully examined either by high-quality TTE or whenever possible with TEE, because their close proximity may result in inoculation or direct extension of infection to the aortic valve leaflets. In summary, when prosthetic valve endocarditis is suspected and TTE is equivocal, TEE should be undertaken. Similarly, TEE is recommended when the diagnosis of prosthetic valve endocarditis is known, but complications, including ring

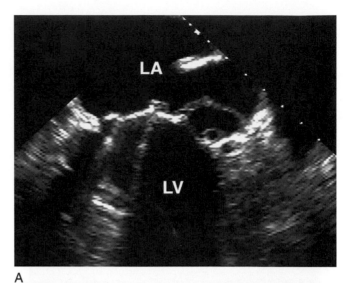

A

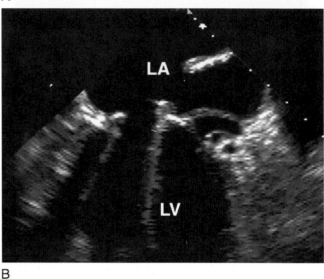

B

FIGURE 11-23. A, Close-up systolic image of a St. Jude prosthetic mitral valve in a patient with a perivalvular abscess caused by *Streptococcus viridans* endocarditis. The mechanical leaflets are closed, but an echolucent area projects from the lateral annulus into the left atrium. A portion of the left atrial prominence is visualized in the left atrium. No definite vegetation is seen attached to the mechanical valve in this view. B, The two leaflets of the mitral prosthesis are open in this diastolic frame. The abscess is again identified as a complex structure with a large echolucent area surrounding the coronary sinus and left circumflex coronary arteries, which are adjacent to each other in the AV groove.

abscess, paravalvular regurgitation, valve obstruction, or dehiscence, are suspected.

AORTIC VALVE DISEASE

Anatomical Evaluation

The structure of the aortic valve is often thought to be less complex than the mitral valve. However, the complete apparatus of the aortic valve includes not only the leaflets of the valve but the surrounding supporting structures.

The junction between the left ventricular outflow tract and the aorta is the fibrous aortic annulus that forms the base of the aortic leaflets. Although most of the annulus consists of fibrous tissue, the posterior aspect of the annulus is ventricular myocardium. The attachment of the aortic leaflets to the wall of the root describes a coronet arrangement (Figure 11-24).[28] The sinotubular junction is the distal extent of the aortic root and is composed primarily of elastic tissue. The sinuses of Valsalva lie between the aortic annulus and the sinotubular junction and have a diameter larger than both. This arrangement holds the coronary artery ostia away from the aortic leaflets in systole. The sinuses are named for the coronary ostium associated with them as are the leaflets (left coronary, right coronary, and noncoronary). The root at the level of the sinuses is not entirely symmetrical, with the noncoronary sinus being slightly larger than the others.[29]

The aortic valve leaflets are nonplanar structures with a small excrescence at the tip of each leaflet. The commissures are defined as the parallel portions of the leaflets that coapt in diastole. The function of the aortic valve apparatus has been shown to be highly complex and asymmetrical in animal studies.[28] The aortic annulus, lies below the valve leaflets, is exposed to ventricular pressures and expands during the isovolumic contraction period. During ejection, however, the aortic annulus contracts, whereas the sinotubular junction expands. This expansion facilitates the opening of the leaflets. The opposing motion of the annulus and sinotubular junction results in torsional deformation of the root that may counteract the strain caused by ventricular contraction.

Assessment of the aortic root size and function is important in evaluation of the causes of valvular dysfunction. Dilation of the aortic root is the most common cause of aortic regurgitation. Other abnormalities of the root, such as a change in wall stiffness, may cause dysfunction of the valve leaflets. Successful surgical procedures to repair the aortic valve have been found to be dependent on the techniques used in addressing the aortic root and its interaction with the leaflets (see later).

Commissures

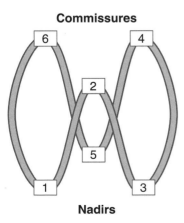

Nadirs

FIGURE 11-24. Diagram of the attachment of the aortic leaflets to the aortic root. (Reprinted with permission from Dagum P, et al. Deformational dynamics of the aortic root: modes and physiologic determinants. *Circulation* 1999; 100(19 Suppl):II54.)

Echocardiography

Echocardiography is the dominant method for anatomical assessment of the aortic valve. Visualization of the valve leaflets is possible with cinefluoroscopy only if the leaflets are calcified and has only been compared with M-mode echocardiography. Orifice-view aortography is a contrast cine technique that allows planimetry of the valve, but it has never been compared with two-dimensional echocardiography and suffers from the need for invasive procedures and the use of contrast agents. Similarly, CMR has undergone a number of technical developments but is routinely indicated in very few situations to assess valvular function. In 1998, the Task Force of the European Society of Cardiology listed no class I or II indications for CMR in the evaluation of valvular heart disease, except for supravalvular pulmonic stenosis.[30] The normal heart valves are thin structures that are difficult to image with conventional CMR pulse sequences. Recent advances may allow visualization of the leaflets, even in normal patients, but it currently remains a research tool. The resolution of CMR is too low to identify small vegetations. In contrast, CMR is the method of choice for evaluation of aortic dissection.[20,30] CMR may be useful in the evaluation of involvement of the aortic root by the dissection flap and has identified aortic root abscess in patients with endocarditis.

Echocardiographically, the aortic valve is best imaged from the parasternal windows. The aortic valve is imaged anterior to the mitral valve in the parasternal long axis (Figure 11-1). In diastole, two of the aortic valve leaflets are imaged in the middle of the aortic root. The leaflets open in systole and appear to approximate the walls of the aorta. The right coronary cusp is always the anterior leaflet, whereas the posterior leaflet is usually the noncoronary cusp. Angulation of the transducer brings the left coronary cusp into view. The left ventricular outflow tract dimension is measured immediately below the attachment of the cusps in this view. The larger diameter at the level of the sinuses of Valsalva is evident, as is the relative narrowing of the root at the sinotubular junction. Only a portion of the aortic root may be imaged on the standard parasternal long-axis view. The transducer may be moved in a cranial direction to a higher interspace to image the proximal ascending aorta. According to the American Society of Echocardiography Standards, measurements should be made perpendicular to the long axis of the aorta from leading edge to leading edge. The parasternal long-axis view also allows assessment of the leaflet structure, including the presence of calcification and leaflet thickening. Systolic doming of the valve leaflets may be due to rheumatic disease or a congenitally abnormal valve. Disruption of coaptation, valve prolapse, and the presence of vegetations are usually best seen in this view. Color flow Doppler imaging will demonstrate aortic regurgitation in the left ventricular outflow tract arising from the level of the aortic valve leaflets in diastole.

The parasternal short axis of the valve images the sinuses of Valsalva, the corresponding coronary arteries, and the leaflets. The right coronary cusp is imaged anteriorly, the left coronary cusp is seen to the right of the screen posteriorly, and the noncoronary cusp is seen to the left of the left coronary cusp. The commissure between the left and noncoronary cusp is at the level of pulmonary valve. The commissure between the noncoronary and the right cusps is adjacent to the tricuspid valve. Apical angulation of the transducer will image the left ventricular outflow tract in short axis, and cranial angulation will bring the ascending aorta into view. Measurements are best taken from the long-axis view to confirm the level of the image.

The aortic valve may also be imaged from the apical five-chamber view and the apical long-axis view. However, the valve is in the far field in these views, and the imaging of leaflet and root structure is rarely optimal. In contrast, Doppler ultrasound evaluation of aortic stenosis and regurgitation is best undertaken from the apical position, because the ultrasound beam is parallel to the blood flow. A short-axis view of the aortic valve can be obtained from the subcostal view (Figure 11-25). The relationship of the commissures to the adjacent structures will allow identification of the leaflets. The subcostal view may be particularly helpful when the parasternal images are suboptimal, whether because of the poor echocardiographic windows or the presence of chest tubes and surgical incisions.

Transesophageal imaging of the aortic valve is an important technique for further evaluation. The short axis of the aortic valve is best seen in the midesophageal views with a multiplane transducer at an imaging angle between 35 degrees and 50 degrees (Figure 11-26). In this image, the most anterior leaflet, the right coronary cusp, is seen at the bottom of the screen, and the noncoronary cusp is seen to the left of the image bisected by the interatrial septum. The structure of the sinuses of Valsalva and the competency of the commissures are best seen in this view. The long-axis view of the valve from the midesophagus at an imaging angle of approximately 130 degrees is similar to the parasternal long-axis view, except that the leaflet at the top of the screen is usually the noncoronary cusp, and the one seen below is the right coronary cusp (Figure 11-27). This view offers the best assessment of the outflow tract and dimensions of the annulus, sinuses, and sinotubular junction. The modified four-chamber view from the transverse plane in the midesophageal position may also allow the demonstration of the left ventricular outflow tract. This is particularly important, because vegetations are generally attached to the ventricular surface of the aortic valve and may be seen in the modified four-chamber view prolapsing into the outflow tract.

Transgastric imaging does not allow visual assessment of the valve but does allow for the Doppler interrogation of the aortic valve gradients and aortic regurgitation. The alignment of the ultrasound beam with the aortic jets may be suboptimal, because the transducer position is limited by the relationship of the gastric lumen to the apex of the heart. In general, the two-dimensional imaging of the aortic valve is best on transesophageal studies, whereas Doppler assessment is more reliable from the transthoracic approach.

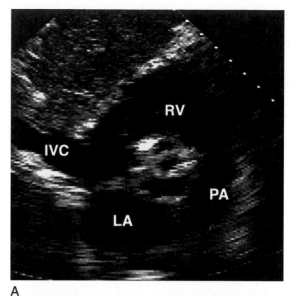

A

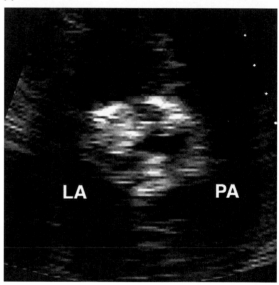

B

FIGURE 11-25. A, Subcostal short axis view at the level of the base of the heart. The inferior vena cava is seen entering the right atrium. The right ventricular outflow tract and the pulmonary artery surround the aortic valve, with the left atrium located in the far field. The subcostal views may provide the only adequate images in some technically difficult patients. **B,** Close-up image of the calcified and stenotic aortic valve imaged in A. IVC, inferior vena cava; RV, right ventricle; PA, pulmonary artery; LA, left atrium.

AORTIC STENOSIS

Pathophysiology and Hemodynamics

Obstruction of the aortic valve is usually a gradual process that allows the ventricle enough time to accommodate to the increasing afterload. The left ventricle undergoes concentric hypertrophy, and the resultant remodeling maintains wall stress at normal levels despite the increased cavity pressure. A number of factors may contribute to the development of symptoms in previously asymptomatic patients. There is a wide overlap in

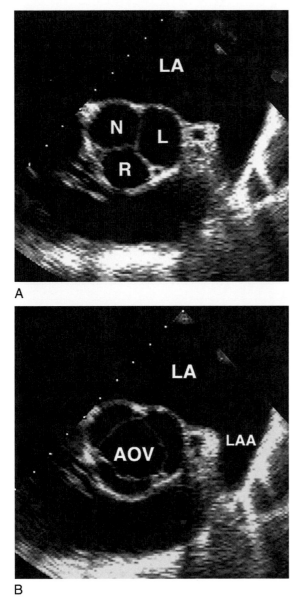

A

B

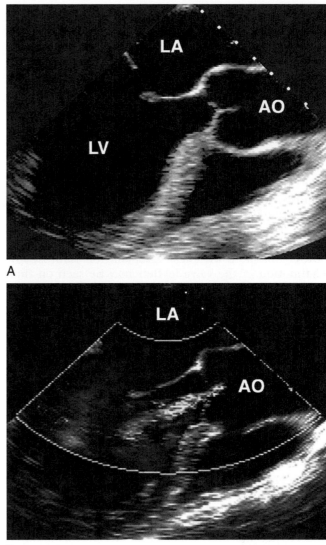

A

B

FIGURE 11-26. A, Transesophageal echocardiogram from the midesophagus, imaging angle approximately 60 degrees. The aortic valve is seen in short axis. In diastole, the valve is closed, and the normal anatomy of the cusps is clearly seen. **B,** Similar view in systole, the cusps are opened and the aortic valve orifice is identified. The relationship of the commissures, leaflets, and the corresponding sinuses of Valsalva is demonstrated. The left atrial appendage is imaged to the right of the screen and appears normal. N, noncoronary cusp; L, left coronary cusp; R, right coronary cusp; LA, left atrium; LAA, left atrial appendage; AOV, aortic valve orifice.

FIGURE 11-27. A, Transesophageal echocardiogram in the longitudinal plane (imaging angle 130 degrees) from the midesophagus. The left ventricular outflow tract, aortic valve, root, and ascending aorta are imaged in this diastolic frame. The view is similar to the parasternal long-axis view. The mitral valve leaflets are partially opened. **B,** Transesophageal echocardiogram from the same transducer position. A high-velocity turbulent jet of aortic regurgitation arises from the aortic leaflets and extends into the left ventricular outflow tract. The ratio of the jet width immediately below the valve leaflets to the outflow tract diameter is much less than 25%, which is diagnostic of mild aortic regurgitation. See also Color Insert.

valve area between patients with and without symptoms. Therefore, other factors must contribute to the development of symptoms in the disease. Significant hypertrophy develops in most but not all patients with severe stenosis. The degree of hypertrophy varies by body size, with patients with low body mass having less hypertrophy. Studies have also shown a variation in the hypertrophic response to the pressure load on the basis of angiotensin-converting enzyme gene polymorphism and gender. Most studies have demonstrated that women

tend to have smaller cavities with larger relative wall thickness and increased ejection fractions than men. MR is frequently associated with aortic stenosis and may be due to concurrent mitral valvular disease or to early left ventricular dysfunction. MR improves in approximately 50% of patients after aortic valve replacement.[31] A larger LV mass, which may be related to high wall stress, predict patients most likely to demonstrate a postoperative decrease in MR.

Eventually, no further compensation is possible, and the cardiac output becomes fixed. At this point, exertional symptoms develop and include dyspnea, angina, and syncope, all manifestations of limited cardiac output. Once symptoms develop, the associated mortality is very high, and the prognosis is measured in months to several years. The development of symptoms at rest of portends a grave prognosis and is a clinical emergency.

Aortic Sclerosis and Calcification

Although physical examination accurately predicts the presence of a significant hemodynamic abnormality of the aortic valve, echocardiography is far more sensitive for assessing the degree of aortic stenosis or regurgitation. Many physical findings correlate with severe stenosis, but there is lack of sensitivity in predicting the presence of severe aortic stenosis in individuals, particularly in patients with depressed systolic function and multivalvular disease.[32] Calcification of the valve may be demonstrated on chest X-ray and on fluoroscopy. The motion of the valve leaflets may be seen on fluoroscopy only if they are calcified. Approximately 31% of patients with aortic stenosis had valve calcification visible by chest X-ray.

The physical examination cannot reliably distinguish between aortic valve sclerosis and calcification. Sclerosis of the valve will result in turbulent flow and an audible murmur without obstruction to flow. The two entities may be easily differentiated on TTE. Nevertheless, the presence of aortic valve sclerosis diagnosed by echocardiography is associated with cardiovascular death. The risk of death has been estimated to be 50% higher in patients with aortic sclerosis in the absence of stenosis than in patients with normal valves. The mechanism of this increased risk is not clear, but aortic valve sclerosis is associated with aortic atheroma[33] and coronary artery disease. Factors associated with the presence of aortic sclerosis include the presence of mitral annular calcification, hypercholesterolemia, and elevated creatinine. Patients with familial hypercholesterolemia may have an accelerated calcification of the aortic root and valve, with a peculiar distribution that can extend into the coronary arteries producing ostial lesions. Presumably, the presence of aortic sclerosis is a marker for atherosclerosis rather than a cause of the associated increased mortality. The calcification of the aortic valve may also be assessed by electron beam computed tomography (EBCT). The rate of progression of calcification of the valve is related to the rate of progression of coronary calcification as well as the level of serum low-density lipoprotein.[34]

Anatomical Evaluation

Echocardiography

The most common cause of significant aortic stenosis in the adult population is senile calcification. The calcific deposits in the bodies of the valve cusps prevent adequate opening. The calcific deposits may be easily visualized in the parasternal long axis or in the short axis at the level of the valve (Figure 11-28). The commissures are free, but the leaflets are restricted in their motion. In contrast, rheumatic valvulitis causes thickening of the

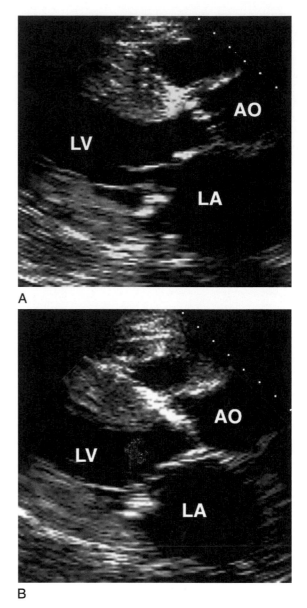

A

B

FIGURE 11-28. **A,** Parasternal long-axis view in diastole. The aortic valve is heavily calcified and closed in this diastolic frame. The left atrium is dilated, and there is severe posterior mitral annular calcification. This calcification extends along the posterior leaflet, restricting its opening. Severe concentric hypertrophy is present. The interventricular septum is almost 2.0 cm thick. **B,** Similar view in systole. There is little detectable motion of the aortic valve in this patient with critical aortic stenosis. Systolic function is preserved.

commissures with fusion and progressive restriction of motion. The degree of opening of the leaflets, best seen on the parasternal long-axis view, correlates with the degree of obstruction but is difficult to interpret, particularly in the heavily calcified valve.

The aortic valve area may be planimetered from the transthoracic short-axis view. In one small study, this approach was feasible in 76% of patients with aortic stenosis and correlated well with invasive measurements. However, the valve orifice is seen better from the transesophageal approach (Figure 11-26, *B*). The valve areas obtained in this manner correlate well with invasively determined valve areas, as well as Doppler echocardiographically derived measurements in most studies but not all. Multiplane imaging allows for better assessment of the true orifice area than biplane imaging. The inner edge of the cusps must be traced to provide the best correlation with other measurements. The aortic valve area as measured by planimetry does not vary with cardiac output, an important difference from the Gorlin equation. Stenotic valves open and close more slowly than normal valves when assessed by serial planimetry in a single ejection cycle. The peak gradients correlate better with maximal opening rather than mean valve area over the ejection period. The duration of maximal valve opening is also less in stenotic valves than normal. Recently, three-dimensional reconstruction of the valve orifice, acquired from the transesophageal approach, have been shown to correlate better with invasively derived measures than two-dimensional planimetry. Preliminary results from intracardiac studies have also yielded good correlation between planimetered valve areas and echocardiographic and invasive measurements.

Quantification of Severity of Stenosis

Echocardiography

Doppler Gradients

Historically, the measurement of the gradients across the aortic valve and the calculation of the aortic valve area were done by cardiac catheterization. Echocardiographic methods have largely replaced catheterization for the routine evaluation of aortic stenosis. Doppler measurements of the gradient across the aortic valve correlate very well with invasive measurements. The Bernoulli equation describes the gradient across the valve in terms of velocities of the jets before and after an obstruction. The increase in blood flow velocity distal to the stenosis is quadratically related to the pressure gradient across the stenosis, as shown by the Bernoulli equation. The modified Bernoulli equation is applied to the aortic valve by measuring the velocity of blood in the outflow tract and at the level of the valve orifice.

$$\Delta P = 4(v_{AV}^2 - v_{LVOT}^2) \qquad \text{(Equation 12)}$$

where ΔP is the pressure gradient between the left ventricular outflow tract and the aorta ($P_{LVOT} - P_{AO}$), v_{AV} is the peak velocity across the obstruction, assumed to be at the level of the orifice and measured by continuous-wave Doppler, and v_{LVOT} is the velocity measured by pulsed-wave Doppler in the left ventricular outflow tract. In aortic stenosis, the velocity in the left ventricular outflow tract is usually less than 1 m/s, and thus the term v_{LVOT} is negligible compared with the square of the velocity of the jet across the obstruction. For this reason, the simplified Bernoulli equation is usually written:

$$\text{Pressure gradient} = 4\,v^2 \qquad \text{(Equation 1)}$$

For example, if the velocity across the valve is measured with continuous-wave Doppler as 4.0 m/s, the peak

aortic valve gradient is 64 mmHg. In some situations, the velocity in the left ventricular outflow tract may be abnormally high and must be taken into account to avoid overestimation of the aortic valve gradient. Severe aortic regurgitation will increase the velocity in the outflow tract, as will dynamic outflow tract obstruction and high cardiac output. In these circumstances, Equation 12 should be used to calculate the valvular gradient. Integration of the spectral Doppler velocity envelope over time yields the mean gradient across the valve. Ultrasound systems allow tracing of the spectral envelope and calculation of the peak and mean gradients on line.

Several caveats exist in determining the peak aortic gradient by Doppler. The beam of the ultrasound must be aligned as closely as possible with the ejection jet. Deviation from the correct incidence angle will cause the peak velocity to be underestimated. In heavily calcified, or congenitally abnormal valves, the ejection jet may be eccentric. It is mandatory to measure the aortic valve gradient from more than one view, and the spectral envelope with the highest velocity should be used. The apical five-chamber view usually provides the closest alignment with the jet, but the gradient should also be measured from the apical long-axis view, the suprasternal notch, and the right parasternal view. In the latter two views, the aortic ejection jet will be toward the transducer (Figure 11-29). Although two-dimensional and color Doppler directed continuous-wave Doppler imaging may seem to provide the best alignment with the aortic jet, the footprint of the transducer is much larger than the dedicated continuous-wave (Pedoff) probe. Assessment of the gradient with a Pedoff probe is recommended in all patients with significant aortic stenosis.

Correlation of Doppler-derived gradients with invasively determined measurements is generally excellent. It should be noted that the gradient obtained in the invasive laboratory is an extrapolated peak-to-peak gradient, whereas the gradient measured by Doppler is the instantaneous gradient across the valve (Figure 11-30). By necessity, the valvular gradient recorded by Doppler will be higher than the peak-to-peak gradient, although the mean gradient should be identical. In addition, invasive measurement of the aortic valve gradient requires a catheter be placed across the aortic valve. This may result in an erroneously high gradient if the valve area is small. Doppler echocardiography avoids this artifactual increase in transaortic gradient.

In clinical studies, Doppler echocardiography may also obtain a higher transvalvular gradient than that measured invasively because of the phenomenon of pressure recovery. The ejection jet achieves its highest velocity at the site of the obstruction, the valvular orifice. The pressure drop at this point is the highest. As the jet enters the aortic root, it loses velocity as kinetic energy is converted to potential energy. In theory, the pressure recovery would be complete if the system were a frictionless, nonturbulent stream. In reality, a number of factors affect the degree of pressure recovery in the aortic root. For invasive measurement of gradients, the pressure transducer catheter is not placed directly at the valve orifice but in the proximal aorta, where some degree of pressure

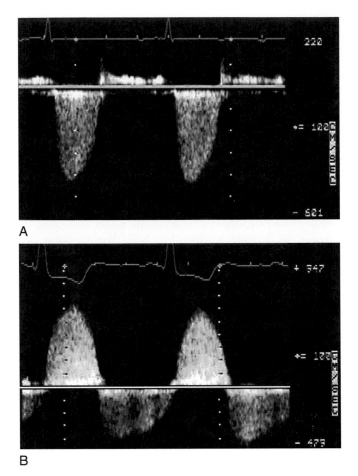

A

B

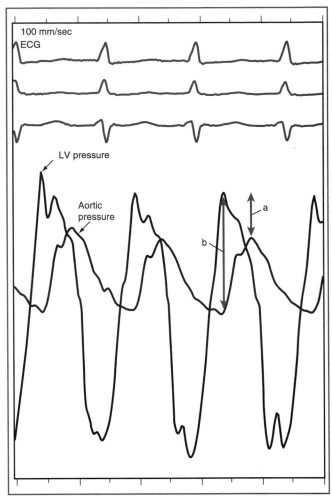

FIGURE 11-29. A, Spectral display of aortic ejection jet measured by continuous-wave Doppler from the apical position. The high-velocity systolic jet is directed away from the transducer. The peak velocity is 4.3 m/s, which predicts a peak gradient of 74 mmHg. **B,** Spectral display of aortic ejection jet measured by continuous-wave Doppler from the suprasternal notch in a different patient. The ejection jet is toward the transducer and so is displayed above the baseline. The peak gradient is more than 130 mmHg. The aortic regurgitation is displayed below the baseline.

FIGURE 11-30. Left ventricular and aortic pressure tracings obtained invasively in a patient with aortic stenosis. The peak to peak is indicated by the small arrow (a) and is the peak gradient reported in the catheterization laboratory. The peak instantaneous gradient, which would be measured by Doppler ultrasound, is indicated by the larger arrow (b).

recovery has occurred. The Doppler gradient will therefore be higher than the catheter gradient, which will explain the discrepancies in many cases. The degree of pressure recovery may be substantial. The phenomenon has been demonstrated in vitro and in vivo. The absolute value of pressure recovery increases with decreasing orifice areas and increased transvalvular gradient. However, the clinical significance of pressure recovery is best measured by the relative pressure recovery or the ratio of recovered pressure to transvalvular gradient. Studies have demonstrated that pressure recovery is a clinically significant phenomenon at moderate degrees of stenosis. Smaller aortic size is also a major contributing factor to significant relative pressure recovery. The phenomenon may be most important in prosthetic aortic valves in patients with aortic diameters <3 cm.[35]

Aortic Valve Area

The principle of conservation of mass is applied to calculate the aortic valve area with Doppler ultrasound. The velocity time integral in the left ventricular outflow tract multiplied by the cross-sectional area of the left ventricular outflow tract is equal to the stroke volume. The stroke volume through the aortic valve must be identical. This is expressed by the equation:

$$CSA_{AV} \times VTI_{AV} = CSA_{LVOT} \times VTI_{LVOT} \qquad \text{(Equation 13)}$$

where CSA_{AV} is the cross-sectional area of the aortic valve orifice, VTI_{AV} is the velocity time integral of the spectral envelope of the continuous-wave Doppler signal across the aortic valve, CSA_{LVOT} is the cross-sectional area of the left ventricular outflow tract, and VTI_{LVOT} is the VTI of the pulsed Doppler signal in the left ventricular outflow tract. The area of the left ventricular outflow tract is assumed to be circular and is obtained by measuring the diameter of the outflow tract in the parasternal long-axis view immediately below the insertion of the valve leaflets. Equation 3 may be rearranged to give the aortic valve area. The equation is referred to as the continuity equation:

$$AVA = \pi\ (D/2)^2 \times VTI_{LVOT}/VTI_{AV} \qquad \text{(Equation 14)}$$

where *AVA* is the aortic valve area and *D* is the diameter of the left ventricular outflow tract. In the continuity equation, the diameter of the left ventricular outflow tract is squared. Any error in this measurement will propagate a significant error in the aortic valve area. The diameter should only be measured in the parasternal long-axis view in midsystole. The measurement is unlikely to change in most patients over time. Use of different left ventricular outflow tract diameters in serial studies may introduce erroneous variation in the aortic valve area. On occasion, the measurement cannot be adequately obtained because of severe calcification of the aortic valve, and in this instance it is reasonable to use the value of 2 cm for the average size patient. The continuity equation also assumes a flat velocity profile in the left ventricular outflow tract. However, there may be significant variability in the velocity profile across the outflow tract, with the highest velocities occurring along the interventricular septum. The left ventricular outflow tract velocity is measured from the apical five-chamber or long-axis view with pulsed-wave Doppler. The sample volume is placed immediately below the valve leaflets in the left ventricular outflow tract. The highest velocity demonstrating laminar flow should be used. Often, the spectral envelope of the continuous-wave Doppler contains a double envelope, with the inner envelope corresponding to the left ventricular outflow tract measurement. The velocity of the inner envelope can be used as a check that the highest outflow tract velocity has been recorded.

The continuity equation has proved to be extremely reliable in calculating aortic valve areas and correlates well with areas determined by the Gorlin equation with invasive measurements. Although some authors have demonstrated poor correlation, the reliability of the continuity equation and Doppler transvalvular gradients has obviated the need for invasive measurements in many centers, although not for the need for preoperative coronary angiography in at-risk patients. TEE may also be used to measure the outflow tract diameter and the velocities across the valve and the outflow tract. Alignment of the ultrasound beam with the ejection jet is more problematic from the esophageal approach but can be performed reliably by experienced operators.

The Gorlin formula, used in the calculation of aortic valve area from invasive measurements is flow dependent. The gradient across an obstruction necessarily increases with an increase in flow rates. However, the Gorlin formula has been shown to yield larger orifice areas for increased flow rates when the orifice size is fixed. It was initially thought that echocardiographically calculated valve areas by means of the continuity equation did not share this flow dependence. Other investigators have questioned the flow independence of the aortic valve area, demonstrating a change in the continuity equation–derived valve area with exercise and pharmacological manipulation of cardiac output. These variations in aortic valve area are most significant in low-flow states.

The question of flow dependence of aortic valve area measurements assumes particular importance in evaluating patients with poor systolic function and low stroke volumes. It is likely that in partially flexible valves, an increase in flow will result in an actual improvement in orifice area. In rigid valves, any increase in calculated valve area with an increase in flow would be considered to be an artifact of the method. A change in valve area during the ejection period has been demonstrated in patients with aortic stenosis.[36] Some investigators have recommended the use of mean valvular resistance as a flow-independent assessment of stenosis severity for both noninvasive and invasive assessments of aortic stenosis. The valvular resistance is calculated by the formula:

$$R = 1.333\ (4\ v_{AV}{}^2)/\ Area_{LVOT} \times v_{LVOT} \qquad \text{(Equation 15)}$$

where *R* is the valvular resistance, *1.333* is the constant for the conversion to units of dyne-sec-cm⁻⁵, v_{AV} is the maximum velocity across the aortic valve measured by continuous-wave Doppler, $Area_{LVOT}$ is calculated by the formula $\pi\ (D/2)^2$ (as in the continuity equation), and v_{LVOT} is the velocity in the LVOT measured by pulsed-wave Doppler. However, the valvular resistance may also vary with flow rate[37] and lacks the clinically validated cutoff values for severity.

Cardiac Catheterization

Cardiac catheterization is required in the evaluation of aortic stenosis if the echocardiographic study is technically limited or if the measurement of valve area is discordant with clinical history or physical examination.[7] As noted previously, the aortic valve gradient measured at catheterization differs from the instantaneous peak gradient across the valve measured by continuous-wave Doppler. In addition, accurate invasive assessment of the gradient is ideally accomplished by simultaneous recordings from two centrally placed catheters, one in the aorta and one passed retrograde into the left ventricle. However, it is usual clinical practice to use the femoral artery pressure in place of the central aortic pressure. In general, the femoral artery pressure has a higher peak that is delayed compared with the central pressure, resulting in an underestimation of the gradient. Temporal alignment of the pressure tracings or pullback across the valve has been used to avoid this problem. Other potential sources of error in the measurement of the gradient and aortic valve area by means of the Gorlin formula include the frequency response of the recording catheters and the use of an assumed Fick method to calculate the cardiac output. Fluid-filled catheters are also commonly used, although high-fidelity manometer-tipped catheters are the most accurate.

CMR

The turbulent flow across the stenotic valve may be detected by CMR by use of cine gradient echo imaging with velocity mapping, and the level of the obstruction may also be identified. Advances in applying velocity mapping to CMR have led to the ability to determine aortic valve gradients. CMR is not limited by acoustic windows and has the ability to align parallel to eccentric jets because of its flexible imaging planes. In the future, CMR, particularly with fast spiral phase-contrast sequences, may permit real-time color assessment of valves and lead to its more frequent use.[21]

Clinical Evaluation

Aortic valve calcification is a common finding in patients, and the frequency increases with age, being present in approximately 30% of patients older than 65 years of age. The development of significant aortic stenosis is less common but also increases in incidence with age. The presence of aortic stenosis (AS) may be suspected by detection of a harsh ejection murmur on auscultation. However, auscultation fails to discriminate patients with moderate or severe aortic stenosis from those with mild obstruction.[32] This may be especially significant in patients with low transvalvular gradients because of systolic dysfunction. Similarly, it is not unusual for the diagnosis of severe AS to be made in the echocardiographic laboratory without clinical suspicion of the lesion before the study. Approximately one third of patients with severe AS are found to have unsuspected stenosis despite previous evaluation by a physician. Appropriate categorization of patients therefore depends on noninvasive assessment with TTE.

Grading of the degree of stenosis relies on identification of the valvular morphology, calcification, and separation of the valve leaflets. Peak Doppler flow velocities across the aortic valve of >4.5 m/s and a mean aortic valve gradient >50 mmHg are specific for severe aortic stenosis. However, these values are not sensitive for the detection of severe stenosis, particularly because of the problem of systolic dysfunction causing low transvalvular gradients. In general, calculation of the aortic valve area by careful application of the continuity equation (see earlier) is a more reliable discriminator. The conventional cutoff values for the severity of the stenosis were derived from the invasive laboratory by use of the Gorlin formula and applied to the echocardiographically determined areas. The area of the normal aortic valve in adults is approximately 3 to 4 cm^2. Mild stenosis is present with a valve area of 1.5 cm^2, moderate with a valve area between 1 and 1.5 cm^2, severe stenosis with a valve area of ≤1 cm^2, and critical aortic stenosis with a valve area of ≤0.7 cm^2. Analysis of the other echocardiographic parameters, including leaflet mobility, peak and mean gradient, and systolic function, must be incorporated into the assessment of the valve area. Occasionally, the two-dimensional images are poor, and the valve motion cannot be adequately assessed. In this instance, if the continuity equation yields a valve area consistent with severe stenosis, it should be viewed with caution and particular attention given to possible errors in the continuity equation calculation.

When systolic dysfunction is present, low transvalvular gradients may coexist with severe or even critical aortic stenosis. The continuity equation would be expected to provide an accurate assessment of the aortic valve area. However, as noted previously, concern that the continuity equation, as well as the Gorlin formula, underestimates the valve area in low-flow states has led to the use of dobutamine echocardiography to increase the transvalvular flow for a confirmation of the valve area. An increase in stroke volume may cause the aortic valve leaflets to open more fully and increase the valve area. Severely calcified valves with significant obstruction have a smaller increase in valve area calculated by the continuity equation than those with spuriously low valve areas because of low cardiac output. An increase in the valve area with dobutamine infusion does not rule out the presence of surgical AS. However, the final valve area tends to be lower in patients with severe stenosis.[38] It should be noted, however, that a valve area of 1.0 cm^2 may cause symptoms in patients with large body mass indices. This has led to the concept of aortic valve area indexed to body surface area as another measurement of the degree of AS. The normal aortic valve area index is 2.02 ± 052 cm^2/m^2.[39] Severe AS is present at valve area indices of <0.6 cm^2/m^2.

For those asymptomatic patients with normal LV function and moderate to severe stenosis, close clinical follow-up is mandatory. The development of symptoms may be subtle and may be missed by a patient who limits exertion and thus fails to recognize the onset of symptoms. Serial echocardiographic studies have demonstrated that moderate AS tends to predictably worsen over time. One study of 123 patients demonstrated an annualized increase in the peak velocity across the valve of 0.3 ± 0.34 m/s, which resulted in an increase in peak gradient of 7 ± 7 mmHg and a yearly decrease in the valve area of 0.12 ± 0.19 cm^2.[40] Another study of 394 patients demonstrated similar findings. In both studies, there was significant individual variation in the rates of progression. Otto et al[40] also demonstrated that a rapid rate of progression of stenosis predicted clinical events (death or valve replacement) in a group of originally asymptomatic patients. Several studies have shown more rapid progression in those with more mild degrees of stenosis.[41] Furthermore, elevated serum cholesterol, tobacco use, elevated serum creatinine, and calcium metabolism abnormalities correlate with more rapid progression.[34,41]

Given the variability in the rate of progression and the difficulty in grading the severity of stenosis on the basis of auscultation alone, serial echocardiograms are undertaken by many practitioners. The natural history of asymptomatic AS does not support yearly echocardiography for every patient with some degree of obstruction. The risk of sudden cardiac death in adults as the first symptom of AS is low. The current recommendations are that patients with severe stenosis have yearly transthoracic echocardiograms, but that patients with moderate or mild degrees of obstruction have echocardiograms performed at intervals of 2 and 5 years, respectively.[7]

The Congenitally Abnormal Valve

Bicuspid aortic valve is the most common congenital abnormality in adults, occurring in up to 1% of the adult population. The morphology of the valve is usually apparent on transthoracic imaging. The coaptation plane of the aortic valve is often not in the midline of the aortic root on the parasternal long-axis image. Systolic doming of the aortic valve is a clue to the presence of a bicuspid valve. In the short-axis view, the direction of the commissure between the two leaflets can be determined (Figure 11-31). The orientation of the commissure is defined by its relationship to the coronary arteries rather than to the chest wall or transducer orientation. Both coronary arteries arise from the anterior sinus with a horizontal commissure and from opposite sinuses with a vertical commissure. Raphe, which represents an incom-

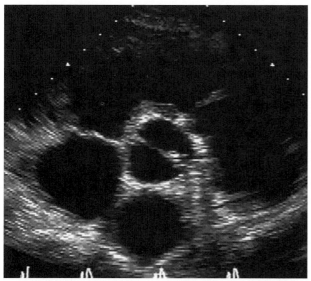

A

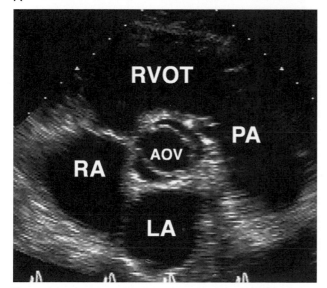

B

FIGURE 11-31. A, Parasternal short axis at the base of the heart in diastole. The aortic valve is bicuspid. The anterior leaflet is slightly larger than the posterior leaflet, and the normal arrangement of three sinuses is not present. The coronary ostia are not clearly visualized on this image, but both arose from the anterior sinus, making this an example of a horizontal commissure. The pulmonary valve is slightly thickened. **B,** Similar view in systole. The characteristic ellipsoid orifice is clearly visualized. The leaflet edges are mildly thickened. This valve was only mildly regurgitant and did not have significant calcification in this young patient.

plete division between the valve leaflets, may be mistaken for a normally placed commissure in diastole. In systole, however, the typical ellipsoid appearance of the valve orifice will distinguish the bicuspid from the tricuspid aortic valve. Occasionally, off-axis visualization of the normal valve will image only two leaflets, usually the noncoronary and the right coronary cusps, giving the appearance of a bicuspid valve. However, the characteristic ellipsoid orifice shape is never present in a normal valve and will help distinguish the two. Multiplane TEE is more sensitive than biplane TEE studies in diagnosing the morphology of the valve. Unicuspid, quadricuspid, and other abnormalities are very rare compared with the incidence of bicuspid valves. Although most bicuspid valves are not functionally normal, the diagnosis is important, even in the absence of valvar AS or regurgitation. After surgery for supravalvar or subvalvar stenosis, which may be associated with a congenitally abnormal valve, failure to replace a bicuspid aortic valve results in a high risk of repeat surgery. In addition, bicuspid aortic valve is associated with a variety of other congenital abnormalities. Left dominance of the coronary arteries with an abnormally short left main is more common in patients with bicuspid valve. Patients with coarctation of the aorta have a high incidence of bicuspid aortic valve on the order of 20% to 50%. Imaging of the aortic arch and descending thoracic aorta should be obtained from the suprasternal notch in all patients, but careful evaluation of the aorta is mandatory in patients with bicuspid aortic valve.

Hemodynamically significant AS may be present at birth in congenitally abnormal valves, with unicuspid valves being more likely to be stenotic than bicuspid valves. Bicuspid valves tend to calcify at an accelerated rate, with significant AS seen in the fourth to fifth decade of life. Horizontal commissures are more common and tend to calcify at a greater rate than valves with vertical commissures. Dense calcification of the valve may obscure the original architecture and make the diagnosis of bicuspid valve difficult. However, calcific aortic stenosis is rare in young adults, except in the setting of end-stage renal disease, in which case it is usually associated with calcification of other structures in the heart, particularly the mitral annulus. Hypercholesterolemia and hypertension also seem to be risk factors for calcification of bicuspid aortic valves, as they are for the development of senile calcification of anatomically normal valves.[42] The ejection jet across the stenosis may be particularly eccentric in bicuspid valves, making it difficult to detect the peak velocity by continuous-wave Doppler across the valve. Occasionally, the bodies of the aortic valve cusps may remain highly mobile, but the actual orifice may be restricted, resulting in significant stenosis. In this case, planimetry of the valve orifice may be misleading if the smallest orifice is not imaged. The presence of an aliased, turbulent color Doppler jet in the ascending aorta may be the clue to obstruction in mobile but highly stenotic congenitally abnormal valves.

In adults, most bicuspid aortic valves are at least mildly regurgitant. Aortic regurgitation is more likely to be severe in patients with bicuspid aortic valves than in patients with congenitally normal valves. The increased prevalence of aortic valve prolapse may contribute to the increased incidence of regurgitant lesions. Endocarditis is not infrequent in patients with congenitally abnormal valves and may precipitate acute worsening of the aortic regurgitation.

There is growing evidence that the congenital abnormality involves the aorta in patients with bicuspid aortic valves. Aortic root dilation associated with normally functioning bicuspid aortic valves has been well documented. Approximately 52% of men with bicuspid aortic valves without hemodynamically significant lesions have aortic root dilation. Pathology of the ascending aorta from surgical cases has demonstrated a high incidence of degenerative changes in the aorta compared with controls. The aortic root dilates out of proportion to the degree of associated hemodynamic lesions compared with controls with the same degree of AS or regurgitation.[43] The associated aortic abnormalities are important from a surgical standpoint, because valve replacement alone could not be expected to prevent the progressive development of aortic dilation in these patients.

Symptomatic Aortic Stenosis

The degree of left ventricular hypertrophy in symptomatic aortic stenosis eventually ceases to be an adequate compensation for the pressure load, and subendocardial ischemia and diastolic dysfunction may develop. Nuclear and echocardiographic studies have demonstrated abnormal diastolic indices in symptomatic patients with AS. Systolic dysfunction may develop as the result of afterload mismatch, subendocardial ischemia, epicardial coronary disease, or an unrelated cardiomyopathy. In some patients, the development of early symptoms may be missed by the patient and the casual questioner. In equivocal cases, exercise testing may be undertaken to evaluate the presence of symptoms. Some apparently asymptomatic patients may be discovered to have symptoms on exercise testing because of a sedentary lifestyle or ineffective communication. Exercise testing may be undertaken with caution in asymptomatic patients with moderate to severe AS, unless they have symptoms of syncope, presyncope, or chest pain. ST depression is a nonspecific finding caused by the presence of left ventricular hypertrophy, but the test should be terminated for a fall in systolic pressure of 10 mmHg or the development of presyncope.[40] Patients with critical AS should not undergo exercise testing.

Although progressive obstruction of the valve is the rule, development of symptoms in previously asymptomatic patients with AS is usually due to failure of the compensatory mechanisms and the development of diastolic or systolic dysfunction. In some patients with systolic dysfunction and symptoms of dyspnea, clinical evaluation cannot distinguish between symptoms caused by valvular stenosis and those caused by decreased ejection fraction. In these patients, the transvalvular gradient may be low because of low stroke volume, and the aortic valve area calculated by the continuity equation may be erroneously small. Invasive evaluation is plagued by the same difficulties given the flow dependence of the Gorlin formula. Dobutamine stress echocardiography has been used to distinguish between patients with severe AS and systolic dysfunction caused by afterload mismatch and those with underlying cardiomyopathy with moderate AS. Infusion of dobutamine in a group of patients with resting aortic valve areas of <0.9 cm^2 and an average left ventricular ejection fraction of 27% distinguished between those patients with true severe AS and those with moderate stenosis. The mean gradient across the valve increased in both groups with dobutamine, but in the group with moderate aortic stenosis, there was an increase in the valve area of >0.3 cm^2 to a valve area >1.0 cm^2.[38] In patients without contractile reserve, the stroke volume will not augment by 20% with dobutamine infusion, and critical AS cannot be distinguished from an artifactually low valve area attributable to the systolic dysfunction. These patients have been noted to have a particularly poor prognosis.[44] Planimetered aortic valve area obtained by multiplane TEE does not vary with dobutamine infusion and resultant changes in cardiac output.

Invasive measurement of aortic valve gradients and area is not usually necessary before surgery, although it may be required in some patients with technically limited echocardiograms. Angina is often caused by the AS rather than epicardial coronary artery disease, and the significance of ST segment depression and perfusion abnormalities in the setting of associated left ventricular hypertrophy is problematic. Exercise testing is also contraindicated in patients who are clearly symptomatic. Therefore, given the association with AS and coronary artery disease, particularly in the elderly population, coronary angiography is mandatory before aortic valve replacement in men older than 35 and women at risk for coronary artery disease.

Surgical Intervention in Aortic Stenosis

It is generally accepted that symptomatic patients with severe AS should undergo aortic valve replacement.[7] The prognosis of unoperated patients with symptoms is poor and improved by surgery. Patients with symptoms discovered on exercise testing should be treated with aortic valve replacement. However, aortic valve replacement in asymptomatic patients with severe AS is usually not indicated. Occasionally, surgery will be recommended for patients with critical AS with gradients >100 mmHg and valve areas <0.7 cm^2. There have been no data to suggest that mortality is improved by surgery for asymptomatic patients with severe AS. However, there is concern that those with severe left ventricular hypertrophy or systolic dysfunction may represent a high-risk group. Patients with severe AS defined by a Doppler peak gradient >64 mmHg became symptomatic and required surgery within 2 years in most cases (Figure 11-32).[40] Asymptomatic patients with severe AS who have the greatest increase in peak jet velocity at 1-year follow-up, >0.3 m/s, had an 80% incidence of surgery or death within the subsequent year.[45] This is the rationale for a more elective approach to surgery in asymptomatic patients rather than waiting for the occurrence of symptoms. Patients with ejection fractions <30% with severe AS have a higher operative mortality than patients with

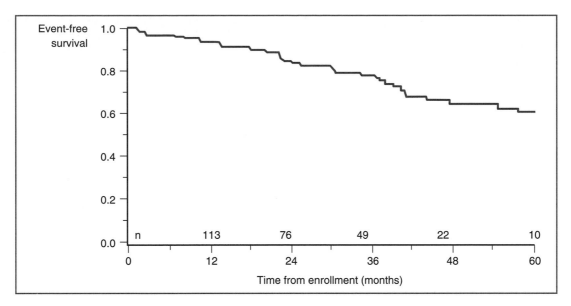

FIGURE 11-32. Kaplan-Meier life-table analysis showing survival without valve replacement for 123 subjects with initially asymptomatic valvular aortic stenosis. (Reprinted with permission from Otto et al. *Circulation* 1997; 95(9): 2262.

less severe left ventricular dysfunction. Larger preoperative left ventricular dimensions and lack of improvement in left ventricular volume and ejection fraction postoperatively portend a particularly poor prognosis.[46] However, improvement in operative techniques and outcomes have led to the use of surgery in this high-risk group and in elderly patients. Patients with severe left ventricular hypertrophy may represent a high-risk group for perioperative mortality in the absence of other risk factors. A high left ventricular outflow velocity has also been associated with higher operative mortality.

Coronary bypass grafting should be undertaken at the time of valve replacement in patients with significant coronary artery lesions detected by angiography. The higher mortality rates in patients undergoing coronary artery bypass grafting during the aortic valve replacement may be due to clinical risk factors associated with significant atherosclerosis rather than the surgery itself. Similarly, patients undergoing other cardiac surgeries who are found to have moderate AS should be considered for aortic valve replacement at the time of the original surgery. Given the known progression of stenosis over time, patients with moderate aortic stenosis require reoperation at a significant rate within several years of bypass surgery. The operative mortality for redo surgery is much higher than for primary valve surgery. Therefore, the risk/benefit ratio favors aortic valve replacement at the time of bypass surgery in these patients.[7]

AORTIC REGURGITATION

Pathophysiology and Hemodynamics

The prevalence of aortic regurgitation (AR) increases in the population with age. Even trace AR is uncommon in healthy young subjects with no history of heart disease. Mild degrees of AR are present in up to 10% to 14% of

middle-aged and elderly patients. Ventricular adaptation to the chronic volume load of severe AR leads to eccentric hypertrophy of the left ventricle. The ventricle frequently dilates in a globular fashion, with the minor axis approaching the length of the major axis. The ventricular geometry may be visualized by left ventriculography and by CMR, but echocardiography is the dominant clinical method, primarily because of the ease of application and the ability to perform serial studies. Radionuclide angiography has also been used to measure left ventricular ejection fraction but gives no information about valvular morphology.

Patients may remain asymptomatic despite severe chronic AR. The initial normalization of the wall stress, provided by left ventricular remodeling, eventually fails, and the left ventricular function declines. Contractile function may not improve after relief of the volume load by valve replacement. The fall in ejection fraction may occur despite an absence of symptoms, even in patients who are not sedentary. Symptoms associated with aortic regurgitation are associated with a poor prognosis, and some patients will not have recovery of left ventricular systolic function after valve replacement.

The physical examination is sensitive for the diagnosis of chronic severe AR but not for more mild degrees. Echocardiography remains the only efficient method for detection of AR and for serial examinations. Similarly, echocardiography is the ideal tool for assessment of left ventricular remodeling and the development of systolic dysfunction.

Anatomical Evaluation

Echocardiography

The mechanism of AR is most easily diagnosed by echocardiography. Aortic root dilation is a frequent cause of AR and is assessed by transthoracic two-dimensional or M-mode examination. The leaflets are unable to coapt, resulting in regurgitation at the center of the valve or, in more severe cases, along all of the commissures. This pattern is most helpful in confirming root dilation as the cause of the regurgitation, whether it is the result of long-standing hypertension or an acute process such as aortic dissection. A 50% dilation of the aortic root may result in a decrease of 18% in leaflet coaptation.[47] Disruption of the supports of the valve leaflets themselves may result in prolapse of the one of the cusps of the valve. Prolapse is best demonstrated in the parasternal long-axis view or on transesophageal imaging of the valve and left ventricular outflow tract in the longitudinal plane at an imaging angle of approximately 130 degrees. Destruction of the annular attachment of a cusp may occur with aortic dissection into the root, traumatic damage to the valve, or in endocarditis. The degree of AR correlates with the extent of disruption of the commissural supports defined by the percentage of the annulus that is dissected.[48] Prolapse may also be seen in severe aortic root dilation. Bicuspid aortic valves may also prolapse into the left ventricular outflow tract. The high-velocity jet from perimembranous ventricular septal defect may, over time, disrupt the valve architecture and result in prolapse of the right coronary cusp. Abnormalities of the commissures themselves may prevent complete coaptation, resulting in various degrees of regurgitation. Nonspecific thickening of the cusps occurs with age and is associated with mild degrees of regurgitation. Similarly, calcific deposits in the valve leaflets and rheumatic valvulitis may result in aortic regurgitation through this mechanism. All of these conditions are usually easily confirmed on TEE examination if the transthoracic image is not adequate.

Assessment of the Severity of AR

Although echocardiography remains the most reliable method of detecting AR, there is more controversy about the most accurate method to quantify AR. Lack of a reliable "gold standard" measurement makes comparison of various modalities problematic, unlike aortic stenosis in which the actual anatomical area can be measured at surgery.

Echocardiography

Doppler Velocity Color Flow Mapping

Aortic regurgitation is detected as a high-velocity turbulent jet arising at the level of the aortic valve cusps and extending into the left ventricular outflow tract for a variable distance. The color Doppler signal is best demonstrated in the parasternal or apical long-axis or in the apical five-chamber view (Figure 11-33). Parasternal or subcostal short-axis views of the aortic valve with color Doppler may also detect the diastolic jet and pinpoint the origin with regard to the aortic valve architecture. The demonstration of AR by continuous-wave Doppler requires interrogation from the apical position, because the jet must be parallel to the ultrasound beam for adequate assessment. The spectral envelope of AR is a high-velocity diastolic

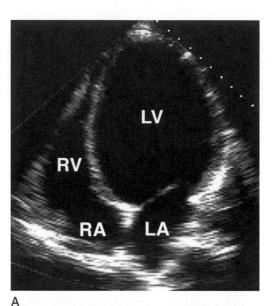

A

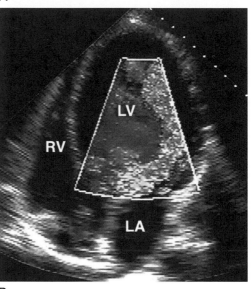

B

FIGURE 11-33. A, Diastolic image from the apical four-chamber view in a patient with severe chronic aortic regurgitation. The typical globular shape of the left ventricle, which has remodeled in response to severe aortic regurgitation, is well demonstrated. The right ventricle is normal. The mitral valve does not seem to have fully opened, which was due to the severe aortic regurgitation. B, Similar view in the same patient with color flow Doppler imaging. The high-velocity, turbulent jet of aortic regurgitation extends almost to the apex of the dilated ventricle. See also Color Insert.

signal toward the transducer displayed above the baseline (Figure 11-34). It can be distinguished from mitral stenosis by its much higher velocity (approximately 4 m/s), earlier onset, and the spectral envelope contour.

A number of echocardiographic measures exist to assess the degree of aortic insufficiency. In the oldest system, the degree of regurgitation is graded by the extent of the regurgitant jet in the left ventricle. Trace regurgitation is visible only immediately below the valves. Grade 1 regurgitant jets are present only in the proximal left ventricular outflow tract, and grade 2 extends to the tips of the mitral valve leaflets. Grade 3

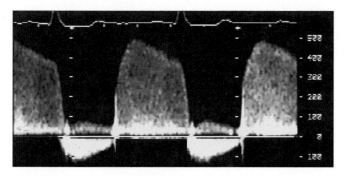

FIGURE 11-34. Spectral display of continuous-wave Doppler across the aortic valve with the transducer in the apical position. The spectral envelope of the aortic regurgitation is holodiastolic, with a peak velocity of 5 m/s and a deceleration slope of 300 cm/s², consistent with moderately severe aortic regurgitation.

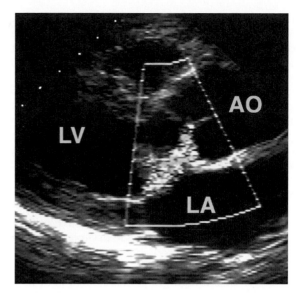

FIGURE 11-35. Parasternal long-axis view in diastole. There is eccentric aortic regurgitation that is directed posteriorly along the anterior mitral valve leaflet. The width of the jet immediately below the aortic valve leaflets is difficult to measure, because the jet runs parallel to the leaflets. The degree of regurgitation was moderate. The mitral valve appears closed in this diastolic frame, but filling was normal. The patient has a dilated root and had mitral valve prolapse in systole (not shown). These findings are consistent with the diagnosis of Marfan's syndrome. See also Color Insert.

and 4 demonstrate jets that extend to the papillary muscle tips and beyond, respectively. A number of factors affect the apparent extent of the regurgitant jet visible on color Doppler besides the actual regurgitant volume. These include not only clinical variables such as the left ventricular compliance and aortic diastolic pressure but also characteristics of the ultrasound machine, including gain settings, pulse repetition frequency, and the transmission frequency. To minimize this variability, a number of other measurements have been proposed. The deceleration slope of the spectral envelope of the aortic regurgitation jet correlates with the change in pressure gradient between the aorta and left ventricle over the course of diastole. A steeper deceleration slope is indicative of more rapid equilibration between the two, and so more severe regurgitation. A slope of <200 cm/s² is considered an indication of mild AR, and a slope >350 cm/s² is considered severe. The slope is also related to the left ventricular compliance and is not as reliable a variable as had been hoped. The presence of left ventricular hypertrophy and relaxation abnormalities makes the deceleration slope an unreliable indicator of regurgitation severity. Detection of reversed diastolic flow in the descending thoracic or abdominal aorta is also an indication of severe AR. However, false-positive results occur if the subclavian artery flow is sampled in diastole, especially if there is a surgical arteriovenous fistula in the left arm.

The width of the regurgitant jet as measured in the left ventricular outflow tract from the parasternal long-axis or the transesophageal long-axis view correlates well with the degree of regurgitation as assessed by aortography. In many studies, the ratio of the jet width to the width of the left ventricular outflow tract is the most useful color Doppler measure of AR. Correlation with angiographic grade has been demonstrated, although as noted, this technique cannot be considered to be a reference standard. The width of the jet must be measured directly below the aortic valve leaflets because of dispersion of the jet as it travels down the outflow tract (Figures 11-27, *B*, and 11-35). A ratio of <25% is consistent with mild AR. Moderate AR has a ratio between 25% and 40%, and a ratio >40% is consistent with severe AR. Markedly eccentric jets may lead to an underestimation

of the width.[49] This measurement may also be made in the transesophageal view, but the apical five-chamber and apical long-axis views have the aortic valve and outflow tract in the far field and are not reliable for measurement. The short-axis view of the aortic valve with color Doppler imaging will allow comparison of the aortic regurgitant jet area to the short axis area of the left ventricular outflow tract. This is not a standard view in most laboratories, and imaging at the level of the aortic root will falsely lower the ratio. Nevertheless, done correctly, this measurement has demonstrated acceptable reproducibility and reliability.[49] The short-axis view does allow assessment of an asymmetrical jet with its major axis oriented perpendicular to the long axis, which would artifactually increase the jet width/outflow tract ratio.

Effective Regurgitant Orifice Area

Effective regurgitant orifice area can be calculated for AR, and the values correlate with the degree of AR measured invasively. By use of the continuity equation, the retrograde diastolic flow in the proximal ascending aorta is assumed to be equal to the diastolic flow through the aortic valve, ignoring the coronary artery diastolic flow. The effective regurgitant orifice area is smaller than the anatomical regurgitant orifice and is the area of the vena contracta that is formed as the regurgitant jet passes through the aortic valve. It is given by the equation:

$$ERO_{area} = AO_{area} \times VTI_{AO}/VTI_{AV} \qquad \text{(Equation 16)}$$

where ERO_{area} is the effective regurgitant orifice, AO_{area} is the area of the ascending aorta measured assuming a circular geometry, VTI_{AO} is the velocity time integral of the diastolic flow in the ascending aorta measured by pulsed-wave Doppler, and VTI_{AV} is the velocity time integral of the aortic regurgitant jet measured by continuous-wave Doppler across the aortic valve. Mild regurgitation is associated with an effective regurgitant orifice of 0.2 to 0.5 cm^2 and severe regurgitation with an orifice area of >1 cm^2. The effective regurgitant orifice area is not a load-independent measure, because the size of the orifice has been shown to vary with aortic distending pressure, and this dependence varies with the location of the regurgitation (central vs. through a defect in the leaflet) and the aortic root diameter. In addition, the effective orifice area varies during the course of a single diastole. However, the method is generally reproducible with good interobserver variability in practiced hands. A simpler method of calculating the effective regurgitant orifice area is to measure the diameter of the vena contracta with color Doppler imaging. Assuming a circular diameter of the regurgitant orifice, the effective regurgitant orifice is calculated as:

$$ERO = \pi \times (\text{vena contracta width}/2)^2 \quad \text{(Equation 17)}$$

The severity of aortic regurgitation measured by electromagnetic flowmeter correlates with the size of effective regurgitant orifice area measured by this method in animal studies and in patients.[50]

Regurgitant Volume and Regurgitant Fraction

Regurgitant volume and regurgitant fraction both depend on loading conditions but can be calculated from Doppler parameters. The regurgitant volume per beat is equal to the difference between the forward flow in systole across the aortic valve and the flow in diastole across the mitral valve. The systolic flow in the pulmonary artery may also be used in place of the mitral valve stroke volume if mitral regurgitation is present. The regurgitant fraction is given by the equation:

$$\text{Regurgitant fraction} = SV_{AO} - SV_{MV}/SV_{AO} \quad \text{(Equation 18)}$$

where SV_{AO} is the stroke volume across the aortic valve and SV_{MV} is the stroke volume across the mitral valve. The aortic stroke volume is relatively easy to measure in clinical practice, but the mitral stroke volume is less reliable. The mitral annulus changes over the course of systole and may not be circular.

The proximal isovelocity surface area method had been used to calculate both the regurgitant volumes and the effective regurgitant orifice area. Flow toward a small orifice accelerates such that at any given radius from the center of the orifice, the velocity of the jet is uniform across the hemisphere formed by the radius. Thus, the flow across the orifice is equal to the flow across the isovelocity hemispheres. The flow rate across the surface area of the hemisphere is calculated by the equation:

$$RF = 2\pi r^2 \times v_r \quad \text{(Equation 9)}$$

where RF is the flow rate in cm^3/s, r is the radius from the center of the orifice, and v_r is the velocity of the flow

at radius r. The aliasing velocity can be adjusted to allow reliable imaging of the PISA surface. The distance from the valvular orifice to the first aliasing velocity can be measured, and the regurgitant flow rate is thus:

$$RF = 2 \pi r^2 \times \text{Nyquist limit velocity} \quad \text{(Equation 9a)}$$

where RF is the regurgitant flow rate and r is the radius from the orifice to the Nyquist limit velocity. The effective regurgitant orifice area is equal to:

$$EROA = RF/V_{max} \quad \text{(Equation 10)}$$

where V_{max} is the maximum velocity of the aortic regurgitant jet in diastole measured by continuous-wave Doppler. The flow convergence method correlates with EROA measured invasively. The PISA method is feasible in most patients. Apical imaging of the aortic flow results in artifacts and difficulty in alignment, reducing the usefulness of the method for aortic regurgitation. Imaging from the high right parasternal edge in the right lateral decubitus position may allow better visualization and alignment of eccentric flow convergence surfaces with the ultrasound beam. Regurgitant volume per beat may be calculated by multiplying the effective regurgitant orifice area by the velocity time integral of the continuous-wave Doppler envelope.[51] Similarly, the regurgitant fraction may be computed as the ratio of regurgitant volume to the LV stroke volume. Regurgitant fraction of <20% correlates with mild aortic regurgitation and of >55% with severe regurgitation.[49]

Cardiac Catheterization

In the catheterization laboratory, AR is usually evaluated by cinefluoroscopy of aortic root injection. The rapidity and degree of left ventricular opacification is used as a semiquantitative measure of AR. Left ventricular diastolic pressures may also be measured at the time of catheterization. Overestimation of AR severity may result from excessive injection speed and catheter interference with aortic valve closure. Invasively, calculated regurgitant fractions vary widely with angiographic grade assessed by aortography. The role of catheterization in the evaluation of AR has been supplanted by echocardiography, and invasive evaluation is reserved for symptomatic patients in whom the noninvasive tests are inconclusive or discordant regarding the need for surgery.[7] As in other valvular lesions, patients at risk for coronary artery disease should undergo coronary angiography before surgical valve replacement.

CMR

CMR has also been used to detect regurgitant jets. Regurgitant lesions cause turbulent flow, which leads to signal loss on cine gradient echo images. The size of the signal void is a good semiquantitative determination of the degree of regurgitation and demonstrates good correlation with color Doppler and cardiac catheterization. The strength of CMR lies in the ability to assess left and right ventricular volumes accurately. Regurgitant volume and regurgitant fraction may be determined by comparing right and left ventricular stroke volumes in patients with no other regurgitant lesions. Phase-velocity mapping encodes the velocity of the blood flow into the phase of the signal. The velocity profile across an entire cross-sectional area of the aorta can be determined. This method has been used to measure regurgitant flow by use of a transverse slice in the ascending aorta. Measurement of the regurgitant volume varies with aortic compliance and the distance of the transverse slice from the valve plane but the optimal position of the imaging plane.

Radionuclide Angiography

Although nuclear angiography cannot be used to diagnose the mechanism of aortic regurgitation, it is a well-established method for calculation of regurgitant fractions and ventricular volumes. Exercise radionuclide angiography has been used to identify patients with depressed ventricular function at rest or patients who fail to increase their systolic function with exercise. Both are indications for valve replacement in patients with AR.

Clinical Evaluation

Patients with severe, chronic regurgitation require frequent assessment of the left ventricular size and function to identify the appropriate timing of surgery and avoid irreversible ventricular dysfunction. Medical therapy with afterload reduction is indicated for asymptomatic patients with chronic severe AR and normal LV systolic function.[7] Afterload reduction reduces the remodeling associated with chronic severe AR and may result in decreased LV volumes and regurgitant fraction in some patients. Others have not found a change in LV volumes with chronic afterload reduction; however, a decrease in LV mass may be seen.[52] Afterload reduction should not be withheld out of concern that it will mask the development of symptoms or the detection of irreversible myocardial dysfunction.

Monitoring of left ventricular size and function is indicated in patients with chronic severe AR even if the patient is asymptomatic. Echocardiograms at an interval of 2 to 3 months will establish the stability of the left ventricular function and size. Subsequently, asymptomatic patients should have echocardiograms performed at least at yearly intervals. Those patients with more severe AR and those with bicuspid valves tend to have faster rates of progression of regurgitation and larger ventricular volumes. The size of the aortic root and ascending aorta should also be assessed during these examinations. Radionuclide angiography can be performed if the patient has inadequate echocardiographic windows or if the change in left ventricular systolic dysfunction identified on echocardiography is equivocal. The onset of symptoms should precipitate immediate evaluation with assessment of left ventricular systolic function and size. Serial testing is not recommended for patients with mild degrees of AR or moderate regurgitation and normal LV dimensions and systolic function (Figure 11-36).

Acute AR is very poorly tolerated if the regurgitant fraction is significantly elevated. The ventricle does not have time to remodel to accommodate the sudden increase in volume, and its ability to increase ejection fraction is limited. The patient may present in cardiogenic shock, and the murmur of AR may be quiet because of the low-pressure gradient between the left ventricle and the aorta or may be obscured by respiratory noise. Acute severe AR may be difficult to diagnose by echocardiography. With severe AR caused by acute flail of one or two leaflets, the pressure in the left ventricle and the proximal aorta may equilibrate rapidly after ventricular contraction has ceased. The color flow jet may encompass the entire outflow tract and occur only in early diastole. The color flow may be difficult to visualize. Other echocardiographic signs of severe decompensated AR include early closure of the mitral valve in the absence of first-degree atrioventricular (AV) block. Diastolic opening of the aortic valve has also been described. However, in some patients, the only echocardiographic sign may be the movement of the aortic cusps, demonstrating a completely flail leaflet. Acute severe AR requires emergency surgical intervention if the patient is to survive.

Surgical Intervention in AR

In clinical practice, asymptomatic patients with an end-systolic dimension of 55 mm or a fall in ejection fraction have been recommended for valve replacement. Other authors have recommended use of an end-systolic diameter of 50 mm as a cutoff. Recently, concern has been raised that women and men with small stature may not achieve ventricular dimensions described in the older series despite severe decompensated AR. End-systolic diameter may be indexed to body surface area, and a value of ≥ 25 mm/m^2 can be considered an indication for surgery. Patients may also eventually have symptoms without any measurable change in their echocardiographic parameters of left ventricular size or function. However, large end-systolic diameters and ejection fraction <40% as assessed by echocardiography and radionuclide ventriculography predict the development of congestive heart failure in long-term follow-up after aortic valve replacement.

Echocardiography is essential in planning the operative approach. The ascending aorta is frequently abnormally dilated in patients with regurgitation because of bicuspid valve, and simultaneous aortic root replacement should be considered. Patients with aortic dissection as the etiology of their AR may benefit from aortic valve resuspension rather than valve replacement.[48] The aortic annulus can be sized from the parasternal long-axis or from the transesophageal long-axis views. This is particularly important in patients with aortoannular ectasia, who may require annuloplasty along with valve replacement. Appropriate homograft sizing may also be determined by echocardiography. Some patients may have annular sizes that exceed available homograft dimensions. The success of the Ross procedure depends on the pulmonary autograft being an appropriately sized replacement for the aortic valve. This should clearly be determined before the start of the procedure. Finally, intraoperative TEE is

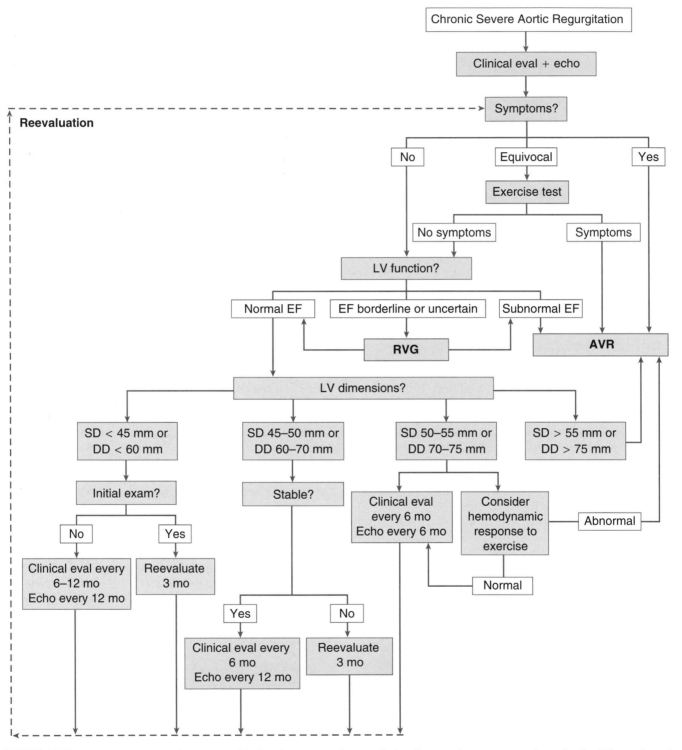

FIGURE 11-36. Management strategy for patients with chronic severe aortic regurgitation. Preoperative coronary angiography should be performed routinely as determined by age, symptoms, and coronary risk factors. Cardiac catheterization and angiography may also be helpful when there is discordance between clinical findings and echocardiography. In some centers, serial follow-up may be performed with RVG or CMR rather than echocardiography to assess LV volume and systolic function. DD, end-diastolic dimension; RVG, radionuclide ventriculography; SD, end-systolic dimension. (Reprinted with permission from Bonow et al. *J Am Coll Cardiol* 1998; 32:1486).

essential for assessment of the surgery and diagnosis of any acute complications.

NORMAL AND ABNORMAL FUNCTION IN PROSTHETIC HEART VALVES

Echocardiographic assessment of prosthetic valves in the aortic position is accomplished in a manner similar to the assessment of native valves. The thickness of the leaflets and the sewing ring, motion of the valve at the sewing ring, and motion of the leaflets should be visually assessed. Mechanical valves may be difficult to image because of shadowing of the valve leaflets by the sewing ring. Reverberation artifacts may also obscure leaflet motion. The posterior aortic root is unlikely to be adequately imaged in a transthoracic study, whereas the anterior root is not well visualized in a transesophageal study. Intense reverberations may also arise from the stents of some bioprosthetic valves, which may prevent visualization of the leaflets. In general, excessive motion of the valve with rocking at the sewing ring because of prosthetic dehiscence can usually be detected in a long-axis view.

Doppler gradients across the valve are generally easily obtained from transthoracic studies with the transducer in the apical position. Normal ranges for various valves have been published. As with native valves, the gradient depends on the stroke volume. All prosthetic aortic valves are mildly stenotic, and the peak systolic gradient is higher than in a normal native valve. Pressure recovery may be most important in cases of mild-to-moderate stenosis, such as the degree of stenosis expected with normally functioning prosthetic valves. This may lead to much higher Doppler gradients than those obtained in the catheter laboratory. Effective orifice area of the valve may be calculated by use of the continuity equation in a manner similar to that for native valves.[53] The effective orifice area is smaller than the anatomical area usually reported by the manufacturers because of flow convergence distal to the valve. The effective orifice area is more likely to be a flow-independent assessment of the prosthetic valve function than the gradients. The range of usual effective orifice areas for various valves has been published (Table 11-2).[27,54] Errors in the calculation of

effective orifice area occur with measurement of the diameter of the LV outflow tract, which may be partially obscured by the artifact created by the prosthetic valve. In addition, the orientation of the valve may not be exactly perpendicular to the LV outflow, introducing another error into the calculation. The effective flow area, defined as the area of the vena contracta distal to the valve probably, has the most clinical significance but is currently best measured in vitro. Bileaflet mechanical valves contain a central orifice and two larger side orifices. The maximum pressure gradient measured in the side orifices is 24% lower than those measured through the central orifice because of a difference in velocity profile and pressure recovery. For bileaflet valves, such as St. Jude valves, the gradient should be measured through the side orifice if feasible.

TEE is important for preoperative or perioperative sizing of the aortic root for homograft placement. Sizing of the aortic root and pulmonary valve annulus is also essential to the successful completion of the Ross procedure (pulmonary autograft). Echocardiographic follow-up after the procedure must include assessment of the pulmonary prosthetic valve for the development of pulmonic stenosis, the aortic valve for development of regurgitation, and the aortic root for dilation.[55]

The size of the prosthetic valve that can be placed in the aortic position is limited by the size of the annulus. Congenital abnormalities, severe LV hypertrophy, dense annular calcification, or the presence of a mitral valve prosthesis may limit the size of the prosthesis that can be placed, necessitating the use of one that is moderately or severely stenotic. Prosthesis-patient mismatch is presumed to be present when the effective orifice area indexed to body surface area is <0.9 cm^2/m^2.[54] Prosthesis-patient mismatch is more likely to occur with prosthetic aortic valves 21 mm in diameter or smaller, in patients with larger body surface areas, and in those with aortic stenosis as the primary indication for valve replacement. In general, stented bioprosthetic valves have lower effective orifice areas than stentless bioprosthetic valves, homografts, and pulmonary autografts. Supraannular placement may also allow for larger prosthesis size. Prosthesis-patient mismatch accounts in part for high transvalvular gradients. The gradients across the prosthetic valves with the smaller effective orifice area

■ ■ ■

TABLE 11-2 NORMAL DOPPLER VALUES FOR AORTIC PROSTHESES

Aortic prostheses	Peak velocity (m/s)	Mean gradient (mmHg)	Area mean (cm²)	Area range (cm²)
Starr-Edwards	3.1 ± 0.5	24 ± 4	*	*
Bjork-Shiley	2.5 ± 0.6	14 ± 5	2.2	1.6-2.9
St. Jude Medical	3.0 ± 0.8	11 ± 6	2.4	1.8-3.4
CarboMedics	2.5 ± 0.5	14 ± 5	2.3	1.8-3.2
Medtronic Hall	2.6 ± 0.3	12 ± 3	*	*
Omniscience	2.8 ± 0.4	14 ± 3	*	*
Aortic Homograft	0.8 ± 0.4	7.1 ±3	2.2	1.7-3.1
Hancock	2.4 ± 0.4	12 ± 2	1.8	1.4-2.3
Carpentier-Edwards	2.4 ± 0.5	14 ± 6	1.8	1.2-3.1

*Insufficient data available.
From Zabalgoitia M, Oraby M, Evaluation of prosthetic heart valves, in Pohost G (ed): *Imaging in Cardiovascular Disease*, Philadelphia, Lippincott, Williams & Wilkins, 2000, p 617.

are higher at rest and with exercise. The clinical significance is less clear, except at extreme values. The incidence of the problem may also be decreasing because of the design of recent mechanical and bioprosthetic valves. LV hypertrophy caused by aortic stenosis regresses after valve replacement.[56] However, there is evidence that there is less long-term regression in patients with valves with smaller effective orifice areas. Early remodeling may not be affected. Patient-prosthesis mismatch has also been invoked to explain abnormal exercise tolerance after valve replacement. Transvalvular gradients with exercise are noted to be higher across valves with smaller effective orifice areas. However, some studies have failed to demonstrate decreased exercise tolerance in patients with small-size prostheses.[57]

Echocardiography is the method of choice for evaluating prosthetic valves and for diagnosing valvular dysfunction. Cardiac catheterization is not an attractive alternative for monitoring and carries unacceptable risks compared with echocardiography in the anticoagulated patient and because of potential complications in crossing the prosthetic valve. An initial postoperative echocardiogram before discharge or on the first outpatient visit is recommended to establish a baseline for future comparisons. There is debate about the importance of routine evaluation of prosthetic valves with no definite recommendation on this topic by the ACC/AHA Guidelines.[7] However, echocardiography is the method of choice in diagnosing prosthetic valve dysfunction and should be undertaken immediately in any patient with symptoms or physical examination signs of dysfunction. Progressive calcification of the leaflets may result in stenosis of bioprosthetic valves that can be detected by two-dimensional and Doppler examination. More commonly, the calcified leaflets tear and result in significant, acute AR. Rarely, large vegetations may also obstruct the valves.

By far, the most common causes of prosthetic valve obstruction are pannus formation and thrombosis of mechanical valves. It is important to distinguish between the two conditions, because subacute valve thrombosis may accelerate and cause hemodynamic instability or death. Echocardiography is the primary method for detecting prosthetic valve obstruction through the demonstration of increasing gradients across the valve and decreased effective orifice area. It may also be possible to visualize decreased leaflet motion or a mass associated with the valve leaflets. TTE is the primary method for demonstrating obstruction by means of Doppler measurements, with catheterization being used uncommonly.[58] TEE may be necessary to determine the exact mechanism of the obstruction. Factors that favor thrombus over pannus as the mechanism of obstruction are the presence of multiple mobile masses, attachment to the occluder of the valve, and elevated gradients. The finding of all three is highly specific for detection of thrombus.[59] Fluoroscopy may also be helpful in the detection of decreased leaflet motion as an adjunct to echocardiographic examination. Although in some cases the use of fluoroscopy obviated the need for transesophageal study, nonocclusive thrombus may be found by TEE in a number of patients with systemic emboli and

a negative transthoracic echocardiogram and cinefluoroscopy. Echocardiography, particularly TEE, can be used to monitor the results of anticoagulant or thrombolytic therapy in patients with prosthetic valve obstruction and may help determine which patients require urgent surgery because of failed medical therapy.[60]

INFECTIVE ENDOCARDITIS

Endocarditis of the aortic valve most commonly occurs in congenital AR. Calcific aortic stenosis is also a risk factor for endocarditis, but infection may occur on normal valves even in patients without other risk factors such as infections of indwelling lines, poor dentition, and diabetes.[61] Echocardiography has revolutionized the diagnosis of endocarditis. The revised Duke diagnostic criteria for endocarditis include valvular vegetations visualized on echocardiography (Box 11-1). The vegetations usually appear as low-density mobile masses attached to the ventricular surface of the valve and are associated with some degree of aortic insufficiency. Vegetations usually demonstrate chaotic, high-frequency oscillation.

TTE is less sensitive for the detection of vegetations. The resolution of an optimal transthoracic image is approximately 2 mm. Image quality may be limited by patient body habitus and in critically ill patients by mechanical ventilation and inability to position the patient. Overall sensitivity for the detection of vegetations is 40% to 60%. The finding of a typical vegetation on TTE is highly specific for endocarditis. However, false-positive results may arise with healed vegetations, nonspecific thickening, and valvular strands. Multiplane TEE is more reliable in demonstrating vegetations and should be performed in any patient with a strong clinical suspicion of endocarditis with a negative transthoracic study.[7,62] The Duke criteria incorporating visualization of vegetations on TEE as a major criteria has a negative predictive value of 90% to 92% for native left-sided valves. However, in a patient with a strong clinical suspicion of endocarditis, a negative TEE does not completely rule out the disease, particularly if it is performed early in the clinical course. High-risk patients with an originally negative TEE include those with ongoing bacteremia and aortic prosthetic valves. Repeat TEE should be considered if the patient is at high risk for endocarditis or continues to have a clinical presentation consistent with the disease.

Similarly, TEE is generally necessary to diagnose the complications of endocarditis, primarily valve ring abscess. Abscess should be suspected on transthoracic studies when thickening of the aortic root to >4 mm is detected. In addition, an echolucent area adjacent to the valve, eccentric regurgitation, and vegetations attached to the annulus of the valve rather than the leaflets are of concern (Figure 11-37). Pericardial effusion may also be a harbinger of annular involvement. TEE may not visualize the anterior aortic root as well as transesophageal studies. Complications such as pseudoaneurysms, compression of the coronary ostia by abscess, involvement of the mitral aortic intervalvular fibrosa, extension of the infection to the mitral valve, and fistula formation may all be visualized by TEE. Abscess formation may occur dur-

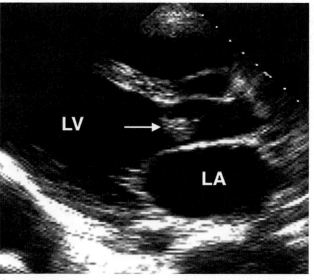

A

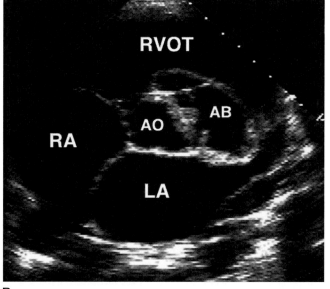

B

FIGURE 11-37. A, Parasternal long-axis view in diastole in a patient with aortic valve endocarditis. A vegetation is attached to the aortic valve leaflets *(arrow)*. Severe aortic regurgitation was present by color flow Doppler (not shown), causing early closure of the mitral valve in diastole. There is an echolucent structure in the anterior aortic root that extends along the ascending aorta. This represents an abscess cavity. **B,** Parasternal short axis of the same patient. The scanning plane is at the level of the ascending aorta, and the aortic valve leaflets are out of plane. The aorta (AO) is dwarfed by the large abscess cavity (Ab) that contains several masses and septae.

ing antibiotic therapy in patients who seem to clinically improve. A high index of suspicion is necessary, and repeat TEE is warranted in any patient with recurrent fever or other evidence of infection while receiving appropriate antibiotics. Catheterization is not recommended in the setting of aortic valve endocarditis. The risk of embolization of the vegetations is increased by the presence of the angiography catheter in the aortic root. The resolution of CMR is generally insufficient to

image vegetations, although the technique may have some use for diagnosing perivalvular complications.

Endocarditis of prosthetic aortic valves poses a special challenge, because even TEE may not visualize the anterior sewing ring and the subvalvular structures. Periannular complications occur more commonly in aortic prosthetic valve endocarditis and are particularly common in early postoperative infections. TEE is 90% sensitive in making the diagnosis. Native valve endocarditis that requires surgical valve replacement because of either severe valvular dysfunction or abscess carries a risk of infecting the prosthetic valve. Intraoperative TEE is essential for baseline comparisons should the patient seem to have ongoing or recrudescent infection after surgery.

TRICUSPID VALVE DISEASE

Anatomical Evaluation

The tricuspid valve is a unit with four components, the valve leaflets, the annulus, the chordae tendineae, and the papillary muscles, which are an integral part of the right ventricular myocardium. The anterior leaflet is the largest of the three leaflets and takes origin from the posterolateral aspect of the AV junction and extends to the membranous septum, where it forms part of the anterior commissure with the smaller septal leaflet. The attachment of the septal leaflet extends from the posterior ventricular wall across the muscular and membranous septum to the anterior septal commissure. The septal leaflet of the tricuspid valve takes origin from the septum more apically ($\approx$6 mm) than the septal leaflet of the mitral valve. The posterior tricuspid leaflet is attached entirely to the free right ventricular wall. The chordae tendineae extend from the papillary muscles and insert into the free margins of the three valve leaflets, preventing them from inverting in systole and creating a vale orifice area of almost 7 cm^2 in diastole.

Echocardiography

The geometry of the tricuspid tensor apparatus, the insertion and location of the papillary muscles, and right ventricular morphology can be determined by TTE images of the right ventricular inflow tract from the left parasternal and apical four-chamber views. The posterior leaflet of the tricuspid valve is imaged only in the right ventricular inflow view. In the setting of a dilated right ventricle, the tricuspid valve may occasionally be seen in short axis from the subcostal position. The anatomy of the tricuspid valve leaflets and the disposition of the commissures can be examined in real time by TEE imaging from the deep gastric view of the right ventricular short axis. There are three papillary muscles, two of which insert into the muscular interventricular septum in contrast to the two papillary muscles in the left ventricle, neither of which insert into the septum. The anterior and septal leaflets are commonly imaged in the modified four-chamber view. Diseases that alter any of the components of the tricuspid valve unit may interfere with valve competence, producing either obstruction (stenosis) or regurgitation.

TRICUSPID STENOSIS

Pathophysiology and Hemodynamics

Partial obstruction of the tricuspid valve orifice occurs when the material properties of the valve leaflet tissue change, causing stiffening of the leaflets that restrict valve opening. Thickening of the tricuspid valve leaflets occurs most commonly in rheumatic heart disease and rarely in carcinoid (Figure 11-38), endomyocardial fibro-

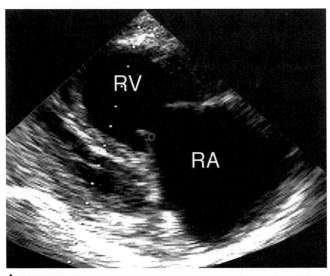

A

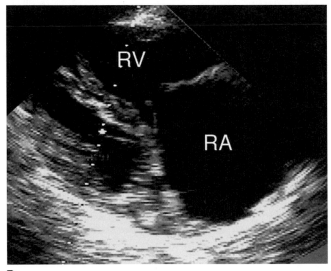

B

FIGURE 11-38. A, Parasternal long-axis right ventricular inflow view in diastole. The tricuspid valve leaflets are thickened and do not open completely, resulting in moderate tricuspid stenosis. The leaflets do not dome and are rigid. The right atrium is dilated. **B,** Parasternal long-axis right ventricular inflow view in systole. There is no significant motion of the tricuspid valve leaflets. The leaflets do not coapt, resulting in severe regurgitation. The right ventricular function is moderately decreased because of the right ventricular volume overload in this patient with carcinoid heart disease.

sis, and with use of ergot alkaloids and anorexic agents. Rheumatic tricuspid stenosis results from fusion of the valve commissures caused by chronic inflammation and restriction of leaflet motion caused by chordal thickening and shortening, both of which are specific for rheumatic heart disease. Rheumatic tricuspid valve stenosis is always associated with mitral and/or aortic valve disease, occurring usually in mild form in approximately 5% of patients with rheumatic valve disease but never as an isolated lesion. Tricuspid stenosis progresses slowly and is usually of less hemodynamic importance than the associated mitral and/or aortic valve lesions. Fibrosis of the valve leaflets related to pacemaker leads has been reported as a rare cause of tricuspid stenosis. As the hemodynamic severity of tricuspid stenosis increases, the diastolic pressure gradient across the valve increases, right atrial pressure increases causing dilation of the right atrium and transmission of the elevated pressure to the systemic veins with jugular vein distention, hepatic enlargement, lower extremity edema, and finally anasarca.

The symptoms of tricuspid stenosis are easy fatigue, abdominal bloating, lower extremity edema, and palpitations that occur when tricuspid stenosis is the dominant hemodynamic lesion. More frequently, the symptoms of coexistent mitral and/or aortic valve disease predominate over those of tricuspid stenosis. The clinical findings of tricuspid stenosis may not be recognized in patients with concomitant mitral stenosis, because the cardiac murmurs may be ascribed to the mitral valve, unless tricuspid obstruction is considered. The diagnostic findings may be obscured in the presence of atrial fibrillation, but in sinus rhythm, there is jugular venous distention with a characteristically prominent "a" wave that is brisk and short duration with a slow "y" descent denoting slow and prolonged rather than the normally rapid right ventricular early filling phase. On auscultation at the left lower sternal border in patients with tricuspid stenosis in sinus rhythm, the typical findings are an opening snap and a middiastolic murmur with presystolic accentuation that increases in amplitude with inspiration and decreases with expiration.

Anatomical Evaluation

The chest radiograph demonstrates cardiomegaly, right atrial enlargement, and prominence of the superior vena cava at the upper right heart border. Cardiac catheterization is rarely performed but reveals an elevated right atrial pressure, a giant "a" wave, and a holodiastolic pressure difference between the right atrium and ventricle, with a mean diastolic gradient of 2 to 5 mmHg.

Echocardiography

Echocardiography is the diagnostic modality of choice in tricuspid stenosis, because the valve leaflet thickness, motion pattern, and hemodynamic severity can all be evaluated. The valve leaflets in rheumatic tricuspid stenosis are thickened, and their opening motion is restricted by commissural fusion, which can be appreciated in images of the tricuspid valve in the left parasternal right ventricular inflow tract view and in the apical four-chamber view. Unlike mitral valve stenosis, the tricuspid orifice area cannot be assessed echocardiographically by direct visualization and planimetry, because the stenotic valve orifice cannot be imaged in a single plane. However, the severity of tricuspid stenosis can be assessed by applying the modified Bernoulli formula to the tricuspid inflow velocity measured by continuous-wave Doppler. The peak and mean velocities downstream of the stenosis are squared and multiplied by 4 to obtain the peak and mean pressure gradients. The normal tricuspid valve area is 6 to 7 cm². Therefore, a mean gradient of even 2 mmHg is sufficient to establish the diagnosis of tricuspid stenosis. A peak gradient of 4 mmHg or more indicates severe tricuspid stenosis. In addition, the tricuspid effective valve orifice area can be determined by the pressure half-time method that was initially derived empirically for assessment of the mitral valve orifice area in mitral stenosis. The gradients measured by Doppler echocardiography correlate closely with those obtained at cardiac catheterization and have been used successfully to guide management, including surgical valve repair and replacement.

TRICUSPID REGURGITATION

Pathophysiology and Hemodynamics

Tricuspid regurgitation may be due to primary involvement of the valve leaflets and subvalve tensor apparatus or more commonly secondary to dilation of the right ventricle and tricuspid annulus. Stretching of the tricuspid annulus distorts the tricuspid valve geometry and prevents coaptation of the normal valve leaflets. Primary causes of tricuspid regurgitation include rheumatic valvulitis, leaflet prolapse, endocarditis, rheumatoid arthritis, carcinoid, chest trauma, radiation therapy, congenital structural abnormalities including Ebstein's anomaly, and connective tissue disorders such as Marfan's syndrome. The tricuspid valve may be injured by blunt chest trauma or by the bioptome forceps during endomyocardial biopsy (Figure 11-39).[63] Secondary causes of tricuspid regurgitation are right ventricular dilation and failure caused by pressure overload associated with discrete outflow tract obstruction at infundibular, valvar, and supravalvar levels. Other causes of secondary tricuspid regurgitation include idiopathic pulmonary hypertension and pulmonary hypertension caused by pulmonary fibrosis; acute and chronic thromboembolism; intracardiac shunts at atrial, ventricular, and great arterial levels; and left heart disease such as mitral stenosis and left ventricular dysfunction. Tricuspid regurgitation is almost ubiquitous when the right ventricular systolic pressure exceeds 40 mmHg, resulting in further ventricular dilation that may progress insidiously and escalate the onset of right ventricular failure.

Symptoms of severe tricuspid regurgitation include easy fatigue, exercise intolerance, satiety, anorexia, abdominal bloating, weight loss, and lower extremity edema. Clinical examination is remarkable for jaundice, cachexia, and even cyanosis in the most severe cases.

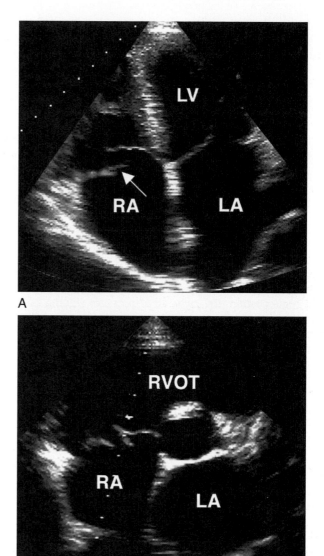

A

B

FIGURE 11-39. A, Apical four-chamber view in a patient who has undergone orthotopic heart transplant. The anterior leaflet of the tricuspid valve *(arrow)* is partially flail and prolapses into the right atrium with attached chordae. The tricuspid valve apparatus had been damaged in a right ventricular biopsy undertaken for surveillance to detect cardiac rejection. The resulting tricuspid regurgitation was severe and directed toward the interatrial septum. The composite atria are enlarged, and the site of the surgical anastomosis is visible as an area of thickening in the interatrial septum. The left ventricular function is near normal in this systolic frame, although the left atrial annulus is dilated and the mitral valve leaflets are tented toward the left ventricular apex. B, Parasternal short-axis view of the same patient. In systole the anterior leaflet of the tricuspid valve is partially flail. RVOT, right ventricular outflow tract.

There is jugular venous distention with prominent "c" and "v" waves and a brisk "y" descent in the jugular venous pulse contour. The right ventricular impulse may cause a left lower parasternal lift. On auscultation there is a holosystolic murmur appreciated best at the left lower sternal border that augments with inspiration. In right heart failure and pulmonary hypertension, there may be a third heart sound and an exaggerated pulmonary component of the second heart sound, respectively. The liver is usually enlarged and palpable below the right costal margin and remarkable for exhibiting systolic pulsation.

Electrocardiographic changes are nonspecific and may include right ventricular conduction delay and right ventricular hypertrophy with repolarization abnormalities in patients with severe pulmonary hypertension from Eisenmenger reaction to intracardiac shunts. Chest radiograph reveals cardiomegaly, right atrial enlargement, and pulmonary vascular markings consistent with pulmonary venous or pulmonary arterial hypertension.

Cardiac catheterization is rarely undertaken nowadays to establish the diagnosis of tricuspid regurgitation or to evaluate its hemodynamic severity, because this can almost always be achieved noninvasively by Doppler echocardiography. The right atrial pressure contour demonstrates a prominent "v" wave that increases in amplitude with increasing severity of regurgitation. In severe tricuspid regurgitation, the right atrial pressure tracing closely simulates the right ventricular pressure waveform. Right ventricular end-diastolic pressure rises with increasing right ventricular contractile dysfunction in response to chronic pressure and volume overload. Right ventricular systolic and pulmonary arterial systolic pressures have prognostic value in terms of the clinical outcome in patients with tricuspid regurgitation. In secondary tricuspid regurgitation caused by pulmonary hypertension, estimates of pulmonary vascular resistance, which can only be obtained by cardiac catheterization, may be useful in directing management of patients with intracardiac shunts.

Transthoracic echocardiography enables the tricuspid valve leaflets, subvalve apparatus, and annulus to be visualized. In rheumatic tricuspid valvulitis, the valve leaflets become thickened, retracted, and tethered with reduced mobility caused by commissural fusion and more often result in predominant regurgitation than stenosis. TTE imaging in the apical four-chamber view shows the restricted motion pattern of the valve leaflets so characteristic of rheumatic disease and the Doppler color flow velocity regurgitant jet in enlarged right atrium during systole. Carcinoid involvement of the tricuspid valve also causes leaflet thickening, reduced mobility, and regurgitation. However, carcinoid can be distinguished from rheumatic valve disease echocardiographically, because the leaflets are usually fixed in the partially opened position. Carcinoid, unlike rheumatic disease, is only rarely associated with involvement of the left-sided heart valves but is frequently accompanied by pulmonic valve thickening, stenosis, and regurgitation. Increased leaflet thickening also occurs because of myxomatous degeneration in tricuspid prolapse in which rather than restricted motion, the leaflets are excessively mobile and prolapse back into the right atrium, resulting in tricuspid regurgitation of varying severity. Transthoracic echocardiograms demonstrate that the systolic prolapse disrupts the coaptation of the three leaflets, allowing blood to regurgitate between the leaflets easily demonstrable by the origin and extent of the Doppler color flow regurgitant jet. A further cause of primary tricuspid regurgitation is vegetative endocarditis in which disruption of the valve leaflets may result in fenestration or avulsion caused by excessive traction on the valve by large mobile vegetations and result in failure of normal leaflet coaptation. Congenital abnormalities of the tricuspid valve that are associated with tricuspid regurgitation include Ebstein's anomaly, which can be diagnosed by either the apical displacement of the insertion of the valve leaflets from the true annulus and/or tethering of the leaflets, which prevents normal leaflet coaptation (see Chapter 14).

Secondary tricuspid valve regurgitation occurs as a consequence of right ventricular dilation and concomitant stretching of the tricuspid annulus in the absence of any intrinsic valve leaflet abnormalities and may vary in severity from mild to severe. Two-dimensional Doppler echocardiography is the method of choice for diagnosis of secondary tricuspid regurgitation, because it demonstrates the abnormal right ventricular geometry and the normal tricuspid valve apparatus. Reversal of right ventricular dilation is associated with attenuation of secondary, but not primary, tricuspid regurgitation in which the leaflets and tensor apparatus are abnormal. Acute right ventricular dilation, contractile dysfunction, and secondary tricuspid regurgitation may result from major pulmonary embolism and/or right ventricular myocardial infarction. All these acute and chronic causes of secondary tricuspid regurgitation can be recognized by Doppler echocardiography.

Assessment of the Severity of Tricuspid Regurgitation

Historically, the severity of tricuspid regurgitation has been assessed clinically in terms of symptoms of fatigue and signs of jugular venous distention with an accentuated "v" wave, right ventricular prominence, a holosystolic murmur at the lower left sternal border that varies in intensity with respiration, pulsatile hepatomegaly, dependent edema, and occasionally anasarca. Causally related pulmonary hypertension is indicated by increased amplitude of the pulmonary closing component of the second heart sound, and clinical examination enables detection of associated pulmonary parenchymal disease or left heart disease.

Chest radiograph demonstrates cardiomegaly with a prominent right heart border caused by right atrial enlargement and other radiographic features associated with tricuspid regurgitation, for example, rheumatic mitral valve disease.

Cardiac Catheterization

Cardiac catheterization is only rarely undertaken for evaluation of primary tricuspid regurgitation, except preoperatively in patients with rheumatic multivalve disease in whom coronary artery disease needs to be documented or in rare patients in whom noninvasive studies are severely technically limited. Right atrial pressure waveforms characteristically shows a prominent "v" wave, and in severe tricuspid regurgitation, the right atrial pressure waveform resembles the right ventricular pressure pulse and does not exhibit the normal variation with inspiration. Right heart catheterization provides accurate measurement of pulmonary artery pressures. Pulmonary artery systolic pressure >40 mmHg is almost invariably associated with some degree of tricuspid regurgitation. However, pulmonary artery pressure per se does not correlate strongly with the severity of tricuspid regurgitation, and this is evidenced by the normal pulmonary artery pressures and free tricuspid regurgitation after surgical tricuspid valvectomy for intractable vegetative endocarditis. Pulmonary artery pressure measurement does not reliably discriminate between primary and secondary causes of tricuspid regurgitation.

Echocardiography

There are a number of semiquantitative and quantitative Doppler echocardiographic methods in use in contemporary cardiology practice for assessing the severity of tricuspid regurgitation noninvasively. Color flow Doppler velocity mapping of the right atrium is exquisitely sensitive for detecting the presence of tricuspid regurgitation but is semiquantitative and is subject to variability from a number of the same factors that influence interpretation of the severity of mitral regurgitation. These confounding factors include the size and compliance of the receiving chamber, initial jet velocity, heart rate, loading conditions, and jet collision/impaction with the atrial wall. The origin and direction of the tricuspid regurgitant jet by color Doppler enables appropriate alignment of the interrogating continuous-wave Doppler for quantitation of the right atrial/right ventricular peak systolic gradient by use of the modified Bernoulli formula (Figure 11-40), to which an estimate of right atrial pressure is added to calculate pulmonary artery systolic pressure. Right atrial pressure has been variously estimated from regression correction of simultaneously recorded pulmonary artery pressure at cardiac catheterization and Doppler echocardiography. Strong correlations have been demonstrated between hemodynamic assessment of pulmonary artery pressure at cardiac catheterization and estimates by Doppler echocardiography.

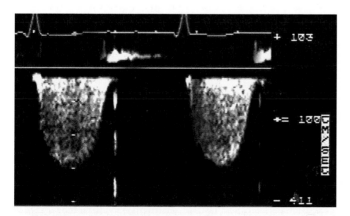

FIGURE 11-40. Spectral display of continuous-wave Doppler of tricuspid regurgitation from the apical position. The peak velocity of the tricuspid regurgitation is 3 m/s. The right atrial pressure was estimated as 10 mmHg, and there was no pulmonic stenosis. Therefore, the peak pulmonary artery pressure was estimated as 46 mmHg.

Hepatic vein Doppler velocity reflects blood flow into the right atrium and may be altered by tricuspid regurgitation. These changes in hepatic flow velocity parallel the changes in blood flow velocity patterns in the pulmonary veins in subjects with mitral regurgitation. Severe tricuspid regurgitation is associated with systolic reversal of flow in the hepatic veins and as such provides a semiquantitative means of discriminating between moderate and severe regurgitation with a high positive predictive value. Reversal of flow during ventricular systole occurs because there is no effective venous valve preventing reflux of blood into the proximal inferior vena cava and hepatic veins with severe tricuspid regurgitation.

An alternative quantitative method of assessing the severity of tricuspid regurgitation on the basis of the conservation of mass that has been validated clinically and experimentally is the EROA, which corresponds to the area of the vena contracta. The EROA is a measure of severity of tricuspid regurgitation that is less influenced by variation in hemodynamics and heart rate than are regurgitant volume or regurgitant fraction. Two refinements for local and geometric factors have been applied to the calculation of regurgitant volume. The first correction is the ratio of (V/V−Vr), in which V is the regurgitant peak velocity and Vr is the aliasing velocity. The second correction is the ratio of (α/180) in which α is the angle of the tricuspid valve funnel. Regurgitant flow (RFlow) was calculated as:

$$RFlow = 2\pi \times r^2 \times Vr \times (V/V-Vr) \times (\alpha/180) \quad \text{(Equation 19)}$$

ERO can be calculated as:

$$ERO = RFlow \div \text{Regurgitant velocity} \quad \text{(Equation 20)}$$

EROA correlates weakly with tricuspid regurgitant jet area by color flow Doppler velocity mapping but less well with the ratio of jet area/right atrial area.[18] A tricuspid effective regurgitant orifice area of 40 mm² and a tricuspid regurgitant volume of more than 45 mL indicate the presence of severe tricuspid regurgitation with sensitivities and specificities of 94% and 89%, and 74% and 95%, respectively. Severe tricuspid regurgitation defined as an ERO >40 mm² was significantly associated with reversal of flow in the hepatic veins.

Management of Tricuspid Valve Disease

The optimal management of patients with tricuspid valve disease relies on the combination of clinical examination together with Doppler echocardiographic examination of the valve leaflets and subvalve apparatus, right ventricular geometry and function, and pulmonary artery pressure. Because tricuspid valve disease is often secondary to associated mitral valve disease or pulmonary hypertension caused by left ventricular disease, careful consideration must be given to the etiology of the tricuspid regurgitation.

Rheumatic tricuspid stenosis can be identified by fusion of the valve commissures and concomitant mitral valve disease. The hemodynamic severity of both valve lesions can be assessed by Doppler echocardiography that determines whether continuing medical therapy or surgical intervention is indicated. In addition, assessment of the leaflet thickness, calcification, and mobility are important determinants of whether successful commissurotomy is feasible or valve replacement is required.

Primary tricuspid regurgitation can be recognized echocardiographically by the presence of abnormalities of the tricuspid leaflets that cause improper leaflet coaptation and regurgitation. In secondary tricuspid regurgitation, the valve leaflets by definition are intrinsically normal, and the regurgitation results from dilation of the tricuspid annulus impairing leaflet coaptation. The importance of distinguishing primary from secondary tricuspid regurgitation is in selecting the optimal therapy for each of the two pathoetiologies. Regardless of whether tricuspid regurgitation is primary or secondary, the EROA and regurgitant volume should be calculated whenever possible to confirm the hemodynamic severity of the regurgitation. In primary tricuspid regurgitation, the hemodynamic severity determines whether therapy should be aggressive medical therapy with diuretics, angiotensin-converting enzyme (ACE) inhibitors, and digoxin or, alternatively, surgical valve repair or replacement when the valve leaflets are diseased. By contrast, when medical therapy with diuretics, vasodilators, and ACE inhibitors fails to reduce regurgitant volume or EROA in secondary tricuspid regurgitation, reduction in tricuspid annular circumference and thereby valve orifice area can be achieved with ring annuloplasty or De Vega technique. Reducing annular area either by afterload reduction or ring annuloplasty restores leaflet coaptation and reduces or abolishes tricuspid regurgitation.[64] When surgical intervention is required for either primary or secondary tricuspid regurgitation, intraoperative transesophageal Doppler echocardiography after repair or replacement should be used to assess the adequacy of repair in terms of the residual regurgitation by Doppler color flow velocity mapping.

ENDOCARDITIS

Tricuspid valve endocarditis occurs most commonly in intravenous drug users or in patients with indwelling central lines. However, it is rarely reported in patients with no predisposing conditions. Tricuspid vegetations are optimally visualized by TTE in the apical four-chamber, the parasternal short-axis view of the aorta, or the right ventricular inflow tract view (Figure 11-41). Vegetations usually appear as echodense mobile masses attached to the leaflets, usually taking origin from the right atrial surface of the tricuspid valve and ranging in size from 2 to 43 mm. Vegetations that are large (>10 mm) and/or mobile are prone to embolization to the lungs, where they may cause multiple lung abscesses. The likelihood of embolization diminishes with administration of antibiotic therapy. Whenever tricuspid valve vegetations are suspected but not demonstrated unequivocally, confirmation must be sought by urgent TEE, which permits visualization of all three leaflets from the apical four-chamber view and the

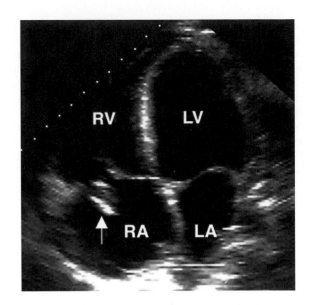

FIGURE 11-41. Apical four-chamber view in a patient with idiopathic dilated cardiomyopathy and tricuspid valve endocarditis. There is a large vegetation *(arrow)* attached to the anterior leaflet of the tricuspid valve that prolapses into the right atrium in systole. The right atrium is dilated, and there is biventricular systolic dysfunction.

transgastric modified short-axis view of the right ventricle.

PULMONARY VALVE DISEASE

Anatomical Evaluation

Echocardiography

The pulmonary valve is the most anterior cardiac structure and may be difficult to visualize because of its substernal location in the adult. The valves are attached in a semilunar manner to the pulmonary annulus, which gives rise to the sinuses in an arrangement similar to the aortic valve. The pulmonary valves are less stiff than the aortic leaflets, possibly because of a lower collagen content. The leaflets of the pulmonary valve are normally thin and are difficult to detect in systole, because the leaflets approximate the walls of the pulmonary artery. The high parasternal long-axis window usually demonstrates the valve and a small portion of the infundibulum and the proximal pulmonary artery. The parasternal short axis affords a better assessment of these structures. It is not possible to demonstrate the normal valve in short axis, and echocardiographic detection of bicuspid pulmonic valves is unreliable. Thickening of the leaflets and doming in systole may be present in both acquired and congenital disease. Historically, right ventriculography was important for visualization of the infundibulum and proximal pulmonary artery. However, echocardiographic assessment of the pulmonary valve has largely replaced this method, although catheterization is still useful for measurement and localization of gradients.

The width of the pulmonary annulus and the pulmonary artery can be measured in most subjects. The main pulmonary artery branches into the right and left main pulmonary arteries, with the right branch passing posterior to the left atrium. The left branch is more difficult to visualize for any length because of its posterior course. The pulmonary valve and artery may also be visualized from the subcostal window in a view perpendicular to the subcostal four-chamber view. The tricuspid valve and high right ventricular outflow tract surround the aortic valve in short axis. The pulmonary artery is seen in long axis with the pulmonary bifurcation in the far field. CMR is more reliable in measurement of pulmonary artery size and has a higher degree of correlation with angiography. CMR also is more accurate than echocardiography in diagnosing nonconfluence of the right and left pulmonary arteries.

Doppler interrogation of the valve may be accomplished in all of the standard echocardiographic views. The upper limit of normal peak systolic velocity in adults is 0.9 m/s. The velocity is lower than that in the aortic root, because the pulmonary valve area index is greater than the aortic valve area. The pulmonary valve area is linearly related to body surface area.[39] Sampling of the infundibulum and main pulmonary artery is best accomplished from the parasternal short-axis view by pulsed-wave Doppler. However, multiple views should be used to ensure the best alignment between the ultrasound beam and the pulmonary outflow jet. The infundibulum separates the inlet and muscular portion of the RV from the pulmonary valve. Hypertrophy of the muscle bundles of the infundibulum may create dynamic subvalvular obstruction. Turbulence and acceleration of velocities can be detected at this level by color flow Doppler.

Transesophageal imaging of the pulmonary valve often adds little to the evaluation, because anterior cardiac structures are in the far field of the transesophageal scanning plane. It is not possible to obtain adequate alignment with the outflow jet to measure velocities with any accuracy. The right pulmonary artery may be seen in short axis in the longitudinal plane and in the long axis in the transverse plane in a high esophageal window. In general, only the proximal left pulmonary artery can usually be visualized.

PULMONARY STENOSIS

Pathophysiology and Hemodynamics

Acquired stenosis of the pulmonary valve is rare, and most abnormalities are caused by congenital disease (see Chapter 14). A distinction has been made between congenital stenosis with pliable leaflets and fusion of the commissures and dysplastic thickened valves associated with annular hypoplasia. The dysplastic valves generally are more severely stenotic and more likely to be symptomatic in infancy. The leaflets appear immobile in systole and diastole. Supra-annular narrowing may also be present (Figure 11-42). Dysplastic valves are uncommon, even in pulmonary stenosis associated with Noonan's syndrome. The frequency of bicuspid pulmonic valves is unknown but is common in tetralogy of Fallot. The annulus is often abnormal in the presence of congenital

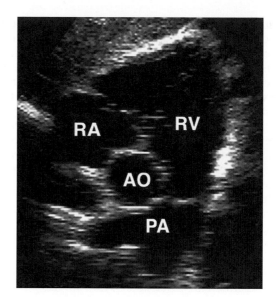

FIGURE 11-42. Subcostal short-axis view at the base of the heart. The right ventricle is dilated. The pulmonary annulus is narrowed, and the pulmonary valve is dysplastic. The leaflets are thickened and did not move significantly in systole.

stenosis, and supra-annular stenosis may also be present. In typical pulmonic stenosis, poststenotic dilation of the pulmonary artery may occur. Unlike congenitally abnormal aortic valves, the calcification of the valve leaflets over time is uncommon.

Acquired pulmonic stenosis may develop in patients with carcinoid disease. In these cases, the valve is usually both stenotic and regurgitant because of thickening and fixation of the leaflets without fusion of the commissures. Pulmonic stenosis may also develop postoperatively in patients after arterial switch and annulus repairs, as well as after correction of anomalous coronary arteries if the annulus does not enlarge with growth of the patient.

Severe pulmonic stenosis presents in infancy with right heart failure or severe cyanosis in the setting of an intracardiac shunt. Systemic hypoxia may be compounded by pulmonary malperfusion. In the adult, mild and moderate levels of pulmonary stenosis are usually asymptomatic. Severe stenosis may by asymptomatic or present with mild levels of effort intolerance.

Anatomical Evaluation

Echocardiography is the best diagnostic test for patients suspected of having pulmonic stenosis. By use of the parasternal windows, it is usually possible to identify the level of the stenosis. Assessment of the morphology of the valves is not always feasible, and the diagnosis of bicuspid leaflet arrangements is unreliable. Nevertheless, it is usually possible to distinguish dysplastic valves by the marked thickening, immobility, and small annular size. Valvular stenosis without dysplastic leaflets often results in poststenotic dilation. The characteristic thickening of the leaflets with fixation suggests carcinoid disease, in which regurgitation is usually present as well as stenosis.

Echocardiography is also essential to evaluate the presence of associated defects, particularly cardiac shunts and pulmonary artery hypoplasia or atresia. Occasionally, tetralogy of Fallot will not be discovered until adulthood. The parasternal long axis demonstrates an overriding aorta with a malalignment ventricular septal defect. Rarely, pulmonic stenosis may be caused by tumor involvement of the pulmonary artery or subvalvular apparatus. Lipoma of the pulmonary valve may also cause obstruction to outflow. Papillary fibroelastomas of the pulmonary valve have been reported but rarely cause stenosis. Spontaneous regression of obstructing pulmonary valve myxomas has been reported in infants.

Poststenotic dilation of the pulmonary artery may occur and has been suggested by some to lead to an eventual decrease in the degree of annular stenosis[65] (Figure 11-43). Dilation of the pulmonary artery is usually a benign condition, although spontaneous dissection has been described in association with severe pulmonary hypertension. Assessment of the main pulmonary artery branches is important in the evaluation of the patient with pulmonic stenosis. CMR may be the most reliable method of evaluating the pulmonary artery anatomy and the presence of aortopulmonary collaterals.[66]

Quantification of Severity of Stenosis

Doppler echocardiography allows assessment of the gradient across the valve. The ultrasound beam should be aligned as closely as possible with the flow across the valve. This is usually accomplished in the parasternal short-axis view at the base that lays out the pulmonary artery in long axis. The subcostal view of the pulmonary valve and artery may also be used if the parasternal windows are technically limited. Pulsed-wave and color Doppler evaluation should be used to identify the level of obstruction. The gradient across the stenosis is calculated from the continuous-wave Doppler spectral envelope by use of the modified Bernoulli equation (Figure 11-44). Mild pulmonic stenosis is classified as a transvalvular gradient of <50 mmHg. Severe stenosis is designated as a transvalvular peak gradient >75 mmHg. The pulmonic valve area is not calculated, because the right ventricular outflow tract does not have circular cross-sectional geometry. The gradients measured with Doppler ultrasound correlate with those measured invasively. In children, pulmonic valve gradients measured by Doppler echocardiography may be significantly higher in the nonsedated patient, particularly if a component of infundibular stenosis is present. The diameter of the annulus may also be measured with a right ventricular angiogram.

Right ventricular hypertrophy is usually present with moderate or severe stenosis. Hypertrophy of the infundibular muscle bundles in the right ventricular outflow tract may result in additional subvalvular stenosis. Assessment of right ventricular function is an important part of the evaluation.

Clinical Evaluation

Studies have demonstrated the relative insensitivity of auscultation for the diagnosis of pulmonic stenosis. Echocardiography is recommended in asymptomatic children and adults with systolic murmurs that do not fit the criteria of an innocent murmur.[7,67,68] In general, mild and moderate degrees of stenosis in older children and adults do not progress. Serial echocardiographic studies are not indicated and may be reserved for the development of symptoms, such as dyspnea or effort intolerance.[67]

Severe pulmonic stenosis may be relieved with balloon valvuloplasty with similar results to those obtained in infants and children. Indications for the procedure vary. Guidelines have been published for the pediatric population.[69] Balloon valvuloplasty is considered a class I intervention in adult asymptomatic patients with a pul-

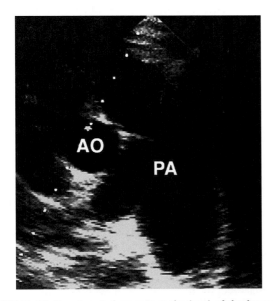

FIGURE 11-43. Parasternal short axis at the level of the base of the heart in systole. The pulmonary valve is not dysplastic but demonstrates restricted motion consistent with severe stenosis. The leaflets are not thickened, and the annulus is dilated rather than narrowed. There is severe poststenotic dilation of the pulmonary artery and the left main pulmonary artery branch.

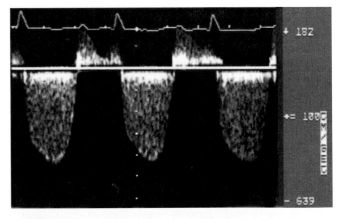

FIGURE 11-44. Spectral display of continuous-wave Doppler across the pulmonic valve. The transducer is in the parasternal location along the long axis of the pulmonary artery. The peak velocity is 4.2 m/s, which is consistent with a gradient of 71 mmHg.

monary valve gradient of >50 mmHg and in patients with lower gradients and symptoms caused by fixed cardiac output.[7] TEE may be performed during the procedure to guide balloon sizing and positioning. The use of intracardiac ultrasound has also been described. The presence of dysplastic valves and the use of undersized balloons are predictors for suboptimal outcome. Restenosis and the development of severe pulmonic regurgitation may be monitored by serial echocardiograms. Excellent long-term outcome is the rule, and regression of both infundibular stenosis and severe tricuspid regurgitation have been reported after balloon valvuloplasty.[7] The persistence of a Doppler gradient of $\geq$40 mmHg after balloon valvuloplasty should initiate close clinical and echocardiographic follow-up.[67] Surgery for open valvuloplasty or replacement may still occasionally be required, especially in patients with dysplastic valves associated with Noonan's syndrome.

PULMONARY REGURGITATION

Pathophysiology and Hemodynamics

Trivial pulmonary regurgitation is detected in virtually all normal patients who undergo color Doppler flow imaging. Significant pulmonary regurgitation is rarely congenital, but a number of secondary causes have been described. Pulmonary artery dilation from any cause may result in pulmonic regurgitation. Pulmonary hypertension may be dynamic and result in pulmonary artery dilation and valvular regurgitation that resolves with the relief of the hypertension. This phenomenon occurs in patients with acute pulmonary embolism and in patients with end-stage renal disease before dialysis. Carcinoid valvular disease, as already mentioned, is a cause of a mixed pulmonary regurgitation and stenosis. Endocarditis of the pulmonary valve is rare. Congenital lesions and intravenous drug use are risk factors for endocarditis. High-velocity pulmonary regurgitation is probably not a significant risk factor for endocarditis in patients with anatomically normal valves. Traction on the pulmonary annulus by the surgical anastomosis of the pulmonary artery in orthotopic heart transplant recipients occasionally results in significant pulmonary regurgitation. Many patients who undergo surgical repair of tetralogy of Fallot and other lesions associated with severe congenital pulmonary stenosis are left with significant pulmonary regurgitation. The degree of regurgitation and the right ventricular diastolic dimensions correlate with the postoperative size of the pulmonary annulus.[70] Balloon valvuloplasty often results in some degree of pulmonary regurgitation but is not a cause of acute hemodynamic decompensation. More severe degrees of regurgitation correlate with lower residual gradient.

Severe pulmonary regurgitation has traditionally been considered a well-tolerated hemodynamic lesion. However, severe pulmonary regurgitation may eventually cause significant right ventricular volume overload.[70] An abnormally low augmentation in cardiac output in response to exercise has been demonstrated in patients with chronic moderate or severe pulmonary regurgitation.

Assessment of the Severity of Pulmonic Regurgitation

The right ventricular outflow tract does not have a circular cross-section and is not coplanar with the proximal pulmonary artery. It is difficult to evaluate the degree of pulmonary regurgitation on the basis of the extent of the pulmonary regurgitation color Doppler jet, because the jet is usually directed out of the imaging plane. The width of the pulmonary regurgitation jet should be measured at the valve orifice. The ratio of the jet width to the diameter of the pulmonary annulus is a better measure of the severity of pulmonary regurgitation and correlates with the angiographic grade.[71] Diastolic retrograde flow in the main branches of the pulmonary artery is associated with at least moderate pulmonic regurgitation. The deceleration slope of the continuous-wave Doppler spectral envelope of the regurgitation velocities may also be helpful. A rapid fall in the diastolic gradient is associated with severe pulmonic regurgitation and right ventricular decompensation. However, right ventricular dysfunction from other causes, such as right ventricular infarction, may cause a similar pattern. Doppler quantification of regurgitant volume and fraction has been more problematic because of the complex geometry of the outflow tract. Recently, digital color Doppler flow measurements in orthogonal planes has shown promise as a more reliable quantitative method.[72] Similarly, three-dimensional reconstruction of color Doppler jets may prove useful in the evaluation.[17] Transesophageal examination adds little incremental information to the evaluation of pulmonary regurgitation by transthoracic imaging.

Difficulties in assessment of right ventricular volumes and functions have led to a search for alternate methods to evaluate both pulmonary regurgitation and right ventricular response to the volume load. CMR has been used to measure pulmonary regurgitant flow and right ventricular volumes and ejection fraction at rest and with exercise.[70,73]

Clinical Evaluation

Patients at risk for the development of significant pulmonic regurgitation, such as those who have undergone repair of pulmonary valve stenosis, should be monitored by serial echocardiograms, although a yearly frequency is probably not necessary. Development of severe tricuspid regurgitation and life-threatening arrhythmias may be associated with the development of right ventricular enlargement.[74] Right ventricular dilation and systolic dysfunction may precede the development of symptoms, which has led some to suggest that pulmonary valve replacement be undertaken earlier than previously recommended. Improvement in right ventricular size and function has been documented after pulmonary valve replacement by CMR imaging.[75] Surgery is generally reserved for patients with significant symptoms, with low operative mortality and good long-term results.

PULMONIC PROSTHETIC VALVE

Prosthetic valves in the pulmonary position have become more frequent as the Ross procedure is used in young patients with aortic valve disease. The native pulmonary valve is used as an autograft in the aortic position, and an allograft is used to replace the pulmonic valve. The prosthetic pulmonary valve is assessed in a similar manner to the native valve. A rise in transvalvular gradients may indicate the development of stenosis from fibrosis or thrombus formation. Pulmonary allograft dysfunction has developed in up to 22% of patients after the Ross procedure in some series and may require reoperation. Endocarditis may also develop. Mechanical valves are generally not recommended for pulmonary valve replacement. The lower velocity flow in this position tends to favor the development of valvular thrombosis. Bileaflet valves may be incompetent because of lower closing pressures than in the aortic position.

REFERENCES

1. Prior DL, Jaber WA, Homa DA, Thomas JD, Mayer Sabik E. Impact of tissue harmonic imaging on the assessment of rheumatic mitral stenosis. *American Journal of Cardiology*. 86(5):573-6, A10, 2001.
2. Pellerin D, Brecker S, Veyrat C. Degenerative mitral valve disease with emphasis on mitral valve prolapse. *Heart (British Cardiac Society)*. 88 Suppl 4:iv20-8, 2002.
3. Irvine T, Li XK, Sahn DJ, Kenny A. Assessment of mitral regurgitation. *Heart (British Cardiac Society)*. 88 Suppl 4:iv11-9, 2002.
4. Rodriguez L, Thomas JD, Monterroso V, Weyman AE, Harrigan P, Mueller LN, Levine RA. Validation of the proximal flow convergence method. Calculation of orifice area in patients with mitral stenosis. *Circulation*. 88(3):1157-65, 1993.
5. Faletra F, Pezzano A Jr., Fusco R, Mantero A, Corno R, Crivellaro W, De Chiara F, Vitali E, Gordini V, Magnani P, Pezzano A Sr. Measurement of mitral valve area in mitral stenosis: four echocardiographic methods compared with direct measurement of anatomic orifices. *Journal of the American College of Cardiology*. 28(5):1190-7, 1996.
6. Binder TM, Rosenhek, R, Porenta G, Maurer G, Baumgartner H. Improved assessment of mitral valve stenosis by volumetric real-time three dimensional echocardiography. *Journal of the American College of Cardiology*. 36(4):1355-61, 2000.
7. Anonymous. ACC/AHA guidelines for the management of patients with valvular heart disease. A report of the American College of Cardiology/American Heart Association. Task Force on Practice Guidelines. *Journal of the American College of Cardiology*. 32(5):1486-588, 1998.
8. Kang DH, Park SW, Song JK, Kim HS, Hong MK, Kim JJ, Park SJ. Long-term clinical and echocardiographic outcome of percutaneous mitral valvuloplasty: randomized comparison of Inoue and double-balloon techniques. *Journal of the American College of Cardiology*. 35(1):169-75, 2000.
9. Cafri C, de la Guardia B, Barasch E, Brink J, Smalling RW. Transseptal puncture guided by intracardiac echocardiography during percutaneous transvenous mitral commissurotomy in patients with distorted anatomy of the fossa ovalis. *Catheterization & Cardiovascular Interventions*. 50(4):463-7, 2000.
10. Salgo IS, Gorman JH 3rd, Gorman RC, Jackson BM, Bowen FW, Plappert T, St John Sutton, MG, Edmunds LH Jr. Effect of annular shape on leaflet curvature in reducing mitral leaflet stress. *Circulation*. 106(6):711-7, 2002.
11. Avierinos JF, Gersh BJ, Melton LJ 3rd, Bailey KR, Shub C, Nishimura RA, Tajik AJ, Enriquez-Sarano M. Natural history of asymptomatic mitral valve prolapse in the community. *Circulation*. 106(11):1355-61, 2002.
12. Lambert AS, Miller JP, Merrick SH, Schiller NB, Foster E, Muhiudeen-Russell I, Cahalan MK. Improved evaluation of the location and mechanism of mitral valve regurgitation with a systematic transesophageal echocardiography examination. *Anesthesia & Analgesia*. 88(6):1205-12, 1999.
13. Grigioni F, Enriquez-Sarano M, Zehr KJ, Bailey KR, Tajik AJ. Ischemic mitral regurgitation: long-term outcome and prognostic implications with quantitative Doppler assessment. *Circulation*. 103(13):1759-64, 2001.
14. Yiu SF, Enriquez-Sarano M, Tribouilloy C, Seward JB, Tajik AJ. Determinants of the degree of functional mitral regurgitation in patients with systolic left ventricular dysfunction: A quantitative clinical study. *Circulation*. 102(12):1400-6, 2000.
15. Kaplan SR, Bashein G, Sheehan FH, Legget ME, Munt B, Li XN, Sivarajan M, Bolson EL, Zeppa M, Arch MZ, Martin RW. Three-dimensional echocardiographic assessment of annular shape changes in the normal and regurgitant mitral valve. *American Heart Journal*. 139(3):378-87, 2000.
16. Messas E, Guerrero JL, Handschumacher MD, Chow CM, Sullivan S, Schwammenthal E, Levine RA. Paradoxic decease in ischemic mitral regurgitation with papillary muscle dysfunction: insights from three-dimensional and contrast echocardiography with strain rate measurement. *Circulation*. 104(16):1952-7, 2001.
17. DeSimone R, Glombitza G, Vahl CF, Meinzer HP, Hagl S. Three-dimensional color Doppler reconstruction of intracardiac blood flow in patients with different heart valve diseases. *American Journal of Cardiology*. 86(12):1343-8, 2000.
18. Tribouilloy CM, Enriquez-Sarano M, Capps, MA, Bailey KR, Tajik AJ. Contrasting effect of similar effective regurgitant orifice area in mitral and tricuspid regurgitation: a quantitative Doppler echocardiographic study. *Journal of the American Society of Echocardiography*. 15(9):958-65, 2002.
19. Thomas L, Foster E, Hoffman JI, Schiller NB. Prospective validation of an echocardiographic index for determining the severity of chronic mitral regurgitation. *American Journal of Cardiology*. 90(6):607-12, 2002.
20. Sondegaard L, Stahlberg F, Thomsen C. Magnetic resonance imaging of valvular heart disease. *Journal of Magnetic Resonance Imaging*. 10(5):627-38, 1999.
21. Nayak KS, Pauly JM, Kerr AB, Hu BS, Nishimura DG. Real-time color flow CMR. *Magnetic Resonance in Medicine*. 43(2):251-8, 2000.
22. Otto CM. Clinical practice. Evaluation and management of chronic mitral regurgitation. *New England Journal of Medicine*. 345(10):740-6, 2001.
23. Yun KL, Sintek CF, Miller DC, Pfeffer TA, Kochamba GS, Khonsari S, Zile MR. Randomized trial comparing partial versus complete chordal-sparing mitral valve replacement: effects on left ventricular volume and function. *Journal of Thoracic & Cardiovascular Surgery*. 123(4):707-14, 2002.
24. Zabalgoitia M, Oraby M. Evaluation of prosthetic heart valves, in Pohost G (ed): *Imaging in Cardiovascular Disease*. P. 617 2000.
25. Fernandes V, Olmos L, Nagueh SF, Quinones MA, Zoghbi WA. Peak early diastolic velocity rather than pressure half-time is the best index of mechanical prosthetic mitral valve function. *American Journal of Cardiology*. 89(6):704-10, 2002.
26. Di Salvo G, Habib G, Pergola V, Avierinos JF, Philip E, Casalta JP, Vailloud JM, Derumeaux G, Gouvernet J, Ambrosi P, Lambert M, Ferracci A, Raoult D, Luccioni R. Echocardiography predicts embolic events in infective endocarditis. *Journal of the American College of Cardiology*. 37(4):1069-76, 2001.
27. Vongpatanasin W, Hillis LD, Lange RA. Prosthetic heart valves. *New England Journal of Medicine*. 335(6):407-16, 1996.
28. Dagum P, Green GR, Nistal FJ, Daughters GT, Timek TA, Foppiano LE, Bolger AF, Ingels NB Jr., Miller DC. Deformational dynamics of the aortic root: modes and physiologic determinants. *Circulation*. 199(19 Suppl):II54-62, 1999.
29. Underwood MJ, El Khoury G, Deronck D, Glineur D, Dion R. The aortic root: structure, function, and surgical reconstruction. *Heart (British Cardiac Society)*. 83(4):376-80, 2000.
30. Anonymous. The clinical role of magnetic resonance in cardiovascular disease. Task Force of the European Society of Cardiology, in collaboration with the Association of European Paediatric Cardiologists. *European Heart Journal*. 19(1):19-39, 1998.
31. Brasch AV, Khan SS, DeRobertis MA, Kong JH, Chiu J, Siegel RJ. Change in mitral regurgitation severity after aortic valve replacement for aortic stenosis. *American Journal of Cardiology*. 85(10):1271-4, 2000.

32. Attenhofer Jost CH, Turina J, Mayer K, Seifert B, Amann FW, Buechi M, Facchini M, Brunner-La Rocca HP, Jenni R. Echocardiography in the evaluation of systolic murmurs of unknown cause. *American Journal of Medicine.* 108(8):614-20, 2000.

33. Adler Y, Vaturi M, Wiser I, Shapira Y, Herz I, Weisenberg D, Sela N, Battler A, Sagie A. Nonobstructive aortic valve calcium as a window to atherosclerosis of the aorta. *American Journal of Cardiology.* 86(1):68-71, 2000.

34. Pohle K, Maffert R, Ropers D, Moshage W, Stilianakis N, Daniel WG, Achenbach S. Progression of aortic valve calcification: association with coronary atherosclerosis and cardiovascular risk factors. *Circulation.* 104(16): 1927-32, 2001.

35. Baumgartner H, Steenelli T, Niederberger J, Schima H, Maurer G. "Overestimation" of catheter gradients by Doppler ultrasound in patients with aortic stenosis: a predictable manifestation of pressure recovery [see comment]. *Journal of the American College of Cardiology.* 33(6):1655-61, 1999.

36. Lester SJ, McElhinney DB, Miller JP, Lutz JT, Otto CM, Redberg RF. Rate of change in aortic valve area during a cardiac cycle can predict the rate of hemodynamic progression of aortic stenosis. *Circulation.* 101(16):1947-52, 2000.

37. Blais C, Pibarot P, Dumesnil JG, Garcia D, Chen D, Durand LG. Comparison of valve resistance with effective orifice area regarding flow dependence. *American Journal of Cardiology.* 88(1):45-52, 2001.

38. Schwammenthal E, Vered Z, Moshkowitz Y, Rabinowitz B, Ziskind Z, Smolinski AK, Feinberg MS. Dobutamine echocardiography in patients with aortic stenosis and left ventricular dysfunction: predicting outcome as a function of management strategy. *Chest.* 119(6):1766-77, 2001.

39. Capps SB, Elkins RC, Fronk DM. Body surface area as a predictor of aortic and pulmonary valve diameter. *Journal of Thoracic & Cardiovascular Surgery.* 119(5):975-82, 2000.

40. Otto CM, Burwash IG, Legget ME, Munt BI, Fujioka M, Healy NL, Kraft CD, Miyake-Hull CY, Schwaegler RG. Prospective study of asymptomatic valvular aortic stenosis. Clinical, echocardiographic, and exercise predictors of outcome. [see comments] *Circulation.* 95(9):2262-70, 1997.

41. Palta S, Pai AM, Gill KS, Pai RG. New insights into the progression of aortic stenosis: implications for secondary prevention. *Circulation.* 101(21):2497-502, 2000.

42. Chan KL, Ghani M, Woodend K, Burwash IG. Case-controlled study to assess risk factors for aortic stenosis in congenitally bicuspid aortic valve. *American Journal of Cardiology.* 88(6):690-3, 2001.

43. Keane MG, Wiegers SE, Plappert T, Pochettino A, Bavaria JE, St. John Sutton MG. Bicuspid aortic valves are associated with aortic dilatation out of proportion to coexistent valvular lesions. *Circulation.* 102:III35-III38, 2000.

44. Monin JL, Monchi M, Gest V, Duval-Moulin AM, Dubois-Rande JL, Gueret P. Aortic stenosis with severe left ventricular dysfunction and low transvalvular pressure gradients: risk stratification by low-dose dobutamine echocardiography. *Journal of the American College of Cardiology.* 37(8):2101-7, 2001.

45. Rosenhek R, Binder T, Porenta G, Lang I, Christ G, Schemper M, Maurer G, Baumgartner H. Predictors of outcome in severe, asymptomatic aortic stenosis. [see comment]. *New England Journal of Medicine.* 343(9):611-7, 2000.

46. Smith RL, Larsen D, Crawford MH, Shively BK. Echocardiographic predictors f survival in low gradient aortic stenosis. *American Journal of Cardiology.* 86(7):804-7, A10, 2000.

47. Grande KJ, Cochran RP, Reinhall PG, Kunzelman KS. Mechanisms of aortic valve incompetence: finite element modeling of aortic root dilatation. *Annals of Thoracic Surgery.* 69(6):1851-7, 2000.

48. Keane MG, Weigers SE, Plappert T, Pochettino A, Bavaria JE, St. John Sutton MG. Aortic regurgitation in Type A dissection: structural determinants and the role of Valvular resuspension. *American Journal of Cardiology.* 85:604-610, 2000.

49. Evangelista A, del Castillo HG, Calvo F, Permanyer-Miralda G, Brotons C, Angel J, Gonzalez-Alujas T, Tornos P, Soler-Soler J. Strategy for optimal aortic regurgitation quantification by Doppler echocardiography: agreement among different methods. *American Heart Journal.* 139(5):773-81, 2000.

50. Tribouilloy Cm, Enriquez-Sarano M, Bailey KR, Seward JB, Tajik AJ. Assessment of severity of aortic regurgitation using the width of the vena contracta: A clinical Doppler imaging study. *Circulation.* 102(5):558-64, 2000.

51. Quinones MA, Otto CM, Stoddard M, Waggoner A, Zoghbi WA. Doppler Quantification Task Force of the Nomenclature and Standards Committee of the American Society of Echocardiography. Recommendations for quantification of Doppler echocardiography. A report from the Doppler Quantification Task Force of the Nomenclature and Standards Committee of the American Society of Echocardiography. *Journal of the American Society of Echocardiography.* 15(2):167-84, 2002.

52. Sondegaard L, Aldershvile J, Hildebrandt P, Kelback H, Stahlberg F, Thomsen C. Vasodilatation with felodipine in chronic asymptomatic aortic regurgitation. *American Heart Journal.* 139(4):667-74, 2000.

53. Bech-Hanssen O, Caidahl K, Wallentin I, Ask P, Wranne B. Assessment of effective orifice area of prosthetic aortic valves with Doppler echocardiography: an in vivo and in vitro study. *Journal of Thoracic & Cardiovascular Surgery.* 122(2):287-95, 2001.

54. Pibarot P, Dumesnil JG. Hemodynamic and clinical impact of prosthesis-patient mismatch in the aortic valve position and its prevention. *Journal of the American College of Cardiology.* 36(4): 1131-41, 2000.

55. Savoye C, Auffray JL, Hubert E, Godart F, Francart C, Goullard L, Deklunder G, Rey C, Prat A. Echocardiographic follow-up after Ross procedure in 100 patients. *American Journal of Cardiology.* 85(7): 854-7, 2000.

56. Ikonomidis I, Tsoukas A, Parthenakis F, Gournizakis A, Kassimatis A, Rallidis L, Nihoyannopoulos P. Four year follow up after aortic valve replacement for isolated aortic stenosis: a link between reduction in pressure overload, regression of left ventricular hypertrophy, and diastolic function. *Heart.* 86(3): 309-16, 2001.

57. Becassis P, Hayot M, Frapier JM, Leclercq F, Beck L, Brunet J, Arnaud E, Prefaut C, Chaptal PA, Davy JM, Messner-Pellene P, Grolleau R. Postoperative exercise tolerance after aortic valve replacement by small-size prosthesis: functional consequence of small-size aortic prosthesis. *Journal of the American College of Cardiology.* 36(3): 871-7, 2000.

58. Girard SE, Miller FA Jr., Orszulak TA, Mullany CJ, Montgomery S, Edwards WD, Tazelaar HD, Malouf JF, Tajik AJ. Reoperation for prosthetic aortic valve obstruction in the era of echocardiography: trends in diagnostic testing and comparison with surgical findings. *Journal of the American College of Cardiology.* 37(2): 579-84, 2001.

59. Lin SS, Tiong IY, Asher CR, Murphy MT, Thomas JD, Griffin BP, Thomas JD. Investigator: Thomas JD. Prediction of thrombus-related mechanical prosthetic valve dysfunction using transesophageal echocardiography. *American Journal of Cardiology.* 86(10): 1097-101, 2000.

60. Ozkan M, Kaymaz C, Kirma C, Sonmez K, Ozdemir N, Balkanay M, Yakut C, Deligonul U. Intravenous thrombolytic treatment of mechanical prosthetic valve thrombosis: a study using serial transesophageal echocardiography. *Journal of the American College of Cardiology.* 35(7): 1881-9, 2000.

61. Mylonakis E, Calderwood SB. Infective endocarditis in adults. *New England Journal of Medicine.* 345(18):1318-30, 2001.

62. Bayer AS, Bolger AF, Taubert KA, Wilson W, Steckelberg J, Karchmer AW, Levison M, Chambers HF, Dajani AS, Gewitz MH, Newburger JW, Gerber MA, Shulman ST, Pallasch TJ, Gage TW, Ferrieri P. Diagnosis and management of infective endocarditis and its complications. *Circulation.* 98(25):2936-48, 1998.

63. Bailey PL, Peragallo R, Karwande SV, Lapunzina P. Mitral and tricuspid valve rupture after moderate blunt chest trauma. *Annals of Thoracic Surgery.* 69(2):616-8, 2000.

64. Gatti G, Maffei G, Lusa AM, Pugliese P. Tricuspid valve repair with the Cosgrove-Edwards annuloplasty system: early clinical and echocardiographic results. *Annals of Thoracic Surgery.* 73(3):764-7, 2001.

65. Guntheroth WG. Causes and effects of poststenotic dilation of the pulmonary trunk. *American Journal of Cardiology.* 89(6):774-6, 2002.

66. Geva T, Greil GF, Marshall AC, Landzberg M, Powell AJ. Gadolinium-enhanced 3-dimenensional magnetic resonance angiography of pulmonary blood supply in patients with complex pulmonary stenosis or atresia: comparison with X-ray angiography. *Circulation.* 106(4):473-8, 2002

67. Driscoll D, Allen HD, Atkins DL, Breener J, Dunnigan A, Franklin W, Gutgesell HP, Herndon P, Shaddy RE, Taubert KA, et al. Guidelines for evaluation and management of common congenital cardiac problems in infants, children, and adolescents. A statement for healthcare professionals from the Committee on Congenital Cardiac Defects of the Council on Cardiovascular Disease in the Young, American Heart Association. *Circulation*. 90(4):2180-8, 1994.

68. Cheitlin MD, Alpert JS, Armstrong WF, Aurigemma GP, Beller GA, Bierman FZ, Davidson TW, Davis JL, Douglas PS, Gillam LD. ACC/AHA Guidelines for the Clinical Application of Echocardiography. A report of the American College Cardiology/ American Heart Association Task Force on Practice Guidelines (Committee on Clinical Application of Echocardiography). Developed in collaboration with the American Society of Echocardiography. *Circulation*. 95(6):1686-744, 1997.

69. Allen HD, Beekman RH 3rd, Garson A Jr., Hijazi ZM, Mullins C, O'Laughlin MP, Taubert KA. Pediatric therapeutic cardiac catheterization: a statement for healthcare professionals from the Council on Cardiovascular Disease in the Young, American Heart Association. *Circulation*. 97(6):609-25, 1998.

70. Uebing A, Fischer G, Bethge M, Scheewe J, Schmiel F, Stieh J, Brossmann J, Kramer HH. Influence of the pulmonary annulus diameter on pulmonary regurgitation and right ventricular pressure load after repair of tetralogy of Fallot. *Heart*. 88(5):510-4, 2002.

71. Williams RV, Minich LL, Shaddy RE, Pagotto LT, Tani LY. Comparison of Doppler echocardiography with angiography for determining the severity of pulmonary regurgitation. *American Journal of Cardiology*. 89(12):1438-41, 2002.

72. Mori Y, Irvine T, Jones M, Rusk RA, Pham Q, Kenny A, Sahn DJ. Validation of a digital color Doppler flow measurement method for pulmonary regurgitant volumes and regurgitant fractions in an in vitro model and in a chronic animal model of postoperative repaired tetralogy of Fallot. *Journal of the American College of Cardiology*. 37(2) 632-40, 2001.

73. Roest AA, Helbing WA, Kunz P, van den Aardweg JG, Lamb HJ, Vliegen HW, van der Wall EE, de Roos A. Exercise MR imaging in the assessment of pulmonary regurgitation and biventricular function in patients after tetralogy of fallot repair. *Radiology*. 223(1):204-11, 2002.

74. de Ruijter FT, Weenink I, Hitchcock FJ, Meijboom EJ, Bennink GB. Right ventricular dysfunction and pulmonary valve replacement after correction of tetralogy of Fallot. *Annals of Thoracic Surgery*. 73(6):1794-800; discussion 1800, 2002.

75. Vliegen HW, van Straten A, deRoos A, Roest AA, Schoof PH, Zwinderman AH, Ottenkamp J, van der Wall EE, Hazekamp MG. Magnetic resonance imaging to assess the hemodynamic effects of pulmonary valve replacement in adults late after repair of tetralogy of fallot. *Circulation*. 106(13):1703, 2002.

Pulmonary Embolism, Pulmonary Hypertension, and Cor Pulmonale

Samuel Z. Goldhaber

Acute Pulmonary Embolism
Pulmonary Hypertension and Cor Pulmonale

ACUTE PULMONARY EMBOLISM

Despite multiple advances in the accurate diagnosis and aggressive management of thrombotic pulmonary embolism (PE), this common cardiovascular illness has both a surprisingly high mortality rate and likelihood of recurrence. Acute PE is difficult to diagnose, and treatment often fails if cardiogenic shock has already occurred.

Epidemiology

A prospective registry that includes all patients can provide a "real-world" perspective. The largest prospective registry is ICOPER: the International Cooperative Pulmonary Embolism Registry, which enrolled 2454 consecutive PE patients from 52 participating hospitals in 7 countries. The aim was to establish the 3-month all-cause mortality rate and to identify factors associated with death.[1] Three-month follow-up was completed in 98% of the patients. The all-cause mortality rate was 11.4% during the first 2 weeks after diagnosis and 17.4% at 3 months. After exclusion of patients in whom PE was first discovered at autopsy, the mortality rate was 15.3% (Figure 12-1). Importantly, most patients who died had succumbed to PE, not to other comorbidities such as cancer. Specifically, regarding the most common causes of death, 45% of deaths were ascribed to PE, 18% were due to cancer, 12% were sudden cardiac deaths (which undoubtedly included some undiagnosed PEs), and 12% were labeled as respiratory failure and probably included deaths caused by PE. Nonfatal recurrent PE occurred in 4% of patients.

Age greater than 70 years increased the likelihood of death by 60%. Six other risk factors independently increased the likelihood of mortality by a factor of twofold to threefold: cancer, clinical congestive heart failure, chronic obstructive pulmonary disease, systemic arterial hypotension with a systolic blood pressure of <90 mmHg, tachypnea (defined as >20 breaths/min), and right ventricular hypokinesis on echocardiogram, an especially useful sign to identify high-risk patients who might be suitable for aggressive interventions such as thrombolysis or embolectomy.

When PE is not fatal, it can cause chronic thromboembolic pulmonary hypertension, with disabling fatigue and breathlessness. It can also exert a psychological toll because of the high risk of recurrence after anticoagulation is discontinued. With 10 years of follow-up, as many as 30% of patients may have a recurrence.[2] Risk factors for recurrence include an initial idiopathic venous thromboembolism (VTE) (not related to surgery or trauma), cancer, and underlying cardiopulmonary disease.

In the Brest District of Western France, with a defined population of 342,000 inhabitants, the incidence of VTE was 1.8/1000 per year.[3] Deep venous thrombosis (DVT) without PE had an incidence of 1.2/1000 per year, whereas PE with or without DVT had an incidence of 0.6/1000 per year. VTE incidence increased markedly with increasing age for both men and women. Among those older than 75 years of age, the incidence was 1/100 per year. VTE occurred at home in 63% of the affected population, 16% of whom had been hospitalized within the previous 3 months.

The etiology of PE is often unknown. However, with an appropriate workup for hypercoagulability, inherited disorders can be identified with increasing frequency.[4] Many patients with PE have a combination of an inherited hypercoagulable state that remains clinically silent until it is exacerbated by an acquired cause of venous thrombosis.

Diagnosis

Clinical Assessment

A high index of clinical suspicion helps to detect this elusive condition. The clinical setting is important for estimating the likelihood of PE. Principal symptoms include otherwise unexplained breathlessness, chest discomfort, or light-headedness. Most patients are initially seen with normal systemic arterial pressure, even if they have impending hemodynamic instability with moderate or severe right ventricular dysfunction. Signs of PE often include anxiety and tachypnea. Occasionally, unilateral leg swelling will provide an especially useful diagnostic clue.

Traditionally, the clinical likelihood of PE has been estimated by "gestalt" as low, moderate, or high. More recently, quantitative clinical scoring systems have been used. These approaches help provide standardization and improve communication among health care

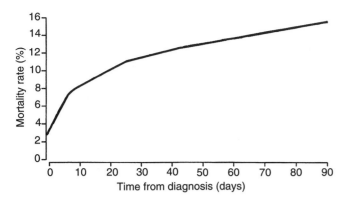

FIGURE 12-1. Overall cumulative mortality caused by PE in the International Cooperative Pulmonary Embolism Registry (ICOPER) of 2454 patients with 11.4% at 2 weeks and 17.4% at 3 months. After exclusion of patients in whom PE was first discovered at autopsy, the mortality rate was 15.3%. (Adapted with permission from Goldhaber SZ, Visani L, DeRosa M, for ICOPER: Acute pulmonary embolism: clinical outcomes in the International Cooperative Pulmonary Embolism Registry [ICOPER]. *Lancet* 1999; 353:1386.)

providers when considering the likelihood of PE. The Canadian Scoring System[5] places greatest emphasis on the signs or symptoms of DVT and whether an alternative diagnosis is unlikely. If the score exceeds 4 points, the overall likelihood of PE confirmed with imaging tests is 41%. However, the likelihood of PE is only 8% if the score is 4 points or less. The Geneva Scoring System[6] is more objective but also more complex and requires obtaining arterial blood gases on all patients suspected of PE. This classic approach is no longer considered standard practice, because data from the Prospective Investigation of Pulmonary Embolism Diagnosis have shown that neither hypoxemia nor an elevated alveolar-arterial oxygen gradient can differentiate patients between those who have angiographically proven PE and those who have normal pulmonary angiograms.

Nonimaging Tests

Among patients with suspected PE, a plasma D-dimer enzyme-linked immunosorbent assay (ELISA) is a useful screening test in patients without active comorbid conditions such as myocardial infarction, pneumonia, cancer, sepsis, or the postoperative state.[7] Endogenous fibrinolysis, although ineffective in preventing PE, almost always causes the release of D-dimers from fibrin clot in patients with established PE. Elevated levels of the D-dimer are highly sensitive as a screening test for PE, whereas normal D-dimer ELISA levels have a high negative predictive value and virtually exclude the diagnosis of acute PE. In patients with a normal D-dimer level, the likelihood of no PE is approximately 95%. The combination of low clinical suspicion, ideally quantified with a validated scoring system and a normal D-dimer ELISA, makes PE exceedingly unlikely.

An electrocardiogram is a universally available and inexpensive rapid bedside test. It can identify coronary ischemia caused by unstable angina or acute myocardial infarction and can suggest right ventricular dysfunction that, in the proper clinical setting, may be due to acute

PE. The most common electrocardiographic abnormality among PE patients is T-wave inversion in leads V_1 to V_4 (Figure 12-2). Other findings occasionally present in PE are also due to right heart strain, such as a deep S in lead I, a Q wave in lead III, and T-wave inversion in lead III.

Chest X-Ray

The chest X-ray is useful for suggesting illnesses that may mimic or accompany PE, such as pneumonia or congestive heart failure. On rare occasions, pneumothorax can present with breathlessness that is suspicious for PE. A normal lung scan occurs in only a minority of patients with PE.[8] Common abnormalities include cardiac enlargement, pleural effusion, elevated hemidiaphragm, pulmonary artery enlargement, atelectasis, infiltrate, and pulmonary congestion. Pulmonary infarction is due to an anatomically small PE and will appear in the periphery of the lung as a small wedge-shaped density. A normal chest X-ray indicates that lung scanning will probably yield a normal ventilation lung scan.

Lung Scanning

Technetium–99m macroaggregated albumin is the radiopharmaceutical agent used for pulmonary perfusion scanning. The pulmonary capillaries temporarily block the particles from entering the pulmonary venous circulation. Only approximately 0.1% of the capillaries are blocked, and >95% of the particles are removed from the circulation after the first pass.

Xenon-133 is the most commonly used ventilation scanning agent. This gas is inert, widely available, relatively inexpensive, and allows acquisition of single-breath, equilibrium, and washout images. At Brigham and Women's Hospital, we inject ^{99m}Tc-macroaggregated albumin first and follow this with a ventilation scan if the perfusion scan is abnormal.

The classic Prospective Investigation of Pulmonary Embolism Diagnosis (PIOPED) compared lung scanning

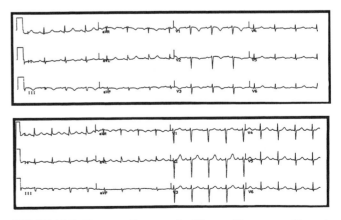

FIGURE 12-2. Electrocardiogram of a 77-year-old woman with acute PE before *(upper panel)* and after *(lower panel)* thrombolytic therapy. The upper panel is notable for T-wave inversions in leads V_1 through V_4, which resolve and normalize in the lower panel after the successful administration of thrombolytic therapy. (From Dr. Goldhaber's private collection.)

with pulmonary angiography among patients suspected of having PE. Clinical suspicion was assessed qualitatively before diagnostic testing was undertaken. In the presence of high clinical suspicion, a lung scan with multiple large perfusion defects and normal ventilation had a high probability, >90%, of being due to PE (Figure 12-3). However, most lung scans were nondiagnostic, despite subsequent extensive revision of the diagnostic and probability criteria for PE. What emerged was a complex and cumbersome set of rules for determining high, intermediate, and low probability for PE (Table 12-1). These have proven difficult to implement in routine practice with wide interobserver variability. With lung scans, there is often failure to obtain a clear-cut answer to the diagnostic dilemma of whether a patient has PE. Therefore, lung scanning is declining in popularity as a diagnostic tool for PE.

Chest CT

Chest CT scanning is diagnostic of PE when an intraluminal pulmonary arterial filling defect is surrounded by contrast material. Less frequently observed is an obstructed artery shown as an unopacified vessel. CT scanning has two major advantages over lung scanning: (1) direct visualization of thrombus, and (2) establishing alternative diagnoses on images of the lung parenchyma that are not evident on chest X-ray.

Conventional chest CT scanning used to rely on imaging a series of consecutive sections of the chest. With the introduction of spiral chest CT scanning, patients suspected of PE can now be scanned continuously.[9] While the patients advance through the scanner, the X-ray

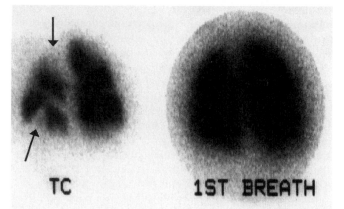

FIGURE 12-3. A 41-year-old woman was seen with sudden onset of shortness of breath and retrosternal chest discomfort. Her heart rate was 168 beats/min, respiratory rate 32/min, oxygen saturation 86%, and blood pressure 112/70 mmHg. She underwent a ventilation *(right panel)*-perfusion *(left panel)* lung scan with xenon-133 gas (26 mCi) in the left posterior oblique position. Numerous scattered segmental *(arrows)* and subsegmental perfusion defects with near normal ventilation were found. This ventilation-perfusion mismatch was interpreted as high probability for pulmonary embolism. (Reproduced with permission from Goldhaber SZ. Pulmonary embolism, in Braunwald E, Zipes DP, Libby P (eds), *Heart Disease*, ed 6, Philadelphia: W.B. Saunders, 2001, p 1886.)

source and single-row detector array rotate around them. These scans are performed during a single breath hold, thereby eliminating respiratory motion, which previously limited thoracic imaging. Complete data volumes are acquired, thus ensuring overlap of data from adjacent slices and reducing the possibility of missed pathology.

■ ▫ ■

TABLE 12-1   REVISED PIOPED LUNG SCAN INTERPRETATION CRITERIA

High Probability

π	≥2 large (>75% of a segment) segmental perfusion defects without corresponding ventilation or CXR abnormalities
π	1 large segmental perfusion defect and ≥2 moderate (25% to 75% of a segment) segmental perfusion defects without corresponding ventilation or CXR abnormalities
π	≥4 moderate segmental perfusion defects without corresponding ventilation or CXR abnormalities

Intermediate Probability

π	1 moderate to <2 large segmental perfusion defects without corresponding ventilation or CXR abnormalities
π	Corresponding V/Q defects and CXR parenchymal opacity in lower lung zone
π	Corresponding V/Q defects and small pleural effusion
π	Single moderate matched V/Q defects with normal CXR findings
π	Difficult to categorize as low or high probability

Low Probability

π	Multiple matched V/Q defects, regardless of size, with normal CXR findings
π	Corresponding V/Q defects and CXR parenchymal opacity in upper/middle lung zone
π	Corresponding V/Q defects and large pleural effusion
π	Any perfusion defects and large pleural effusion
π	Any perfusion defects with substantially larger CXR abnormality
π	Defects surrounded by normally perfused lung (Stripe sign)
π	Single or multiple small (<25% of a segment) segmental perfusion defects with a normal CXR
π	Nonsegmental perfusion defects (cardiomegaly, aortic impression, enlarged hili)

Normal

π	No perfusion defects and perfusion outlines the shape of the lung seen on CXR

Adapted with permission from Gottschalk A, Sostman HD, Coleman RE, Juni JE, Thrall J, McKusick KA, et al. Ventilation-perfusion scintigraphy in the PIOPED study. Part II. Evaluation of the scintigraphic criteria and interpretations. *J Nucl Med* 1993; 34:1119.

Because scans are performed in <30 seconds, excellent vascular opacification of the pulmonary arteries with contrast agent can usually be achieved (Figure 12-4). However, the major limitation has been failure to detect PEs beyond third-order pulmonary arterial branches.

Further innovations occurred with the use of multi-row detector CT scanners. This newer technology permits four slices to be acquired simultaneously during each rotation of the X-ray source. The gantry rotates around the patient in <1 second, and the total examination time can be eight times faster than with single-row detector systems. Fewer motion artifacts occur, and resolution is improved from 5 mm to 1.25 mm. Subsegmental vessels can generally be well visualized with multirow detector scanners. With these newer scanners, the combination of shorter scan times, narrow collimation, and narrow reconstruction intervals greatly enhances accuracy. Compared with conventional spiral CT, sensitivity of multirow detector scanners increases from approximately 70% to >90% for the diagnosis of acute PE.

Venous Ultrasonography

Most PEs are caused by leg or pelvic DVT that embolizes. Identification of DVT with venous ultrasonography is used at times as an inexpensive and often more readily available surrogate for establishing the diagnosis of PE as compared with lung or chest CT scanning. It may not always be necessary to differentiate DVT from PE, because anticoagulation is the foundation of therapy for both conditions. However, the absence of DVT cannot be construed as excluding the diagnosis of PE. In at least two thirds of patients in recent series, venous ultrasound was normal in patients with proven PE.

The principal noninvasive test to detect DVT is duplex venous ultrasonography, which combines pulsed-wave Doppler interrogation and measurement of blood flow velocity with direct visualization of thrombus (Figure 12-5) and assessment of vein compressibility by ultrasound examination. The cardinal criterion for diagnosing venous thrombosis by ultrasonography is loss of venous compressibility with the ultrasound transducer held transverse to the artery and vein. Color Doppler flow is evaluated in longitudinal axis images as an adjunct to the gray-scale compression technique. Color Doppler may improve the detection of venous thrombosis by (1) differentiating arteries from veins, (2) diagnosing nonocclusive thrombus when flow is detected around an anechoic mass within the veins, and (3) helping to find deep calf veins. These tiny veins are often difficult to distinguish from other structures when examined solely by gray-scale ultrasound compression technique.

Echocardiography

Echocardiography should not be used routinely to diagnose suspected PE, because approximately 50% of patients with PE have normal echocardiograms.[10] Nevertheless, imaging a normal left ventricle and dilated, hypokinetic right ventricle may serendipitously suggest the diagnosis (Figure 12-6). Echocardiography is useful diagnostically in hemodynamically unstable patients in whom the differential diagnosis includes pericardial tamponade, right ventricular infarction, and dissection of the aorta, as well as PE.

Perhaps the most useful role for echocardiography in PE is to help assess risk and prognosis (Table 12-2). As

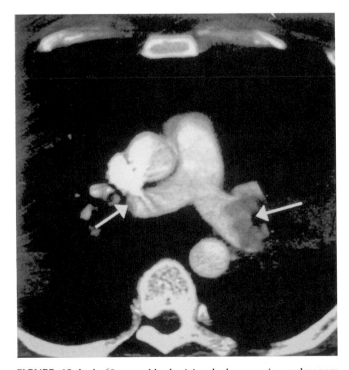

FIGURE 12-4. A 62-year old physician had a massive pulmonary embolism 2 weeks after prostatectomy. Spiral chest CT with contrast provided a definitive diagnosis, with a large thrombus burden apparent in the right and left main pulmonary arteries *(arrows)*. (Reproduced with permission from Goldhaber SZ. Pulmonary embolism, in Braunwald E, Zipes DP, Libby P (eds): Heart disease, ed 6, Philadelphia, W.B. Saunders, 2001, p 1886.)

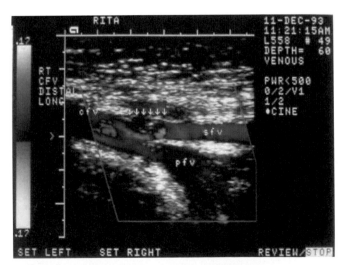

FIGURE 12-5. Longitudinal axis view of a color Doppler ultrasound examination demonstrating an extensive superficial femoral vein thrombosis. The "superficial" femoral vein, despite its name, is a deep vein. The superficial femoral vein (SFV) and the profunda femoral vein (PFV) join to form the common femoral (CF) vein. (From Dr. Goldhaber's private collection.)

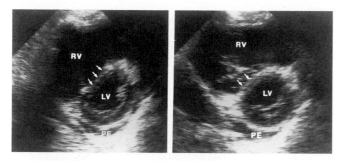

FIGURE 12-6. Parasternal short-axis views of the right ventricle (RV) and left ventricle (LV) in diastole *(left)* and systole *(right)*. Diastolic and systolic bowing of the interventricular septum *(arrows)* into the LV is compatible with RV volume and pressure overload, respectively. The RV is appreciably dilated and markedly hypokinetic, with little change in apparent RV area from diastole to systole. PE, Small pericardial perfusion. (Adapted with permission from Come PC. Echocardiographic evaluation of pulmonary embolism and its response to therapeutic interventions. *Chest* 1992; 101:151S.)

many as 40% of patients with PE may have a normal systemic arterial pressure and heart rate, despite impending hemodynamic instability caused by moderate or severe right ventricular dysfunction. Despite intensive anticoagulation, these patients are at high risk of recurrent PE. They may benefit from adjunctive thrombolysis or embolectomy in addition to anticoagulation.

The pulmonary arterial systolic pressure can be estimated by measuring the peak velocity of the tricuspid regurgitant jet obtained with Doppler echocardiography (Table 12-2). The gradient across the tricuspid valve can be estimated by use of the modified Bernoulli equation, where V in the equation $P = 4V^2$ is the peak velocity of the regurgitant jet. P represents the peak pressure difference between the right atrium and right ventricle. The estimated right atrial pressure is added to the gradient to obtain an estimate of pulmonary arterial systolic pressure. If necessary, agitated saline contrast can be used to enhance the tricuspid regurgitant Doppler tracing. In the absence of tricuspid regurgitation, the time to peak velocity in the right ventricular outflow tract is reduced in the presence of elevated pulmonary arterial pressures. However, this measurement is less precise than the modified Bernoulli equation.

Despite moderate or severe right ventricular free wall hypokinesis, PE patients with abnormal echocardiograms often have relatively normal contraction and "sparing" of the right ventricular apex. McConnell and colleagues quantified this abnormality[11] (Figures 12-7 and 12-8), and this finding has become widely known as the "McConnell sign." The McConnell sign had a 77% sensitivity, 94% specificity, 71% positive predictive value, and 96% negative predictive value for PE. The McConnell sign seems to be useful as a screening test to help distinguish between right ventricular dysfunction caused by PE and dysfunction caused by other conditions such as primary pulmonary hypertension.

Transesophageal echocardiography for suspected PE is best reserved for critically ill patients in whom inadequate imaging is obtained with transthoracic views. This imaging technique diagnoses PE by direct visualization of thrombus, assesses its extent, and helps to determine whether the thrombus is surgically accessible. Transesophageal echocardiography is easiest to perform in the unconscious patient. Conscious patients virtually always require topical anesthesia of the pharynx and often benefit from small, sedating doses of midazolam or fentanyl. In general, the main pulmonary artery and then the right pulmonary artery are first visualized. The right pulmonary artery can be followed until it branches to the right lobar pulmonary arteries. The transducer is then rotated to examine the left pulmonary artery (Figure 12-9). At times, interposition of the left main bronchus may interfere with the ultrasound beam in the middle portion of the left pulmonary artery.

■ ■ ■

TABLE 12-2 ABNORMAL ECHOCARDIOGRAPHIC FINDINGS IN PULMONARY EMBOLISM

Abnormal finding	Description
Right ventricular dilation and hypokinesis	Associated with leftward septal shift; the ratio of the RVEDA to LVEDA exceeds the upper limit of normal (0.6); associated with right atrial enlargement and tricuspid regurgitation.
Septal flattening and paradoxical septal motion	Right ventricular contraction continues even after the left ventricle starts relaxing at end-systole; therefore, the interventricular septum bulges toward the left ventricle.
Diastolic left ventricular impairment with a small difference between left ventricular area during diastole and systole, indicative of low cardiac output	Because of septal displacement and reduced left ventricular distensibility during diastole; consequently, Doppler mitral flow exhibits a prominent A wave, much higher than the E wave, with an increased contribution of atrial contraction to left ventricular filling.
Direct visualization of pulmonary embolism	Only if pulmonary embolism is large and centrally located; much more easily visualized on transesophageal than on transthoracic echocardiography.
Pulmonary arterial hypertension detected by Doppler flow velocity in the right ventricular outflow tract	Shortened acceleration time, with peak velocity occurring close to the onset of ejection. Biphasic ejection curve, with midsystolic reduction in velocity.
Right ventricular hypertrophy	With mildly increased right ventricular thickness (often about 6 mm, with 4 mm as upper limit of normal); clear visualization of right ventricular muscle trabeculations.
Patent foramen ovale	When right atrial pressure exceeds left atrial pressure, the foramen ovale may open and cause worsening hypoxemia or stroke.

RVEDA, right ventricular end-diastolic area; LVEDA, left ventricular end-diastolic area.

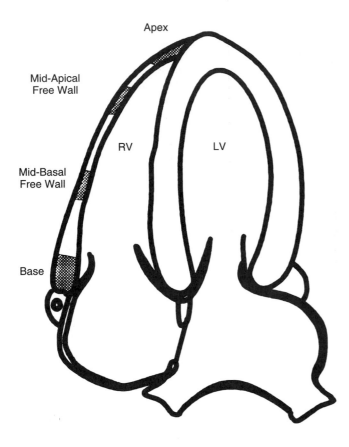

Apical Four-Chamber View

FIGURE 12-7. Schematic diagram of the apical four-chamber view from a transthoracic two-dimensional echocardiogram. Qualitative wall motion scores were assigned at four locations of the right ventricular free wall *(shaded areas)*. The excursion of the right ventricular free wall was measured from end-diastole to end-systole, and a centerline was defined midway between the diastolic and systolic curves. Chord lengths were then defined perpendicular to the centerline extending from the diastolic to the systolic curve. Forty measurements were obtained from the right ventricular base to the right ventricular apex. LV, Left ventricle; RV, right ventricle. (Reprinted with permission from McConnell MV, Solomon SD, Rayan ME, Come PC, Goldhaber SZ, Lee RT. Regional right ventricular dysfunction detected by echocardiography in acute pulmonary embolism. *Am J Cardiol* 1996; 78:469.)

Transesophageal echocardiography may have a uniquely valuable role in identifying patients who have unexplained sudden cardiac arrest and pulseless electrical activity caused by acute PE. PE represented 5% of those who were seen with cardiac arrest in a series of 1246 patients in Vienna.[12] Of those with PE, 63% presented with pulseless electrical activity. Therefore, occult PE should be considered when patients present with pulseless electrical activity.

Pulmonary Angiography

Pulmonary angiography has traditionally been considered the "gold standard" for the diagnosis of PE. Although, chest CT scanning has virtually replaced pulmonary angiography at most hospitals.[13] Vascular access is usually obtained by way of the right common femoral vein. Right heart and pulmonary arterial pressures are measured before contrast

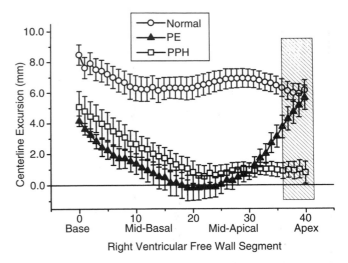

FIGURE 12-8. Segmental right ventricular free wall excursion (mean ± SEM) by centerline analysis as a function of right ventricular free wall segment. The 40 right ventricular free wall segments were arbitrarily numbered from 1 at the base to 40 at the apex. The centerline excursion was then plotted at each of these 40 intervals. This process generated a curve for normal right ventricular function in which the centerline excursion remained fairly constant at 7 to 8 mm. Centerline excursion in patients with acute pulmonary embolism (PE) was near normal at the apex *(hatched area)* but abnormal at the mid-free wall and base ($P < 0.02$ vs. normal). Centerline excursion in patients with primary pulmonary hypertension (PPH) was reduced compared with that in normal subjects in all segments ($P < 0.03$). (Reprinted with permission from McConnell MV, Solomon SD, Rayan ME, Come PC, Goldhaber SZ, Lee RT. Regional right ventricular dysfunction detected by echocardiography in acute pulmonary embolism. *Am J Cardiol* 1996; 78:469.)

injection. For a complete study, selective right and left pulmonary artery injections are usually performed with two views of each lung. If an embolus is discovered at angiography, no further injections are necessary.

The primary criterion for diagnosing acute PE is visualization of an intraluminal filling defect in the column of

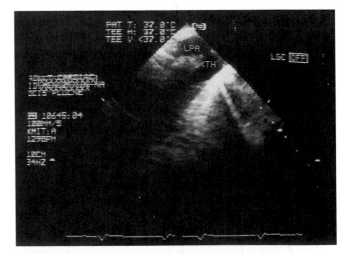

FIGURE 12-9. Transesophageal echocardiogram demonstrating a mobile thrombus (TH) in the left pulmonary artery (LPA) of a patient with acute pulmonary embolism. (Donated from the private collection of Adam Torbicki, MD, Chairman, Department of Chest Medicine, Institute of Tuberculosis and Lung Diseases, Warsaw, Poland.)

contrast dye (Figure 12-10). Secondary signs reflect decreased perfusion and consist of abrupt occlusion of vessels, oligemia or avascularity of a segment, a prolonged arterial phase with slow filling and emptying of veins, and tortuous tapering peripheral vessels. Angiography can detect emboli as small as 1 to 2 mm.

Low-osmolar contrast agent is used preferentially. It reduces coughing and other forms of involuntary motion. The right and left main pulmonary arteries usually require 40 to 50 mL of contrast at 20 to 25 mL/s. Conventional X-ray filming rates are usually three images per second for 3 seconds and then one image per second for 6 seconds. We now perform all our filming with digital acquisition. The filming rate is 7.5 frames per second for 1 second before injection (to obtain mask images for digital subtraction), followed by 7.5 frames per second for the first 3 seconds after the beginning of the injection. The filming rate can then be decreased to one to two frames per second for about 5 seconds. It is important to view the images in the unsubtracted mode, because subtraction may lead to artifacts that can mimic PE.

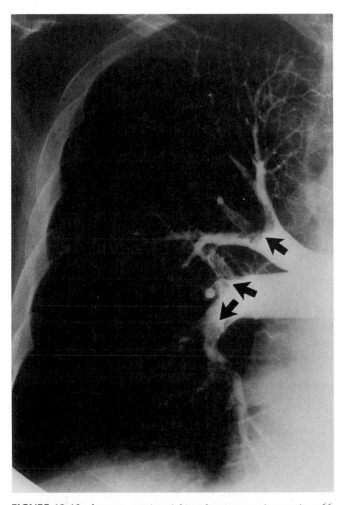

FIGURE 12-10. Anteroposterior right pulmonary angiogram in a 66-year-old man with thromboemboli in the right upper, right middle, and right lower lobes (*arrows*). (From Dr. Goldhaber's private collection.)

As with any invasive procedure, there is a "learning curve" to optimize technical quality, patient comfort, and safety. With fewer pulmonary angiograms being performed, this diagnostic test is often considered uncomfortable and hazardous. Instead of proceeding to pulmonary angiography, often the workup for PE concludes by accepting a chest CT result as normal, even if the technical quality of the CT scan is poor and the clinical suspicion for PE is high. In the series of 1111 patients who underwent pulmonary angiography in PIOPED, 5 patients (0.5%) died and 9 (1%) had major nonfatal complications, primarily respiratory or renal failure.[14] When undertaken by properly trained individuals for legitimate indications, pulmonary angiography can be carried out safely and can be of immense benefit in forging a clinical management plan.

Cardiac Magnetic Resonance (CMR)

Early two-dimensional phase-contrast and time-of-flight sequences without the use of contrast agents were time consuming and were limited by imaging and motion artifacts. With the introduction of stronger gradients and contrast-enhanced gradient echo techniques, imaging of the pulmonary vasculature with a single breath hold is possible. Magnetic resonance pulmonary angiography currently has adequate spatial resolution to allow imaging of the pulmonary arteries to the segmental level.[15]

Gadolinium-enhanced magnetic resonance angiography (MRA) is a new technique that shows promise as an accurate noninvasive diagnostic method. It does not require ionizing radiation or iodinated contrast material. To date, there are a few prospective blinded studies on the detection of PE with contrast-enhanced three-dimensional MRA compared with conventional or digital subtraction pulmonary angiography. On the basis of consensus viewing of the blinded readers, Meaney et al reported a sensitivity of 100% and specificity of 95% in detecting PE to the segmental level compared with conventional contrast pulmonary angiography.[16] In a more recent reported, with high interobserver correlation, a sensitivity of 87% and specificity of 100% compared with digital subtraction pulmonary angiography in detecting PE to the segmental level. Sensitivity declined to 68% when subsegmental emboli were included. These preliminary results seem very promising. Cine cardiac CMR can also assess right ventricular function in the same imaging session. This means that in the future, CMR may supplant the common current combination of tests, which often includes chest CT scanning to determine the anatomical extent of the PE and echocardiography to assess the physiological effect of the PE. MR pulmonary angiography may also become the ideal imaging test when PE is suspected during pregnancy.

Integrated Diagnostic Approach

We have many diagnostic tools available to help investigate patients with suspected PE. Of paramount importance is maintaining clinical suspicion for venous thromboembolism. Unless this diagnosis is considered, PE and DVT will not be detected. As contemporary clinicians, we should begin our workup by quantitating the clinical likelihood of PE on the basis of one of the available algorithms and point scoring systems. This includes taking a relevant history, including asking about family history of venous thromboembolism; performing a physical examination that focuses on the cardiopulmonary system and the deep leg veins; and obtaining both a chest X-ray and an electrocardiogram. The next step is to obtain a D-dimer ELISA. If this screening test is normal, we can be virtually assured that the patient does not have PE. Ordinarily, the workup for PE should stop at this point (Figure 12-11). In a Canadian study of 930 consecutive patients suspected of PE, 437 had a low clinical probability of PE and a normal D-dimer. These patients underwent follow-up at 3 months, and only 1 of the 437 patients had PE develop during that period.[17]

Clinicians who are triaging patients do not necessarily follow the protocols, despite the existence of many protocols that are promulgated for evaluating PE. For example, at Brigham and Women's Hospital, our emergency department ordered 1172 plasma D-dimer ELISAs during 2000. The negative predictive value of a normal D-dimer was 99% (95% CI, 98% to 99%). Of the 1172 tests, 581 (50%) were <500 ng/mL and were, by definition, within normal limits. Nevertheless, 143 of these 581 patients (25%) underwent lung scanning, chest CT, or pulmonary angiography. Of these 143, only 3 (2%) were positive for PE. Thus, in our emergency department, normal D-dimer ELISAs were often disregarded, despite an extremely low rate of diagnosis of PE on subsequent imaging studies. Our findings indicate that streamlined diagnostic workups and important cost savings can be achieved by screening for acute PE with D-dimer ELISAs. However, successful educational interventions must accompany normal D-dimer ELISAs to prevent the ordering of subsequent and costly low-yield imaging tests for PE.

The next step for patients with an elevated D-dimer is to choose an appropriate imaging test. With increasing frequency, the imaging test of choice will be chest CT scanning with contrast. For patients allergic to contrast agent or for patients with renal insufficiency, lung scanning is a suitable alternative. If these tests are equivocal, a venous ultrasound can be undertaken to look for DVT, a surrogate marker of PE. Finally, if these tests are negative or equivocal, and if clinical suspicion is extremely high, patients can be treated empirically for PE or can undergo contrast pulmonary angiography.

Therapy

Risk Stratification

Acute PE spans a wide range of risk, from small asymptomatic emboli to massive thromboembolism with catastrophic cardiovascular collapse and death caused by right ventricular failure. Therapy must be geared to patient risk. Low-risk patients will do well with anticoagulation alone, whereas high-risk patients may require thrombolysis, embolectomy, or placement of an inferior vena caval filter in addition to anticoagulation.

The Geneva Prognostic Index predicts adverse outcomes after PE.[6] Other nonimaging markers of poor prognosis include hypoxemia despite oxygen, physical examination evidence of pulmonary hypertension or right ventricular strain (accentuated pulmonic component of the second heart sound, a left parasternal heave, or distended neck veins), or an elevated troponin level.

The most important imaging test for risk stratification is echocardiographic assessment of right ventricular function.[18] In a cohort of 209 consecutive PE patients, 65 (31%) were initially seen with the combination of normal systemic arterial pressure and echocardiographic evidence of right ventricular dysfunction. Of this group,

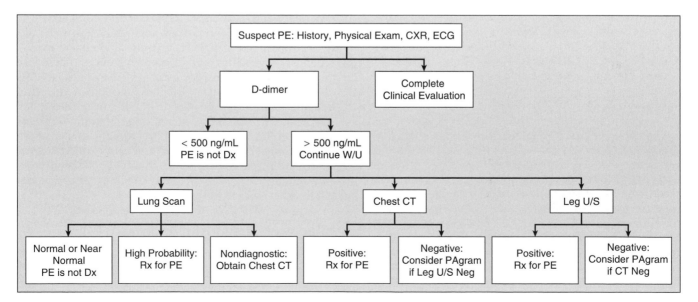

FIGURE 12-11. Integrated PE diagnostic workup. Please refer to text.

six (10%) had cardiogenic shock develop within 24 hours of diagnosis, and three (5%) died during the initial hospitalization. Conversely, none of the 97 normotensive patients with normal right ventricular function on echocardiography had PE-related mortality.

Pulmonary hypertension, as estimated by Doppler echocardiography, that persists for more than 5 weeks after the diagnosis of PE is also associated with an adverse long-term prognosis.[19] Among 78 patients with PE who were followed prospectively, those with persistent pulmonary hypertension and right ventricular dysfunction were nine times more likely to die during the ensuing 5 years than those whose pulmonary arterial pressures and right ventricular function had normalized.

Anticoagulants

Continuous intravenous unfractionated heparin or subcutaneously administered low molecular weight heparin is used for 5 to 7 days in the initial treatment of PE until a therapeutic effect has been achieved with oral anticoagulants such as warfarin. Although unfractionated heparin has served as the standard foundation of PE treatment for many years, its variable protein binding leads to an often unpredictable dose response and makes it difficult to administer properly. Subtherapeutic levels of heparin increase the risk of recurrent PE, whereas excessive levels increase the risk of major bleeding.

Unfractionated heparin for PE treatment is usually ordered as an intravenous bolus followed by a continuous intravenous infusion. The required dose is unpredictable and must be adjusted according to the activated partial thromboplastin time (PTT), which is not well standardized among different hospital laboratories. In general, the target PTT is 60 to 80 seconds. Heparin can be dosed by weight-based nomograms, but none of the nomograms provides a consistent dose response. An alternative approach is to initiate unfractionated heparin in an arbitrary dosing regimen, such as a 5000 to 10,000 U bolus, followed by 1250 U/hour.

Low molecular weight heparins have revolutionized the initial management of venous thromboembolism.[20] They have a much more predictable dose response than unfractionated heparin. In the absence of renal insufficiency or massive obesity, low molecular weight heparins can be administered to treat PE with a fixed dose on the basis of weight, without any blood testing to adjust the dose. In the United States, enoxaparin and tinzaparin are approved for treatment of patients with symptomatic DVT, with or without (asymptomatic) PE, on the basis of results from several trials. The Food and Drug Administration has not approved any low molecular weight heparin for patients seen primarily with symptomatic PE.

Warfarin is the standard oral anticoagulant used in the United States. It is limited by a narrow therapeutic index. Too little anticoagulant effect leads to thromboembolism, and excessive anticoagulation leads to bleeding. The drug is plagued by a long list of interactions with other drugs that either decrease or increase warfarin's anticoagulant effect. The consumption of vitamin K–containing foods such as green leafy vegetables decreases the anticoagulant effect, whereas the ingestion of alcohol increases the likelihood of hemorrhage. Warfarin dosing is adjusted according to a standardized prothrombin time by use of the international normalized ratio (INR). For PE treatment, the target INR is ordinarily between 2.0 and 3.0. However, the optimal duration of anticoagulation is extremely controversial.

Thrombolysis

Cardiovascular imaging can assist in selecting appropriate patients for PE thrombolysis and for gauging their response to therapy (Figures 12-12, *A* to *C*, 12-13, and 12-14, *A*,*B*). Echocardiography helps identify a subgroup of PE patients with impending right ventricular failure who seem to be at high risk of adverse clinical outcomes if treated with anticoagulants alone. Successful thrombolysis reverses right heart failure rapidly and safely, thereby preventing death from ensu-

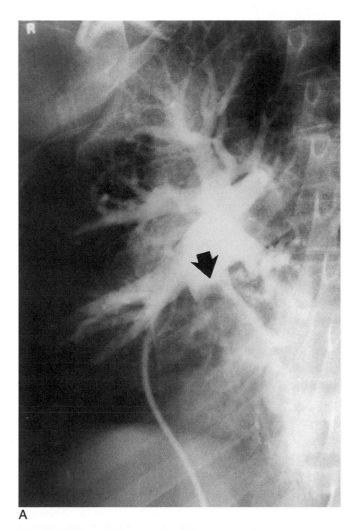

A

FIGURE 12-12. **A,** Right posterior oblique right pulmonary angiogram in a 30-year-old man, demonstrating a large embolus occluding the right lower lobe distal to the superior segmental artery (*arrow*).

Continued

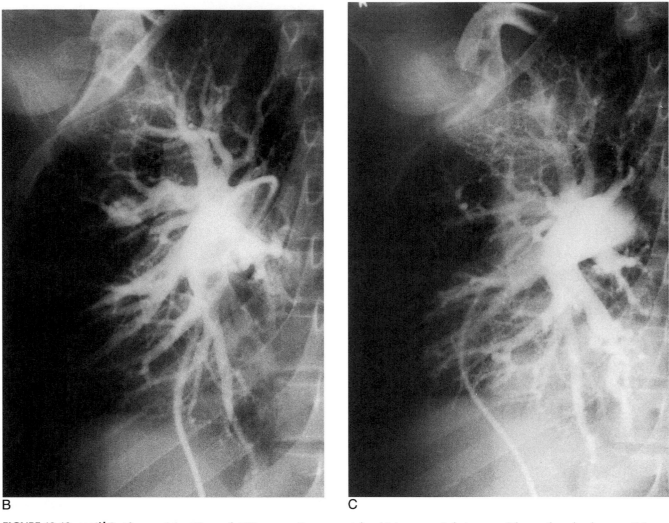

B   C

FIGURE 12-12. cont'd B, After receiving 50 mg of rt-PA as a continuous peripheral intravenous infusion over 2 hours, there has been partial resolution, with reperfusion of the anterior basal, medial basal, and lateral basal segments. **C,** After an additional 40 mg of rt-PA administered over the ensuing 4 hours, there has been complete resolution of the emboli. (From Dr. Goldhaber's private collection.)

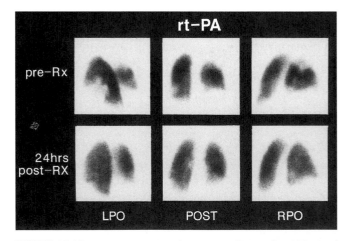

FIGURE 12-13. Improvement in pulmonary perfusion after 100 mg of rt-PA administered as a continuous peripheral intravenous infusion over 2 hours. The top row demonstrates perfusion lung scanning before thrombolytic therapy and shows multiple segmental perfusion defects in the left posterior oblique (LPO), posterior (POST), and right posterior oblique (RPO) views. The bottom rows demonstrate the marked improvement and near normalization of pulmonary perfusion in a follow-up perfusion scan obtained 24 hours after therapy with rt-PA. (From Dr. Goldhaber's private collection.)

ing cardiogenic shock. Thrombolysis may also prevent the development of chronic pulmonary hypertension long term and thus improve exercise tolerance and quality of life.

We tested the hypothesis that among hemodynamically stable PE patients, rt-PA followed by anticoagulation accelerates the improvement of right ventricular function, assessed by echocardiography, and pulmonary perfusion, assessed by lung scanning, more rapidly than anticoagulation alone.[22] In this multicenter, controlled trial, 101 patients were randomly assigned: 46 to rt-PA 100 mg/2 hours followed by heparin and 55 to heparin alone. No clinical episodes of recurrent PE occurred among rt-PA patients, but there were five (two fatal and three nonfatal) clinically suspected recurrent PEs within 14 days in patients randomly assigned to heparin alone ($P = 0.06$). All five initially were seen with right ventricular hypokinesis on echocardiogram, despite normal systemic arterial pressure at baseline.

Right ventricular wall motion was assessed qualitatively, and right ventricular end-diastolic area from the apical four-chamber view was planimetered on serial echocardiograms at baseline, 3 hours, and 24 hours. At

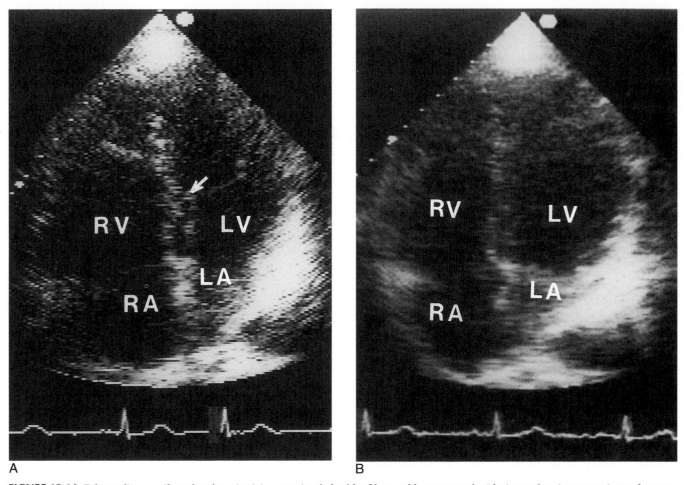

A   B

FIGURE 12-14. Echocardiogram (four-chamber view) in a previously healthy 53-year-old man treated with tissue plasminogen activator for acute PE. **A,** Enlargement and dysfunction of the right ventricle before treatment. The right ventricular end-diastolic area was 42.9 cm², and the interventricular septum (*arrow*) was displaced toward the left ventricle. There was moderately severe right ventricular hypokinesis. **B,** One hour after completing a continuous peripheral intravenous infusion of 100 mg of tissue plasminogen activator over 2 hours, the size of the right ventricle normalized, with a decrease in the planimetered area to 25.7 cm². Right ventricular wall motion also normalized. (Reproduced with permission from Goldhaber SZ. Treatment of acute pulmonary embolism, in Goldhaber SZ, Cardiopulmonary diseases and cardiac tumors, in Braunwald E [series ed], *Atlas of Heart Diseases,* Vol. 3, Philadelphia, Current Medicine, 1995, p 3.1.)

baseline, slightly more than half the patients with PE had entirely normal right ventricular function. Qualitative assessment of right ventricular wall motion at baseline vs. 24 hours demonstrated that 39% of the rt-PA patients improved and 2.4% worsened, compared with 17% improvement and 17% worsening among those who received heparin alone ($P = 0.005$). Quantitative assessment showed that rt-PA patients had a significant decrease in right ventricular end-diastolic area, indicating improved right ventricular function, during the 24 hours after randomization, compared with none among those allocated to heparin alone ($P = 0.01$).

We have subsequently demonstrated quantitatively that most patients who receive thrombolytic therapy for PE achieve recovery of regional and global right ventricular function. At baseline, right ventricular areas were significantly larger than normal at end-diastole and at end-systole. Diastolic and systolic right ventricular areas decreased after thrombolysis. The area of the right ventricle most severely affected (and most

improved after therapy) was the mid-right ventricular free wall (Figure 12-15).

Inferior Vena Caval Filters

There are two indications for placing an inferior vena caval (IVC) filter for patients with acute PE: (1) major bleeding that requires active transfusion or conditions such as postoperative craniotomy that preclude anticoagulation, and (2) recurrent PE despite prolonged intensive anticoagulation. Although filters reduce the frequency of PE, they do not halt the thrombotic process and are associated with a doubling of the rate of DVT.[23]

Embolectomy

Patients with moderate or severe right ventricular enlargement, who are not improving with anticoagulation alone, should be considered for embolectomy if they have contraindications to thrombolytic therapy.

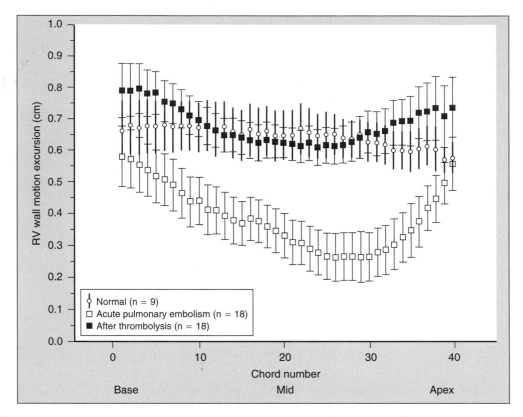

FIGURE 12-15. Right ventricular wall motion excursion and range for normal subjects *(open circles with gray bars)*, patients with acute PE *(open squares)*, and after thrombolysis *(solid squares)*. Wall motion excursion was significantly different from normal in chords 9 to 37, representing the entire right ventricle except the apex and base, in patients with acute PE. After thrombolysis, there were no differences in wall motion when comparing normal individuals and those who had PE. (Reproduced with permission from Nass N, McConnell MV, Goldhaber SZ, Chyu S, Solomon SD. Recovery of regional right ventricular function after thrombolysis for pulmonary embolism. *Am J Cardiol* 1999; 83:804.)

Embolectomy can be performed as a catheter-based procedure in the interventional laboratory or in the operating room. Catheter embolectomy has a very limited application; it is not suitable for patients in cardiogenic shock nor can it successfully remove large amounts of thrombus, because of limitations in available catheter devices.

Surgical embolectomy for acute PE is best performed on a warm beating heart with continuous transesophageal echocardiographic monitoring, after performing a median sternotomy and placing the patient on cardiopulmonary bypass.[24] The embolus should be removed under direct visualization, never "blindly." With experience, all lobar and most segmental pulmonary artery branches can be visualized. Ideally, high-risk PE patients will be referred for embolectomy before the development of cardiogenic shock as soon as their prognosis with anticoagulation has been established. At Brigham and Women's Hospital, we have formed an interdisciplinary clinical team to evaluate and refer patients for open surgical embolectomy (Figure 12-16). We have recently performed 26 emergency embolectomies, with a survival rate of 92% (95% CI, 75% to 99%). One of these patients had paradoxical arterial embolism, as well as acute PE (Figure 12-17, *A, B*).

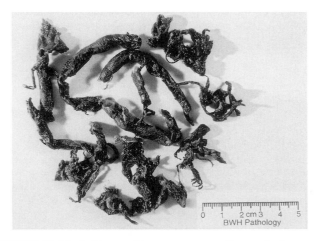

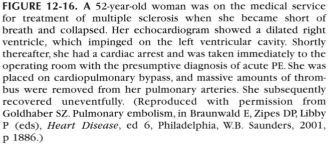

FIGURE 12-16. A 52-year-old woman was on the medical service for treatment of multiple sclerosis when she became short of breath and collapsed. Her echocardiogram showed a dilated right ventricle, which impinged on the left ventricular cavity. Shortly thereafter, she had a cardiac arrest and was taken immediately to the operating room with the presumptive diagnosis of acute PE. She was placed on cardiopulmonary bypass, and massive amounts of thrombus were removed from her pulmonary arteries. She subsequently recovered uneventfully. (Reproduced with permission from Goldhaber SZ. Pulmonary embolism, in Braunwald E, Zipes DP, Libby P (eds), *Heart Disease*, ed 6, Philadelphia, W.B. Saunders, 2001, p 1886.)

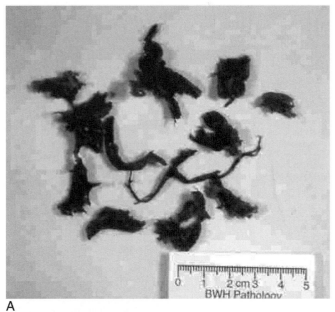

A

B

FIGURE 12-17. This 34-year-old woman was initially seen with chest discomfort, shortness of breath, and left arm discomfort and numbness. Chest CT scan suggested both pulmonary embolism and aortic thrombus. Further workup included transesophageal echocardiography, which showed moderately severe right ventricular dysfunction, bidirectional color flow across the interatrial septum, and a thrombus at the proximal origin of the left subclavian artery. We diagnosed pulmonary and paradoxical arterial thromboembolism and referred her for urgent embolectomy. At surgery, a 15- to 20-mm patent foramen ovale was closed with two layers of sutures. A, Multiple fragments of acute pulmonary embolus were removed from both proximal pulmonary arteries. The thromboembolus measured 4 × 3 × 2 cm in aggregate. B, Two large arterial thromboemboli, measuring 11 cm and 16 cm, were then removed. The 11-cm embolus extended from the left subclavian artery to the descending aorta. The 16-cm embolus extended from the left subclavian artery to the right subclavian artery by way of the innominate artery. (From Dr. Goldhaber's private collection.) See also Color Insert.

To manage severe chronic pulmonary thromboembolic hypertension caused by prior PE, a completely different and more technically challenging operation, pulmonary thromboendarterectomy, can be performed. The center with the largest experience is the University

of California at San Diego, where more than 1000 of these operations have been performed.[25] Such patients may be virtually bedridden with breathlessness caused by high pulmonary arterial pressures. If successful, this operation can reduce and possibly cure pulmonary hypertension. This surgery requires dissecting old thrombus, which has turned whitish and hardened, from the walls of the pulmonary arteries (Figure 12-18). Complications include pulmonary arterial perforation and hemorrhage, pulmonary "steal syndrome" in which blood rushes from previously well-perfused lung tissue to newly perfused tissue, and reperfusion pulmonary edema. For patients in whom surgery is not feasible, especially because of inaccessible distal thrombus, balloon pulmonary angioplasty can be considered.[26] These patients may achieve long-term functional improvement (Figure 12-19, *A, B*).

PULMONARY HYPERTENSION AND COR PULMONALE

This chapter has focused on PE and pulmonary hypertension as a consequence of PE. However, there are a multitude of nonthromboembolic etiologies of pulmonary hypertension. When no etiology can be detected, patients are labeled as having primary pulmonary hypertension (Figure 12-20, *A, B*). Patients with pulmonary hypertension have joined forces to advocate for themselves and to support each other through the emotional and physical challenges of this condition. They have created an excellent web site for their Pulmonary Hypertension Association, with a web address of www.phassociation.org.

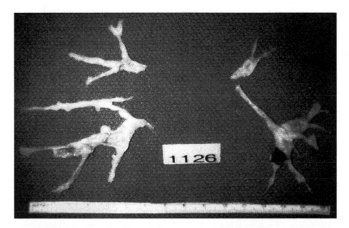

FIGURE 12-18. A 30-year-old man with chronic PE complained of exercise intolerance. His echocardiogram showed mild to moderate right ventricular dysfunction and enlargement. Lung scan, chest CT scan, and pulmonary angiogram showed numerous thrombi. He underwent pulmonary thromboendarterectomy after insertion of a prophylactic inferior vena caval filter. At surgery, a moderate amount of thromboembolic material was removed from both lungs. His pulmonary artery pressure decreased from a baseline of 35/10 mmHg to 18/9 mmHg before the pulmonary artery catheter was removed. He has enjoyed an excellent and uncomplicated recovery. (Reproduced with permission from Goldhaber SZ. Pulmonary embolism, in Braunwald E, Zipes DP, Libby P (eds), *Heart Disease,* ed 6, Philadelphia, W.B. Saunders, 2001, p 1886.)

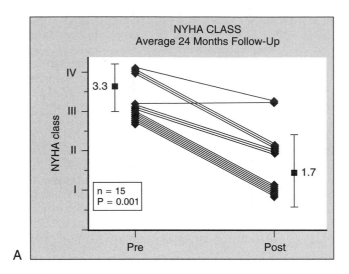

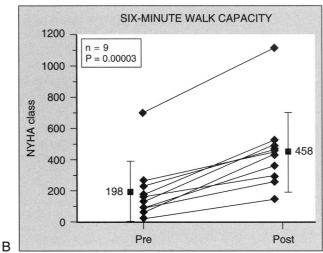

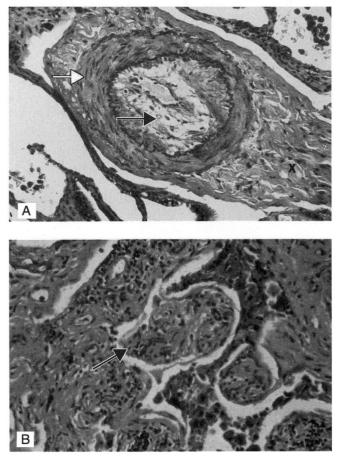

FIGURE 12-19. Functional improvement after balloon angioplasty in chronic thromboembolic pulmonary hypertension. **A,** Improvement in New York Heart Association Class. **B,** Improvement in 6-minute walk capacity. (Reproduced with permission from Feinstein JA, Goldhaber SZ, Lock JE, Fernandes SM, Landzberg MJ. Balloon pulmonary angioplasty for treatment of chronic thromboembolic pulmonary hypertension. *Circulation* 2001; 103:10.)

FIGURE 12-20. Characteristic lung pathology in primary pulmonary hypertension. **A,** Muscular pulmonary artery with medical hypertrophy *(white arrow),* luminal narrowing by intimal proliferation *(black arrow),* and proliferation of adventitia *(X).* **B,** Characteristic plexiform lesion from an obstructed muscular pulmonary artery *(arrow).* (Reproduced with permission from Gaine SP, Rubin LJ. Primary pulmonary hypertension. *Lancet* 1998; 352:719.) See also Color Insert.

Primary Pulmonary Hypertension

This is a syndrome of dyspnea, chest pain, and syncope that occurs in the presence of increased pulmonary vascular resistance and in the absence of a known cause.[27] Its familial form is linked to genes on chromosome 2. The lumen in primary pulmonary hypertension is prothrombotic. The endothelium produces excessive vasoconstrictors relative to vasodilators. The smooth muscle cells are depolarized and overloaded with calcium. The adventitia displays excessive remodeling that is associated with endothelial dysfunction. Despite contemporary therapy, the 5-year survival rate is only 50%.

For the past decade, patients with primary pulmonary hypertension have routinely received chronic anticoagulation to minimize the development of in situ thrombosis. About one fifth of patients have had a clinical response to high-dose calcium channel blocking agents. A typical dose for a responder is nifedipine SR, 270 mg once daily. These measures were supplemented with oxygen, diuresis, and at times digoxin for patients with cor pulmonale.

The advent of long-term treatment with intravenous epoprostenol (prostacyclin) led to unprecedented symptomatic, hemodynamic, and clinical improvement, including improved survival. The mechanism remains enigmatic. However, a consensus has emerged that epoprostenol therapy leads to beneficial remodeling, because pulmonary vascular resistance decreases even though there is no apparent pulmonary vasodilation. Continuous-infusion epoprostenol is inconvenient, because it requires a permanent indwelling central venous catheter. An aerosolized prostacyclin analogue, iloprost, seems to be safe and has sustained beneficial effects on exercise capacity and pulmonary hemodynamics.[28]

Secondary Pulmonary Hypertension

Secondary pulmonary hypertension with defined nonthromboembolic causes such as collagen-vascular etiologies may improve with continuous intravenous epoprostenol in a manner similar to primary pulmonary hypertension. For patients with cor pulmonale caused by secondary pulmonary hypertension, it seems that both impaired nitric oxide availability and increased endothelin expression result in pulmonary vascular endothelial dysfunction. These secondary forms of pulmonary hypertension may respond to inhaled iloprost[29] or inhaled nitric oxide,[30] with improvement of hemodynamics, physical function, and cor pulmonale.

REFERENCES

1. Goldhaber SZ, Visani L, De Rosa M. Acute pulmonary embolism: clinical outcomes in the International Cooperative Pulmonary Embolism Registry (ICOPER). *Lancet* 1999; 353:1386.

2. Heit JA, Mohr DN, Silverstein MD, Petterson TM, O'Fallon WM, Melton LJ 3rd. Predictors of recurrence after deep vein thrombosis and pulmonary embolism: a population-based cohort study. *Arch Intern Med* 2000; 160:761.

3. Oger E. Incidence of venous thromboembolism: a community-based study in Western France. EPI-GETBP Study Group. Groupe d'Etude de la Thrombose de Bretagne Occidentale. *Thromb Haemost* 2000; 83:657.

4. Seligsohn U, Lubetsky A. Genetic susceptibility to venous thrombosis. *N Engl J Med* 2001; 344:1222.

5. Wells PS, Anderson DR, Rodger M, et al. Derivation of a simple clinical model to categorize patients' probability of pulmonary embolism: increasing the models utility with the SimpliRED D-dimer. *Thromb Haemost* 2000; 83:416.

6. Wicki J, Perneger TV, Junod AF, Bounameaux H, Perrier A. Assessing clinical probability of pulmonary embolism in the emergency ward: a simple score. *Arch Intern Med* 2001; 161:92.

7. Bates SM, Kearon C, Crowther M, et al. A diagnostic strategy involving a quantitative latex D-dimer assay reliably excludes deep venous thrombosis. *Ann Intern Med* 2003; 138:787.

8. Kruip MJ, Leclercq MG, Heul CV, Prins MH, Buller HR. Diagnostic strategies for excluding pulmonary embolism in clinical outcome studies. A systematic review. *Ann Intern Med* 2003; 138:941.

9. Perrier A, Nendaz MR, Sarasin FP, Howarth N, Bounameaux H. Cost-effectiveness analysis of diagnostic strategies for suspected pulmonary embolism including helical computed tomography. *Am J Respir Crit Care Med* 2003; 167:39.

10. Bova C, Greco F, Misuraca G, et al. Diagnostic utility of echocardiography in patients with suspected pulmonary embolism. *Am J Emerg Med* 2003; 21:180.

11. McConnell MV, Solomon SD, Rayan ME, Come PC, Goldhaber SZ, Lee RT. Regional right ventricular dysfunction detected by echocardiography in acute pulmonary embolism. *Am J Cardiol* 1996; 78:469.

12. Kurkciyan I, Meron G, Sterz F, et al. Pulmonary embolism as a cause of cardiac arrest: presentation and outcome. *Arch Intern Med* 2000; 160:1529.

13. Ruiz Y, Caballero P, Caniego JL, et al. Prospective comparison of helical CT with angiography in pulmonary embolism: global and selective vascular territory analysis. Interobserver agreement. *Eur Radiol* 2003; 13:823.

14. Stein PD, Athanasoulis C, Alavi A, et al. Complications and validity of pulmonary angiography in acute pulmonary embolism. *Circulation* 1992; 85:462.

15. Olin JW. Pulmonary embolism. *Rev Cardiovasc Med* 2002; 3 Suppl 2:S67.

16. Meaney JF, Weg JG, Chenevert TL, Stafford-Johnson D, Hamilton BH, Prince MR. Diagnosis of pulmonary embolism with magnetic resonance angiography. *N Engl J Med* 1997; 336:1422.

17. Wells PS, Anderson DR, Rodger M, et al. Excluding pulmonary embolism at the bedside without diagnostic imaging: management of patients with suspected pulmonary embolism presenting to the emergency department by using a simple clinical model and d-dimer. *Ann Intern Med* 2001; 135:98.

18. Grifoni S, Olivotto I, Cecchini P, et al. Short-term clinical outcome of patients with acute pulmonary embolism, normal blood pressure, and echocardiographic right ventricular dysfunction. *Circulation* 2000; 101:2817.

19. Ribeiro A, Lindmarker P, Johnsson H, Juhlin-Dannfelt A, Jorfeldt L. Pulmonary embolism: one-year follow-up with echocardiography Doppler and five-year survival analysis. *Circulation* 1999; 99:1325.

20. Merli GJ. Low-molecular-weight heparins versus unfractionated heparin in the treatment of deep vein thrombosis and pulmonary embolism. *Am J Phys Med Rehabil* 2000; 79:S9.

21. Simonneau G, Sors H, Charbonnier B, et al. A comparison of low-molecular-weight heparin with unfractionated heparin for acute pulmonary embolism. The THESEE Study Group. Tinzaparine ou Heparine Standard: Evaluations dans l'Embolie Pulmonaire. *N Engl J Med* 1997; 337:663.

22. Goldhaber SZ, Haire WD, Feldstein ML, et al. Alteplase versus heparin in acute pulmonary embolism: randomised trial assessing right-ventricular function and pulmonary perfusion. *Lancet* 1993; 341:507.

23. Decousus H, Leizorovicz A, Parent F, et al. A clinical trial of vena caval filters in the prevention of pulmonary embolism in patients with proximal deep-vein thrombosis. Prevention du Risque d'Embolie Pulmonaire par Interruption Cave Study Group. *N Engl J Med* 1998; 338:409.

24. Ullmann M, Hemmer W, Hannekum A. The urgent pulmonary embolectomy: mechanical resuscitation in the operating theatre determines the outcome. *Thorac Cardiovasc Surg* 1999; 47:5.

25. Archibald CJ, Auger WR, Fedullo PF, et al. Long-term outcome after pulmonary thromboendarterectomy. *Am J Respir Crit Care Med* 1999; 160:523.

26. Feinstein JA, Goldhaber SZ, Lock JE, Ferndandes SM, Landzberg MJ. Balloon pulmonary angioplasty for treatment of chronic thromboembolic pulmonary hypertension. *Circulation* 2001; 103:10.

27. Runo JR, Loyd JE. Primary pulmonary hypertension. *Lancet* 2003; 361:1533.

28. Hoeper MM, Schwarze M, Ehlerding S, et al. Long-term treatment of primary pulmonary hypertension with aerosolized iloprost, a prostacyclin analogue. *N Engl J Med* 2000; 342:1866.

29. Olschewski H, Ghofrani HA, Schmehl T, et al. Inhaled iloprost to treat severe pulmonary hypertension. An uncontrolled trial. German PPH Study Group. *Ann Intern Med* 2000; 132:435.

30. Krasuski RA, Warner JJ, Wang A, Harrison JK, Tapson VF, Bashore TM. Inhaled nitric oxide selectively dilates pulmonary vasculature in adult patients with pulmonary hypertension, irrespective of etiology. *J Am Coll Cardiol* 2000; 36:2204.

chapter 13

The Role of Cardiac Imaging and Hemodynamic Assessment in Pericardial Disease

Sharon Coplen Reimold

Pericardial disease may be manifest as four principal types of physiological disorders: congenital abnormalities of the pericardium, pericarditis, pericardial effusion with or without hemodynamic compromise, and pericardial constriction. Infections, tumors, connective tissue disorders, surgery, and renal disease account for a significant proportion of pericardial diseases, but there are many other potential etiologies of pericardial diseases. Identification and characterization of pericardial disorders may be achieved by a variety of noninvasive cardiac imaging modalities. Often these imaging modalities are complementary, offering different anatomical and physiological information. The application of chest radiography, transthoracic and transesophageal echocardiography, computed tomography (CT scanning), and cardiac magnetic resonance (CMR) to the diagnosis and management of pericardial disease is described.

ANATOMY AND FUNCTION OF THE PERICARDIUM

The pericardium is composed of two layers of connective tissue. The inner layer, or visceral pericardium, is serous and is attached to the epicardial surface of the heart. The outer layer, known as the parietal pericardium, is fibrous tissue containing both elastin and collagen fibers. The two layers of the pericardium are attached by elastin. A a microscopic level, villi and cilia are present on these surfaces, allowing for transport and resorption of fluids. The thickness of the pericardium ranges from 0.4 to 1.9 mm.

The anatomical distribution of the pericardium is shown in Figure 13-1. Reflections of the pericardium are present anteriorly around the left atrial appendage in a region known as the transverse sinus and posteriorly around the aortic root in a region known as the obtuse sinus. The pericardium is attached by means of ligamentous processes to the sternum, xiphoid process, diaphragm, and the vertebral column. The pericardial space might contain up to 50 mL of fluid. The normal characteristics of this fluid are consistent with an ultra-filtrate of plasma. The pericardial space drains by the thoracic duct and the right lymphatic duct. Development of pericardial effusions can occur with excess production of pericardial fluid, decreased clearance of fluid by way of the thoracic and lymphatic ducts, or some combination of these abnormalities.

One role of the pericardium is to produce a restraining effect on the heart that is more pronounced during volume overload. The pericardium also serves as protection for the heart, limiting friction and adverse interactions between the heart and adjacent organs. The pericardium seems to have biochemical functions, producing prostaglandins that might modulate cardiac sympathetic stimulation and electrophysiological properties.[1]

CONGENITAL ABNORMALITIES OF THE PERICARDIUM

Pericardial cysts are developmental abnormalities of the pericardium. Typically they are located at the right costophrenic angle, but they may be found in a variety of other locations, including the left costophrenic angle and superior mediastinum near the aortic arch.[2] Because these cysts tend to be asymptomatic, the presence of an abnormality is most frequently detected on chest radiograph, demonstrating a round mass adjacent to the right cardiac border. These cysts tend to be filled with clear fluid and are rarely loculated or multilobar. The biochemical characteristics of cysts are usually transudative. Intrapericardial teratomas or bronchial cysts may occur in a similar distribution. Differentiation of a pericardial cyst from a tumor or aneurysm is usually possible with echocardiography or CT scanning.[3,4] Although these tend to be benign structures and need no further therapy, successful aspiration of right costophrenic angle cysts has been performed by use of fluoroscopy.[5] Cysts located in this position can also be drained with echocardiographic or CT guidance. Angiography and hemodynamic assessment do not play a significant role in the evaluation of pericardial cysts.

Pericardial agenesis is an uncommon form of pericardial anomaly that exists in two forms, total absence of the left pericardium and partial absence of the right or left pericardium. Patients with total absence of the left pericardium have leftward displacement of the heart, because the pericardium is not present to "hold" the heart in its

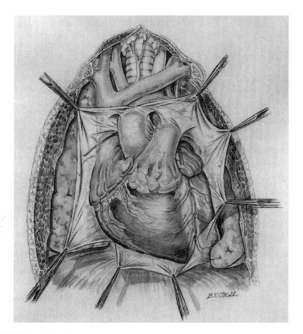

FIGURE 13-1. A depiction of the opened pericardium and heart is shown. Reflections of the heart can be seen along the great vessels. A probe is placed in the transverse sinus. (From Spodick DH. *Acute Pericarditis*, New York, Grune and Stratton, 1959.)

typical medial position. This may be apparent on a posteroanterior chest radiograph. Chest radiography findings include leftward displacement of the heart and prominence of the main pulmonary artery. In this disorder, lung tissue is interposed between the pulmonary artery and the aorta. This abnormally positioned lung tissue, as well as absent left pericardium and preaortic recess, may be suspected on standard radiography and confirmed by CT or CMR.[6,7] Transthoracic echocardiography of total absence of the pericardium is associated with the appearance of right ventricular volume overload with paradoxical septal motion. The position of the heart is displaced laterally, requiring nonstandard imaging windows for image acquisition.

Partial absence of the left pericardium, the most common congenital pericardial abnormality, is associated with herniation of part of the left heart through the defect. This can include herniation of the left atrial appendage, left ventricle, or atrium and can occasionally produce diastolic compression of the coronary arteries. As a result, herniation of a portion of the heart may be associated with chest discomfort, syncope, and death.[8,9] A chest radiogram may demonstrate protuberance of the left atrial appendage adjacent to the left pulmonary artery. Transthoracic echocardiography and CMR may identify herniation of the appendage through the pericardium. Herniation of the atrial appendage through the pericardium is classically identified by pulmonary arteriography, with attention focused on opacification of the left heart and extension of left atrial appendage contrast beyond the left heart border.

Partial absence of the right pericardium results in herniation of the right atrium or the right ventricle through the defect. This uncommon abnormality might be manifest as a protuberant right heart on chest radiography.

Right atrial angiography has traditionally been the diagnostic mode of choice for identifying portions of the right heart that extend beyond the typical pericardial border. Because of the potential for cardiac strangulation, surgical repair of the defect is recommended in patients with partial absence of the right or left pericardium.

COMPARISON OF IMAGING TECHNIQUES FOR EVALUATING CONGENITAL ABNORMALITIES OF THE PERICARDIUM

Congenital abnormalities of the pericardium are uncommon. Although these abnormalities might be suspected from chest radiography, echocardiography, CT, CMR, and angiography are useful to confirm the diagnosis. Because of the uncommon nature of these disorders, no comparative data are available in the literature. Standard transthoracic echocardiography may be adequate to define a pericardial cyst but may be inadequate to provide specific anatomical detail in partial absence of the pericardium. The advantage of CT and CMR as opposed to the other imaging options is better definition of the relationship between the pericardium and adjacent vascular and pulmonary tissues.

In the era of advanced noninvasive imaging techniques, angiography and invasive hemodynamics are infrequently needed to establish the diagnosis of congenital abnormalities of the pericardium.

PERICARDITIS

Pericarditis is inflammation of the pericardium that occurs in response to a variety of stimuli. The clinical syndrome includes the development of chest pain consistent with pericarditis, the presence of a pericardial friction rub, and the development of serial electrocardiographic abnormalities. The inflammatory response results in increasing pericardial vascularity, fibrin deposition, and migration of inflammatory cells into the pericardium. The visceral pericardium may produce excess fluid, resulting in a pericardial effusion. The cardiac imaging findings in a patient with pericarditis are variable. Pericarditis might result in no visible abnormalities with any cardiac imaging technique. Variable increased pericardial thickness and pericardial effusions might be seen in individuals with pericarditis.

Pericardial Thickness

The pericardium may become thick because of inflammation. Transthoracic echocardiography can detect increased pericardial thickness. Small relative increases in pericardial thickness (4 to 5 mm) may be difficult to detect with conventional echocardiographic methods, unless this increased thickness is associated with constrictive physiology. Extreme increases in pericardial thickness may be detected by transthoracic imaging (Figure 13-2). Transesophageal echocardiographic

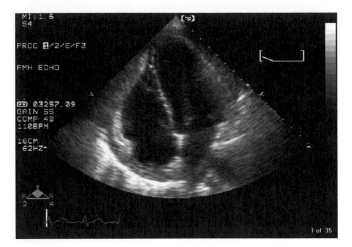

FIGURE 13-2. Apical transthoracic image demonstrating normal chamber dimensions and dramatic pericardial thickening.

imaging enables more precise measurement of pericardial thickness.[10] Measurements of pericardial thickness by use of transesophageal echocardiography are similar to those obtained by CT scan.[11]

CT scanning has been used for assessment of pericardial thickness and calcification.[12] The pericardium may be visualized as a thin line between the epicardium and the mediastinal fat. Conventional CT scanners do not have electrocardiographic gating and have a long acquisition time.[13] These features may lead to blurring of interfaces between the pericardium and adjacent structures. This blurring might lead to an overestimation of pericardial thickness. Electron beam X-ray CT (EBCT) offers the advantage of shorter acquisition times. Therefore, EBCT can provide a more accurate representation of pericardial thickness. In addition, EBCT is extremely sensitive in identifying calcification within the body and is the best imaging technique for evaluating pericardial calcification.

The presence of pericardial effusions may complicate measurement of pericardial thickness. A precise estimation of pericardial thickness by CT may be difficult in the setting of an exudative pericardial effusion because attenuation often leads to overestimation of pericardial thickness.[12,14] In individuals with suspected exudative effusions, assessment of pericardial thickness by an alternative imaging technique might be helpful.

The pericardium is a low-intensity band located between the epicardium and mediastinal fat by use of CMR T1-weighted spin-echo imaging. Both the fat and epicardium appear bright compared with the pericardium. The parietal pericardium might be nonuniform and is thicker around sites of pericardial attachments. The pericardium is seen prominently around the right ventricle, as well as the inferior and apical aspects of the left ventricle.[13] The average thickness of this low-intensity area is 1 to 2 mm by CMR compared with 0.4 to 1 mm on pathological studies.[15] Thicknesses of >3 mm are considered abnormal by CMR.

Several technical issues may lead to the "overestimation" of pericardial thickness by CMR. These issues include cardiac motion during image acquisition, inclusion of pericardial fluid in the measurement, and partial volume averaging. Chemical shift effects can occur, because fat and water have different resonant frequencies. A low signal intensity border may be present at transition zones between tissues with high fat content (mediastinal fat) and low fat content (myocardium).[13] This can lead to an apparent increase in pericardial thickness relative to pathological measurement.

Transudative pericardial effusions have low intensity on T1-weighted spin-echo CMR images. It is therefore difficult to distinguish between a transudative effusion and pericardial thickening with this technique. ECG-gated gradient-echo CMR can be used to assess pericardial thickness in transudative pericardial effusions. Pericardial effusions have a high-signal intensity with gradient-echo CMR, but the pericardium itself has low-signal intensity.[16] Because the biochemical characteristics of the pericardium are not typically known before imaging, pericardial images should be obtained with both spin-echo and gradient-echo CMR techniques to distinguish more precisely pericardial thickening from effusion. Similar to the spin-echo techniques, cardiac motion and chemical shift effects can lead to an increase in apparent pericardial thickness. Newer techniques, such as the steady-state free precession method, may minimize the apparent increases in pericardial thickness.[17]

Chest radiography, angiography, and hemodynamic assessment are not valuable tools in the detection of pericardial thickness. Routine radiography and fluoroscopy are useful ways to detect pericardial calcification that may occur together with a thickened pericardium.

Comparison of Imaging Techniques for Evaluating Pericardial Thickness

Echocardiography, CT, and CMR offer the ability to identify pericardial thickening (Table 13-1). In the absence of pericardial fluid, transesophageal echocardiography, CT, and CMR provide the most accurate quantitation of peri-

■ ■ ■

TABLE 13-1 ROLE OF CARDIAC IMAGING MODALITIES FOR QUANTITATION OF PERICARDIAL THICKNESS

Method	Pericardial thickness	Pericardial thickness (in presence of pericardial effusion)
Chest radiography and fluoroscopy	–	–
Transthoracic echocardiography	+	–
Transesophageal echocardiography	+++	++
CT	+++	+ (difficult with exudative effusions)
CMR	+++	+++
Cardiac catheterization and hemodynamic assessment	–	–

–, Not useful; +, minimally useful; ++, moderately useful; +++, most useful.

cardial thickening. CT and CMR offer the advantage of a broader imaging window, which might facilitate identification of localized pericardial thickening. The presence of a pericardial effusion might lead to overestimation of pericardial thickness, depending on the biochemical characteristics of the effusion. New CMR methods provide insight into drug delivery to the pericardial space, which may prove useful in gene therapy approaches to cardiac disorders.[18]

Pericardial Effusion

When a pericardial effusion is identified, several features should be characterized. These features include the size of the pericardial effusion, the anatomical distribution of the effusion, the imaging characteristics of the effusion, and the presence or absence of identifiable hemodynamic effects of the effusion. Pericardial effusions may be evaluated with a variety of imaging modalities, including chest radiography, echocardiography, CT, and CMR.

Chest Radiography and Fluoroscopy

The cardiac silhouette normally occupies <50% of the thoracic width on a posteroanterior chest film. In the presence of a pericardial effusion, the size of the cardiac silhouette enlarges. The shape of the heart changes with a large effusion and might appear flask-shaped on the posteroanterior projection. In some patients, the epicardial fat separates the cardiac and the pericardial shadows, highlighting the presence of a pericardial effusion as opposed to significant cardiac chamber enlargement. On the lateral chest film, the fat lines may appear lucent within the cardiac shadow, suggesting the presence of an effusion. In asymptomatic patients, the lung fields generally appear clear without increased lung markings. Pleural effusions, especially on the left are frequently associated with pericardial effusions.

In the absence of clinical suspicion, pericardial effusions may be difficult to diagnose. The chest radiographs of 17 individuals without pericardial effusions were compared with 83 patients with various sizes of pericardial effusion.[19] The four radiographic signs of possible pericardial effusion included enlarged cardiac silhouette, pericardial fat stripe, predominant left-sided pleural effusion, and an increase in transverse cardiac diameter. The most sensitive parameter, enlarged cardiac silhouette (71%), was not specific (41%) for an effusion. The other parameters were more specific for pericardial effusion (fat stripe 94%, left-sided pleural effusion 100%, and increase in transverse cardiac diameter 80%), but the sensitivities were <50%.[19] The most suggestive signs of a pericardial effusion were a predominant left-sided effusion and a pericardial fat stripe. These signs were not adequate to confirm or exclude the presence of an effusion. Therefore, additional imaging studies are needed to evaluate the pericardium in more depth if an effusion is suspected on chest radiography.

In the presence of a pericardial effusion, the cardiac silhouette does not change in shape or size with the respiratory cycle by use of fluoroscopy. The hemodynamic assessment of pericardial effusions typically does not reveal abnormalities unless tamponade or constriction is present.

Echocardiography

Echocardiography is the most reliable means of evaluating pericardial effusions. On the parasternal long-axis projection, an anterior clear space may be seen because of fat in the epicardial space. When a very small amount of pericardial fluid is present, it is often noted as an echolucent space posteriorly. Approximately 25 mL of fluid is necessary for this space to be visualized throughout the cardiac cycle.[20] Pericardial effusions might be differentiated from pleural effusions by echocardiography because of their location. Posterior fluid collections represent a left pleural effusion if they extend posterior to the descending aorta and pericardial fluid if the fluid extends between the left atrium and descending aorta into a reflection of the pericardium.

Effusions are semiquantitated as small, moderate, and large. Small pericardial effusions range up to 1 cm in diameter. Moderate pericardial effusions are 1 to 2 cm in diameter, and large pericardial effusions are >2 cm in diameter. The diameter should be measured in several locations from different imaging windows to completely characterize the effusion. Cardiac motion might be abnormal, with large effusions resulting in swinging of the heart within the pericardial sac. This abnormal motion is consistent with tamponade physiology, which can be further evaluated by Doppler echocardiography (see later).

The distribution of pericardial fluid should be described as circumferential or localized. Localized effusions are almost always loculated, because normally there is free communication within the pericardial space. Localized effusions occur after cardiac surgery or in purulent pericarditis, settings in which fibrin deposition may develop and wall off the normal pericardial space.

The appearance of the pericardial fluid might be characterized by ultrasound. Typical pericardial fluid appears lucent, with separation of the visceral and parietal pericardial layers. Pericardial inflammation and organization of the pericardial effusion might lead to echogenic fibrinous debris identified as strands within the pericardium. Occasionally, fluid in a purulent pericardial effusion may appear echogenic as in this case of tuberculous pericarditis (Figure 13-3).

Blood in the pericardial space might be seen because of postinfarction free wall rupture and aortic dissection. Fresh blood in the pericardial space appears echogenic and gelatinous. Pericardial hematomas can develop after cardiac surgery and appear as a mass with increased density adjacent to the heart. Organized hematomas will appear more dense than nonclotted blood within the pericardium, with the consistency of liver. Often the clinical scenario is helpful in elucidating the underlying etiology of hemopericardium. Suspicion of blood in the pericardial space is important, because disorders associated with this finding include left ventricular rupture and aortic dissection. These disorders are associated

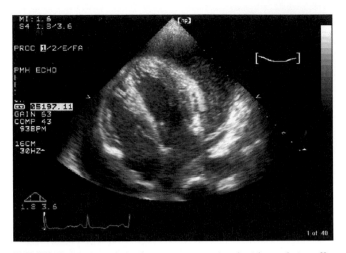

FIGURE 13-3. Pericardial infections are associated with exudative effusions. In this patient with an exudative pericardial effusion caused by tuberculosis, the pericardium appears grainy compared with a transudative effusion.

with an extremely high mortality rate and require emergent cardiac surgery.

Malignant pericardial effusions may be associated with masses attached to the pericardium or the epicardial surface of the heart. Pericardial studding may be difficult to distinguish from epicardial fat. The anatomical distribution of the pericardial mass can be helpful. Fat is located predominantly in the atrioventricular grooves and along the inferior aspect of the heart. Tumor studding may appear in different locations and appear globular or less uniform. No other echocardiographic aspects are helpful in distinguishing fat from malignancy.

Transesophageal echocardiography is rarely needed to establish the presence of a pericardial effusion. Transthoracic images usually provide sufficient information to establish the diagnosis. In some patients in whom transthoracic images are extremely difficult to obtain, transesophageal images might be a useful adjunct.

CT Scan

Pericardial effusions may be visualized by CT. Detection of a pericardial effusion is often an incidental finding on CT scan. On these images, the size of the effusion may be estimated by the distance between the parietal pericardium and myocardium. Long-acquisition times might lead to an overestimation of effusion size on conventional CT scanning. Better estimates of effusion size can be obtained with EBCT. Exudative effusions have low signal intensity on conventional imaging, whereas transudative effusions will have higher intensity.

CMR

The presence and the size of a pericardial effusion can be estimated by cardiac magnetic resonance. Estimated volumes of pericardial effusions correlate well with echocardiographic estimates and pericardial drainage volume.[21,22] Estimates of pericardial volume may be made using Simpson's rule. Pericardial fluid may be detected in the

transverse sinus by this technique.[23] The transverse sinus itself is a normal finding and should not be confused with abnormal pathology. Semiquantitative estimates of pericardial size can be made by measuring the diameter of the effusion in different projections.

Small effusions of all types have low signal intensities on spin-echo images. This is due to motion artifact. Characterization of these effusions is difficult by CMR. Larger effusions may be characterized by CMR. Chylous fluid, blood, transudative effusions, and exudative effusions exhibit differing T1 values. Chylous effusions have T1 values similar to fat. They have a short T1 time and have signal intensity similar to fat. Transudative effusions with a small number of cells and a low protein content have a long T1 time and low signal intensity. Exudative effusions have a T1 intermediate between transudative effusions and chylous fluid and with medium intensity. Methods are available to measure the T1 of an effusion to aid in the characterization of the effusion. This T1 measurement can be compared with standard values for serum with various cell concentrations.[21,22]

T2-weighted sequences have been used in extracardiac imaging to characterize hemorrhagic areas and hematomas. Conventional T2-weighted spin-echo sequences do not resolve effusions, making application of these methods to the heart and paracardiac structures problematic. Newer fast spin-echo methods might be better suited for classification of hemorrhagic effusions.[24] Pericardial hematomas may be differentiated from simple hemorrhagic effusions by their signal characteristics and the changes in T1 and T2, which occur with time after hematoma formation. These changes in signal intensity are readily evident with CMR.[25]

Malignant pericardial effusions may be accompanied by pericardial masses. These effusions are typically exudates and exhibit intermediate T1. Tumors may be difficult to distinguish from fat. Sequences that identify fat (fat saturation) may be used to distinguish between fat and tumor. In addition, many malignant tumors enhance with the administration of gadolinium-diethylenetriaminepentaacetic acid (DTPA).[26]

Comparison of Imaging Techniques for Evaluating Pericardial Effusions

The presence of a pericardial effusion may be suspected on the basis of radiographic or fluoroscopic images. The absolute size of an effusion is not assessable with these techniques. Echocardiography, CT scanning, and CMR may be used to assess pericardial effusions (Table 13-2). The advantages of echocardiography are portability and ease of use in identifying and quantifying pericardial effusions. In addition, echocardiography provides a practical means of noninvasively assessing the hemodynamic effects of an effusion. Although CT provides a wide window in the assessment of pericardial disease, the blurring of pericardial borders with conventional imaging limits the quantitative assessment of effusions. CMR is an excellent noninvasive technique to assess effusions and offers discriminatory capabilities in terms of effusion content.

■ ■ ■

TABLE 13-2 COMPARISON OF IMAGING TECHNIQUES FOR DETECTING AND QUANTIFYING PERICARDIAL EFFUSIONS

Method	Identifying effusions	Quantitating effusion	Characterizing effusions
Chest radiography	+	-	-
TTE	+++	++	++
CT	+++	+	+
CMR	+++	+++	+++
Cardiac catheterization and hemodynamic assessment	+	+	-

–, Not useful; +, minimally useful; ++, moderately useful; +++, most useful.

PERICARDIAL TAMPONADE

Pericardial tamponade occurs when pericardial pressure exceeds intracardiac pressures, leading to a constellation of clinical findings, including dyspnea, decreased cardiac output, and hypotension. The finding of pulsus paradoxus (decrease in systolic blood pressure of >10 mmHg with inspiration) on examination is suggestive of tamponade physiology. In tamponade, the pericardial effusion constrains cardiac filling. With inspiration, there is a drop in intrathoracic pressure, allowing increased blood to enter the right heart. Decreased blood flow in the left heart leads to a decrease in stroke volume during inspiration. This correlates with an inspiratory decrease in systolic blood pressure.

Chest Radiography and Fluoroscopy

Routine chest radiography and fluoroscopy play no role in establishing the diagnosis of pericardial tamponade.

Echocardiographic Findings

There are several two-dimensional and Doppler echocardiographic findings in tamponade (Box 13-1). Tamponade might occur with all sizes of pericardial effusions. A pericardial effusion can develop acutely because of perforation of a cardiac chamber during an invasive cardiac procedure such as an electrophysiological study or angioplasty. Rapid accumulation of a small amount of pericardial fluid can result in tamponade, because the pericardium is not distensible, and a large increase in intrapericardial pressure relative to pericar-

■ ■ ■

BOX 13-1 MAJOR ECHOCARDIOGRAPHIC FINDINGS IN TAMPONADE

Right atrial collapse
Right ventricular diastolic indentation
Respirophasic flow velocity changes
Dilated, nonpulsatile inferior vena cava
Abnormal ventricular septal motion
Rocking or swinging motion of heart in pericardial space
Respiratory variation in ventricular size

dial volume will occur. Most cases of tamponade, however, are associated with moderate to large pericardial effusions.

Right atrial inversion is a sensitive but nonspecific sign of tamponade.[27,28] Right atrial pressure normally exceeds pericardial pressure, leading to a convex right atrial free wall. Fluid in the pericardial space leads to elevation in pericardial pressure. Pericardial pressure can exceed right atrial pressure, leading to right atrial notching or inversion.[29] Underlying right heart pathology such as pulmonary hypertension or tricuspid regurgitation associated with elevation of the right atrial pressure may obscure the development of right atrial inversion.

Right ventricular diastolic indentation represents a similar phenomenon.[30] The free wall of the right ventricle becomes indented when the pericardial pressure exceeds right ventricular pressure. This occurs most commonly in early diastole when right ventricular pressure is at its lowest.[31] The duration and extent of diastolic indentation is directly related to increasing severity of tamponade. Although right ventricular indentation may be detected with two-dimensional and M-mode echocardiography, M-mode tracings have better temporal resolution and can identify this abnormality more easily. Performing M-mode tracings in the parasternal and subcostal windows allows detection of right atrial diastolic indentation. Right atrial and right ventricular inversion are more apparent in individuals with decreased intravascular volume.

Respirophasic variation in ventricular size is observed in tamponade.[32] Normally, flow into the right heart is enhanced during inspiration. All walls of the ventricles can expand during this time. In the presence of a significant pericardial effusion, the right ventricular free wall cannot expand in diastole. A shift of the interventricular septum from right to left occurs, resulting in a decrease in left ventricular volume. The heart may swing in the pericardial space with tamponade. This swinging of the heart within the pericardial space gives rise to electrical alternans noted on electrocardiography.

Exaggerated respirophasic flow velocities are important findings in tamponade.[33] In the normal heart, there is a mild increase in inspiratory flow velocities in the right heart and a mild decrease in inspiratory flow velocities in the left heart. Echocardiographic signs of tamponade include a 50% increase in tricuspid and pulmonic velocities during inspiration, with a decrease in velocities during expiration. On the left side, a 25% decrease in transvalvar velocities is seen during inspiration, with an increase during expiration. An example of significant respirophasic changes is presented in Figure 13-4. Respirophasic changes in hepatic and pulmonary vein velocities mirror those of the right-sided and left-sided valves, respectively. Respirophasic flow velocity changes may be seen in patients without pericardial effusions, most prominently in those patients on positive-pressure ventilation and those with chronic lung disease, acute pulmonary embolism, and right ventricular infarction.

During inspiration, the inferior vena cava normally collapses with inspiration. In the setting of a large

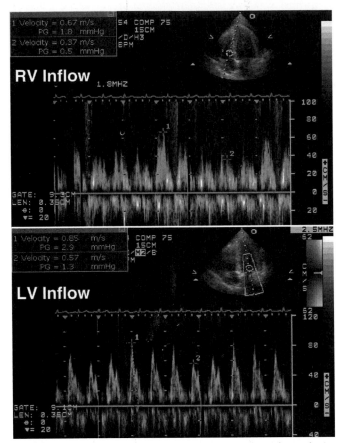

FIGURE 13-4. The respirophasic pulsed-wave Doppler velocity changes across the mitral and tricuspid valve indicate physiology.

pericardial effusion, the inferior vena cava does not collapse and is plethoric.[34] This is a sensitive sign of tamponade.

Transesophageal Echocardiography

Transthoracic echocardiography is adequate to image the pericardium in most instances. In patients in whom transthoracic imaging is suboptimal, transesophageal echocardiography may be used to evaluate the pericardial space. Pericardial fluid in the transverse and oblique sinus might be visualized by transesophageal echocardiography, CT, and CMR. Transesophageal echocardiography may be necessary to evaluate the pericardium in patients early after cardiac surgery and after placement of a left ventricular assist device. These patients are more likely to have loculated effusions that can result in regional tamponade.

CT Scanning

CT currently has limited ability to assess the hemodynamics associated with anatomical abnormalities. Therefore, if a large pericardial effusion is identified and tamponade is suspected, echocardiography is generally performed. Uncommon causes of pericardial tamponade such as posterior pericardial abscesses might be detected with CT techniques.[35]

CMR

CMR is able to identify the size and location of pericardial fluid collections. By use of cine imaging techniques, localized diastolic compression of cardiac chambers may be detected, suggesting a hemodynamically important effusion. Respirophasic variation in flow cannot be assessed by CMR, because current techniques assess flow by averaging several cardiac cycles. CMR is rarely used for the identification of tamponade physiology, because these patients may be unstable and difficult to manage in the magnet.

Pulmonary Artery Catheterization/ Hemodynamic Assessment

Cardiac tamponade is diagnosed in the catheterization laboratory with a pulmonary artery catheter when there is pressure equilibration between diastolic atrial and ventricular pressures. These pressures are essentially the same as intrapericardial pressure, and in most cases are elevated (16 to 20 mmHg). Right atrial waveforms typically demonstrate loss or a blunted "y" descent. Placement of a pulmonary artery catheter to assess cardiac filling pressures raises the suspicion of tamponade in hospitalized patients in the intensive care unit. Full hemodynamic assessment of tamponade is performed less commonly in the current era, because the combination of echocardiography and clinical presentation is usually sufficient to suggest the diagnosis. Use of a pulmonary artery catheter at the time of pericardial drainage is the only method to identify persistent elevation in intracardiac pressures after pericardial pressure has fallen. This occurs in a small, but important, subset of patients with tamponade.

Special Situations—Hemopericardium

Hemopericardium might occur in several circumstances, including trauma, left ventricular free wall rupture, aortic dissection, and after cardiac surgery. Hemopericardium consists of free-flowing blood in the pericardial space and organized thrombi in the pericardium. By two-dimensional echocardiography, these effusions appear gelatinous and granular. Detection of hemopericardium constitutes a medical emergency. Mortality rates for this condition are exceedingly high without prompt surgical intervention.

Patients who have undergone cardiac surgery may have postoperative effusions and local thrombi develop in the pericardial space. These thrombi generally occur because of bleeding at a suture site or pacemaker wire site and may result in localized tamponade. The classic echocardiographic signs of tamponade might not be present in the postoperative patient, because the pericardium is opened during the operative procedure. Localized diastolic compression might be the only sign of a hemodynamically important effusion. This diastolic abnormality may include compression of the left heart, an unusual manifestation of important pericardial disease. Suspicion of an important pericardial effusion should be raised in the postoperative cardiac patient who develops dyspnea.

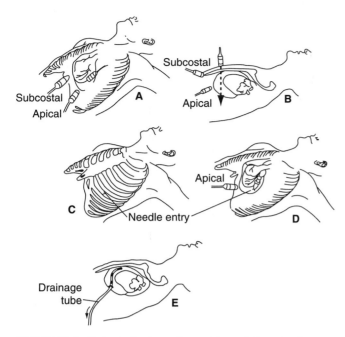

FIGURE 13-5. Method of echocardiographic-guided pericardiocentesis. Step 1. Identify the echocardiographic window on the chest where the largest amount of effusion can be identified. Mark this area **(A-C)**. Step 2. Determine the depth and angle of the effusion relative to the marked position. Step 3. Prepare and anesthetize the area for pericardial drainage **(D)**. Step 4. Inject saline solution through the needle to help localize the needle if necessary. Step 5. Use echo to monitor the success of the drainage. Step 6. Consider placement of a pigtail catheter in the pericardial space to decrease recurrent development of effusion **(E)**. (Modified from Callahan J, Seward J, Tajik A. Pericardiocentesis assisted by two-dimensional echocardiography. *J Thorac Cardiovasc Surg* 1983; 85:877.)

Special Situations–Pericardial Drainage

Pericardial fluid may be drained percutaneously in the catheterization laboratory with fluoroscopic guidance, surgically by use of a subxiphoid or lateral thoracotomy approach, or percutaneously with echocardiographic guidance. The technique for echo-guided pericardiocentesis is shown in Figure 13-5.[36-38] Echocardiography is used to identify the best approach for draining the effusion, localizing the optimal position and angle for tapping the fluid. With this strategy, there have been few serious complications (risk of death <0.1%).[36] The use of percutaneous drainage has been described in 977 consecutive patients.[39] The percutaneous approach was successful in 97% of cases. From 1979 to 2000, the use of pericardial catheters for extended drainage increased to decrease recurrence of effusion. Limited transthoracic echocardiographic imaging is used frequently to evaluate residual or recurrent pericardial fluid.

Comparison of Techniques for Diagnosing Tamponade

Although the "gold standard" for establishing the diagnosis of tamponade is pulmonary artery catheterization, sufficient echocardiographic data are available to support its use for making the diagnosis of tamponade when combined with clinical data. Other radiographic methods play little role in diagnosing tamponade. The clini-

cian and imaging specialists must be aware of clinical processes, such as recent cardiac surgery, which might alter the sensitivity and specificity of standard echocardiography for making the diagnosis.

Constriction

Cardiac constriction is typified by abnormalities of diastolic filling in the presence of preserved left ventricular systolic function. These diastolic filling abnormalities result in elevation of the venous pressures. Although cardiac constriction is typically associated with marked thickening of the pericardium, maximal pericardial thickness ranged from 1 to 17 mm in 344 cases of surgically confirmed constriction.[40]

Chest Radiography and Fluoroscopy

The pericardium may become calcified in patients with constrictive pericarditis. Calcification is more common in patients with tuberculosis and chronic constriction. This may be visualized best on the lateral chest film and takes the shape of a ring. This calcification may be seen on fluoroscopy. Bilateral pleural effusions are common in constriction. In some patients, dilation of the superior vena cava and azygous vein can be detected. Pulmonary vascular redistribution may be present as a consequence of elevated left-sided filling pressures.

Echocardiography

The echocardiographic findings in constriction include a thickened pericardium, abnormal ventricular septal motion, decreased or absence posterior wall motion during diastole, respiratory variation in ventricular size, and dilated inferior vena cava. These findings have inadequate sensitivity and specificity as single findings. The Doppler findings of constriction are important in differentiating constrictive from restrictive physiology.[41] In pericardial constriction, exaggerated ventricular interdependence in diastolic filling is seen (as in tamponade), and there is dissociation between intrathoracic and intracardiac pressures.

In the presence of an inflamed or thickened pericardium, total diastolic filling of the left and right ventricles becomes fixed. As decreased left ventricular filling occurs during inspiration, increased filling of the right ventricle occurs, leading to a leftward septal shift. This is accompanied by an increase in tricuspid and hepatic vein diastolic velocities. Echocardiographic criteria for constriction are respiratory variation of 25% in the mitral inflow velocity and increased diastolic flow reversal with expiration in the hepatic veins. This degree of respiratory variation in mitral flow velocities might be attenuated by increases in left atrial pressures. Significant respirophasic flow velocity variation might be more apparent in these individuals in the sitting position as opposed to the supine position.[42]

Patients with chronic obstructive lung disease may also exhibit respirophasic changes in atrioventricular valve flow. Constriction can be distinguished from chronic lung disease by several features. In lung disease, the mitral E velocity is highest at end expiration. In constriction, the E velocity is highest at the onset of expiration. Superior vena caval flow shows marked increases in velocities with inspiration in the patient with lung disease. In patients with constriction, little change in superior vena caval flow is seen with respiration.

Distinguishing constriction from restriction may be challenging. Both entities exhibit restrictive ventricular filling patterns. The ventricular interdependence seen with constriction is not seen with restriction.[41] Therefore, respiratory variation is seen in constriction but not in restrictive cardiomyopathies. The absence of respiratory variation on baseline imaging, however, does not exclude the diagnosis of constriction (see earlier). In restriction, there might be more prominent inspiratory flow reversal in the hepatic veins. In addition, by Doppler tissue imaging, the E'diastolic velocity in construction is ≥ 8 cm/s versus < 8 cm/s in resttriction. A comparison between Doppler findings in constriction and restriction is given in Table 13-3.

CT

In normal subjects, the pericardium measures 0.4- to 1.9-mm thick. Constriction can result in an increase in pericardial thickness of >1 cm. This increased pericardial thickness and calcification can be visualized with CT.[43] A small proportion of cases of constriction might occur with a fibrotic visceral pericardium in the absence of significant parietal pericardial thickening. The role of CT scanning in the evaluation of constriction is primarily in the identification of pericardial thickening. EBCT may be used to establish the degree of pericardial calcification.

CMR

Pericardial thickness may be optimally determined by CMR.[44,45] Pericardial thickening does not necessarily imply constrictive physiology. In the patient with clinical evidence of constriction, CMR is useful in defining the distribution of pericardial thickening and may serve as a guide for surgical stripping. Both spin-echo and gradient-echo images should be obtained to distinguish between pericardium and adjacent effusion.

CMR can provide some physiological details regarding the hemodynamic effects of the pericardial thickening. Methods to assess early diastolic filling are available and may allow detection of brisk early diastolic filling in constriction.[46] Myocardial tagging may distinguish between constriction and thickened pericardium without hemodynamic evidence for constriction. Normally, the heart slides within the pericardial sac. In constriction, the pericardium is tethered to the myocardium throughout the cardiac cycle. This may be evident by tagged cine CMR images.[47] In a normal heart, the "tags" of the myocardium move independently of the pericardium. In a heart with constriction, the "tags" do not move and appear to be adherent to the pericardium.

Ascites, pleural effusions, and dilation of the superior and inferior vena cavae frequently accompany pericardial constriction and may be overlooked, because the search may initially focus on liver disease as the cause of ascites and abnormal liver function tests in these patients.[48] These findings may be imaged by CMR and by CT scanning. In addition, CMR allows assessment of underlying left ventricular global and regional function. CMR may also be useful in detecting constrictive physiology in unique situations, such as after a pericardiectomy associated with an extrapleural pneumonectomy.[49] Despite the complicated anatomy, CMR is able to distinguish the constraining influence of the postoperative bandlike adhesions that may form under these circumstances.

Cardiac Catheterization and Hemodynamic Assessment

Constrictive physiology is classically identified by simultaneous right-heart and left-heart catheterization, demonstrating elevated and equal end-diastolic pressures (within 5 mmHg) in the atria and the ventricles. The

■ ■ ■

TABLE 13-3 COMPARISON OF DOPPLER FINDINGS IN CONSTRICTION AND RESTRICTION

	Normal	Constriction	Restriction
Mitral inflow	≤10% respiratory variation in E DT ≥160 ms	Inspiratory E less than expiratory # (≥25%) DT ≤ 160 ms	No respiratory variation DT≤ 160 ms Increased E velocity (≥ 1.0 m/s) Decreased A velocity (≤ 0.5 m/s)
Tricuspid inflow	Mild (≤ 15%) respiratory variation in E DT ≥ 160 ms	Inspiratory E greater than expiratory E (≥ 40% change) DT ≤ 160 ms	Mild (≤ 15%) respiratory variation in E DT ≤ 160 ms
Hepatic vein	Systolic forward flow greater than diastolic forward flow (sinus rhythm) Systolic forward flow less than diastolic forward flow (atrial fibrillation)	Decreased diastolic forward flow with expiration Marked decrease in diastolic forward flow and increase in diastolic flow reversals	Systolic forward flow less than diastolic forward flow Increase in systolic and diastolic flow reversals with
inspiration			
	Increase in systolic and diastolic reversals with expiration	with expiration	(greater than seen in normal subjects)

DT, Deceleration time.
From Hatle L, Appleton C, Popp R. Differentiation of constrictive pericarditis and restrictive cardiomyopathy by Doppler echocardiography. *Circulation* 1989; 79:357.

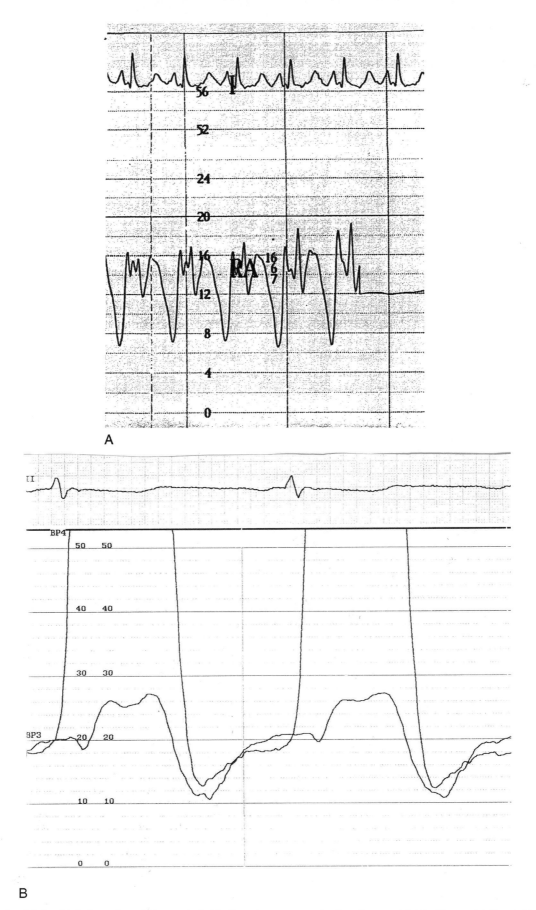

FIGURE 13-6. Constrictive hemodynamics are demonstrated in these two pressure tracings from a patient with constriction secondary to radiation. In the right atrial waveform (**A**), the right atrial pressure is mildly elevated with prominent x and y descents. In another patient (**B**), there is diastolic equilibration of wedge and left ventricular pressures.

■ ■ ■

TABLE 13-4 COMPARISON OF CARDIAC IMAGING TECHNIQUES IN THE EVALUATION OF CARDIAC CONSTRICTION

Imaging modality	Detection of pericardial thickness	Detection of pericardial calcification	Detection of hemodynamics associated with constriction	Detection of associated findings*
Chest radiography and fluoroscopy	–	+++	–	++
Echocardiography	+	–	+++	+
CT	+++	+++ (EBCT)	–	+++
CMR	+++	–	++	+++
Cardiac catheterization and hemodynamic assessment	–	++	+++	+

*Includes pleural effusions, ascites, and dilated caval structures.
–, Not useful; +, minimally useful; ++, moderately useful; +++, most useful.

right atrial pressure contour shows well-developed x and y descents compared with tamponade (Figure 13-6). Right and left ventricular pressure tracings demonstrate a dip and plateau pattern frequently referred to as the "square root" sign. Right ventricular and pulmonary pressures are generally minimally elevated, and right ventricular end-diastolic pressure is greater than one third of right ventricular systolic pressure. Left ventricular systolic function and right ventricular systolic function by angiography are normal. It might be difficult to differentiate constrictive from restrictive physiology, and the use of multiple imaging methods may be necessary to establish the definitive diagnosis of constriction.

Comparison of Noninvasive Cardiac Imaging Techniques in the Evaluation of Pericardial Constriction

Most cases of pericardial constriction are accompanied by significant pericardial thickening, as well as hemodynamic derangements associated with impaired ventricular filling and fixed cardiac volumes. Echocardiography is limited in assessing pericardial thickness but is able to identify hemodynamic derangements by the use of Doppler echocardiography (Table 13-4). CT is limited in providing hemodynamic correlates of constriction but can accurately assess pericardial thickening and provide the best measure of pericardial calcification. CMR offers the best anatomical and functional information concerning pericardial constriction and provides a useful "roadmap" for guiding surgical pericardiectomy. Constrictive hemodynamics may be suggested by echocardiographic and CMR parameters and should be confirmed in most cases by catheterization.

REFERENCES

1. Miyazaki T, Pride H, Zipes D. Prostaglandins in the pericardial fluid modulate neural regulation of cardiac electrophysiological properties. *Circ Res* 1990; 66:163.
2. Feigin D, Fenoglio J, McAllister H, et al. Pericardial cysts: a radiologic-pathologic correlation and review. *Radiology* 1977; 125:15.
3. Hynes J, Tajik A, Osborn M . Two-dimensional echocardiographic diagnosis of pericardial cyst. *Mayo Clinic Proc* 1983; 58:60.
4. Song H, Choi Y, Jang I, et al. Pericardium: anatomy and spectrum of disease on computed tomography. *Curr Prob Diagn Radiol* 2002; 31(5):198.
5. Klatte E, Yune H. Diagnosis and treatment of pericardial cysts. *Radiology* 1972; 104:541.
6. Gutierrez F, Shackelford G, McKnight R. Diagnosis of congenital absence of left pericardium by MR imaging. *J Comput Assist Tomogr* 1985; 9:551.
7. Gatzoulis M, Munk M, Merchant N, et al. Isolated congenital absence of the pericardium: clinical presentation, diagnosis, and management. *Ann Thorac Surg* 2000; 69(4):1209.
8. Auch-Schweik W, Bonzel T, Krause T. Differential diagnosis of chest pain and diagnostic findings in pericardial defects combined with coronary artery disease. *Clin Cardiol* 1988; 11:650.
9. Jones J, McManus B. Fatal cardiac strangulation by congenital partial pericardial defect. *Am Heart J* 1984; 107:183.
10. Izumi C, Iga K, Sekiguchi K, et al. Usefulness of the transgastric view by transesophageal echocardiography in evaluating thickened pericardium in patients with constrictive pericarditis. *J Am Soc Echocardiogr* 2002; 15(9):1004.
11. Ling L, Oh J, Tei C. Pericardial thickness measured with transesophageal echocardiography: feasibility and potential clinical usefulness. *J Am Coll Cardiol* 1997; 29:1317.
12. Stanford W, Thompson B. Cardiac masses and pericardial disease: imaging by electron-beam computed tomography. W. B. Saunders, Philadelphia in Cardiac Imaging. Marcus ML, Schelbert HR, Skorton DJ , Wolf GL (Eds.) *A Companion to Braunwald's Heart Disease* 1996. 96.
13. Vick III G, Rokey R. Cardiovascular magnetic resonance evaluation of the pericardium in health and disease. In Manning WJ, Pennell DJ (Eds.): Cardiovascular Magnetic Resonance. New York, Churchill Livingstone, 2002, p. 355.
14. Oren R, Grover-McKay M, Stanford W. Accurate preoperative diagnosis of pericardial constriction using cine computed tomography. *J Am Coll Cardiol* 1993; 22:832.
15. Ferrans V, Ishihara T, Roberts W. Anatomy of the pericardium. In Keddy PS, Leon DP, Sharer Saleas, Pericardial Disease. New York, Raven Penn, 1982, p.15.
16. Bogaert J, Duerinckx A. Appearance of the normal pericardium on coronary MR angiograms. *J Magn Reson Imaging* 1995; 5:579.
17. Kovanlikaya A, Burke L, Nelson M, et al. Characterizing chronic pericarditis using steady-state free-precession cine MR imaging. *Am J Roentgenol* 2002; 179(2):475.
18. Gleason J, Nguyen K, Kissinger K, et al. Myocardial drug distribution pattern following intrapericardial delivery: an CMR analysis. *J Cardiovasc Magn Reson* 2002; 4(3):311.
19. Eisenberg M, Dunn M, Kanth N, et al. Diagnostic value of chest radiography for pericardial effusion. *J Am Coll Cardiol* 1993; 22:588.
20. Oh J, Seward J, Tajik A. Pericardial disease. *Echo Manual* 1999; 1999:181.

21. Rokey R, Vick III G, Boli R. Assessment of experimental pericardial effusion using nuclear magnetic resonance imaging techniques. *Am Heart J* 1991; 121:1161.

22. Mulvaugh S, Rokey R, Vick III G. Usefulness of nuclear magnetic resonance imaging for evaluation of pericardial effusions, and comparison with two-dimensional echocardiography. *Am J Cardiol* 1989; 64:1002.

23. Im J, Rosen A, Webb W. MR imaging of the transverse sinus of the pericardium. *Am J Roentgenol* 1988; 150:79.

24 Seelos K, von Smekal A, Vahlensieck M. Cardiac abnormalities: Assessment with T2 weighted turbo spin-echo MR imaging with electrocardiogram gating at 0.5 T. *Radiology* 1993; 189:517.

25. Arata M, Reddy G, Higgins C. Organized pericardial hematomas: magnetic resonance imaging. *J Cardiovasc Magn Reson* 2000; 2:1.

26. Ohnishi J, Shiotani H, Ueno H. Primary pericardial mesothelioma demonstrated by magnetic resonance imaging. *Jpn Circ J* 1996; 60:898.

27. Kronzon I, Cohen M, Winer H. Diastolic atrial compression: a sensitive echocardiographic sign of cardiac tamponade. *J Am Coll Cardiol* 1983; 2:770.

28. Gillam L, Guyer D, Gibson T. Hydrodynamic compression of the right atrium: a new echocardiographic sign of cardiac tamponade. *Circulation* 1983; 68:294.

29. Singh S, Wann L, Schuchard G. Right ventricular and right atrial collapse in patients with cardiac tamponade: a combined echocardiographic and hemodynamic study. *Circulation* 1984; 70:966.

30. Schiller N, Botvinick E. Right ventricular compression as a sign of cardiac tamponade: an analysis of echocardiographic ventricular dimensions and their clinical impressions. *Circulation* 1977; 56:774.

31. Leimgruber P, Klopfenstein H, Wann L. The hemodynamic derangement associated with right ventricular diastolic collapse in cardiac tamponade: an experimental echocardiography study. *Circulation* 1983; 68:612.

32. Settle H, Adolph R, Fowler N. Echocardiography study of cardiac tamponade. *Circulation* 1977; 56:951.

33. Appleton C, Hatle L, Popp R. Cardiac tamponade and pericardial effusion: respiratory variation in transvalvular flow velocities studied by Doppler echocardiography. *J Am Coll Cardiol* 1988; 11:1020.

34. Himelman R, Kircher B, Rockey D. Inferior vena cava plethora with blunted respiratory response: a sensitive echocardiographic sign of cardiac tamponade. *J Am Coll Cardiol* 1988; 12:1470.

35. Groves A, Tasker A. Computed tomography imaging of cardiac tamponade secondary to a posterior pericardial abscess. *Heart* 2003; 89(4):364.

36. Callahan J, Seward J. Pericardiocentesis guided by two-dimensional echocardiography. *Echocardiography* 1997; 14:497.

37. Callahan J, Seward J, Tajik A. Pericardiocentesis assisted by two-dimensional echocardiography. *J Thorac Cardiovasc Surg* 1983; 85:877.

38. Callahan J, Seward J, Tajik A. Cardiac tamponade: pericardiocentesis directed by two-dimensional echocardiography. *Mayo Clinic Proc* 1985; 60:344.

39. Tsang T, Enriquez-Sarano M, Freeman W. Consecutive 1127 therapeutic echocardiographically guided pericardiocenteses: clinical profile, practice patterns, and outcomes and spanning 21 years. *Mayo Clinic Proc* 2002; 77:429.

40. Oh K, Shimizu M, Edwards W, et al. Surgical pathology of the parietal pericardium: a study of 344 cases. *Cardiovasc Pathol* 2001; 10:157.

41. Hatle L, Appleton C, Popp R. Differentiation of constrictive pericarditis and restrictive cardiomyopathy by Doppler echocardiography. *Circulation* 1989; 79:357.

42. Oh J, Tajik A, Seward J. Preload reduction to unmask the characteristic Doppler features of constrictive pericarditis: a new observation. *Circulation* 1997; 95:796.

43. Isner J, Carter B, Bankoff M. Differentiation of constrictive pericarditis from restrictive cardiomyopathy by computed tomographic imaging. *Am Heart J* 1983; 105:1019.

44. White C. MR evaluation of the pericardium. *Topics Magn Reson Imaging* 1995; 7:258.

45. Smith W, Beacock D, Goddard A, et al. Magnetic resonance evaluation of the pericardium. *Br J Radiol* 2001; 74:384.

46. Hariala J, Mostbeck G, Foster E. Velocity-encoded cine CMR in the evaluation of the left ventricular diastolic function. Measurement of mitral valve and pulmonary vein flow velocities and flow volume across the mitral valve. *Am Heart J* 1993; 125:1054.

47. Kojima S, Yamada N, Goto Y. Diagnosis of constrictive pericarditis by tagged cine magnetic resonance imaging. *N Engl J Med* 1999; 341:373.

48. Van der Merwe S, Dens J, Daenen W, et al. Pericardial disease is often not recognised as a cause of chronic severe ascites. *J Hepatol* 2000; 32(1):164.

49. Byrne J, Karava, Colson Y, et al. Cardiac decortication (epicardiectomy) for occult constrictive cardiac physiology after left extrapleural pneumonectomy. *Chest* 2002; 122(6):2256.

Imaging of the Adult with Congenital Heart Disease

Roger Andrew O. de Freitas
Gerald Ross Marx
Michael J. Landzberg

Atrial Septal Defects
Ventricular Septal Defects
Tetralogy of Fallot
Common Atrioventricular Canal
Isolated Patent Ductus Arteriosus
Truncus Arteriosus
Aortopulmonary Window
Ebstein's Anomaly
Pulmonic Stenosis
Anomalous Pulmonary Venous Connections
Cor Triatriatum
Congenital Mitral Stenosis
Aortic Stenosis
Segmental Approach to Cardiac Anatomy
Transposition of the Great Arteries
Double Outlet Right Ventricle
Coarctation of the Aorta
Coronary Anomalies
Single-Ventricle Physiology

The key to effective imaging of adult congenital heart disease is to provide insight into the mechanism of disease and the appropriate clinical management strategy. This poses challenges distinct from those encountered in the investigation of acquired heart disease. An understanding of embryologically based anatomy, physiology, defect natural history, and techniques of repair is necessary for planning an investigation. This chapter will emphasize the clinical implications for a cardiologist planning a study or series of studies for an adult with congenital heart disease. After a brief review of a lesion or group of lesions with similar structure and physiology, imaging techniques will be reviewed in detail, emphasizing practical suggestions to help the reader to answer the most relevant management questions. This chapter is intended as a foundation for the cardiologist inexperienced in congenital heart disease. A more detailed review of the preprocedural complications of specific underlying lesions and its associations is expected. We will begin with a discussion of shunt lesions: atrial septal defects (ASDs), ventricular septal defects (VSDs), tetralogy of Fallot (TOF), atrioventricular canal defects (AVC), and the patent ductus arteriosus (PDA). After this, we will follow the course of blood through the heart, describing the more common

defects of structures encountered along the way. More complex congenital heart diseases that typically result in single-ventricle physiology will be saved for a general discussion at the end of the chapter.

Before starting an analysis of specific lesions, a few basic principles of congenital heart disease imaging are worth reviewing. Echocardiography remains the mainstay of noninvasive imaging. In acquired heart disease, emphasis is placed on obtaining images and measurements in standardized views and planes that maximize the cardiologist's ability to relate the information to established norms. In congenital heart disease, complete initial definition of anatomy typically requires imaging with sweeps of the transducer to demonstrate the lesion in its full extent. At times, the anatomy is best defined by moving the transducer to a nonstandard view (e.g., a sinus venosus septal defect may be best imaged from a right parasternal view). The echocardiography laboratory standard at the Children's Hospital in Boston is to perform a complete examination of cardiovascular anatomy unless this has previously been detailed or reviewed by our own laboratory. If a full evaluation is not possible, absent details are noted in the report for further evaluation on subsequent examinations. A study must also evaluate the effects of the anomaly on the rest of the cardiac system. Congenital defects often associate with other defects, and so it is essential to search for associated lesions, particularly if surgical repair is contemplated.

Poor acoustic windows in the adult with congenital heart disease often limit transthoracic images, particularly if the patient has undergone surgical repair. As a result, transesophageal echocardiography and cardiac magnetic resonance (CMR) imaging techniques are discussed for each lesion. Three-dimensional (3D) echocardiography and radionuclide angiography are less widely used at present. They will be discussed when they seem to offer significant additional benefit in answering specific questions.

CMR imaging plays an essential role in our noninvasive imaging of adults with congenital heart disease. We expect that this role will grow as techniques and imaging sequences continue to develop. CMR offers the advantage of excellent image quality that does not degrade with advancing patient age or after surgical repair. However, it is limited to varying degrees by artifacts produced by implanted metal. Sternal wires produce a local artifact that usually does not limit the usefulness of CMR. The metallic supporting structure of an implanted valve, even a tissue valve, also produces local artifact that may prevent evaluation of the valve but allows examination of the rest of the heart. Intravascular stents likewise prevent assessment of the lumen with sequences presently available. In contrast, stainless steel intravascular coils, which are often used to occlude undesirable collateral vessels, produce extensive artifact that prevents imaging of structures within several centimeters of the coil. Use of alternate materials (e.g., platinum coils) may allow continued CMR imaging in a patient who requires coil occlusion of collaterals. Pacemaker implantation is a strong relative contraindication to CMR imaging.

CMR is typically our preferred technique for initial noninvasive imaging of extracardiac structures such as the aorta or the pulmonary veins and arteries. Because CMR provides tomographic views of the irregularly shaped right ventricle, it allows quantitation of right ventricular volume and function. We therefore rely on CMR for serial evaluation of anomalies that place pathological loads on the irregularly shaped right ventricle, such as TOF, or the Mustard or Senning atrial baffle repairs of transposition of the great arteries. The quantitation of flow volumes by phase-contrast velocity mapping allows noninvasive quantitation of valvar regurgitant lesions, such as pulmonary regurgitation. Although valve anatomy is being visualized in greater detail as imaging sequences and scanner technology improves, echocardiography (transesophageal echocardiography in particular) is usually the technique of choice for evaluating valve structure and valve leaflet malfunction. Similarly, CMR techniques to measure pressure gradients across stenoses have significant limitations. For this reason, CMR and Doppler echocardiography may be used together as complementary procedures for noninvasive assessment of valvar abnormalities and their effects on myocardial function.

CMR examinations begin with fast "localizer" sequences that orient the heart within the thorax. Subsequent studies are prioritized to answer the questions of greatest clinical value during the time-limited CMR examination. Typically, cardiac structure and function are first assessed with cine images of the heart in short axis ("bread loafing" the heart) and in the long axis of the ventricle. These images are obtained with ECG-gated cine fast gradient-echo sequence with segmented K-space filling. New, more rapid, techniques that use steady-state free precession sequences are in development. The pulmonary and systemic circulations are typically imaged with 3D fast-spoiled gradient echo with intravenous gadolinium contrast (3D-CMRA). This imaging sequence provides a 3D data set that can be manipulated and reconstructed after the data have been acquired to allow optimal definition of anatomy. Phase-velocity cine (also known as phase-contrast cine) CMR allows quantitation of blood flow within a vascular structure. Combining measurements from different vascular structures allows quantitative estimation of relative blood flows to different structures, valvar regurgitant fraction, and shunt ratios.

The importance of cardiac catheterization for imaging congenital heart disease evolves as noninvasive techniques grow in accuracy and precision. One of the most challenging tasks in the catheterization of congenital heart disease can be achieving a catheter position that allows controlled hemodynamic assessment and angiography of the region of interest. This typically requires a combination of a guide wire with a flexible tip and a tracking catheter, which uses biplane angiography to obtain orthogonal views. After measurement of hemodynamics, a flexible-tipped guide wire is left in place to secure position. An angiographic catheter with multiple side holes, such as a pigtail that has been cut off after the first 90 degrees of the pigtail loop (a "cutoff pigtail," also available commercially as a Royal Flush II, Cordis Corp.) is advanced over the guide wire to the desired location. Power injection of contrast through the angiographic catheter is performed with the guide wire secured in place. Angiography often involves structures that receive the full cardiac output and therefore require a substantial amount of contrast for opacification. To avoid excessive contrast loads, the structures of greatest interest that cannot be seen noninvasively are imaged first. This chapter attempts to familiarize the practicing adult cardiologist with pertinent questions and the role of catheterization in answering them. It does not attempt to provide a handbook for performing congenital catheterizations. Catheterization of congenital heart disease requires sufficient knowledge and experience that, similar to noninvasive imaging, consideration should be given to referring a patient to an adult congenital cardiologist when imaging is desired.

Atrial Septal Defects

Defects in the atrial septum are second only to bicuspid aortic valve disease in frequency of presentation of congenital heart disease in adulthood. Although an ASD with a large left-to-right shunt may show a classic presentation, a lesser degree of shunting may be hemodynamically significant over decades and yet not manifest a classic physical examination. A patent foramen ovale (PFO) is normally found in up to 20% to 30% of the population and may offer no clinical findings until it allows a paradoxical embolus to cause a stroke. This section will emphasize typical secundum ASDs and PFOs. The sinus venosus septal defect is not truly a defect of the atrial septum, but rather embryologically is the result of incomplete division of the vena cava from a pulmonary vein. It will be discussed in this section, because its physiology is similar to that of a secundum ASD, and its occurrence is one of the more common mimics of a secundum ASD. Coronary sinus septal defects are rare and will be discussed only briefly. Primum ASDs are part of the continuum of atrio-ventricular canal (AVC) defects and very frequently have associated defects of the atrioventricular valves or ventricular septum. They will be contrasted with secundum ASDs, although they will be more fully discussed separately as a form of AVC. Partial anomalous pulmonary venous return also is seen with a left-to-right shunt at the atrial level, but because the focus of the imaging is different from that of the atrial septum, it will be discussed separately.

The atrial septum normally develops from the joining of three structures. The semicircular muscular septum secundum meets the endocardial cushions (which will divide a common atrioventricular valve into two valves), leaving a central fossa ovalis, which is normally closed by the thin, fibrous "flap valve" of septum primum after birth. Before birth, right atrial (RA) pressures exceed those in the left atrium (LA), allowing blood from the placenta to cross through the foramen ovale, pushing back septum primum and proceeding to the left side of the heart and the systemic arteries. After birth, left atrial pressures and resistance to emptying rise and close the flap valve of septum primum against the surrounding septum secundum. In approximately 70% to 80% of adults, the septum primum fuses with the septum secundum, resulting in an intact atrial septum. However, in the 20% to 30% of adults with a PFO, the two septa are not fused, and septum primum is held shut against septum secundum during those phases of the cardiac cycle when left atrial pressure exceeds that in the right atrium. However, when the relative pressures and resistance to emptying are reversed (e.g., with changes in intrathoracic pressure, such as with a Valsalva or Mueller maneuver), blood may flow across the atrial septum from right to left. A secundum ASD results when the central portion of the atrial septum (within the fossa ovalis) is deficient. A central defect in atrial septation may also occur when dilation of the atria pulls the flap valve of septum primum away from septum secundum, which is sometimes referred to as a "stretched PFO."

A primum ASD occurs when there is incomplete development of the endocardial cushion that will septate the atrioventricular valves and is a deficiency of the atrial septum adjacent to the atrioventricular valves. Because this hole in the atrial septum occurs earliest in embryological development, it carries the name ostium primum, and the defect caused by incomplete closure is known as a primum ASD. Sinus venosus septal defects occur when there is incomplete development of the walls that separate the superior vena cava (SVC) from the right upper or middle pulmonary veins. The pulmonary veins may override the atrial septum, resulting in partial anomalous pulmonary venous drainage into the right atrium (creating a left-to-right shunt). A "coronary sinus septal defect" occurs when there is incomplete development of the wall of the coronary sinus, "unroofing" the sinus so that (1) desaturated blood from the coronary sinus will drain into the left atrium, causing a small right-to-left shunt, and (2) blood may shunt left to right across the ostium of the coronary sinus (which becomes the structurally normal "defect" in the atrial septum). An "unroofed" coronary sinus may also provide drainage to a persistent left SVC that is draining the left upper extremity.

In the presence of a large ASD, blood returning to the left atrium may flow either to the systemic circulation or back again through the ASD to the pulmonary circulation. The degree of shunting varies with many factors, including the size of the defect, the relative compliance of the two ventricles, and the capacitance of the pulmonary vs. the systemic circulation. With a large shunt, right-sided volume, as well as changes in pulmonary vasculature, cause enlargement of the right atrium, right ventricle, and left atrium. Standard repair of a secundum ASD involves either primary suture closure or placement of a patch, usually of glutaraldehyde-treated autologous pericardium. Repair of a defect diagnosed in childhood is usually performed electively at the age of 4 to 5 years. Septal defect closure devices delivered by means of cardiac catheterization currently offer an alternative to surgical repair. Successful deployment of a transcatheter device requires an adequate rim of septal tissue against which the arms can hold.

Imaging Essentials, Unrepaired ASD

1. Anatomy of the defect: dimensions, location, rim of septal tissue
2. Direction and degree of shunting
3. Right ventricular response to volume load: function, dilation, evidence of pressure or volume overload
4. Pulmonary vascular response to increased flow: evidence of elevated right-sided pressure
5. Presence of associated lesions: anomalous pulmonary venous return
6. Full anatomical survey

Imaging Essentials, Repaired ASD

1. Residual shunt
2. Change in dimensions of right atrium, right ventricle, and left atrium
3. Estimate of right ventricular and pulmonary artery pressures

Imaging Essentials, Postdevice Closure

1. Residual shunt
2. Position of umbrella arms (double-umbrella device) and device disks (double-disk device): evaluate for possible prolapse of arm or disk through ASD to opposite side to the atrial septum
3. Atrioventricular valve function: evaluate for possible distortion of the leaflet, causing valvar insufficiency
4. Venous inflow: of both systemic and pulmonary veins; rule out obstruction (possibly seen with larger devices)

Echocardiography

Transthoracic echocardiography remains the primary technique for diagnosing ASDs but presents important limitations and pitfalls. Structures are best seen by echocardiography when the ultrasound beam is aimed perpendicular to their surface. For the atrial septum, this implies that the subcostal view will provide optimal imaging (Figure 14-1, A). Although this is usually true, many adults have limited subcostal acoustic windows. Sweeping the transducer from posterior to anterior in the subcostal long axis and from right to left in subcostal short axis usually demonstrates the dimensions of the

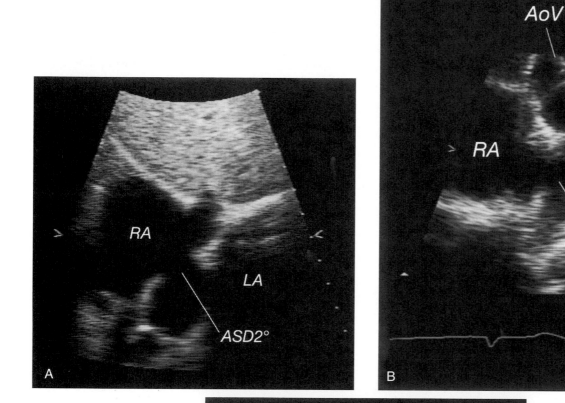

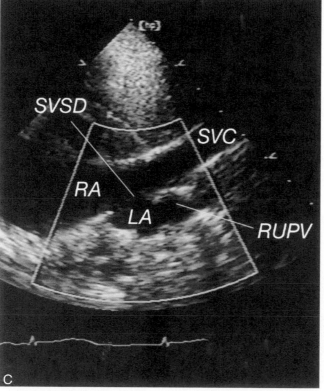

FIGURE 14-1. Secundum ASD and sinus venosus septal defect. **A,** Note how subcostal imaging of the atrial septum places the septum more perpendicular to the plane of ultrasound and the flow across the ASD more parallel to the transducer. **B,** Typical appearance of a secundum ASD from parasternal short axis. **C,** Sinus venosus septal defect from a right parasternal window with the transducer oriented in a vertical plane.

defect and the rim of the atrial septum. An "in-between" view allows imaging of the rightward and superior portion of the atrial septum, where the SVC and right upper pulmonary vein (RUPV) pass adjacent to each other. Sweeping through this view with a focus on the SVC and RUPV may demonstrate a sinus venosus septal defect. Color-flow mapping may identify a defect when the 2D imaging is equivocal. Because flow across a nonrestrictive ASD has a lower velocity than flow across a VSD or regurgitant jet, setting the scale to a lower velocity may accentuate its appearance. Color-flow Doppler demonstrates the predominant direction of flow across the ASD, but pulsed-wave Doppler may bring out short, transient periods of reversal of flow (e.g., brief right to left flow). If the defect is small and restrictive, Doppler techniques may also allow estimation of the pressure gradient across the atrial septum.

If subcostal windows are limited, a rightward sweep from parasternal short axis may demonstrate the atrial septum, in particular the region under the aortic valve (Figure 14-1, B). Because the septum is parallel to the beam of ultrasound, resolution is often poor and subject to distortion from "false dropout." However, because the atrial septum is closer to the transducer than in the apical view, resolution is usually better. A superior sinus venosus septal defect may sometimes be optimally imaged by rolling the patient onto the right side and imaging from a right parasternal short-axis view (Figure 14-1, C).

A PFO may be visualized if good subcostal imaging demonstrates the "flap valve" of the fossa ovalis lifting off the muscular septum secundum during a portion of the cardiac cycle. However, transthoracic imaging is typically so limited that it is important to verify that, in addition to an apparent small defect in 2D imaging, appropriate color flow is seen crossing the atrial septum at the site of the PFO. Right-to-left shunting at the PFO may be brief, yet significant. Injection of agitated saline contrast through an intravenous line into the right side of the heart, along with either the Mueller or Valsalva maneuver during imaging, may demonstrate the shunt, because "bubbles" appear in the left atrium before six cardiac cycles. Trendelenburg position, injection of contrast into the femoral vein during cardiac catheterization,[1] and transmitral Doppler techniques[2] may aid in the recognition of right-to-left shunting. Left-to-right shunting may be identified during contrast injection as a flow of contrast-free blood across the atrial septum into the contrast-filled right atrium. Of note, streaming of contrast-free inferior vena cava blood may give a similar negative contrast appearance.

Assessing the volume of left-to-right shunt is difficult and, in our experience, imprecise. In practice, our laboratory uses short-axis views to look for evidence of right ventricular volume overload causing bowing of the septum from the right toward the left ventricle in diastole as an indicator of RVVO. RVVO may also be caused by other lesions that present a volume load to the RV, including tricuspid and pulmonic regurgitation or anomalous pulmonary veins. These lesions should be sought before interpreting RVVO as indicative of a large shunt across the atrial septum. Right ventricular dilation is commonly seen in patients with an ASD and suggests the effect of a large shunt. Right ventricular systolic function is difficult to assess quantitatively by echocardiography, and usually a qualitative assessment is given. Radionuclide angiography and newer noninvasive techniques such as CMR imaging offer promise in the quantitative assessment of right ventricular function.[3,4] RV pressure is assessed by tricuspid regurgitation and verified by interventricular septal position during systole, with systolic septal flattening suggesting that RV pressure is at least 50% of systemic (left ventricular; LV) pressure.

Because the esophagus is adjacent to the left atrium, the atria and vessels draining into it are well seen by transesophageal echocardiography (TEE), and TEE should be considered whenever a PFO or ASD is suspected but not demonstrated by transthoracic echocardiography (e.g., unexplained RVVO or embolic stroke).[5] TEE examination begins with visualization of the atrial septum from 0 degrees (Figure 14-2, A), sweeping cranially and then caudally to demonstrate the pulmonary veins.

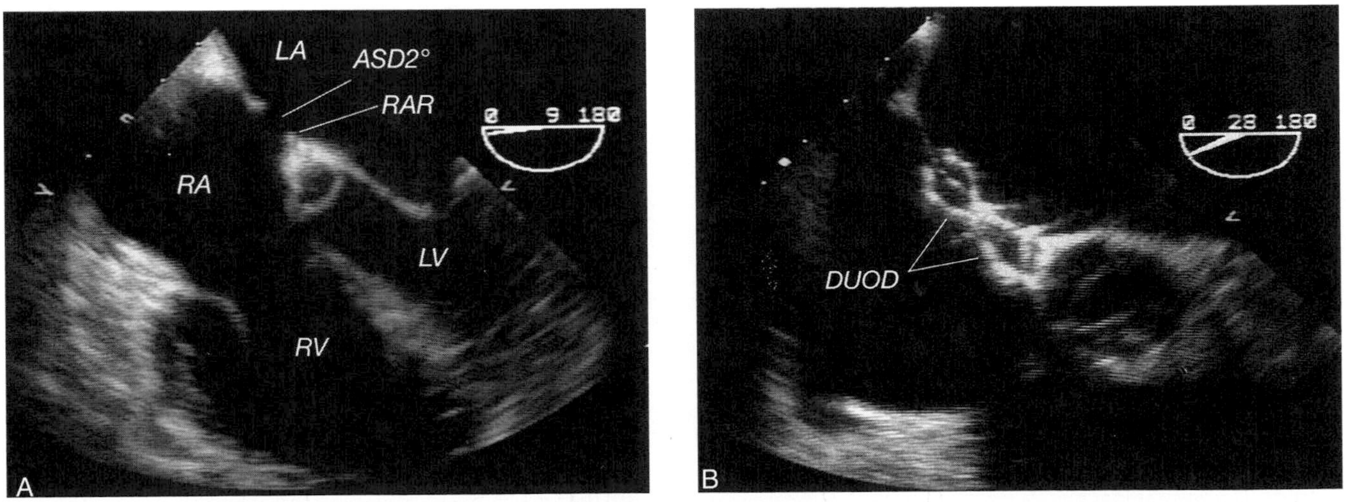

FIGURE 14-2. Transesophageal echo imaging of ASD and occlusion device. **A,** Secundum ASD (ASD2°) with a deficient retroaortic rim (RAR) that was still adequate to allow implantation of a double-umbrella occlusion device (DUOD) **(B)**.

Ventricular structure and function are also surveyed from 0 degrees. The retroaortic atrial septum is well visualized with an imaging plane of 30 degrees. Further rotation to 90 degrees provides a long-axis view of the venae cavae ("caval view"), particularly useful for demonstration of sinus venosus septal defects adjacent to the superior and inferior venae cavae.[6] If a PFO is identified, agitated saline contrast injection is performed to evaluate for right-to-left shunting (if paradoxical embolus is suspected). If the patient is receiving mechanical ventilation, a sustained positive-pressure breath hold, followed by release, mimics the effects of the Valsalva maneuver on the atrial septum and may facilitate imaging of right-to-left shunting. The connections of right and left pulmonary veins to the left atrium are identified.

TEE is invaluable for evaluating the details of atrial septal anatomy before transcatheter device closure. Although devices are constantly being redesigned, stable placement requires an adequate rim surrounding most of the ASD. The rim may be deficient, particularly in the retroaortic region, but if the deficiency lies in only a small "arc" of the circumference of the defect, a device may be stably implanted. The retroaortic region is well seen with a transducer angle of approximately 30 to 45 degrees. Selection of the proper-sized device requires precise sizing of the diameter of the defect. At present, ASDs (but not necessarily PFOs) are usually evaluated with TEE before device placement, and deployment is performed under TEE guidance to ensure position of the device arms on the appropriate septal surface (Figure 14-2, *B*). The role of intracardiac echocardiography in device implantation is promising and in evolution.[7-9]

CMR

CMR imaging is rarely required for assessment of the anatomy of the atrial septum and does not allow estimation of intracardiac pressures. However, CMR offers optimal assessment of RV function. Flow analysis of pulmonary arterial compared with aortic flow offers a quantitative assessment of left-to-right shunting (Q_p/Q_s).[10] Pulmonary venous connections may also be imaged by CMR. If this information is not adequately assessed by echocardiography, CMR may complement other imaging modalities.[11]

Radionuclide Angiography

Radionuclide angiography (RNA) is capable of providing a quantitative analysis of both the amount of left-to-right shunting and RV ejection fraction. However, because echocardiography usually answers the requisite questions, RNA is rarely used in the evaluation of an ASD in our institution.

Cardiac Catheterization

Cardiac catheterization is almost never required for imaging of atrial septal defects. However, if catheterization is carried out for hemodynamic evaluation or intended device implantation, angiography may be performed to assess the ASD. The defect can be demon-strated by following a contrast injection into the pulmonary artery into levophase as it returns to the left atrium. With cameras in the "four-chamber view" (25 to 45 degrees left anterior oblique [LAO], 15 to 45 degrees cranial, adjusted to the individual), flow is seen crossing over the atrial septum. Alternately, contrast may be injected through a catheter that crosses the ASD, reaching to the orifice of the RUPV.

VENTRICULAR SEPTAL DEFECTS

VSDs are the most common congenital heart defect, presenting in the first three decades of life. In contrast to ASDs, their physical examination findings are usually readily apparent. As a result, they are typically diagnosed in childhood and repaired surgically. In some instances, they may be managed medically, if the defect is small or if the VSD resulted in pulmonary vascular disease that contraindicates surgical repair. The anatomy of VSDs will be reviewed, partly because there is no universally accepted classification scheme. Anatomically, the septum can be divided into four or five parts (Figure 14-3). The membranous septum is most easily considered from the perspective of the left ventricle, where it is visualized as a small fibrous portion of the septum lying in the left ventricular outflow tract (LVOT) under the aortic valve. On the right ventricular surface, it is situated beneath the anterior aspect of the septal leaflet of the tricuspid valve, with part on the atrial side and part on the ventricular side of the leaflet. The other components of the septum can be considered as radiating from the membranous

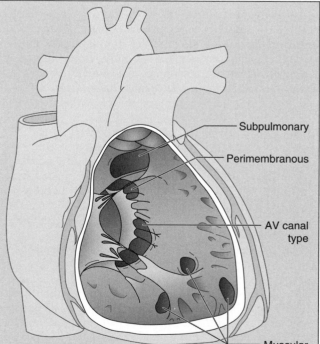

FIGURE 14-3. VSD types. (From Fyler DC. Ventricular septal defects, in *Nadas' Pediatric Cardiology*, Philadelphia, Hanley & Belfus, 1992, p 437, with permission).

septum like the spokes of a wheel.[12] The inlet septum extends from the tricuspid valve to the chordal attachments of the septal leaflet and has a smooth surface. Some divide this more precisely into the "atrioventricular septum," which is truly smooth walled, and the "inlet" septum, which is finely trabeculated but lies beneath the attachments of the septal leaflet. The trabecular muscular septum extends from the chordal attachments to the apex and anteriorly to the septal band. The infundibular or outlet muscular septum lies between the septal band and the pulmonary valve and also has a smooth septal surface.

The term "membranous VSD" refers to a defect in the membranous septum. However, because it usually extends into the adjacent muscular septum, many favor the term "perimembranous VSD." One can further describe the location by specifying the portion of the muscular septum into which the VSD extends, giving perimembranous inlet, perimembranous trabecular, or perimembranous outlet VSDs. "AVC"-type VSDs are a form of endocardial cushion defect, lie adjacent to the tricuspid annulus, and are associated with defects of the atrioventricular valves. "Muscular" VSDs are bounded on all sides by muscular septum (Figure 14-4, A, B). The presence of multiple muscular defects in different portions of the septum should be distinguished from a defect in which blood flow arises from a single defect on the left ventricular surface and is broken up into multiple jets by trabeculations in the right ventricle.

A terminology based on the surgeon's view and approach to the defects has also been suggested.[13] "Conoventricular" VSDs are located at the junction of the inlet and outlet portion of the RV. "Trabecular" defects are muscular and bordered by the trabecular septum and possibly the anterior wall. "Outlet" VSDs lie in the RVOTs and LVOTs. Inlet VSDs occur between the atrioventricular valve annulus and the chordal attachments of the septal leaflet. The practice in our noninvasive laboratory has been to describe the defect by its location in the long axis (base to apex), as well as its anterior-posterior position (e.g., a posterior apical muscular VSD). Defects beneath the pulmonary valve are distinguished, because they result in deficient structural support of the right coronary cusp. This may cause prolapse of the leaflet into the VSD and possibly aortic regurgitation as a result. These defects have been described as "supracristal," "subpulmonic," and "doubly committed subarterial." Perimembranous VSDs may occur as a result of malalignment of outlet portions of the septum, with encroachment on the RVOTs, as in TOF.

The hemodynamic effect of a VSD is determined by the size (and resistance to flow) of the defect, as well as the pulmonary vascular resistance. Small defects offer a very high resistance; the additional resistance to flow offered by the pulmonary vasculature is negligible. Large defects, on the other hand (with diameters close to the diameter of the aortic valve), offer little resistance to flow and allow equalization of ventricular pressures. The relative flow through the pulmonary and systemic vasculature is determined by their relative resistances. Moderately large VSDs result in an increase

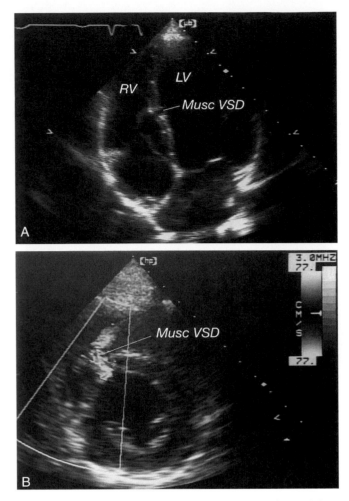

FIGURE 14-4. Muscular VSD. **A,** Midmuscular VSD with apical four-chamber imaging. **B,** Color-flow Doppler interrogation from parasternal short axis demonstrates left-to-right flow.

in RV pressure without equalization. The amount of shunting is determined by a combination of the resistance offered by the VSD and that of the pulmonary vessels.

VSDs typically are seen as pulmonary resistance drops and offers a pressure gradient across the ventricular septum within the first days to months of life. A typical murmur, possibly accompanied by symptoms of congestive heart failure, prompts a referral to a pediatric cardiologist, where a patient may be medically managed with the expectation of some degree of spontaneous closure or referred for surgical closure. Rarely, but most commonly occurring with atrioventricular canal defects in patients with Down syndrome, the pulmonary vascular resistance (PVR) may never drop enough to allow sufficient left-to-right shunting to bring out a typical murmur or other physical findings. This subclinical presentation allows these defects to go undetected, with progression of pulmonary vascular disease until patients finally are irreversibly cyanotic. This scenario and the prevalence of AVC defects in Down syndrome are the basis for recommendations for echocardiographic screening of all Down syndrome patients.

Essentials of Imaging, Unrepaired Ventricular Septal Defect

1. VSD anatomy: location (perimembranous, inlet, muscular, outlet), relation to adjacent structures (subpulmonary), dimensions, morphology (e.g., malalignment, single defect in left ventricle with jet broken up by trabeculations in right ventricle vs. multiple defects)
2. VSD physiology: direction of shunt, gradient, Q_p/Q_s
3. Estimate of right ventricular pressure: secondary to nonrestrictive VSD or elevated pulmonary vascular resistance
4. Estimate of left ventricular volume load: left ventricular dilation
5. Effect on adjacent structures: potential prolapse of aortic valve cusp with membranous VSD or partial closure of VSD with tricuspid valve tissue
6. Effect on pulmonary vasculature: assessment of pulmonary vascular resistance by catheterization, if indicated
7. Associated lesions: multiple VSDs, pulmonary stenosis, PDA, ASD, subaortic membrane, aortic stenosis, aortic regurgitation
8. Full anatomical survey: if not previously performed

Essentials of Imaging, Repaired Ventricular Septal Defect

1. Patch leak: size, gradient, direction of shunt
2. Pulmonary and right ventricular pressures: possible pulmonary vascular disease if a long-standing, large, left-to-right shunt had been present before repair
3. Left ventricular size and systolic function: possible regression of dilation after removal of volume load
4. Possible development of subaortic membrane
5. Progression of previously noted complications (e.g., aortic cusp prolapse and aortic regurgitation)

Echocardiography

Transthoracic echocardiography usually provides all of the information necessary to medically manage, refer for surgery, or to follow patients postoperatively. The exception is the patient with a moderate to large VSD and elevated pulmonary pressures, in whom it is unclear whether the elevated right-sided pressures reflect the unrestrictive shunt flow or elevated PVR. Large defects are typically visualized with a 2D survey. Small defects may only be identified by sweeps with color-flow Doppler imaging. If RV pressure is elevated because of pulmonary vascular disease or presence of a large, unrestrictive VSD, the velocity of flow across small additional VSDs may be low. Color-flow Doppler imaging will be improved if the scale is set to a lower velocity.

Optimal acoustic windows vary with the type of defect. Perimembranous VSDs are typically well seen from parasternal long and short axes, with complementary images from an apical five-chamber view. Inlet VSDs under the septal leaflet of the tricuspid valve may be visualized with long-axis imaging from the apex, sub-costal long axis, or parasternal long axis angled posteriorly. Complementary orthogonal images in the short-axis plane are always obtained. Muscular VSDs are usually well seen from a combination of imaging in long axis from the apex and short-axis imaging from either the parasternal or subcostal windows (Figure 14-4, A, B). If a VSD is suspected but eludes observation, placement of the transducer where the murmur is loudest may facilitate imaging.[14]

Doppler interrogation is performed from whatever location brings the ultrasound beam parallel to the VSD jet, often involving a nonstandard window (e.g., low parasternal). Color-flow Doppler will show the predominant direction of blood flow. Dimensions of the defect are taken with 2D imaging if image quality allows; otherwise, the width of the color-flow jet is reported. Continuous-wave Doppler interrogation allows assessment of transeptal gradient and estimated RV pressure, provided a simultaneous brachial blood pressure is obtained and there are no stenoses from the left ventricle to the brachial artery.

Estimated RV pressure may be verified qualitatively by ventricular septal position. Systolic septal flattening suggests right ventricular pressure greater than one-half systemic, and systolic bowing into the left ventricle suggests suprasystemic right ventricular pressure. Left ventricular dimensions are best assessed quantitatively from the parasternal window. Unless other etiologies of LV dilation are present (e.g., aortic regurgitation), LV dilation usually suggests a chronic, pathological degree of left-to-right shunting warranting repair.

The aortic valve is examined from parasternal long axis to identify potential prolapse of the right or non-coronary cusp into the VSD, with or without associated aortic regurgitation. The VSD may be partly or completely occluded by a "windsock" of tricuspid valve tissue that adheres to the margin of the defect, creating the appearance of a thin-walled aneurysm in the center of the defect. Of import, the LVOT should be interrogated from parasternal long-axis and apical five-chamber views for development of a subaortic membrane. This rare complication carries a murmur that can be confused with a residual VSD and should be sought on all echocardiography evaluations.

Cardiac Magnetic Resonance

Assessment of hemodynamics (gradient or flow) is a necessary component to deciding about the need for VSD repair. This is typically well addressed by echocardiography. Therefore, CMR is typically not a primary method of imaging a VSD. However, CMR offers increasingly accurate and precise noninvasive quantitation of shunt flow (Q_p/Q_s) and may be of assistance when echocardiography is unable to provide sufficient detail.

Cardiac Catheterization

Catheterization is performed when necessary to evaluate PVR, to quantitate shunt flow, when coronary evaluation is required before surgery, or when multiple VSDs are suspected but not sufficiently ruled out by noninvasive imaging. Left ventriculography typically demonstrates the VSD, with differing camera angles depending on VSD location (see Table 14-1). If aortic regurgitation is suspected, an aortic root injection is performed.

TETRALOGY OF FALLOT

Patients with TOF with a wide spectrum of anatomy, physiology, and repairs are seen by the cardiologist caring for adults. Tetralogy involves the combination of an anteriorly malaligned VSD, some degree of stenosis of the RVOT and pulmonary valve, an aortic valve that overrides the RVOT, and right ventricular hypertrophy (RVH). All four findings may be considered to arise from the anterior malalignment of the conal septum, which narrows the infundibulum and the pulmonary annulus, "pulling" the aortic valve anteriorly over the RVOT and preventing the subpulmonary septum from joining the rest of the muscular septum. The equalization of pressures allowed by the large VSD combined with RVOT obstruction result in RVH.

The variation seen in tetralogy lies mostly in the degree of malalignment of the conal septum and subsequent underdevelopment of the pulmonary valve and pulmonary arteries. Acyanotic patients with tetralogy may have nearly normal pulmonary annulus size, and in childhood they may be seen with symptoms of a large VSD, showing congestive heart failure from pulmonary overcirculation. In most patients with TOF, a hypoplastic RVOT leads to a pulmonary valve typically with dysplastic leaflets, resulting in both subvalvar and valvar pulmonary stenosis. The main and branch pulmonary arteries may be hypoplastic or may contain discrete stenoses. In the most severe form of tetralogy, the pulmonary valve is atretic (TOF with pulmonary atresia, or TOF-PA, also called pulmonary atresia with VSD). Pulmonary blood flow is supplied by systemic arterial collaterals. The collateral blood supply often includes a large "ductlike" collateral that arises from the aorta at the usual location of the ductus arteriosus, as well as numerous other collaterals from systemic arteries, most often the aorta (aortopulmonary collaterals, or APCs). These collaterals may join a central pulmonary artery, a lobar pulmonary artery deeper within the lung parenchyma, or may supply lung parenchyma directly. Collaterals and the vessels they supply often have stenoses, which may preserve a patient's candidacy for eventual repair. An APC without stenoses may supply systemic pressure to a pulmonary vascular bed and could induce pulmonary vascular disease over time.

In addition to the anterior malalignment VSD, patients may have additional, muscular VSDs. Imaging of the additional defects may be subtle, because the large malalignment VSD equalizes pressures and reduces the velocity of flow across the defects. In addition, these VSDs may be in the anterior or apical portion of the septum, which may be difficult to discern by echocardiographic imaging in older patients. A right aortic arch is seen in 8% to 20% of patients with TOF. Coronary anomalies are present in from 5% to 19% of patients with TOF. Such anomalies include a left anterior descending coronary artery (LAD) arising from the right coronary artery (RCA), an LAD arising from the right coronary cusp, bilateral LADs arising from the RCA and left main coronary artery, an RCA arising from the LAD, and a large conus coronary artery arising from the RCA. Identification is important before surgery, because the usual incision for enlargement of the infundibulum would transect a large coronary that crossed the RVOT.

Initial surgical palliation of TOF treated cyanosis by augmenting pulmonary blood flow with a shunt from the systemic arterial circulation (Figure 14-5). In a "classic" Blalock-Taussig shunt (BTS), the subclavian artery is transected and anastomosed end-to-side to the pulmonary artery either on the right or left side. Most centers use the modified Blalock Taussig shunt (MBTS)

■ ■ ■

TABLE 14-1 VENTRICULAR SEPTAL DEFECTS: ANGIOGRAPHIC PROJECTIONS

Location	Camera angulation
Perimembranous	LAO + orthogonal RAO
Muscular	
Infundibular septum	RAO
Anteroconal septum	RAO
Midtrabecular septum	LAO
Posterior-trabecular septum	4-chamber
Inflow septum	4-chamber or cranially angled shallow LAO
	4-chamber + reciprocal cranially angled RAO
Atrioventricular septum	

LAO, Long axial oblique: 70 degrees left anterior oblique, 30 degrees cranial; RAO, 30 degrees right anterior oblique; 4-chamber: 30 to 45 degrees left anterior oblique, 15 to 45 degrees cranial.

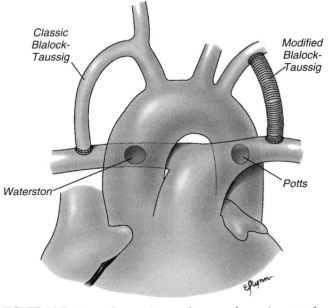

FIGURE 14-5. Types of systemic to pulmonary shunts (see text for details).

consisting of a Gore-Tex tube anastomosed from the subclavian to the pulmonary artery. Two shunts that may still be seen in older patients are the Waterston and Potts shunts. The Waterston shunt connects the ascending aorta to the right pulmonary artery (RPA); the Potts shunt connects the descending aorta to the left pulmonary artery. Both may result in excessive circulation and kinking of the pulmonary arteries. The Potts shunt, in particular, has been associated with the development of pulmonary vascular occlusive disease.

Anatomical repair of TOF with pulmonary stenosis requires patch closure of the VSD, relief of RVOT stenosis, and may require enlargement of the pulmonary valve and patch augmentation of the pulmonary arteries if significant central stenoses are present. In our institution, this is usually accomplished with an infundibulotomy, which provides access to the VSD for patch closure and allows patch augmentation of the outflow tract to treat the RVOT stenosis. If the pulmonary valve is stenotic, the incision and patch may be extended through the annulus (a transannular patch), and pulmonary valve leaflets may be resected if they are thick and dysplastic on inspection. Severe pulmonary regurgitation usually results. Similarly, hypoplastic or stenotic central pulmonary arteries may require patch augmentation. A useful means of assessing the degree of hypoplasia of the pulmonary annulus and arteries in children has been to index the dimension to body surface area (BSA) and to calculate its standard deviation from the mean for BSA, expressed as a Z score. If the Z score is more negative than −2, the annulus is likely to require augmentation. Repair is also performed by means of a transatrial approach.[15]

Repair of TOF-PA is much more complicated and obviously varies greatly with the specific anatomy and age of the patient. The goal is creation of a RV-dependent pulmonary circulation by anastomosing a conduit from the RV to central pulmonary vessels. One key to determination of the ability to repair in TOF-PA is the anatomy of the central pulmonary arteries. If the hilar main and branch pulmonary arteries are well developed and continuous, it may be straightforward for the surgeon to anastomose a valved conduit from the RVOT to the central pulmonary artery. However, if the hilar pulmonary arteries are poorly developed, anatomical repair requires "unifocalizing" the aortopulmonary collaterals to join a conduit that is then joined to the central conduit. Assessing a patient's candidacy requires a detailed definition of a patient's pulmonary artery anatomy, which includes the presence and anatomy of central pulmonary arteries, as well as a detailed evaluation of aortopulmonary collaterals. Each pulmonary vascular bed supplied by an APC must also be evaluated for the presence of pulmonary vascular disease, indicated by pressures within the bed and angiographic appearance. If a collateral duplicates flow provided by an adequate central pulmonary artery, it may not aid pulmonary blood flow but rather create a volume load on the left ventricle (in a manner analogous to a PDA). Such collaterals may be excluded from the final repair either by intravascular occlusion coils or by surgical ligation. On occasion, a patient is seen with a prior decision that no

surgical therapy is possible, yet they have anatomy that allows unifocalization and repair, with subsequent dramatic improvement in their functional capacity. The precise definition of pulmonary artery anatomy allowed by CMR, combined with hemodynamic assessment by cardiac catheterization, has been key to identifying patients with a favorable risk/benefit profile.

Each form of repair or palliation presents several potential anatomical problems that should be sought during an examination. Inadequate relief of RVOT stenosis presents a pressure load to the right ventricle. Leaks at the margin of the VSD patch may be hemodynamically insignificant or may also create a pressure load. Stenoses of the central or peripheral pulmonary arteries (either native or related to the site of insertion of a previous shunt) may either provide a pressure load to the right ventricle or cause unbalanced pulmonary blood flow and ventilation-perfusion mismatching. Free pulmonary regurgitation presents a volume load to the right ventricle, which typically results in ventricular dilation. Over a period of decades, this may also result in ventricular failure and tricuspid regurgitation related to annular dilation. Aneurysmal dilation of the RVOT may occur at the site of the infundibular patch and also rarely in the pulmonary arteries (Figure 14-6). An RV-PA conduit may be compressed against the sternum, causing a right ventricular outflow obstruction.

Essentials of Imaging, Unrepaired Tetralogy of Fallot

1. Anatomical diagnosis: anterior malalignment VSD
2. Levels and degree of sub- and pulmonic stenosis: assessment of RVOT anatomy (dimensions),

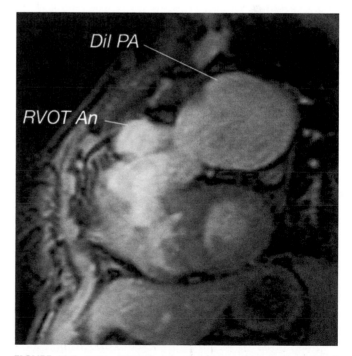

FIGURE 14-6. CMR of RVOT and pulmonary aneurysms in repaired tetralogy of Fallot.

degree of obstruction (gradient), pulmonary valve morphology (leaflet dysplasia, commissural fusion)

3. Pulmonary artery anatomy: size of main and branch pulmonary arteries, presence of central stenoses, with pulmonary atresia, presence of central pulmonary arteries, possible continuity between bilateral branch pulmonary arteries, and dimensions

4. Coronary anatomy: rule out significant branches crossing RVOT

5. Search for additional VSDs

6. Aortic valve: for aortic regurgitation

7. Aortic arch anatomy: evaluate for right aortic arch

8. Detailed evaluation of aortopulmonary collaterals, specifically their full course and anatomy, presence of stenoses, region of lung supplied (and potential overlap with lung supplied by central pulmonary arteries), distal pulmonary artery pressures (indicating likelihood of pulmonary vascular disease), and appearance of pulmonary vascular bed ("pruned tree" appearance suggesting vascular disease)

9. Evaluation of previous shunts: for patency (including leakage through a shunt despite previous attempts at ligation), pressures in the pulmonary vascular bed supplied by the shunt, appearance of the vascular bed, and possible stenosis or distortion caused by the shunt

10. Ventricular function

11. Complete anatomical evaluation

Imaging Essentials, Repaired Tetralogy of Fallot

1. Causes of possible residual right ventricular hypertension
   a. Residual stenoses within RVOT, typically caused by residual obstructive muscle bundles
   b. Residual valvar pulmonary stenosis (gradient, size of pulmonary annulus)
   c. Main, branch, or peripheral pulmonary artery stenoses

2. Causes of possible right ventricular volume overload and dilation
   a. Pulmonary regurgitation
   b. Tricuspid regurgitation: tricuspid annulus dimension, leaflet morphology

3. Causes of possible residual left ventricular volume load and left ventricular dilation
   a. Residual VSD (additional VSD or patch leak)
   b. Residual aortopulmonary collaterals (duplicating blood flow supplied by the right ventricle)
   c. Residual central (Waterston or Potts) shunt
   d. Aortic regurgitation

4. Right ventricular pressure: if elevated, may indicate subvalvar, valvar, or pulmonary artery stenosis, or presence of a large residual VSD

5. Right ventricular size and function

6. Anatomy of repaired right ventricular outflow tract: definition of stenoses if present (dimensions, location within RVOT, pressure gradient), search for RVOT aneurysms

7. Pulmonary valve function: presence and severity of valvar stenosis or regurgitation

8. Tricuspid valve function: severity of TR, mechanism (annular dilation with dilated RV)

9. Evaluation for residual VSD: either secondary to patch leak or presence of additional muscular VSD; gradient across the patch leak VSD (combined with systemic blood pressure allows another estimation of right ventricular pressure)

10. Pulmonary artery anatomy: evidence of stenoses, and their anatomy and severity (dimensions, gradient, and effect on perfusion)

11. Coronary anatomy: if reoperation is considered and either this had not been previously documented (previous echocardiography, catheterization, or operative report) or documentation is unavailable

12. Residual shunts: may be present despite prior attempted ligation

13. Aortic valve function

14. Left ventricular function

Echocardiography

The anatomy of the ventricular outflow tracts and the ventricular septum is typically well demonstrated with imaging from a combination of parasternal and apical windows. In the unrepaired patient, long-axis imaging from either window clearly shows the aorta overriding the ventricular septum (Figure 14-7, *A, B*). Color-flow Doppler imaging demonstrates how right ventricular blood flows through its outflow tract to the overriding aorta, causing cyanosis. After repair, the RV outflow tract is often well visualized from a low parasternal short-axis view (Figure 14-8, *A*), unless the patient required implantation of a RV-to-pulmonary artery conduit. The outflow tract should be assessed for aneurysmal dilation (which may require repair [Figure 14-8, *B*]) or residual obstruction (Figure 14-8, *C*), which may be secondary to obstruction within the ventricle (from hypertrophic muscle bundles) or at the level of the pulmonary valve (if a transannular patch was not used despite an inadequate pulmonary annulus). Typically, free pulmonary regurgitation will be seen if a transannular patch was used for repair. Its appearance may be subtle, because the lack of restriction to regurgitant flow may produce a smooth, laminar color-flow signal that is unusual for regurgitant jets. Pulsed-wave Doppler may be helpful if the color-flow signals are confusing. Visualization of structures deeper within the thorax may be difficult because of calcification of a homograft conduit. Although the subcostal window is often limited in adult patients, it orients the ultrasound beam parallel to the direction of blood flow as it enters the conduit. It may therefore be useful for Doppler interrogation of suspected conduit stenosis, even if the conduit cannot be visualized with either 2D or color-flow Doppler imaging.

RV size and systolic function are assessed with a combination of parasternal short-axis and apical four-chamber imaging. In the unrepaired patient, the right ventricle is notably hypertrophied, in contrast to the repaired patient, in whom the right ventricle usually demonstrates moderate to severe dilation (if a transannular

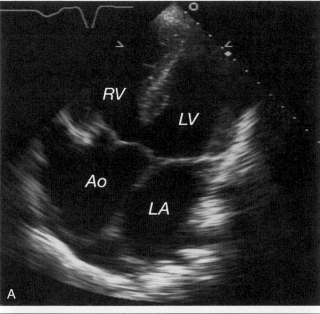

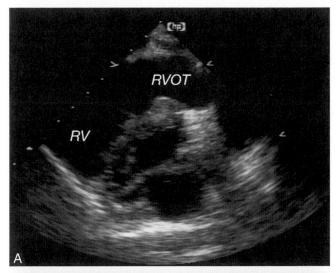

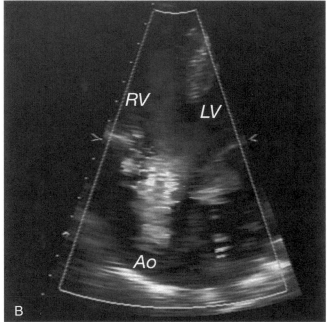

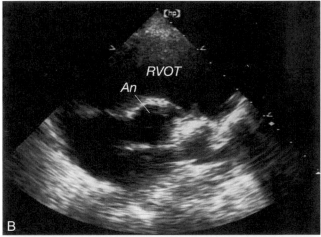

FIGURE 14-7. Overriding aorta in tetralogy of Fallot. **A,** Aorta overriding the right ventricular overflow tract (RVOT). Color-flow Doppler imaging **(B)** shows laminar flow of both desaturated right ventricular and left ventricular blood through the aortic valve, causing systemic desaturation.

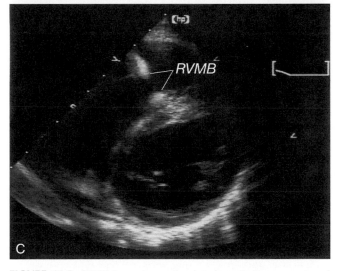

FIGURE 14-8. RVOT in postoperative tetralogy. **A,** Low parasternal short-axis image may give a good view of the RVOT. **B,** An aneurysmally dilated RVOT. **C,** Residual, obstructive right ventricular muscle bundles (RVMB).

patch repair produced free pulmonary regurgitation). Systolic function is assessed qualitatively. The main and most proximal branch pulmonary arteries may be assessed from a parasternal window. However, the suprasternal notch, "looking down" at the pulmonary arteries, may offer a long-axis image of the proximal branch pulmonary artery that allows assessment of the dimensions of a stenosis, although it rarely provides an optimal angle for Doppler interrogation. The mechanism and severity of tricuspid stenosis are evaluated from parasternal long-axis and apical four-chamber win-

dows, as in acquired heart disease. VSD patch repairs are evaluated as described previously. The aortic annulus and root are evaluated for dilation, which may result in aortic regurgitation. Although annulus and root dimensions are typically larger than those seen in unaffected individuals, progressive dilation and increasing aortic regurgitation may require repair.[16-18]

Unrepaired patients who are considered for repair should be assessed for additional VSDs. Reducing the velocity scale and wall filter enhances visualization of these defects, despite the reduced velocity of shunt flow. Although proximal coronary anatomy is routinely evaluated by echocardiography in pediatric patients, cardiac catheterization is almost always required in unrepaired adults. An attempt should be made to visualize previous shunts, even if ligation has been reported, because of occasional failure of ligation. Very large aortopulmonary collaterals may occasionally be visualized from the suprasternal notch ("arch") view, but other imaging modalities are almost always required for complete evaluation.

TEE is not frequently used for evaluation of tetralogy at our institution, partly because CMR imaging has proven so useful. TEE is mainly used in patients with a contraindication to CMR, including patients with a pacemaker or defibrillator, but also if patients have had implantation of vascular coils, which may cause a large artifact in the region of interest. A four-chamber view from 0 degrees yields an initial view of the right ventricle's response to either the pressure load of an unrepaired defect or the volume load usually seen after repair. The tricuspid valve is evaluated for both severity and mechanism (e.g., annular dilation) of tricuspid regurgitation. A transducer angle of 60 to 80 degrees gives a long-axis image of the RVOT that allows assessment of residual obstruction or dilation. Doppler interrogation of the RVOT may be performed from a deep transgastric view, with the probe fully anteflexed to "look back" up the outflow tract. Residual VSDs are assessed from transesophageal imaging, starting at 0 degrees, but with modification as needed to determine the necessary characteristics of the VSD (e.g., site along patch margin, relation to adjacent structures). Apical and anterior muscular VSDs may be best imaged from transgastric short-axis and long-axis views. The aortic valve, LVOT, and aortic root are imaged with usual short-axis and long-axis imaging planes, with measurement of aortic annulus and root dimensions and attention to potential mechanism of aortic regurgitation. Finally, the central pulmonary arteries are assessed from a high transesophageal location, although imaging is often limited.

CMR

After localizing sequences, cine images of the heart in short axis and in the long axis of the right ventricle (equivalent to an echocardiographic four-chamber view) are obtained by use of retrospectively ECG-gated cine fast gradient-echo sequence with segmented K-space filling. Tracing these images and summing the "stack" of "slices" allows estimation of RV dimensions and quantitative description of systolic function, measured as ejection fraction.[19] Phase-contrast encoding of blood flow within the pulmonary artery allows quantitative assessment of pulmonary regurgitant fraction in a patient with repaired tetralogy and free pulmonary regurgitation.[20] Pulmonary artery anatomy, including the presence and course of APCs is well visualized with 3D-MRA (Figure 14-9, A, B).[21] The data set may be reconstructed off-line (after the data has been acquired) to optimally demonstrate APCs.

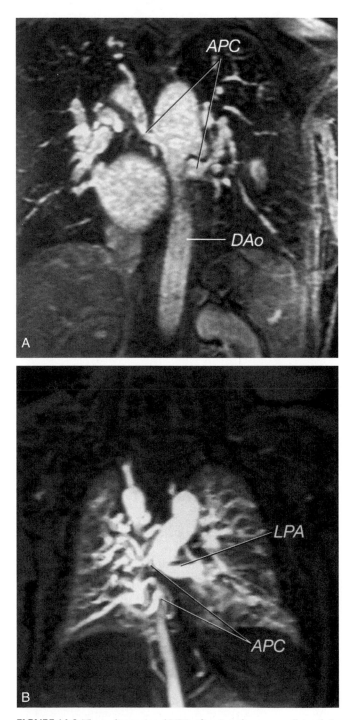

FIGURE 14-9. Three-dimensional MRA of aortopulmonary collaterals in tetralogy with pulmonary atresia. **A,** APCs arising from the descending aorta. **B,** A collateral supplying a central, hilar pulmonary artery. (Images courtesy of Tal Geva, MD.)

Cardiac Catheterization

Catheterization was once our only method of visualizing tetralogy outside of the operating room. Although many pediatric patients no longer require catheterization before complete repair, angiography and invasive hemodynamic assessment may still play an important role in the evaluation of the adult patient with tetralogy. Most unoperated or palliated patients with tetralogy and pulmonary stenosis require catheterization only when anatomy is not seen by noninvasive imaging or if there are hemodynamic questions. Typically, this may involve the anatomy of the coronary arteries (possible anomalous coronaries) or the pulmonary arteries (stenoses, their contribution to right ventricular obstruction, and suitability for patch repair by the surgeon). TOF-PA, on the other hand, routinely requires preoperative catheterization to evaluate the pulmonary vascular bed as mentioned previously. This includes measurement of distal pressures and selective angiography of the collateral vessels. After repair of tetralogy with pulmonary stenosis, the adult patient requires catheterization when (1) RV hypertension is noted noninvasively, (2) symptoms occur, and residual shunting is present, either at the VSD patch margin or at the site of a previously ligated shunt or by way of aortopulmonary connections, or (3) when coronary artery disease is suspected.

Once hemodynamic measurements have been obtained, exchange for an angiographic catheter is performed and appropriate images obtained, typically by power injection through a cutoff pigtail over a guide wire. Angiography of the branch and lobar PAs with degrees of LAO and RAO angulation defines proximal LPA or RPA obstruction (Table 14-2). The most proximal branch pulmonary obstruction may require steep caudal or cranial angulation to open up the junction of the branch pulmonary artery with the conduit or main pulmonary artery. Collaterals that provide a dual supply to a region perfused from the right ventricle may be identified as "negative contrast" (flow of unopacified blood from the collateral "washing into" a stream of contrast opacified blood from the central injection). Angiography of the right ventricle and the RVOT is typically performed with a Berman catheter (a balloon-tipped catheter with side holes proximal to the balloon), with straight AP and lateral camera orientations.

Aortopulmonary collaterals and systemic-pulmonary shunts are accessed retrograde from the aorta with a guiding catheter and floppy wire. Selective angiography of each collateral is performed after hemodynamics have been obtained. Left ventriculography may be helpful as an additional means of viewing a patch leak VSD but is rarely required to demonstrate the unrepaired, anterior malalignment VSD, which is usually well seen by noninvasive imaging.

COMMON ATRIOVENTRICULAR CANAL

Like many diagnoses in congenital heart disease, the term "atrioventricular canal defect" encompasses a very broad anatomical and physiological spectrum, with varying childhood presentations. Patients with a milder form of this defect (primum ASD with a cleft mitral valve) typically are seen in childhood but may occasionally experience few symptoms until their adult years. Alternately, others with the most severe form, a complete common atrioventricular canal, typically are seen either in infancy with congestive heart failure or have pulmonary vascular disease develop, precluding later repair. Although a wide spectrum of anatomical variation exists, the underlying structural similarities unify our understanding of the potential complications and surgical approach to therapy. As with VSDs, there is a wide range of descriptive terminology applied to AVC defects. This discussion will review the underlying anatomy of the defect, introducing commonly used terms. It is worth noting that even the term common atrioventricular canal is not used universally; some prefer the designation "atrioventricular septal defect," whereas others refer to this same group of abnormalities as "endocardial cushion defects."

During the embryological development of the heart, the superior and inferior endocardial cushions grow in from the edge of the primitive heart tube, eventually joining the atrial septum primum and muscular ventricular septum in partitioning the heart into the right and left sides. The lateral endocardial cushions contribute to development of the atrioventricular valves. When endocardial cushion development is incomplete, the resulting defects may include some combination of deficiency of the apical portion of the atrial septum (ostium primum ASD), the basal portion of the ventricular septum ("atrioventricular canal type" VSD), and the atrioventricular valves. Common to all is deficiency of the most basal portion of ventricular septum, causing it to look "scooped out" and bringing the atrioventricular valve annulus closer to the apex. This carries several anatomical consequences. First, rather than the tricuspid and mitral annuli appearing offset, with the tricuspid annulus slightly closer to the apex than the mitral, both seem to be at the same

TABLE 14-2 TETRALOGY OF FALLOT: ANGIOGRAPHIC PROJECTIONS

Location	Camera angulation
RVOT and PA bifurcation	15° left anterior oblique + 30° cranial or 15° right anterior oblique + 30° caudal and Left lateral ± 20° caudal
RPA branches (proximal)	RAO ± 10-15° cranial and Left lateral ± 20° caudal
(distal)	AP ± RAO and Left lateral
LPA branches (proximal)	30-60° left anterior oblique + 30-40° cranial and Left lateral ± 20° caudal
(distal)	AP ± 30° left anterior oblique and Left lateral
VSDs	See earlier sections

level. Pulling the left-sided atrioventricular valve annulus apically also prevents the LVOT from lying wedged in between the anterior portions of the right and left ventricles. Instead, it is pushed more anteriorly. The combination of shortening the left ventricular inflow-apex dimension, while leaving the left ventricular outflow dimension the same and "unwedging" the outflow tract, causes the outflow tract to look narrow and elongated and results in the classic "gooseneck" deformity of the LVOT seen on angiography. Although subaortic obstruction is an uncommon association, this "gooseneck" deformity may exacerbate the obstruction caused by structures in the outflow tract, such as chordal attachments from the atrioventricular valves.

In a less severe form, an atrioventricular canal defect may consist of an ostium primum ASD and a "cleft" mitral valve, described by some as a "partial atrioventricular septal defect." Separate right and left atrioventricular valve annuli are present. The ventricular septum is "scooped out," but there is no VSD because of the close proximity of the atrioventricular valve annuli and dense chordal attachments to the crest of the septum. The anterior mitral leaflet appears to have a "cleft" extending from the free edge of the leaflet to its base against the septum. The cleft mitral valve may be competent or regurgitant. If regurgitant, flow may be directed through the primum ASD, giving the appearance of a left ventricular-to-right atrial shunt. Mitral regurgitation may exacerbate left-to-right shunting through the ASD and accelerate presentation of symptoms.

As the deficiency of the inlet portion of the ventricular septum increases and chordal attachments become less dense, small VSDs occur. Some refer to this form of atrioventricular canal defect as a "transitional" canal. With a "complete" canal defect, not only are there large, unrestrictive, confluent ASDs and VSDs (the common atrioventricular canal), but there is also a common atrioventricular valve. Details of valve morphology vary, but typically there are large anterior (or superior) and posterior (inferior) bridging leaflets extending across the atrioventricular septum (Figure 14-10, A, B). There are two additional leaflets in the right ventricle, which may be referred to as the right anterosuperior and inferior (mural) leaflets and, in the left ventricle, a left lateral (mural) leaflet. The anterior bridging leaflet may be divided and have chordal attachments to the ventricular septum (Rastelli type A). It may also be divided without septal attachments (type B) or undivided and unattached ("floating," type C). This complicated terminology attempts to communicate to the surgeon the elements crucial to planning repair. The valve leaflets may be thin and coapt well but may also be thickened with rolled edges, making repair more difficult. The left-sided atrioventricular valve apparatus typically consists of two papillary muscles that are oriented anterior and posterior, rather than anterolateral and posteromedial. If these are too closely spaced, or if there is a single papillary muscle, a repair in which the "cleft" between the anterior and posterior leaflets is closed may create a stenotic, "parachute" left-sided atrioventricular valve. Valve chordae may also "straddle" the septum, crossing to insert into the opposite ventricle.

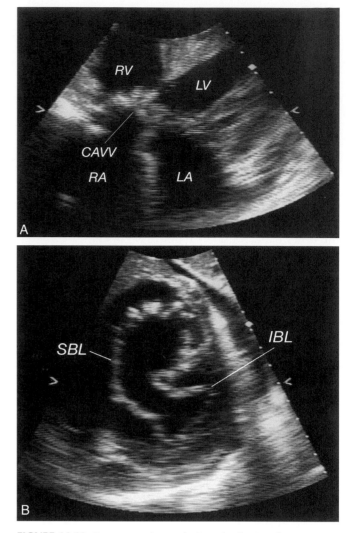

FIGURE 14-10. Common atrioventricular valve in complete common atrioventricular canal. A, The common AV valve (CAVV) is seen from an apical four-chamber window B, Short-axis imaging of the valve from either a parasternal or subcostal window demonstrates the superior (anterior) bridging leaflet (SBL) and the inferior (posterior) bridging leaflet (IBL) of the common AV valve.

Uncommonly, an atrioventricular canal defect may occur with a relatively isolated abnormality outside of the spectrum presented previously, for example, just a cleft mitral valve or a VSD. An AVC defect may also show relative hypoplasia of one of the ventricles, described as an "unbalanced" canal. With severe hypoplasia, a single ventricle approach to repair may be necessary. Patients with AVC defects may also have a large variety of associated abnormalities at all levels: left SVC, secundum ASD, additional VSDs (usually posterior muscular), deviation of the conal septum to the right (creating TOF) or to the left (creating left ventricular outflow obstruction), and coarctation. Down syndrome is commonly associated with canal defects. Up to 50% of patients with Down syndrome have congenital heart disease, and more than half of the affected patients have AVC lesions.

Patients with a primum ASD and a cleft mitral valve may be seen in childhood or adolescence with a murmur and RV volume overload, but if the cleft mitral valve is regurgitant, they may show more severe symptoms of pulmonary overcirculation. When minimal regurgitation occurs, presentation is occasionally first seen during adult years. Patients with complete common atrioventricular canals typically have congestive heart failure in infancy. Pulmonary vascular disease commonly develops in the setting of an unrepaired complete common AVC, in part secondary to the effects of pressure and volume load on the pulmonary vasculature created by the large VSD. Rarely, a patient may have little regression of pulmonary pressures after birth and thereby avoid pulmonary overcirculation and congestive heart failure. However, PVR progresses with time, with increasing cyanosis and eventual exclusion of surgical repair options. Today, repair is undertaken when symptoms are observed or at approximately 6 months of age.

Surgical repair of a cleft mitral valve and a primum ASD involves suturing closed the cleft, with additional annuloplasty if needed, and pericardial patch closure of the ASD, with the coronary sinus commonly draining to the left atrium. Because many surgeons leave the coronary sinus on the left atrial side of the patch, it is essential to identify an anomalous left SVC draining to the coronary sinus to avoid a large right-to-left shunt. At our institution, repair of a complete AVC requires division of the common atrioventricular valve and creation of competent, but not stenotic, right and left atrioventricular valves. The small VSD of a transitional canal may allow closure with simple or pledgetted sutures to draw together subvalvar attachments. Larger ASDs require closure with either a single or two patches extending from the ventricular septal crest to the atrial septum, possibly with resuspension of chordae from the patch.

Postoperative sequelae primarily involve residual ASDs, VSDs, and, more commonly, atrioventricular valve regurgitation. Mild left-sided regurgitation without stenosis is considered an excellent outcome. With longer-term follow-up, progressive atrioventricular valve regurgitation may result from poor coaptation, progressive "rolling" of the leaflets, annular dilation, or dehiscence of the sutures closing the "cleft." Septal patch leaks may also occur. Pulmonary hypertension present before repair may not regress after repair or may continue to progress despite surgery.

Essentials of Imaging, Unrepaired AVC Defect

1. Atrioventricular valve anatomy: bridging leaflets vs. cleft mitral valve, leaflet morphology (potential thickening and rolling of leaflet edges), chordal attachments to the septum, number and separation of papillary muscles (potential for creation of stenotic, parachute mitral valve with closure of cleft), possible second mitral orifice (potentially creating a stenotic double orifice mitral valve with cleft repair, or mitral regurgitation if the bridging tissue is divided)

2. Atrioventricular valve function: competence, degree of regurgitation, mechanism of regurgitation (e.g., regurgitation through cleft vs. poor coaptation secondary to annular dilation, or deficient leaflet tissue)

3. ASD anatomy: possible additional secundum defect or confluent primum and secundum defects

4. VSD anatomy: size of defect, restriction to flow (gradient), possible additional defects (multiple-inlet VSDs or additional posterior muscular VSDs)

5. Left ventricular outflow: possible obstruction, degree, and mechanism of obstruction (discrete fibromuscular ring, chordal attachments, diffuse narrowing)

6. Ventricular size and function: possible hypoplasia of right or left ventricle (unbalanced canal), right ventricular pressure

7. Associated anomalies: left SVC, TOF, anomalous pulmonary venous drainage, coarctation

Imaging Essentials, Repaired AVC Defect

1. Left atrioventricular valve function: degree of stenosis or regurgitation, mechanism (residual cleft, annular dilation, leaflet dysplasia)

2. Right atrioventricular valve function

3. Residual septal defects: location, size, restriction to flow (gradient)

4. Ventricular function

5. Estimate of right ventricular and pulmonary artery pressure: directly (catheterization) or from right ventricular pressure (echo) to assess for pulmonary vascular disease

6. LVOT: possible stenosis

Echocardiography

Long-axis imaging, either from a subcostal window (in a child) or apical four chamber (in an adult), should quickly orient one to the essentials of anatomy and one to the relative size of the ASDs and VSDs, the relation of the atrioventricular valve, and whether the anatomy is more consistent with a partial, transitional, or complete common AVC defect. Short-axis imaging from left parasternal or subcostal windows provides a complementary view and shows the atrioventricular valve to have either a single, common orifice (with anterior and posterior bridging leaflets [Figure 14-11, *B*]) or two separate orifices. Leaflet morphology is well seen from long-axis imaging, particularly from the parasternal window. The apical four-chamber view provides optimal Doppler assessment of valvular stenosis or regurgitation. Sweeping anteriorly and posteriorly is important to define the nature of regurgitation. Regurgitation through a cleft will show as a color-flow jet extending into the anterior mitral valve leaflet toward the septum. Parasternal short axis will usually demonstrate the cleft with 2D imaging (Figure 14-11, *A*). Color-flow Doppler will confirm regurgitant flow and may show a residual leak in a repaired cleft or along the leaflet coaptation margin, resulting from annular dilation. The subvalvar apparatus is examined from a combination of short-axis and long-axis imaging. Starting at the valve leaflets and sweeping apically will demonstrate the papillary

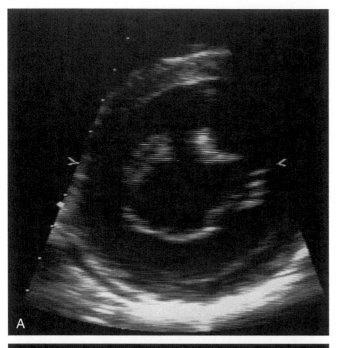

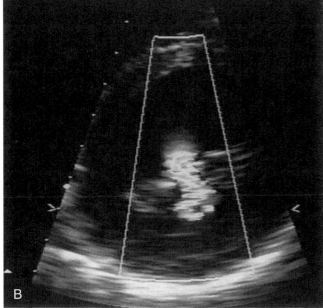

FIGURE 14-11. "Cleft" mitral valve in a partial atrioventricular septal defect. **A,** Parasternal short-axis imaging demonstrates the defect in the formation of the anterior mitral valve. **B,** Mitral regurgitation through this defect is seen with color-flow Doppler imaging.

muscles, which are usually anterior and posterior but may be single or very closely spaced, suggesting risk of mitral stenosis if the cleft is closed. Chordal attachments to the septum may be seen from parasternal short-axis, long-axis, and apical four-chamber imaging. Atrial and ventricular septal defects are imaged with 2D and color-flow Doppler, and the gradient across the VSD is measured. Chordal attachments to the septum or straddling the septum are noted.

After repair, residual septal defects are imaged with color-flow Doppler sweeps from apical four-chamber and parasternal short-axis windows. Gradients are measured, if possible. The LVOT normally looks somewhat elongated (the "gooseneck" appearance described previously) but is interrogated for significant obstruction by Doppler interrogation from the apical four-chamber view. RV pressure is estimated by Doppler assessment of the tricuspid regurgitation jet. In the unrepaired patient, elevated right ventricular pressure may reflect an unrestrictive VSD. However, particularly in the repaired patient or one with a smaller VSD, pulmonary hypertension may reflect increased PVR potentially related to elevated left atrial pressures from a stenotic left atrioventricular valve or to the development of pulmonary vascular disease.

TEE of the adult with an unrepaired AVC defect is most commonly performed to assess RV volume caused by a primum ASD and mitral regurgitation caused by a cleft mitral valve. From an imaging plane of 0 degrees, the four chambers are examined, followed by examination of the atrial septum. The deficiency in the atrial septum is seen adjacent to the atrioventricular valves with a primum ASD. Color-flow Doppler examination of the cleft mitral valve in a four-chamber view of the heart will show the jet of mitral regurgitation extending to the base of the valve, against the atrioventricular septum. Short-axis transgastric imaging of the mitral valve will show the defect in the anterior leaflet of the mitral valve. The focus of a TEE examination in patients with AVC defect after repair is on atrioventricular valve function and residual septal defects.

3D reconstructions have shown promise in pediatric patients and may prove useful in adults with AVC defects.[22]

CMR

CMR is helpful when transthoracic acoustic windows are limited but does not typically give detailed images of the atrioventricular valves or the subvalvar apparatus, which is usually the focus of investigation before or after a repair. Quantitation of regurgitant fraction by phase-contrast cine may complement information obtained by other modalities when assessing an incompetent valve.

Cardiac Catheterization

Cardiac catheterization is most helpful to evaluate hemodynamics, especially PVR, either preoperatively or in long-term follow-up. Catheterization is rarely required in infantile repairs. Angiography may include left ventriculography to evaluate for atrioventricular valve regurgitation, with the frontal camera at 30 degrees RAO and the lateral in the hepatoclavicular (four-chamber) view. The frontal camera will best image the "gooseneck" shape of the LV outflow and any significant atrioventricular valve regurgitation. The lateral camera will demonstrate a VSD and the LVOT.

ISOLATED PATENT DUCTUS ARTERIOSUS

A typical PDA presenting in adulthood arises from the junction of the aortic arch and descending aorta at roughly the level of the left subclavian artery. It passes somewhat cranially to insert at the junction of the main and left pulmonary arteries. The shape of the PDA is highly variable. Often it is somewhat conical, with the larger base at the aortic end, variably tapering to the pulmonic end. However, a PDA may also have a long, thin, tortuous shape or a short, widely opened configuration. When a PDA supplies pulmonary blood flow in patients with pulmonary atresia, it may arise from the underside of the aortic arch.

The physiology and presentation of an isolated PDA vary widely. Most commonly, a PDA that is seen in adulthood is restrictive, with continuous left-to-right shunt flow from the aorta to the lower-resistance pulmonary artery. This results in the typical high-pitched, continuous murmur that envelopes the second heart sound and extends into diastole. The shunt flow rarely causes pulmonary vascular disease, and when pulmonary hypertension is seen in the presence of a small PDA, alternate causes of pulmonary hypertension (e.g., obstruction to left heart inflow from cor triatriatum or mitral stenosis) should be ruled out. A large PDA typically causes significant left-to-right shunting that places a volume load on the left ventricle, resulting in dilation and eventual diastolic and systolic dysfunction. The pressure and volume load caused by a large PDA may also result in development of pulmonary vascular disease and pulmonary hypertension. With elevated pulmonary pressures, the velocity across the PDA may drop, causing the PDA murmur to become softer or absent, and shunt flow may become bidirectional or right to left. When a continuous murmur is heard but investigation fails to reveal a PDA, other etiologies such as a ruptured sinus of Valsalva aneurysm, coronary fistula, APCs, and systemic (chest wall) arteriovenous fistulae should be considered.

Although it is rare, endocarditis is one of the more frequent complications of a PDA, and its relatively high incidence in patients with a clinically apparent (i.e., audible) PDA justifies subacute bacterial endocarditis (SBE) prophylaxis. Closure of a PDA in a patient with a small, but clinically apparent, PDA may be indicated to eliminate the need for long-term prophylaxis. However, the incidence of SBE in tiny PDAs that do not produce an audible murmur is not known. There are no clear therapeutic recommendations, and benefit of closure of the inaudible ductus has not been shown. Rarely, a ductal aneurysm may form, usually at the aortic end of the duct, which may have a larger caliber than the rest of the duct.

Repair may be performed either surgically by way of a lateral thoracotomy and ligation of the duct or by video-assisted thoracoscopic surgical (VATS) ligation, in which the PDA is occluded with an external clip. VATS ligation is typically monitored with transesophageal echocardiography. Devices delivered in the cardiac catheterization laboratory have also been used to occlude PDAs and are the treatment of choice for audible PDAs in adult patients. Vascular occlusion coils may be pushed through a catheter that has been passed retrograde (typically) through the PDA. The coil is extruded from the catheter until approximately one and a half loops have formed on the pulmonary artery side of the duct. The catheter is

then withdrawn as the remainder of the coil loops in the aortic ampulla of the PDA. Residual flow can be addressed with delivery of additional coils. Larger ducts may require use of double-umbrella or double-disk devices, such as those developed for septal defect occlusion.

Imaging Essentials

1. Anatomy of PDA: minimum dimension, general structure (long and tortuous vs. short and wide)
2. Direction of shunting and restriction to flow: gradient across PDA
3. RV pressure
4. Hemodynamic significance of left-to-right flow: LV dilation, retrograde flow in the descending aorta
5. Full survey on initial study

Echocardiography

A PDA is usually best seen from a high left parasternal window. Typically, a PDA is identified first by interrogating with color-flow Doppler. Rarely, the PDA may be visualized with 2D echocardiography after turning off color-flow Doppler. From a high left parasternal short-axis view, sweeping the transducer to the patient's left brings the main and left pulmonary arteries into view (Figure 14-13). If a PDA is present, it usually runs from the descending aorta and inserts at the junction of the middle pulmonary artery (MPA) and LPA. Sweeping the transducer from right to left offers one a sense of the anatomy, demonstrating whether the PDA is thin and tortuous or short and wide. Interrogation by pulsed-wave Doppler demonstrates the direction of flow. The gradient across a restrictive PDA may be estimated by continuous-wave Doppler. A PDA may also sometimes be identified from the suprasternal notch, sweeping right to left with the aorta in long axis.

Apical views may allow quantitative estimation of RV pressure by tricuspid regurgitation jet. Imaging from the usual parasternal short-axis window may demonstrate ductal flow in the MPA moving toward the transducer. It also allows assessment of LV dimensions and septal position. The subcostal window allows pulsed-wave Doppler assessment of flow in the descending aorta, which may have a large retrograde component in diastole (because of "runoff" of systemic blood into the lower–resistance pulmonary circuit). Lowering the wall filter aids in assessing retrograde flow.

TEE is almost never required for evaluation of a PDA. However, intraoperative TEE is used during VATS ligation of a PDA. The PDA is visualized from a high transesophageal position, with the angle of ultrasound adjusted to produce the optimal signal for that particular PDA. Ligation of the PDA with a surgical clip eliminates the color-flow Doppler signal.

CMR

CMR is rarely required to evaluate a PDA but can be helpful in the presence of poor acoustic windows and a high clinical suspicion of occurrence or to evaluate the

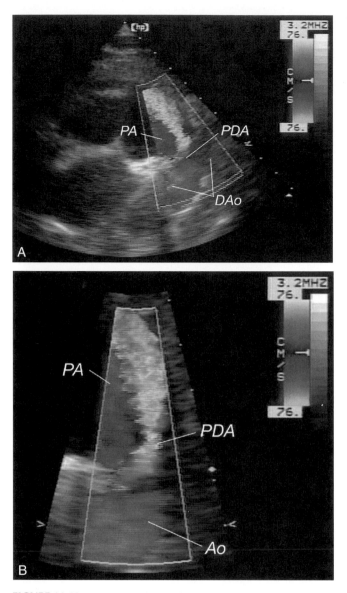

FIGURE 14-12. "Duct view" (high right parasternal) of a PDA. **A,** Color-flow sweep from side to side may allow one to follow the course of ductal flow from the descending aorta to the pulmonary artery. **B,** Magnification of the image is helpful in assessing the duct's minimum dimensions.

adjacent aorta if aortic complications (e.g., ductal aneurysm) or associated anomalies are suspected.

Cardiac Catheterization

Catheterization offers definitive assessment of PDA anatomy and physiology and may also offer a method of closing the PDA. Angiography is typically performed in retrograde approach, either with a pigtail catheter in the descending aorta, just at the level of the PDA, or with a cutoff pigtail spanning the PDA, anchored over a guide wire placed retrograde from the descending aorta into the pulmonary artery. A power injection recorded with cameras initially straight anteroposterior and lateral typically best demonstrates ductal anatomy. Commonly, the PDA is wider where it arises from the descending aorta (the ductal diverticulum), then narrows centrally before

it inserts into the pulmonary artery. Dimensions (diameter, length) are estimated relative to the width of the catheter. Percutaneous closure by occlusion coils or devices may than be carried out according to the practice and protocol of the catheterization laboratory.

TRUNCUS ARTERIOSUS

Truncus arteriosus is an uncommon lesion that usually is seen in infancy and requires early repair for survival. It is, therefore, rare to see an unrepaired adult patient with truncus arteriosus. Those who have survived to adulthood will almost certainly have pulmonary vascular disease and are not candidates for repair. We will, therefore, focus on repaired patients and the long-term complications they experience.

This lesion occurs when the embryological truncus arteriosus fails to divide into two separate arteries, a process that normally occurs at 4 to 5 weeks of development. The aorta may give rise to a short main pulmonary artery from which the branch pulmonary arteries arise (Collett and Edwards type I), or each branch pulmonary artery may arise separately from the aorta with their origins either close together (type II) or widely separated (type III). What was once described as a type IV or "pseudotruncus" lesion (pulmonary blood supply arising from the descending aorta) is now described as tetralogy with pulmonary atresia and APCs. A large, outlet VSD is almost always present. Additional muscular VSDs may also be seen. The single semilunar valve, termed the "truncal valve," usually has three distinct cusps but may have either two or four, and, very rarely, five cusps. Truncal valve cusps may be thickened and dysplastic, causing truncal valve regurgitation (more commonly) or stenosis (less commonly), both of which hasten deterioration after birth. The truncal valve usually overrides the interventricular septum because of malalignment of the conal septum. Aortic arch anomalies are common and include a right aortic arch in approximately one third and an interrupted arch in 10% to 20% of affected patients. When the arch is interrupted, a PDA connects the pulmonary artery to the descending aorta, creating a "ductal arch." Coronary artery anomalies include a left coronary that arises high on the sinus of Valsalva, close to the origin of the LPA, as well as a LAD from the right coronary and a large conus coronary, both of which run across the usual location of a ventriculotomy into which a conduit is placed.

The large typically unobstructive communication between the high-pressure systemic and pulmonary arterial circulations causes a large left-to-right shunt, with pulmonary overcirculation and respiratory distress. This progression often occurs in the first 2 weeks of life as the PVR falls. Infants typically fail from progressive congestive heart failure. Unrepaired survival is 15% at 1 year. Repair is now generally performed shortly after diagnosis or as soon as congestive symptoms appear. Surgery involves excision of the pulmonary artery origins from the aorta with adjacent tissue, which can be sewn into a conduit from the right ventricle. When valved conduits are used, the valves typically degenerate rapidly and may contribute to obstruction within the conduit. Conduit stenosis and regurgitation present pressure and volume loads to the right ventricle.

Imaging Essentials: After Repair

1. Degree of RV-PA conduit stenosis and regurgitation
2. RV pressure: potential pressure load caused by conduit stenosis, pulmonary artery stenoses, or pulmonary vascular disease
3. Ventricular function: RV function (given potential pressure and volume loads discussed above) and LV function (in the setting of truncal valve abnormalities)
4. Truncal valve structure and function: number and function of cusps, mobility, degree of stenosis and regurgitation, mechanism of regurgitation (potential for repair vs. replacement)
5. Pulmonary artery structure: possible branch PA stenoses contributing to pressure load
6. Residual VSDs: possible patch leak contributing to pressure load on RV
7. Sites of aortic repair: patch repair where pulmonary arteries excised
8. Coronary artery anatomy: if conduit revision is considered and prior documentation describing coronary anatomy (imaging study, operative note) is not available

Echocardiography

The truncal valve is examined with a combination of long-axis imaging from the left parasternal and apical five-chamber views and short-axis imaging from left parasternal short axis. Long-axis imaging demonstrates the truncal valve overriding the outlet VSD and the structure (thickening, dysplasia) and mobility of the cusps. Color-flow Doppler provides an estimate of the severity of truncal valve (the neoaortic valve after repair) regurgitation. Parasternal short axis offers a cross-sectional view of the truncal valve, allowing assessment of structure (number of cusps) and potentially the mechanism of regurgitation (e.g., poor coaptation related to a dilated annulus).

Ventricular size and function is assessed from a combination of long-axis and short-axis imaging. The ventricular septum and site of a VSD patch should be interrogated with color-flow Doppler from both parasternal short-axis and the apical four-chamber and five-chamber views. Any VSDs identified should be assessed for size (jet width as flow passes through the defect), preferably in two dimensions. Flow velocity across the defect allows estimation of the gradient between the right and left ventricle. Combined with knowledge of systemic arterial pressure, and in the absence of aortic stenosis, this allows an alternate means of estimating RV pressure. The conduit from the right ventricle to the pulmonary artery is imaged in a fashion similar to that in patients with TOF.

TEE may be useful when transthoracic windows are limited and may offer detailed images of the trun-cal valve when repair is considered, imaging the truncal valve in planes similar to those used for the aortic valve. Imaging is similar to that described for TOF.

CMR

As in TOF, CMR offers advantages in assessing the right ventricle and extracardiac structures such as the aorta, conduit, and pulmonary arteries. Imaging of a repaired truncus is largely the same as that in tetralogy, except that additional imaging of the aortic arch should be performed to evaluate for possible aneurysm formation at the site of repair (as described under "Coarctation of the Aorta").

Cardiac Catheterization

Angiography, when performed, should include left ventriculography from long axial oblique angulation to assess the left ventricular outflow tract for obstruction and residual VSDs. Aortic root injection from the same angle will further demonstrate the truncal valve and allow assessment of the degree of regurgitation. In repaired patients, the right ventricle, conduit, and branch pulmonary arteries are imaged in a fashion similar to that in patients with TOF.

AORTOPULMONARY WINDOW

An aortopulmonary (AP) window is an extremely rare defect. It is discussed primarily to distinguish it from PDA. The AP window occurs when there is incomplete development of the aorta and pulmonary arteries, resulting in a communication between the two. Rarely, the defect is small, restrictive, and circular and may be seen as a small PDA. More commonly, it is large and may have a helical shape as the aorta joins the adjacent main and even RPA.

The patient with an AP window typically is seen in infancy with pulmonary congestion resulting from a large left-to-right shunt. Repair involves sewing a patch of pericardium or Gore-Tex into the defect to separate the two vessels, although they remain contiguous at the borders of the defect. Surgery is usually carried out in infancy to treat symptomatic congestive hart failure.

Imaging Essentials: Unrepaired Aortopulmonary Window

1. Anatomy of defect: location, relation to aortic and pulmonary valves
2. Estimate of pulmonary pressures: PVR
3. Coronary anatomy: assessment for an anomalous coronary artery that might require altered placement of the patch
4. Associated defects: ASD, VSD, PDA, peripheral PA stenoses, interrupted aortic arch, TOF, complex congenital heart disease

Imaging Essentials: Repaired Aortopulmonary Window

1. Assessment for patch leak: degree of shunting if seen
2. Structure of main and branch pulmonary artery and ascending aorta: possible distortion, degree of stenosis if present
3. RV pressure

Echocardiography

The AP window is usually best visualized from parasternal short axis. After assessment of its dimension, the distance from the aorta and pulmonary valves is ascertained. The extent of the defect distally (e.g., possible extension to the RPA) is obtained. The ostia and course of the proximal coronary arteries should also be assessed from the parasternal short axis if the acoustic windows permit.

Subcostal long-axis imaging displays the aorta and pulmonary artery at the location of an AP window. The atrial septum should be interrogated for an associated ASD. Subcostal short axis allows Doppler interrogation of the aorta, which should confirm retrograde diastolic flow seen when systemic blood is allowed to "run off" to the lower-resistance pulmonary circuit. Apical imaging rarely provides useful views of the defect in the adult. Sweeping very anteriorly may provide a view of the defect in a young child. RV pressure can be estimated by tricuspid regurgitant jet velocity but should be systemic or near systemic in the typically large window. Estimation of PVR requires cardiac catheterization. A color sweep should be performed to search for VSDs. Because RV pressure is near systemic, resulting in lower-velocity flow across the VSD, setting the scale to a lower-velocity may facilitate visualization of the VSD. High parasternal imaging allows a search for an associated PDA. Suprasternal notch imaging provides assessment of arch anatomy.

In the repaired patient, parasternal short-axis windows once again give a good view of the main pulmonary arteries and may allow imaging of the proximal branch pulmonary arteries. The position of the septum allows qualitative estimation of RV pressure. Imaging from the apex should allow estimation of RV pressure by tricuspid regurgitation jet, as well as assessment of aortic valve function. Doppler assessment of aortic flow in the aorta or distal arch allows qualitative assessment of the magnitude of a patch leak, assuming there are no other lesions to account for the retrograde flow (e.g., aortic regurgitation, PDA). TEE may provide an additional view of the aorta and main pulmonary artery if transthoracic windows are especially poor, but imaging of the branch pulmonary arteries is limited by the intervening bronchus.

CMR

In the repaired patient, CMR provides imaging of the anatomy of the two great vessels. A patch leak may be identified as a jet of turbulent flow in the main pulmonary artery. Phase-contrast imaging of the descending aorta and branch pulmonary arteries may allow estimation of the degree of left-to-right shunting. CMR is not typically required before repair but may be useful if initial studies suggest questions, particularly regarding extracardiac anatomy (possible coronary, aortic arch, or pulmonary artery abnormalities).

Cardiac Catheterization

Catheterization is rarely required for anatomical definition of an AP window, unless intervention is considered for closure of a residual leak.

EBSTEIN'S ANOMALY

Ebstein's anomaly is an uncommon defect with a spectrum of presentations ranging from cyanosis with low cardiac output in the newborn to a lack of symptoms through adulthood. Embryologically, the tricuspid valve forms as a layer lifting off the endocardial surface of the right ventricle in a process known as "delamination." The anterior leaflet forms first, followed at 3 to 4 months of gestation by the posterior and septal leaflets. It has been suggested that Ebstein's anomaly results from arrested delamination. The anatomical result is a tricuspid valve with septal and posterior leaflets that are displaced toward the RV apex. These leaflets may be dysplastic and fused to the myocardium or atretic. The degree of apical displacement necessary to diagnose Ebstein's anomaly has been defined as 15 mm in children and 20 mm in adults ($8 mm/m^2$, indexed to BSA[23]). The anterior leaflet is typically large and redundant and is often described as "sail-like" (Figure 14-13). It may be fenestrated and have chordal attachments to the ventricular wall, limiting its mobility. Apical displacement of the tricuspid valve results in two ventricular chambers: a "true RV" apical to the valve and an "atrialized" RV that combines with the "true" right atrium to create a large atrial chamber. The atrialized RV is typically composed of thin and often poorly contractile myocardial tissue.

Ebstein's anomaly varies in the degree of apical displacement of the tricuspid valve and in the size and function of both the true and atrialized RV. A true RV with preserved dimensions may dilate as a result of chronic tricuspid regurgitation. Alternately, severe displacement of the tricuspid valve may result in a tiny true RV and a large atrialized RV that joins the true RA. The tricuspid valve is typically regurgitant and occasionally stenotic. The RV typically has a thin wall, and its systolic and diastolic function may be abnormal, with occasional left ventricular functional abnormalities. Displacement of the tricuspid valve into the RV outflow tract may cause outflow tract obstruction. The mitral valve is occasionally redundant and regurgitant. An interatrial communication is present in most patients.

The combination of deficient capacitance and function of an RV pumping chamber, regurgitant AV valve, and inefficient atrial pumping results in elevated right atrial pressures that produce right-to-left shunting across the atrial septum. In neonates with elevated PVR, this can pose an exceptionally challenging and often lethal prob-

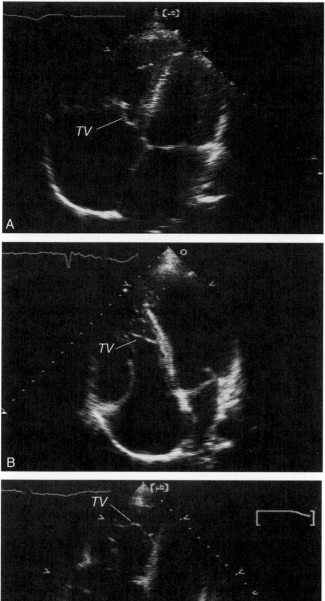

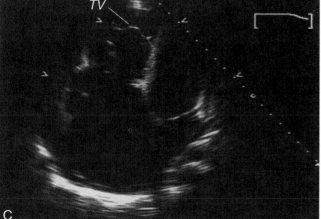

FIGURE 14-13. Ebstein's anomaly. These apical four-chamber images demonstrate mild **(A)**, moderate **(B)**, and severe **(C)** apical displacement of the tricuspid valve. **B,** The "sail-like" anterior leaflet of the tricuspid valve.

lem. However, if the infant can be supported until PVR falls, the infant may markedly improve and have a much more favorable longer-term prognosis. However, many affected patients are asymptomatic or have mildly decreased exercise capacity early in life but have progressive cyanosis or right heart failure develop as RV function fails later in life. Tricuspid regurgitation may

cause a systolic murmur at the left sternal border and even a diastolic rumble, both of which vary with respiration.

The goals and approach to surgery vary depending on the affected patient's age and presentation. There is growing consensus as to the appropriate surgical timing and approach to surgical repair in patients with cyanosis, functional limitation, and Ebstein's anomaly. In an older cohort with functional limitation or progressive cyanosis, Danielson and colleagues[24] describe a repair that involves reduction right atrioplasty, tricuspid annuloplasty, and ablation of accessory pathways, producing a more competent tricuspid valve and a less capacitant atrium. Recently, a side-to-side anastomosis of the SVC to PA (variation of a Glenn shunt) in addition to tricuspid valve repair or replacement has been suggested for some patients in an attempt to decrease the volume load on the RV.[25] As a complementary strategy, when cyanosis is incapacitating but tricuspid regurgitation is not considered sufficiently severe to warrant surgical repair, we have closed atrial communications with transcatheter-deployed occlusion devices with dramatic improvement. The optimal management of patients with Ebstein's anomaly continues to evolve.

Essentials of Imaging

1. Tricuspid valve function: degree of regurgitation or (less commonly) stenosis
2. Anterior leaflet anatomy: size, structure (dysplasia), chordal attachments (potentially creating tricuspid or RVOT stenosis), adherence to myocardium, and presence of fenestrations within leaflet
3. Septal and posterior leaflet anatomy: degree of apical displacement, degree of leaflet dysplasia, adherence of leaflets to underlying myocardium
4. Anatomy of atrial septum: presence of ASD or PFO and degree and direction of shunting.
5. Anatomy of right atrium: degree of overall enlargement, size of atrialized portion of RV
6. RVOT: degree of subvalvar obstruction by tricuspid valve attachments, rare pulmonary valve stenosis
7. RV function
8. LV anatomy and function: possible compression of the LV by a massively enlarged RV, with bowing of the septum into the LV and compromise of LV systolic function, possible primary LV dysfunction
9. Mitral valve function: potential redundant leaflet; degree of regurgitation.

Echocardiography

Echocardiography is the mainstay of imaging to assist in the diagnosis and management of Ebstein's anomaly, in part because most adult patients have not required repair and therefore have preserved acoustic windows. Subcostal short-axis imaging provides an intuitive cross-sectional view of the tricuspid valve leaflets. Its view of the proximal RVOT complements that seen from parasternal short axis. The apical four-chamber view demonstrates the relations and anatomy of the different leaflets of the tricuspid valve (specifically the apical displacement of the septal leaflet and the large, "sail-like" anterior leaflet [Figure 14-13, A, B]). Doppler interrogation allows assessment of tricuspid valve function (stenosis, regurgitation), as well as evaluation of defects (fenestration) within the anterior leaflet. LV function and the degree of paradoxical ventricular septal motion can also be evaluated from the apical window. A sweep for a rare associated VSD should be performed. Parasternal short axis may provide useful cross-sectional views of the tricuspid valve leaflets and their attachments and assessment of mobility. In particular, this window allows imaging of the RVOT and pulmonary valve, any obstruction caused by the tricuspid valve attachments, and a cross-sectional view of the ventricles and ventricular septum. Parasternal short-axis imaging also allows assessment of RV volume overload, the degree to which the septum impinges on the LV, and RV diastolic and systolic function. If the atrial septum cannot be well seen from subcostal windows, scanning rightward from a parasternal short-axis window may demonstrate a potential ASD or PFO, although image quality is limited by the nearly parallel angle of the ultrasound beam to the atrial septum. Agitated saline contrast injection may assist in identifying an ASD.

TEE from multiple imaging planes may be required for the detailed evaluation of tricuspid valve anatomy, particularly in the intraoperative setting. The combination of transesophageal views from multiple imaging planes allows assessment of the tricuspid valve. A long-axis view of the RVOT is best obtained from a 40- to 80-degree transesophageal imaging plane. Transgastric views allow short-axis "slices" through the tricuspid valve and also show the change in ventricular septal position and ventricular function with repair.

CMR

CMR complements other imaging techniques with its ability to quantitate the size and function of the irregularly shaped right ventricle, as well as the degree of tricuspid valve regurgitation. However, at present, it does not offer the precise imaging of tricuspid leaflet morphology allowed by other modalities, such as echocardiography. After localizer sequences, cine short-axis images are obtained and analyzed to give RV and LV dimensions and ejection fraction as described earlier. Phase-contrast cine imaging of the tricuspid inflow and pulmonary artery is performed to assess regurgitant fraction.

Cardiac Catheterization

Aside from preoperative coronary angiography, cardiac catheterization is uncommonly used in the anatomical evaluation of Ebstein's anomaly. However, catheter-based techniques offer a nonsurgical route for closure of ASDs in the cyanotic patient. Angiography of the right ventricle can be performed with a Berman angiographic catheter, typically performed from straight frontal and lateral projections. Left ventriculography may be performed from the 30-degree RAO and LAO views to assess ventricular function and the presence and degree of mitral regurgitation.

PULMONIC STENOSIS

Diagnosis and surgical and transcatheter therapies of valvar pulmonary stenosis have earned great success for affected patients. Anatomical morphology of the stenotic valve may vary. Partial or complete fusion of one or more commissures, with varying degrees of leaflet thickening, and an orifice that may be either central or eccentric may cause variable degrees of stenosis and poststenotic dilation of the main and branch pulmonary arteries (usually the left more than the right). Of note, the degree of poststenotic dilation does not correlate well with the severity of stenosis. Pulmonary valve leaflets may be dysplastic or thickened, with minimal mobility, and may be associated with supravalvar narrowing rather than dilation. Flow through the right ventricle may also be obstructed by hypertrophied, anomalous muscle bundles, which separate the right ventricular sinus from the infundibulum. This creates high-and-low pressure chambers and is referred to as a "double-chambered right ventricle" (DCRV). DCRV is frequently associated with a VSD. Unlike TOF, there is no malalignment of the infundibular septum, and the obstruction to flow through the right ventricle occurs between the sinus and the infundibulum rather than at the level of the infundibulum.

Depending on the severity of stenosis, patients may be seen in infancy with cyanosis or with no symptoms and a murmur noted on routine examination. With critical stenoses, the infant is resuscitated with prostaglandin E to reopen the ductus arteriosus and then brought to the cardiac catheterization laboratory for balloon dilation of the pulmonary valve. With severe but noncritical stenoses, the infant may experience fatigue and dyspnea and less commonly cyanosis because of intracardiac shunting at atrial level. The second natural history study showed that most patients with transvalvar peak gradients of at least 50 mmHg eventuated in surgical repair.[26] Percutaneous balloon valvuloplasty has become the procedure of choice for valvar pulmonary stenosis, unless a patient requires surgery for other cardiac lesions. Balloon valvuloplasty creates a tear either along a fused commissure or within a leaflet and results in stable, mild pulmonic stenosis (a peak gradient of <36 mmHg) in most patients (>85%).[27] Although procedural success was lower with dysplastic valves, the lack of precision in assessment of dysplasia and the presence of commissural fusion (that responds to balloon valvuloplasty) in some dysplastic valves are suggestions that the indication for surgery is a failure of balloon valvuloplasty.

Surgical repair techniques include valvotomy, valvectomy, and placement of a transannular patch (when a small annulus restricts flow). The two latter procedures typically result in moderate to severe pulmonary regurgitation. Although this is typically well tolerated throughout childhood, there is concern about longer-term effects on RV function on the basis of the natural history of TOF repaired with a transannular patch. Surgery is the treatment of choice for DCRV. A transatrial approach typically allows adequate access for resection of obstructive muscle bundles.

Essentials of Imaging, Pulmonary Stenosis

1. Level of stenosis: distinction between DCRV, infundibular stenosis, valvar stenosis, pulmonary artery stenosis
2. Anatomy of pulmonary valve: number of leaflets and commissures, degree of thickening and dysplasia of leaflets
3. Degree of obstruction: gradient across stenosis
4. RV pressure and systolic function
5. Main pulmonary artery structure: "poststenotic dilation" vs. possible supravalvar stenosis
6. Evidence of transatrial shunting: especially right-to-left shunting across a PFO or ASD in the setting of severe pulmonary stenosis or RV failure
7. Associated anomalies: particularly a VSD

Echocardiography

The pulmonary valve and main and branch pulmonary arteries are typically well seen from parasternal short axis, particularly if the transducer is dropped one or two rib spaces (to a low parasternal window). 2D imaging may show "doming" of the valve leaflets or poorly mobile, dysplastic leaflets. Color-flow Doppler interrogation will demonstrate turbulence at the valve, and pulsed-wave Doppler assessment will verify that flow acceleration starts at the level of the valve in valvar pulmonary stenosis. Continuous-wave Doppler allows assessment of the transvalvar gradient. The low parasternal window usually gives an optimal angle of interrogation. The pulmonary valve and its commissures may sometimes be seen in cross section from a high parasternal or a suprasternal notch window. The main and branch pulmonary arteries are imaged from parasternal short axis, and dimensions are noted for each. Slight clockwise rotation may open up the proximal right pulmonary artery. A high parasternal window may allow visualization of a greater length of the branch pulmonary artery.

Subcostal short-axis and long-axis views may provide optimal imaging of the junction of the body and infundibulum of the RV, where hypertrophic muscle bundles could produce a DCRV. RV function is evaluated from parasternal short- and apical four-chamber views. Septal flattening may suggest RV hypertension. RV pressure should be estimated from the tricuspid regurgitation jet and correlated with estimates of the pulmonary valve gradient. A color-flow sweep of the ventricular septum from parasternal short-axis and apical four-chamber view should identify any associated VSD. If RV pressures are elevated, flow across the VSD may be lower velocity and may be better visualized with a lower-velocity scale on color-flow Doppler. Flow across the atrial septum is ideally seen from subcostal long-axis and short-axis sweeps, or from parasternal short axis, angled to the patient's right.

CMR

At present, an estimate of the transvalvar gradient cannot be provided by CMR, and, therefore, it is rarely used in the primary evaluation of pulmonic stenosis. However, CMR is ideal for evaluation of RV function, pulmonary regurgitation, and assessment of pulmonary artery anatomy as described earlier.

Cardiac Catheterization

Catheterization offers a verification of the hemodynamic effects of the stenotic valve, as well as potential for definitive intervention. Right ventriculography is typically performed by use of orthogonal views, including a frontal projection with 30 degrees of cranial angulation and a straight lateral projection. Imaging should provide optimal images of the right ventricle, infundibulum, pulmonary valve, and main and branch pulmonary arteries. If balloon dilation will be performed, the pulmonary annulus is typically measured in the lateral projection, guiding selection of an appropriate-sized dilation balloon.

ANOMALOUS PULMONARY VENOUS CONNECTIONS

Anomalous pulmonary venous connections are usually seen by the adult cardiologist either as a cause of left-to-right shunting in a patient without a septal defect or as a patient with repaired total anomalous connections. A brief review of the anatomical background helps to understand the spectrum of defects. In embryological development, the lungs drain to a splanchnic plexus of veins, which in turn drain to the umbilicovitelline vein and the left cardinal vein of the systemic venous circulation. The splanchnic plexus develops a common pulmonary vein, which joins an outpouching from the left atrium. The developing pulmonary veins may connect anomalously with nearby systemic veins, causing a partial anomalous pulmonary venous connection (PAPVC). The common pulmonary vein may not connect with the outpouching from the left atrium, in which case it will maintain its connections with the primitive systemic veins. This may result in a "vertical vein" coursing superiorly to connect to the innominate vein or, less commonly, to the right SVC or the azygous vein, described as the "supracardiac" form of total anomalous pulmonary venous connection (TAPVC). The common pulmonary vein may also connect to the coronary sinus or, less commonly, the right atrium ("cardiac" forms of TAPVC) (Figure 14-14, A). A vertical vein may also descend, usually passing beneath the diaphragm, to connect with the ductus venosus or some part of the portal circulation ("infracardiac" TAPVC).

The physiology and presentation of anomalous pulmonary venous drainage depend on the nature of the anomalous connections and, most importantly, the degree of obstruction to pulmonary venous drainage. Patients with a single anomalously draining vein may remain asymptomatic and undiagnosed until later in life.

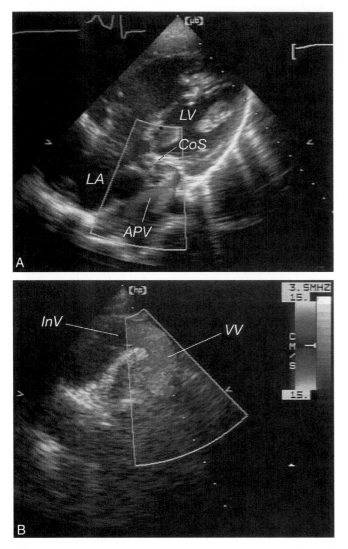

FIGURE 14-14. Anomalous pulmonary venous connections. **A,** Total anomalous pulmonary venous connections (APV) to the coronary sinus (CoS) seen from a modified apical four-chamber view. **B,** An anomalous left pulmonary vein (ALPV) carries flow superiorly to the innominate vein (InV).

However, PAPVC is usually associated with an ASD, and the combined left-to-right shunting of both lesions may produce sufficient RV volume overload to indicate repair. Just as with ASDs, the degree of left-to-right shunting may change with time, as the relative resistances of the native and anomalous pathways change. With increasing left atrial pressure, the resistance to blood flow through the normally connected lung may rise, increasing the proportion of blood flowing through the anomalously connected lobe draining to the right atrium.

In the infant with TAPVC, systemic and pulmonary venous drainage all return to the right atrium. Some blood will flow across an ASD to the left heart, and the rest will be pumped through the pulmonary circuit. Such patients may be seen with congestive heart failure caused by pulmonary overcirculation but with minimal cyanosis. Alternately, obstruction to pulmonary venous return will raise pulmonary venous pressure and PVR and limit pulmonary blood flow. The cyanosis and aci-

dosis that result have no effective medical therapy and must be treated with emergent surgical repair.

The most common form of PAPVC involves drainage of the right upper and middle pulmonary veins to the SVC, often through separate connections. PAPVC is often associated with a sinus venosus septal defect. The entire right lung may also drain anomalously through two or three separate connections to the right atrium, frequently associated with a sinus venosus septal defect as well. The most common form of partial anomalous drainage from the left lung involves drainage of the left upper lobe to a vertical vein that ascends to the innominate vein (Figures 14-14, *B*, and 14-15). The left lower pulmonary vein rarely drains anomalously to the coronary sinus. Scimitar syndrome results from abnormal development of the right lung and includes not only anomalous drainage of the right pulmonary veins to the junction of the right atrium and inferior vena cava but also hypoplasia of the RPA and the right lung parenchyma. Right lung hypoplasia results in dextrocardia, because the heart is "pulled" into the right side of the thorax.

Supracardiac connections are the most frequently occurring form of TAPVR. Obstruction may occur as a result of the vertical vein passing between the LPA and the left mainstem bronchus. Obstruction may also occur as veins connect to the azygous vein or the SVC. Drainage to the coronary sinus was once thought to be rarely associated with obstruction, but more recent reviews suggest otherwise. Infracardiac drainage is almost always associated with varying degrees of obstruction, which may occur as the descending vein passes through the diaphragm, because of the length of the vein, or because of the high resistance of the portal venous system after the ductus venosus has closed.

Repair of PAPVC to the SVC usually involves transection of the SVC superior to the entrance of the highest pulmonary vein. The proximal SVC, therefore, carries only pulmonary venous drainage and is baffled with a pericardial patch to the left atrium by means of the sinus venosus septal defect. The superior portion of the SVC is reanastomosed to the right atrial appendage to reestablish systemic venous drainage from the upper body.[28] This form of repair is believed to minimize trauma to the sinus node and to decrease the risk of subsequent sinus node dysfunction.

Repair of total anomalous pulmonary venous drainage usually involves anastomosis of the common pulmonary vein to the posterior aspect of the left atrium with ligation of the vertical vein. Exceptions include drainage of the common pulmonary vein to the coronary sinus. In this circumstance, unroofing the coronary sinus and patching its orifice and the ASD will return pulmonary venous flow to the left atrium. However, if flow from the common pulmonary vein to the left atrium is obstructed, a direct anastomosis is required. Another exception is drainage of the pulmonary veins to the right atrium, in which case a baffle may be placed to direct pulmonary venous flow across the ASD. The primary concern in longer-term follow-up is occurrence of pulmonary venous stenoses, either at the site of anastomosis or where the individual pulmonary veins meet the common pulmonary vein. Surgical repair of the former is usually straightforward. The latter is usually a difficult management problem and typically responds only transiently to angioplasty, stent implantation, or patch venoplasty, with rapid development of restenosis.

Essentials of Imaging, Unrepaired

1. Pulmonary venous anatomy: site of drainage of all pulmonary veins, possible presence of a common pulmonary vein, connection of pulmonary veins to systemic venous pathway
2. Assessment of pulmonary venous pathway obstruction: possibly at the site of anastomosis of the individual pulmonary veins to the common pulmonary vein, along the route of a vertical vein, or at the site of connection with a systemic vein
3. Anatomy of atrial septum: possible presence of sinus venosus septal defect with PAPVC, size and restriction to flow of ASD/PFO in TAPVC (rarely restrictive)
4. RV structure and function: possible dilation, RV volume overload
5. Estimate of pulmonary artery pressure and/or pulmonary vascular resistance: noninvasively by septal position or tricuspid regurgitation jet or direct invasive measurement

Essentials of Imaging, Repaired

1. Anatomy of pulmonary venous pathway: possible stenoses, especially at junction of individual pulmonary veins with the common pulmonary vein or anastomosis of the common pulmonary vein with the left atrium in TAPVC
2. Assessment of pulmonary artery pressure

Echocardiography

One indication of unsuspected PAPVC may be the presence of RV volume overload in a heart that appears otherwise structurally normal, without identifiable ASD or tricuspid or pulmonary regurgitation. The primary focus of any study in which anomalous connection is known or suspected is identification of all pulmonary veins. Especially with poor acoustic windows, pulmonary veins are usually first identified with color-flow Doppler. Imaging is enhanced by lowering the velocity scale to accentuate the lower-velocity venous flow.

From a left parasternal short-axis window, clockwise rotation (so that the descending aorta is seen in cross section between the two lower pulmonary veins) and sometimes moving up a rib space usually demonstrate the left upper and lower, as well as the right lower pulmonary veins. A "crab view," taken from the suprasternal notch or a high parasternal window, angled downward so that the imaging plane is almost coronal, often shows three or all four of the pulmonary veins simultaneously. If the right upper pulmonary vein is not seen from the "crab view," subcostal imaging may be helpful. Starting anteriorly, with the SVC flow moving toward the transducer, a slow sweep inferiorly will usually demonstrate the right upper pulmonary vein as it enters the superior

aspect of the left atrium. After identifying the location of the pulmonary vein with color-flow Doppler, it can usually be evaluated with 2D imaging.

If all pulmonary veins cannot be identified, sites of anomalous drainage should be imaged carefully. The superior vena cava is interrogated with color-flow Doppler from the right parasternal window and suprasternal notch, looking for anomalous flow entering the vein. The right atrium is well seen from the subcostal long-axis view and may also show an anomalous venous flow signal from its right lateral wall or at the junction of the IVC or SVC. Imaging the innominate vein from beneath the left clavicle may show a vertical vein carrying flow superiorly from the lung field to drain into the innominate vein (Figure 14-14, B). This is contrasted with a persistent LSVC to coronary sinus, in which flow is carried away from the innominate vein down to the heart. A supracardiac connection typically results in a dilated SVC at its right atrial border. Drainage to the coronary sinus will cause a dilated coronary sinus, seen on apical four-chamber (Figure 14-14, A) and parasternal long-axis images. Following the source of flow using a modified parasternal short-axis window may identify it as coming from a pulmonary vein in PAPVC or from the left subclavian vein, if the coronary sinus is receiving a left SVC. The source of flow to the coronary sinus may be further evaluated by agitated saline contrast injection into the left arm. A persistent LSVC to coronary sinus will opacify immediately with contrast injection; an anomalous pulmonary vein should not. Obstructed pulmonary venous flow shows continuous turbulence rather than the usual triphasic Doppler pattern.

The course of pulmonary venous flow is followed from the individual pulmonary veins, through the common pulmonary vein, until its connection with the left atrium, which may be by a direct anastomosis, by way of the coronary sinus, or possibly along a baffle from the right atrium. Stenosis may occur at any of these levels. If flow acceleration is identified on color-flow Doppler, it is interrogated with pulsed-wave Doppler. A phasic venous flow pattern may be replaced with a continuous, higher-velocity flow pattern with significant obstruction. Dimensions of structures that appear stenotic should be obtained. TEE may be used to visualize the pulmonary veins with either of two approaches.[29] From an esophageal position and a transducer array angle of 70 degrees, the transducer is rotated to the patient's right, which should demonstrate the pulmonary veins entering the right atrium in a "Y" configuration. The left pulmonary veins are imaged with a transducer array angle of 110 degrees and rotating the probe to the patient's left. Alternately, with the transducer array at 0 degrees, the probe is rotated to the patient's right. From the level of the pulmonary artery, the right upper pulmonary vein will be seen in cross section. Advancing the probe will demonstrate the vein as it courses toward and enters the left atrium. The right lower pulmonary vein will be seen as the probe is advanced further. The left upper pulmonary vein is identified with leftward rotation of the probe, starting at the level of the left atrial appendage and advancing the probe as before. An anomalous right upper pulmonary vein entering the SVC may be identified by imaging the SVC in short axis (0 degrees) and withdrawing the probe above the level of the right atrium. Connections to the inferior vena cava are more difficult to visualize but may be seen by advancing the probe past the level of the right atrium.

CMR

CMR is ideal for evaluating anomalous pulmonary venous connections.[30] After axial, coronal, and sagittal localizers, the heart is imaged in short and long axis to establish its response to the abnormal flow (e.g., right ventricular dilation and volume overload in PAPVC). Gadolinium-enhanced 3D CMRA provides a data set that can be reconstructed and manipulated to follow the vascular course and connections of the veins (Figure 14-15). Phase-contrast cine assessment of the pulmonary artery and ascending aorta allows quantitation of shunt ratios (Q_p/Q_s) for PAPVR. This technique may offer greater accuracy than cardiac catheterization because of the difficulty, at catheterization, of obtaining an appropriate mixed venous saturation when a pulmonary vein connects to a systemic vein.

Cardiac Catheterization

Cardiac catheterization is particularly useful for demonstrating the hemodynamic significance of a shunt

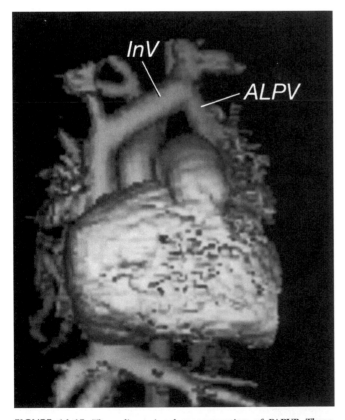

FIGURE 14-15. Three-dimensional reconstruction of PAPVR. Three-dimensional MRA generated a three-dimensional data set that allows models of the pulmonary venous drainage to be built. An anomalous left pulmonary vein (ALPV) drains to the innominate vein (InV; images courtesy of Tal Geva, MD.).

(Q_p/Q_s) in PAPVC and for identifying anomalous connections not demonstrable by echocardiography. Selective angiography of the right and left pulmonary arteries is followed into levophase to demonstrate the path of the anomalous vein. Imaging is performed with straight anteroposterior and lateral camera angles. Catheterization of the repaired patient primarily looks for evidence of stenosis within the pulmonary venous pathway. Selective pulmonary angiography in frontal and lateral projections should identify stenoses. Alternatively, pulmonary artery wedge angiograms may provide more detailed images of the pulmonary veins.

COR TRIATRIATUM

Cor triatriatum is a very uncommon lesion, but one that is occasionally be seen for the first time in adulthood. Embryologically, it results from failure of incorporation of the common pulmonary vein into the left atrium during the fifth week of development. As a result, the pulmonary veins drain into a chamber that was the embryological common pulmonary vein, which may be separated from the true left atrium by either a fibromuscular "diaphragm" (which often has the appearance of a thin "windsock" that bulges down close to the mitral valve [Figure 14-16, A]), a "constriction" that appears to encircle and compress the left atrium and is visible from outside the heart, or a "tubular" connection. Anatomically, the key distinction between this and a mitral supravalvar stenosing ring (SVSR) (Figure 14-16, B) is that, in cor triatriatum, the left atrial appendage is on the same side of the membrane as the mitral valve. In SVSR, the membrane comes between the appendage and the mitral valve. Cor triatriatum is commonly associated with an ASD, which may drain into either the common pulmonary venous chamber or, more often, into the true left atrium. There may also be anomalous pulmonary venous connections, a VSD, or a PDA. "Partial" cor triatriatum occurs when some of the pulmonary veins drain into the common accessory chamber, and others drain normally into the left atrium.

The physiology of cor triatriatum is usually similar to that of mitral stenosis. Restriction to flow from the pulmonary veins into the left ventricle results in pulmonary venous congestion, typically without elevated LV end-diastolic pressures. If an ASD communicates with the pulmonary venous chamber, it may decompress the pulmonary venous chamber. Pulmonary hypertension typically results from elevated pulmonary venous pressures.

The age of presentation in patients with cor triatriatum varies with the severity of obstruction to flow. Surgical repair involves curative resection of the membrane and is indicated for symptoms in the setting of significant obstruction.

Imaging Essentials

1. Structure of atrium and restriction: fibromuscular "diaphragm" vs. "constriction" vs. "tubular" connection; number and size of communications from

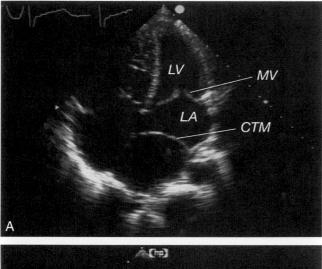

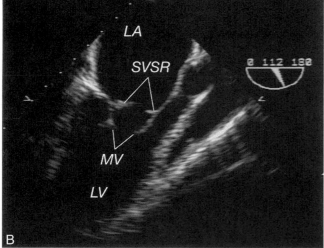

FIGURE 14-16. Cor triatriatum vs. supravalvar stenosing ring. **A,** A cor triatriatum membrane (CTM) in the left atrium, seen with apical four-chamber imaging. **B,** TEE demonstrates a supravalvar stenosing ring adherent to the mitral valve.

common pulmonary venous chamber to true left atrium

2. Degree of restriction to flow
3. Presence of PFO or ASD and communicating chambers: communication with either pulmonary venous or true left atrial chamber
4. Estimation of pulmonary artery pressure
5. Evaluation for associated anomalies: full survey of anatomy, with particular attention to possible anomalous pulmonary venous drainage, left SVC draining to the coronary sinus, VSD, PDA

Echocardiography

Parasternal long-axis imaging reveals the defect dividing the left atrium. Left parasternal short axis allows assessment of pulmonary venous drainage and estimation of RV systolic pressure from septal position. Color-flow interrogation of the atrial and ventricular septum should be performed to assess for associated septal defects. Apical imaging provides the optimal angle for Doppler assessment of restriction to flow across the orifice of the membrane. It also allows Doppler estimation of RV pressure by tricuspid regurgitation jet, which will likely reflect pulmonary pressures. Color-flow Doppler interrogation should also be performed from apical windows to evaluate for apical VSDs. Subcostal imaging provides an optimal look at the atrial septum and an additional view of the defect.

TEE imaging allows a detailed assessment of the structure and function of the defect when these are not well seen with transthoracic imaging. The membrane should be assessed from multiple angles, so that multiple orifices, when present, can be identified. Evaluation of the atrial septum and pulmonary venous anatomy is essential.

CMR

CMR provides an additional noninvasive means of assessing cardiovascular structure that may be particularly helpful if questions regarding vascular structure (e.g., pulmonary venous drainage) remain after echocardiography. CMR will not provide an assessment of degree of restriction to flow other than showing turbulent flow at the site of restriction.

Cardiac Catheterization

Cardiac catheterization is often carried out to assess the elevation of PVR present before surgery. Angiography may be performed by injection into the pulmonary arteries, with imaging continued until contrast enters the left atrium in levophase. Optimal imaging may involve positioning the anterior camera at 30 degrees RAO and 30 degrees caudal, with the lateral camera in the "hepato-clavicular" or "four-chamber" view (25 to 30 degrees LAO and 30 to 40 degrees cranial).

CONGENITAL MITRAL STENOSIS

Congenital mitral stenosis most often presents in childhood, when the greatest challenge in the symptomatic infant is supporting growth until the child is of sufficient size to accept a prosthetic mitral valve. However, some varieties of congenital mitral stenosis are amenable to repair (e.g., isolated supravalvar stenosing ring). We will review the variety of congenital abnormalities that can create congenital mitral stenosis, realizing that it may be an exceptional patient that survives to adulthood without valve replacement. Congenital mitral stenosis most commonly occurs with other defects, typically in the left heart. The most severe end of the spectrum is the hypoplastic left heart syndrome, a surgical challenge that typically requires a single ventricle approach to repair. This discussion will be confined to congenital mitral anomalies that could conceivably present to the adult cardiologist in a patient with two functional ventricles.

Congenital mitral stenosis may result from obstruction above the level of the leaflets (a supravalvar stenosing ring), at the level of the leaflets (e.g., congenital commissural fusion or leaflet dysplasia), or from the subvalvar apparatus (various structural abnormalities of the chordae or papillary muscles). An SVSR or supravalvar mitral membrane (SVMM) very rarely presents as an isolated defect. The ring of connective tissue usually adheres to the atrial surface of the anterior leaflet of the mitral valve but is separate from and basal to the posterior leaflet. Obstruction at the level of the leaflets may be caused by fusion of thickened, dysplastic leaflets, which typically occurs with thickened, distorted chordae. The most common form of congenital mitral stenosis is a "parachute mitral valve," in which normal leaflets attach to short, thickened chordae tendineae, which insert onto a single or two very closely spaced papillary muscles (Figure 14-17, *A-C*). Stenosis is at the subvalvar level, with flow obstructed by the narrow interchordal spaces.

A small piece of tissue joining the anterior and posterior mitral leaflets will produce a double-orifice mitral valve (DOMV) (Figure 14-17, *D*). Both stenosis and regurgitation may result from this abnormal connection, but many double-orifice valves function well and may present as an incidental finding in an adult referred for other indications. Disruption of the connection can produce significant mitral regurgitation. Repair is undertaken when indicated by symptoms or hemodynamics.

Hemodynamic sequelae are the same as for acquired mitral stenosis in adults, including the development of pulmonary hypertension with chronically elevated left atrial pressures. Clinical experience suggests that pulmonary hypertension typically resolves with resolution of the mitral stenosis (i.e., valve replacement or repair). Presentation and course vary with the degree of stenosis. More severe stenoses present with tachypnea in infancy and usually result in mitral valve replacement in childhood or adolescence. However, if left-sided struc-

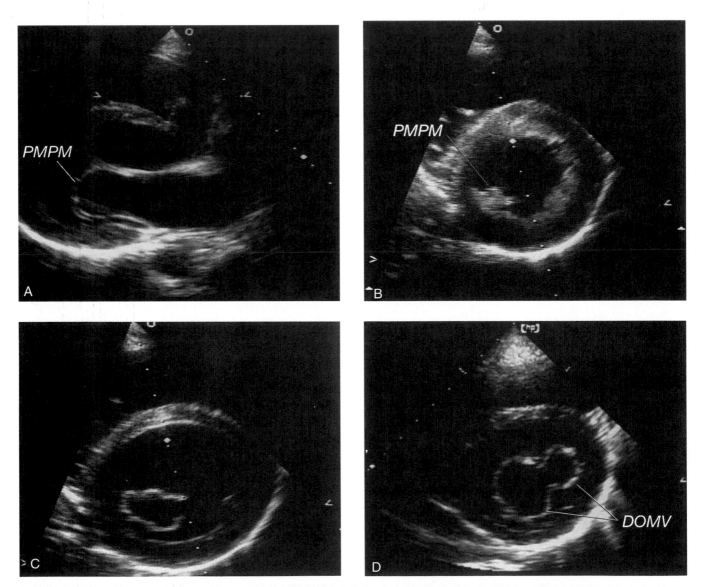

FIGURE 14-17. Parachute mitral valve and double-orifice mitral valve. **A-C,** A parachute mitral valve. **A,** Parasternal long-axis imaging demonstrates how the chordal apparatus "funnels" into a dominant papillary muscle. **B,** Parasternal short-axis imaging shows the dominant posteromedial papillary muscle (PMPM), to which the mitral orifice is oriented **(C). D,** A double-orifice mitral valve.

tures are too small to allow a two-ventricle repair, the patient may instead receive a cavopulmonary anastomosis (single-ventricle repair). Less severe stenoses may result in dyspnea on exertion during childhood or adolescence. If symptoms are mild and pulmonary hypertension does not become excessive, patients may be managed medically.

Surgical repair varies with the anatomical defect. Supravalvar stenosing rings may be resected by the surgeon, restoring improved mobility to the mitral valve leaflets. Because of the frequency of associated defects (e.g., subvalvar aortic stenosis), resection often occurs in the course of surgery for other anomalies. Repair of subvalvar defects is generally less successful. The surgeon may attempt to widen interchordal spaces by judicious resection of tissue but often falls back on mitral valve replacement.

Imaging Essentials

1. Mitral valve leaflet structure: assessment for possible supravalvar stenosing ring, commissural fusion, thickening of mitral valve leaflets with restricted motion, tissue bridging anterior and posterior mitral valve leaflets (creating a double-orifice mitral valve)
2. Papillary muscle structure: possible single papillary muscle or two closely spaced or fused papillary muscles (parachute mitral valve)
3. Chordal apparatus: possible short, thickened chordae with obstruction caused by narrowed interchordal spaces
4. Assessment of restriction to flow: flow acceleration or gradient across the mitral valve
5. Estimation of pulmonary artery pressure: to evaluate for reactive pulmonary hypertension
6. Left ventricular structure and function
7. Associated left heart lesions: coarctation, subvalvar and valvar aortic stenosis
8. Full anatomical survey

Echocardiography

Parasternal long-axis imaging offers an initial view of the mitral valve, supravalvar area, and subvalvar apparatus, often in higher resolution than possible from other windows (Figure 14-17, A). Left parasternal short-axis windows give a complementary view of the valve and papillary muscles (Figure 14-17, B-D). Synthesis of the two views should demonstrate the level and cause of obstruction (e.g., parachute mitral valve vs. interchordal obstruction). Apical imaging offers an additional long-axis view, optimized for Doppler color-flow imaging and assessment of the degree and site of flow acceleration (above, at the level of, or below the leaflets). The LVOT and aortic valve should be assessed for possible subvalvar or valvar stenosis. The aorta should be assessed for possible associated coarctation from both a subcostal window, with the aorta in long axis (for blunted abdominal aortic Doppler flow profile), and from the suprasternal notch (long-axis imaging and Doppler interrogation).

TEE provides ideal views of much of the mitral valve and is particularly useful intraoperatively to further assess anatomy before repair and to evaluate the results of repair.

CMR

At present, CMR does not provide the detailed imaging necessary to evaluate mechanism and therapeutic options for congenital mitral stenosis. However, questions regarding associated lesions may be well suited for CMR assessment.

Cardiac Catheterization

Cardiac catheterization provides additional hemodynamic information that may assist in deciding the need for surgery. Angiography of the mitral valve and its subvalvar apparatus is performed by injection of contrast into the left atrium or ventricle. Cine angiography with the frontal camera at 30 degrees RAO and 30 degrees caudal, and the lateral camera at 30 degrees LAO and 40 degrees cranial, provides optimal imaging.

AORTIC STENOSIS

Congenital aortic stenosis shows a wide range of variability of both structure and presentation. At one extreme is critical aortic stenosis seen in infancy, when closure of the ductus arteriosus removes the only source of systemic blood supply, and the infant is seen with shock. As long as the rest of the left heart has developed sufficiently to supply systemic needs, emergent percutaneous balloon or surgical aortic valvuloplasty can allow the infant to survive with residual mild or moderate aortic stenosis. In contrast, children with mild to moderate aortic stenosis may be relatively asymptomatic until later in childhood, diagnosed when a murmur is noted on routine examination. When the gradient becomes more significant, they may be referred for balloon valvuloplasty, which usually leaves them with mild residual aortic stenosis and some degree of aortic insufficiency, usually mild. Some will ultimately require aortic valve replacement, either with a pulmonary autograft and prosthetic pulmonary valve replacement (Ross procedure) or with a homograft or prosthetic valve. Less commonly, patients may also have been seen in childhood with either subvalvar or supravalvar aortic stenosis, which may have required repair. This wide spectrum of patients, obviously with different issues, can be seen by the adult cardiologist.

Most congenital aortic stenosis (60% to 75%) occurs at the valvar level. The aortic valve develops when three tubercles become excavated to form the separate, thin mobile aortic valve cusps. Incomplete development may result in a valve with incomplete development of the commissures, resulting in a bicuspid (or bicommissural) aortic valve or a unicuspid (unicommissural) valve. Incomplete development or fusion of the intercoronary commissure, which is most common, results in an anterior leaflet (the fused left and right cusps) and a posterior leaflet. Fusion of the right noncoronary or the left noncoronary cusps results in rightward and leftward leaflets.

Subaortic stenosis may result from a spectrum of abnormalities, including a thin, discrete fibrous membrane around the LVOT, a broader fibromuscular ridge, and a "tunnel-like" stenosis below the valve. Subaortic stenosis is usually associated with other anomalies, including complex congenital heart disease (such as the hypoplastic left heart), VSDs, double-chamber right ventricle, and coarctation of the aorta. Interestingly, in multiple instances, the development of subvalvar obstruction has been observed in patients previously followed for other defects (e.g., a VSD). Subaortic stenosis may be seen years after VSD repair with a murmur of increasing intensity (mistaken clinically for a patch leak VSD). Studies have suggested that children who have subaortic membranes develop have a more acute septal-left ventricular outflow tract angle, which may result in turbulence that stimulates endothelial activity and fibroblast development.[31]

Supravalvar stenosis is the least common form of obstruction. It is commonly found in Williams syndrome. The stenosis may occur as a discrete band at the sinotubular junction, or it may extend more broadly up the ascending aorta ("hourglass" form). It may also occur with diffuse hypoplasia of the aortic arch. The coronary arteries may be compromised either by nonatherosclerotic ostial stenoses (caused when disorganized tissue narrows the ostium) or by adherence of the free edge of a cusp to the aorta, causing obstruction to coronary flow. When diffuse hypoplasia of the arch is present, the ostia of the brachiocephalic vessels are often stenotic as well. Supravalvar stenosis may be associated with pulmonary artery stenoses, usually at the level of the branch and peripheral pulmonary arteries. These stenoses may be discrete but are often longer and more diffuse.

Therapy varies with the site and severity of obstruction, as well as with the associated lesions, but in the pediatric population it is typically performed when peak gradients of 50 mmHg are observed with symptoms or when peak gradients rise above 80 mmHg.[32] Percutaneous balloon aortic valvuloplasty results in tearing of the stenotic valve structure at the site of fused commissures or even within the valve tissue itself. Successful dilation typically results in no more than mild to moderate aortic insufficiency. Surgical valvuloplasty usually is performed by commissurotomy of fused commissures. If aortic valve replacement is required, a pulmonary autograft with prosthetic pulmonary valve replacement (Ross procedure) may be performed or a homograft or prosthetic aortic valve implanted.

Subaortic membranes are resected surgically. Extension and adherence of the membrane to the anterior leaflet of the mitral valve or the aortic valve cusps requires further resection. Tunnel-like subaortic stenosis may require patch enlargement of the LVOT, which is done with a right ventriculotomy. A patch is applied to a longitudinal incision in the outlet septum to increase the diameter of the LVOT. Supravalvar stenoses are amenable to patch aortoplasty, with the extent of the stenosis determining the extent of the patch.

Preoperative Imaging Essentials

1. Valve anatomy: number of leaflets, fusion of commissures, leaflet structure (thickening, dysplasia in valvar stenosis or as a consequence of subvalvar stenosis), leaflet mobility, annulus diameter
2. LVOT anatomy: presence of discrete stenoses vs. "tunnel-like" obstruction, extension of fibrous membranes to adjacent valves (anterior leaflet of mitral valve or ventricular surface of aortic valve)
3. Anatomy of aortic root and ascending aorta: supravalvar stenosis (discrete vs. diffuse), poststenotic dilation of ascending aorta in valvar stenosis, and less commonly subvalvar stenosis
4. Degree of obstruction to flow: gradient and location of obstruction (contribution of subvalvar, valvar, and supravalvar components)
5. Aortic valve competence: possible aortic regurgitation because of leaflet dysplasia or resulting from subvalvar stenosis
6. Left ventricular response to pressure load: degree of LV hypertrophy
7. Aortic arch anatomy: possible associated coarctation, diffuse hypoplasia of the arch (supravalvar stenosis), ostial stenoses of brachiocephalic vessels (supravalvar stenosis)
8. Associated right heart lesions: DCRV (subvalvar stenosis), stenoses or hypoplasia of the branch or more peripheral pulmonary arteries (supravalvar stenosis)
9. Coronary anatomy: with supravalvar stenosis to assess for ostial stenoses
10. Full anatomical survey: with initial study or if not performed previously

Imaging Essentials, Postprocedure

1. Residual or recurrent obstruction: site, degree, and mechanism (recurrence of subaortic membrane, thick dysplastic leaflets that respond poorly to attempted balloon dilation)
2. Aortic valve incompetence: degree and mechanism (poor coaptation, leaflet dysplasia, tear in leaflet, cusp perforation secondary to endocarditis or surgery)
3. Anatomy and dimension of aortic root and ascending aorta
4. Change in associated lesions

Echocardiography

Left parasternal imaging typically provides the most detailed imaging of the outflow tract, valve, and proximal ascending aorta. Long-axis views show leaflet structure and mobility and allow assessment of dimensions of each area (LVOT, annulus, root, sinotubular junction, and pro-ximal ascending aorta). If discrete subvalvar stenosis is present (Figure 14-18), its dimensions (distance from the valve, extension into the LVOT) should be noted. Angling the transducer more inferiorly may identify a membrane that extends across the LVOT to the anterior leaflet of the mitral valve. Short-axis imaging (Figure 14-19, A, B) demonstrates the valve orifice

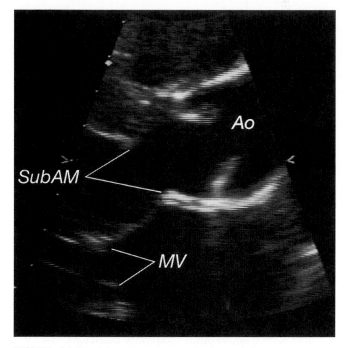

FIGURE 14-18. Subaortic stenosis. Parasternal long-axis imaging demonstrates a subaortic membrane (SubAM) that is seen to attach to the anterior mitral leaflet as well as the interventricular septum.

and fusion of the commissures, if present. Color-flow Doppler imaging in short axis demonstrates the mechanism of aortic valve incompetence, if present. Apical windows offer another long-axis view of the outflow tract and valve. Doppler interrogation shows the level of obstruction and allows calculation of the severity of obstruction by the modified Bernoulli continuity equations, which are discussed elsewhere. Continuous-wave Doppler interrogation is routinely performed from the apex, suprasternal notch, and sometimes the right parasternal window. If gradients vary widely depending on the site of interrogation, more than one value is reported.

The aortic arch is evaluated from the suprasternal notch with 2D and color-flow Doppler imaging. In patients with supravalvar aortic stenosis, particular attention is paid to flow in the brachiocephalic vessels for potential ostial stenoses. An attempt should also be made to image the coronary ostia from parasternal short axis, although this will rarely be successful with transthoracic echocardiography in the adult. The distal arch is interrogated with pulsed- and continuous-wave Doppler signals to assess for possible co-existant coarctation. This is confirmed by abdominal aortic Doppler imaging, which will display a blunted flow signal if significant stenosis is present. Associated right heart anomalies including DCRV and pulmonary artery stenosis may be seen from subcostal and parasternal windows. Color-flow sweeps from the left parasternal and the apical locations assess for associated VSDs or a residual defect (if one was previously closed or if the outflow tract was enlarged with a patch).

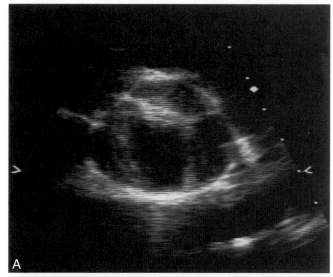

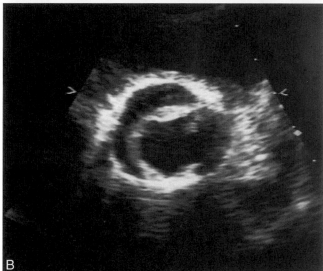

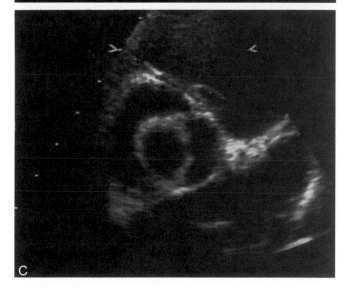

FIGURE 14-19. Valvar aortic stenosis. **A,** A bicuspid aortic valve resulting from fusion of the intercoronary commissure. **B,** The right-noncoronary commissure is fused. **C,** A unicuspid valve, with fusion of both the intercoronary and right-noncoronary commissures.

TEE offers detailed images of the LVOT, aortic valve, proximal ascending aorta, and may offer imaging of coronary ostia as well. Intraoperative TEE is used routinely in valve repair.

CMR

CMR is particularly valuable in imaging the aorta and arch in supravalvar aortic stenosis and presents an alternate means of assessing LV function and the LVOT in subvalvar stenosis. Although the basic morphology of the aortic valve may be seen by CMR, imaging is not sufficiently precise with this technique, compared with TEE, to offer additional insight into mechanisms of valve dysfunction. CMR may assist in the assessment of regurgitant fraction when aortic regurgitation is present (e.g., after valvuloplasty).

Cardiac Catheterization

Cardiac catheterization is carried out as for valvar aortic stenosis, with hemodynamic assessment of the primary and secondary lesion and possible balloon aortic valvuloplasty therapy. Angiography should include ventriculography to assess the LVOT and aortic valve and an aortic root injection, which offers both a complementary view of the aortic valve leaflets and an assessment of aortic regurgitation. Ventriculography is typically performed with the frontal camera at 30 degrees RAO and the lateral camera in the "long axial oblique" orientation. This should demonstrate not only the LVOT but also any associated VSDs. Even if the angiograms appear to present an image of a discrete membrane some distance from the valves (aortic and mitral), such membranes are sometimes found to extend to the valves at the time of surgery, presenting the surgeon with a greater challenge than anticipated. Aortic root angiography may be performed with the same camera angles. An "orifice view," looking at the valve en face, may be obtained from a camera angle of 10 degrees LAO and 40 degrees caudal. Coronary angiography is performed in patients with supravalvar aortic stenosis to evaluate for possible ostial stenoses, as well as in adult patients at risk for coronary atherosclerosis in whom surgery is contemplated. Selective catheter intubation of the orifice may undistort the narrowed proximal portion. Ostial stenoses may best be visualized with nonselective cusp angiography. If there is hemodynamic evidence of a DCRV, right ventriculography should be considered, by use of an angiographic catheter placed in the apex of the right ventricle, with the frontal camera aligned in the straight anterior-posterior plane with some cranial angulation (20 to 30 degrees) and with the lateral camera placed in straight lateral position.

SEGMENTAL APPROACH TO CARDIAC ANATOMY

Discussion of transposition of the great arteries (TGA) and abnormal ventriculoarterial alignments (such as double-outlet right ventricle) requires a more precise system of terminology. The "segmental approach" describes cardiac chambers independently of their connecting structures. The heart is broken down into several "segments" and their connections or, more appropriately, "alignments." The segments include the atria, ventricles, and great arteries. The alignments are the atrioventricular and ventriculoarterial alignments. The atria and ventricles have morphological features that usually allow identification of their morphology by noninvasive imaging. These are related to their location establishing a "set" of descriptions that, along with a statement of alignments, allow the heart to be described precisely. The types of "visceroatrial situs" (anatomical organization of the atria) are *solitus* ("S," normal, with a right-sided right atrium, left-sided left atrium), *inversus* ("I," left-sided right atrium), and *ambiguus* ("A," atrial morphology cannot be diagnosed by imaging).

The ventricles are more easily identified with noninvasive imaging. The RV is identified by its coarse trabeculations, trabeculated septal surface, and numerous papillary muscles that attach both to the septum and the free wall ("septophilic" papillary muscles). The left ventricle, in contrast, has a smooth septal surface, fine trabeculations, and papillary muscles that do not arise from the septum ("septophobic" papillary muscles). Formation of the ventricles involves a "looping" process that normally occurs in a "right-handed" fashion but may occur in an anomalous, "left-handed" manner. The direction of looping can be determined by imagining one's hand with the thumb in the inflow, the palm against the septum, and the fingers in the outflow tract of the right ventricle being imaged (Figure 14-20). If the right hand would fit, the ventricle was formed by "D" looping; if the left hand fits, the ventricle was formed by "L" looping. Finally, the great arteries may be normally related with either the usual anatomy (*solitus*) or normally related in a mirror image anatomy (*inversus*). They may also be abnormally related, transposed, or malposed, so that the aorta lies more anterior than usual and either to the right of the pulmonary valve ("D-transposition"), to the left ("L-transposition"), or anterior ("A-malposition"). Abnormal alignments are described verbally.

Typical transposition of the great arteries is described as "{S,D,D} transposition of the great arteries," whereas the atria and ventricles are normal; morphologically, an abnormal alignment of the ventricles and great arteries is present, with the aortic valve to the right of the pulmonic valve. In contrast, "congenitally corrected transposition" is described as "{S,L,L} transposition of the great arteries" because "L" looping of the ventricles results in ventricular inversion, with discordant alignment of both the atrioventricular and ventriculoarterial connections; and an aortic valve that lies to the left of the pulmonary valve. This "double discordance" results in a "physiological correction" that sends systemic venous blood to the pulmonary arteries. The position of the heart within the chest is described separately and may be described as showing normal *levocardia* (left-sided), *dextrocardia* (right-sided), or *mesocardia* (within the center of the thorax).

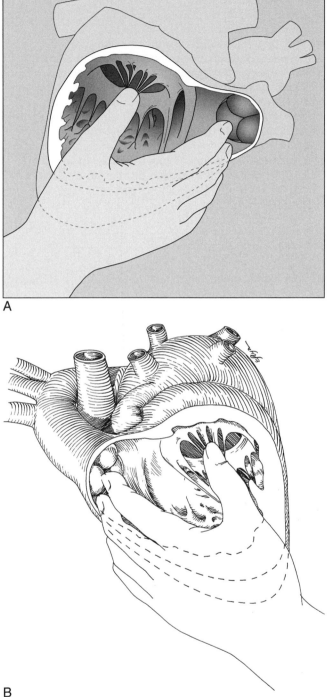

FIGURE 14-20. Ventricular looping. The type of loop is determined by imaging placing one's hand with the thumb in the inflow (atrioventricular valve), fingers in the outflow tract, and palm against the septum. If the right hand fits the observed anatomy (A), the ventricles are "D looped." If the left hand fits (B), the ventricle was formed by "L looping"

TRANSPOSITION OF THE GREAT ARTERIES

Evolution in the management of TGA has been met by tremendous success in the past decades. Lesions that previously were associated with early mortality are now amenable to surgery that leaves patients "repaired"

(anatomically corrected), with good long-term function. An important interim step was the development of atrial baffle procedures (Mustard and Senning) that left patients "physiologically corrected" (i.e., with pulmonary and systemic circuits in series, rather than parallel), but with the right ventricle functioning as the systemic pump. This produced a cohort of adult atrial baffle patients who experience the complications of this physiology. As with most congenital heart disease, patients with transposition cover a wide spectrum of structural abnormalities, with different approaches to categorizing, naming, and discussing them. This discussion will initially focus on patients with normal "D-looped" ventricles and ventriculoarterial discordance, with or without a VSD. The next section will discuss "congenitally corrected" TGA ("isolated ventricular inversion" with an "L-looped" ventricle, or "L-TGA"). This will be followed by a brief discussion of double-outlet right ventricle (DORV), an abnormality that frequently includes transposed great arteries and whose repair may require techniques developed in the management of D-TGA.

D-TGA may occur with a VSD, but other significant intracardiac defects are uncommon. Transposed great arteries result in systemic venous return being pumped by the right ventricle back to the aorta and pulmonary venous return pumped by the left ventricle to the pulmonary artery. If no mixing occurred between these parallel circuits, death would result from hypoxemia and progressive acidosis. Limited mixing may occur through a PFO, an ASD, an associated VSD, or a PDA. Mixing may not be reliable, and enlargement of the atrial communication is frequently performed in the first hours of life by means of a balloon atrial septostomy (BAS).

Atrial Baffle (Mustard or Senning) Repair

The Mustard and Senning atrial baffle procedures create separate pulmonary and systemic arterial circuits. After resecting the atrial septum, systemic venous return is baffled from the venae cavae to the mitral valve with either atrial tissue (Senning) or a prosthetic or pericardial patch (Mustard). The baffle has been described as a "pair of pants," with each leg attached to one of the venae cavae, leading systemic venous blood along the "leg" of the pant, to the "waist," which lies at the opening of the mitral valve, and then to the left ventricle and pulmonary artery (Figure 14-21). Pulmonary venous return enters the atrial chamber that has been excluded from the baffle and flows in between the "pant legs" and around the "crotch" of the pant-like baffle to the systemic tricuspid valve, right ventricle, and aorta. Potential complications of the atrial baffle procedures include narrowing or stenosis of the baffled pathways, which usually involves one of the systemic venous "pant legs." Such stenoses are often amenable to percutaneous dilation and stent implantation. Obstruction to pulmonary venous flow is less common. Atrial baffle repair may also be complicated by development of a patch leak where the baffle was sutured to the atrial wall. Such a leak will act as an ASD, with the direction of shunting determined by the pressures of each atrial chamber (most commonly from

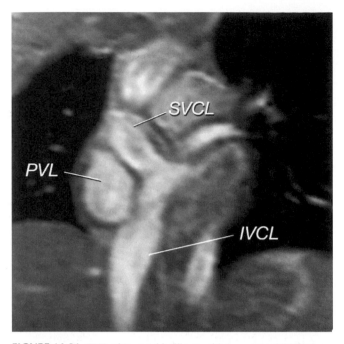

FIGURE 14-21. CMR of Mustard baffle. An oblique coronal CMR image of a Mustard pathway. This demonstrates how the baffle appears as two "pant legs," with the SVC limb (SVCL) and the IVC limb (IVCL) carrying flow from the venae cavae to the orifice of the mitral valve (the "waist" of the pants). Pulmonary venous blood flows between the two systemic limbs to the tricuspid valve, in the pulmonary venous limb (PVL).

the pulmonary venous to the systemic venous chamber). This shunting results in pulmonary overcirculation and a volume load on the pulmonary left ventricle. However, if filling pressures are elevated in the pulmonary left ventricle (which may occur because of dynamic LVOT obstruction, creating functional subpulmonary stenosis), shunting may be bidirectional and may result in systemic desaturation.

Late systemic RV failure is not uncommon,[33] although there has been debate as to how much of this is a result of insults experienced before surgery and how much is due to a mismatch between RV structure and its function as a systemic pump. With failure, the right ventricle dilates, resulting in worsened coaptation of the systemic tricuspid valve, progressive systemic tricuspid regurgitation, and accelerating symptoms and decline in function. Treatment of such patients remains challenging. The "double-switch" procedure (takedown of the atrial baffle and arterial switch) requires either natural or surgical "preparation" of the left ventricle to face the markedly increased afterload of the systemic vasculature. Atrial baffle patients commonly have atrial arrhythmias, which may behave quite differently from typical adult arrhythmias and may result in ventricular dysfunction if sustained.

Imaging Essentials, Status Post Atrial Switch (Mustard or Senning) Operation

1. Systemic venous pathway: presence and degree of obstruction

2. Pulmonary venous pathway: presence and degree of obstruction
3. Atrial baffle leak: location, estimate of dimensions, estimate of shunt flow
4. Systemic (tricuspid) atrioventricular valve function: degree and mechanism of regurgitation (often caused by dilation of ventricle and annulus, resulting in poor leaflet coaptation)
5. Systemic RV function
6. Pulmonic or subpulmonic stenosis: degree of obstruction and mechanism (bowing of septum from the systemic right ventricle into pulmonary left ventricle, causing subpulmonic stenosis vs. fixed stenosis)
7. LV pressure: by MR jet, for estimation of pulmonary artery pressure (accounting for any subpulmonic stenosis)
8. VSD patch: if repair included patch closure of a VSD

Echocardiography

In unrepaired or atrially palliated D-TGA, the right ventricle is the systemic pumping chamber and, therefore, is larger and more hypertrophied than the normal right ventricle. Unless there is significant subpulmonary LVOT obstruction raising LV pressure, the interventricular septum typically bows from right to left, which may contribute to dynamic LVOT obstruction. The other notable difference lies in the outflow tracts and great arteries. In the normal heart, the RVOT, pulmonary valve, and pulmonary artery twist around the LVOT, aortic valve, and ascending aorta. Transposing the two great arteries allows them to follow a parallel course as they curve posteriorly. This produces long-axis images that show the "side-by-side great arteries" characteristic of D-TGA. Corresponding short-axis imaging will show side-by-side cross sections of the two arteries.

The flow of blood through the atrial baffle can be confusing, but apical windows offer some of the more intuitive initial views. The use of color-flow Doppler early to follow the flow of blood also helps to sort out the chambers and to clarify signals that may represent abnormal flow, such as a baffle leak. When images are obtained from a standard four-chamber view, angling anteriorly toward the SVC with slight clockwise rotation will produce a long-axis view of the superior limb of the baffle (the "upper pant leg" along its length) (Figures 14-22, A, 14-23, A). Sweeping more posteriorly into the "middle" of the chambers will show the "crotch" of the baffle, with pulmonary venous flow passing around the baffle (within the pulmonary venous atrium), to the systemic tricuspid valve (Figures 14-22, B, 14-23, B). Continuing inferiorly with slight counterclockwise rotation may (with good windows) demonstrate the inferior limb of the baffle, directing flow within from the inferior vena cava toward the mitral valve in the pulmonary pathway. In our laboratory, an initial anterior-posterior sweep with 2D imaging is performed, followed by a sweep with color-flow Doppler. Color-flow Doppler imaging should be obtained with a lowered velocity scale to enhance imaging of lower-velocity pulmonary venous flow. Turbulence may indicate areas of stenosis along the baffle, which should be further interrogated with pulsed- or

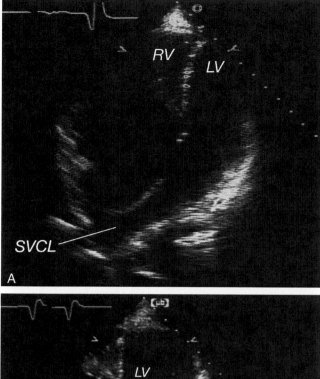

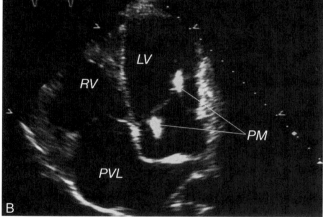

FIGURE 14-22. Transthoracic echo of Mustard baffle. Imaging from the apex with anterior angulation and slight clockwise rotation (**A**) may demonstrate the SVC limb (SVCL) of the Mustard baffle connecting to the mitral valve. Angling more posteriorly demonstrates the pulmonary venous limb (PVL, **B**). **B**, A pacemaker wire is seen crossing the sub-pulmonary mitral valve.

FIGURE 14-23. Color-flow Doppler imaging of a Mustard baffle. Because transthoracic windows are usually very limited, baffle pathways may be visualized only with color-flow Doppler interrogation, which demonstrates the SVC limb (**A**) and the pulmonary venous chambers (**B**). See also Color Insert.

continuous-wave Doppler to obtain a mean gradient. Stenosis is most common in the SVC limb of the baffle but may be seen in any portion of systemic or pulmonary venous baffles. The color-flow Doppler sweep should also be closely examined for baffle leaks and residual VSDs. Baffle leaks typically result in bidirectional flow. Agitated saline contrast injection may be helpful in verifying small baffle leaks that allow right-to-left shunting (particularly if a source of systemic desaturation is being sought).

The SVC and superior limb of the baffle may also be interrogated from the suprasternal notch (SSN), "looking down" the SVC as it carries blood away from the transducer to the heart. Turbulence at the distal portion of the SVC may indicate stenosis where the SVC joins the baffle. Right parasternal imaging may supplement imaging of the superior limb of the pathway.

Subcostal windows in a modified long axis may offer a view of the IVC as it joins the inferior limb of the systemic venous baffle. Pulmonary venous drainage is usually well seen from parasternal short-axis imaging, but flow through the pulmonary venous atrium is best shown from the apical views.

RV size and systolic function are demonstrated in the apical and parasternal short-axis views. RV systolic function is judged qualitatively in our laboratory; CMR is used when more quantitative evaluation is desired. Systemic tricuspid valve function is evaluated from apical and parasternal long-axis and short-axis imaging. Long-axis imaging allows evaluation of the width of the vena contracta. Cross-sectional imaging from parasternal short-axis and potentially subcostal short-axis views may demonstrate the mechanism of tricuspid regurgitation (e.g., poor central coaptation related to dilation of the annulus). The LVOT (in the pulmonary pathway) is evaluated with long-axis imaging from the left parasternal and apical windows. Fixed obstruction should be differentiated from dynamic obstruction caused by bowing of the septum into the LVOT. Doppler assessment from the apex may demonstrate the typical Doppler flow signal of a dynamic outflow tract gradient and allows assessment of the severity of obstruction.

TEE is particularly useful for assessment of the atrial baffle. With the probe rotated clockwise and advanced to the level of the liver and the transducer array at 0 degrees, the probe is withdrawn, identifying the IVC in short axis as it enters the atrium. As the imaging plane enters the atrium, the inferior limb of the systemic venous pathway is seen to baffle the flow of blood to the mitral valve. As the probe is withdrawn to the level of the atrial appendage, the superior limb of the systemic venous pathway is seen and followed superiorly with clockwise rotation of the probe. Both 2D and color-flow Doppler imaging are performed to look for baffle leaks at the suture lines between the baffle and the atrium. Pulsed-wave Doppler interrogation of the systemic venous pathways may demonstrate turbulent, continuous (rather than phasic) flow. The pulmonary venous flow is followed from the pulmonary veins through the pulmonary venous chamber to the right-sided, systemic tricuspid valve. Agitated saline contrast may be used as described previously. The LVOT (subpulmonary) is assessed for dynamic outflow tract obstruction with long-axis imaging and possible patch repair of a VSD is assessed.

CMR

CMR has become a mainstay of noninvasive imaging of atrial baffle patients in our institution because of their frequently limited echocardiographic windows. The greatest limitation is its contraindication in patients with pacemakers in this group with frequent sinus node dysfunction. CMR offers clear views of the venous baffle pathways,[34] and although gradients cannot be estimated at present, stenoses are visualized as turbulent flow at sites of stenosis. If baffle leaks are present, phase-velocity mapping will provide an estimate of the pulmonary/systemic flow ratio (Q_p/Q_s). As discussed previously, CMR provides a quantitative assessment of systemic RV function (ejection fraction) and dimensions, as well as systemic tricuspid valve regurgitation (regurgitant fraction).[35]

ECG-gated fast-gradient recalled echo images are obtained in the short axis for assessment of ventricular dimensions and ventricular function, followed by imaging prescribed in multiple oblique planes in the long axis of the ventricle to visualize the baffle pathways (Figure 14-21). Gadolinium-enhanced 3D-MRA allows visualization of larger defects in the atrial baffle or interventricular septum but may not detect smaller defects. Phase-contrast cine imaging of the pulmonary artery and ascending aorta is performed, if indicated, to evaluate systemic-to-pulmonary shunting.

Cardiac Catheterization

Catheterization is most often performed to assess the hemodynamic significance of findings on noninvasive imaging or to perform potential intervention. Angiography may include contrast injection in both the superior and inferior venae cavae to evaluate for baffle obstruction. If obstruction is seen, dilated collateral veins (azygous and vertebral veins) may carry systemic venous blood around the obstruction. Power injection in the region of a baffle leak may produce flow of contrast through the defect into the pulmonary venous pathway, even though the direction of shunting is predominantly from the pulmonary to the systemic venous baffle (functionally "left-to-right"). Left ventriculography performed in the long-axial oblique view should provide an image of the LVOT and any dynamic or fixed obstruction (which will produce subpulmonic stenosis), as well as identify residual VSDs.

Passing an angiographic catheter retrograde to the systemic right ventricle allows retrograde right ventriculography, usually performed with straight anteroposterior and lateral imaging. Selective coronary angiography to demonstrate possible anomalous coronary anatomy should be performed if an arterial switch is considered (e.g., late atrial baffle takedown with arterial switch).

Arterial Switch Operation

Jatene described the arterial switch in 1975. It was modified in 1981 by LeCompte by bringing the distal main and branch pulmonary arteries anterior to the aorta (the LeCompte maneuver), allowing direct anastomosis without need for a bridging conduit. Initially, high early mortality declined with improvement in techniques of coronary artery transfer. In D-TGA with usual coronary anatomy (68%), the right and left coronary arteries arise from the two sinuses that face the pulmonary artery (dominant right coronary and left coronary arteries dividing into LAD and circumflex [LCx]). In this scenario, the coronary arteries are explanted with a generous "button" of aortic tissue, mobilized, and moved posteriorly to the facing sinus of the previous pulmonary artery (neoaorta). In the next most common coronary artery pattern (20%), the circumflex coronary artery arises from the RCA. More rare patterns include a single right or left coronary artery and intramural coronary arteries. The main significance of these variations lies in planning surgical repair. Development of coronary stenoses is an increasingly recognized potential complication of the arterial switch operation, and the cardiologist investigating coronary anatomy should be aware of potential anatomical variations. Other complications include development of supravalvar pulmonic stenosis at the site of anastomosis and dilation of the root of the neoaorta.

Imaging Essentials, Status Post Arterial Switch Operation

1. Great artery anastomoses: presence and severity of possible stenoses at pulmonary artery and aortic suture lines
2. Aortic root dimensions: possible aortic root dilation
3. Left ventricular function and segmental wall motion abnormalities: possibly related to stenoses of transplanted coronary arteries

4. RV function and estimated pressure: indicator of possible supravalvar PS at site of anastomosis
5. VSD patch: if required at time of original surgery

Echocardiography

The arterial switch operation leaves the patient with near normal intracardiac anatomy. The atria and ventricles do not appear unusual, with the exception that the semilunar valves have an almost parallel orientation. Exterior to the heart, the LeCompte maneuver pulls the bifurcation of the main and branch pulmonary arteries anterior to the ascending aorta, and the aorta no longer loops around the right pulmonary artery.

The proximal great arteries at the level of their anastomoses are seen well from views similar to those used for imaging the normal heart. Parasternal long-axis and apical five-chamber views demonstrate the aortic root and ascending aorta at the level of the anastomosis. A modified parasternal short-axis view demonstrates the supravalvar area of the main pulmonary artery. Because of the unusual orientation of the valve and proximal artery, Doppler assessment of flow acceleration should be performed from a variety of windows, including low left parasternal, subcostal, and apical (because the plane of the pulmonary valve faces more toward the apex in D-TGA than in the normal heart). The main and branch pulmonary arteries should be assessed for stenoses as well.

Biventricular function is assessed as in adults with acquired heart disease, with particular attention to regional wall motion abnormalities, given the potential for compromised coronary flow related to coronary artery translocation. The atrial and ventricular septa are assessed by color-flow Doppler from apical and parasternal windows.

CMR

CMR is ideal for imaging the great arteries, allowing detection of distortion, anastomotic stenosis (more commonly at the pulmonary anastomosis), and aortic root dilation. Cine imaging of the ventricles allows assessment of wall motion abnormalities that may suggest coronary arterial compromise. Protocols for detailed assessment of the anatomy of the proximal coronary arteries are under development. Evaluation begins with short-axis assessment of ventricular wall motion and function. Gadolinium-enhanced 3D-MRA allows evaluation of the great arteries. Fast-spin echo sequences may be useful for evaluation of proximal coronary artery anatomy.

DOUBLE OUTLET RIGHT VENTRICLE

In DORV complexes, both great arteries arise from the right ventricle. However, the actual relations of the great arteries show great variation: side-by-side (with the aorta to the right, the "classic" form); aorta rightward and anterior; aorta leftward and anterior; and aorta rightward and posterior. DORV complexes almost always include a VSD, adding to variation. The VSD may be subaortic, subpul-

monary, "doubly committed" (i.e., adjacent to both great arteries), or "remote" from the great arteries (usually either a muscular or inlet VSD). If a VSD lies immediately beneath the aorta, the defect could be repaired by sewing a patch or baffle that would lead LV blood to the aorta, restoring normal physiology. Alternately, if the defect were immediately beneath the pulmonic valve (e.g., the Taussig-Bing anomaly), one might achieve the same physiology with an arterial switch operation, baffling blood from the VSD to the neoaortic valve. However, if the VSD is not immediately beneath the aortic valve, one runs the risk that, if the distance between the VSD and aorta was too great, placing an intraventricular baffle could obstruct flow within the RVOT. An alternative repair includes division of the main pulmonary artery and reanastomosis to the right ventricle either with an interposed conduit (Rastelli procedure) or directly without a pulmonic valve with a pericardial patch (Reparation a l'Etage Ventriculaire, or REV[36]). If significant subaortic stenosis exists, detaching the proximal main pulmonary artery from the branch pulmonary arteries and joining it with the aorta allows creation of an aortic outflow that uses both semilunar valves (the Damus-Kaye-Stansel anastomosis), with the branch pulmonary arteries connected to the right ventricle by a conduit. Possible chordal attachments of the mitral valve to the septum affect surgical options as well. These more complicated forms of DORV could even require a different approach to repair, such as pursuit of a single-ventricle form of palliation.

The clinical presentation of DORV reflects the wide spectrum of physiology accompanying different anatomical variations. These include presentations typical of (1) VSD (if the VSD is subaortic, so that the streaming of blood preserves a normal physiology), (2) TOF (if there is pulmonic stenosis), (3) TGA (if the VSD is subpulmonic, so that LV blood streams to the pulmonary artery), or (4) single ventricle (if the VSD is doubly or noncommitted, resulting in complete mixing of systemic and pulmonary venous blood). Most cardiac lesions can be associated with a DORV, including abnormal systemic or pulmonary venous connections, AVC defects, multiple VSDs, pulmonary and subpulmonary stenosis, subaortic stenosis, coarctation of the aorta, interrupted aortic arch, and coronary anomalies.

Most patients with DORV are seen for repair in childhood; therefore, imaging of the adult with DORV emphasizes assessment of the repair. Long-term sequelae vary with the underlying anatomy and type of repair and can be seen in all parts of the cardiopulmonary circuit. Tricuspid valve chordae sometimes require division and reattachment as part of a repair, potentially compromising tricuspid valve function. Pulmonary and subpulmonary stenosis may progress or recur at multiple levels. Development of a double-chambered right ventricle has been described. A large intraventricular baffle might create subpulmonic obstruction as could infundibular stenosis that was inadequately relieved at the time of surgical repair. Right ventricle-to-pulmonary artery conduits develop stenotic obstruction. A "tetralogy-like" repair (with a right ventriculotomy that transected the pulmonary artery to relieve pulmonary stenosis) might leave an affected patient with free pulmonary regurgitation. A left ventricle to aorta baffle/patch may be obstructed either at the level of the VSD (which will sometimes grow smaller with time) or within the baffle channel. Conversely, the VSD patch may have leaks, allowing a left-to-right shunt, particularly if growth places tension on the patch. Associated defects also require follow-up evaluation.

Imaging Essentials, Status Post Repair of DORV

1. VSD baffle/patch: potential obstruction, level of obstruction (VSD, within the baffle), leaks (location, size, direction of flow, evidence of volume load on left ventricle).
2. RV outflow: possible obstruction by DCRV, VSD baffle/patch, or infundibular stenosis; RV-PA conduit obstruction
3. Tricuspid valve function: particularly if chordal reattachment required in repair
4. Pulmonary valve function: particularly if original anatomy included pulmonary stenosis, and transannular patch was required
5. Aortic valve function
6. Biventricular function: response to pressure and/or volume load presented by various lesions
7. Aortic arch anatomy: particularly if associated coarctation or interrupted arch was repaired

Echocardiography

Given the variation in anatomy, the optimal imaging needs to be individualized to a patient's anatomy. General recommendations follow. The VSD patch initially may be interrogated from parasternal windows to assess baffle leaks. Evaluation of flow through the baffle to the aortic valve is performed from an apical window with Doppler interrogation, although acoustic shadowing from the VSD patch may limit imaging at the level of the aortic valve. Suprasternal notch imaging may be helpful for assessment of the aortic valve. Subcostal imaging may demonstrate patch leak VSDs typically at the inferior margin of the patch. Subcostal short-axis imaging may also provide an optimal angle for Doppler assessment of the pulmonary artery. The pulmonary artery may also be well seen from apical and parasternal views, depending on its orientation. Ventricular function is assessed from parasternal short-axis and apical windows. Tricuspid valve and mitral valve function is assessed from the usual acoustic windows.

CMR

CMR offers images that can be invaluable in understanding intracardiac and extracardiac anatomy and the relations of various structures in patients with DORV. The ability to orient the imaging planes in an infinite variety of angles also allows a detailed assessment of structures that may be critical to assessment of surgical options.

CMR is, at most, complementary to other imaging modalities in that it does not provide the anatomical detail to allow identification of valve chordae or their attachments, which may preclude certain surgical options. Techniques that provide quantitative assessment of the effects of stenoses on blood flow are under development and not widely available.

Cine fast gradient echo sequences are obtained in short axis for assessment of ventricular structure and function. Cine imaging is then performed in oblique long-axis planes of appropriate structures, such as an intraventricular baffle. Gadolinium-enhanced 3D-MRA allows identification of larger baffle leaks or residual VSDs. Phase-contrast cine imaging of the aorta and pulmonary arteries is performed if noninvasive assessment of pulmonary/systemic flow ratios is indicated (e.g., to quantitate the severity of a baffle leak).

Cardiac Catheterization

Catheterization provides hemodynamic information on the significance of stenoses, PVR, and assessments of shunts (e.g., patch leaks) that may be present. It also provides an alternative mode of imaging, which complements echocardiography, particularly if CMR is not available. Angiography of the right ventricle and the origins of the great arteries is usually accomplished by beginning with angle choices of straight frontal and lateral camera positions, with modification as necessary depending on individual anatomy. The lateral view may be particularly helpful in identifying intraventricular obstructions. Angiography of conduits, the main pulmonary artery, and its tributaries is similar to techniques used for patients with TOF. Left ventriculography is typically performed from a "long axial oblique" orientation. This should demonstrate VSD patch leaks and any stenoses along the VSD baffle. Aortic root angiography is indicated if there are questions of aortic valve incompetence or aortic root dilation. Aortic arch angiography should be performed if hemodynamic assessment raises the possibility of stenoses or if coarctation or an interrupted aortic arch was previously diagnosed or repaired.

COARCTATION OF THE AORTA

Coarctations typically occur at the junction of the aortic arch and the descending aorta, at the level of the insertion of the ductus arteriosus. The subclavian artery usually arises proximal to the coarctation segment and is dilated. Occasionally, the subclavian artery arises at the level of the coarctation, with compromised perfusion to the left arm. Anatomically, the coarctation typically is a "shelf" of tissue in the posterolateral aorta, which some believe represents ductal tissue that has encircled or "lassoed" the aorta. Externally, the aorta appears to be "indented" in the area of the coarctation (Figure 14-24). There is often poststenotic dilation of the descending aorta. The prominent knob, indented coarctation, and dilated descending aorta may give the upper left cardiac silhouette the contour of a "3" on chest x-ray. In the neonate, the aorta proximal to the coarctation (distal

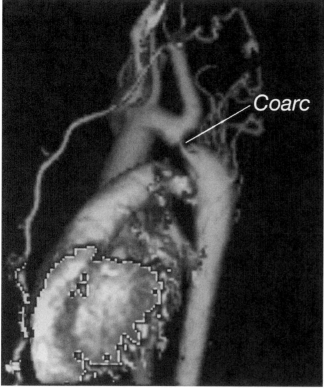

Coarc

FIGURE 14-24. CMR of coarctation. A reconstruction of data obtained from a three-dimensional data set, which can be "rotated" at the workstation to examine the coarctation from different perspectives.

arch) may be hypoplastic and require intervention during surgery. A completely interrupted aortic arch may be seen in the same manner as a critical coarctation and receives similar surgical correction. The designation of types A, B, and C refer to whether the aortic interruption occurs after the left subclavian artery, between the left common carotid and left subclavian, or between the left common carotid and innominate arteries.

Coarctation of the aorta is frequently associated with other cardiac lesions, most typically a bicuspid aortic valve. Poststenotic dilation of the ascending aorta may occur, placing a second part of the aorta at risk for dissection, particularly in the setting of upper body hypertension. Association with VSDs is common. The increased afterload created by the coarctation may increase the degree of left-to-right shunting and accelerate the presentation of pulmonary overcirculation and congestive heart failure. Also associated with coarctation are left-sided obstructive lesions both of the mitral valve (supramitral ring, parachute mitral valve) and of the aortic valve (subvalvar or valvar aortic stenosis), which in more extreme forms occur with a hypoplastic left ventricle that may require a single-ventricle approach to repair. In the extracardiac circulation, the occurrence of berry aneurysms in the circle of Willis is associated with an increased risk of intracranial hemorrhage.

Initial attempts at surgical repair included resection of the coarcted segment and end-to-end anastomosis.

However, before the development of prostaglandin E_1, many infants were seen in shock and benefited from prosthetic patch aortoplasty, because this more rapid procedure did not require extensive dissection to mobilize the aorta for anastomosis. Prosthetic patch aortoplasty has been complicated by a high incidence of aneurysm formation on the wall of the aorta opposite the area of the patch. Concern about the ability of a circumferential anastomosis to grow with the child led to subclavian flap repairs, in which the left subclavian artery is divided and its proximal end used to patch open the aorta in the region of the coarctation. This repair compromises flow to the left arm, with variable effects on its growth. As well, it does not remove the coarctation tissue that some believe will not grow normally as the affected patient continues to grow. With the availability of prostaglandin E_1 as a pharmacological temporizing agent, surgical preference has returned to resection of the coarctation and end-to-end anastomosis. When the distal arch is hypoplastic, more extensive dissection of the distal arch and an end-to-side anastomosis of the descending aorta to the underside of the arch may be carried out. As well, the descending aorta may require patch augmentation. In our institution, elective repairs are performed between the ages of 3 and 6 months in asymptomatic patients. Balloon angioplasty of the coarctation has been attempted, augmented more recently by stent implantation. The incidence of aneurysm formation after dilation of native lesions is estimated to be 5% to 15%.[37,38] Dilation of recurrent coarctation after surgical repair seems to pose a lower risk of rupture and aneurysm formation.

Long-term complications of unrepaired coarctation include aortic dissection or rupture, which occurs most often in the ascending aorta but may also occur in the aorta distal to the coarctation. Other potential complications include increased risk of endocarditis, intracranial hemorrhage, and accelerated complications of hypertension, such as atherosclerosis, congestive heart failure, and sudden death. Repaired patients are observed for development of recurrent coarctation and aneurysm formation. Recurrent coarctation is more common with repairs done earlier in life. Hypertension may persist after coarctation repair, more commonly when repair is performed later in life.

Imaging Essentials, Prerepair

1. Coarctation anatomy: discrete vs. longer segment, degree of restriction to flow (gradient)
2. Arch anatomy: size of distal arch (need for augmentation), relation of adjacent vessels (subclavian artery)
3. Assessment for associated intracardiac defects: especially VSD, mitral valve anomalies, subaortic or aortic stenosis, bicommissural aortic valve
4. Ascending aorta: potential development of aneurysmal dilation with risk of dissection or rupture
5. Left ventricular structure and function: development of left ventricular hypertrophy or depressed systolic function
6. Coronary artery anatomy (if cardiac catheterization is performed): possible accelerated atherosclerosis

Imaging Essentials, Postrepair

1. Site of repair: development of restenosis or aneurysm
2. Dilation of the aorta: potentially the descending, as well as ascending aorta
3. Associated lesions: potential development of aortic stenosis in a bicommissural aortic valve, patch leaks in a repaired VSD, progressive enlargement or dissection of a dilated ascending aorta
4. Coronary arteries (if undergoing catheterization): especially in patients who received later repairs, who are more likely to have persistent hypertension and its complications

Echocardiography

The aortic arch is best visualized from the suprasternal notch or beneath the left clavicle with long-axis imaging (Figure 14-25). Dimensions are taken of the ascending aorta, transverse arch, isthmus (portion of the aortic arch between the left subclavian artery and ductus or coarctation), and descending aorta. In addition to imaging the arch in long axis, the transducer should be "swept" from side to side to identify aneurysms that may lie outside of the plane of the long axis of the arch. Color-flow Doppler imaging reveals flow acceleration at the site of the native or recurrent coarctation. Because some flow acceleration is common proximal to the site of the coarctation, pulsed-wave Doppler should be used to assess the velocity in the arch well proximal to the coarctation. If the velocity is greater than 1 m/s, this should be subtracted from the velocity within the coarctation, using the expanded Bernoulli equation, $\Delta P = 4(V_2{}^2 - V_1{}^2)$. Continuous-wave Doppler assessment of flow acceleration within the coarctation will show a blunted upstroke with flow that may continue throughout diastole if the coarctation is severe. Use of the "blind" continuous-wave probe placed in the suprasternal notch may be helpful if assessment with an imaging transducer yields limited information. Complementary information can be obtained from pulsed-wave Doppler assessment of flow in the descending aorta, which will show low-velocity flow that may be continuous and not return to the baseline, again with a blunted upstroke.

The aortic root and ascending aorta should be imaged from parasternal long-axis windows to identify dilation or aneurysm formation. The mitral valve and its subvalvar apparatus are assessed for a supravalvar stenosing ring and a parachute mitral valve. Imaging of the LVOT and aortic valve investigates for possible subvalvar stenosis and bicommissural aortic valve, which may become stenotic. The septum is assessed by color-flow Doppler for presence of a VSD or a patch leak of a repaired VSD.

TEE rarely provides adequate images of the coarctation segment and is not used routinely in its imaging.

CMR

CMR has become our procedure of choice for noninvasive assessment of both repaired and unrepaired adult aortic coarctation.[39] It offers screening for long-term complications of repair (aneurysm formation, dissection, or restenosis) and an assessment of the effects of any residual defect on ventricular function. Information about the restriction to flow presented by the coarctation is limited with the imaging sequences available in most centers. However, the anatomical detail offered by CMR allows optimal selection and planning of interventions. Of particular interest to the interventional cardiologist is the relationship of the coarctation to adjacent head and neck vessels and the diameters of the aorta proximal to, distal to, and at the narrowest portion of the coarctation. The presence of large collateral vessels may offer insight to the restriction caused by a coarctation.[40] MRA may be used to screen for associated renal artery stenosis during the same examination.

Initial imaging typically includes cine fast-gradient echo imaging of ventricular structure and function in short axis. The aortic arch and coarctation site are then assessed with either fast-spin echo or cine fast-gradient echo sequences prescribed in the long axis of the distal arch. Gadolinium-enhanced 3D-CMRA provides a data set for off-line 3D analysis. Phase-contrast cine assessment of flow in the descending aorta may suggest significant restriction to flow if a blunted flow pattern is seen.

Cardiac Catheterization

Noninvasive imaging usually provides adequate information to guide clinical decisions if a patient has adequate acoustic windows. If windows are limited, CMR may provide the necessary information, but catheterization may also be helpful. When indicated by hemodynamic data, angiography may include a left ventriculogram to assess for a VSD and subaortic stenosis. Aortic root angiography is performed as indicated to assess for aortic root dilation, aortic valve structure, and may visualize the coarctation site. Typically, additional detail is necessary, and angiography is performed at the coarctation site

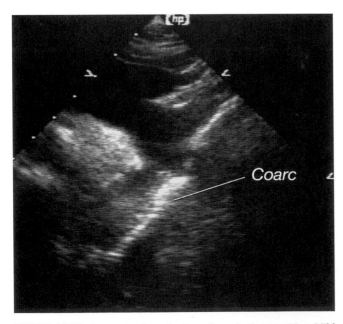

FIGURE 14-25. Suprasternal notch view of repaired coarctation. Mild residual narrowing at the site of coarct repair (Coarc).

with a side-hole catheter (e.g., cutoff pigtail) over a guide wire, with orthogonal views emphasizing lateral and semioblique projections. Left ventriculography is performed with a long axial oblique projection. The aortic arch is typically well seen from the same angles, but removal of the cranial angulation may improve imaging.

CORONARY ANOMALIES

Coronary artery anomalies have been mentioned as associations with different congenital heart defects, usually because of their impact on surgical strategy (e.g., potential transection during right ventriculotomy). They also may pose a primary anomaly, with several different presentations.

A coronary artery may arise anomalously from the pulmonary artery rather than the aorta. Usually, it emerges from the coronary sinus of the pulmonary artery that "faces" the "normal" coronary sinus of the aorta. However, the coronary artery may also arise from another coronary sinus, the main pulmonary artery, or rarely a branch pulmonary artery. The anomalous artery is most frequently the left main coronary, abbreviated as ALCAPA (anomalous left coronary artery from the pulmonary artery). After birth, as pulmonary vascular resistance and pulmonary artery pressure drop, coronary artery perfusion pressure and the saturation of the blood perfusing the coronary artery decrease. Collaterals from the RCA typically develop, but as the resistance and pressure in the pulmonary artery continue to decrease, blood from right coronary collaterals begins to flow retrograde up the left coronary, draining to the lower-pressure pulmonary artery rather than perfusing the higher-resistance left coronary circulation. The right coronary artery dilates in response to this shunt flow. Presentation may be with heart failure symptoms in early infancy, or throughout adult life, depending on the degree of collateral formation, ischemic injury, and development of mitral regurgitation.

Early repairs included ligation of the LCA where it drained into the pulmonary artery (allowing all of the collateral flow from the RCA to perfuse the left coronary circulation), as well as placement of a pulmonary artery band to increase perfusion pressure. The Takeuchi repair includes formation of an aortocoronary tunnel running through the pulmonary artery to the coronary ostium to provide aortic blood to the coronary artery. This repair has been complicated by baffle obstruction and leaks. Grafts from the systemic circulation (internal mammary artery, subclavian artery, saphenous vein grafts) have also been performed. With experience gained from the arterial switch operation, coronary transfer to the aorta, when feasible, has become the procedure of choice. After restoration of aortic flow, patients may experience significant improvement in ventricular function.[41]

A coronary artery may also arise anomalously from the aorta, typically from the opposite coronary sinus. When an RCA arises from the left coronary sinus, it often arises tangentially from the aorta rather than perpendicular to it. Such coronary arteries may have a "slitlike" orifice and may course through the wall of the aorta ("intramural coronary"). Patients with this anatomy may be seen with exertional chest pain or syncope, typically in teenage years, and may be at increased risk of sudden death.[42,43] Postulated mechanisms of ischemia include restriction to flow by the slitlike orifice, compression of the intramural coronary artery by the aortic root as it dilates with exercise, and compression between the two great arteries. The left coronary artery may arise from the right sinus of Valsalva, with several different possible courses. The left main coronary artery has been visualized passing posterior to the aorta, anterior to the pulmonary artery (like a conus coronary), through the ventricular septum, or between the aorta and pulmonary artery. In particular, a course between the aorta and pulmonary artery is associated with a slitlike orifice and intramural course and has been seen in patients with exertional ischemia, syncope, and in victims of sudden death. Different approaches to repair have been described, including "unroofing" of the intramural coronary artery with removal of the ostial membrane (when the ostium is not adjacent to an aortic valve commissure). In our institution, adolescents with an appropriate history of exertional syncope or exertional chest pain typically require noninvasive imaging to assess proximal coronary anatomy.

As well, coronary arteriovenous (also described as coronary-cameral) fistulas may be seen at various ages, either with a continuous murmur or as an incidental finding at noninvasive or invasive cardiac imaging. Draining of coronary blood into such a low-pressure sink can produce a coronary steal phenomenon and may place the affected patient at risk of endocarditis and development of congestive heart failure. Such fistulae may be ligated surgically or occluded with devices delivered in the cardiac catheterization laboratory.

Essentials of Imaging

1. Coronary ostia and proximal coronary anatomy: possible anomalous origin from the opposite coronary sinus or pulmonary artery, tangential takeoff, intramural course, dilated coronaries when the RCA provides collateral flow to ALCAPA or with coronary-cameral fistulae
2. Proximal coronary course: anomalous coronaries passing between the aorta and pulmonary artery
3. Site of drainage of enlarged coronaries: drainage to pulmonary artery (ALCAPA) or within cardiac chambers (coronary-cameral fistula)
4. Ventricular function: possible regional wall motion abnormalities vs. diffusely depressed function
5. Mitral valve function: possibly regurgitant as a result of ischemia
6. Full anatomical survey: if not performed previously

Echocardiography

In pediatric patients, the normal coronary ostia may be imaged from parasternal short axis, "zoomed" on the aortic root. Identification of the arteries is facilitated by the use of the highest transducer frequency possible for that patient, low gains, and low compression, creating a black blood pool. With cardiac motion, the coronary artery will be seen to "flash" through the transducer's imaging plane. The coronary artery can be demonstrated by freezing and scrolling back to the frame that caught the coronary artery in long-axis imaging. Capturing good images requires experimentation with small variations in transducer rotation and position. Imaging the LCA may require slight counterclockwise rotation and movement caudally on the chest from a typical parasternal short axis. It may also be seen from parasternal long axis. Optimal views of the RCA may require slight counterclockwise transducer rotation. The transverse pericardial sinus may sometimes be erroneously identified as the LCA. Color-flow Doppler helps to verify that an apparent vessel is a coronary artery by visualizing appropriate flow. With ALCAPA, flow in the proximal LCA may be retrograde, because the coronary artery will drain into its origin from the pulmonary artery.

The origin of a coronary artery from the pulmonary artery may be demonstrated from a parasternal short-axis view, angled rightward to the pulmonary artery, parasternal long axis view, or from a high parasternal short-axis view. Color-flow Doppler (with a low-velocity scale) may identify the ostium by flow draining into the pulmonary artery.

TEE may demonstrate proximal coronary anatomy when this is not visible on transthoracic echocardiography. This is well seen from a short-axis view of the aortic valve.

Catheterization

Catheterization of children with ALCAPA is not required before surgical intervention but is a standard part of the evaluation of cardiomyopathy in older adolescents and adults. Absence of an LCA ostium in the left coronary sinus and typical RCA dilation are routine. Septal perforating collaterals and retrograde filling by collaterals of the LAD and left circumflex coronary arteries are common and may be associated with dilated, aneurysmal LCA anatomy or systolic decompression of the LCA or collateral segments (similar to that seen in intramyocardial coursing of the coronary arteries). These aneurysmal and compression findings may be first noted or appear to worsen after repair. Postoperative catheterization may identify obstruction or development of baffle leak after Takeuchi repair. Selective coronary artery imaging angles are similar to those used in imaging the proximal left main coronary artery for acquired coronary artery disease.

Various imaging techniques have been suggested for identifying the course of anomalous origin of the coronary arteries within the aortic root by means of standard projections of selective coronary angiography. However, the usefulness and precision of standard views in obtaining nonstandard information is limited. We have found that selective coronary angiography performed in steep cranial or caudal anterior projections ("laid-back view") with a means of identifying the limits of the anterior pulmonary artery (typically with a pulmonary artery catheter sitting within its lumen) is most useful and

accurate in suggesting a coronary course between the aorta and pulmonary artery. However, differentiating an intramyocardial or extramyocardial course between the aorta and pulmonary artery remains less accurate, although it may be suggested by the location of a coronary artery course relative to the pulmonary valve annulus on nonangulated anterior imaging. Use of these views may demonstrate rest-induced or exercise-induced compression of the coronary artery by the RVOT throughout its proximal course.

Concerns regarding a compromised orifice of a coronary artery cannot typically be addressed by selective coronary angiography because of alleviation of stenosis by direct intubation of the ostium by the angiographic catheter. This remains a significant limitation of catheter-based angiography, although nonselective angiography in the affected coronary artery cusp may be suggestive of ostial compromise.

CMR

CMR offers a 3D view of the proximal coronary arteries and their course relative to other structures.[44,45] This is particularly helpful in identifying some coronary arterial anomalies (such as an anomalous LAD from the right coronary cusp coursing between the aorta and pulmonary artery) that carry an increased risk of sudden death. CMR is presently less reliable (at most centers) for assessment of luminal stenoses. CMR sequences to optimally define proximal coronary anatomy are in evolution, as discussed elsewhere.

SINGLE VENTRICLE PHYSIOLOGY

Single-ventricle repair has been typically offered to patients with hypoplasia of one of the ventricles, including tricuspid atresia, some forms of pulmonary atresia with intact ventricular septum (PA-IVS), and hypoplastic left heart syndrome (HLHS). However, other anatomical abnormalities may preclude a two-ventricle repair. Examples in patients without ventricular hypoplasia include (1) mitral valve anatomy that would have to be disrupted in the formation of two ventricles, and (2) PA-IVS with coronary fistulae to the right ventricle and proximal coronary stenoses. The coronary artery is perfused retrograde from the right ventricle, and perfusion depends on high pressures in the right ventricle caused by obstructed pulmonary outflow. Decompression of the right ventricle with a two-ventricle repair would typically drop perfusion pressure and bring lethal ischemia to RV-dependent coronary circulation.

This section reviews the most common examples of ventricular hypoplasia that may lead to a single-ventricle repair. We recognize that within each group there is a wide spectrum of abnormalities and that the surgical approach is individualized for a patient's anatomy. Discussion will emphasize a "final common pathway," in the various stages of a single-ventricle palliation that the practicing adult cardiologist may encounter. The end result of this pathway, the Fontan palliation, places the pulmonary and systemic circulations in series.

In patients with tricuspid atresia, the right ventricle receives no inflow from the tricuspid valve as a stimulus for development. All blood flow to the right ventricle comes by way of a VSD (bulboventricular foramen). The right ventricle is typically hypoplastic, without an inflow portion, but with a sinus and an infundibulum. The great arteries may have a concordant alignment or may be transposed, with the aorta arising from either the left or right ventricle. The VSD and infundibulum may restrict blood flow. If the pulmonary artery arises from the right ventricle, this restriction in the subpulmonary outflow may result in cyanosis or, rarely, a circulation that is temporarily balanced and prevents pulmonary overcirculation and congestive heart failure. With transposed great arteries, progressive narrowing of the VSD and infundibulum may produce subaortic stenosis. Coarctation of the aorta may be seen, typically in association with subaortic obstruction.

In patients with pulmonary atresia with intact ventricular septum (PA-IVS), as well as in patients with HLHS, ventricular dimensions are critical in determining the feasibility of a two-ventricle repair. Indices have been developed that relate surgical outcome to tricuspid annulus dimension and right ventricular volume. Of note, the right ventricle is not always diminutive in PA-IVS. On occasion, a freely regurgitant tricuspid valve allows the development of a large but thin-walled right ventricle that may have difficulty ejecting blood against the newborn's elevated PVR (similar to severe Ebstein's anomaly), carrying a dismal prognosis. Severe RV hypoplasia, an RV-dependent coronary circulation, or a dilated, poorly contractile right ventricle with free tricuspid regurgitation may all require a single-ventricle palliation.

In patients with HLHS, the mitral and aortic valves may be either severely hypoplastic or atretic. The left atrium is typically small and poorly compliant, relying on an ASD to return blood to the systemic right ventricle. The ascending aorta is typically hypoplastic and receives retrograde blood flow from a PDA, allowing perfusion of the coronary arteries. The hypoplastic ascending aorta and arch must be addressed at the time of surgery. Development or recognition of aortic coarctation after the first stage of repair has not been uncommon.

The path to ultimate single-ventricle repair typically involves three stages. Initially, reliable blood flow from the heart is established by addressing any obstruction to outflow from the single ventricle. At the same time, a reliable source of pulmonary perfusion is provided, usually by means of a modified Blalock-Taussig shunt (MBTS). The placement of systemic/pulmonary artery shunts comes at the cost of a volume load on the single ventricle, with resultant ventricular dilation and hypertrophy. In the second stage of a single-ventricle repair, a bidirectional Glenn shunt is created, anastomosing the SVC to the pulmonary arteries and taking down the MBTS. Usually, the pulmonary circuit is perfused solely with venous return from the upper body, removing part of the volume load on the single ventricle and allowing for regression of some of the ventricular dilation and hypertrophy that had occurred in the first stage of repair. This results in systemic arterial saturations in the high 70% to mid-80% range because of mixing of systemic venous (from the IVC) and pulmonary venous return within the single ventricle. Before bidirectional Glenn repair, it is essential to know the pattern of systemic venous drainage (e.g., the possible presence of bilateral SVCs and whether they are joined by a connecting vein) and whether there are any distortions or stenoses of the pulmonary arteries. If present, pulmonary artery stenoses are typically addressed either in the interventional catheterization laboratory before surgery or with patch augmentation at the time of surgery. Possible obstruction to outflow within the ventricle or in the aortic arch must be reassessed and may require revision at the time of the second stage of surgical repair.

In the third stage (the Fontan procedure), anastomosis of the remaining systemic venous return from the inferior vena cava directly to the pulmonary circulation is performed. The volume load on the single ventricle is eliminated, and the circulation relies on systemic venous return and intrathoracic dynamics to facilitate pulmonary blood flow. Both before creation of the Fontan circulation and in longer-term follow-up of Fontan patients, there is potential for development of systemic/pulmonary venous collaterals and pulmonary arterial/pulmonary venous malformations that bypass the pulmonary capillary bed and cause systemic desaturation. When identified, these require occlusion.

Additional reparative strategies may be necessary when tricuspid atresia is present with transposed great arteries, narrowing of the VSD, and subaortic infundibulum, creating subaortic stenosis. Enlargement of the VSD carries a risk of injury to the conduction system. An alternative is to divide the main pulmonary artery and anastomose it side-to-side to the aorta, allowing creation of a "dual outflow" from the single ventricle to the aorta (the Damus-Kaye-Stansel anastomosis). Similarly, in HLHS, the aortic valve and ascending aorta may be too small to carry the cardiac output. The main pulmonary artery can be divided and anastomosed to the aorta, and the hypoplastic aortic arch is patch augmented with an aortic homograft in a similar Damus-Kaye-Stansel repair. Of note, despite extension of the patch past the level of a coarctation, obstruction may develop at that site.

Early Fontan anastomoses connected the right atrium to the pulmonary artery by means of a prosthetic conduit. Experience showed that these anteriorly placed conduits often became obstructed by a combination of tissue ingrowth and external, sternal compression. As atrial pressures and wall tension rose, the right atrium became severely dilated, occasionally with associated posterior compression of pulmonary venous return to the left atrium. Newer approaches to completing the Fontan anastomosis have included (1) the "lateral tunnel," in which a patch is placed along the lateral wall of the atrium, carrying blood up from the IVC, through the atrium to the SVC, where it continues to flow upward until it reaches the anastomosis with the pulmonary arteries; and (2) placement of an extracardiac conduit.

Placement of a "fenestration" in the systemic venous pathway allows decompression of elevated systemic venous pressures at the cost of some right-to-left shunting and cyanosis, which is typically well tolerated. In the lateral tunnel version of the Fontan, a 4-mm punch may be used to create a hole in the patch, allowing flow from the systemic venous baffle to the pulmonary venous atrium. With suitable postconvalescent hemodynamics, the fenestration can be occluded with a transcatheter occlusion device or with a transcutaneously modifiable suture, raising saturations and potentially lowering the risk of paradoxical embolus.

Imaging Essentials

Postarterial Shunt, Pre-Glenn

1. Pulmonary artery anatomy: presence and degree of stenoses
2. Systemic venous return: identification of possible left superior vena cava (LSVC); if present, evaluation for a "connecting vein" linking the LSVC to the RSVC
3. ASD: presence of a widely patent ASD without restriction to venous return
4. Systemic atrioventricular valve function: presence and degree of regurgitation
5. Ventricular function
6. Ventricular outflow tract and semilunar valve structure and function: potential subvalvar or valvar stenosis
7. Aortic arch anatomy: possible stenoses at the Damus-Kaye-Stansel anastomosis or at the usual site of a coarctation
8. Evaluation for aortopulmonary collaterals

Post-Glenn, Pre-Fontan

As described previously (pre-Glenn), with additional attention focused on:
1. Glenn pathway: evaluation for patency, possible stenoses at the site of anastomosis or caused by distortion of the branch pulmonary artery, Glenn pathway pressures
2. Assessment for venovenous collaterals or pulmonary artery to pulmonary venous collaterals: as a potential source of systemic desaturation
3. Complete hemodynamics

Post-Fontan

1. Fontan pathway: patency, presence of stenoses or possible thrombus, baffle leaks (allowing right-to-left shunting and systemic desaturation)
2. Fontan fenestration: patency (spontaneous closure possible), gradient from Fontan pathway to pulmonary venous atrium (candidacy for transcatheter device closure)
3. Atrioventricular valve function: degree of regurgitation
4. Ventricular function
5. Outflow tract, semilunar valve, aortic arch structure, and function: presence and degree of possible obstruction to flow, potentially at the level of the bulboventricular foramen (VSD) if this is part of the outflow tract
6. Assessment for collaterals: venovenous (bypassing the pulmonary capillary bed and causing systemic desat-

uration) or aortopulmonary (creating a volume load on the single ventricle, and potentially increasing pulmonary arterial and Fontan pathway pressures and predisposing to hemoptysis)
7. Complete hemodynamics: especially in the symptomatic patient

Echocardiography

The suprasternal notch often provides the optimal window for imaging the pulmonary arteries and their source of blood flow in the single-ventricle patient. A right Blalock-Taussig shunt is seen by angling the transducer toward the patient's right. Initial imaging with color-flow Doppler techniques helps to identify the right pulmonary artery and a systemic-to-pulmonary artery shunt with continuous flow entering from the right subclavian artery. Once identified, 2D imaging can be attempted if acoustic windows allow. Doppler interrogation should be performed to estimate the gradient from the subclavian artery to the pulmonary artery. If a right arm blood pressure is obtained, this allows estimation of pulmonary artery pressure.

Glenn and Fontan anastomoses may be imaged in a similar manner. Color-flow Doppler imaging can be used to follow the SVC to its anastomosis with the RPA (Figure 14-26, B). However, because the venous source of blood flow has low velocity, color-flow Doppler imaging is improved if the velocity scale is decreased. Stenoses are seen as an area of flow acceleration and may occur at the site of anastomosis or in the adjacent pulmonary artery, which may be distorted. The intracardiac Fontan baffle may be seen from a subcostal short-axis view (Figure 14-27, B), as well as an apical four-chamber, which demonstrates the baffle in cross section against the lateral wall of the atrium (Figures 14-26, A, 14-27, A). The apical four-chamber view often gives an ideal angle for Doppler interrogation of the fenestration, which usually faces the apex (Figure 14-27, A). Baffle leaks may be identified as color-flow signals leading from the baffle into the atrium, separate from the fenestration.

The atrial septum may be imaged from the subcostal, apical, or parasternal short-axis windows, and defects should demonstrate no restriction to blood flow. If flow acceleration is noted, a gradient should be measured. The atrioventricular valve and ventricular functions are assessed from apical and parasternal windows. Assessment of the hypoplastic chamber, particularly its inflow and outflow, is individualized to the specific defect. In tricuspid atresia, the VSD (bulboventricular foramen), right ventricle, and particularly the RV outflow are evaluated with a combination of parasternal long-axis and short-axis, as well as apical imaging. With HLHS, patency and flow through the mitral and aortic valves is assessed primarily from parasternal and apical windows.

The proximal aorta and the Stansel anastomosis, when used, are evaluated from apical, parasternal long-axis, and suprasternal notch views. The Stansel anastomosis is examined for evidence of stenosis. Dimensions are taken of the semilunar valves, ascending aorta, arch, and descending aorta. The junction of the arch and

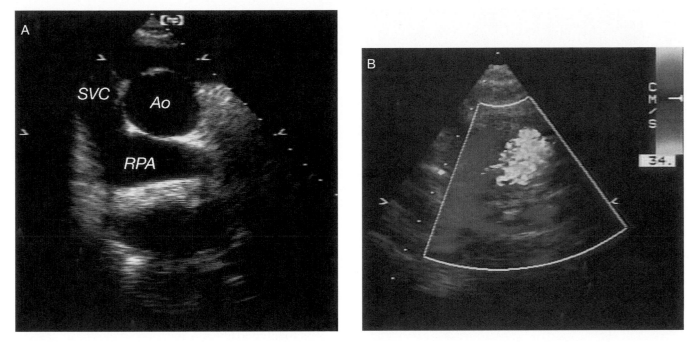

FIGURE 14-26. Cavopulmonary anastomosis in Fontan circulation. **A,** Imaging from the suprasternal notch with a "left-right" transducer orientation demonstrates the cavopulmonary anatomosis. **B,** Color-flow Doppler is used to assess for flow acceleration indicating possible stenoses. See also Color Insert.

descending aorta is examined carefully for development of a coarctation. After surgery, and with removal of the thymus, the suprasternal notch may not offer an effective view for definitive evaluation of the arch, and catheterization may be required to rule out arch obstruction.

TEE offers particularly good imaging of the atria and the interatrial Fontan baffle when it is present. It is frequently used in the evaluation of intraatrial thrombus in a Fontan patient at risk for thrombus. Spontaneous echo contrast ("smoke") may be seen in many Fontan patients, especially those with dilated atria.

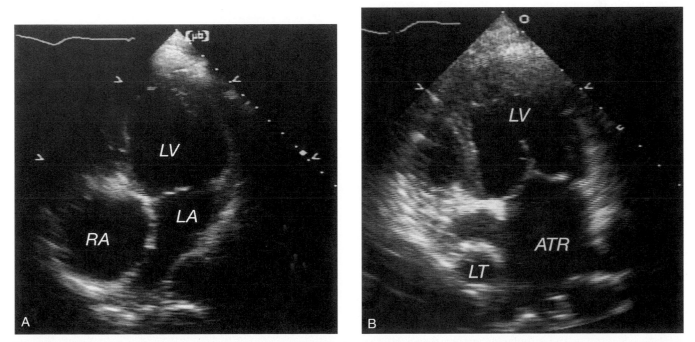

FIGURE 14-27. Fontan in tricuspid atresia vs. hypoplastic left heart syndrome. **A,** Tricuspid atresia was addressed with a right atrium-to-pulmonary artery anastomosis, resulting in right atrial dilation. **B,** A lateral tunnel (LT) was used to bring IVC flow up to the pulmonary artery.

Continued

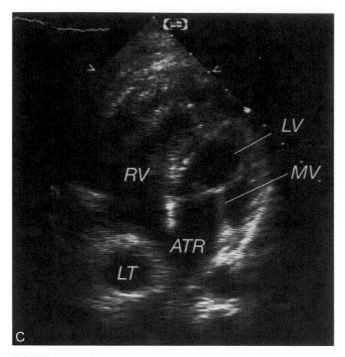

FIGURE 14-27. CONT'D C, Hypoplastic left heart syndrome, treated with a lateral tunnel Fontan. The atrial septum is taken down to create a common atrium (ATR).

CMR

CMR offers many advantages in noninvasive assessment of single-ventricle physiology, making it central to our approach to imaging the adult patient. Tomographic imaging allows quantitative assessment of ventricular function, even when the single ventricle is irregularly shaped (as in HLHS). CMR is optimal for imaging the extracardiac vascular anatomy that is critical to assessment of single-ventricle physiology (aortopulmonary collaterals, residual systemic-to-pulmonary artery shunts, cavopulmonary anastomoses, and pulmonary artery and aortic arch anatomy). Stainless steel intravascular occlusion coils prevent CMR imaging of structures in their vicinity. Use of platinum coils circumvents this restriction.

Ventricular size and systolic function are evaluated with cine fast-gradient echo sequence imaging in a short-axis plane. Further cine images are obtained in the long axis of pathways of particular interest described previously (cavopulmonary anastomosis, pulmonary arteries, etc). 3D-CMRA provides further images of the various vascular pathways. Atrioventricular valve regurgitation may be quantified with phase-contrast cine sequences, if indicated.

Cardiac Catheterization

After hemodynamic evaluation, angiography of the shunt or cavopulmonary anastomosis is performed to identify stenoses, baffle leaks, and patency of a Fontan fenestration. Power injection through a side-hole (e.g., pigtail) catheter in the subclavian artery (for a MBTS), distal SVC (for a Glenn shunt), or in the Fontan baffle will demonstrate the pathway. Selective angiography of each branch pulmonary artery, as indicated, is typically performed using a side-hole catheter (e.g., cutoff pigtail) advanced over a guide wire. Retrograde ventriculography demonstrates ventricular function and possible atrioventricular valve regurgitation. Axial oblique projections are typically used. Ascending aortography evaluates a Stansel anastomosis, if performed, and may also demonstrate APCs. Balloon occlusion of distal venous flow and injection of contrast in the subclavian vein may identify a left SVC or venovenous collaterals that are candidates for coil occlusion.

CONCLUSIONS

As we have emphasized, optimal cardiac imaging of the adult with congenital heart disease requires intense preprocedural knowledge of underlying defects and their associations, physiology, untreated and treated natural history, therapeutic options, and posttherapeutic sequelae. An intimate understanding of the usefulness and limits of all forms of cardiopulmonary imaging and access to all modalities is therefore requisite to answering the questions necessary for the development of an optimal therapeutic plan for affected individuals. We continue to advocate that imaging of the adult with congenital heart disease be performed in centers that maintain sufficient expertise and volume in congenital heart disease imaging, as well as access to therapeutic options for patients, in accordance with recommendations of the 32nd Bethesda Conference concerning the "Care of the Adult With Congenital Heart Disease."[46]

We would like to thank several colleagues for their assistance: Tal Geva, MD, for CMR images; Megan C. Sherwood, MD, for three-dimensional reconstructions; and Ravin Davidoff, MD, B. Talbot Joziatis, RDCS, and Ruthanne Pepin, RDCS, for comments and suggestions.

REFERENCES

1. Gin KG, Huckell VF, Pollick C. Femoral vein delivery of contrast medium enhances transthoracic echocardiographic detection of patent foramen ovale. *J Am Coll Cardiol* 1993; 22:1994.
2. Kerr AJ, Buck T, Chia K, Chow CM, Fox E, Levine RA, Picard MH. Transmitral Doppler: a new transthoracic contrast method for patent foramen ovale detection and quantification. *J Am Coll Cardiol* 2000; 36:1959.
3. Mohiaddin RH, Underwood R, Romeira L, Anagnostopoulos C, Karwatowski SP, Laney R, Somerville J. Comparison between cine magnetic resonance velocity mapping and first-pass radionuclide angiocardiography for quantitating intracardiac shunts. *Am J Cardiol* 1995; 75:529.
4. Rominger MB, Bachmann GF, Pabst W, Rau WS. Right ventricular volumes and ejection fraction with fast cine magnetic resonance imaging in breath-hold technique: applicability, normal values from 52 volunteers, and evaluation of 325 adult cardiac patients. *J Magn Reson Imaging* 1999; 10:908.
5. Pascoe RD, Oh JK, Warnes CA, Danielson GK, Tajik AJ, Seward JB. Diagnosis of sinus venosus atrial septal defect with transesophageal echocardiography. *Circulation* 1996; 94:1049.
6. Oliver JM, Gallego P, Gonzalez A, Dominguez FJ, Aroca A, Mesa JM. Sinus venosus syndrome: atrial septal defect or anomalous venous connection? A multiplane transesophageal approach. *Heart* 2002; 88:634.

7. Hijazi Z, Wang Z, Cao Q, Koenig P, Waight D, Lang R. Transcatheter closure of atrial septal defects and patent foramen ovale under intracardiac echocardiographic guidance: feasibility and comparison with transesophageal echocardiography. *Cathet Cardiovasc Intervent* 2001; 52:194.

8. Mullen MJ, Dias BF, Walker F, Siu SC, Benson LN, McLaughlin PR. Intracardiac echocardiography guided device closure of atrial septal defects. *J Am Coll Cardiol* 2003; 41:285.

9. Bartel T, Konorza T, Arjumand J, Ebradlidze T, Eggebrecht H, Caspari G, Neudorf U, Erbel R. Intracardiac echocardiography is superior to conventional monitoring for guiding device closure of interatrial communications. *Circulation* 2003; 107:795.

10. Petersen SE, Voitglander T, Kreitner KF, Kalden P, Wittlinger T, Scharhag J, Horstick G, Becker D, Hommel G, Thelen M, Meyer J. Quantification of shunt volumes in congenital heart disease using a breath-hold magnetic resonance phase contrast technique-comparison with oximetry. *Int J Cardiovasc Imaging* 2002; 18:53.

11. Greil GF, Powell AJ, Gildein HP, Geva T. Gadolinium-enhanced three dimensional magnetic resonance angiography of pulmonary and systemic venous anomalies. *J Am Coll Cardiol* 2002; 39:335.

12. Hagler DJ, Edwards WD, Seward JB, Tajik AJ. Standardized nomenclature of the ventricular septum and ventricular septal defects, with applications for two-dimensional echocardiography. *Mayo Clinic Proc* 1985; 60:741.

13. Soto B, Ceballos R, Kirklin JW. Ventricular septal defects: a surgical viewpoint. *J Am Coll Cardiol* 1989; 14:1291.

14. Acar P, Abdel-Massih T, Douste-Blazy MY, Dulac Y, Bonhoeffer P, Sidi D. Assessment of muscular ventricular septal defect closure by transcatheter or surgical approach: a three dimensional echocardiographic study. *Eur J Echocardiogr* 2002; 3:185.

15. Atallah-Yunes NH, Kavey RE, Bove EL, Smith FC, Kveselis DA, Byrum CJ, Gaum WE. Postoperative assessment of a modified surgical approach to repair of tetralogy of Fallot. Long-term follow-up. *Circulation* 1996; 94(9 Suppl):II22.

16. Dodds GA III, Warnes CA, Danielson GK. Aortic valve replacement after repair of pulmonary atresia and ventricular septal defect or tetralogy of Fallot. *J Thorac Cardiovasc Surg* 1997; 113:736.

17. Niwa K, Siu SC, Webb GD, Gatzoulis MA. Progressive aortic root dilatation in adults late after repair of tetralogy of Fallot. *Circulation* 2002; 106:1374.

18. Warnes CA, Child JS. Aortic root dilatation after repair of tetralogy of Fallot: pathology from the past? *Circulation* 2002; 106:1310.

19. Davlouros PA, Kilner PJ, Hornung TS, Li W, Francis JM, Moon JC, Smith GC, Tat T, Pennell DJ, Gatzoulis MA. Right ventricular function in adults with repaired tetralogy of Fallot assessed with cardiovascular magnetic resonance imaging: Detrimental role of right ventricular outflow aneurysms or akinesia and adverse right to left ventricular interaction. *J Am Coll Cardiol* 2002; 40:2044.

20. Vliegen HW, Van Straten A, DeRoos A, Roest AA, Schoof PH, Zwinderman AH, Ottenkamp J, Vanderwall EE, Hazekamp MG. Magnetic resonance imaging to assess the hemodynamic effects of pulmonary valve replacement in adults late after repair of tetralogy of Fallot. *Circulation* 2002; 106:1703.

21. Gera T, Greil GF, Marshall AC, Landzberg M, Powell AJ. Gadolinium enhanced three-dimensional magnetic resonance angiography of pulmonary blood supply in patients with complex pulmonary stenosis or atresia: comparison with x-ray angiography. *Circulation* 2002; 106:473.

22. Acar P, Laskari C, Rhodes J, Pandian N, Warner K, Marx G. Three-dimensional echocardiographic analysis of valve anatomy as a determinant of mitral regurgitation after surgery for atrioventricular septal defects. *Am J Cardiol* 1999; 83:745.

23. Ammash NM, Warnes CA, Connolly HM, Danielson GK, Seward JB. Mimics of Ebstein's anomaly. *Am Heart J* 1997; 134:508.

24. Danielson GK, Driscoll DJ, Mair DD, Warnes CA, Oliver WC. Operative treatment of Ebstein's anomaly. *J Thorac Cardiovasc Surg* 1992; 104:1195.

25. Marianeschi SM, McElhinney DB, Reddy VM, Silverman NH, Hanley FL. Alternative approach to the repair of Ebstein's malformation: intracardiac repair with ventricular unloading. *Ann Thorac Surg* 1998; 66:1546.

26. Hayes CJ, Gersony WM, Driscoll DJ, Keane JF, Kidd L, O'Fallon WM, Pieroni DR, Wolfe RR, Weidman WH. Second natural history study of congenital heart defects. Results of treatment of patients with pulmonary valvar stenosis. *Circulation* 1993; 87(Suppl):128.

27. McCrindle BW, Kan JS. Long-term results after balloon pulmonary valvuloplasty. *Circulation* 1991; 83:1915.

28. Gaynor JW, Burch M, Dollery C, Sullivan ID, Deanfield JE, Elliott MJ. Repair of anomalous pulmonary venous connection to the superior vena cava. *Ann Thorac Surg* 1995; 59:1471.

29. Ammash NM, Seward JB, Warnes CA, Connolly HM, O'Leary PW, Danielson GK. Partial anomalous pulmonary venous connection: diagnosis by transesophageal echocardiography. *J Am Coll Cardiol* 1997; 29:1351.

30. Ferrari VA, Scott CH, Holland GA, Axel L, Sutton MS. Ultrafast three-dimensional contrast-enhanced magnetic resonance angiography and imaging in the diagnosis of partial anomalous pulmonary venous drainage. *J Am Coll Cardiol* 2001; 37:1120.

31. Kleinert S, Geva T. Echocardiographic morphometry and geometry of the left ventricular outflow tract in fixed subaortic stenosis. *J Am Coll Cardiol* 1993; 22:1501.

32. Keane JF, Driscoll DJ, Gersony WM, Hayes CJ, Kidd L, O'Fallon WM, Pieroni DR, Wolfe RR, Weidman WH. Second natural history study of congenital heart defects. Results of treatment of patients with aortic valvar stenosis. *Circulation* 1993; 87(2 Suppl):I16.

33. Sarkar D, Bull C, Yates R, Wright D, Cullen S, Gewillig M, Clayton R, Tunstill A, Deanfield J. Comparison of long-term outcomes of atrial repair of simple transposition with implications for a late arterial switch strategy. *Circulation* 1999; 100(19 Suppl):II176.

34. Fogel MA, Hubbard A, Weinberg PM. A simplified approach for assessment of intracardiac baffles and extracardiac conduits in congenital heart surgery with two- and three-dimensional magnetic resonance imaging. *Am Heart J* 2001; 142:1028.

35. Hechter SJ, Webb G, Fredriksen PM, Benson L, Merchant N, Freeman M, Veldtman G, Warsi MA, Siu S, Liu P. Cardiopulmonary exercise performance in adult survivors of the Mustard procedure. *Cardiol Young* 2001; 11:407.

36. Lecompte Y, Batisse A, Di Carlo D. Double-outlet right ventricle: a surgical synthesis [review]. *Adv Cardiac Surg* 1993; 4:109.

37. Harrison DA, McLaughlin PR, Lazzam C, Connelly M, Benson LN. Endovascular stents in the management of coarctation of the aorta in the adolescent and adult: one year follow up. *Heart* 2001; 85:561.

38. Marshall AC, Perry SB, Keane JF, Lock JE. Early results and medium-term follow-up of stent implantation for mild residual or recurrent aortic coarctation [see comments]. *Am Heart J* 2000; 139:1054.

39. Godart F, Labrot G, Devos P, McFadden E, Rey C, Beregi JP. Coarctation of the aorta: comparison of aortic dimensions between conventional magnetic resonance imaging, 3D MR angiography, and conventional angiography. *Eur Radiol* 2002; 12:2034.

40. Gutberlet M, Hosten N, Vogel M, Abdul-Khaliq H, Ehrenstein T, Amthauer H, Hoffman T, Teichgraber U, Berger F, Lange P, Felix R. Quantification of morphologic and hemodynamic severity of coarctation of the aorta by magnetic resonance imaging. *Cardiol Young* 2001; 11:511.

41. Schwartz ML, Jonas RA, Colan SD. Anomalous origin of left coronary artery from pulmonary artery: recovery of left ventricular function after dual coronary repair. *J Am Coll Cardiol* 1997; 30:547.

42. Taylor AJ, Rogan KM, Virmani R. Sudden cardiac death associated with isolated congenital coronary artery anomalies. *J Am Coll Cardiol* 1992; 20:640.

43. Basso C, Maron BJ, Corrado D, Thiene G. Clinical profile of congenital coronary artery anomalies with origin from the wrong aortic sinus leading to sudden death in young competitive athletes [review]. *J Am Coll Cardiol* 2000; 35:1493.

44. McConnell MV, Ganz P, Selwyn AP, Li W, Edelman RR, Manning WJ. Identification of anomalous coronary arteries and their anatomic course by magnetic resonance coronary angiography. *Circulation* 1995; 92:3158.

45. Taylor AM, Thorne SA, Rubens MB, Jhooti P, Keegan J, Gatehouse PD, Wiesmann F, Grothues F, Somerville J, Pennell DJ. Coronary artery imaging in grown up congenital heart disease: complementary role of magnetic resonance and x-ray coronary angiography. *Circulation* 2000; 101:1670.

46. Landzberg MJ, Murphy DJ Jr, Davidson WR Jr, Jarcho JA, Krumholz HM, Mayer JE Jr, Mee RB, Sahn DJ, Van Hare GF, Webb GD, Williams RG. Task force 4: organization of delivery systems for adults with congenital heart disease. *J Am Coll Cardiol* 2001; 37:1187.

Cardiac Imaging of Masses, Tumors, and Thrombi

Bernhard L. Gerber

David A. Bluemke

John A. Rumberger

Karen M. Horton

João A.C. Lima

Although detection of a cardiac or pericardial mass is an infrequent event in clinical practice, its correct diagnostic evaluation is of great importance. Cardiac masses constitute a wide spectrum of diseases, ranging from clinically benign incidental findings, which do not require any intervention, to highly malignant tumors with a rapidly fatal outcome (Table 15-1). Therefore, a goal-directed diagnostic approach leading to accurate diagnosis and treatment of cardiac masses is mandatory. Although the precise diagnosis of many malignant conditions may require histopathological examination of a specimen obtained by direct tissue sampling, such an aggressive approach may not be warranted in many patients with benign conditions. Noninvasive imaging techniques frequently provide the correct diagnosis and may direct further management in terms of aggressiveness of intervention for the individual patient.

CONTRIBUTION OF IMAGING TECHNIQUES IN THE DIAGNOSIS OF CARDIAC MASSES

Echocardiography

Echocardiography has many important functions in the evaluation of cardiac masses. Two-dimensional (2D) transthoracic (TTE) and transesophageal (TEE) echocardiography are usually the primary modalities that reveal the presence of a cardiac or paracardiac mass (Figure 15-1). Often the discovery of a cardiac mass is an incidental finding on a transthoracic echocardiographic examination performed for routine screening or a finding in the workup of a specific complaint such as heart failure or chest pain. Transesophageal echocardiography is now the preferred modality for evaluation of patients with stroke or systemic thromboembolism. In this context, it may often reveal the presence of a left atrial mass that cannot be identified by TTE imaging alone.

TTE and TEE are typically used for the initial diagnostic workup of cardiac masses. In many cases, they may provide useful information about anatomical localization and appearance, which may be useful for the diagnosis. TTE has a limited field of view restricted by the presence of few acoustic windows that may be accessible and of sufficient quality, especially in obese or emphysematous patients. TTE often also fails to reveal structures within the atria with sufficient spatial resolution. A comprehensive examination of a suspected mass by TTE may also be difficult, because the extension of lesions to the pericardium, to the mediastinum, or to the vena cava cannot be visualized. TEE offers wider acoustic windows and has higher resolution with better definition of lesions, especially in the atria. Because of this, it has better sensitivity than TTE to detect small intraatrial lesions, especially small tumors, laminated thrombi, and thrombi that are limited to the left or right atrial appendage. TEE is more effective in demonstrating compression of the heart or the great vessels by mediastinal tumors. More importantly, however, TEE is more accurate in describing the morphology of cardiac masses, allowing differentiation of abnormal masses from normal variants and detecting the necessary criteria for tumor malignancy.[1]

Tumor growth in and outside the heart, infiltration, and invasion, as well as characterization of the border zone between normal tissue and tumor, can be significantly better identified by TEE than by TTE. Echocardiography may not be sufficient to make the final diagnosis concerning the nature of a cardiac mass and provides little useful information for tissue characterization. The acoustic density of the tissue is dependent on the transmitting power and receiver gain settings and on the distance that the ultrasound travels in the tissue. Most cardiac masses have a uniform appearance of increased echo density, and the differential diagnosis relies on anatomical information alone. Therefore, the

TABLE 15-1 FREQUENCY OF DISTRIBUTION OF CARDIAC MASSES IN ALL AGE GROUPS

Mass	Estimated absolute frequency	Relative frequency
Thrombus	1-3%	
Secondary tumors (metastasis)	3-5%	
Primary benign tumors	0.001-0.02%	
Myxoma		41%
Lipoma		14%
Papillary fibroelastoma		13%
Rhabdomyoma		11%
Fibroma		5%
Hemangioma		5%
Teratoma		4%
Paraganglioma		<1%
Primary malignant tumors	0.001-0.0075%	
Angiosarcoma		31%
Rhabdomyosarcoma		20%
Other sarcomas		16%
Mesothelioma		15%
Primary lymphoma		6%

Adapted from McAllister et al. *Curr Prob Cardiol* 1999; 24:57; and Fyke et al. *J Am Coll Cardiol* 1983; 1:1352.

use of additional noninvasive techniques, such as computed tomography (CT) or cardiac magnetic resonance imaging (CMR) may be warranted. TEE can be performed during fluoroscopy to guide the transvenous biopsy of a cardiac mass and intraoperatively to help delineate the precise location of a tumor and to assess the surgical approach for resection. Finally, echocardiography is used for follow-up of patients during treatment to ensure the absence of tumor recurrence after surgery or chemotherapy or to document regression of thrombus during anticoagulation treatment.

Conventional CT and Electron Beam CT

Conventional CT and electron beam CT (EBCT) may provide useful information about cardiac masses. CT is

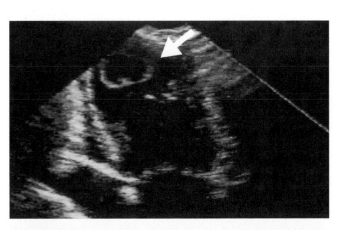

FIGURE 15-1. Transthoracic echocardiogram of a patient with hepatic echinococcosis, showing a cystic mass *(arrow)* in the apex of the left ventricle. This mass corresponded to a ventricular location of the echinococcosis.

readily available, fast, and provides high-quality tomographic images of the heart and the pericardium. CT allows for volumetric images representing a true 3D display of the mass, which cannot be obtained with echocardiography. CT has fewer contraindications than CMR and can be performed in patients with pacemakers and automatic defibrillation devices. A particular advantage of conventional, and especially helical, CT is the high image quality of nonmoving body parts. Therefore, CT is best used for providing information on structures such as the mediastinum, the great vessels, and the pericardium, which can be less well explored by echocardiography. The X-ray transmission measurements collected by CT allow for digitized determination of tissue attenuation coefficients. These attenuation coefficients are expressed relative to the value for water as "Hounsfield units (HU)." The analysis of these attenuation coefficients provides information that may prove useful for tissue characterization of various cardiac masses. CT is generally not a primary modality for screening of cardiac masses or tumors. However, it may sometimes incidentally reveal cardiac or pericardial masses in patients who have presented with nonspecific symptoms and undergo this test for diagnostic exploration of the thorax and mediastinum. CT may confirm the presence of a mass suspected by echocardiography and improve definition of the extent of the mass and its relation to other cardiac structures, especially to the mediastinum and the pericardium. By allowing some tissue characterization, CT is also helpful in the differential diagnosis of cardiac masses and is the most accurate test to identify calcification within masses. By measuring the attenuation characteristics of a mass, CT may identify whether its nature is lipomatous or aqueous. Enhancement patterns after contrast administration provide additional information. Generally, tumors are enhanced more intensely than the surrounding uninvolved myocardium. Because CT provides spatially well-localized images, which can be easily reproduced, it may allow more precise follow-up of masses over time than echocardiography.

CMR

CMR produces high-resolution tomographic images of the heart with excellent delineation of cardiac and intravascular spaces and of the high tissue signal of the different surrounding soft tissue structures[2] (Table 15-2). Because of the ability of CMR to directly acquire images in multiple orthogonal or oblique orientations, views unavailable by other imaging modalities can be obtained. CMR provides superior differentiation of soft tissue structures and better tissue characterization, facilitating the correct diagnosis of cardiac masses.[3] In particular, it may help to define whether a suspected tumor is well delineated and encapsulated, suggesting a benign lesion, or demonstrate invasion of surrounding tissue, suggesting malignancy. CMR allows cine and functional imaging of the heart, providing information about the mobility of the mass and its influence on cardiac function. Finally, when contrast agents are used for CMR, they are usually better tolerated and cause less allergic reaction than CT contrast agents.

■ ■ ■

TABLE 15-2   SPECIFIC PURPOSES OF CARDIAC IMAGING TECHNIQUES IN THE EVALUATION OF CARDIAC MASSES

	TE	TEE	CT	MRI
Diagnosis				
First identification	+++	++	+	+
Confirm the presence of mass	+	+++	+++	+++
Delineation of anatomical extent	+	++	+++	+++
Relation to other structures				
Differential diagnosis of cardiac masses	+	++	++	+++
Follow-up				
Response to treatment	++	+	+++	+++

+, Some value; ++, higher value; +++, highest value.

These attributes make CMR especially useful for the evaluation of suspected cardiac masses. CMR may also define the type and the origin of intraatrial masses, for example, discriminating atrial myxoma, which typically presents with a narrow insertion on the septum, from sarcoma, which typically has a large insertion originating from other parts of the atria. CMR has the potential for tissue characterization by identifying T1 and T2 relaxation times of masses, which may be diagnostic in the case of lipomas, fibromas, angiomas, or pericardial cysts. T1 and T2 characteristics may also identify whether masses are solid or fluid, thereby differentiating cystic from solid tumors. By use of gradient echo sequences, CMR may allow the identification of hemorrhage or calcification within the mass, and by use of contrast-enhanced techniques it may identify the degree of vascularization, another factor used to distinguish benign from malignant lesions.

Technical Considerations

Echocardiography

Cardiac masses constitute 3D objects, which need to be carefully examined in several orientations. It is, therefore, mandatory that acquisitions be performed from several echocardiographic windows and with different probe angles. In many cases, much additional information may be obtained from "nonconventional" echographic windows. The subcostal view particularly may provide valuable information on the localization of cardiac masses by use of TTE examinations. Similarly, for TEE, multiplane probes have improved the capabilities of exploring multiple orientations. Harmonic tissue imaging has significantly enhanced imaging quality and border definition for TTE. This may be especially important in patients with poor echographic windows and low image quality. Intravenous echo contrast agents may also be useful to improve delineation of left ventricular mural thrombi and to estimate the perfusion and vascularity of a mass. Three-dimensional echocardiographic imaging may provide better visualization of the exact location and extent of a mass[4] and may be especially important in tumor staging and in preoperative surgical planning.[5] However, this technique still remains experimental.

CT

With respect to cardiovascular imaging, CT scan acquisition times equivalent to about one cardiac cycle still represent a limitation, because image quality depends on patient cooperation in avoiding movement. The latest generation of scanners use a rotating X-ray source with a circular, stationary detector array and continuous scanning (spiral or helical CT). In addition, they use "slip-ring technology" for scan acquisition times on the order of 0.75 to 1.0 second with shortened interscan delay. Algorithms have also been implemented that enable volumetric imaging, and multiple high-quality reconstructions of various volumes of interest can be performed retrospectively. However, precise movement of the X-ray tube, high tube currents, and the continuous X-ray exposure impose physical limits on the capacity of helical CT for achieving short scan acquisition times and the maximum number of scans per series. Typical parameters for cardiac CT image acquisition include 3-mm collimator with 5 to 6 mm/s table speed and 2 to 3 mm reconstruction. Multidetector CT offers the latest advantage in CT technology by combining multiple rows of detectors and faster gantry rotation speeds. Multidetector CT offers a distinct advantage over traditional spiral CT for imaging the beating heart. Although multidetector scanners offer a rotation speed of only 500 ms, advanced reconstruction algorithms may increase temporal resolution to 250 ms, which provides additional benefit for reduction of cardiac motion artifacts. This may potentially obviate the need for cardiac gating.

EBCT enables ultrafast scan acquisition times of 50 to 100 ms. The main advantage of EBCT over other CT techniques is its short acquisition time, which provides cardiac imaging free of motion blurring. Other advantages are its high heat capacity and wide gantry, allowing the patient table to be tilted, so that short-axis and long-axis views of the heart can be acquired. By the use of such orthogonal contrast images, EBCT can identify structures as small as 1 to 2 mm, including left atrial appendage thrombus formation. Because EBCT combines high spatial resolution and speed, it has gained interest as a tool for functional cardiac imaging. Ultrafast EBCT allows cardiac imaging in several modes. In "cine" or movie mode, tomographic scans 8-mm thick can be acquired every 50 ms; as many as 80 scans in rapid sequence can be taken during one contrast injection. Thus, it is possible to obtain multislice movies spanning from the base of the heart to the apex during a single study. In "volume" mode, images of 3, 6, or 10 mm can be obtained. The images are acquired when the system is triggered at an operator-selected point on the ECG. As many as 20 multilevel scans can be obtained in one contrast injection. Thus, this acquisition mode produces multilevel contiguous images of the entire heart at a specific point in the cardiac cycle. The full usefulness of EBCT for evaluation of cardiac tumors is, however, still incompletely understood at present. Specific limitations of EBCT relate to the more complex technology compared with conventional or spiral CT, requiring more intense maintenance and quality control. Furthermore, the availability of EBCT is limited to relatively few sites in North America, Europe, and Asia.

CT scanning protocols for evaluation of cardiac masses generally require intravenous injections of iodinated contrast material to reveal the atrial and ventricular cavities. The amounts used per diagnostic examination range from 50 to 200 mL. Generally, side effects from contrast administration tend to be minor. Patients experience a hot "flush" as contrast passes through the circulation. However, severe allergic reactions and exacerbations of hyperthyroidism are rare, but serious, complications. Also, renal function can deteriorate in patients with compromised baseline renal function. Caution must also be exercised in patients with congestive heart failure, which may undergo fluid overload during such contrast administration protocols.

CMR

CMR of the heart is technically somewhat more challenging than CMR of other organs because of the combined existence of cardiac and respiratory motion. At present, electrocardiographic gating is mandatory for all cardiac imaging to avoid artifacts caused by cardiac motion. In addition, it is highly desirable to perform imaging during breath holds if possible to minimize respiratory motion artifacts. Alternately, newly developed respiratory navigator sequences or multiple excitations may be used to minimize respiratory motion. To provide maximal signal/noise ratio, CMR should be performed on high-field (1.5 T) scanners with dedicated surface coils for cardiac and thoracic imaging. Newer scanners have improved hardware with higher gradient strengths optimized for cardiac imaging, which allow fast imaging. The delineation of different structures and tissue contrast by CMR is highly dependent on the choice of the pulse sequence and of the imaging parameters. Different sequences may provide complementary information on the mass by revealing different characteristics of a given structure. Therefore, a comprehensive examination of suspected cardiac masses by CMR should include the use of different pulse sequences performed in different spatial orientations.[2,6]

Anatomical Imaging and Tissue Characterization

T1- and T2-weighted sequences provide detailed morphological information of the heart, the great vessels, and the adjacent structures. Turbo–spin-echo is now preferred over conventional spin-echo to acquire these images because of its higher acquisition speed. New turbo–spin-echo sequences with multiple echoes per excitation allow the acquisition of one single slice in 12 to 16 heartbeats during a single breath hold. This minimizes respiratory motion artifacts. The use of a double-inversion recovery pulse results in black blood, which facilitates differentiation of heart from blood within the vascular cavities. For gated turbo–spin-echo acquisitions, repetition time (TR) is determined by the R-R interval of the electrocardiogram and thus heart rate. T1-weighted images can be obtained by choosing a relatively short repetition time (1 R-R interval) and short excitation time (TE) (<20 ms). T1-weighted images have excellent imaging contrast and high signal/noise ratio and are, therefore, generally used to obtain images evaluating the anatomical extent of masses and tumors. In addition, T1-weighted imaging provides important information allowing the diagnostic differentiation of masses. In general, cysts and lipomas have very high signal intensity on T1-weighted images. Fibromas and hemangiomas have also somewhat higher signal intensity than normal myocardium, whereas solid tumors are generally isointense on T1-weighted imaging. T2-weighted imaging is achieved by choosing a longer TR (two R-R intervals) and longer TE (60 to 90 ms). Compared with T1-weighted imaging T2-weighted images have increased image contrast but less signal/noise ratio. T2-weighted images usually contribute significantly to the diagnostic differentiation of cardiac masses. Typically, tumors appear brighter than normal myocardium on T2-weighted images. Acute and subacute hematomas have even higher signal on T2-weighted images.

Additional tissue differentiation can be obtained with fat-suppression techniques and with gradient echo imaging. Fat suppression may be obtained by adding a short inversion recovery pulse (STIR) to a T1-weighted turbo–spin-echo sequence. Because of the third inversion pulse, the sequence is often also termed triple-inversion recovery. Application of this short inversion recovery pulse allows signal nulling of fat but not of tissues with longer T1. Applications of the STIR technique include the distinct recognition of fatty tissues such as lipomas and the improved visualization of structures surrounded by fatty tissue.

Gradient echo imaging may also be useful in providing some tissue characterization. Gradient echo, which is also called fast low-shot angle (FLASH) imaging, uses small flip angles (10 to 20 degrees), allowing for shorter TRs (4 to 10 ms) and faster image acquisition. Gradient echo imaging is, therefore, mostly used to acquire localizer or cine imaging. Gradient echo images are characterized by lower soft tissue contrast, which is mainly determined by proton density, making them generally less valuable for imaging of cardiac masses relative to spin-echo techniques. Yet, specific features of gradient echo images may be used to provide additional differentiation of cardiac masses. Gradient echo images are characterized by bright signal intensity because of the inflow of nonexcited protons (they are therefore also called bright blood images). Because spin-echo images can often present artifacts when blood is flowing slowly, gradient echo images may be more useful for the differentiation of intravascular structures, in particular for the differentiation of thrombus from flowing blood. Gradient echo images are more prone to magnetic susceptibility artifacts than spin-echo images, because T2* effects are not refocused with a 180-degree radiofrequency pulse. Signal void can occur in areas of hemorrhage caused by hemosiderin deposition or around calcified areas. These features may be useful for identification of certain tumors (i.e., myxoma or osteoblastoma).

Cine Images

Cine imaging may be obtained either with gated segmented K-space gradient echo techniques or with newer true fast imaging in steady-state precession (FISP) sequences. Gradient echo sequences have a repetition time of typically 6 to 8 ms, which typically allows the acquisition of one cine slice with a temporal resolution of 40 to 50 ms within one breath hold of a 12- to 16-heartbeat duration. As previously discussed, gradient echo sequences demonstrate bright blood and intermediate tissue signal. True FISP sequences are gradient echo sequences with balanced refocusing gradients. This allows the generation of supplementary echoes per excitation and therefore faster image acquisitions (TR 2 to 3 ms and typical breath-hold duration of six to eight heartbeats for a temporal resolution of 40 to 50 ms per image) can be achieved. True FISP sequences show less cardiac signal but better contrast between the myocardium and flowing blood. Because true FISP sequences rely on a steady state of constant excitation and gradient balance, they are more prone to motion artifacts and also to chemical shift artifacts than conventional gradient echo sequences. Cine imaging allows the assessment of cardiac mass mobility and the appreciation of their hemodynamic consequences, such as prolapse from the atrium into the left ventricle and partial obstruction of mitral inflow. Tumor mobility is also an important criterion for identification of certain masses such as thrombi and myxomas. In addition, cine imaging allows the evaluation of global cardiac function in patients with cardiac tumors and masses. This may be important for preoperative risk stratification of patients with cardiac masses.

Cardiac tagging may be an additional useful method for the evaluation of cardiac tumors.[6] Tagging relies on the application of a pattern of selective presaturation pulses to the myocardium in end-diastole. The tags persist during a period of approximately 500 ms on the tissue and can be visualized as black bands on subsequent cine gradient echo images during systole. Because myocardial tags reflect an intrinsic property of the tissue, they deform with myocardial motion during the cardiac cycle. Deformation of tag lines can thus allow the differentiation of contractile from noncontractile tissue. This may be useful to determine whether a cardiac mass is intramyocardial or pericardial, as well as to define the exact limit of an intramyocardial mass.

Contrast-Enhanced CMR

The use of paramagnetic contrast agents is also beneficial for the differential diagnosis of cardiac masses.[7] The most commonly used contrast agent, gadolinium-diethylene-triamine-pentaacetic acid (Gd-DTPA), has low molecular weight and mainly extracellular distribution. Because of this extracellular diffusion, the behavior of this contrast agent in tissue is rather complex and has different behavior over time. Although few authors have reported on the influence of time between contrast injection and image acquisition, contrast-enhanced studies in infarcted myocardium and studies of tumors in

other organs, such as the liver, suggest that the time when images are acquired may be an important factor that has to be taken into account for the correct interpretation of contrast-enhanced images. Early images during the first passage of the contrast agent reflect primarily tissue perfusion. Images acquired at later time points (5 to 15 minutes after contrast injection) have been shown to reveal myocellular necrosis and also fibrosis. It is likely that as for solid tumors and infarct characterization, these characteristics also apply to imaging of cardiac masses. First-pass images are likely to provide information about vascularity, whereas later images will provide information about necrosis and fibrosis.

Imaging Protocol

To allow comprehensive examination of a typical cardiac mass, first, plain scout images in coronal or sagittal direction are performed to localize the mass (Table 15-3), then a set of axial T1- and T2-weighted turbo–spin-echo images are prescribed to cover the entire area of the mass. To allow precise anatomical evaluation of the extent of the mass in three-dimensions, additional coronal and sagittal T1 images should be performed. A set of axial or short-axis cine gradient echo images can be performed next to evaluate tumor mobility. Finally, perfusion of the mass can be evaluated by first-pass and delayed gadolinium-enhanced sequences.

NORMAL VARIANTS AND MASSES OF UNKNOWN SIGNIFICANCE

Normal Anatomical Variants

Several normal anatomical structures may sometimes be confused with cardiac tumors. The crista terminalis is a fibromuscular ridge, which extends along the posterolateral aspect of the right atrium between the openings of the superior and inferior vena cava. It is derived from the regression of the septum separating the sinus venosus from the atrium proper. Inferiorly, the crista terminalis merges with the valve of the inferior vena cava (Eustachian valve) and the valve of the coronary sinus (thebesian valve). The Eustachian valve may often be identified as highly mobile structures floating inside the right atrial chamber at the level of junction with the inferior vena cava. The Chiari network may be seen in the right atrium of 2% to 3% of normal subjects. All these structures may sometimes be confused with right atrial cardiac masses when they are extensive. They are most often visualized by TEE but can also frequently be seen on CMR images as nodular thickening of the posterior right atrial wall. In the left atrium, pectinate muscles are a series of normal muscle ridges that can frequently be visualized as parallel echogenic densities protruding into the lumen of the lateral atrial wall. They may sometimes be confused with left atrial thrombus.[8] In the right ventricle, the moderator band is a muscular structure through which the fibers of the right bundle-branch run. It typically extends from the midventricular septum through the

TABLE 15-3 COMPONENTS OF A TYPICAL CMR PROTOCOL FOR COMPREHENSIVE ASSESSMENT OF CARDIAC TUMORS AND MASSES

Description	Orientation	Pulse sequence	Repetition time	Echo time	Excitation flip angle	Echo train length	Other
Anatomical							
T1 weighted	Axial and oblique	Turbo–spin-echo with black blood (double IR)	1 RR interval (600-1000 ms)	30 ms	90˚	24-32	
T2 weighted	Axial or *oblique*	Turbo–spin-echo with black blood (double IR)	2 RR interval (1200-2000 ms)	60 ms	90˚	24-32	
T1 *fat-suppressed*	Axial or *oblique*	Turbo–spin-echo with fat suppression (triple IR)	1 RR interval (600-1000 ms)	30 ms	90˚	24-32	Inversion time 200-250 ms
Cine							
Regular cine	Axial and/or short-axis	Cine fast-gradient echo or cine true-FISP	6 ms / 3 ms	2-3 ms / 1-2 ms	10-20˚ / 40-50˚	–	Segmented K-space cine
Tagged cine	*Short-axis*	*Cine fast-gradient echo with SPAMM*	6 ms	2-3 ms	10-20˚	–	Segmented K- space cine
Contrast-enhanced							
First pass	Axial	Saturation recovery fast-gradient echo with echo-planar readout	6 ms	2-3 ms	10-20˚	4	Recovery time 150 ms
Late images (5 min)	Axial	Inversion recovery fast-gradient echo	6 ms	2-3 ms	10-20˚	–	Inversion time 200-300 ms

Elements marked in bold are part of the standard protocol. Elements in italics are optional and can be used to obtain additional diagnostic information in selected cases. Times are approximate, and parameters are as used on the authors' system.
Adapted from Hoffman et al. *Eur Heart J* 1998; 19:553.

cavity of the right ventricle and attaches near the base of the anterior tricuspid papillary muscle. This structure is present in most normal individuals but is more prominent in patients with right ventricular hypertrophy and dilation. It may sometimes be mistaken for a right ventricular tumor or thrombus. False tendons and muscular bridges are mobile structures, which connect trabeculations in the apex of the left ventricle. These structures are more commonly identified in patients with left ventricular hypertrophy and/or dilation and may cause confusion with apical thrombus. Lambl's excrescences are fine filamentous deposits of thrombus and connective tissue covered by a single layer of endothelium, which form on the surface of the heart valves after endothelial damage. They are 1-cm long and 1-mm thick and typically arise from the ventricular surface of the aortic valve, particularly along the closure margins of the aortic valve cusps. They sometimes may be confused with vegetations or papillary fibroelastoma.

Mitral Annulus Calcification

Calcification of the mitral annulus is a common abnormality observed in elderly patients and in patients with hypertension and diabetes. The incidence of mitral annulus calcification is also increased in patients with chronic renal failure and secondary hyperparathyroidism. Mitral annulus calcification usually involves the posterior aspect of the annulus, and the entire valve ring may become calcified with extension to involve the posterior mitral valve leaflet. In most cases, mitral annular calcification is of little functional consequence. However, when the calcification becomes extensive, it may interfere with the normal mitral valve closure and become a cause of mitral regurgitation. It may be associated with an increased risk for stroke according to data from the Framingham study and has also been associated with embolization of calcium debris. Last, in patients with severe calcification of the cardiac skeleton, the conduction system may become involved with development of atrioventricular or intraventricular conduction defects.

Echocardiography

Mitral annular calcification is commonly identified on TTE as brilliant immobile enhancement of the mitral annulus and the proximal insertion of the posterior mitral valve leaflet. The immobility of the calcification helps to differentiate this condition from calcified mitral vegetations and echodense tumors. Echocardiography also allows investigation of the consequences of this condition on mitral valve dynamics, such as the presence and severity of mitral regurgitation or stenosis.

CT

Mitral annular calcification can readily be identified on non–contrast-enhanced images CT imaging as an intense radiopacity (>130 HU) in the posterior annulus region.

CMR

On CMR imaging, mitral valve calcification appears as an area of profound signal void in the posterior valve region that can be better appreciated on gradient echo images but is usually also visible on T1- and T2-weighted images. Mitral valve regurgitation can be best appreciated as a systolic jet of signal void in the atrium on cine gradient echo or true FISP images.

Lipomatous Infiltration of the Intraatrial Septum

Lipomatous hypertrophy of the intraatrial septum is defined as any deposit of fat in the atrial septum that exceeds 2 cm in transverse dimension. This abnormality results from epicardial fat infiltration into the intraatrial septum and is more common in obese and elderly patients. This is considered to be a hyperplasia of primordial fat in the interatrial septum rather than a cardiac tumor, and it is generally a benign condition. It has been associated with supraventricular arrhythmias. The mass of accumulated fat frequently causes the atrial septal endocardium to bulge and may grow up to 8 cm in diameter and become confused with a true atrial tumor. A typical feature of lipomatous infiltration of the interatrial septum is its anterior location, which typically spares the fossa ovalis.

Echocardiography

Two-dimensional echocardiography can identify lipomatous infiltration of the intraatrial septum as increased thickening and echodensity. The thickened interatrial septum and thin fossa ovalis create a distinctive "dumbbell" appearance, and with TTE, this is best identified from the subcostal four-chamber view.[9] Because of its better spatial resolution, higher diagnostic accuracy is achieved with TEE than with TTE. If the "dumbbell" configuration is not visualized, then to distinguish it from other tumors, additional workup by CT or CMR may be warranted. Lipid deposition in the atrioventricular groove, particularly between right atrium and right ventricle, may be mistaken as an intracavitary (intraatrial) mass on echocardiography.

CT

CT can readily identify the interatrial septum in normal subjects and precisely evaluate its thickness. Abnormal thickening is present when the septum is >10 mm in either the region anterior or posterior to the fossa ovalis.[10] The fatty nature of the infiltrate is suggested by hypointensity relative to water with an attenuation coefficient between −60 and −100 HU.

CMR

The tissue characterization capabilities of CMR make it the diagnostic test of choice for this condition.[11] The nature of the infiltrate in the interatrial septum can be documented as being fatty by the identification of a high signal intensity signal on T1- and T2-weighted images.

Selective reduction of the signal intensity on fat-suppressed images provides definite confirmation of the lipomatous nature of the infiltrate.

Pericardial Cysts

Pericardial cysts are developmental abnormalities of the pericardium that are found in <1:100,000 of the general population. They occur when a portion of the pericardium is isolated during embryonic development, resulting in a fluid-containing cystic mass not connected to the pericardial sac. Pericardial cysts are the most common benign pericardial tumors and are most commonly located in the right costophrenic angle. One fourth of the cysts can be present at the heart border. Pericardial cysts can grow to sizes of >16 cm in diameter and are usually unilocular and filled with a clear liquid. They are usually asymptomatic and are most often discovered as incidental findings on routine chest films. Rarely, chest pain may occur because of cyst torsion. Dyspnea may also occur with cyst enlargement and cardiac compression.

Echocardiography

The echocardiographic appearance of a pericardial cyst is that of an ovoid extracardiac mass that is free of internal echoes and is clearly separated from the ventricular cavities. Pericardial cysts may often be difficult to diagnose with conventional TTE views because of their location behind the right atrium. Visualization may be better with a subcostal view.[12] TEE may provide better visualization of pericardial cysts because of larger imaging windows of the pericardium (Figure 15-2).

CT

CT is the method of choice for the diagnosis of pericardial cyst, because it can determine the liquid nature of the cyst by demonstrating an attenuation coefficient near zero HU. A benign cyst is usually well circumscribed and is located in the right costophrenic angle

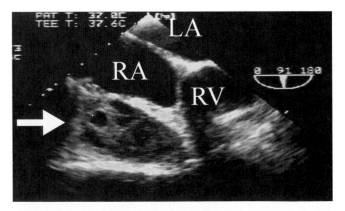

FIGURE 15-2. TEE demonstrating a multiloculated mass *(arrow)* with numerous echo-free spaces bordering the right atrium (RA). The mass was revealed to be a pleuropericardial cyst. LA, left atrium; RV, right ventricle.

along the pericardium. A pericardial cyst does not enhance with intravenous contrast. Positional gravity drainage with a Valsalva maneuver has been recommended to differentiate between a cyst and diverticulum. A diverticulum may change in shape and volume during such maneuvers.

CMR

CMR will identify pericardial cysts. The liquid nature of the cyst is revealed by a typical pattern of homogeneous low signal intensity on T1-weighted images and high signal intensity on T2-weighted images (Figure 15-3).[13]

Intracardiac Thrombi

Intracardiac thrombi are the most commonly occurring cardiac mass. Thrombus can be located in all four cardiac chambers but is more frequently found in left heart chambers. Thrombi in the left atrium occur frequently in patients with chronic atrial fibrillation, mitral stenosis, mitral prostheses, or cardiomyopathy and are a common cause of embolic stroke or systemic embolization.[14] Approximately 50% to 70% of left atrial thrombi originate from the left atrial appendage (Figure 15-4), but they also arise from the left atrial posterior wall (Figure 15-5). They can be mural or protruding. Less commonly, left atrial thrombi become detached and freely mobile. This most often occurs in patients with valve obstruction. Mobile thrombi have the highest risk for systemic embolization and may obstruct the mitral valve, causing electromechanical dissociation or sudden cardiac death. Mobile left atrial thrombi (Figure 15-6) may require emergent surgical removal.

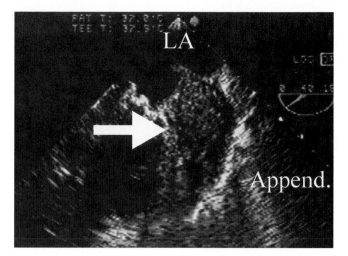

FIGURE 15-4. TEE showing a left atrial appendage *(Append.)* clot *(arrow)* in a patient with atrial fibrillation and stroke.

Ventricular thrombi occur most frequently in the left ventricle, usually in areas of reduced contractility, particularly in patients with acute myocardial infarction or dilated cardiomyopathy. These thrombi are typically mural and located in the apex of the left ventricle. Ventricular thrombi are more common in patients with anterior than with inferior infarction. They are frequent and may occur in up to 60% of patients with acute infarction and in about 20% to 40% with end-stage cardiomyopathy. In such patients, intraventricular thrombi are a common source of cerebral and systemic embolization.

Right atrial thrombus is found less often than left atrial thrombus and occurs in patients with low cardiac output states, such as cardiomyopathy, or from conditions resulting in stasis of blood in the right atrium, such as rheumatic tricuspid stenosis, tricuspid valve replacement, or chronic atrial fibrillation. Such in situ right atrial clots most commonly adhere to the atrial wall and are relatively immobile. Right atrial thrombus frequently forms

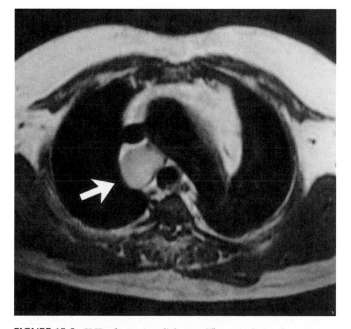

FIGURE 15-3. CMR of a pericardial cyst. The cyst *(arrow)* appears as a well-defined homogeneous mediastinal mass. Its liquid nature is suggested by its high signal intensity on the T2-weighted images.

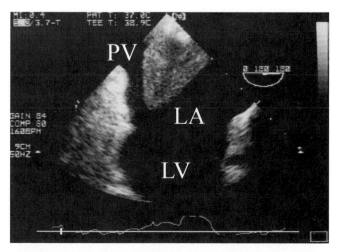

FIGURE 15-5. TEE of a patient with a prosthetic mitral valve and a large mural thrombus attached to the posterior wall of the left atrium (LA). PV, pulmonary vein; LV, left ventricle.

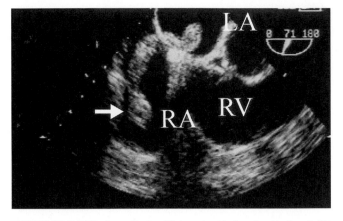

FIGURE 15-6. TEE of a patient with transient ischemic attacks. A fili-form thrombus is entrapped in the foramen ovale of the interatrial septum impending paradoxical embolism.

on indwelling catheters or pacemaker leads (Figure 15-7) and may become large and fragile. Venous thromboemboli may become transiently entrapped in the right atrium and are mobile and often not attached to the atrial wall (so-called ball thrombi) and are shaped as elongated filamentous structures. Such mobile right atrial or ventricular thrombi have high potential for pulmonary embolism, right heart failure, and sudden death and may require surgical removal.

Echocardiography

Left atrial thrombi may appear as discrete well-circumscribed mobile masses that are fairly homogeneous and somewhat more echodense than normal myocardium. Typically, they arise from the tip of the left atrial appendage, and they may be serpentine, dangling into the left atrial cavity. Left atrial thrombi are often accompanied by spontaneous left atrial echo contrast. This has been described as dynamic smoke-like echoes within the

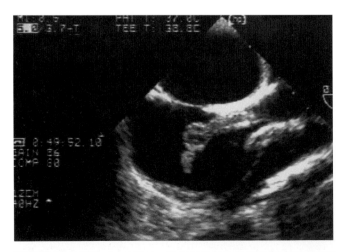

FIGURE 15-7. TEE of a patient with breast cancer who had recurring episodes of fever and positive blood cultures because of infection of a subcutaneous central venous access port. TEE revealed the presence of a mobile thrombus attached to the tip of the catheter.

atrial cavity and left atrial appendage that have a characteristic swirling motion that cannot be eliminated by changes in gain setting (Figure 15-4). The identification of left atrial thrombus is sometimes possible on TTE, especially when thrombi are large and mural. Mobile left ventricular thrombi are generally recognized on TTE. However, because the visualization of the left atrial appendage is poor by TTE, most left atrial thrombi cannot be visualized by this technique, and the overall diagnostic sensitivity of TTE is low, approximately 30% to 40%. TEE provides superior visualization of the left atrial appendage and has excellent sensitivity and specificity for detection of left atrial thrombus, close to 100% against surgical inspection. Therefore, it is currently considered the "gold standard" for detection of left atrial thrombus in patients with stroke or systemic embolism and in patients with chronic atrial fibrillation before percutaneous mitral balloon dilatation or cardioversion.[15,16] The echocardiographic presentation of left ventricular thrombus is that of an echodense apical mass, with well-defined margins, which is associated with hypokinetic myocardium and is identifiable throughout the cardiac cycle and distinguishable from chordal structures and muscle trabeculations.[17,18] Left ventricular thrombus can most commonly be revealed by TTE, with a sensitivity of >90% but with false-positive rates as high as 28%, especially for thrombi located in the apical region, because near-field artifacts may limit satisfactory imaging in this region. False-positive identification of thrombi is reduced if the abnormalities are identified in at least two different views, are found to have clear margins, and are clearly associated with regional wall motion abnormalities. Newer harmonic imaging techniques and contrast administration have improved the delineation of the endocardium and facilitated the diagnosis of left ventricular thrombus, and after administration of contrast, the clot appears as a contrast defect within the cavity clearly distinguished from the surrounding myocardium. In doubtful cases, CT and CMR may be helpful to confirm the diagnosis. Protruding and mobile thrombi (Figure 15-6) are more prone to embolization than mural nonmobile thrombi. Right atrial thrombi are sometimes visualized with TTE, especially when they are large and free floating.[19] TEE (Figure 15-7) provides superior visualization of the superior and inferior vena cavae, the interatrial septum, and the right atrial appendage. TTE may be unable to distinguish right atrial thrombi from other normal intracardiac structures, such as muscular trabeculations, papillary muscles, or false tendons or in differentiating intraventricular thrombus from tumor, and the improved image resolution provided by TEE helps.

CT

The use of blood-enhancing contrast agents allows the detection of thrombi by CT as relatively homogeneous, smooth filling defects within the atrial and ventricular cavities. The absorption rate is variable and dependent on the age of the thrombus. Fresh thrombi have low absorption rate of about + 40 HU. As thrombi organize, they become denser, and their absorption rate increases.

Old thrombi may develop calcification, which can also be identified by CT. Organization of old thrombi may be more difficult to distinguish from cardiac tumors such as cardiac myxoma and sarcoma.

CT is well suited for the detection of left ventricular mural thrombi, and a higher sensitivity and specificity of CT compared with conventional TTE has been reported. CT imaging of the left ventricular apex is better than echocardiography, because it may allow better distinction between thrombi, blood and myocardium. In screening patients with acute myocardial infarction for the presence of left ventricular thrombus, 2D echocardiography is performed more easily, safely, and economically than CT, which may be used to confirm doubtful findings. CT is also capable of detecting right and left atrial mural thrombi (Figure 15-8). However, high-speed EBCT is superior for detecting atrial thrombi, especially within the left atrial appendage. A greater sensitivity for evaluation of left and right atrial thrombi by EBCT over standard TTE has been suggested, but this advantage has been obviated by the introduction of TEE into accepted and widespread clinical practice.

CMR

The age and degree of organization of cardiac thrombus affects CMR images. Fresh thrombi may have a homogeneous appearance with higher signal intensity than myocardium on both T1- and T2-weighted imaging. The high signal intensity on T2-weighted images is consistent with a high amount of hemoglobin. After 1 to 2 weeks, the thrombus begins to organize, undergoing changes, such as loss of water and condensation of paramagnetic iron complexes. This results in a more heterogeneous appearance on CMR imaging and in reduced signal intensity on both T1- and T2-weighted imaging. Old organized thrombi have low signal intensity because of more pronounced water loss. Chronic thrombi may also present areas of calcification, resulting in more heterogeneous signal intensity. Thrombus may

be difficult to distinguish from slow-flowing blood on T1-weighted spin-echo images, but slow-flowing blood shows increased signal intensity on T2-weighted imaging compared with thrombus. Gradient echo images can distinguish between flowing blood, which has high signal intensity, and thrombus, which has low signal intensity. Cine imaging may demonstrate mobility of the thrombus, which typically corresponds to higher fragility and greater risk of embolization. Finally, contrast administration can be useful to differentiate thrombus from tumor. Tumors usually have enhanced signal intensity after contrast administration because of their high vascularization and thrombi are usually not vascularized and thus do not display enhancement after contrast administration.

Although the value of CMR is limited for the diagnosis of left atrial thrombi in the left atrial appendage, which are usually correctly identified with TEE, it may have some role in confirming the diagnosis of doubtful cases of mural atrial and ventricular thrombi. For ventricular thrombus, CMR provides better contrast and spatial resolution than TTE. In addition, the identification of infarcted regions to which a thrombus usually attaches by contrast-enhanced CMR may also facilitate the differentiation of ventricular thrombi.

SECONDARY MALIGNANT CARDIAC TUMORS

Secondary malignant cardiac tumors or metastasis to the heart are 20 to 40 times more common than primary cardiac tumors, and at autopsy, their presence can be detected in 20% of patients with malignancies. A solitary metastasis to the heart is rare. The most common tumors producing cardiac metastasis in adults are carcinoma of the lung and breast, malignant melanoma, lymphoma, and leukemia. In children, the most common secondary tumors are Wilms' tumor, neuroblastoma, and lymphoma. Tumor spread to the heart may occur by three fundamental mechanisms: direct extension, venous extension, or hematogenous spread. Contiguous spread of tumors in the chest cavity is the mechanism most often involved in cardiac metastasis from lung and breast cancer (Figures 15-9 and 15-10). Renal cell carcinoma, adrenal carcinoma, hepatocarcinoma, and uterine leiomyosarcoma reach the heart through the inferior vena cava. Thyroid carcinoma can grow through the superior vena cava. Carcinoma of the lung can invade the pulmonary veins and extend into the left atrium (Figure 15-11). Hematogenous metastatic spread is the third and most common mechanism of tumor invasion of the heart (Figure 15-12). This typically results in metastasis in the ventricles. Both the right and left cardiac chambers are affected by hematogenous metastasis with equal frequency.[20]

Cardiac metastases may be clinically silent and only discovered at autopsy. Because metastasis to the heart occurs relatively late in the course of cancer, symptoms caused by invasion of other organs may be more prominent. Malignant pericardial invasion is the most frequent presentation of metastasis and may cause

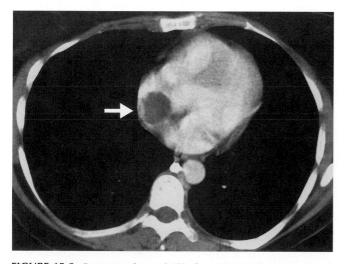

FIGURE 15-8. Contrast-enhanced CT of a patient with recurrent pulmonary embolism. There is a filling defect *(arrow)* corresponding to mural thrombus within the right atrium.

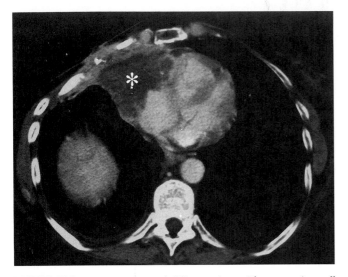

FIGURE 15-9. Contrast-enhanced CT in a patient with metastatic small cell lung cancer. The tumor (∗) has invaded the chest wall and sternum and has metastasized to the right ventricle by contiguous spread and direct invasion through the pericardium.

pericardial effusion and tamponade or symptoms of pericardial inflammation with typical chest pain. Invasion of the myocardium by the tumor itself occurs in only 5% of cardiac metastasis (Figure 15-11) and may result in arrhythmia, congestive heart failure, and peripheral emboli. Invasion or compression of the superior vena cava may lead to its thrombosis and may present as a typical syndrome of superior vena cava occlusion characterized by facial plethora, edema of the face and of the superior extremities, and by collateral vessel development. Because cardiac metastases are rarely the initial manifestation of metastatic cancer, the diagnosis of cardiac metastatic disease vs. primary cardiac tumor only rarely poses a serious dilemma. Differentiation of thrombus vs. intracavitary tumor extension may be more difficult to resolve and sometimes requires histological confirmation.

Echocardiography

Cardiac metastasis may have numerous echocardiographic manifestations. Pericardial effusion is easily identified on TTE imaging, and pericardial metastases present as echodense protrusions and thickening of either the visceral or parietal pericardium.

Tumor extension into the vena cavae or atria is usually not well detected by TTE, but TEE, which has better acoustic windows and closer location to these structures, can usually demonstrate tumor extension.

Malignant invasion of the myocardium may present as intracavitary or intramural masses. Intracavitary masses can be readily identified by both TTE and TEE as echodense protrusions into the cardiac chambers (Figure 15-13). Neoplastic infiltrative masses may show a peculiar echogenicity and ultrasound texture, which is different from that of normal myocardium.

Paracardiac infiltration of tumors is usually poorly identified by TTE but can be better visualized by TEE. Although paracardiac infiltration of tumors is typically investigated by CT or CMR, TEE was found to provide additional information, which was useful for the diagnosis or staging of tumors, which could not be obtained by other techniques.

CT

CT is useful in demonstrating pericardial and paracardiac mediastinal metastasis (Figures 15-9, 15-11, and 15-12). Pericardial effusions can be detected with similar accuracy to echocardiography. However, CT is clearly superior to echocardiography to delineate pericardial thickening and infiltration associated with metastatic tumor invasion (Figure 15-11). The precise demarcation of the pericardium on CT and CMR imaging is of value in determining the extent of mediastinal tumor invasion and may be helpful for the staging of certain mediastinal tumors such as lymphoma.

Contrast-enhanced CT is necessary to determine the presence of intramyocardial metastasis. Intracavitary and intravascular metastases are revealed as filling defects in

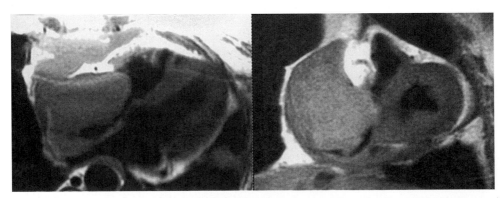

FIGURE 15-10. CMR of a 64-year-old woman with mediastinal non-Hodgkin's lymphoma. **A,** Transaxial T1-weighted image view showing the invasion of the mediastinal mass into the right atrium and ventricle. **B,** Sagittal T1-weighted image showing compression of the right atrium and inferior vena cava.

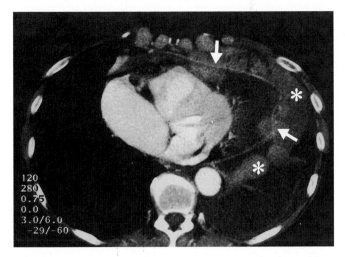

FIGURE 15-11. Contrast-enhanced CT of a patient with advanced lung cancer. The tumor (∗) presents higher contrast enhancement than the neighboring tissue and completely encases the left and right ventricle. The pericardium can clearly be identified as a fine line between the heart and the tumor. Tumor invasion through the pericardium occurs at two distinct locations (arrows). In addition, there is an important pericardial effusion that compresses the left and right ventricle.

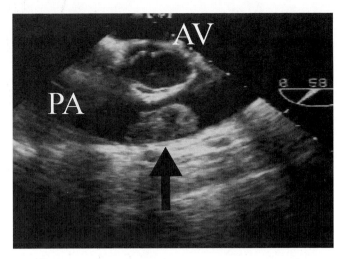

FIGURE 15-13. TEE of a patient with metastatic melanoma. The axial view at the level of the aortic valve (AV) shows a metastasis (arrow) protruding into the lumen of the pulmonary artery (PA).

the atria or vena cavae. Contrast-enhanced CT may also identify intramural metastases. Usually, they present as hypervascular masses surrounded by normal myocardium. Heterogeneity corresponding to necrosis is also often present. Detection of cardiac metastasis by conventional CT may be limited by poor image quality because of motion artifacts. Ultrafast EBCT imaging or gated multidetector spiral imaging may be superior for this purpose.

CMR

CMR may be used to demonstrate pericardial metastases. Thickening and disruption of the pericardium

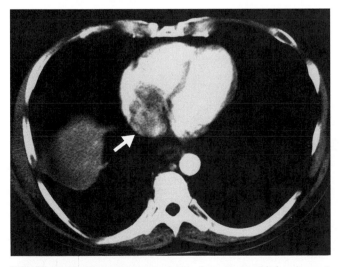

FIGURE 15-12. Contrast-enhanced CT of a patient with hepatocarcinoma. The tumor (arrow) has metastasized to the right atrium by extension through the inferior vena cava.

may be optimally visualized with weighted images. Pericardial metastases are often associated with an exudative pericardial effusion with a high protein content and associated high signal intensity on T1-weighted images. Hemorrhagic pericardial effusions will present with even higher signal intensity on T1-weighted images. Because these hemorrhagic pericardial effusions often contain blood of variable age, the imaging will be more heterogeneous. Conversely, benign transudative nonhemorrhagic effusions have low intensity on T1-weighted and high intensity on T2-weighted spin-echo and gradient echo images.

Tumor extension into the vena cavae and atria is readily identified on both CT and CMR, but CMR may allow better delineation of anatomical relations between the tumor and vascular structures in oblique and sagittal cuts. The best tissue contrast is obtained with CMR, which can be used to identify the presence of intramural metastases. Signal intensity on T1- and T2-weighted images varies with the type of the tumor but is usually distinct from normal myocardium (Figure 15-10). Whereas certain tumors, such as melanoma, may have specific signal intensity patterns (hyperintense on T1-weighted and hypointense on T2-weighted images), determination of the type of metastasis from T1 and T2 characteristics is usually not possible. Contrast-enhanced CMR is useful for delineation of intramural metastasis and manifests intense hyperenhancement of metastases because of high vascularity.

PRIMARY BENIGN CARDIAC TUMORS

Primary tumors of the heart are rare, with an incidence of 0.001% to 0.03% of patients. Three quarters of primary tumors are benign, and the remainder are malignant. In adults, nearly half of all benign tumors are myxoma. The remainder are mostly lipomas, papillary fibroelastomas, and rhabdomyomas. Fibromas, hemangiomas, teratomas, and mesotheliomas of the atrioventricular node are found less frequently. In children, rhabdomyomas, fibromas, and teratomas are the most common primary cardiac tumor.

Myxoma

Cardiac myxoma can occur in all age groups but is particularly frequent in patients between 30 and 60 years old.[21,22] Myxomas usually occur as isolated tumors, but rare cases of multiple myxomas have been reported. Although most cardiac myxomas are sporadic, they may be part of an autosomal-dominant familial syndrome, know as Carney complex.[23] Myxomas present generally as solitary intracavitary polypoid, pedunculated tumors of the atria. Seventy-five percent of all myxomas originate in the left atrium; 15% to 20% originate in the right atrium. Right and left ventricular locations are rare, with less than 4% in each side. Most myxomas arise from the interatrial septum at the border of the fossa ovalis, but they can originate from the posterior atrial wall, the anterior atrial wall, and the atrial appendage. Multiple tumors and atypical locations are more frequent in cases of familiar myxoma. The clinical presentation of myxomas depends on their location. Left-sided myxomas typically produce a classic triad of symptoms similar to mitral valve stenosis with dyspnea, progressive congestive heart failure, systolic and diastolic murmurs, and atrial arrhythmias. Systemic embolism is common. Patients with right-sided myxomas have more variable signs. Right-sided myxoma may cause pulmonary embolism or mimic tricuspid or pulmonary stenosis. Occasionally, myxomas may be associated with fever of unexplained origin or arthralgias.

Echocardiography

TTE is the primary noninvasive technique for the diagnosis of cardiac myxoma. Myxomas generally appear as a heterogeneous roughly globular interatrial masses with a gelatinous aspect, typically attached to the interatrial septum by a small stalk. The appearance of an atrial myxoma is typically frondlike, with multiple speckles so that the body of the tumor is as reflective as its margins. Echo-

free spaces may appear within the mass, corresponding to hemorrhage or necrosis. Areas of calcification, presenting as intense echo signals, may also be identified. Two-dimensional echocardiography can usually identify left and right atrial myxomas with high accuracy if the mass is of sufficient size. Large myxomas may prolapse into or through the mitral valve during diastole and may cause partial inflow obstruction, and Doppler echocardiography can provide hemodynamic information by demonstrating the transvalvular gradient produced by mitral valve obstruction and the degree of regurgitation caused by tumors that interfere with normal valve closure. Better delineation of atrial myxomas can be provided by TEE (Figure 15-14), which can identify small myxomas and further delineate the point of insertion of the stalk. The morphology of a left atrial myxoma seen by TEE is predictive of the frequency of embolic events. Polypoid morphology is more frequently associated with systemic embolization than rounded morphology.

CT

Myxomas viewed by CT characteristically present as large lobulated and more rarely as smooth intraatrial masses (Figure 15-15) . The attachment of the mass to the septum and its stalk can usually be identified on gated cine images but not on ungated CT images. EBCT cine imaging allows visualization of mass mobility. Attenuation of myxoma is generally heterogeneous because of hemorrhage and necrosis, and in some cases, tissue attenuation is less than blood, or myxomas are calcified and can be identified with noncontrast-enhanced imaging. Intravenous administration of contrast may improve myxoma definition as a low enhancing mass surrounded by the enhancing intracardiac blood (Figure 15-15).

CMR

Myxomas are seen with CMR as heterogeneous intraatrial masses characteristically attached to the interatrial septum, and visualization of the stalk is usually not possible. T1-weighted images of atrial myxomas show heterogeneous tissue of intermediate signal intensity compared with normal myocardium.[24,25] With T2-weighted images, myxomas usually have higher signal intensity than neighboring

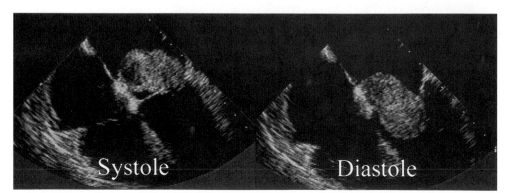

FIGURE 15-14. Perioperative TEE of a large left atrial myxoma. The tumor prolapses through the mitral valve into the left ventricle during diastole.

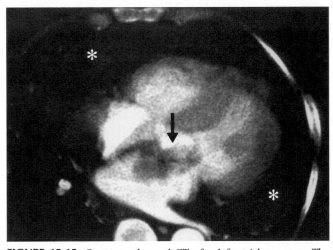

FIGURE 15-15. Contrast-enhanced CT of a left atrial myxoma. The tumor *(arrow)* appears as a large filling defect in the left atrium. Its attachment to the atrial septum can be clearly identified. In addition, a large pericardial effusion (∗) is present.

myocardium. Gradient echo images differentiate tumor from flowing blood better than turbo–spin-echo images, and they present characteristically as a low signal intensity mass, clearly separated from surrounding bright blood (Figure 15-16). The low signal intensity on gradient echo images has been postulated to occur because of the high iron content of the tumor, causing susceptibility artifacts. Myxomas also often have tumor hemorrhage, and acute hemorrhage may appear as heterogeneous areas of low signal intensity on T2-weighted and gradient echo images. Subacute and chronic hemorrhages are seen as heterogeneous areas of high signal intensity on T1- and T2-weighted images. Calcification of a myxoma can be identified as a signal void on T2-weighted images. Gradient echo images typically demonstrate myxomas as hypointense masses, which can be clearly distinguished from flowing blood. Cine images of myxomas are useful to demonstrate the mobility of the tumor in the atrium. Contrast-enhanced studies generally show contrast enhancement of the tumor because of its high vascularity, and this feature helps differentiation between myxoma and thrombus. Contrast enhancement of myxoma can be homogeneously intense but is often inhomogeneous. Enhanced areas correspond histologically to inflammatory changes within the tumor; nonenhanced areas correspond to cystic or necrotic lesions within the tumor.

Lipoma

Cardiac lipomas are the second most common benign cardiac tumor in adults and occur at all ages with equal gender frequency. Lipomas can occur in various regions. The most common locations are the left ventricle, right atrium, and interatrial septum. Usually, lipomas present as sessile tumors growing from the subepicardium into the pericardial space or from the subendocardium into the cardiac cavity. One fourth of all lipomas are completely intramuscular. Lipomas are often clinically asymptomatic and may be discovered as incidental findings on chest X-ray or echocardiograms. Subendocardial tumors may cause cavitary obstruction and shortness of breath. Subepicardial lipomas can cause cardiac compression and pericardial effusion. Cardiac lipomas have also been associated with a variety of arrhythmic events, including atrial fibrillation, ventricular tachycardia, and atrioventricular block.

Echocardiography

Endocardial lipomas appear as echodense homogeneous sessile masses protruding into the left ventricular cavity. Pericardial lipomas may appear relatively echolucent and may be confused with pericardial fluid. Because of the lack of tissue characterization by echocardiography, the differential diagnosis of lipoma compared with other cardiac masses is difficult. Typically, lipomas appear somewhat less mobile and more echodense than myxomas. Because the echocardiographic appearance may mimic other tumors such as fibroma, fibroelastoma, or thrombus, further diagnostic testing by CT or CMR imaging is generally warranted.

CT

CT can identify fat and, therefore, can be used to diagnose cardiac lipoma with a high degree of specificity. By use of CT, cardiac lipomas appear as homogeneous, low-attenuation masses, with an attenuation coefficient of less than −50 HU. Contrast administration increases the density differences between the nonenhancing tumor, the myocardium, and the cardiac chambers. Contrast administration may further define the anatomy and explain the relationship between coronary arteries to allow surgical planning.

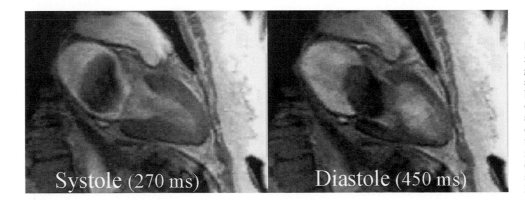

Systole (270 ms)   Diastole (450 ms)

FIGURE 15-16. CMR of a left atrial myxoma. On these bright blood gradient echo images, the myxoma appears dark relative to the blood because of its high iron content. The cine imaging mode allows one to appreciate the motion of the tumor during the cardiac cycle. During diastole, the tumor prolapses through the mitral valve into the left ventricle. (Images supplied by Dr. Anna John and Dr. Thorsten Dill from Bad Neuheim, Germany).

CMR

CMR has the ability to specifically identify fat and is the test of choice to diagnose cardiac lipomas. Lipomas present as homogeneous masses of high signal intensity on both T1- and T2-weighted images. Sometimes, fine septations can be identified within the lipoma. The signal intensity of lipomas is similar to that of mediastinal fat and characteristically can be reduced by fat-suppression techniques. Lipomas are slightly hyperintense on gradient echo images and do not enhance after contrast injection.

Rhabdomyoma

Rhabdomyomas are congenital tumors that present at birth, in early infancy, or in young childhood. Adult cases are rare. There is a well-described association of rhabdomyomas with tuberous sclerosis. Approximately 40% of patients with pathologically confirmed cardiac rhabdomyoma have tuberous sclerosis; conversely, 50% of patients with tuberous sclerosis have evidence of rhabdomyoma on echocardiography. In most cases, rhabdomyomas present as multiple tumors. They occur with equal frequency in the right and left ventricle. Rarely, they can also involve the atria but never the cardiac valves. The clinical presentation is variable, and patients are often asymptomatic.

The tumor may cause a mass effect and protrude into the ventricular cavities and cause obstruction. Rhabdomyomas may also cause a wide variety of cardiac arrhythmias. They are slow-growing tumors and may often regress spontaneously. Noninvasive imaging techniques may be useful to monitor the evolution of the tumor in asymptomatic patients.

Echocardiography

With 2D TTE, rhabdomyomas appear as nodular intracavitary and intramural masses with greater echodensity than the surrounding myocardium. The presence of such multiple masses in several chambers in the heart in a young child, especially with a history of tuberous sclerosis, is highly suggestive for rhabdomyoma. When only one mass is present, or when presentation occurs in adults, the differential diagnosis with other tumors such as fibroma or lipoma is difficult and may require additional noninvasive tests and biopsy. Presence of rhabdomyomas can sometimes be diagnosed on prenatal echograms in utero. Echocardiography is a useful noninvasive method for screening asymptomatic children with tuberous sclerosis for presence of cardiac tumors and useful for serial follow-up.

CT

Few studies of imaging rhabdomyomas by CT have been reported, but identification on noncontrast-enhanced images is difficult, because these tumors present attenuation similar to normal myocardium and blood. After contrast injection, rhabdomyomas can be identified as protruding intracavitary masses, with homogeneous enhancement similar to normal myocardium.

CMR

Using T1-weighted CMR, rhabdomyomas present as a slightly hyperintense or isointense homogeneous intramural mass.[26] On T2-weighted images, rhabdomyomas also appear isointense. Gradient echo images are poorly suited to differentiate rhabdomyoma from neighboring normal myocardium. Tagged cine imaging or contrast-enhanced imaging may be used to distinguish the limits of the tumor from normally contracting myocardium. CMR and echocardiography are complementary for the detection of rhabdomyoma, because rhabdomyomas detected by echocardiography may be missed with CMR and vice versa. In general, echocardiography demonstrates small, or entirely intramural, lesions better than CMR.

Papillary Fibroelastoma

Papillary fibroelastomas are rare benign tumors.[27,28] Most commonly, these tumors affect patients older than 60 years of age. Papillary fibroelastomas may occur anywhere in the heart but most frequently arise from the valves. Left-sided and right-sided tumors occur with nearly equal frequency. Most often the ventricular surface of the semilunar valves and the atrial side of the atrioventricular valves are affected. The tricuspid valve is most commonly involved in children; the mitral and aortic valves more commonly in adults. Papillary fibroelastoma can also involve the chordae tendineae, the endocardium of the right atrium or the papillary muscles, or either side of the ventricular septum. The tumors are usually isolated, although some descriptions of multiple tumors have been made. Calcification rarely occurs. The tumors are characteristically of small size (<1.5 cm) and have an appearance like a "sea anemone," because they consist of multiple papillary fronds attached to the endocardium by a short stalk. Fibroelastomas are usually discovered in asymptomatic patients as incidental findings. When symptoms are present, they relate to systemic or coronary embolization from thrombi that collect on the tumor.

Echocardiography

Echocardiography is the principal imaging technique for the identification and diagnosis of papillary fibroelastoma. By use of 2D echocardiography, papillary fibroelastomas appear as homogeneous, rounded, well-demarcated masses attached to the cardiac valves, and dynamic 3D echocardiography may provide improved assessment.[29] The most characteristic ultrasound features that identify an endocardial mass as a papillary fibroelastoma are small size, their pedicle attachment, high mobility, and refractive appearance.[30] Often, areas of echolucency can be seen within the tumor. The peripheral edge of tumor characteristically has a stippled edge and a vibration or shimmer. These features are all clearer with TEE. Typically, these valvular tumors are not associated with valvular insufficiency or stenosis.

CT

Because of its low temporal resolution, conventional CT is not useful for the diagnosis of these valvular tumors.

CMR

CMR is of little value for diagnostic imaging of papillary fibroelastoma. Because of their mobility, these tumors are usually not well visualized on T1- or T2-weighted CMR images. Cine sequences, especially with thin slices, may allow visualization of the valves and sometimes identification of fibroelastoma, but these are not used routinely clinically. This, however, provides little additional diagnostic information compared with echocardiographic imaging.

Fibroma

Cardiac fibromas are tumors that primarily affect children. They constitute the second most common type of primary tumor in children. Presentation typically occurs before the age of 10 years, and 40% are diagnosed in infants <1 year old. Almost all fibromas occur within the ventricular myocardium, most frequently within the anterior free wall of the left ventricle or the intraventricular septum. More rarely, fibromas may occur in the posterior wall of the left ventricle or in the right ventricle. Fibromas are usually large well-circumscribed tumors with a mean diameter of 5 cm. Calcification is common; focal cystic changes, hemorrhage, or necrosis are absent.

Cardiac fibromas are often associated with arrhythmias and may be a cause of sudden cardiac death. They may also be associated with heart failure, atypical chest pain, murmurs, and pulmonary or aortic infundibular stenosis.

Echocardiography

The typical presentation of cardiac fibroma is that of a large intramural lesion identified in a young child. Echocardiography reveals these tumors as echodense, usually homogeneous and well circumscribed. Fibroma, in contrast to rhabdomyoma, usually presents as a single tumor. The characteristic location within the intraventricular septum or the ventricular free wall helps in the diagnosis, and the affected wall segment is usually hypokinetic and heterogeneous in ultrasonic texture. Central tumor calcification may be identified as intense echodensity with shadowing or may be seen on a chest X-ray, and the presence of such calcification is relatively characteristic.

CT

By unenhanced CT, fibromas appear as homogeneous intramural tumors. After contrast injection, fibromas appear as a low-attenuation masses with homogenous or more rarely heterogeneous enhancement, similar to normal myocardium.

CMR

With CMR imaging, fibromas are homogeneous tumors that are isointense or slightly hypointense on T1-weighted images compared with the surrounding myocardium. On T2-weighted images, fibromas are hypointense relative to myocardium (Figure 15-17). Contrast enhancement is typically absent, so that fibromas are usually hypointense relative to the surrounding myocardium. However, they may exhibit a hyperenhanced core or homogeneous or heterogeneous enhancement.

Hemangioma/Lymphangioma

Hemangiomas are rare, accounting for <5% of all cardiac tumors and are usually discovered incidentally. They may occur in any part of the heart but are usually intramural more commonly in right heart chambers. Hemangiomas may also present in the visceral pericardium. Clinical manifestations of hemangiomas include dyspnea, arrhythmias, or pericardial effusion, sometimes with hemopericardium.

Echocardiography

The typical echocardiographic presentation of cardiac hemangioma is that of an echodense but nonhomogeneous mass with multiple echo-free spaces, resulting in a granular spongy appearance.[31] They may also present as solid echodense masses or as unilocular cysts, mimicking a pericardial cyst. Typically, hemangiomas are subendocardial, nonmobile, and nonpedunculated. Partial calcification may occur and present as an echodense structure. Such calcification, especially when associated with a cavernous aspect, is very suggestive of hemangioma. Right ventricular location is also suggestive for hemangioma but not typical. Characterization of the tumor by echocardiography alone is unusual. The best identification of hemangiomas is provided by coronary angiography, where a discrete vascular supply arising from the coronary arteries can be identified. The high vascularization results in a typical "tumor blush" after contrast injection. CT and CMR imaging may reveal the vascular nature of the mass.

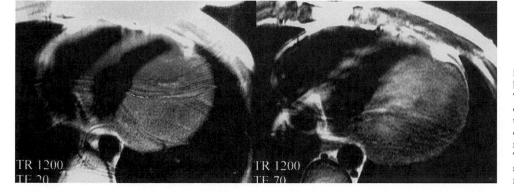

FIGURE 15-17. MR in a 14-year-old boy with a left ventricular fibroma. T1-weighted images *(left panel)* demonstrate a homogeneous mass in the lateral free wall of the left ventricle, which is isointense relative to neighboring normal myocardium. On T2-weighted images, the mass is slightly hyperintense relative to neighboring myocardium.

CT

With unenhanced CT imaging, hemangiomas present as heterogeneous masses, which approximately have the same intensity as cardiac muscle. After contrast administration, they characteristically demonstrate intense enhancement, a finding that can be diagnostic.

CMR

With CMR, hemangiomas are characterized as heterogeneous regions of increased signal intensity of T1-weighted images because of slow-flowing blood. On T2-weighted images, they also present high signal intensity. Hemangiomas typically present pronounced contrast enhancement because of their high vascularity.

Paraganglioma/Pheochromocytomas

Cardiac paragangliomas or pheochromocytomas are very rare neuroendocrine tumors.[32] These tumors are most often located in the posterior mediastinum, in the posterior wall of the left atrium, or the left atrial roof. More rarely, they may also arise from the interatrial septum. Paragangliomas can be nonfunctional or functional, secreting catecholamines and therefore associated with signs and symptoms characteristic of a pheochromocytoma. Localization of secreting tumors is best performed by ^{131}I-MIBG scintigraphy. Echocardiography, CT, and CMR may localize secreting and nonsecreting tumors in the heart and mediastinum.

Echocardiography

Paragangliomas can be identified as echodense masses on 2D TTE imaging when atrial location is the case. More rarely, TTE may reveal mediastinal lesions. Better identification of mediastinal and intraatrial location is obtained with TEE.

CT

By use of unenhanced CT, paragangliomas appear as circumscribed heterogeneous masses with low attenuation. Dynamic imaging after contrast administration reveals marked contrast enhancement. Often central areas of low attenuation can be observed, corresponding to central necrosis. Tumor calcification may also be identified. Small cardiac paragangliomas may be missed on unenhanced, or poorly enhanced, chest CT scans because of their isointensity with normal tissue.

CMR

With CMR, paragangliomas are usually isointense or hypointense on T1-weighted images. However, increased signal intensity has been reported, presumably because of hemorrhage within the tumor. With T2-weighted images, they usually have markedly increased signal intensity. Paragangliomas demonstrate intense contrast enhancement because of their vascularity, which may be heterogeneous, with central nonenhancing areas caused by tumor necrosis. CMR seems to be superior to CT for the detection and accurate localization of paraganglioma.

Teratomas

Teratomas are rare primary cardiac tumors usually diagnosed in neonates and infants. They occur more frequently in the anterior mediastinum than in the heart. Cardiac locations are more frequently pericardial. Symptoms may arise from pericardial compression.

Echocardiography

The typical echocardiographic aspect of intrapericardial teratoma is that of a multilocular intrapericardial cyst. Intracardiac teratomas present generally as right-sided masses with heterogeneous echogenicity.

CT

CT can readily identify teratomas. A teratoma typically presents as a heterogeneous multiloculated cyst with low-density fluid content and calcification. Pericardial effusions are often associated with cardiac teratomas.

CMR

T1-weighted CMR imaging shows teratomas as heterogeneous multiloculated masses of the pericardium.[33] A case observed in our hospital demonstrated both a heterogeneous aspect on T2-weighted imaging and a heterogeneous contrast enhancement on T1-weighted CMR (Figure 15-18).

PRIMARY MALIGNANT CARDIAC TUMORS

Primary cardiac malignancies are rare. They constitute only 25% of all primary cardiac tumors. Nearly all of these are sarcomas. Angiosarcomas and undifferentiated sarcomas are the most common, followed by rhabdomyosarcomas, fibrosarcomas, and osteosarcomas. Other types of primary cardiac sarcomas such as leiomyosarcoma, liposarcoma, and synovial sarcoma have also been described but are extremely uncommon.

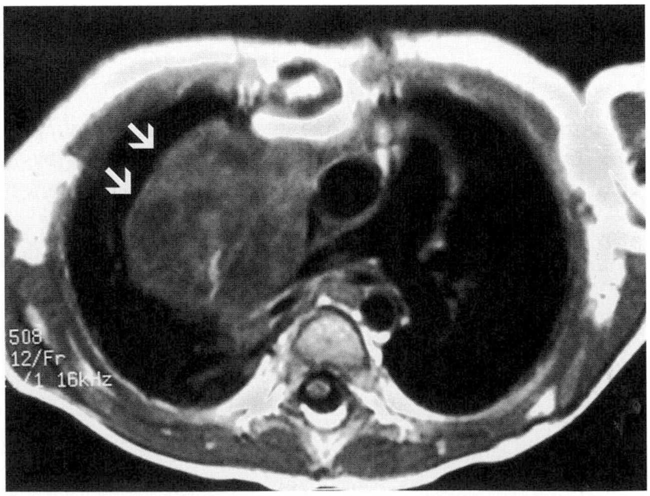

FIGURE 15-18. MR of a pericardial teratoma. The tumor (arrows) appears as a multiloculated anterior mediastinal mass originating from the pericardium and presents with heterogeneous signal intensity on T1-weighted images.

Sarcomas may occur at any age but are most common between the third and fifth decade. Symptoms for sarcomas are determined primarily by the location of the tumor and the extent of cardiac involvement. Typical presentations may include progressive congestive heart failure, pericardial effusion and tamponade, precordial pain, obstruction of the venae cavae, and arrhythmias. Primary malignant tumors of the heart typically have rapid growth and short survival time after diagnosis. Approximately 75% of patients have evidence of metastasis at the time of death, and the most frequent locations for metastasis are the lungs, thoracic lymph nodes, mediastinum, and vertebral bodies. Sarcomas are most commonly detected by echocardiography. CT and CMR are helpful for the evaluation and stratification of sarcomas and may be required to determine myocardial, pericardial, and mediastinal extension, as well as extension into the great vessels and lungs.[34]

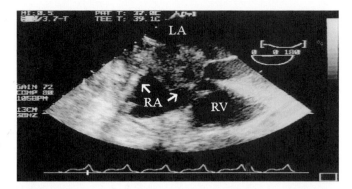

FIGURE 15-19. Transesophageal echocardiogram in a 51-year-old man with right atrial angiosarcoma. The tumor can be seen as a large mass with irregular contours and heterogeneous echogenicity in the intraatrial septum. The malignancy of the mass is suggested by its large base of implantation and by its invasive character toward the free wall of the atrium and the tricuspid valve *(arrows)*.

Angiosarcoma

Angiosarcoma is the most common cardiac sarcoma and usually occurs in middle-aged men, who seem to be affected two to three times more frequently than women. Angiosarcoma has a striking predilection for the right atrium, and two main presentations have been described. The first presentation is as a well-defined polypoid mass with a wide base of implantation that protrudes into the right atrial cavity and typically spares the atrial septum. The other presentation of angiosarcoma is as a diffuse invasion of the epicardial atrial wall, which extends into the pericardium and obliterates the pericardial space. This presentation can be associated with cutaneomucous lesions of Kaposi's sarcoma and AIDS. The clinical signs of angiosarcoma are often related to right atrial inflow obstruction and include distended jugular veins, positive Kussmaul sign, peripheral and facial edema, pulsus paradoxus, and hepatomegaly. Approximately half of the patients have hemopericardium or tamponade. In rare cases, cardiac rupture may occur. Angiosarcoma is a rapidly progressing tumor with a rapidly fatal outcome. Typically, patients are detected at stages when the disease has progressed so far that tumor resection is unwarranted.[35]

Echocardiography

The typical echocardiographic features of angiosarcoma are presence of a right atrial tumor associated with a pericardial effusion. Characteristically, the mass is ill defined and infiltrates the right atrium toward the right ventricle or the vena cava. Such a presentation is highly suspicious of angiosarcoma and when identified mandates further diagnostic investigation. This typical presentation can only be identified in approximately 40% of all patients by TTE, and in many other cases, atrial involvement is not identified. One may see enlargement of the right atrial chamber, thickening of the cardiac wall, and/or pericardial effusion. Therefore, TTE is often nondiagnostic for angiosarcoma. TEE is better suited to demonstrate the atrial mass or atrial infiltration (Figure 15-19). Usually, correct identification of the condition may require CT and CMR, which allow better delineation of atrial infiltration by a small tumor mass than echocardiography, and these techniques may be more useful for staging the tumor and determining its operability. Echocardiography, on the other hand, may be useful to follow patients during the course of chemotherapy.

CT

With noncontrast-enhanced CT, angiosarcoma may appear as a hypodense nodular heterogeneous mass in the right atrium. Pericardial effusion is often present. After contrast administration, angiosarcoma typically appears as a filling defect in the right atrium with broad implantation and heterogeneous enhancement (Figure 15-20). CT allows the appreciation of the malignant character of the tumor by showing pericardial and mediastinal invasion, as well as extension into the vena cava.

CMR

With T1-weighted CMR images, angiosarcoma typically has a heterogeneous aspect. This appears as a cauliflower-like appearance and consists of areas of focal or peripheral increases in signal intensity, which correspond to intratumoral hemorrhage, interspersed within a tumor of intermediate signal intensity. A similar appearance can also be identified on T2-weighted images (Figure 15-21). The malignant character of the lesion on CMR is suggested by infiltration of the tumor into the myocardium, the pericardium, or the great vessels. Contrast-enhanced images may show intense enhancement in a heterogeneous pattern because of the presence of tumor hemorrhage and necrosis. In cases with diffuse pericardial infiltration, linear contrast enhancement along vascular lakes has been described to present a "sunray" appearance.

Rhabdomyosarcoma

Rhabdomyosarcomas account for only 4% to 7% of cardiac sarcomas but are the most common cardiac malignancy in infants and children. This tumor has a slight male preponderance. Rhabdomyosarcomas may arise anywhere in the myocardium and involve the left and

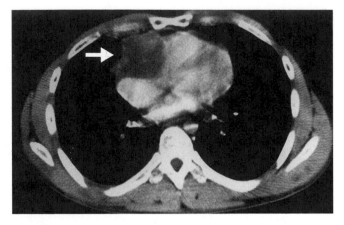

FIGURE 15-20. Contrast-enhanced CT in a 27-year-old woman with angiosarcoma. The tumor *(arrow)* can be seen as a large filling defect with wide base of implantation in the right atrium.

right side of the heart with similar frequency; they are often multiple and may invade the pericardium. Rhabdomyosarcoma is also more likely than any other sarcoma to arise from the cardiac valves but typically is an infiltrating tumor of the myocardium or may present as polypoid extensions into the cardiac chambers.

Echocardiography

With echocardiography, rhabdomyosarcomas typically present as solitary or multiple echodense cardiac masses with broad attachment. The malignant character of the mass is suggested by its wide base of attachment, its

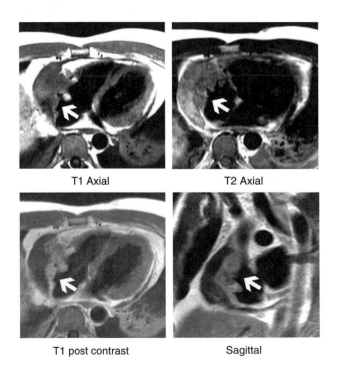

T1 Axial   T2 Axial

T1 post contrast   Sagittal

FIGURE 15-21. CMR image of a 40-year-old man with right atrial angiosarcoma. T1-weighted images show a heterogeneous mass protruding into the right atrial cavity and into the pericardial space. There is presence of a large pericardial effusion. The tumor invades into the right atrial appendage and into the inferior and superior vena cavae. On T2-weighted images, the tumor is slightly hyperintense and heterogeneous. After contrast administration, there is intense and heterogeneous enhancement of the tumor mass.

nonhomogeneous appearance, and its infiltrative character. Pericardial effusion is often observed. Valvular extension is best visualized on echocardiography.

CT

Rhabdomyomas can be identified on contrast-enhanced CT imaging as smooth or irregular low-attenuation masses with heterogeneous contrast enhancement, and wide point of attachment. Pericardial invasion and effusion, as well as extracardiac extension, are also clearly depicted at CT imaging.

CMR

With CMR, rhabdomyosarcomas appear as isointense or heterogeneous intracardiac masses with a wide point of attachment.[34] CMR may also demonstrate pericardial involvement and necrosis of the tumor. Similar to other sarcomas, rhabdomyosarcomas may also present contrast enhancement after Gd-DTPA injection.

Fibrosarcoma and Malignant Fibrous Histiocytomas

Fibrosarcoma and malignant fibrous histiocytomas are rare malignant mesenchymal tumors. Fibrosarcoma can occur in patients of all ages and has no predilection for a single site in the heart. The left and right sides of the heart are affected with similar frequency. Involvement of multiple sites is present in half of all patients.

Fibrosarcoma frequently protrudes into the cardiac chambers and involves the cardiac valves in approximately 50% of cases. Pericardial invasion is also common.

Echocardiography

No typical echocardiographic appearance of fibrosarcoma has been described. The presentation of this tumor resembles that of rhabdomyosarcoma. Single or multiple cardiac masses with typically broad attachment may be identified protruding in different cardiac chambers. Pericardial effusion may be present. Valvular invasion can be visualized on 2D TTE or TEE as valvular thickening with abnormal motion. This suggests the malignant character of the lesion.

CT

The appearance of fibrosarcoma resembles that of other sarcomas on CT imaging, and it appears as a low-attenuation soft tissue mass in a cardiac chamber, which is associated with pericardial effusion and invasion.

CMR

The appearance of fibrosarcomas on CMR resembles that of other sarcomas. With T1-weighted images, they have isointense and slightly heterogeneous signal intensity. T2-weighted images show increased signal intensity. The malignant character of the tumor is suggested by a wide point of attachment and invasion of the pericardium or cardiac valves.

Osteosarcoma

Osteosarcoma is another rare malignant cardiac tumor that can affect patients of all ages and most commonly arises from the left atrium. Because of this left atrial location, osteosarcomas are likely to be confused with benign myxomas. The site of origin from the nonseptal atrial walls and tumor extension into the pulmonary veins are useful in distinguishing osteosarcoma from myxomas and other left atrial tumors. Osteosarcomas often present with calcifications, which may be identified by different imaging modalities.

Echocardiography

Osteosarcoma can usually be identified with echocardiographic images as a left atrial echodense mass. Other than their nonseptal broad point of attachment, typical characteristics allowing the differentiation from myxomas are the absence of systolic and diastolic motion, the presence of pulmonary vein invasion, and sometimes pericardial effusion. Calcification can sometimes be identified as intense echo reflections. These features are usually better identified on TEE than on TTE.

CT

CT may identify osteosarcoma as a low-attenuation left atrial filling defect with a nonseptal insertion. CT has the highest sensitivity of all imaging techniques for revealing calcifications in osteosarcoma (Figure 15-22). Such calcifications, however, may sometimes be minimal or in early stages and be mistaken for benign dystrophic calcifications, which may delay the diagnosis of osteosarcoma.

CMR

Two descriptions of osteosarcomas by CMR have been reported. Similar to other sarcomas, these tumors were reported to have an intermediate heterogeneous intensity on T1-weighted images and high signal intensity on T2-weighted images. Contrast enhancement was intense and heterogeneous. As for other primary sarcomas, CMR may be useful in determining the malignant character and extension of the tumor.

Mesotheliomas

Primary mesotheliomas are the most common primary malignant tumors of the pericardium. They represent approximately 5% of all primary pericardial tumors. Mesotheliomas can occur in a wide age range among adults but are uncommon in children. Mesotheliomas diffusely involve both the visceral and parietal pericardia. The tumor spreads by direct extension into contiguous structures, including the epicardial layers of the myocardium, but unlike cardiac sarcomas, they do not invade the endocardium or spread into a cardiac chamber. The clinical presentation of mesothelioma is often similar to acute pericarditis and includes chest pain, cough, dyspnea, and palpitations. Pericardial effusion is often present. Patients with mesotheliomas may also have signs of constrictive pericarditis including right-sided heart failure.

Echocardiography

With TTE the appearance of a mesothelioma may be difficult to distinguish from a pericardial effusion. Mesotheliomas appear as diffuse pericardial thickening with thick intense echoes separated by echo-free spaces, corresponding to loculated effusion. Typically, the tumor invasion stiffens the pericardium, so that there is less motion of the entire heart in comparison with uncomplicated pericardial effusion. Absence of regional wall thickening may also occur. This may be better appreciated on M-mode echo. In addition, the tumor may sometimes be directly visualized as an echodense mass encasing the heart. TEE may offer better pericardial imaging, but the best visualization of this tumor can be achieved on chest CT and CMR.

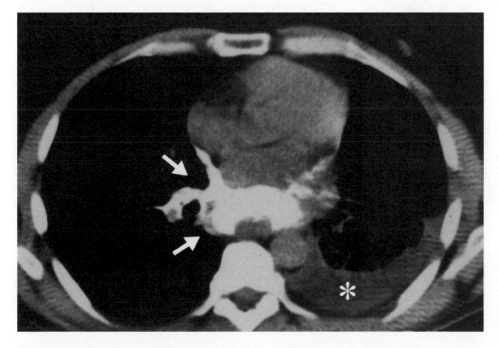

FIGURE 15-22. Noncontrast-enhanced CT in a patient with primary cardiac osteosarcoma. The tumor is revealed by extensive calcification *(arrows)* of the left atrium extending into the pulmonary veins. In addition, a small left pleural effusion (∗) can be observed.

CT

Because it allows excellent visualization of the pericardium, CT is the primary imaging technique to diagnose this tumor. It presents as a localized tumor associated with pericardial effusion or as a diffuse, irregular, thickening of the pericardium encasing the heart.[36]

CMR

CMR can readily demonstrate the presence of pericardial thickening and effusion associated with a mesothelioma. The image intensity characteristics of the pericardial tumor are, however, nonspecific on T1- and T2-weighted imaging, making differentiation of this condition from benign chronic pericarditis difficult.

Lymphoma

Primary lymphoma of the heart by definition involves only the heart and the pericardium. Primary cardiac lymphomas are very rare. They are much less frequent than cardiac metastases from non-Hodgkin's lymphomas, although there is an increased prevalence of primary cardiac lymphomas in immunocompromised patients. The tumor most commonly arises in the right side of the heart, with the right atrium being reported as the most common site. Pericardial effusions may be the only manifestation of a primary lymphoma of the heart, which may also present as circumscribed polypoid or ill-defined infiltrative cardiac masses.[37]

Echocardiography

Primary cardiac lymphomas can usually be identified as right atrial or right ventricular masses on TTE or TEE. The malignant nature of the mass is suggested by the atypical location and invasion of neighboring tissues. Intramyocardial infiltration by the tumor may cause focal wall thickening, hypokinesis, and heterogeneous echo reflectivity.

CT

CT can reveal the presence of cardiac lymphoma as a pericardial effusion or filling defect within one of the cardiac chambers. Cardiac lymphomas are typically hypoattenuating or isoattenuating relative to the myocardium and demonstrate heterogeneous enhancement after the intravenous administration of contrast agents.

CMR

CMR offers superior anatomical details of myocardial and pericardial infiltration, making it more useful than echocardiography or CT for detection of cardiac lymphomas. With CMR, primary cardiac lymphomas have a typical appearance of isointensity relative to normal myocardium on both T1- and T2-weighted images. Hyperintensity relative to myocardium on T2-weighted images has also been reported. Contrast enhancement is usually heterogeneous and intense.

USE OF ECHOCARDIOGRAPHY, CT, AND CMR IN THE DIFFERENTIAL DIAGNOSIS OF CARDIAC MASSES

The differential diagnosis of cardiac masses requires the correlation of clinical parameters, such as patient demographic and clinical presentation, together with the imaging features of the mass. Important imaging features are the specific location of the lesion, its morphology, and distinctive imaging findings with the use of different imaging modalities. Complex presentations may require the combination of anatomical information and tissue characterization from echocardiography, CT and CMR to obtain the diagnosis (Figure 15-23, Table 15-4). Often, the final diagnosis can only be provided by histology. Indicators of malignancy of a mass include a broad base of attachment, rapid growth, and infiltration or invasion into neighboring myocardium, pericardium, or blood vessels.

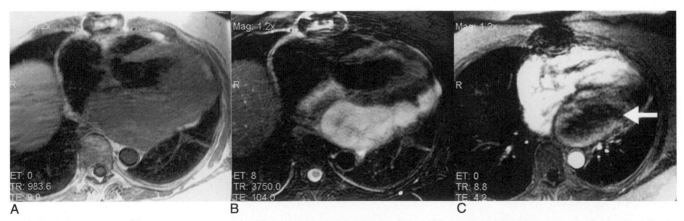

FIGURE 15-23. CMR in a 66-year-old woman with hemangiopericytoma, a malignant form of hemangioma. CMR demonstrates a large tumor involving the pericardium and the posterior wall of the left atrium. On T1-weighted images **A,** the tumor is isointense to the myocardium. On T2-weighted CMR images **B,** the tumor is hyperintense relative to the neighboring myocardium. After gadolinium administration **C,** there is intense hyperenhancement in the rim of the tumor, reflecting the intense vascularization of this tumor. In contrast, the center of the tumor remains unenhanced *(arrow)* likely because of central tumor necrosis.

■ ■ ■

TABLE 15-4 TYPICAL APPEARANCES OF THE MOST COMMON CARDIAC MASSES ON CARDIAC IMAGING TECHNIQUES

	Presentation	Location	Typical appearance by echocardiography	CT		MRI	
Thrombus							
	1. Chronic AF	Left atrial appendage	Echodense masses	NCE	Old thrombi sometimes calcified	T1 W	Fresh thrombi: hyperintense, homogeneous
	2. Post MI	Left ventricular apex					Old thrombi: isointense
	3. Heart failure	Right atrium		CE	Homogeneous filling defect	T2 W	Fresh thrombi: hyperintense Old thrombi: isointense No enhancement
Benign tumors							
Myxoma	Adults	LA 75% Septal insertion small stalk	Globular, gelatinous Multiple speckles Highly mobile	NCE CE	Low attenuation Sometimes calcified Heterogeneous Homogeneous	T1W T2W GRE Cine CE	Heterogeneous, intermediate Heterogeneous hyperenhanced Hypoenhanced Highly mobile Homo- or heterogeneous
Lipoma	Adults	Subendo- or subepicardial LV, RA, septum	Echodense Atypical appearance Low mobility	NCE CE	Low attenuation Homogeneous No enhancement	T1W T2W CE	Very bright, homogeneous Very bright, homogeneous No enhancement
Rhabdomyoma	Infants <1 y	Multiple tumors LV, RV Intramural or subendo	Echodense	NCE CE	Not visible Homogeneous CE	T1W T2W CE	Homogeneous, isointense Homogeneous
Papillary fibroelastoma	Adults >60 y	Valves "sea-anemone" like	Mobile masses Shimmering	Not visible			Usually not visible
Fibroma	Infants <10 y	Single tumor Intramural, LV	Echodense, well circumscribed	NCE CE	Often calcified Homogeneous CE	T1W T2W CE	Homogeneous, isointense Hypointense No enhancement
Hemangioma	All ages	Intramural, RA, RV	Echodense Spongeous aspect	NCE CE	Heterogeneous Vascular "blush"	T1W T2W CE	Hyperintense, heterogeneous Hyperintense Intense enhancement
Malignant tumors							
Angiosarcoma	Adults 40-60 y Male>female	RA, broad implantation, invasive behavior	Echodense, heterogeneous mass	NCE CE	Hypodense Heterogeneous CE	T1W T2W CE	Heterogeneous, cauliflower aspect Cauliflower aspect Heterogeneous CE
Osteosarcoma	All ages	LA, broad implantation invasive behavior	Echodense, heterogeneous calcification sometimes visible	NCE CE	Often calcified Heterogeneous CE	T1W T2W CE	Intermediate heterogeneous Hyperintense Heterogeneous
Mesothelioma	Adults	Pericardial effusion and densening	Pericardial effusion and densening	CE	No typical aspect	T1W T2W	No typical aspect No typical aspect

AF, Atrial fibrillation; MI, myocardial infarction; LA, left atrium; LV, left ventricle; RA, right atrium; RV, right ventricle; CE, contrast-enhanced; NCE, noncontrast-enhanced; GRE, gradient echo; Cine, cine imaging; T1W, T1-weighted MR image; T2W, T2-weighted MRI.

Valvular Masses

The differential diagnosis of valvular masses are Lambl's excrescences, vegetation, thrombus, papillary fibroelastoma, and fibroma. Lambl's excrescences typically arise along the closure margins of the aortic valve cusps. They are uniform in aspect and in length and are usually about 1 mm in diameter and <1 cm long. Vegetations have a variable appearance. They are usually attached on the regurgitant side of the valve (i.e., on the atrial aspect of the mitral and tricuspid valve and the ventricular aspect of the aortic valve) and may arise from any part of the valve. Fibroelastomas are generally attached to the ventricular surface of the aortic valve, arise from areas of valvular apposition, and cause no valvular dysfunction. Moreover, they are usually of smaller size and higher refractive appearance than vegetations. Thrombi most often occur on the ring of prosthetic valves. They appear as echodense material superimposed on the mechanical valve. Fibromas, rhabdomyosarcomas, and fibrosarcomas may all cause valvular tumors with increased thickness of the entire valve and presence of tumor in neighboring cardiac locations. The differential diagnosis of valvular tumors is best accomplished by TEE imaging. Because of their lower temporal resolution and poor visualization of cardiac valves, CT and CMR play a less important role.

Solitary Intraatrial Cardiac Masses

Left Atrium

The differential diagnosis of a solitary left atrial mass includes thrombus, myxoma, and osteosarcoma. Thrombus is the most common left atrial mass and is suggested by a history of atrial fibrillation or mitral valve disease. Typically, left atrial thrombi are highly mobile and originate from the left atrial appendage. Echocardiographic features of left atrial thrombi include a laminated appearance, irregular or lobulated borders, microcavitations, and absence of a pedicle. Myxoma is suggested by insertion on the interatrial septum and a small stalk; it is usually highly mobile within the left atrium and has a typical gelatinous appearance with multiple speckles seen with echocardiography. Both thrombi and myxoma exhibit heterogeneous signal intensity on spin-echo images and low signal intensity on gradient echo CMR images. Thrombi usually do not enhance with contrast material by either CT or CMR. Imaging features that may suggest osteosarcoma include a broad base of attachment and atypical origination from locations other than the atrial septum, tumor extension into the pulmonary veins, invasion of the left atrial wall, or infiltrative growth along the epicardium. These anatomical features can usually be observed by TEE. Tissue invasion may be better defined by CT or CMR. Contrast enhancement is heterogeneous on both CT and CMR and may help to differentiate osteosarcoma from myxoma and thrombus. Finally, intratumor calcification is best identified on CT images and may be very helpful in the diagnosis of osteosarcoma.

Right Atrium

The differential diagnosis of right atrial masses includes thrombus, metastasis, and angiosarcoma. Myxoma may also present in the right atrial location in 25% of cases and has similar characteristics as in the left atrium, that is, a small stalk and septal attachment. Thrombus may be associated with heart failure, venous thromboembolism, atrial fibrillation, and foreign objects such as catheters or pacemaker leads in the right atrium. The diagnosis of metastases can usually be made on clinical grounds with knowledge of a patient's history. Sarcoma is suggested by rapid progression of disease. Diagnostic differentiation among these entities may be difficult by echocardiography, because all these masses can appear with a wide point of attachment inserted to the posterior wall of the atrium. Thrombus is suggested by homogeneous aspect and absence of tissue invasion with CT and CMR images. Also, CT and CMR demonstrate absence of contrast enhancement in thrombus, whereas angiosarcoma or metastasis commonly present with intense but heterogeneous contrast enhancement.

Intramural Ventricular Mass

In infants, the primary differential diagnosis for an intramural mass is rhabdomyoma or fibroma. Rhabdomyoma is suggested by a history of tuberous sclerosis and evidence of multilocular tumors. Fibroma is suggested by solitary location in the septum or lateral free ventricular wall. Calcification and cystic degeneration does not occur in rhabdomyoma but may be present in fibroma. The characteristic CMR signal intensity of rhabdomyomas and fibromas differ. Although both tumors are typically isointense on T1-weighted images, rhabdomyomas are hyperintense on T2-weighted images, whereas fibromas are dark. Rhabdomyosarcoma does not calcify, it is frequently cystic or necrotic, and may invade the pulmonary veins, the pericardial space, and adjacent structures.

In adults, the differential diagnosis of an intramural ventricular mass is more difficult and may include metastasis, fibroma, lipoma, hemangioma, myxoma, and sarcoma. Metastasis is the most common intramural ventricular mass in adults and generally occurs in multiple sites and in the context of malignancies in other organs. Fibromas and lipomas have an encapsulated homogeneous appearance on echocardiography and are usually single tumors. CMR allows accurate identification of these two tumors. Lipomas have characteristic high signal intensity on T1-weighted images. Fibromas may be identified by low signal intensity on T1- and T2-weighted images. Also fibromas characteristically do not present contrast enhancement by either CT or CMR. Hemangiomas present intense and homogenous enhancement by both these techniques. Sarcoma is suggested by a heterogeneous mass, which presents with signs of malignancy such as ragged borders and invasion of neighboring tissue. Pericardial effusion is often present. This is usually best identified by CT or CMR. Characteristically, sarcomas and other malignant tumors have a heterogeneous appearance with nonenhanced CMR, resulting from intratumoral necrosis and hemorrhage. They also present intense but heterogeneous contrast enhancement with both CT and CMR imaging.

Pericardial Mass

The differential diagnosis of pericardial masses include teratoma, lipoma, pericardial cyst, metastasis, and mesothelioma. Cardiac CT or CMR provides the best images. Teratoma typically presents as a multilocular heterogeneous tumor. Lipoma may be identified by a reduced signal on CT imaging and hyperintense signal on T1-weighted CMR images. Pericardial cysts are usually unilocular and fluid filled. This can best be appreciated by measuring the absorption coefficient on CT imaging or by demonstrating typical patterns of homogeneous low signal intensity on T1-weighted CMR images combined with high signal intensity on T2-weighted images. Solid pericardial masses, by opposition, are highly suspicious of malignancy and require biopsy for diagnosis.

CONCLUSIONS

Cardiac masses are caused by a wide spectrum of diseases. The identification and differential diagnosis of these conditions requires multiple imaging techniques, including TTE and TEE, CT, and CMR. These techniques provide complementary diagnostic information.

REFERENCES

1. Geibel A, et al. Diagnosis, localization and evaluation of malignancy of heart and mediastinal tumors by conventional and transesophageal echocardiography. *Acta Cardiol* 1996; 51:395.
2. Hoffmann U, Globits S, Frank H. Cardiac and paracardiac masses. Current opinion on diagnostic evaluation by magnetic resonance imaging. *Eur Heart J* 1998; 19:553.
3. Schvartzman PR, White RD. Imaging of cardiac and paracardiac masses. *J Thorac Imaging* 2000; 15:265.
4. Ahmed S, et al. Volume quantification of intracardiac mass lesions by transesophageal three-dimensional echocardiography. *Ultrasound Med Biol* 2002; 28:1389.
5. Borges AC, et al. Preoperative two-and three-dimensional transesophageal echocardiographic assessment of heart tumors. *Ann Thorac Surg* 1996; 61:1163.
6. Bouton S, et al. Differentiation of tumor from viable myocardium using cardiac tagging with MR imaging. *J Comput Assist Tomogr* 1991; 15:676.
7. Matsuoka H, et al. Morphologic and histologic characterization of cardiac myxomas by magnetic resonance imaging. *Angiology* 1996; 47:693.
8. Orsinelli DA, Pearson AC. Usefulness of multiplane transesophageal echocardiography in differentiating left atrial appendage thrombus from pectinate muscles. *Am Heart J* 1996; 131:622.
9. Pochis WT, Saeian K, Sagar KB. Usefulness of transesophageal echocardiography in diagnosing lipomatous hypertrophy of the atrial septum with comparison to transthoracic echocardiography. *Am J Cardiol* 1992; 70:396.
10. Broderick LS, Conces DJ Jr, Tarver RD. CT evaluation of normal interatrial fat thickness. *J Comput Assist Tomogr* 1996; 20:950.
11. Basso C, Barbazza R, Thiene G. Images in cardiovascular medicine. Lipomatous hypertrophy of the atrial septum. *Circulation* 1998; 97:1423.
12. Hynes JK, et al. Two-dimensional echocardiographic diagnosis of pericardial cyst. *Mayo Clin Proc* 1983; 58:60.
13. Frank H, Globits S. Magnetic resonance imaging evaluation of myocardial and pericardial disease. *J Magn Reson Imaging* 1999; 10:617.
14. Kaymaz C, et al. Location, size, and morphologic characteristics of left atrial thrombi as assessed by transesophageal echocardiography in relation to systemic embolism in patients with rheumatic mitral valve disease. *Am J Cardiol* 2003; 91:765.
15. Irani WN, Grayburn PA, Afridi I. Prevalence of thrombus, spontaneous echo contrast, and atrial stunning in patients undergoing cardioversion of atrial flutter. A prospective study using transesophageal echocardiography. *Circulation* 1997; 95:962.
16. von der Recke G, et al. Use of transesophageal contrast echocardiography for excluding left atrial appendage thrombi in patients with atrial fibrillation before cardioversion. *J Am Soc Echocardiogr* 2002; 15(10 Pt 2):1256.
17. Gupta S, Kahn RA. Image in clinical medicine. Left ventricular thrombus. *N Engl J Med* 2002; 346:e5.
18. Hamilton A, et al. Left ventricular thrombus enhancement after intravenous injection of echogenic immunoliposomes: studies in a new experimental model. *Circulation* 2002; 105:2772.
19. Schwartzbard AZ, et al. The role of transesophageal echocardiography in the diagnosis and treatment of right atrial thrombi. *J Am Soc Echocardiogr* 1999; 12:64.
20. Case records of the Massachusetts General Hospital. Weekly clinicopathological exercises. Case 45-1992. A 75-year-old man with carcinoma of the colon and a right ventricular mass. *N Engl J Med* 1992; 327:1442.
21. Reynen K. Cardiac myxomas. *N Engl J Med* 1995; 333:1610.
22. Acebo E, et al. Clinicopathologic study and DNA analysis of 37 cardiac myxomas: a 28-year experience. *Chest* 2003; 123:1379.
23. Edwards A, et al. Carney's syndrome: complex myxomas. Report of four cases and review of the literature. *Cardiovasc Surg* 2002; 10:264.
24. Araoz PA, et al. CT and MR imaging of benign primary cardiac neoplasms with echocardiographic correlation. *Radiographics* 2000; 20:1303.
25. Grebenc ML, et al. Primary cardiac and pericardial neoplasms: radiologic-pathologic correlation. *Radiographics* 2000; 20:1073; quiz 1110.
26. Matsumura M, et al. Evaluation of cardiac tumors in tuberous sclerosis by magnetic resonance imaging. *Am J Cardiol* 1991; 68:281.
27. Evans AN, et al. Cardiac papillary fibroelastoma. *Eur J Cardiothorac Surg* 2002; 21:1120.
28. Eslami-Varzaneh F, Brun EA, Sears-Rogan P. An unusual case of multiple papillary fibroelastoma, review of literature. *Cardiovasc Pathol* 2003; 12:170.
29. Dichtl W, et al. Images in cardiovascular medicine. Improved preoperative assessment of papillary fibroelastoma by dynamic three-dimensional echocardiography. *Circulation* 2002; 106:1300.
30. Klarich KW, et al. Papillary fibroelastoma: echocardiographic characteristics for diagnosis and pathologic correlation. *J Am Coll Cardiol* 1997; 30:784.
31. Ruygrok PN, et al. Myocardial haemangioma: echocardiographic, CMR, and anatomical correlation. *Heart* 2000; 84:117.
32. Somasundar P, et al. Paragangliomas? a decade of clinical experience. *J Surg Oncol* 2000; 74:286.
33. Beghetti M, et al. Images in cardiovascular medicine. Intrapericardial teratoma. *Circulation* 1998; 97:1523.
34. Araoz PA, et al. CT and MR imaging of primary cardiac malignancies. *Radiographics* 1999; 19:1421.
35. Sinatra R, et al. Integrated approach for cardiac angiosarcoma. *Int J Cardiol* 2003. 88:301
36. Quinn DW, Qureshi F, Mitchell IM. Pericardial mesothelioma: the diagnostic dilemma of misleading images. *Ann Thorac Surg* 2000; 69:1926.
37. Ceresoli GL, et al. Primary cardiac lymphoma in immunocompetent patients: diagnostic and therapeutic management. *Cancer* 1997; 80:1497.

Peripheral Arterial, Aortic, Renal Artery, and Carotid Artery Diseases

Mark A. Creager
Joshua A. Beckman
Andrew C. Eisenhauer
Marie D. Gerhard-Herman
Satyendra Giri
Piotr Sobieszczyk

Peripheral Arterial Disease
Aortic Diseases
Renal Artery Stenosis
Carotid Artery Disease

Arterial diseases, especially secondary to atherosclerosis, are common in Western society and contribute importantly to morbidity and mortality; they coexist with, or occur independent of, coronary artery disease. Clinical manifestations of peripheral arterial disease, aortic disease, renal artery stenosis, and carotid artery disease will be reviewed with the diagnostic tests used to evaluate each of these conditions.

PERIPHERAL ARTERIAL DISEASE

Peripheral arterial disease (PAD) is defined as a vascular disorder in which the arteries of the limb are narrowed or obstructed. PAD affects 8 to 10 million persons in the United States, with an age-related prevalence of 12% to 20% in middle-aged and older populations. The most common cause is atherosclerosis. Other causes include thrombosis in situ, embolism, vasculitides such as Takayasu's arteritis or giant cell arteritis, fibromuscular dysplasia, extrinsic compression such as popliteal artery entrapment, and adventitial cysts. Intermittent claudication occurs in approximately one third of persons with PAD, and others have functional limitations that reduce walking speed and distance and cause difficulty with gait and balance.[1] In primary care patients older than 70 years of age (or in patients older than 50 years of age with a smoking history or diabetes), nearly a third have PAD, and they have a substantially greater risk of myocardial infarction and stroke, and a threefold to sixfold increase in mortality. Approximately 4% to 5% patients with PAD die annually.

Clinical Evaluation

The cardinal symptom of PAD is intermittent claudication. Typically, claudication is described as an ache, cramp, pain, or sense of weakness or fatigue that occurs in an exercising limb and resolves within 5 minutes of rest. The location of the symptoms depends on the site of stenosis or occlusion. Patients with atherosclerosis of the aorta and iliac arteries may complain of buttock and thigh claudication, whereas those with femoral and popliteal artery stenoses may experience calf claudication. Pedal claudication can occur in patients with tibial and peroneal artery disease. Questionnaires are available to assist the clinician in eliciting symptoms of claudication and assessing its severity (Figures 16-1 and 16-2). Lower extremity claudication is classified according to the level of debilitation and or restriction in activities. A current scale used to group patients is the Rutherford-Baker scale, which is a 7-point scale (Table 16-1) extending from 0 to 6.[2] Classic claudicants usually are scales 2 or 3, whereas more debilitated patients with more rest symptoms are in the 4 to 5 range. Patients with major tissue loss are scale 6. It is important to select the appropriate patients for angiography, given that the morbidity from vascular access may be as high as 2.9% in patients with significant peripheral occlusive disease. Generally, patients with Rutherford scale 2 or higher and positive noninvasive studies will benefit from angiography.

Critical limb ischemia is defined as a condition in which the metabolic requirements of the resting limb are not met by the available blood supply, and it is manifested as paresthesias, pain, and skin lesions. Typically, the pain occurs in the most distal parts of the limb, such as the foot or toes. Often, the pain is sharp and lancinating, and the affected area is exquisitely sensitive to touch. The pain is worsened by leg elevation and improved when the leg is placed in a dependent position. It may be worst at night when the patient is in bed. Relief is sought by

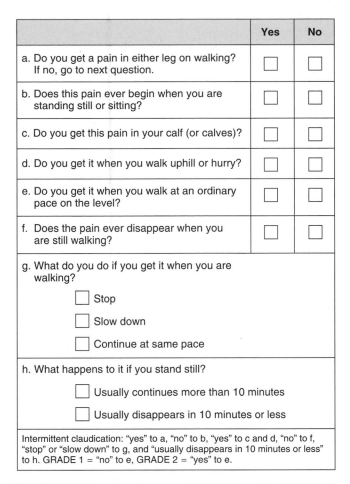

	Yes	No
a. Do you get a pain in either leg on walking? If no, go to next question.	☐	☐
b. Does this pain ever begin when you are standing still or sitting?	☐	☐
c. Do you get this pain in your calf (or calves)?	☐	☐
d. Do you get it when you walk uphill or hurry?	☐	☐
e. Do you get it when you walk at an ordinary pace on the level?	☐	☐
f. Does the pain ever disappear when you are still walking?	☐	☐

g. What do you do if you get it when you are walking?

☐ Stop

☐ Slow down

☐ Continue at same pace

h. What happens to it if you stand still?

☐ Usually continues more than 10 minutes

☐ Usually disappears in 10 minutes or less

Intermittent claudication: "yes" to a, "no" to b, "yes" to c and d, "no" to f, "stop" or "slow down" to g, and "usually disappears in 10 minutes or less" to h. GRADE 1 = "no" to e, GRADE 2 = "yes" to e.

FIGURE 16-1. Rose Questionnaire. (Adapted from Criqui MH, et al. *Vasc Med* 1996; 1:65.)

hanging the leg over the bed or sitting in a chair. With acute limb ischemia, usually from thrombosis or embolism, the onset and severity of symptoms are much more flagrant. Pain, numbness, and/or weakness occur distal to the site of arterial occlusion and, depending on location, may involve extensive portions of the limb.

The physical examination is important in confirming PAD. Loss of pulses implicates PAD, although the dorsalis pedis pulses are absent in up to 5% of healthy individuals. A competent examiner may be able to localize a stenosis to the femoropopliteal segment if the femoral pulse is present, but the popliteal pulse is not. A palpable right femoral pulse and absent left femoral pulse suggests the presence of left iliofemoral artery disease. A useful test is to elevate the legs and ask the patient to repeatedly dorsiflex and plantar flex the feet. Pallor often develops on the soles of the feet in patients with significant PAD. The severity of disease and the presence of collateral vessels can be assessed further by gauging the time required for the feet to redden and their veins to distend after the resumption of a dependent position.

Chronic limb ischemia may be manifested by muscle or subcutaneous atrophy, hair loss, petechiae, cool, smooth and shiny skin, and thickened, yet brittle, toenails. In patients with critical limb ischemia, the affected foot may be pale or cyanotic when examined in the neu-

tral (horizontal) position and even reddened when placed in a dependent position because of reactive dilation of peripheral resistance vessels. Tissue lesions indicative of critical limb ischemia include fissures, ulcers, and necrosis on the heel, between the toes, or on the tips of toes. Arterial ulcers are characterized by exquisite tenderness when touched, and they typically have a pale base and either well-demarcated or irregular borders. In patients with acute limb ischemia, the limb may be pale or mottled, cold, hypesthetic, weak, and/or paralyzed.

Noninvasive Vascular Tests

Noninvasive vascular tests are divided into those that give physiological information, such as limb perfusion pressure, or anatomical information, such as lesion location and severity. Commonly used physiological tests include limb segmental blood pressure measurements, pulse volume recordings, and treadmill exercise testing. Noninvasive imaging techniques used to acquire anatomical information include color-assisted duplex ultrasonography, magnetic resonance angiography, and computed tomographic angiography.

Segmental Pressure Measurements and the Ankle/Brachial Index

To measure arterial pressure along segments of the leg, appropriately sized pneumatic cuffs are placed on the upper and lower segments of the thighs, the calves, and above each ankle. Reference cuffs are placed also on each arm. The cuffs are sequentially inflated to suprasystolic pressure either manually or by an automated instrument and then gradually deflated. The onset of systole is detected by a Doppler ultrasound probe placed over the dorsalis pedis or posterior tibial artery. Normally, the systolic pressure along the segments of the leg should be the same as that of the brachial arteries. Indeed, leg systolic pressure may be slightly higher, because the amplitude of the pressure wave increases as it travels distally. A limb arterial stenosis >70% in cross-sectional area can create a pressure gradient, and a 20-mmHg fall in perfusion pressure between successive cuffs is indicative of a significant intervening stenosis (Table 16-2). For example, an upper thigh systolic pressure of 160 mmHg and a lower thigh systolic pressure of 108 mmHg would indicate a stenosis of the superficial femoral artery (SFA) as it courses through the thigh.

A simplified version of limb segmental pressure measurements is calculation of the ankle/brachial index (ABI) (Table 16-2). The ABI is the ratio of the systolic pressure measured at the ankle to that measured at the brachial artery. The higher of the two brachial artery measurements is used as the denominator in this calculation. The ABI is calculated at the right and left dorsalis pedis and posterior tibial pulses (four sites). A normal ABI is 1.0 or slightly higher. A significant stenosis anywhere along an artery perfusing the leg may decrease the ankle pressure and cause a corresponding fall in the ABI. An ABI of ≤0.9 is considered diagnostic of PAD, and, with contrast angiography as a "gold standard," an ABI of ≤0.9

		R	L
1. Do you get pain in either leg or either buttock on walking? (if no or uncertain, stop)	**No** **Yes** **Uncertain**	1 2 9	1 2 9
2. Does this pain ever begin when you are standing still or sitting?	**No** **Yes** **Uncertain**	1 2 9	1 2 9
3. In what part of the leg or buttock do you feel it?			
a. Pain includes calf/calves	**No** **Yes**	1 2	1 2
b. Pain includes thigh/thighs	**No** **Yes**	1 2	1 2
c. Pain includes buttock/buttocks	**No** **Yes**	1 2	1 2
4. Do you get it when you walk uphill or hurry?	**No** **Yes** **Never walks uphill/hurries**	1 2 3	1 2 3
5. Do you get it when you walk at an ordinary pace on the level?	**No** **Yes** **Uncertain**	1 2 9	1 2 9
6. Does the pain ever disappear when you are walking?	**No** **Yes** **Uncertain**	1 2 9	1 2 9
7. What do you do if you get it when you are walking?	**Stop or slow down** **Carry on**	1 2	1 2
8. What happens to it if you stand still? (If unchanged, stop)	**Lessens or relieved** **Unchanged**	1 2	1 2
9. How soon?	**10 minutes or less** **More than 10 minutes**	1 2	1 2

Coding
1) **No pain**–1 = 1 *or* 9
2) **Pain at rest**–1 = 2 *and* 2 = 2
3) **Non-calf**–1 = 2 *and* 2 = 1 or 9 *and* 3 = 1 *and* 3b = 2 or 3c = 2
4) **Non-Rose calf**–1 = 2 *and* 2 = 1 or 9 *and* 3a = 2, *and* not Rose
5) **Rose**–1 = 2 *and* 2 = 1 or 9 *and* 3a = 2 *and* 4 = 2 or 3 (*and* if 4 = 3, then 5 = 2), *and* 6 = 1 or 9 *and* 7 = 1 *and* 8 = 1 *and* 9 = 1

FIGURE 16-2. San Diego Claudication Questionnaire. (Reproduced from Criqui MH, et al. *Vasc Med* 1996; 1:65.)

■ ■ ■

TABLE 16-1 RUTHERFORD-BAKER SCALE OF SEVERITY OF PAD

Grade	Category	Clinical description	Objective criteria
0	0	Asymptomatic	Normal treadmill test Ankle pressure after exercise <50 mmHg but >25 mmHg less than brachial
	1	Mild claudication	
I	2	Moderate claudication	More moderate symptoms Does not complete treadmill test ankle pressure after exercise <50 mmHg
	3	Severe claudication	Resting ankle pressure <60 mmHg, decreased pulse volume recording
II	4	Ischemic rest pain	
	5	Minor tissue loss, nonhealing ulcers	Resting ankle pressure <40 mmHg PVR moderately decreased
III	6	Major tissue loss above the metatarsal limb no longer salvageable	As noted in category 5

Adapted from Rutherford RB et al. *J Vasc Surg* 1997; 26:517. PAD: peripheral arterial disease.

■ ■ ■

TABLE 16-2 LEG SEGMENTAL PRESSURE MEASUREMENTS IN A PATIENT WITH LEFT THIGH AND CALF CLAUDICATION

	Right (mmHg)	Left (mmHg)
Brachial artery	154	152
Upper thigh	164	160
Lower thigh	162	108
Calf	158	106
Ankle	160	70
Ankle/Brachial index	1.01	0.44

In the right leg, the pressure measurements are normal. There are no pressure gradients between upper and lower thigh and between the calf and ankle. In the left leg, there are pressure gradients between upper and lower thigh and between the calf and ankle. These are indicative of stenoses in the superficial femoral artery and in the tibioperoneal arteries.

has 95% sensitivity and specificity for diagnosing PAD. A typical ABI range for patients with intermittent claudication is 0.5 to 0.8 and for patients with critical limb ischemia is <0.5. The simplicity of the ABI lends itself readily to be used as an office-based procedure.[3]

Segmental pressures and the ABI cannot be used to assess PAD in patients with calcified, noncompressible vessels. Vascular calcification occurs in patients with diabetes or severe renal insufficiency, in the very elderly, and in idiopathic medial calcinosis. The inability to compress the artery by inflating the pneumatic cuff yields falsely high systolic blood pressure recordings and inaccurate ABI calculations. An ABI >1.3 should be regarded as inaccurate and raises the possibility of vascular calcification. In these circumstances, great toe pressures can be measured by placing an appropriately sized cuff on the proximal phalanx. Toe systolic pressures can be determined with plethysmographic recording devices. A normal toe/ brachial index is ≥0.6.

Pulse Volume Recordings

The pulse volume is defined as the volumetric displacement of a segment of the limb with each heartbeat. Plethysmographic instruments that use strain gauge and air transducers can detect changes in limb volume and display pulse volume waveforms. The normal pulse volume waveform is composed of a rapid systolic upstroke (increase in volume) rising to a relatively sharp peak and a more gradual downstroke (decrease in volume that contains a dicrotic wave) (Figure 16-3). The pulse volume is determined by flow and is affected by vessel distensibility and perfusion pressure. Recordings can be acquired at multiple segments of the limbs, including the upper and lower portions of the thighs, calves, ankles, metatarsal regions, and digits. If a flow-limiting stenosis is present proximal to the recording site, the contour of the pulse volume waveform will change. The dicrotic wave will be lost, the rate of rise will decrease, and the overall amplitude will diminish (Figure 16-3). In severe ischemia, in which flow and pressure are very low, there may be no detectable pulse volume. Unlike segmental pressure measurements, the pulse volume recording does not provide quantitative information, but it can be useful, especially if calcified vessels limit the accuracy of pressure measurements.

Treadmill Exercise Testing

The functional capacity of patients with PAD can be assessed by treadmill testing. Protocols are broadly categorized as fixed load and incremental work load tests. The times to the onset of claudication symptoms and the maximal time walked are recorded. Fixed load protocols use a constant speed (e.g., 2.5 mph) and a constant incline (e.g., 10% grade). Dynamic protocols increase the speed and/or grade every 2 to 3 minutes, analogous to protocols used in cardiac testing. The measurements may be less in dynamic than fixed load protocols after therapeutic interventions. Treadmill testing can be used to assess functional limitations and as a diagnostic tool to determine whether claudication is limiting the patient. In patients with PAD and intermittent claudication, the ABI should decrease by at least 20% when measured immediately after symptom-limited exercise. For example, a patient with a resting ABI of 0.9 would have a postexercise ABI of <0.7 and typically much lower, if claudication was the cause of walking cessation. Diseases with symptoms that may mimic claudication, such as spinal stenosis or hip arthritis, would not cause a fall in ABI after exercise.

Duplex Ultrasonography

Duplex ultrasonography is a test that combines B-mode ultrasound imaging with pulse Doppler velocity analysis. B-mode imaging provides information about the morphological characteristics of the vessel wall, including the appearance of the intima, wall thickness, and the presence and nature of atherosclerotic plaques and thrombi. Distinct plaque characteristics such as ulceration or calcification can be detected. B-mode imaging also enables the examiner to set the pulse Doppler and interrogate the velocity of blood flow at specific locations along the artery to estimate the severity of stenoses. Color formatting of the Doppler velocity profile is helpful in identifying stenotic segments, because both color intensity and hue are affected by turbulence at stenotic sites.

Duplex imaging of peripheral arteries is a time-consuming process that requires a skilled ultrasonographer.[4] The patient is placed in the supine, oblique, or prone position to image all of the arteries perfusing the leg. The ultrasound probe (with a frequency appropriate for the depth of the artery) is gradually moved from the pelvis along the entire length of the leg to image the iliac, common femoral, superficial femoral, popliteal, tibial, and peroneal arteries. Frequency shift information, derived from pulse Doppler interrogation at selected sites along the arteries, is processed in real time. Velocity measurements are made whenever plaque is identified by B-mode imaging. The normal velocity waveform is triphasic (Figure 16-4). Rapid forward flow occurs during systole. Peak systolic flow is antegrade and normally <150 cm/s. Transient flow reversal occurs during early diastole. Antegrade flow, at a low velocity, occurs during

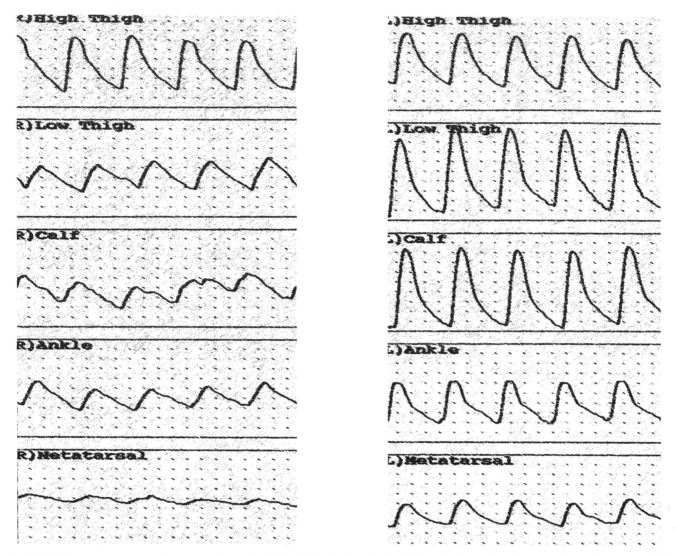

FIGURE 16-3. Pulse volume recording of a patient with right calf claudication. In the left leg *(right panel)*, pulse volume recordings are normal. In comparison, the pulse volume recordings in the right leg *(left panel)* are abnormal, characterized by loss of the dicrotic wave, decreased amplitude, and reduced rate of rise noted particularly in the low thigh, calf, ankle, and metatarsal segments.

the remainder of diastole. Red blood cells are moving together at a relatively uniform speed, yielding a thin envelope when the velocity profile is displayed. Color imaging reveals a homogenous color scheme indicative of normal laminar flow (Figure 16-5).

When a stenosis is present, the velocity increases at the stenotic site. The increase in velocity may be detected by color imaging, which displays a desaturation of color at the highest velocities (e.g., from red to yellow to white, as well as mixtures of colors, red and blue, indicative of directional disturbances caused by turbulence). The velocity at the stenosis is proportional to its severity unless there is total or near total occlusion of the artery. A twofold or greater increase in velocity at the stenosis compared with the velocity measured just proximal to the stenosis is indicative of a 50% or greater decrease in the cross-sectional diameter of the artery (Figure 16-6). Absence of flow, detected by loss of color or recordable velocity profiles, is indicative of a total or subtotal occlusion. With conventional contrast angiogra-

phy as a standard, the sensitivity and specificity of color-assisted duplex ultrasonography for diagnosing iliac, femoral, and popliteal artery stenoses range between 90% and 95%. The specificity and sensitivity of duplex ultrasonography for diagnosing tibial and peroneal artery stenoses are less, particularly if there are proximal stenoses that would decrease flow downstream.

Color-assisted duplex ultrasonography is useful for assessing infrainguinal vein bypass grafts (Figure 16-7) and detecting development of stenoses postoperatively. Several duplex ultrasound criteria have been used to diagnose vein graft stenoses of 50% or greater. A twofold or greater increase in peak systolic velocity, or a peak systolic velocity >200 cm/s, are two such criteria. The sensitivity and specificity of duplex ultrasound for detecting vein graft stenoses each range between 80% and 90%. The effectiveness of this noninvasive test has led to the recommendation for surveillance programs that include vein graft scans 3, 6, and 12 months after surgery and then annually thereafter. The usefulness of duplex ultrasonography for

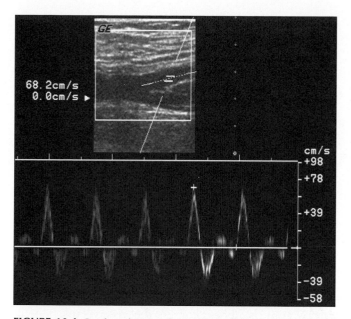

FIGURE 16-4. Duplex ultrasound recording of the common femoral artery bifurcation with pulse Doppler velocity analysis of the superficial femoral artery. This normal pulse velocity waveform demonstrates rapid forward flow during systole, transient flow reversal during early diastole, and antegrade flow at a low velocity during the remainder of diastole. See also Color Insert.

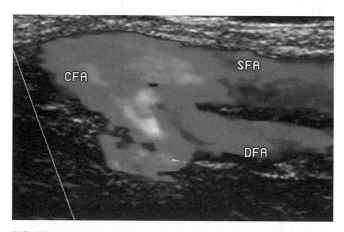

FIGURE 16-5. Color duplex ultrasound examination of a normal common femoral artery bifurcation. The homogeneous red color is indicative of laminar flow. See also Color Insert.

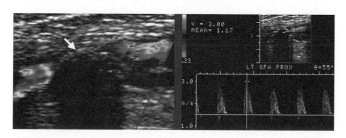

FIGURE 16-6. Duplex ultrasound examination of the proximal portion of a superficial femoral artery. Acoustic shadowing is indicative of a calcified atherosclerotic plaque *(arrow) (left panel)*. The pulse Doppler velocity profile is 300 cm/s, greater than twofold more than that recorded in a more proximal normal section of this artery *(right panel)*. This finding is consistent with a stenosis of at least 50%. See also Color Insert.

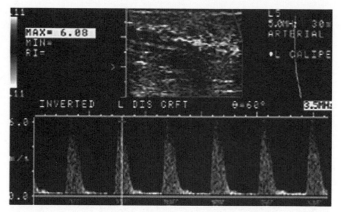

FIGURE 16-7. Color duplex ultrasound examination of the distal anastomosis of a saphenous vein bypass graft. Color discordance and increased pulse Doppler velocity profile is consistent with a stenosis of >50%.

identifying infrainguinal synthetic bypass graft stenoses is less well established. Duplex ultrasonography may be used also to determine whether restenosis has occurred at the site of an endovascular intervention (i.e., angioplasty and stents). A twofold increase in peak systolic velocity is indicative of a restenosis of 50% or greater.

Magnetic Resonance Angiography

Magnetic resonance angiography (MRA) provides images that resemble conventional contrast angiography (Figures 16-8 and 16-9). Contrast-enhanced MRA evaluates the distribution of an intravenously administered paramagnetic contrast medium instead of flowing blood alone. The development of hardware with wide bandwidths allows selective depiction of arterial vessels with contrast-enhanced MRA imaging without venous superimposition or disturbing motion artifacts and has improved diagnostic accuracy. MRA can be used to

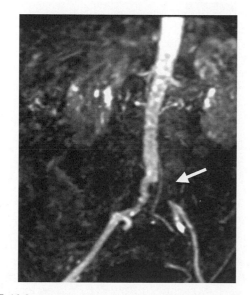

FIGURE 16-8. Contrast-enhanced magnetic resonance angiogram of the abdomen and pelvis. There is a complete occlusion of the left common iliac artery *(arrow)*.

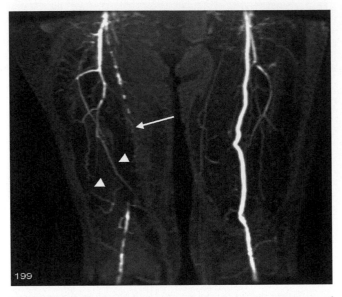

FIGURE 16-9. Contrast-enhanced magnetic resonance angiogram of the right and left thighs. The right superficial femoral artery is totally occluded *(arrow)*. Collateral vessels originating from the right profunda femoral artery are visualized *(arrowheads)*.

image the aorta, iliac, femoral, popliteal, tibial, peroneal, and pedal arteries with resolution similar, or possibly superior, to conventional angiography (Figure 16-10). A meta-analysis found that the sensitivity of MRA for detecting peripheral stenoses was greater than duplex ultrasonography.[5] With conventional angiography as a standard, the sensitivity and specificity of MRA to detect stenoses of 50% or greater are each in excess of 90%.[6] Three-dimensional MRA is more accurate than two-dimensional MRA.[7]

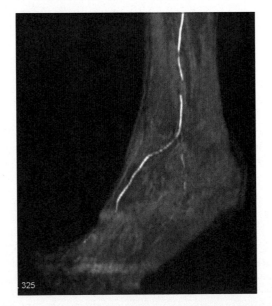

FIGURE 16-10. Contrast-enhanced magnetic resonance angiogram of the foot in a patient with critical ischemia. The dorsalis pedis artery is visualized.

Computed Tomographic Angiography

Computed tomographic angiography (CTA) can be used to image peripheral arteries but requires administration of iodinated contrast. Single-detector technology limits the area that can be imaged, requiring longer study times and greater volumes of contrast. Moreover, the sensitivity of single-detector CTA for diagnosing significant stenoses is <60%, although for complete occlusion may exceed 90%. Therefore, it is not used as a routine diagnostic test in most institutions. In development are multidetector scanners that allow the acquisition of multiple cross-sectional images simultaneously.[8]

Contrast Angiography

The purpose of peripheral angiography is to define the vascular anatomy and to identify significant arterial narrowing requiring revascularization (either percutaneously or surgically). The appropriateness of peripheral angiography is dependent on the risk versus benefits involved in obtaining peripheral imaging, and this should be evaluated.[2]

Contrast angiography is the current diagnostic standard for imaging blood vessels in patients with PAD, and it is indicated primarily for mapping and localizing sites of significant arterial lesions to plan and assess endovascular and open surgical revascularization procedures. Angiography is not useful for delineating properties of the vascular wall. The main contraindications to peripheral angiography include bleeding diathesis, renal failure (true or impending), fever, ongoing infection, or severe anemia.

Imaging of peripheral vascular structures differs from imaging of the coronary tree in several important ways. Peripheral angiography commonly uses a larger image intensifier field (14 inch or 36 cm) to encompass larger regions of interest. Digital (not film-based) angiography allows online display of acquired images, as well as advanced processing techniques to enhance brightness, contrast, or shift of underlying bony structures to enhance the final image. Frequently, digital subtraction angiography is used. With this method a "mask" or baseline background image is obtained immediately before contrast injection to "subtract" any bone, calcifications, air, or soft tissues from the final image, enhancing image quality. Digital subtraction angiography may reduce the volume of contrast and imaging acquisition time required.

Iliac Angiography

The iliac vessels originate at the termination of the abdominal aorta, usually at the L4-5 level. They remain retroperitoneal throughout their course until they cross the inguinal ligament and become the common femoral artery. Angiography of the iliac arteries is best achieved in the anteroposterior (AP) and oblique positions (LAO for the right iliac artery and RAO for the left iliac artery). The imaging catheter, usually a pigtail or flush catheter, is positioned just above the aortic bifurcation to allow the best opacification of the iliac arteries. In general,

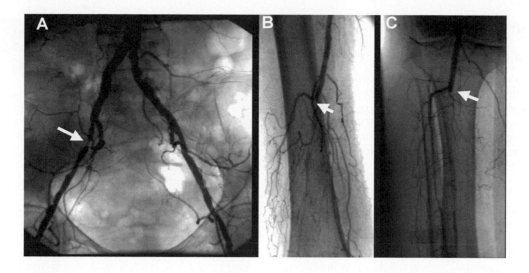

FIGURE 16-11. Conventional contrast angiogram demonstrating significant stenosis of the right external iliac artery (**A**), total occlusion of the right superficial femoral artery (**B**), and reconstitution of the popliteal artery with occlusion of the tibioperoneal artery trunk (**C**).

15 to 30 mL of contrast injected at 20 to 30 mL/s is sufficient to provide adequate opacification. Once a lesion is identified with angiography, its functional significance and suitability for intervention can be further assessed with pressure wire measurements. Currently, a mean gradient of >10 mmHg at rest, or after hyperemia, after vasodilatation with some form of vasodilator (TNG, papaverine) is considered significant. The presence of symptoms, positive noninvasive studies, a significant stenosis on angiography, and a gradient of this magnitude indicates that the lesion may merit revascularization. Various revascularization techniques are available. Intravascular stenting has been associated with improved long-term patency compared with conventional balloon angioplasty, and clinical outcomes after stent placement seem to be similar to long-term outcomes after vascular surgery, although direct comparative data are lacking.

Infrainguinal Angiography

The arterial tree below the inguinal ligament begins with the common femoral artery. This vessel bifurcates early at the level of the femoral head into the profunda femoral artery and the superficial femoral artery (SFA). The SFA is the main vessel supplying the lower extremity. It courses anteriorly through the proximal 60% of its length and then begins to course posteriorly entering the adductor canal (Hunter's canal). This canal exits posteriorly, and the artery becomes the popliteal artery when it exits. The popliteal artery then terminates at the level of the tibial plateau into the anterior tibial artery and tibial-peroneal trunk vessels that terminally bifurcate into the posterior tibial artery and the peroneal artery. Percutaneous interventions to the infrainguinal vessels remain associated with poor long-term patency. Generally, lesions in the SFA are best treated percutaneously if the lesion is focal and <3 cm long. As the

lesion length increases, there is an increase in restenosis after angioplasty. Stenting of the SFA has not been associated with improved patency. Percutaneous intervention of the infrapopliteal arteries is more difficult to maintain patency, given the small diameter of the vessels and their dynamic properties at the level of the lower extremity.

Lower Extremity Angiography

Lower extremity angiography can be performed several ways. There has been increased use of digital angiography and bolus chase techniques, in which the table "steps" at various points of the run to mask the image then returns to the same location and follows the original bolus of contrast throughout the course. These methods allow a single contrast injection to define the anatomy. The main problem with this technique occurs when there is significant patient motion from the mask to the contrast "bolus-chase," and the images become "out of register" and of poor quality. Small amounts of patient motion may be digitally "shifted" in the final angiogram to remove the underlying bony structures and enhance the final angiographic image. In general, contrast volumes for the lower extremity bolus-chase technique range from 30 to 40 mL at 8 to 10 mL/s. Other techniques include static images or older "cut-film" changers. In the static image technique, a focal area is evaluated with single bolus contrast injections of 15 to 30 mL at 8 to 10 mL/s. One unique aspect of peripheral angiography is the antegrade puncture of the femoral artery. The common femoral artery is entered as with standard retrograde access, but it is entered in the antegrade (in the direction of blood flow to the leg) direction. The entry is less steep (about 45 degrees) but should enter the common femoral artery over the femoral head and below the inguinal ligament. This access allows direct intervention for the infrainguinal vessels.

AORTIC DISEASES

Aortic Dissection

Aortic dissection is a rare, but life-threatening, condition most commonly characterized by an intimal tear with pulsating blood propagating within the tear and separating the intima and media from the rest of the vascular wall. Blood commonly causes anterograde separation but may dissect retrograde as well. Most patients will be seen for medical attention with abrupt onset of severe pain. In nearly 70% of patients with aortic dissection, pain will be the only symptom. Up to one fifth of patients with aortic dissection will be seen with evidence of aortic branch vessel compromise. The most commonly involved arteries are the left subclavian and iliac arteries. Physical examination may reveal a pulse deficit. Blood pressure variations of >20 mmHg between arms should be considered suspicious. Depending on the location of vascular disruption, patients may have evidence of cerebrovascular ischemia, paraplegia, or myocardial infarction. Disruption of the aortic leaflets may cause aortic regurgitation, and rupture into the pericardial space may result in pericardial tamponade. Less commonly, renal and mesenteric vessels may be involved, potentially causing renal or mesenteric ischemia.

The result of aortic and branch vessel compromise in aortic dissection has a high mortality rate. In the absence of appropriate therapy, mortality reaches 1%/hour over the first day, 50% by 1 week, and 90% at 3 months. An important contributor to this mortality is lack of recognition. In-hospital mortality rates range between 15% and 25%, and 5-year survival ranges between 50% and 70%. Because the history, physical examination, and routine laboratory examinations, including an electrocardiogram and chest radiograph, are frequently nonspecific, imaging of the aorta becomes crucial for diagnosis and management. Three modalities are predominantly used in the diagnosis of aortic dissection: echocardiography, computed tomography, and magnetic resonance imaging. Aortography is used less frequently. The purpose of diagnostic imaging is to locate the intimal tear and the extent of medial-adventitial separation to define the type of aortic dissection. The type of aortic dissection is defined by areas of involvement, not initial intimal rent site. The Stanford Classification scheme separates dissections into two types, A and B. Type A dissections involve the aorta proximal to the left subclavian artery and typically require urgent surgical repair,[9] whereas type B dissections do not involve the ascending aorta and arch.

Chest Radiography

Abnormalities that are rarely diagnostic can be detected in 60% to 90% of chest X-rays in patients who are seen with aortic dissection. The most common finding, a widened mediastinum, and other suggestive findings include an abnormal aortic contour, an enlarged cardiac silhouette, pleural effusion (left greater than right), and disruption of calcium within the aortic arch (Figure 16-12).

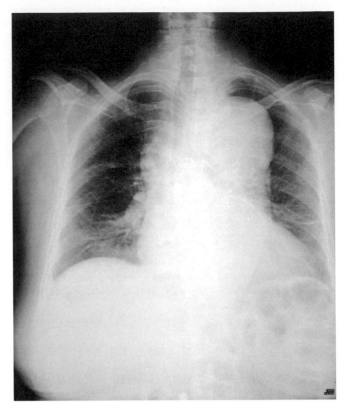

FIGURE 16-12. Posteroanterior chest radiograph demonstrating a widened mediastinum in a patient with aortic dissection.

Echocardiography

Although transthoracic echocardiography (TTE) provides an accurate assessment of ventricular and valvular function, the visualization of the proximal portion of the ascending and the descending aorta provided by TTE is limited. Therefore, the sensitivity of TTE ranges from 59% to 90% in type A and 30% to 40% in type B aortic dissections. Because of the low sensitivity of this test, its use may actually delay the time to diagnosis by providing a false sense of security.

Transesophageal echocardiography (TEE) (Figure 16-13), performed by means of insertion of the sonographic probe into the esophagus, provides high-fidelity imaging of the heart and aorta. As a result of the improved proximity of the probe to the heart, image clarity dramatically increases the sensitivity and specificity for visualization of the intimal flap to 90% to 100% and 70% to 80%, respectively. TEE can be used to identify true and false aortic channels and channel flow patterns. It can determine the presence of a pericardial effusion and assess the left ventricle and aortic valve. TEE does carry some disadvantages: the trachea and left mainstem bronchus limit imaging of the aortic arch. Improvements in TEE probes, including biplane and omniplane imaging, have reduced in scope the area unable to be visualized. Qualified personnel may not be available immediately to perform the test.

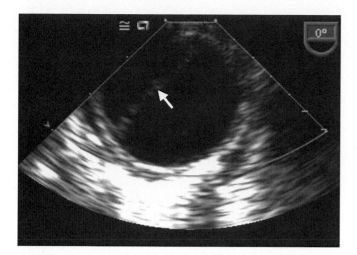

FIGURE 16-13. Transesophageal image of descending thoracic aortic dissection. Note the intimal flap *(arrow)* dividing the true and false aortic lumens.

Computed Tomography

The greatest advantage of computed tomography (CT) is its common, round-the-clock availability in many emergency departments.[10] CT accurately defines the location of the intimal tear and extent of the false lumen (Figure 16-14). In contrast to the sonographic techniques described previously, CT provides a cross-sectional evaluation of the entire aorta. CT can also provide information concerning the presence of a pericardial effusion and of luminal thrombosis. The diagnostic sensitivity and specificity for aortic dissection is similar to that of TEE, ranging from 90% to 100% and 80% to 90%, respectively. Drawbacks to the use of CT include the administration of iodinated contrast and limited ability to evaluate aortic branch vessels.

Cardiac Magnetic Resonance

Cardiac Magnetic resonance (CMR) imaging (Figures 16-15 and 16-16) is considered the current "gold standard" for the diagnosis of aortic dissection, with sensitivity and specificity reaching 100%.[11] CMR does not require the use of contrast agents, can delineate pathology in aortic branch vessels, and with electrocardiographic gating, can provide information about left ventricular function. The major drawbacks to CMR include the difficulty of monitoring a patient in a scanner and limited availability of CMR units for emergency purposes. Therefore, CMR is not recommended for unstable patients. CMR is used when initial investigations are inconclusive and for follow-up examinations of patients with known aortic dissection. MR virtual vascular endoscopy is a new technique allowing endoluminal views of the aorta.[12]

Aortography

Until the advent of rapid, noninvasive testing, aortography was the standard method of diagnosis. Thoracic aortography is used to define the anatomical relation of the aortic arch and the great vessels to determine the diameter of the thoracic aorta, to obtain evidence of dissection, and to evaluate trauma or other vascular injuries. The optimal view of the aortic arch is obtained in the LAO projection at 30 to 40 degrees oblique. The injec-

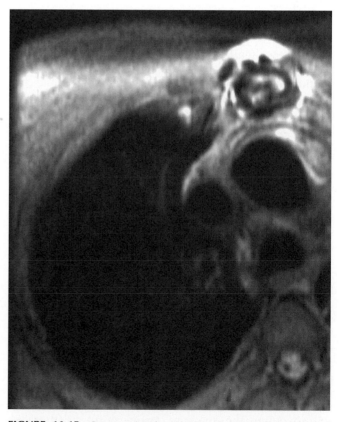

FIGURE 16-15. Cross-sectional magnetic resonance image of the descending thoracic aorta. CMR provides a clear image of the aorta, allowing for sizing and definition of the dissection flap.

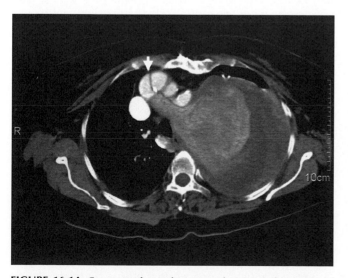

FIGURE 16-14. Contrast-enhanced computed tomographic image of the thoracic aorta demonstrating a chronic aortic dissection.

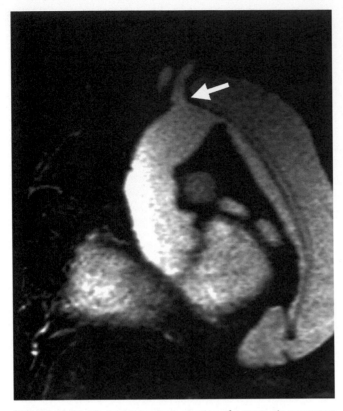

FIGURE 16-16. Maximal intensity projection of a magnetic resonance angiogram demonstrating a type B aortic dissection. The CMRA clearly demonstrates the origin of the dissection beyond the left subclavian artery *(arrow)*.

tion of 30 to 40 mL of contrast at 20 to 30 mL/s generally opacifies the vessels for adequate imaging. If digital subtraction angiography is used, the patient should be instructed to hold the breath to avoid artifacts caused by motion or breathing. Adequate contrast should be injected to ensure that the arch and the great vessels are well opacified. Aortography allows the definition of the intimal flap site, provides good visualization of branch vessels, and can reveal aortic valve insufficiency. The sensitivity and specificity for the examination are 80% to 90% and 90% to 96%, respectively. The requirements for specialized personnel, procedural preparation time, and iodinated contrast have eliminated this test as a first-line diagnostic modality. Moreover, aortography does not allow examination of the vascular wall and may miss important aortic dissection variants, including intramural hematoma and penetrating atherosclerotic ulcer.

Indications to image the abdominal aorta include evaluation of abdominal aortic aneurysm (AAA), dissection, lower extremity claudication, mesenteric ischemia, and renal vascular disease. AP and lateral imaging of the abdominal aorta are usually sufficient to delineate all anatomical areas of interest in the abdominal aorta and mesenteric vessels. In general 20 to 40 mL of contrast, injected at 15 to 30 mL/s, will adequately opacify the vessels to define the anatomy. Again, as in the thoracic aorta, it is critical to fully opacify the lumen and the vessels of interest. If selected conduits require further visualization, then a soft-tipped catheter (i.e., SosOmni, RDC, or

hockey stick) may provide selective angiography without requiring large contrast loads to fully define the anatomy. Mesenteric angiography is best obtained in the AP and lateral projections. Nonselective angiography with a pigtail or tennis racquet catheter can provide information regarding all mesenteric vessels. Selective mesenteric angiography can be performed with a hockey stick or SosOmni catheter.

Aortic Dissection Variants

Intramural Hematoma

Intramural hematoma (IMH) represents the most important aortic dissection variant. First described in 1988, it is characterized by hematoma formation within the medial layer of the aorta, possibly as a result of vaso vasorum rupture. The clinical presentation and prognosis of IMH is quite similar to classic aortic dissection, and most data suggest it should be treated similarly. Recent evidence, however, suggests a more conservative approach that uses medical therapy and frequent imaging may be a viable option.[13,14]

IMH is typically described as a crescentic collection of blood in the aortic wall during cross-sectional imaging. Both CMR and CT provide excellent cross-sectional images of the aorta and are useful modalities. TEE can also detect IMH with a high sensitivity and specificity. In contrast, aortography can fail to image IMH because of the absence of an intimal flap and false channel.

Penetrating Atherosclerotic Ulcer

Severe, ulcerating atheromatous lesions may penetrate the internal elastic lamina into the media or adventitia, yielding dissection, pseudoaneurysm formation, or even aortic rupture.[15] Patients with a penetrating atherosclerotic ulcer may be seen with symptoms similar to aortic dissection. Information about the natural history of this disease is limited, but management should be similar to that for aortic dissection. Patients with penetrating atherosclerotic ulcer are more likely than patients with aortic dissection or IMH to have aneurysmal formation and aortic rupture.[15] Diagnosis can be made with TEE, CT, or CMR. Typical imaging features include a focal lesion with adjacent subintimal hematoma and aortic thickening or enhancement. CMR can differentiate a large atheromatous ulcerated plaque from chronic luminal thrombus and IMH.

Imaging Algorithm

The acute life-threatening nature of the clinical syndrome makes selection of the diagnostic imaging modality particularly important in patients with suspected aortic dissection. The modality of choice is the test that can be obtained most rapidly at the point of care while ensuring adequate patient monitoring. In most centers, this means TEE or CT. Both are appropriate initial diagnostic procedures with a high sensitivity and specificity. Moreover, TEE can be used during surgery to provide supplemental information about ventricular and aortic function if the initial diagnosis is made by CT.

Aortic Aneurysm

An aortic aneurysm is defined as an increase in size of the aorta of >50% compared with an adjacent normal segment. Aneurysmal disease occurs throughout the aorta, and aneurysms are typically classified according to the area of involvement and include thoracic, thoracoabdominal, and abdominal aortic aneurysm (AAA). Most aortic aneurysms develop in the abdomen. In the Cardiovascular Health Study of men and women older than 65 years of age, the prevalence of AAA was 8.8%, with most being smaller than 3.5 cm in diameter. In the Aneurysm Detection and Management Study, AAA of 4.0 cm or larger was found in 1.4% of the participants. AAAs are estimated to cause the death of 1.2% of men and 0.6% of women in the United States. The most important risk factors for AAA formation include cigarette smoking, hypertension, and a family history of aortic aneurysms. The incidence of thoracic aortic aneurysms is less common, approximating 5.9/100,000 person-years. Of these, ascending aorta (51%) is most commonly affected, followed by the descending aorta (38%), and the aortic arch (11%) aneurysms.

Most patients with aortic aneurysm are asymptomatic. The aneurysm is discovered incidentally during evaluation for an unrelated set of complaints. Less commonly, patients may report back or abdominal pain. Physical examination of the abdomen may demonstrate an enlarged, pulsating aorta, but the likelihood of making a diagnosis on the basis of palpation decreases as the abdominal girth increases. The presence of a pulsatile mass in the abdomen in the setting of hypotension should prompt emergent surgical intervention without initial imaging, because any delay increases the risk of death.

Appropriate management of aneurysmal disease requires early diagnosis and careful surveillance to identify those patients who should undergo repair to reduce the risk of rupture. Aneurysmal rupture is a medical emergency with a very high mortality, despite improvements in operative technique.[16] Patients who survive long enough to reach the hospital will complain of severe pain at the location of the rupture. For patients who survive long enough to reach the hospital alive, mortality after AAA rupture is as high as 61%. The risk of rupture should prompt surgical repair when the diameter of the abdominal aorta reaches 5.0 to 5.5 cm and when the thoracic aorta reaches 6 cm.[17,18] Thus, careful follow-up must be performed to ensure that patients are properly identified when the size of the aortic aneurysm merits repair. Appropriate imaging of the aneurysm is therefore crucial to the timing of surgery and operative planning.

Ultrasonography

The simplest method to detect, size, and follow an AAA is ultrasonography (Figure 16-17). The diagnostic sensitivity and specificity each approach 100%. Ultrasound can

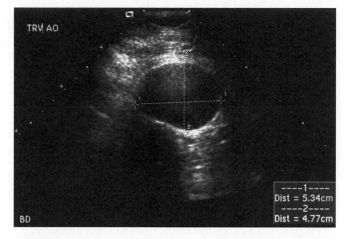

FIGURE 16-17. Duplex ultrasonographic imaging of an abdominal aortic aneurysm. This technique allows for adequate sizing and follow-up over time.

accurately size aneurysm diameters to within tenths of millimeters. Large studies of observation vs. early surgery in small AAAs have demonstrated that abdominal ultrasonography provides accurate sizing of the aortic diameter and can be used to determine the timing of surgery.[19] Ultrasound is adequate for initial sizing and follow-up, but it cannot adequately define the linear extent of the aneurysm and does not provide the anatomical detail required for surgical planning. Echocardiography may be used to assess and follow ascending thoracic aortic aneurysms, but the aortic arch and the descending thoracic aorta cannot be assessed adequately by ultrasound.

CT and CMR

Both CT and CMR (Figures 16-18 and 16-19) can be used to diagnose aortic aneurysms. Often, these imaging tests are ordered for other reasons, and the presence of an aneurysm is an incidental finding. Tomographic measurements made by CT (Figure 16-20) or CMR accurately measure the abdominal aortic diameter to within tenths of a millimeter. They are both accurate in defining the proximal and distal extent of the aneurysm as well, allowing for appropriate surgical planning. Improvements in resolution of both modalities have increased their sensitivity for detecting renal and mesenteric artery involvement. These imaging methods are typically used only during surgical planning, because the increase in cost, study discomfort, and requirement for iodinated contrast for CT imaging makes them less practical than ultrasound for routine examinations. These techniques are necessary for adequate imaging of the thoracic aorta because of the limitations in ultrasonographic evaluation.[11]

Angiography

Angiography delineates the lumen within the aneurysm, but because most aneurysms contain thrombus, the true diameter is not well demarcated. Angiography can define the proximal and distal extent

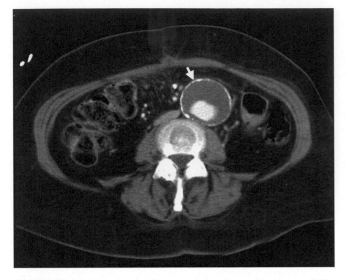

FIGURE 16-18. Cross-sectional computed tomographic image of the abdominal aorta. The aorta is enlarged and has extensive calcification (*arrow*) in the vessel wall. The gray area within the aneurysm is thrombus.

of the lesion. Moreover, it provides the most definition of branch vessel involvement and occlusive disease.

Atheroembolism

The presence of severe atherosclerosis may result in the embolization of components of the atherosclerotic plaque.[20] The composition of the emboli also varies and includes cholesterol crystals, platelets, and fibrin. Cholesterol crystal may accumulate at the base of atherosclerotic lesions and after plaque rupture, millions of these crystals may be liberated to occlude many downstream arterioles, including vessels in the kidneys and lower extremities. The cutaneous manifestation of cho-

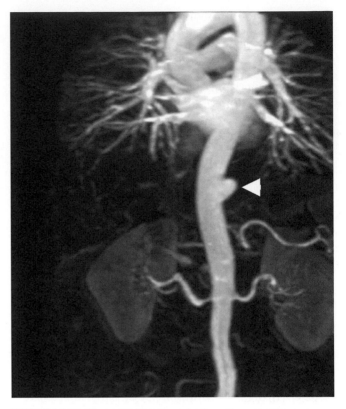

FIGURE 16-19. Maximal intensity projection of a magnetic resonance angiogram demonstrating a saccular aneurysm (*arrowhead*) of the descending thoracic aorta.

lesterol embolization is blue toe syndrome, which may be accompanied by livedo reticularis. When the atheroembolism is composed of fibrin-platelet mass, it may be large enough to occlude muscular conduit arteries and may cause stroke, acute visceral ischemia, or limb ischemia.

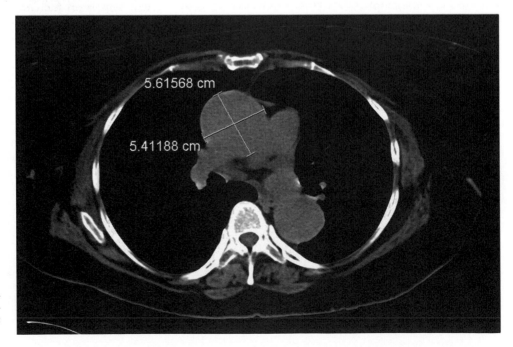

FIGURE 16-20. Computed tomographic angiogram showing and sizing a large ascending aortic aneurysm.

Diagnostic imaging of the aorta in this clinical scenario is primarily performed to provide information concerning the likelihood of recurrence. For example, TEE and CT can show atherosclerotic lesions 4 mm in size or larger in the aortic arch that confer increased risk for embolic stroke (Figure 16-21). In the setting of repeated atheromatous embolization, CT and CMR can be used to identify an area of plaque rupture that may be amenable to surgical correction. Contrast angiography should be avoided when possible, because it may independently cause cholesterol embolization.

Aortitis

Diagnosis of large-vessel vasculitides is difficult and commonly results in a therapeutic delay. Two vasculitides cause the most aortitis: Takayasu's arteritis and giant cell arteritis. These large-vessel inflammatory arteritides have a wide range of clinical presentations varying from nonspecific, constitutional symptoms to specific symptoms resulting from arterial insufficiency to an organ or limb.[21,22] For example, patients may report arm, leg, or jaw claudication with involvement of the subclavian, iliac, or external carotid arteries, respectively. There is typically a long delay between symptom onset and diagnosis because of the nonspecific nature of the complaints, particularly if the predominant symptom is constitutional and the patients report fatigue, malaise, fevers, sweats, and weight loss. Physical examination may reveal subclavian, carotid, or femoral arterial bruits, diminished pulses, aneurysmal dilation, or evidence of arterial hypoperfusion with muscle wasting.

Arterial imaging has become an important adjunct to the diagnosis of aortitis. In contrast to the typical appearance of atherosclerosis, the inflammation within the vascular wall tends to cause generalized wall thickening. The vessel appears narrowed, the stenoses are long and smooth and commonly described as "rat tailed," not irregular as in atherosclerosis. Standard and digital subtraction angiography can demonstrate the compromise of the vascular lumen as a result of these inflammatory changes. Both Takayasu's arteritis and giant cell arteritis may also cause aneurysmal dilation of the aorta. Imaging in this setting is as described previously for other causes of aortic aneurysm.

Both CT and CMR (Figure 16-22) allow examination of the vessel wall, as well as the vessel lumen. Thus, in the absence of lumen compromise, typical vascular wall changes such as uniform thickening may be demonstrated and support the diagnosis.[23] CMR techniques can also provide insight into disease activity. T2 imaging is sensitive to tissue water content, so that mural edema can be visualized in these sequences. In one small series, both diagnostic sensitivity and specificity of 100% was reported in patients suspected of having Takayasu's arteritis on the basis of clinical criteria of disease activity. Furthermore, the reduction of this vessel wall enhancement, a bright area within the wall, may correlate with a decrease in the active inflammation, although the usefulness of CMRA in assessing disease activity has been questioned. Magnetic resonance evaluation for giant cell arteritis has not been as well studied, but evidence of enhancement has been reported in temporal arteries. CMRA provides information useful in the diagnosis of aortitis, including luminal stenosis, aneurysmal dilation, and disease activity.

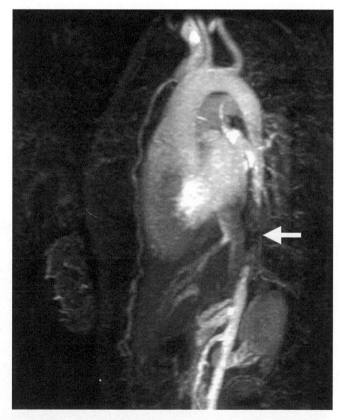

FIGURE 16-22. Maximal intensity projection of a magnetic resonance angiogram illustrating a complete aortic occlusion (arrow) as a result of Takayasu's aortitis. Note the generalized, smooth narrowing of the vessel until the site of occlusion.

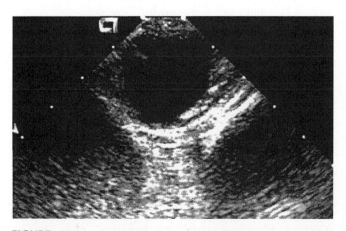

FIGURE 16-21. Transesophageal echocardiogram demonstrating descending aortic atherosclerosis. There is an atherosclerotic plaque at the 10-o'clock position.

Mesenteric Ischemia

Mesenteric ischemia as a result of visceral arterial stenosis or occlusion can be separated into two types: acute and chronic.[24] In situ thrombosis or, more commonly, embolic events to the celiac or superior mesenteric artery may acutely limit blood flow and cause severe abdominal pain. Yet, patients initially may present with few physical signs or laboratory evidence of this vascular catastrophe. In contrast to the rapidity of an embolic event, atherosclerosis of the mesenteric vessels may cause more gradually developing flow-limiting stenoses in the vessels. The extensive collateralization of the visceral vasculature mandates that at least two and commonly all three of the mesenteric arteries (celiac, superior mesenteric, and inferior mesenteric) have significant stenoses or occlusions before the onset of symptoms. Patients with mesenteric insufficiency secondary to atherosclerosis report postprandial abdominal pain, food fear, and a >10% weight loss.

Imaging is prominent in patient evaluation for both acute and chronic mesenteric ischemia, because symptoms of each condition may be subtle and nonspecific. Acute mesenteric ischemia, in particular, requires urgent imaging and surgical intervention to prevent bowel infarction. The two imaging modalities commonly used are CT angiography and contrast angiography. CTA provides visualization of the proximal mesenteric vessels and can be performed rapidly. Contrast angiography has been used successfully for decades to diagnose mesenteric artery disease. In a recent series, CT angiography had similar diagnostic efficacy in this situation.

Chronic mesenteric ischemia does not carry the same level of urgency. The diagnostic modalities may be used over the course of days to weeks. In this setting, determining the presence of mesenteric arterial stenosis or occlusion can be accomplished with both CTA and CMRA.[25,26] Both modalities define the proximal and secondary branches well. Visualization of the distal tertiary vessels is better accomplished with contrast angiography.

RENAL ARTERY STENOSIS

The presence of atherosclerotic renal artery stenosis in a hypertensive patient does not necessarily establish causation, because essential hypertension may coexist with, and also accelerate, the development of atheroma. Similarly, the association of renal artery obstruction and renal insufficiency may be coincidental. Thus, patients with hypertension or renal insufficiency *and* atherosclerotic renal artery stenosis may often have hypertension or renal insufficiency *and* renovascular disease but not hypertension and renal insufficiency because of renovascular disease. True renovascular hypertension is thought to affect 4% to 10% of the hypertensive population. Of all new cases of end-stage renal disease, 10% to 25% are now being categorized as related to hypertensive nephropathy and renal vascular disease. The diagnostic paradigm has shifted toward identifying patients with atherosclerotic renal artery stenosis who are "at risk" for the development of direct consequences of renovascular obstruction and ischemic nephropathy and treatment that is directed toward preserving renal function.

Etiologies of Renovascular Disease

Approximately 80% of renal artery stenoses are caused by atherosclerosis, and plaques are mostly observed in the proximal third of the renal artery, and occasionally perirenal aortic plaques may encroach on the ostium of the renal artery.[27] Atheromatous involvement is bilateral in one third of cases and has a high probability of progressing to complete occlusion. Worsening of stenoses occurs in half the patients with renal artery stenosis of >60% with progression to complete arterial occlusion in 7% to 37%. In one series, the mean rate of progression of percent diameter stenosis was 1.5% per month. Only 3% to 16% of patients have total renal artery occlusion develop, but renal atrophy occurs in 21% of patients with atherosclerotic renal artery stenosis of >60%. By present estimates, renovascular disease is considered to be the primary cause of end-stage renal disease in 15% of patients.

Fibromuscular dysplasia of the renal arteries includes four types of pathological conditions, the most common being medial fibroplasias, which accounts for 70% of cases. Medial fibroplasia predominantly causes renal artery stenosis in women <50 years of age and affects the middle or distal third of the main renal artery trunk. It is bilateral in approximately 60% of cases and, when unilateral, has a predilection toward the right kidney. Its classic "beaded appearance" on angiography is due to thickening of media interspersed by areas of aneurysmal dilation and almost never leads to complete occlusion.

Miscellaneous and uncommon causes of renovascular disease and renal ischemia include atheromatous emboli, neurofibromatosis, coarctation of the aorta, aortic dissection, radiation injury, and rare vasculitides. In the presence of diffuse atherosclerosis, fragments of plaque or associated thrombus can break and embolize into the distal renal vascular bed. This may happen spontaneously or as a consequence of manipulation during surgery, angiography, or an angioplasty. These microemboli are composed of cholesterol crystals and amorphous debris that later get replaced by giant cells and fibrous tissue. Clinical manifestations of such embolization include worsening of renal function and hypertension and may be accompanied by signs and symptoms of mesenteric ischemia, acute pancreatitis, digital infarction, eosinophilia, or livedo reticularis of the lower extremities. The overall mortality of atheromatous embolic has been reported to be as high as 64%. Takayasu's arteritis is an uncommon disease that occurs mainly in young women, causing discrete stenosis of aorta and its major branches, including the renal arteries.

Clinical Manifestations of Renovascular Disease

Renovascular hypertension by way of renin-angiotensin-aldosterone system activation is the most common cause of secondary hypertension and accounts for approximately 5% of the general hypertensive population. Atherosclerotic renal artery stenosis has also been reported in normotensive patients. In patients undergoing coronary angiography, significant atherosclerotic renal artery stenosis has been detected in approximately 20% and is equally common among hypertensive and normotensive patients. In patients being investigated for peripheral vascular disease, up to 60% may have significant atherosclerotic renal artery stenosis of at least one artery. In patients who are seen with accelerated hypertension, atherosclerotic renal artery stenosis has been identified in 43% of white and 7% of black patients. The diagnosis of bilateral renal artery stenosis should be entertained in hypertensive patients with poorly controlled blood pressure who have acute pulmonary edema. Many believe that chronic renal hypoperfusion can lead to renal dysfunction or ischemic nephropathy and may cause one or both kidneys to atrophy. In one series, approximately 70% of surgical revascularizations were carried out in an attempt to salvage renal function caused by atheroma of renal arteries.[27] In the last decade, a sixfold increase in the proportion of new cases of renal failure attributable to hypertension has been described, and although the degree to which ischemic nephropathy has contributed to this is uncertain, it has been estimated to be present in approximately 15% of new cases of end-stage renal disease.

Diagnosis

The age of presentation may be the first clue to the diagnosis of renovascular hypertension. Fibromuscular dysplasia is the most common cause of renal artery stenosis in younger patients, particularly in women. In contrast, the finding of hypertension in an older man with other evidence of atherosclerosis, such as coronary artery disease, should raise the possibility of atherosclerotic renal artery stenosis.[28] Important physical findings that may be clues to the diagnosis of renovascular hypertension are those of generalized atherosclerosis, particularly, the findings of aortic branch vessel disease such as subclavian, carotid, visceral, and iliofemoral obstruction. In the US Cooperative Study of Renovascular Hypertension, 15% of patients with atherosclerotic renal artery stenosis had an elevated creatinine compared with 11% of patients with essential hypertension and only 2% of fibromuscular dysplasia patients. A flow-limiting unilateral renal artery stenosis of >70% may cause reduction in the glomerular filtration rate in the involved kidney without a change in serum creatinine levels until overall renal function is half normal.

Low serum potassium as a result of hyperreninemia can be a marker of renal artery stenosis and is present in approximately 15% of such patients. In the absence of underlying renal parenchymal disease, or other causes of proteinuria, renal artery stenosis and resultant hyperreninemia may be the underlying cause and can be reversible with timely revascularization. Plasma renin activity level is found to be high in approximately 75% of patients with diagnosed renovascular hypertension, and although it may be normal in the presence of renovascular hypertension, it should not be low. Generally, this single "blood test" has not proved to be an appropriate screening tool.

The reactive rise of renin after administration of an angiotensin converting enzyme inhibitor is greater in patients with renovascular hypertension than in those with essential hypertension who may also have an exaggerated renin response to captopril challenge. A post-captopril renin of >12 ng/ mL/hour, an absolute increase of >10 ng/mL/hour, or an increase of >150% (400% if baseline renin <3 ng) is considered positive for renovascular hypertension. The captopril test carries an overall sensitivity of approximately 75% and a specificity of 90%. The positive predictive value is related to the population prevalence of renal artery stenosis, and at this sensitivity the value of the test in a low prevalence population is limited.[29]

In unilateral renal artery stenosis, the increased quantity of renin secreted by the ischemic kidney suppresses the renin secretion by the contralateral kidney, although the systemic renin levels are typically high. This asymmetry can be determined as a ratio of plasma renin activity between the two renal veins (1.5:1 or 2:1) or the increase in the plasma renin activity between the renal vein (V) and the renal artery (A) measured separately on each side $[(V - A)/A]$. The normal increment is 25%, but in people with renovascular hypertension, it can be >50% in the ischemic kidney and zero in the contralateral kidney. In patients with bilateral renal artery stenosis, renal vein renin levels often show asymmetry, and lateralize to the kidney with greatest degree of stenosis in the arteriogram. The lateralization of the renin levels is highest in patients with complete occlusion of one renal artery.

Renal Scintigraphy

Renal scintigraphy with compounds such as ^{131}I hippuran can measure both renal size and blood flow. Tc–diethylene triamine- penta-acetic acid (DTPA) can measure glomerular filtration rate (GFR). The uptake of isotope is highest 1.5 to 2.5 minutes after the radiopharmaceutical injection, and an asymmetry of uptake more than 60:40 is considered abnormal. Time-to-peak-activity should also be evaluated, because it may be delayed in the presence of renal artery stenosis. When the renal artery stenosis is less severe, a delay in excretion of isotope may be the only abnormality present. Renal scintigraphy alone is insufficient to assess renal artery stenosis and is now performed with adjunctive captopril administration.[30] Both GFR and renal blood flow of an ischemic kidney depend on angiotensin and its effect on the efferent glomerular arterioles. In the presence of significant renal artery stenosis, angiotensin-converting enzyme (ACE) inhibition will result in considerable reduction of both GFR and renal blood flow. So administration of captopril in the setting of renal artery stenosis will reduce the uptake of isotopes such as Tc-DTPA, I hippuran, or ^{99m}Tc-mercapto-acetyltriglycerine[31] (Figure 16-23). In selected series of patients with moderate renal artery stenosis, captopril renography has been shown to have a sensitivity of 92%. The changes induced by captopril are somewhat specific for renal artery stenosis and help distinguish it from parenchymal disease. However, in a

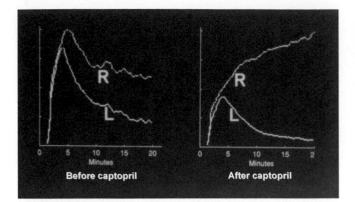

FIGURE 16-23. Renal scintigraphy of a patient with right renal artery stenosis demonstrating radioisotope activity in the right and left kidney before *(left side)* and after *(right side)* captopril administration. The time to peak activity and the excretion rate is delayed in the right kidney, particularly after captopril.

general population likely to be encountered in clinical practice, the sensitivity is low (45% to 80%), especially in cases of severe stenosis, when even the precaptopril scintigram has low isotope uptake.

Intravenous Pyelogram

The sensitivity of the intravenous pyelogram to detect renal artery stenosis is approximately 75% and the specificity 85%. Given the associated dose of radiation and potentially nephrotoxic contrast agent, it is not recommended as a screening test.

Intravenous Digital Subtraction Angiography

Although intravenous digital subtraction angiography enables visualization of renal arteries, it is not used extensively. A large bolus of iodinated contrast agent poses a hazard for patients with impaired renal function, the resolution of the technique is significantly less than arteriography, and proximal renal artery stenosis may be completely missed. Resolution is further impaired in obese patients or patients with impaired cardiac function. A sensitivity of 88% and a specificity of 90% have been reported in selected populations.

CMRA

A contrast-enhanced CMRA examination of vessels in the abdomen and thorax requires a breath-holding technique. Short imaging times are necessary for the acquisition of the data and, when coupled with high flow rates, lead to a higher concentration of the paramagnetic contrast medium in the arteries, resulting in improved contrast/noise ratio in the vessels compared with surrounding tissues. CMRA is now a well-established diagnostic procedure that allows noninvasive visualization of the renal artery (Figure 16-24).[32] Although CMRA of renal arteries does not achieve the high resolution of conventional angiography, a potential advantage is the depiction of the lumen as well as the vessel wall, and the ability to demonstrate parenchymal findings and renal

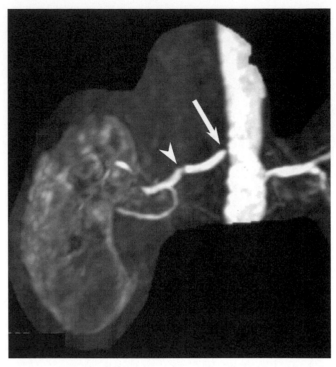

FIGURE 16-24. Reformatted two-dimensional reconstruction of gadolinium-enhanced MRA images that suggests a severe ostial stenosis *(long arrow)* and a stenosis in the midportion of the main right renal artery.

size and volume. CMRA does not use ionizing radiation, and larger vessel sections are well seen. Gadolinium-enhanced CMRA reliably images the main renal arteries.[33] Both the sensitivity and specificity of CMRA in the detection of atherosclerotic renal artery stenosis have been reported to be >90%. The quality of CMRA depends on equipment, personnel, and expertise, and there is no other noninvasive test that offers better or safer anatomical definition.

The disadvantage of CMRA is its inability to accurately characterize more distal renal vasculature and segmental branches. A cooperative patient with the ability to remain motionless is required for the optimal application of this technique, and it has been estimated that approximately 5% of patients do not complete the test because of claustrophobia. For follow-up examinations after renal artery stent implantation, the results of CMRA can be impossible to interpret because of magnetic dephasing effects at the stent site. Additional contraindications to CMRA such as the presence of ferromagnetic foreign bodies, intracranial or spinal vascular clips, or cardiac pacing/defibrillator systems can limit its use.

Ultrasound

Transabdominal Doppler ultrasound scanning to image and record velocity profiles from the renal arteries can demonstrate stenosis (Figure 16-25). In the presence of renal artery obstruction, an acceleration of flow across the stenosis is noted (Figure 16-26). There are three generally accepted criteria for the presence of a severe

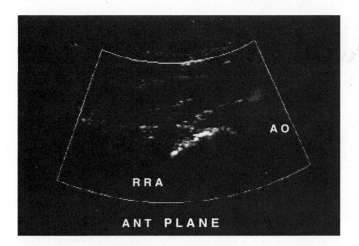

FIGURE 16-25. Color duplex ultrasound examination of the right renal artery. (Courtesy of Dr. Jeffrey Olin, Mt. Sinai Medical Center, New York, NY.) See also Color Insert.

(>60%) stenosis: (1) an aortic-to-renal peak systolic flow velocity flow velocity ratio >3.5; (2) A maximal renal artery end-diastolic velocity of >150 cm/s; or (3) a renal peak systolic velocity of >180 cm/s. Several problems with the technique have limited its usefulness as a routine diagnostic procedure. In the hands of an experienced operator, renal duplex sonography has a sensitivity of 98%, a specificity of 98%, and a negative predictive value of 97%.[34] However, these studies are extremely operator dependent, and in 15% to 40% of studies, it is not technically feasible to obtain an optimal scan. Detection of polar renal artery branches or an accessory renal artery may be difficult, and because 14% of patients being evaluated for renovascular hypertension may have a polar branch artery stenosis, a negative duplex ultrasound may not necessarily eliminate the possibility of renal artery stenosis. Preliminary studies

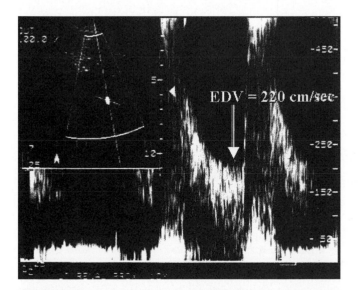

FIGURE 16-26. Continuous-wave Doppler interrogation of a stenosed left renal artery. The peak systolic velocity is >450 cm/s, and the end-diastolic velocity is 200 cm/s, each indicative of a severe stenosis. (Courtesy of Dr. Jeffrey Olin, Mt. Sinai Medical Center, New York, NY.) See also Color Insert.

with relatively small numbers of patients report successful visualization of the renal artery in 80% to 90% of cases, and others claim success in only 60%. Ultrasound is very helpful in the detection of transplant renal artery stenosis, in which the superficial location of the renal artery makes it easier to image. The precision of this technique depends on equipment, personnel, and experience, and problems may be encountered in patients with obesity, bowel gas, recent surgery, and the presence of multiple renal arteries.

CTA

CTA is used to diagnose renal artery stenosis.[35] It offers the theoretical advantage of being noninvasive, easily applied in an ambulatory setting, and not limited by metallic artifact as is CMRA. CTA has been reported to be superior to Doppler ultrasound in detecting the presence of renal artery stenosis. The sensitivity and specificity of CTA compared with conventional angiography is approximately 95% and 98%, respectively.

For hemodynamically relevant renal artery stenosis (>50%), the sensitivity and specificity may be even greater. Technical details such as scan delay after contrast injection or the use of volume-rendered vs. maximum-intensity projection suggests that volume rendering is simpler and more accurate. A normal optimized CTA may virtually rule out renal artery stenosis. A particularly attractive use of CTA may be the evaluation of patients suspected of having "in-stent" restenosis after renal artery intervention (Figure 16-27). This is a setting in which the magnetic effects of the stent renders interrogation of the stented segment impossible with CMRA. Anatomical definition, including stent position and wall apposition in the renal artery, correlates well with catheter angiography.[36] CTA in patients with renal insufficiency has been limited by concerns over the administration of large amounts of iodinated contrast. In a small group of patients randomly assigned to either CTA or digital subtraction angiography (DSA), renal function as determined by inulin clearance did not differ between groups after imaging.[37] CTA, despite its need for iodinated contrast, may have an increasing role in the poststent evaluation of renovascular disease. Eventually this technique may replace conventional catheter-based angiography in the routine anatomical evaluation of the renal circulation in transplant donors.

Angiography

Contrast angiography is described as the diagnostic "gold standard" for the detection of renal artery stenosis.[38] With technological advances, DSA has replaced the traditional cut-films in most institutions. To cause renal ischemia and renovascular hypertension, a stenosis must be at least 70% of the arterial reference diameter. However, the correlation between the angiographic stenosis and the degree of ischemia is poor (Figures 16-28 and 16-29). Truly mild and very severe lesions may be obvious, but the weakness of our current anatomical standard is the unknown individual significance of most moderate (50% to 70%) lesions. If a borderline stenosis is detected, further functional assessment may be appropriate before

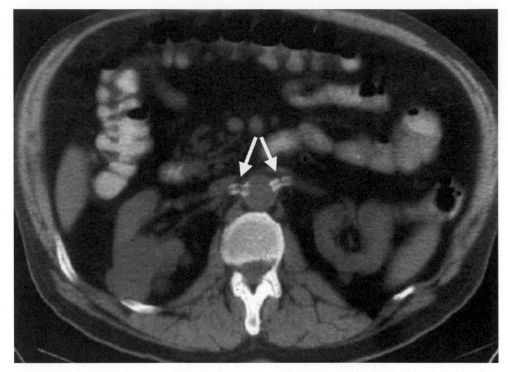

FIGURE 16-27. Cross-sectional CT scan demonstrating stents in the right and left renal arteries *(arrows).*

intervention. Balloon angioplasty currently has a modest, but significant, role in reducing blood pressure in patients with atherosclerotic renal artery stenosis and poorly controlled hypertension.[39]

Digital subtraction technology enables the acquisition of high-resolution pictures with significantly reduced dye loads, and three-dimensional angiographic reconstruction can permit the physician to interrogate the

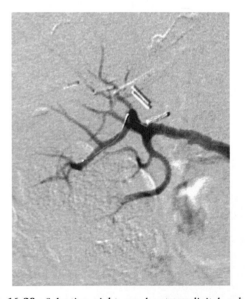

FIGURE 16-28. Selective right renal artery digital subtraction angiograms. A very severe renal artery stenosis is present. In this case, the distal renal arteries within the kidney appear small, irregular, and underfilled. The anatomical appearance of the distal vessels may be difficult to evaluate in the presence of very severe main renal artery stenosis.

renal arteries in views preventing aorto-ostial overlap. The use of smaller-lumen catheters reduces the problems associated with the arterial puncture and cholesterol emboli. In many cases, a renal angiogram can be performed as an outpatient procedure.

After arterial access has been obtained, abdominal aortography is performed with a "tennis-racquet," "pigtail," or "halo" catheter in proper position (Figure 16-30, left panel). Renal arteries are imaged in multiple views with obliquity to profile the renal ostium and segmental branches. An abdominal aortogram should provide adequate visualization of the body of the renal artery; its various branches; yield a good estimation of the renal size, contour, cortical thickness; and rate of appearance of "blush" bilaterally. When possible, a selective renal angiogram should be performed (Figure 16-30, right panel). Selective engagement of the renal artery and subsequent injection allow better visualization and measurement of the pressure gradient and Doppler flow patterns. Use of digital angiography significantly lessens contrast volume.

In an effort to avoid the nephrotoxicity of iodinated contrast agents, alternative imaging media have been sought for renal angiography. Gaseous media such as carbon dioxide (CO_2) have been used and, despite the inability to image distal renal branches, have proved useful in evaluating the main renal arteries for the presence of atherosclerotic renal artery stenosis (Figure 16-31). CO_2 has been used as the primary contrast medium when it is appropriate to eliminate or reduce the need for iodinated media. The technique is particularly sensitive to the presence of bowel gas, motion artifact, and fragmentation of the bolus, but it has been successful in large numbers and is usually well tolerated. Gadolinium-

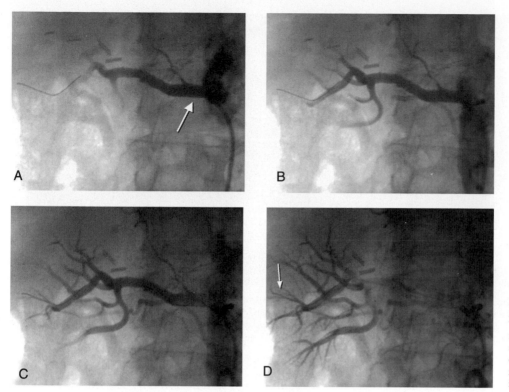

FIGURE 16-29. Renal angiograms of the same patient in Figure 16-26 after percutaneous revascularization and placement of a stent. This series of views from a selective study shows resolution of the severe near-ostial stenosis (*large arrow*, **A**), rapid filling of the distal vasculature (**B**), and normally branching smooth distal intrarenal vasculature (**C** and **D**).

containing paramagnetic contrast agents can also be used as iodinated-contrast–sparing agents in renal angiography (Figure 16-31). Typicaliy, the agent is used for selective angiography with a subtraction technique. There is some evidence that gadolinium may be angiographically superior to CO_2, and the two techniques may be combined to obviate the need for any iodinated contrast. Neither the use of CO_2 nor gadolinium agents is complete assurance against procedure-related renal failure or cholesterol embolization. Nevertheless, the use of these alternative agents has facilitated the safe performance of angiography and intervention in patients with impaired renal function.

Choosing the Appropriate Tests

The relatively low prevalence of renovascular hypertension in the general population of hypertensive individuals, together with the cost and imperfect accuracy of the available screening tests for its diagnosis, means that universal screening of all hypertensive patients is inappropriate. A clinical algorithm (Figure 16-32) is suggested on the basis of the level of clinical suspicion. A thorough history and physical examination looking for clinical clues linked to renal artery stenosis should precede any testing. If clinical clues raise the index of suspicion, patients should be considered for further evaluation (Box

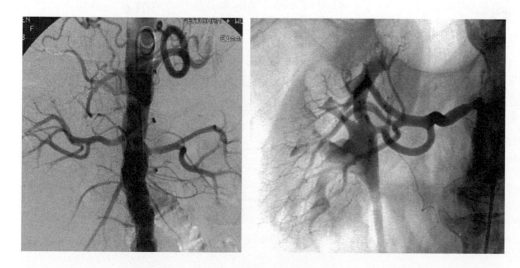

FIGURE 16-30. The left panel is an abdominal aortogram in which the origin of the left renal artery is well seen and has only mild irregularity. The angulation of this view obscures the origin of the right renal artery but does demonstrate wide patency of the midportion of the vessel. A selective angiogram (*right panel*) confirms this finding and shows a very mild lesion at the origin of the right artery with no gradient measured by pressure wire.

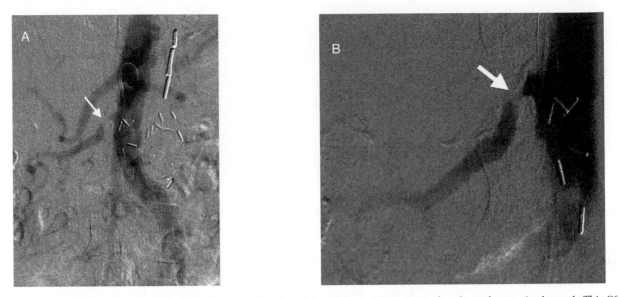

FIGURE 16-31. A, Carbon dioxide contrast can be used to pinpoint the origins of the renal arteries and evaluate the proximal vessels. This CO_2 aortogram clearly demonstrates absence or occlusion of the left renal artery and identifies both the location of the right renal artery and the presence of a severe proximal stenosis *(arrow)*. **B,** In the same patient, angiography was carried out by injecting gadolinium by hand. Digitally subtracted images of the gadolinium injection clearly demonstrate the location and severity of the right renal artery stenosis.

16-1). The evaluation can include assessment of overall renal function, physiological studies to assess the renin-angiotensin-aldosterone system, perfusion studies to evaluate differential blood flow, and imaging studies to image the renal arteries.

For patients with a low index of clinical suspicion, no further evaluation is needed. These would include patients with mild or borderline hypertension in whom the clinical signs and symptoms favoring renovascular

hypertension are absent and patients with a low renin hypertension. In such cases, the prevalence of renovascular hypertension is likely <1%, hence the screening tests that are positive are likely to be false-positive results.

For patients associated with a moderate level of suspicion, in whom the clinical signs and symptoms are present but the evidence of renovascular disease is not overwhelming, the prevalence is likely to be 5% to 15%.

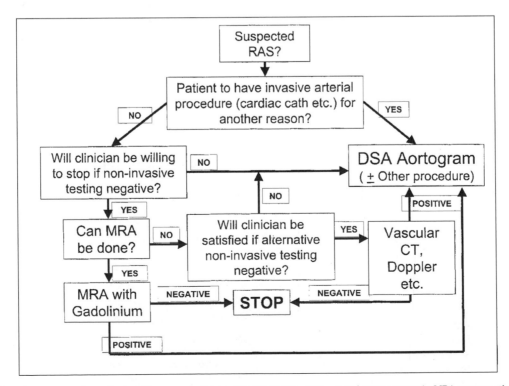

FIGURE 16-32. Imaging strategy for patients with suspected renovascular disease. RAS = renal artery stenosis; MRA = magnetic resonance angiography; DSA = digital substraction angiography.

BOX 16-1 CLINICAL AND HISTORICAL FACTORS ASSOCIATED WITH RENAL ARTERY STENOSIS

Hypertension
New onset after the age of 50 years (suggestive of atherosclerotic renal artery
    stenosis)
Newly refractory hypertension
Accelerated or malignant hypertension
Requirement of three antihypertensive drugs
Renal
Elevated creatinine levels (>2.5 mg/dL)
Increase in creatinine level induced by angiotensin-converting enzyme inhibitor
    therapy
Mild proteinuria without diabetes (<1 g/day)
Disparate kidney size (one normal, one small)
Unexplained hypokalemia
Evidence of systemic atherosclerosis
Coronary atherosclerosis
Carotid artery or cerebrovascular atherosclerosis (stroke, TIA, prior endarterectomy)
Known aortic branch vessel (brachiocephalic/mesenteric) atherosclerosis
Abdominal or flank bruit
Peripheral intermittent claudication
Others
Acute pulmonary edema or congestive heart failure not explained by cardiac
    dysfunction
Severe retinopathy
History of smoking

In such cases, the negative predictive value of a screening test with a sensitivity and specificity of 90% would exceed 98%, and the positive predictive value would be 32%, justifying proceeding to a renal angiogram.

Last, there are patients in whom the index of suspicion is so high that an angiogram could be justified even if all noninvasive diagnostic tests were negative. A typical example would be a patient without diabetes with generalized atherosclerosis, an abdominal bruit, the sudden acceleration of hypertension, and in whom renal function deteriorates when treated with an ACE inhibitor. Such patients have been reported to have a prevalence of renal artery stenosis of >30%.

Early recognition of renal artery stenosis and revascularization may be important to ameliorate hypertension, prevent loss of functional renal mass, and avoid progression to advanced renal failure. The available diagnostic and imaging modalities ultimately are of value only if they serve that purpose.

CAROTID ARTERY DISEASE

Stroke is the third leading cause of death in the United States, and carotid artery disease is an important cause of transient ischemic attacks (TIA) and stroke. Strokes are attributed to ischemia (85%) or hemorrhage (15%). The three major categories of ischemic stroke are atherosclerosis, small-vessel occlusive disease, and cardioembolism. Carotid atherosclerosis is estimated to account for 10% to 20% of all strokes, and carotid stenosis >50% is present in up to 10% of men and 7% of women older

than 65 years of age. Cerebral ischemic events can occur with stenoses of any degree but are more likely in patients with stenoses >75% and progressing stenosis. The annual risk of stroke is up to 4% in selected populations with asymptomatic carotid stenosis and up to 13% in patients with symptomatic carotid stenosis. Patients who have had a stroke continue to be at risk for stroke at the rate of up to 9% per year, with the highest risk in the first few weeks after a stroke. Reducing, or eliminating, risk factors by cigarette smoking cessation and cholesterol-lowering therapies has a direct effect on the carotid artery wall and is likely to decrease the risk of plaque formation and progression.

Etiologies of Carotid Artery Disease

Atherosclerosis is the cause of most cases of carotid artery stenosis and develops preferentially at the bifurcations (Figure 16-33), and the resulting plaque protrudes into the lumen. Plaque rupture leads to thrombus formation with distal embolization to the cerebral circulation or occasionally total occlusion. Other etiologies of carotid disease or thrombosis are much less common and include Takayasu's arteritis, giant cell arteritis, fibromuscular dysplasia, carotid artery dissection, carotid body tumor, radiation arteriopathy, and hypercoagulable conditions.

Takayasu's arteritis is a chronic inflammatory disease affecting the aorta and its branches, most often occurring in women younger than 40 years of age. It is a periarteritis that begins with inflammation throughout the vessel wall, which thickens and progressively encroaches on the carotid lumen. Sonography of the carotid and subclavian arteries demonstrates a characteristic, homogeneous, echoic, circumferential thickening of the wall (Figure 16-34).[40] The pathology includes giant cells present at sites of elastic lamina destruction, and fibrosis of

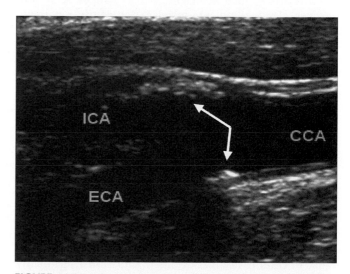

FIGURE 16-33. Ultrasound of the carotid bifurcation. The common carotid artery (CCA) bifurcates into the internal (ICA) and external (ECA) carotid arteries. The physical bifurcation results in disruption of laminar flow, with atherosclerosis most likely to develop in the areas of turbulence. Mild atherosclerosis is evident in the region of the bifurcation (*arrows*).

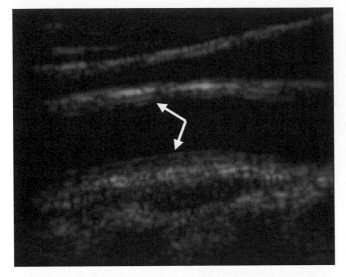

FIGURE 16-34. Ultrasound demonstrating thickened intima in the common carotid artery of a patient with Takayasu arteritis. Arrows indicate the mildly thickened intima on both sides of the vessel.

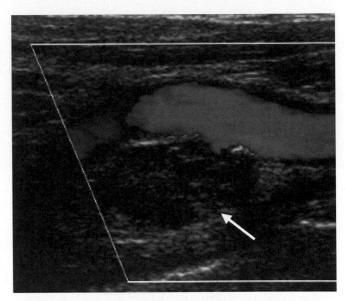

FIGURE 16-35. Duplex ultrasound of the carotid bifurcation. The arrow indicates the carotid body tumor posterior to the carotid artery. See also Color Insert.

the vessel occurs in the chronic phase. In time, arterial insufficiency may develop and with involvement of the brachiocephalic arteries may be seen as cerebrovascular ischemia or arm claudication. Takayasu's arteritis should be suspected in young women with carotid and subclavian bruits.

Giant cell (temporal) arteritis occurs in older individuals. The mean age of onset is 70 years. It begins with both lymphocyte infiltration of the arterial wall and intimal thickening. Classic pathological findings include areas with multinucleated giant cells, focal necrosis, and disrupted elastic lamina interspersed with unaffected areas, resulting in a pattern of "skip" lesions. Carotid, vertebral, temporal, subclavian, brachial, and coronary arteries, and the aorta may be involved.[41] Symptoms of giant cell arteritis include headache, visual changes, scalp tenderness, claudication, and malaise. Half of these patients will have polymyalgia rheumatica.

Noninflammatory diseases of the carotid arteries include fibromuscular dysplasia, carotid dissection, radiation arteriopathy, and carotid body tumor. Fibromuscular dysplasia of the carotid arteries is characterized by intimal and medial fibroplasia and typically affects the distal internal carotid artery. It occurs predominantly in women. The natural history of cervicocranial fibromuscular dysplasia is unknown, but the incidence of stroke is estimated to approach 25%. Asymptomatic carotid fibromuscular dysplasia cases are identified when sought in patients with known renal artery fibromuscular dysplasia. Carotid artery dissections are categorized as spontaneous, secondary to trauma, or extending from aortic arch dissections. The incidence of carotid artery dissection is not known, but it is increasingly recognized as a cause of cerebrovascular events.[42] Radiation arteriopathy results from high-dose irradiation of the neck and fibrosis of the carotid artery. The frequency with which it may result in stroke is unknown. Carotid body tumors are paragangliomas arising on the posterior aspect of the carotid bifurcation (Figure 16-35). They are usually

incorporated into the adventitia of the vessel wall. Most symptoms from carotid body tumor result from involvement of local nerves rather than from narrowing of the carotid artery lumen and cerebrovascular ischemia.

Clinical Presentation

Patients with cerebrovascular insufficiency can present with a wide variety of focal neurological deficits, including amaurosis fugax or transient monocular visual loss, and to contralateral sensorimotor loss and language difficulty (if the dominant hemisphere is affected) or neglect (if the nondominant hemisphere is affected). Ischemic stroke is the most feared presentation of carotid artery lesions.

Tests used in the diagnostic evaluation of carotid artery disease include duplex ultrasonography, MRA, spiral CT, and conventional angiography.[41]

Diagnostic Tests

Duplex Ultrasonography

Duplex ultrasonography detects carotid artery stenosis with sensitivity and specificity of 94% and 96%, respectively. Duplex ultrasound testing consists of both gray scale imaging and flow analysis. Progressive narrowing of arterial segments perturbs the normal laminar pattern of blood flow. Color Doppler is used to identify areas of disturbed flow. Thereafter, the velocity of blood flow in these areas is carefully characterized with pulsed-wave Doppler. It is recommended that the angle between the ultrasound beam and the vessel wall (or flow jet) be ≤ 60 degrees for reproducible velocity measurements. As the severity of the stenosis worsens, the most consistent measurable change is an increase in peak systolic velocity. Pulse Doppler interrogation at the site of carotid artery stenosis (Figure 16-36) detects higher systolic and dias-

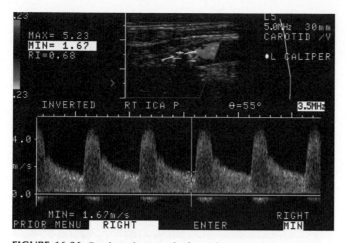

FIGURE 16-36. Duplex ultrasound of a right internal carotid artery. Color Doppler is used to identify areas of turbulence and aliasing. The spectral waveform is notable for the elevated peak systolic velocity of 523 cm/s and the end-diastolic velocity of 167 cm/s. These findings indicate diameter reduction of 95% or greater. See also Color Insert.

tolic velocities compared with those from a nonstenotic artery. Grading the severity of stenosis requires measurement of the peak systolic velocity, end-diastolic velocity, and/or velocity ratios (Table 16-3).[43] The Doppler assessment is more difficult in tortuous vessels where the fastest moving blood is typically located at the outer aspect when it exits the bend rather than in a typical central parabolic laminar distribution.

B flow is a technique to encode gray scale signals from moving red blood cells by use of a high pulse repetition frequency. The vessel wall remains visible as the surrounding gray scale image is obtained simultaneously; therefore, there is no "bleed" artifact as is seen with the color flow data being written over the gray scale image. B flow imaging increases the ability to identify flow jets with ultrasound and to evaluate the blood flow–vessel wall interface (Figure 16-37). Both color Doppler and B flow improve detection of subtotal occlusion by ultrasound. However, ultrasound is more likely to miss a "trickle" of flow than any of the angiographic techniques. Gray scale imaging is used to characterize plaque echolucency, smooth or irregular surface characteristics, and calcification (Figure 16-38). Plaque is defined as (1)

TABLE 16-3 CRITERIA FOR GRADING THE SEVERITY OF CAROTID ARTERY STENOSIS BASED ON PEAK SYSTOLIC VELOCITY AND END-DIASTOLIC VELOCITY

Diameter reduction	PSV (cm/s)	EDV (cm/s)	PSV ICA/PSV CCA
0-29	<100	<40	<3.2
30-49	110-130	<40	<3.2
50-59	>130	<40	<3.2
60-69	>130	40-100	3.2-4.0
70-79	>230	110-140	>4.0
80-95	>230	>140	>4.0
96-99	String flow		
100	No flow		

PSV, Peak systolic velocity; EDV, end-diastolic velocity; CCA, common carotid artery; ICA, internal carotid artery.

hyperechoic (brightness comparable to the adventitia) or hypoechoic (almost as dark as flowing blood), (2) homogenous (uniform density) or heterogeneous (mixed density), (3) calcified (with acoustic shadowing) or noncalcified, and (4) smooth, irregular (undulating surface) or ulcerated (surface crater with flow reversal). The dichotomous categories for grading plaque reduce variability in interpretation. Extensive clinical and laboratory studies over the past decade have demonstrated that the critical features predicting vascular events lie within the plaque itself. Plaque characteristics on ultrasound can predict plaque histology. Ulcerated plaques are associated with an increased risk of TIA/stroke. The ultrasound appearance of an ulcer is a divot in the plaque surface, with flow reversal within the divot. Echolucent plaques have been associated with an increased risk of vascular events. In the Tromso study, subjects with echolucent carotid plaque on ultrasonography had a relative risk of 13.0 for future cerebrovascular events. Ultrasound is also useful in the assessment of carotid stents (Figure 16-39) and can be used to evaluate the artery proximal and distal to the stent. Strict blood flow velocity criteria for stenosis are less reliable in the carotid artery immediate after stent than in the native arteries. All blood flow velocity criteria for stenosis overestimate the degree of stenosis in the immediate

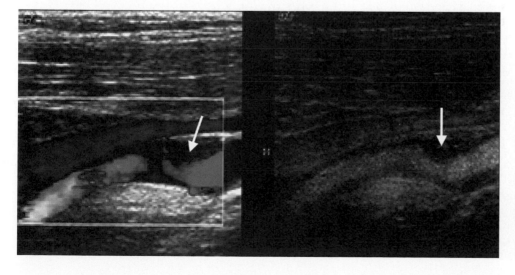

FIGURE 16-37. Blood flow to vessel wall interface of the same vessel evaluated with color Doppler (left) and B flow (right). Relatively hypoechoic plaque (P) is evident on the near wall in both images. The color Doppler is written over the gray scale image, resulting in less definition of the blood flow vessel wall interface than is evident in the B flow image. The B flow image is a gray scale image that uses very high pulse repetition frequency. The internal jugular vein (IJ) is seen above the carotid. See also Color Insert.

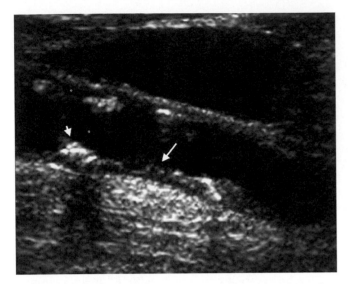

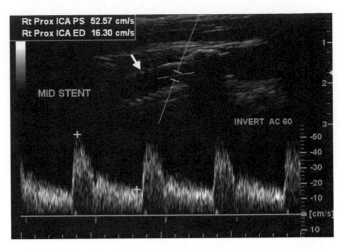

FIGURE 16-38. Gray scale carotid ultrasound illustrating plaque characteristics. A markedly irregular surface protrudes into the lumen. Bright areas of calcified plaque *(small arrow)* and hyperechoic plaque *(large arrow)* are evident.

FIGURE 16-39. Duplex carotid ultrasound of a patent carotid artery with a stent *(arrow)*. The peak systole and end-diastole velocities are normal.

poststent period. These velocities should be obtained to serve as a reference value for future follow-up examinations. An increase in peak systolic velocity of 80% or more at a follow-up examination is consistent with significant restenosis.[44] Duplex ultrasound may be used to diagnose a dissection of the carotid artery, but this test is less reliable than other imaging modalities. Small intimal flaps are difficult to detect with ultrasound. Dissections extending from the arch are more easily imaged (Figure 16-40). Duplex ultrasonography may identify indirect features of dissection, such as a Doppler waveform suggestive of distal internal carotid artery occlusion (Figure 16-39).

CMRA

CMRA can characterize carotid stenosis (Figure 16-41).[45] The sensitivity and specificity for detecting a 70% to 99% stenosis by CMRA are up to 96% and 95%, respectively, with conventional angiography as the "gold standard."[46] The sensitivity and specificity are generally less for determining moderate stenoses of 30% to 70%. Several studies have looked at the ability of CMR to detect lipid cores and fibrous caps within plaque in both animal models and human atherosclerosis, but this aspect of CMR should still be considered investigational. CMR, like ultrasound, has the advantage of permitting direct visualization of plaque and is useful in detection and quantification of mild atherosclerotic changes of carotid arteries compared with intravascular ultrasound and contrast angiography.

CTA

CTA enables imaging of the carotid arteries most effectively by moving the X-ray source and table and the use of multiple detectors to acquire the data in spiral or helical fashion (i.e., multidetector-row CT [MD-CTA]). The high spatial resolution and soft tissue delineation possible with contrast-enhanced MD-CTA may provide some information on noncalcified carotid artery lesions and allow noninvasive imaging of the vessel wall. CT angiography of the carotid arteries is particularly useful to

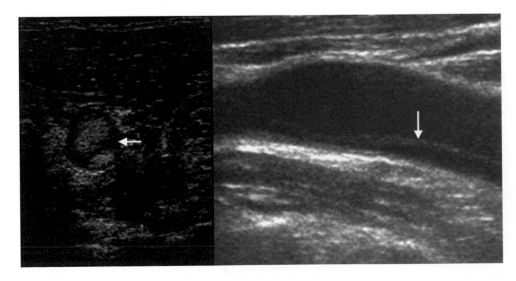

FIGURE 16-40. A, Gray scale ultrasound of the common carotid artery in cross section with B flow. The arrow indicates the dissection flap. Flow is evident on both sides of the flap. **B,** The dissection flap *(arrow)* is also evident on the longitudinal gray scale images in this patient. There is also aneurysm formation in the region of the dissection.

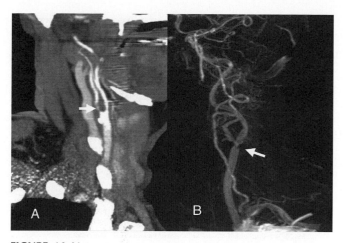

FIGURE 16-41. Magnetic resonance angiography of the carotid. **A,** Arrow indicates region of stenosis in the proximal internal carotid artery. **B,** Complex plaque of the carotid bifurcation.

define diameter stenosis in the presence of calcification (Figure 16-42). CT compares well with conventional angiography and intravascular ultrasound for the detection of stenosis. CTA has a sensitivity of 96% to 100% for the detection of lesions with reference to both IVUS and conventional angiography.[47]

Conventional Contrast Angiography

Conventional contrast angiography is the "gold standard" for the detection of carotid artery stenosis caused by atherosclerosis (Figure 16-43). The three primary branches radiating from the aortic arch are the brachiocephalic, left common carotid, and left subclavian arteries. The right subclavian and carotid arteries are branches off the brachiocephalic trunk. The most common variant of this anatomy is the "bovine" arch, where the left carotid and brachiocephalic share a common origin; it occurs in 10% of the general population. Subclavian stenosis, or occlusion, is manifested by either posterior circulation

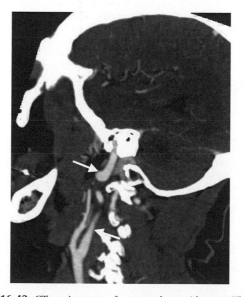

FIGURE 16-42. CT angiograms of a normal carotid artery. The entire course of a tortuous internal carotid artery cannot be seen in a single frame *(arrows)*.

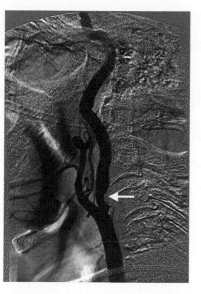

FIGURE 16-43. Conventional angiography of the carotid artery demonstrating a mild stenosis *(arrow)* at the proximal internal carotid artery.

events (flow is reversed in the ipsilateral vertebral artery with upper extremity activity), which are rare, or anterior ischemia (coronary steal syndrome) in the patient who has been treated with left internal mammary artery (IMA) bypass grafting and continues to experience ischemia despite surgery. Subclavian artery angiography is optimally performed by use of both AP and ipsilateral oblique views. Selective angiography can be performed with any straight or slightly angulated catheters (multipurpose, JR4, or IMA). Nonselective angiography in general requires 30 to 40 mL of contrast injected at 20 to 30 mL/s to adequately opacify all vessels in the arch. Selective angiography can be performed with hand injections through the previous catheters. The vessels are usually accessed with the use of the guide wire as a rail, and then the catheter is advanced over the wire. Access to the brachiocephalic, carotid, or subclavian arteries usually requires a counterclockwise movement of the catheter in the ascending aorta for it to engage the vessel of interest. The "J" wire is then advanced into the vessel, and ultimately the catheter is advanced over the wire. Once the wire has been removed and the catheter flushed, angiography can be performed safely. There is usually some shoulder and neck discomfort with moderate contrast injections, and the patient should be forewarned of the "warm" feeling that will follow injections. Discomfort can be minimized if necessary with the use of half-diluted contrast. Excessively vigorous injections should be avoided to prevent subintimal injection or dye staining. Atherosclerosis of the subclavian artery is generally proximal at the origin or within the first few millimeters from the aortic origin. The origin of the internal mammary artery and vertebral artery are usually spared of atherosclerosis. The origin of the vertebral artery may be involved with atherosclerotic lesions, but the need for intervention is low because of the dual blood supply to the posterior circulation that arises from both the contralateral vertebral and ipsilateral carotid arteries.

The carotid arteries generally bifurcate at the level of the fourth cervical vertebra into the internal and external carotid arteries. The internal carotid artery usually has no major branches and becomes tortuous below the petrous bone called the carotid siphon. Once the vessel enters the petrous bone, it is considered the intracranial internal carotid artery. Once the vessel exits the petrous bone, it bifurcates early into the anterior and middle cerebral arteries. The external carotid artery has several branches that supply the face. The most accepted criterion to determine carotid stenosis is by comparison of the diameter measured at the stenosis site to a diameter measurement of the artery distal to the stenosis, which were used in the North American Symptomatic Carotid Endarterectomy Trial (NASCET).[48] However, conventional angiography provides information only about lumen diameter and not about the arterial wall itself. In this respect, angiography is also useful in the diagnosis of fibromuscular dysplasia, in which tubular narrowing may be evident in the distal internal carotid artery. Contrast angiography is also used in the evaluation of cerebral vasculitis. Angiography is useful in the diagnosis of arterial dissections, because it can show the arterial lumen and allows extensive characterization of dissections of the carotid and vertebral arteries. Pathognomonic features of dissection, such as an intimal flap or a double lumen, are not always detected in dissected arteries. The stenosis of carotid artery dissection is typically irregular, starts about 2 to 3 cm distal to the carotid bulb, and extends for various lengths along the artery but not past its entry into the petrous portion of the temporal bone, where the lumen is abruptly reconstituted. Occlusions characteristically have a tapered, flamelike appearance, particularly in the acute phase of the dissection.

Comparison of Imaging Techniques to Evaluate Carotid Stenosis

Prevention of stroke is aided by determination of the degree of carotid artery stenosis and progression of atherosclerosis.[49] Important considerations of the carotid artery evaluation include: (1) estimating degree of stenosis; (2) evaluation of irregularities in arterial walls, including calcification, intimal thickening, ulcers and plaque; and (3) planning for revascularization. All four imaging modalities are accurate for detecting stenosis. An advantage of CMRA is the ability to scan the carotid siphon to the middle cerebral artery at one time. A disadvantage is the tendency to overestimate stenosis with CMRA. Ulceration of the artery wall can be evaluated by duplex ultrasound, CT, and CMRA. Collateral vessels (circumventing occlusions) and flow (e.g., across the circle of Willis) are best evaluated with standard angiography. All these diagnostic modalities can identify carotid stenosis, and test selection must be guided by the specific case and local availability.

REFERENCES

1. McDermott MM, Greenland P, Liu K, et al. The ankle brachial index is associated with leg function and physical activity: the Walking and Leg Circulation Study. *Ann Intern Med* 2002; 136:873.

2. Rutherford RB, Baker JD, Ernst C, et al. Recommended standards for reports dealing with lower extremity ischemia: revised version. *J Vasc Surg* 1997; 26:517.

3. Higgins JP, Higgins JA. Epidemiology of peripheral arterial disease in women. *J Epidemiol* 2003; 13:1.

4. Alexander JQ, Leos SM, Katz SG. Is duplex ultrasonography an effective single modality for the preoperative evaluation of peripheral vascular disease? *Am Surg* 2002; 68:1107.

5. Visser K, Hunink MG. Peripheral arterial disease: gadolinium-enhanced MR angiography versus color-guided duplex US: meta-analysis. *Radiology* 2000; 216:67.

6. Khilnani NM, Winchester PA, Prince MR, et al. Peripheral vascular disease: combined 3D bolus chase and dynamic 2D MR angiography compared with X-ray angiography for treatment planning. *Radiology* 2002; 224:63.

7. Cronberg CN, Sjoberg S, Albrechtsson U, et al. Peripheral arterial disease. Contrast-enhanced 3D MR angiography of the lower leg and foot compared with conventional angiography. *Acta Radiol* 2003; 44:59.

8. Visser K, Kock MC, Kuntz KM, Donaldson MC, Gazelle GS, Myriam Hunink MG. Cost-effectiveness targets for multi-detector row CT angiography in the work-up of patients with intermittent claudication. *Radiology* 2003; 227:647.

9. Tan ME, Dossche KM, Morshuis WJ, et al. Operative risk factors of type A aortic dissection: analysis of 252 consecutive patients. *Cardiovasc Surg* 2003; 11:277.

10. Moore AG, Eagle KA, Bruckman D, et al. Choice of computed tomography, transesophageal echocardiography, magnetic resonance imaging, and aortography in acute aortic dissection: International Registry of Acute Aortic Dissection (IRAD). *Am J Cardiol* 2002; 89:1235.

11. Pereles FS, McCarthy RM, Baskaran V, et al. Thoracic aortic dissection and aneurysm: evaluation with nonenhanced true FISP MR angiography in less than 4 minutes. *Radiology* 2002; 223:270.

12. Glockner JF. Navigating the aorta: MR virtual vascular endoscopy. *Radiographics* 2003; 23:E11.

13. Kaji S, Akasaka T, Horibata Y, et al. Long-term prognosis of patients with type A aortic intramural hematoma. *Circulation* 2002; 106:I248.

14. Ganaha F, Miller DC, Sugimoto K, et al. Prognosis of aortic intramural hematoma with and without penetrating atherosclerotic ulcer: a clinical and radiological analysis. *Circulation* 2002; 106:342.

15. Timperley J, Banning AP. Prognosis of aortic intramural hematoma with and without penetrating atherosclerotic ulcer: a clinical and radiological analysis. *Circulation* 2003; 107:e63.

16. Bown MJ, Sutton AJ, Bell PR, Sayers RD. A meta-analysis of 50 years of ruptured abdominal aortic aneurysm repair. *Br J Surg* 2002; 89:714.

17. Davies RR, Goldstein LJ, Coady MA, et al. Yearly rupture or dissection rates for thoracic aortic aneurysms: simple prediction based on size. *Ann Thorac Surg* 2002; 73:17; discussion 27.

18. Lederle FA, Wilson SE, Johnson GR, et al. Immediate repair compared with surveillance of small abdominal aortic aneurysms. *N Engl J Med* 2002; 346:1437.

19. Long-term outcomes of immediate repair compared with surveillance of small abdominal aortic aneurysms. *N Engl J Med* 2002; 346:1445.

20. Doty JR, Wilentz RE, Salazar JD, Hruban RH, Cameron DE. Atheroembolism in cardiac surgery. *Ann Thorac Surg* 2003; 75:1221.

21. Johnston SL, Lock RJ, Gompels MM. Takayasu arteritis: a review. *J Clin Pathol* 2002; 55:481.

22. Salvarani C, Cantini F, Boiardi L, Hunder GG. Polymyalgia rheumatica and giant-cell arteritis. *N Engl J Med* 2002; 347:261.

23. Tso E, Flamm SD, White RD, Schvartzman PR, Mascha E, Hoffman GS. Takayasu arteritis: utility and limitations of magnetic resonance imaging in diagnosis and treatment. *Arthritis Rheum* 2002; 46:1634.

24. Chang JB, Stein TA. Mesenteric ischemia: acute and chronic. *Ann Vasc Surg* 2003; 17:323.

25. Vosshenrich R, Fischer U. Contrast-enhanced MR angiography of abdominal vessels: is there still a role for angiography? *Eur Radiol* 2002; 12:218.

26. Foley WD. Special focus session: multidetector CT: abdominal visceral imaging. *Radiographics* 2002; 22:701.

27. Bredenberg CE, Sampson LN, Ray FS, Cormier RA, Heintz S, Eldrup-Jorgensen J. Changing patterns in surgery for chronic renal artery occlusive diseases. *J Vasc Surg* 1992; 15:1018; discussion 1023.

28. Safian RD. Atherosclerotic renal artery stenosis. *Curr Treat Options Cardiovasc Med* 2003; 5:91.

29. Huot SJ, Hansson JH, Dey H, Concato J. Utility of captopril renal scans for detecting renal artery stenosis. *Arch Intern Med* 2002; 162:1981.

30. Ong YY, Cohn D, Wijaya J, Roach P. The importance of renal localization with MIBG scintigraphy. *Clin Nucl Med* 2002; 27:479.

31. Krijnen P, Oei HY, Claessens RA, Roos JC, van Jaarsveld BC, Habbema JD. Interobserver agreement on captopril renography for assessing renal vascular disease. *J Nucl Med* 2002; 43:330.

32. Nicholson T. Magnetic resonance angiography for the diagnosis of renal artery stenosis. *Clin Radiol* 2003; 58:257.

33. Qanadli SD, Soulez G, Therasse E, et al. Detection of renal artery stenosis: prospective comparison of captopril-enhanced Doppler sonography, captopril-enhanced scintigraphy, and MR angiography. *AJR Am J Roentgenol* 2001; 177:1123.

34. Nchimi A, Biquet JF, Brisbois D, et al. Duplex ultrasound as first-line screening test for patients suspected of renal artery stenosis: prospective evaluation in high-risk group. *Eur Radiol* 2003; 13:1413.

35. Willmann JK, Wildermuth S, Pfammatter T, et al. Aortoiliac and renal arteries: prospective intraindividual comparison of contrast-enhanced three-dimensional MR angiography and multi-detector row CT angiography. *Radiology* 2003; 226:798.

36. Behar JV, Nelson RC, Zidar JP, DeLong DM, Smith TP. Thin-section multidetector CT angiography of renal artery stents. *AJR Am J Roentgenol* 2002; 178:1155.

37. Lufft V, Hoogestraat-Lufft L, Fels LM, et al. Contrast media nephropathy: intravenous CT angiography versus intraarterial digital subtraction angiography in renal artery stenosis: a prospective randomized trial. *Am J Kidney Dis* 2002; 40:236.

38. Aqel RA, Zoghbi GJ, Baldwin SA, et al. Prevalence of renal artery stenosis in high-risk veterans referred to cardiac catheterization. *J Hypertens* 2003; 21:1157.

39. Nordmann AJ, Woo K, Parkes R, Logan AG. Balloon angioplasty or medical therapy for hypertensive patients with atherosclerotic renal artery stenosis? A meta-analysis of randomized controlled trials. *Am J Med* 2003; 114:44.

40. Raninen RO, Kupari MM, Hekali PE. Carotid and femoral artery stiffness in Takayasu's arteritis. An ultrasound study. *Scand J Rheumatol* 2002; 31:85.

41. Long A, Lepoutre A, Corbillon E, Branchereau A. Critical review of non- or minimally invasive methods (duplex ultrasonography, MR- and CT-angiography) for evaluating stenosis of the proximal internal carotid artery. *Eur J Vasc Endovasc Surg* 2002; 24:43.

42. Albuquerque FC, Han PP, Spetzler RF, Zabramski JM, McDougall CG. Carotid dissection: technical factors affecting endovascular therapy. *Can J Neurol Sci* 2002; 29:54.

43. Filis KA, Arko FR, Johnson BL, et al. Duplex ultrasound criteria for defining the severity of carotid stenosis. *Ann Vasc Surg* 2002; 16:413.

44. Ringer AJ, German JW, Guterman LR, Hopkins LN. Follow-up of stented carotid arteries by Doppler ultrasound. *Neurosurgery* 2002; 51:639; discussion 643.

45. Luccichenti G, Cademartiri F, Lucidi V, Marchesi G, Ugolotti U, Pavone P. MR angiography of the carotid arteries: parameters affecting image quality. *Acad Radiol* 2003; 10:520.

46. Nederkoorn PJ, Van Der Graaf Y, Hunink MG, Forsting M, Wanke I. Duplex ultrasound and magnetic resonance angiography compared with digital subtraction angiography in carotid artery stenosis: a systematic review. *Stroke* 2003; 34:1324.

47. Berg MH, Manninen HI, Rasanen HT, Vanninen RL, Jaakkola PA. CT angiography in the assessment of carotid artery atherosclerosis. *Acta Radiol* 2002; 43:116.

48. Staikov IN, Arnold M, Mattle HP, et al. Comparison of the ECST, CC, and NASCET grading methods and ultrasound for assessing carotid stenosis. European Carotid Surgery Trial. North American Symptomatic Carotid Endarterectomy Trial. *J Neurol* 2000; 247:681.

49. Johnston DC, Goldstein LB. Utility of noninvasive studies in the evaluation of patients with carotid artery disease. *Curr Neurol Neurosci Rep* 2002; 2:25.

Page numbers followed by "f" denote figures; "t" denote tables; and "b" denote boxes